PDR® Concise Drug Guide for PEDIATRICS

FIRST EDITION

PDR® Concise Drug Guide for Pediatrics

FIRST EDITION

Senior Director, Editorial & Publishing: Bette LaGow
Manager, Professional Services: Michael Deluca, PharmD, MBA
Drug Information Specialists: Anila Patel, PharmD; Nermin Shenouda, PharmD; Greg Tallis, RPh
Contributing Editor: Cathy Kim, PharmD
Project Editors: Kathleen Engel, Lori Murray
Associate Editors: Sabina Borza, Elise Philippi
Senior Director, Client Sevices: Stephanie Struble
Project Manager: Christina Klinger
Manager, Production Purchasing: Thomas Westburgh
Manager, Art Department: Livio Udina
Electronic Publishing Designers: Deana DiVizio, Carrie Faeth, Jaime Pinedo
Production Associate: Joan K. Akerlind
Traffic Assistant: Kim Condon

Senior Director, Copy Sales: Bill Gaffney
Senior Product Manager: Richard Buchwald

THOMSON PDR

Executive Vice President, PDR: Kevin D. Sanborn
Vice President, Client Services & Publishing: Christopher Young
Vice President, Clinical Relations: Mukesh Mehta, RPh
Vice President, Operations: Brian Holland
Vice President, Strategic Marketing: Valerie E. Berger
Vice President, Pharmaceutical Sales: Anthony Sorce

THOMSON Copyright © 2007 and published by Thomson Healthcare Inc. at Montvale, NJ 07645-1725. All rights reserved. None of the content of this publication may be reproduced, stored in a retrieval system, resold, redistributed, or transmitted in any form or by any means (electronic, mechanical, photocopying, recording, or otherwise) without the prior written permission of the publisher. Physicians' Desk Reference®, PDR®, Pocket PDR®, PDR Family Guide to Prescription Drugs®, PDR Family Guide to Women's Health and Prescription Drugs®, and PDR Family Guide to Nutrition and Health® are registered trademarks of Thomson Healthcare Inc. PDR® for Ophthalmic Medicines; PDR® for Nonprescription Drugs, Dietary Supplements, and Herbs; PDR® Guide to Drug Interactions, Side Effects, and Indications; PDR® Pharmacopoeia; PDR® Drug Guide for Mental Health Professionals; PDR® Concise Drug Guide for Advanced Practice Clinicians; PDR® Concise Drug Guide for Pediatrics; PDR® Concise Drug Guide for Pharmacists; PDR® for Herbal Medicines; PDR® for Nutritional Supplements; PDR® Medical Dictionary; PDR® Nurse's Drug Handbook™; PDR® Nurse's Dictionary; PDR® Family Guide Encyclopedia of Medical Care; PDR® Family Guide to Natural Medicines and Healing Therapies; PDR® Family Guide to Common Ailments; PDR® Family Guide to Over-the-Counter Drugs; PDR® Family Guide to Nutritional Supplements; and PDR® Electronic Library are trademarks of Thomson Healthcare Inc.

Officers of Thomson Healthcare Inc.: *President and Chief Executive Officer:* Robert Cullen; *Chief Medical Officer:* Alan Ying, MD; *Senior Vice President and Chief Technology Officer:* Frank Licata; *Chief Strategy Officer:* Courtney Morris; *Executive Vice President, Payer Decision Support:* Jon Newpol; *Executive Vice President, Provider Markets:* Terry Cameron; *Executive Vice President, Marketing and Innovation:* Doug Schneider; *Senior Vice President, Finance:* Phil Buckingham; *Vice President, Human Resources:* Pamela M. Bilash; *General Counsel:* Darren Pocsik

ISBN: 1-56363-676-X   Printed in Canada

Contents

FOREWORD vii

HOW TO USE THIS BOOK ix

PDR DRUG MONOGRAPH KEY xi

PDR CONCISE DRUG MONOGRAPHS .1-420

NEOFAX DRUG MONOGRAPHS ..421-552

BRAND/GENERIC INDEX I-1–I-16

THERAPEUTIC CLASS INDEX ...I-17–I-28

VISUAL IDENTIFICATION GUIDE ..V1-V16

APPENDIX: REFERENCE TABLES

Abbreviations, Measurements and Calculations
Abbreviations, Acronyms and Symbols ..A1
Calculations and Formulas A7

Drug Information and Poison Control
Drug Information Centers A15
Poison Antidote Chart A23
Poison Control Centers A29

OTC Drug Comparison Charts

Dermatology
Acne Products A35
Antiseborrheal Products A39
Contact Dermatitis Products A43
Dandruff Products A45
Diaper Rash Products A47
Dry Skin Products A49
Psoriasis Products A57
Wound Care Products A59

Gastrointestinal
Antacid and Heartburn Products A61
Antidiarrheal Products A65
Antiflatulant Products A67
Laxative Products A69

Respiratory
Allergic Rhinitis Products A73
Is it a Cold, Flu, or an Allergy? A77
Cough-Cold-Flu Products A78
Nasal Decongestant/
  Moisturizing Products A91

Miscellaneous
Analgesic Products A93
Antipyretic Products A99

RX Drug Comparison Charts
Acne Management:
  Topical Therapies A103
Acne Management:
  Systemic Therapies A105
Antibiotic Sensitivity Chart
  Aminoglycosides A106
  Carbapenems/Monobactams A110
  Cephalosporins A114
  Fluoroquinolones A119
  Macrolides and Clindamycin A123
  Penicillins A127
  Sulfonamides A131
  Tetracyclines A131
  Miscellaneous A135
Antibiotics: Oral A139
Antibiotics: Neonatal Recommended
  Concentrations for Administration ..A141
Antibiotics: Systemic A142
Asthma Management A177
Asthma Treatment Plan A179
HIV/AIDS Pharmacotherapy A181
Insulin Formulations A185
Oral Contraceptives A187
Topical Corticosteroids A189

Immunization Charts
Recommended Immunization
  Schedule for Persons Aged
  0-6 Years A191
Recommended Immunization
  Schedule for Persons Aged
  7-18 Years A193
Catch-up Immunization Schedule for
  Persons Aged 4 Months–18 Years
  Who Start Late or Who Are More
  Than 1 Month Behind A195
Recommended Adult Immunization
  Schedule, by Vaccine and
  Age Group A197
Recommended Adult Immunization
  Schedule, by Vaccine and Medical
  and Other Indications A201

Miscellaneous

Drugs Excreted in Breast Milk A205
Use-in-Pregnancy Ratings A207
Vitamin Comparison Table A214

CDC Growth Charts

Boys Length-for-age and Weight-for-age,
Birth to 36 months
(5th-95th percentile) A219
Boys Head Circumference-for-age and
Weight-for-length, Birth to 36 months
(5th-95th percentile) A221
Girls Length-for-age and Weight-for-age,
Birth to 36 months
(5th-95th percentile) A223
Girls Head Circumference-for-age and
Weight-for-length, Birth to 36 months
(5th-95th percentile) A225
Boys Stature-for-age and
Weight-for-age, Children 2 to
20 years (5th-95th percentile) ...A227
Boys BMI-for-age, Children 2 to
20 years (5th-95th percentile) A229
Girls Stature-for-age and
Weight-for-age, Children 2 to
20 years (5th-95th percentile) ...A231
Girls BMI-for-age, Children
2 to 20 years (5th-95th percentile) .A233
Boys Weight-for-stature,
(5th-95th percentile) A235
Girls Weight-for-stature,
(5th-95th percentile) A237
Boys Length-for-age and
Weight-for-age, Birth to 36 months
(3rd-97th percentile) A239
Boys Head Circumference-for-age and
Weight-for-length, Birth to 36 months
(3rd-97th percentile) A241
Girls Length-for-age and
Weight-for-age, Birth to 36 months
(3rd-97th percentile) A243
Girls Head Circumference-for-age
and Weight-for-length, Birth to
36 months (3rd-97th percentile) ...A245
Boys Stature-for-age and
Weight-for-age, Children 2 to
20 years (3rd-97th percentile) A247
Boys BMI-for-age, Children 2 to
20 years (3rd-97th percentile) A249
Girls Stature-for-age and
Weight-for-age, Children 2 to
20 years (3rd-97th percentile) A251
Girls BMI-for-age, Children
2 to 20 years (3rd-97th percentile) ..A253
Boys Weight-for-stature
(3rd-97th percentile) A255
Girls Weight-for-stature
(3rd-97th percentile) A257

Foreword

What's changing rapidly in the practice of Pediatrics? The answer, of course, is broad and would vary depending on which pediatricians were asked. Nonetheless, I believe a few constants are inarguable, particularly the number of new drugs and vaccines that are continually emerging and the time pressures on physicians as they face more and more electronic tasks.

Are there really that many recently released pharmaceutical agents in Pediatrics? Although the number of new treatments for infants and children pales in comparison to the wave that confronts our colleagues in internal medicine, the trend is both significant and growing. Just a few examples from the last year or so include Gardasil (human papilloma virus vaccine), Adacel (diphtheria, acellular pertussis, and tetanus vaccine for adolescents), and Altabax (topical antibacterial for impetigo). On top of this, old favorites either appear in new formulations, such as Suprax (cefixime) at 200mg/5mL, or acquire concerning warnings, such as the risk of suicidality with Strattera.

How severe is the impact of electronic medical records (EMR) on a practice? Difficult to quantify, not well studied, perhaps controversial, but *real* is the response that I would offer. The clamor for EMR arises from regulatory agencies, insurance companies, and academicians, who will benefit from access to huge data repositories. The burden of implementation, however, falls on clinicians. To date, no available EMR decreases the amount of time required for charting the information from encounters in office settings.

What can help confront both of these onslaughts? Obviously, no single resource will neutralize completely the "chronophages" that infiltrate the lives of pediatricians with ever greater frequency, but I am convinced that the *PDR® Concise Drug Guide for Pediatrics* can play some role. This publication provides ready reference to those pharmaceuticals that pediatricians prescribe most frequently, thereby eliminating the need to sift through myriad monographs that apply almost exclusively to adults. In addition, the format highlights the newest products and the most updated information for both neonates and children. Thus, I believe that the *PDR Concise Drug Guide for Pediatrics* will find a home on the desk of many pediatricians.

Gary R. Fleisher, MD
Egan Family Foundation Professor
Department of Pediatrics, Harvard Medical School
Pediatrician-in-Chief and Chairman
Department of Medicine, Children's Hospital Boston

HOW TO USE THIS BOOK

The *PDR® Concise Drug Guide for Pediatrics* allows you to quickly prescribe medications with confidence. With over 800 monographs providing current, organized information from *PDR®*, and more than 150 monographs from *NeoFax®*, this handy reference is the perfect companion for the busy healthcare professional involved in pediatric care.

This compact guide is divided into five discrete sections. The first section consists of over 800 concise drug monographs with FDA-approved pediatric indications. All information provided in these monographs is based on FDA-approved prescribing information. These monographs are organized alphabetically by brand name. When a brand is no longer available, the generic name is used. Monographs consist of:

- Brand name
- Generic name
- Manufacturer
- FDA/DEA schedule
- Black Box Warnings
- Therapeutic Class
- Indications
- Dosage (adults, pediatrics, special populations)
- How Supplied (dosage form/strength)
- Contraindications
- Warnings/Precautions
- Interactions
- Adverse Reactions
- Pregnancy category/Nursing considerations

The second section is comprised of more than 150 drug monographs with evidence-based uses for neonatal patients. These monographs are organized alphabetically by product name. Monographs consist of:

- Product Name
- Dose and Administration
- Uses
- Monitoring
- Adverse Effects/Precautions
- Pharmacology
- Special Considerations/Preparation
- Selected References

An explanatory note about NeoFax antibiotic dosing charts
The antibiotic dosing charts reflect the fact that renal function and drug elimination are most strongly correlated with Postmenstrual Age ("PMA," equivalent to Gestational Age plus Postnatal Age). Postmenstrual Age is therefore used as the primary determinant of dosing interval, with Postnatal Age as secondary qualifier.

Example: A baby born at 28 weeks gestation is now 21 days old. To determine the dosing interval for cefotaxime, first go to the row on the chart containing the Postmenstrual Age of 31 weeks (30 to 36) and then the Postnatal Age of 21 days (>14) to reach the dosing interval of 8 hours.

How to Use This Book

The third section is an extensive collection of tables and key references to help healthcare professionals care for pediatric patients. Tables provided include recommended immunization schedules, growth charts, poison control centers, drug comparisons (both Rx and OTC), and much more. Within the drug comparison tables, drugs are organized alphabetically and by class for effortless access. Tables and references may include, but are not limited to:

- Brand/generic name
- How Supplied (dosage form/strength)
- Initial and Max dosages
- Usual dosage range

The fourth section contains indices—all of the drugs are indexed by brand and generic name, as well as pharmacologic category, for quick location and investigation.

The final section of the *PDR® Concise Drug Guide for Pediatrics* contains a Visual Identification Guide featuring hundreds of product images, listed by brand name. This section helps you quickly verify the identity of many forms of medications, from tablets to oral solutions. Each product image will contain both the generic and brand name, strength, and the name of its supplier. Other strengths and dosage forms may be available; please check FDA-approved prescribing information for a complete listing of all strengths and dosage forms.

Important Information About Product Labeling

Entries in the *PDR® Concise Drug Guide for Pediatrics* are drawn from either FDA-approved product labeling as published in *Physicians' Desk Reference®* or supplied by the manufacturer, or in the case of NeoFax, from reliable sources believed to be in accord with good medical practice. The PDR entries are compiled and updated on a regular basis by a staff of experienced pharmacists. While diligent efforts have been made to ensure the accuracy of each entry, it is essential to bear in mind that the information presented here is merely a synopsis of key points in the official labeling, and that the complete labeling contains additional precautionary information that may be of significance in specific cases. Similarly, please remember that only common and dangerous adverse reactions and interactions are included here, and that numerous less-prevalent adverse effects may be reported in the complete labeling. If an entry leaves any question unanswered, be sure to consult *Physicians' Desk Reference* or the manufacturer for additional information.

The function of the publisher is the compilation, organization, and distribution of this information. In organizing and presenting the material in the *PDR Concise Drug Guide for Pediatrics*, the publisher does not warrant or guarantee any of the products described, or perform any independent analysis in connection with any of the product information contained herein.

The *PDR® Concise Drug Guide for Pediatrics* assumes no obligation to obtain and include any information in the PDR entries other than that provided by the manufacturer. The publisher does not warrant, guarantee, or advocate the use of any product described herein. The publisher and editors do not assume, and expressly disclaim, any liability for error, omissions, or typographical errors in the information contained herein or for misuse of any of the products listed.

PDR® DRUG MONOGRAPH KEY

BRAND NAME
Combined Generic (Manufacturer)

FDA/DEA Class*

> Black Box Warning: A brief description of the black box warning(s) that appear in the beginning of the official FDA-approved labeling for the monograph.

OTHER BRAND NAMES: Brand name drugs that have the same generic components as monograph drug.

THERAPEUTIC CLASS: Based on the active ingredients and their mechanism of action.

INDICATIONS: Only includes FDA-approved indications.

DOSAGE: Dosages for adults and pediatrics as indicated in the official FDA-approved labeling.

HOW SUPPLIED: Product description including strength, formulation, (package size), and scored tablet information.

CONTRAINDICATIONS: Details harmful conditions related to the use of the drug and disease states or patient populations where the use of the monograph drug should be avoided.

WARNINGS/PRECAUTIONS: Details harmful conditions related to the use of the drug and disease states or patient populations where caution is dictated.

ADVERSE REACTIONS: Denotes side effects and adverse reactions listed in the official FDA-approved labeling as occurring with greater frequency (generally at a rate of ≥3%) or deemed significant based on the clinical judgment of the editors. Other side effects may be included if deemed serious or life-threatening. For complete prescribing information please refer to the official FDA-approved labeling.

INTERACTIONS: Includes the effects and implications of other drugs and food on the monograph drug based on official FDA-approved labeling.

PREGNANCY: Indicated pregnancy and nursing considerations and, when available, the FDA pregnancy rating system category.†

---

*FDA/DEA CLASS

OTC: Available over-the-counter.
RX: Requires a prescription.
CII: Controlled substance; high potential for abuse.
CIII: Controlled substance; some potential for abuse.
CIV: Controlled substance; low potential for abuse.
CV: Controlled substance; subject to state and local regulation.

---

†FDA USE-IN-PREGNANCY RATINGS

The FDA use-in-pregnancy rating system weighs the degree to which available information has ruled out risk to the fetus against the drugs potential benefit to the patient. The ratings, and the interpretation, are as follows:

CATEGORY	INTERPRETATION
A	**CONTROLLED STUDIES SHOW NO RISK.** Adequate, well-controlled studies in pregnant women have failed to demonstrate a risk to the fetus in any trimester of pregnancy.
B	**NO EVIDENCE OF RISK IN HUMANS.** Adequate, well-controlled studies in pregnant women have not shown increased risk of fetal abnormalities despite adverse findings in animals, or, in the absence of fetal risk. The chance of fetal harm is remote, but remains a possibility.
C	**RISK CANNOT BE RULED OUT.** Adequate, well-controlled human studies are lacking, and animal studies have shown a risk to the fetus or are lacking as well. There is a chance of fetal harm if the drug is administered during pregnancy; but the potential benefits may outweigh the potential risk.
D	**POSITIVE EVIDENCE OF RISK.** Studies in humans, or investigational or post-marketing data, have demonstrated fetal risk. Nevertheless, potential benefits from the use of the drug may outweigh the potential risk. For example, the drug may be acceptable if needed in a life-threatening situation or serious disease for which safer drugs cannot be use or are ineffective.
X	**CONTRAINDICATED IN PREGNANCY.** Studies in animals or humans, or investigational or post-marketing reports, have demonstrated positive evidence of fetal abnormalities or risk which clearly outweighs any possible benefit to the patient.

PDR® Concise Drug Monographs

1-Day OTC
tioconazole (Personal Products Company)

THERAPEUTIC CLASS: Azole antifungal

INDICATIONS: Treatment of recurrent vaginal yeast infections.

DOSAGE: *Adults:* Insert contents of applicator intravaginally once hs.
Pediatrics: ≥12 yrs: Insert contents of applicator intravaginally once hs.

HOW SUPPLIED: Oint: 6.5% (4.6g)

WARNINGS/PRECAUTIONS: Do not use if abdominal pain, fever (>100°F), chills, nausea, vomiting, diarrhea, or foul smelling discharge. Avoid tampons. Do not rely on condoms or diaphragm to prevent STDs or pregnancy until 3 days after last use.

ADVERSE REACTIONS: Vulvovaginal burning.

PREGNANCY: Safety in pregnancy and nursing not known.

Abelcet RX
amphotericin B (lipid complex) (Enzon)

THERAPEUTIC CLASS: Polyene antifungal

INDICATIONS: Treatment of invasive fungal infections in patients refractory or intolerant to conventional amphotericin B therapy.

DOSAGE: *Adults:* 5mg/kg IV at 2.5mg/kg/h.
Pediatrics: 5mg/kg IV at 2.5mg/kg/h.

HOW SUPPLIED: Inj: 5mg/mL

WARNINGS/PRECAUTIONS: Anaphylaxis reported. D/C if respiratory distress occurs. Monitor SCr, LFTs, serum electrolytes, CBC during therapy.

ADVERSE REACTIONS: Chills, fever, increased SCr, multiple organ failure, nausea, hypotension, respiratory failure, vomiting, dyspnea, sepsis, diarrhea, headache, heart arrest, HTN, hypokalemia, infection, kidney failure, pain, thrombocytopenia.

INTERACTIONS: Antineoplastics may potentiate renal toxicity, bronchospasm, hypotension. Corticosteroids and corticotropin may potentiate hypokalemia predisposing patients to cardiac dysfunction. May potentiate digitalis toxicity. Increased risk of flucytosine toxicity. Acute pulmonary toxicity reported with leukocyte transfusions. Nephrotoxic drugs (eg, aminoglycosides, pentamidine) enhance potential for renal toxicity. Cyclosporine within several days of bone marrow ablation associated with nephrotoxicity. Hypokalemia effect may enhance curariform effect of skeletal muscle relaxants.

PREGNANCY: Category B, not for use in nursing.

Abreva OTC
docosanol (GlaxoSmithKline Consumer)

THERAPEUTIC CLASS: Antiviral

INDICATIONS: To treat cold sore/fever blisters on the face or lips.

DOSAGE: *Adults:* Apply to affected area on face or lips at 1st sign of cold sore/fever blister (tingle). Use 5x/day until healed.
Pediatrics: ≥12 yrs: Apply to affected area on face or lips at 1st sign of cold sore/fever blister (tingle). Use 5x/day until healed.

HOW SUPPLIED: Cre: 10% (2g)

WARNINGS/PRECAUTIONS: Avoid in or near eyes, and inside mouth. Discontinue if sore worsens or does not heal in 10 days.

PREGNANCY: Safety in pregnancy and nursing is not know.

Accolate RX
zafirlukast (AstraZeneca LP)

THERAPEUTIC CLASS: Leukotriene receptor antagonist

INDICATIONS: Prophylaxis and chronic treatment of asthma.

AccuNeb

DOSAGE: *Adults:* 20mg bid. Administer 1 hr ac or 2 hrs pc.
Pediatrics: ≥12 yrs: 20mg bid. 5-11 yrs: 10mg bid. Administer 1 hr ac or 2 hrs pc.

HOW SUPPLIED: Tab: 10mg, 20mg

WARNINGS/PRECAUTIONS: Not for treatment of acute asthma attacks. Bioavailability decreases with food. Hepatic dysfunction and systemic eosinophilia reported.

ADVERSE REACTIONS: Headache, infection, nausea, diarrhea, hypersensitivity reactions including angioedema.

INTERACTIONS: Potentiates warfarin. Caution with drugs metabolized by CYP2C9 (eg, tolbutamide, phenytoin, carbamazepine) or CYP3A4 (eg, dihydropyridine calcium-channel blockers, cyclosporine, cisapride, astemizole). Increased levels with ASA. Decreased levels by erythromycin, theophylline. May increase theophylline levels.

PREGNANCY: Category B, not for use in nursing.

AccuNeb
albuterol sulfate (Dey)
RX

THERAPEUTIC CLASS: Beta$_2$ agonist

INDICATIONS: Relief of bronchospasm with asthma.

DOSAGE: *Pediatrics:* 2-12 yrs: Initial: 0.63mg or 1.25mg tid-qid via nebulizer. 6-12 yrs with severe asthma, >40kg or 11-12 yrs: Initial: 1.25mg tid-qid.

HOW SUPPLIED: Sol: 1.25mg/3mL, 0.63mg/3mL (3mL, 25^s)

WARNINGS/PRECAUTIONS: Hypersensitivity reactions reported. Fatalities reported with excessive use. Caution with cardiovascular disorders, especially coronary insufficiency, arrhythmias and HTN. May need concomitant anti-inflammatory agents. Can produce paradoxical bronchospasm. Caution with DM. May cause hypokalemia.

ADVERSE REACTIONS: Asthma exacerbation, otitis media, allergic reaction, gastroenteritis, cold symptoms.

INTERACTIONS: Avoid other short-acting sympathomimetic bronchodilators and epinephrine. Extreme caution within 2 weeks of MAOI or TCA use. Monitor digoxin. ECG changes and/or hypokalemia with non-K$^+$-sparing diuretics may worsen. May be antagonized by β-blockers.

PREGNANCY: Category C, not for use in nursing.

Accutane
isotretinoin (Roche Labs)
RX

> Not for use by females who are or may become pregnant, or if breast feeding. Birth defects have been documented. Approved for marketing only under special restricted distribution program called iPLEDGE™. Must have 2 (-) pregnancy tests. Repeat pregnancy test monthly. Use 2 forms of contraception at least 1 month prior, during, and 1 month following discontinuation. Must fill written prescriptions within 7 days; refills require new prescriptions. May dispense maximum of 1 month supply. Prescriber and patient must be registered with iPLEDGE.

OTHER BRAND NAMES: Claravis (Barr) - Sotret (Ranbaxy) - Amnesteem (Genpharm)

THERAPEUTIC CLASS: Retinoid

INDICATIONS: Severe recalcitrant nodular acne unresponsive to conventional therapy, including systemic antibiotics.

DOSAGE: *Adults:* Initial/Usual: 0.5-1mg/kg/day given bid for 15-20 weeks. Max: 2mg/kg/day (for very serious cases). Adjust for side effects and disease response. May discontinue if nodule count reduced by >70% prior to completion. Repeat only if necessary after 2 months off drug. Take with food.
Pediatrics: ≥12 yrs: Initial/Usual: 0.5-1mg/kg/day given bid for 15-20 weeks. Max: 2mg/kg/day (for very serious cases). Adjust for side effects and disease response. May discontinue if nodule count reduced by >70% prior to completion. Repeat only if necessary after 2 months off drug. Take with food.

HOW SUPPLIED: Cap: 10mg, 20mg, 40mg

CONTRAINDICATIONS: Pregnancy, paraben sensitivity (preservative in gelatin cap).

WARNINGS/PRECAUTIONS: Acute pancreatitis, impaired hearing, anaphylactic reactions, inflammatory bowel disease, elevated TG and LFTs, hepatotoxicity, premature epiphyseal closure, and hyperostosis reported. May cause depression, psychosis, aggressive and/or violent behaviors, rarely suicidal ideation/attempts and suicide; may need further evaluation after discontinuation. May cause decreased night vision, and corneal opacities. Associated with pseudotumor cerebri. Check lipids before therapy, and then at intervals until response established (within 4 weeks). D/C if significant decrease in WBC, hearing or visual impairment, abdominal pain, rectal bleeding, or severe diarrhea occurs. Monitor LFTs before therapy, weekly or biweekly until response established. May develop musculoskeletal symptoms. Avoid prolonged UV rays or sunlight, and donating blood up to 1 month after discontinuing therapy. Caution with genetic predisposition for age-related osteoporosis, history of childhood osteoporosis, osteomalacia, other bone metabolism disorders (eg, anorexia nervosa). Spontaneous osteoporosis, osteopenia, bone fractures, and delayed fracture healing reported; caution in sports with repetitive impact.

ADVERSE REACTIONS: Cheilitis, dry skin and mucous membranes, conjunctivitis, blood dyscrasias, epistaxis, decreased HDL, elevated cholesterol and TG, elevated blood sugar, arthralgias, back pain, hearing/vision impairment, rash, photosensitivity reactions, psychiatric disorders.

INTERACTIONS: Avoid Vitamin A. Limit alcohol consumption. Tetracyclines increase incidence of pseudotumor cerebri. Pregnancy reported with oral and injectable/implantable contraceptives. Avoid St. John's Wort; may cause breakthrough bleeding with oral contraceptives. Caution with drugs that cause drug-induced osteoporosis/osteomalacia and affect vitamin D metabolism (eg, corticosteroids, phenytoin).

PREGNANCY: Category X, not for use in nursing.

ACLOVATE
alclometasone dipropionate (GlaxoSmithKline)

RX

THERAPEUTIC CLASS: Corticosteroid

INDICATIONS: Corticosteroid responsive dermatoses.

DOSAGE: *Adults:* Apply bid-tid. Reassess if no improvement after 2 weeks.
Pediatrics: ≥1 yr: Apply bid-tid. Reassess if no improvement after 2 weeks.

HOW SUPPLIED: Cre, Oint: 0.05% (15g, 45g, 60g)

WARNINGS/PRECAUTIONS: May produce reversible HPA axis suppression, manifestations of Cushing's syndrome, hyperglycemia, and glucosuria. Use appropriate antifungal or antibacterial agent with dermatological infections. Peds may be more susceptible to systemic toxicity. Avoid occlusive dressings. Avoid diaper area. Not for use in diaper dermatitis. D/C if irritation occurs. Caution in peds.

ADVERSE REACTIONS: Itching, burning, erythema, dryness, irritation, papular rash.

PREGNANCY: Category C, caution in nursing.

ACTHIB
haemophilus B conjugate (Sanofi Pasteur)

RX

THERAPEUTIC CLASS: Vaccine

INDICATIONS: Solo or combined with DTP (Aventis Pasteur) for active immunization of children 2-18 months for prevention of invasive disease caused by H.influenzae type B and/or diphtheria, tetanus, and pertussis. Combined with Tripedia® (TriHIBit®) for active immunization of children 15-18 months for prevention of invasive disease caused by H.influenzae type B and diphtheria, tetanus, and pertussis.

DOSAGE: *Pediatrics:* Reconstituted with DTP or Saline: 0.5mL IM in deltoid or thigh at 2, 4, and 6 months old; 4th dose at 15-18 months; 5th dose at 4-6 yrs. Reconstituted with Tripedia® (as 4th dose in series): 0.5mL IM in deltoid or thigh given at 15-18 months; 5th dose at 4-6 yrs. Previously Unvaccinated: 7-11 months old: 2 doses at 8 week intervals with a booster at 15-18 months. 12-14 months: 1 dose followed by a booster 2 months later.

HOW SUPPLIED: Inj: 10mcg

Acticin

WARNINGS/PRECAUTIONS: Immunosuppressed patients may not obtain expected antibody response. Have epinephrine injection (1:1000) available.

ADVERSE REACTIONS: Local: tenderness, erythema, induration. Systemic: fever, irritability, drowsiness, anorexia, nausea, diarrhea, vomiting.

INTERACTIONS: Immunosuppressive therapies may reduce effectiveness.

PREGNANCY: Category C, safety in nursing not known.

Acticin   RX
permethrin (Mylan Bertek)

THERAPEUTIC CLASS: Pyrethroid scabicidal agent

INDICATIONS: Treatment of scabies.

DOSAGE: *Adults:* Massage into skin from head to soles of feet. Wash off after 8-14 hrs. One treatment should be adequate. Retreat if living mites present after 14 days.

Pediatrics: ≥2 months: Massage into skin from head (scalp, temples and forehead) to soles of feet. Wash off after 8-14 hrs. One treatment should be adequate. Retreat if living mites present after 14 days.

HOW SUPPLIED: Cre: 5% (60g)

CONTRAINDICATIONS: Allergy to synthetic pyrethroid or pyrethrin.

WARNINGS/PRECAUTIONS: May temporarily exacerbate infection (eg pruritus, edema, erythema). Avoid eyes. D/C if hypersensitivity occurs.

ADVERSE REACTIONS: Burning, stinging, pruritus, erythema, numbness, tingling, rash.

PREGNANCY: Category B, not for use in nursing.

Actiq   CII
fentanyl citrate (Cephalon)

> May cause life-threatening hypoventilation in opioid non-tolerant patients. Only for cancer pain in opioid tolerant patients with malignancies. Keep out of reach of children and discard properly. Concomitant use with moderate and strong CYP3A4 inhibitors may cause fatal respiratory depression.

THERAPEUTIC CLASS: Narcotic agonist analgesic

INDICATIONS: Management of breakthrough cancer pain in patients with malignancies who are already receiving and are tolerant to opioid therapy.

DOSAGE: *Adults:* Initial: 0.2mg (consume over 15 minutes). Titrate: Redose 15 minutes after previous dose is completed. No more than 2 units per breakthrough pain episode. May increase to next higher available strength if several breakthrough episodes (1-2 days) require more than 1 unit per pain episode. Repeat titration for each new dose. Max: 4 units/day. Prescribe 6 units with each new titration. The lozenge should be sucked, not chewed, and consumed over 15 minutes.

Pediatrics: ≥16 yrs: Initial: 0.2mg (consume over 15 minutes). Titrate: Redose 15 minutes after previous dose is completed. No more than 2 units per breakthrough pain episode. May increase to next higher available strength if several breakthrough episodes (1-2 days) require more than 1 unit per pain episode. Repeat titration for each new dose. Max: 4 units/day. Prescribe 6 units with each new titration. The lozenge should be sucked, not chewed, and consumed over 15 minutes.

HOW SUPPLIED: Loz: 0.2mg, 0.4mg, 0.6mg, 0.8mg, 1.2mg, 1.6mg

CONTRAINDICATIONS: Opioid non-tolerant patients and management of acute or postoperative pain.

WARNINGS/PRECAUTIONS: Caution with COPD, hepatic or renal dysfunction. Risk of clinically significant hypoventilation. Extreme caution with evidence of increased intracranial pressure or impaired consciousness. Can produce morphine-like dependence. Increased risk of dental decay; ensure proper oral hygiene. Caution with bradyarrhythmias, liver or kidney dysfunction. Patients on concomitant CNS depressants must be monitored for a change in opioid effects. May impair mental and/or physical status.

ADVERSE REACTIONS: Respiratory depression, circulatory depression, headache, hypotension, shock, nausea, vomiting, constipation, dizziness, dyspnea, anxiety, somnolence.

INTERACTIONS: Concomitant use with other CNS depressants, including opioids, sedatives, hypnotics, general anesthetics, phenothiazines, tranquilizers, skeletal muscle relaxants, sedating antihistamines, potent inhibitors of CYP3A4 (eg, erythromycin, ketoconazole, itraconazole, ritonavir, troleandomycin, clarithromycin, nelfinavir and nefazodone) or moderate inhibitors (eg amprenavir, aprepitant, diltiazem, erythromycin, fluconazole, fosamprenavir, and verapamil) and alcohol may result in increased plasma concentrations. Avoid grapefruit juice. Avoid within 14 days of MAOIs.

PREGNANCY: Category C, not for use in nursing.

Acular
ketorolac tromethamine (Allergan)
RX

THERAPEUTIC CLASS: NSAID

INDICATIONS: Ocular itching due to seasonal allergic conjunctivitis. Postoperative inflammation in cataract extraction.

DOSAGE: *Adults:* 1 drop qid. Post-op Inflammation: Begin 24 hrs post-op and continue for 2 weeks.

Pediatrics: ≥3 yrs: 1 drop qid. Post-op Inflammation: Begin 24 hrs post-op and continue for 2 weeks.

HOW SUPPLIED: Sol: 0.5% (3mL, 5mL, 10mL)

WARNINGS/PRECAUTIONS: May increase ocular tissue bleeding in conjunction with ocular surgery. Avoid use with contact lenses. D/C if corneal epithelium breakdown occurs. Caution in known bleeding tendencies, complicated ocular surgeries, corneal denervation, corneal epithelial defects, DM, ocular surface diseases (eg, dry eye syndrome), rheumatoid arthritis, or repeat ocular surgeries within a short period of time. Caution if used >24 hrs prior to surgery and use beyond 14 days post-surgery.

ADVERSE REACTIONS: Transient stinging/burning, superficial keratitis or infections, allergic reactions, ocular inflammation, corneal edema, iritis.

INTERACTIONS: Potential for cross-sensitivity to acetylsalicylic acid, phenylacetic acid derivatives, and other NSAIDs. Caution with agents that may prolong bleeding time. Increased potential for healing problems with topical steroids.

PREGNANCY: Category C, caution in nursing.

Adacel
tetanus toxoid - diphtheria toxoid, reduced - pertussis vaccine acellular, adsorbed (Sanofi Pasteur)
RX

THERAPEUTIC CLASS: Vaccine

INDICATIONS: Active booster immunization against tetanus, diphtheria, and pertussis in persons 11-64 years of age.

DOSAGE: *Adults:* ≤64 yrs: 0.5mL IM (deltoid).

Pediatrics: ≥11 yrs: 0.5mL IM (deltoid).

HOW SUPPLIED: Inj: (Tetanus-Diphtheria-Pertussis) 5 LF- 2 LF-2.5mcg/0.5mL

CONTRAINDICATIONS: Encephalopathy not attributable to another identifiable cause within 7 days from initial vaccination. Progressive neurological disorder, uncontrolled epilepsy, or progressive encephalopathy.

WARNINGS/PRECAUTIONS: Evaluate risks/benefits of subsequent doses if temperature ≥105°F within 48 hrs not due to another identifiable cause; if collapse/shock occurs; persistent crying for ≥3 hrs within 48 hrs; and convulsions with or without fever within 3 days of vaccine. Continue with Td vaccine if pertussis must be withheld. Have epinephrine (1:1000) available. May not achieve expected immune response in immunosuppressed patients. Avoid injection into blood vessel. Should not be administered into the buttocks nor by the intradermal route.

ADVERSE REACTIONS: Injection site reactions, fever, headache, body aches, tiredness, chills, sore joints, nausea, lymph node swelling, diarrhea, and vomiting.

INTERACTIONS: Immunosuppressives (eg, irradiation, antimetabolites, alkylating agents, cytotoxic drugs, and corticosteroids) may reduce the immune response to vaccines.

PREGNANCY: Category C, caution in nursing

ADDERALL
amphetamine salt combo (Shire US) [CII]

> High potential for abuse; avoid prolonged use. Misuse of amphetamine may cause sudden death and serious cardiovascular adverse events.

THERAPEUTIC CLASS: Sympathomimetic amine

INDICATIONS: Treatment of attention deficit disorder with hyperactivity (ADHD) and narcolepsy.

DOSAGE: *Adults:* Narcolepsy: Initial: 10mg/day. Titrate: May increase by 10mg/day every week. Usual: 5-60mg/day. Give 1st dose upon awakening, and additional doses q4-6h.

Pediatrics: ADHD: 3-5 yrs: Initial: 2.5mg qd. Titrate: May increase by 2.5mg weekly. ≥6 yrs: 5mg qd-bid. May increase by 5mg weekly. Max (usual): 40mg/day. Narcolepsy: 6-12 yrs: Initial: 5mg/day. May increase by 5mg weekly. ≥12 yrs: Initial: 10mg/day. Titrate: May increase by 10mg/day every week. Usual: 5-60mg/day. Give 1st dose upon awakening, and additional doses q4-6h.

HOW SUPPLIED: Tab: 5mg*, 7.5mg*, 10mg*, 12.5mg*, 15mg*, 20mg*, 30mg* *scored

CONTRAINDICATIONS: Advanced arteriosclerosis, symptomatic cardiovascular disease, moderate to severe HTN, hyperthyroidism, glaucoma, agitated states, history of drug abuse, during or within 14 days of MAOI use.

WARNINGS/PRECAUTIONS: May exacerbate symptoms of behavior disturbance and thought disorder in psychotic patients. Caution when using stimulants to treat patients with comorbid bipolar disorder because of concern for possible induction of mixed/manic episode in such patients. Stimulants at usual doses can cause treatment emergent psychotic or manic symptoms (eg, hallucinations, delusional thinking, mania) in children and adolescents without prior history of psychotic illness. Aggressive behavior or hostility reported in clinical trials and the postmarketing experience of some medications indicated for the treatment of ADHD. Monitor growth in children. May lower convulsive threshold; d/c in presence of seizures. Visual disturbances reported with stimulant treatment. May exacerbate Tourette's syndrome and phonic or motor tics. Caution with HTN and monitor BP. Interrupt occasionally to determine if patient requires continued therapy. Sudden death reported in children with structural cardiac abnormalities; avoid use in children or adults with structural cardiac abnormalities.

ADVERSE REACTIONS: HTN, tachycardia, palpitations, CNS overstimulation, dry mouth, GI disorders, anorexia, impotence, urticaria, rash, angioedema, anaphylaxis, Stevens Johnson Syndrome.

INTERACTIONS: GI acidifying agents (guanethidine, reserpine, glutamic acid, etc) and urinary acidifying agents (ammonium chloride, etc) decrease efficacy. MAOIs may cause hypertensive crisis. Potentiated by GI and urinary alkalinizers, propoxyphene overdose. Potentiated effects of both agents with TCAs. May delay absorption of phenytoin, ethosuximide, phenobarbital. Potentiates meperidine, norepinephrine, phenobarbital, phenytoin. Antagonized by haloperidol, chlorpromazine, lithium. Antagonizes adrenergic blockers, antihistamines, antihypertensives, veratrum alkaloids (antihypertensive). Avoid co-administration with alkalinizing agents (eg, antacids).

PREGNANCY: Category C, not for use in nursing.

ADDERALL XR
amphetamine salt combo (Shire US) [CII]

> High potential for abuse; avoid prolonged use. Misuse of amphetamine may cause sudden death and serious cardiovascular adverse events.

THERAPEUTIC CLASS: Sympathomimetic amine

INDICATIONS: Treatment of attention deficit hyperactivity disorder (ADHD).

DOSAGE: *Adults:* Initial: 20mg qam. Currently Using Adderall: Switch to Adderall XR at the same total daily dose, taken once daily. Titrate at weekly intervals as needed. Swallow cap whole or open cap and sprinkle contents on applesauce; do not chew beads.

Pediatrics: ≥6 yrs: Initial: 10mg qam. Titrate: May increase weekly by 5-10mg/day. Max: 30mg/day. 13 to 17 yrs: Initial: 10mg/day. Titrate: May increase to 20mg/day after one week. Currently Using Adderall: Switch to Adderall XR at the same total daily dose, taken once daily. Titrate at weekly intervals as needed. Swallow cap whole or open cap and sprinkle contents on applesauce; do not chew beads.

HOW SUPPLIED: Cap, Extended-Release: 5mg, 10mg, 15mg, 20mg, 25mg, 30mg

CONTRAINDICATIONS: Advanced arteriosclerosis, symptomatic cardiovascular disease, moderate to severe HTN, hyperthyroidism, glaucoma, agitated states, history of drug abuse, during or within 14 days of MAOI use.

WARNINGS/PRECAUTIONS: May exacerbate symptoms of behavior disturbance and thought disorder in psychotic patients. Caution when using stimulants to treat patients with comorbid bipolar disorder because of concern for possible induction of mixed/manic episode in such patients. Stimulants at usual doses can cause treatment emergent psychotic or manic symptoms (eg, hallucinations, delusional thinking, mania) in children and adolescents without prior history of psychotic illness. Aggressive behavior or hostility reported in clinical trials and postmarketing experience of some medications indicated for the treatment of ADHD. Monitor growth in children. May lower convulsive threshold; d/c in presence of seizures. Visual disturbances reported with stimulant treatment. May exacerbate Tourette's syndrome and phonic or motor tics. Caution with HTN and monitor BP. Interrupt occasionally to determine if patient requires continued therapy. Sudden death reported in children with structural cardiac abnormalities; avoid use in children or adults with structural cardiac abnormalities. May decrease appetite.

ADVERSE REACTIONS: Abdominal pain, asthenia, fever, infection, viral infection, loss of appetite, diarrhea, nausea, vomiting, emotional lability, insomnia, nervousness, weight loss, dry mouth, headache, urticaria, anaphylaxis.

INTERACTIONS: GI acidifying agents (guanethidine, reserpine, glutamic acid, etc) and urinary acidifying agents (ammonium chloride, etc) decrease efficacy. MAOIs may cause hypertensive crisis. Potentiated by GI and urinary alkalinizers, propoxyphene overdose. Potentiated effects of both agents with TCAs. May delay absorption of phenytoin, ethosuximide, phenobarbital. Potentiates meperidine, norepinephrine, phenobarbital, phenytoin. Antagonized by haloperidol, chlorpromazine, lithium. Antagonizes adrenergic blockers, antihistamines, antihypertensives, veratrum alkaloids (antihypertensive). Avoid co-administration of alkalinizing agents (eg, antacid).

PREGNANCY: Category C, not for use in nursing.

Adenocard

adenosine (Astellas)

RX

THERAPEUTIC CLASS: Endogenous nucleoside

INDICATIONS: Conversion of paroxysmal supraventricular tachycardia (including Wolff-Parkinson-White syndrome) to sinus rhythm (SR).

DOSAGE: *Adults:* 6mg rapid IV bolus infusion over 1-2 seconds. If not converted to SR within 1-2 minutes, give 12mg rapid IV bolus; may give 2nd 12mg dose if needed. Max: 12mg/dose.

Pediatrics: <50kg: 0.05-0.1mg/kg rapid IV bolus. If not converted to SR within 1-2 minutes, give additional bolus doses incrementally increasing amount by 0.05-0.1mg/kg. Follow each bolus with a saline flush. Continue process until SR or a maximum single dose of 0.3mg/kg is used. ≥50kg: 6mg rapid IV bolus infusion over 1-2 seconds. If not converted to SR within 1-2 minutes, give 12mg rapid IV bolus; may give 2nd 12mg dose if needed. Max: 12mg/dose.

HOW SUPPLIED: Inj: 3mg/mL (2mL, 4mL)

CONTRAINDICATIONS: 2nd- or 3rd-degree AV block (except with pacemaker), sinus node disease such as sick sinus syndrome or symptomatic bradycardia (except with pacemaker).

WARNINGS/PRECAUTIONS: May produce short-lasting heart block. Transient or prolonged asystole, respiratory alkalosis, ventricular fibrillation reported. Caution with obstructive lung disease (eg, emphysema, bronchitis). Avoid with bronchoconstriction/bronchospasm (eg, asthma). D/C if severe respiratory difficulties develop. New arrhythmias may appear on ECG at time of conversion. Caution in elderly.

Adipex-P

ADVERSE REACTIONS: Facial flushing, dyspnea/shortness of breath, chest pressure, nausea.

INTERACTIONS: Antagonized by methylxanthines (eg, theophylline, caffeine); may need larger adenosine dose. Potentiated by dipyridamole; use lower adenosine dose. Caution with digoxin, verapamil; ventricular fibrillation reported and potential for additive/synergistic depressant effects on the SA and AV nodes. Possible higher degrees of heart block with carbamazepine.

PREGNANCY: Category C, safety in nursing not known.

Adipex-P
phentermine HCl (Gate)

CIV

THERAPEUTIC CLASS: Anorectic sympathomimetic amine

INDICATIONS: Short term adjunct for exogenous obesity if initial BMI ≥ 30 kg/m^2 or ≥ 27 kg/m^2 with other risk factors (eg, hypertension, diabetes hyperlipidemia).

DOSAGE: *Adults:* Usual: 37.5mg before breakfast or 1-2 hrs after breakfast. Alternate Schedule: 18.75mg qd-bid. Avoid late evening dosing.
Pediatrics: >16 yrs: Usual: 37.5mg before breakfast or 1-2 hrs after breakfast. Alternate Schedule: 18.75mg qd-bid. Avoid late evening dosing.

HOW SUPPLIED: Cap: 37.5mg; Tab: 37.5mg* *scored

CONTRAINDICATIONS: Advanced arteriosclerosis, cardiovascular disease, moderate to severe HTN, hyperthyroidism, glaucoma, agitated states, history of drug abuse, within 14 days of MAOI use.

WARNINGS/PRECAUTIONS: Only for short-term therapy. Primary pulmonary HTN and valvular heart disease reported. Abuse potential. Caution with mild HTN. Tolerance may develop.

ADVERSE REACTIONS: Primary pulmonary hypertension, regurgitant valvular heart disease, palpitation, tachycardia, BP elevation, CNS overstimulation, dry mouth, impotence, urticaria.

INTERACTIONS: May alter insulin requirements. Avoid alcohol and other weight loss products including SSRIs. Valvular heart disease and primary pulmonary hypertension reported with fenfluramine and dexfenfluramine. May decrease effects of guanethidine.

PREGNANCY: Category C, not for use in nursing.

Adriamycin
doxorubicin HCl (Bedford)

RX

> Severe local tissue necrosis will occur if extravasation occurs. Do not give IM/SC route. Myocardial toxicity may occur during or after therapy. Increased risk of CHF with high cumulative doses, previous anthracycline/anthracenedione therapy, pre-existing heart disease, radiotherapy to mediastinal/pericardial area, concomitant cardiotoxic drugs. Increased risk of delayed cardiotoxicity in pediatrics. Secondary acute myelogenous leukemia reported. Reduce dose in hepatic impairment. Severe myelosuppression may occur.

THERAPEUTIC CLASS: Anthracycline

INDICATIONS: To produce regression in disseminated neoplastic conditions such as acute lymphoblastic and myeloblastic leukemias, Wilms' tumor, neuroblastoma, soft tissue/bone sarcomas, carcinomas of the breast, ovary, bladder and thyroid, gastric and bronchogenic carcinomas, Hodgkin's disease, malignant lymphoma in which the small cell histologic type is the most responsive compared to other cell types.

DOSAGE: *Adults:* Monotherapy: 60-75mg/m^2 IV every 21 days. Use the lower dose with inadequate bone marrow reserves due to old age, prior therapy, or neoplastic marrow infiltration. Concomitant Chemotherapy: 40-60mg/m^2 IV every 21-28 days. Hyperbilirubinemia: Reduce dose by 50% if 1.2-3mg/dL; reduce dose by 75% if 3.1-5mg/dL.
Pediatrics: Monotherapy: 60-75mg/m^2 IV every 21 days. Use the lower dose with inadequate bone marrow reserves due to old age, prior therapy, or neoplastic marrow infiltration. Concomitant Chemotherapy: 40-60mg/m^2 IV every 21-28 days.

Hyperbilirubinemia: Reduce dose by 50% if 1.2-3mg/dL; reduce dose by 75% if 3.1-5mg/dL.

HOW SUPPLIED: Inj: 2mg/mL, 10mg, 20mg, 50mg

CONTRAINDICATIONS: Marked myelosuppression induced by previous treatment with other antitumor agents or radiotherapy. Previous therapy with complete cumulative doses of doxorubicin, daunorubicin, idarubicin, or other anthracyclines and anthracenes.

WARNINGS/PRECAUTIONS: Irreversible myocardial toxicity may occur. Bone marrow depression and arrhythmias reported. Enhanced toxicity with hepatic impairment; evaluate hepatic function before dosing. Imparts a red coloration to urine for 1-2 days after administration. May induce "tumor lysis syndrome" and hyperuricemia with rapidly growing tumors. Periodically monitor CBC, hepatic function, and radionuclide left ventricular ejection fraction. May cause prepubertal growth failure and gonadal impairment.

ADVERSE REACTIONS: Myelosuppression, cardiotoxicity, alopecia, nausea, vomiting, mucositis, ulceration and necrosis of colon, fever, chills, urticaria, phlebosclerosis, facial flushing.

INTERACTIONS: May potentiate toxicity of other anticancer therapies. May exacerbate cyclophosphamide-induced hemorrhagic cystitis. May enhance hepatotoxicity of 6-mercaptopurine. May increase radiation induced toxicity of the myocardium, mucosae, skin, and liver. Acute "recall" pneumonitis in pediatrics with actinomycin-D. Paclitaxel infused before doxorubicin may decrease clearance of doxorubicin and increase neutropenia and stomatitis episodes, than the reverse sequence of administration. Enhanced neutropenia and thrombocytopenia reported with IV progesterone. Cyclosporine may prolong and exacerbate hematologic toxicity. Phenobarbital increases elimination. May decrease phenytoin levels. Streptozocin may inhibit hepatic metabolism. Live vaccines may be hazardous in those undergoing cytotoxic chemotherapy. Necrotizing colitis reported with cytarabine. Seizures and coma reported with cyclosporine, cisplatin or vincristine. Possible increased risk of cardiotoxicity with calcium channel blockers. Increased risk of CHF with radiotherapy to mediastinal/pericardial area or cardiotoxic drugs.

PREGNANCY: Category D, not for use in nursing.

Advair
salmeterol xinafoate - fluticasone propionate (GlaxoSmithKline)   RX

> Long-acting β_2-adrenergic agonists, such as salmeterol, may increase the risk of asthma-related deaths.

THERAPEUTIC CLASS: Corticosteroid/beta$_2$ agonist

INDICATIONS: For long-term, maintenance treatment of asthma. (250/50mcg only): Treatment of COPD with chronic bronchitis.

DOSAGE: *Adults:* Asthma: 1 inh q12h. Without Prior Inhaled Corticosteroid (CS): Initial: 100/50 bid. Max: 500/50 bid. Current Inhaled CS: Beclomethasone: ≤160mcg/day use 100/50 bid, 320mcg/day use 250/50Bid, 640mcg/day use 500/50 bid. Budesonide: ≤400mcg/day use 100/50 bid, 800-1200mcg/day use 250/50 bid, 1600mcg/day use 500/50 bid. Flunisolide: ≤1000mcg/day use 100/50 bid, 1250-2000mcg/day use 250/50 bid. Flunisolide HFA: ≤320mcg/day use 100/50 bid, 640mcg/day use 250/50 bid. Fluticasone HFA: ≤176mcg/day use 100/50 bid, 440mcg/day use 250/50 bid, 660-880mcg/day use 500/50 bid. Fluticasone Powder: ≤200mcg/day use 100/50 bid, 500mcg/day use 250/50 bid, 1000mcg/day use 500/50 bid. Mometasone: 220mcg/day use 100/50 bid, 440mcg/day use 250/50 bid, 880mcg/day use 500/50 bid. Triamcinolone: ≤1000mcg/day use 100/50 bid, 1100-1600mcg/day use 250/50 bid. If no response within 2 weeks, increase to higher strength. COPD: (250/50 only): 1 inh q12h. Rinse mouth after use.

Pediatrics: ≥12 yrs: 1 inh q12h. Without Prior Inhaled CS: Initial: 100/50 bid. Max: 500/50 bid. Current Inhaled CS: Beclomethasone: ≤160mcg/day use 100/50 bid, 320mcg/day use 250/50 Bid, 640mcg/day use 500/50 bid. Budesonide: ≤400mcg/day use 100/50 bid, 800-1200mcg/day use 250/50 bid, 1600mcg/day use 500/50 bid. Flunisolide: ≤1000mcg/day use 100/50 bid, 1250-2000mcg/day use 250/50 bid. Flunisolide HFA: ≤320mcg/day use 100/50 bid, 640mcg/day use 250/50 bid. Fluticasone HFA: ≤176mcg/day use 100/50 bid, 440mcg/day use 250/50 bid, 660-880mcg/day use 500/50 bid. Flu-

Advair HFA

ticasone Powder: ≤200mcg/day use 100/50 bid, 500mcg/day use 250/50 bid, 1000mcg/day use 500/50 bid. Mometasone: 220mcg/day use 100/50 bid, 440mcg/day use 250/50 bid, 880mcg/day use 500/50 bid. Triamcinolone: ≤1000mcg/day use 100/50 bid, 1100-1600mcg/day use 250/50 bid. If no response within 2 weeks, increase to higher strength. 4-11 yrs: (100/50mcg only): Symptomatic on Inhaled CS: 1 inh q12h. Rinse mouth after use.

HOW SUPPLIED: Disk (Inhalation): (Fluticasone-Salmeterol) (100/50) 0.1mg-0.05mg/inh, (250/50) 0.25mg-0.05mg/inh, (500/50) 0.5mg-0.05mg/inh (60 blisters)

CONTRAINDICATIONS: Status asthmaticus or other acute asthma or COPD episodes.

WARNINGS/PRECAUTIONS: See Contraindications. Deaths due to adrenal insufficiency have occurred with transfer from systemic corticosteroids to inhaled corticosteroids. Resume oral corticosteroids during stress or severe asthma attack. Observe for adrenal insufficiency, systemic corticosteroid withdrawal effects, hypercorticism, reduction in growth velocity (pediatrics). More susceptible to infection. Not for acute bronchospasm. Discontinue if bronchospasm occurs after dosing. Caution with TB; untreated systemic fungal, bacterial, viral or parasitic infections; or ocular herpes simplex. *Candida* infection of mouth and pharynx, glaucoma, hypersensitivity reactions, increased IOP, cataracts reported. Monitor for increasing use of β_2 agonists. QTc interval prolongation reported with large doses. Discontinue if paradoxical bronchospasm occurs. Caution with cardiovascular disorders.

ADVERSE REACTIONS: Upper respiratory tract inflammation, pharyngitis, sinusitis, cough, hoarseness, headaches, GI effects, musculoskeletal pain, palpitations.

INTERACTIONS: Extreme caution with TCAs or MAOIs during or within 14 days of use. Antagonized by β-blockers. Caution with non-potassium sparing diuretics; ECG changes, hypokalemia may develop. Potentiated by ketoconazole, other CYP3A4 inhibitors.

PREGNANCY: Category C, caution in nursing.

Advair HFA RX
salmeterol xinafoate - fluticasone propionate (GlaxoSmithKline)

> Long-acting β_2-adrenergic agonists, such as salmeterol, may increase the risk of asthma-related deaths.

THERAPEUTIC CLASS: Corticosteroid/beta$_2$ agonist

INDICATIONS: For long-term, maintenance treatment of asthma.

DOSAGE: *Adults:* Asthma: 2 inh q12h. Without Prior Inhaled Corticosteroid (CS): Initial: 2 inh of 45/21 bid or 1 inh of 115/21 bid. Max: 2 inh of 230/21 bid. Current Inhaled CS: Beclomethasone: ≤160mcg/day use 2 inh of 45/21 bid, 320mcg/day use 2 inh of 115/21 bid, 640mcg/day use 2 inh of 230/21 bid. Budesonide: ≤400mcg/day use 2 inh of 45/21 bid, 800-1200mcg/day use 2 inh of 115/21 bid, 1600mcg/day use 2 inh of 230/21 bid. Flunisolide: ≤1000mcg/day use 2 inh of 45/21 bid, 1250-2000mcg/day use 2 inh of 115/21 bid. Flunisolide HFA: ≤320mcg/day use 2 inh of 45/21 bid, 640mcg/day use 2 inh of 115/21 bid. Fluticasone Aerosol: ≤176mcg/day use 2 inh of 45/21 bid, 440mcg/day use 2 inh of 115/21 bid, 660-880mcg/day use 2 inh of 230/21 bid. Fluticasone Powder: ≤200mcg/day use 2 inh of 45/21 bid, 500mcg/day use 2 inh of 115/21 bid, 1000mcg/day use 2 inh of 230/21 bid. Mometasone Powder: 220mcg/day use 2 inh of 45/21 bid, 440mcg/day use 2 inh of 115/21 bid, 880mcg/day use 2 inh of 230/21 bid. Triamcinolone: ≤1000mcg/day use 2 inh of 45/21 bid, 1100-1600mcg/day use 2 inh of 115/21 bid. If no response within 2 weeks, increase to higher strength.

Pediatrics: ≥12 yrs: Asthma: 2 inh q12h. Without Prior Inhaled Corticosteroid (CS): Initial: 2 inh of 45/21 bid or 1 inh of 115/21 bid. Max: 2 inh of 230-21 bid. Current Inhaled CS: Beclomethasone: ≤160mcg/day use 2 inh of 45/21 bid, 320mcg/day use 2 inh of 115/21 bid, 640mcg/day use 2 inh of 230/21 bid. Budesonide: ≤400mcg/day use 2 inh of 45/21 bid, 800-1200mcg/day use 2 inh of 115/21 bid, 1600mcg/day use 2 inh of 230/21 bid. Flunisolide: ≤1000mcg/day use 2 inh of 45/21 bid, 1250-2000mcg/day use 2 inh of 115/21 bid. Flunisolide HFA: ≤320mcg/day use 2 inh of 45/21 bid, 640mcg/day use 2 inh of 115/21 bid. Fluticasone Aerosol: ≤176mcg/day use 2 inh of 45/21 bid, 440mcg/day use 2 inh of 115/21 bid, 660-880mcg/day use 2 inh of 230/21 bid. Fluticasone Powder: ≤200mcg/day use 2 inh of 45/21 bid, 500mcg/day use 2 inh of 115/21 bid, 1000mcg/day use 2 inh of 230/21 bid. Mometasone powder: 220mcg/day use 2 inh of 45/21 bid, 440mcg/day use 2 inh of 115/21 bid, 880mcg/day use 2 inh of 230/21 bid. Triamcinolone: ≤1000mcg/day use 2 inh of 45/21 bid, 1100-1600mcg/day use 2 inh of 115/21 bid. If no response within 2 weeks, increase to higher strength.

HOW SUPPLIED: MDI: (Fluticasone-Salmeterol) (45/21) 0.045mg-0.021mg/inh, (115/21) 0.115mg-0.021mg/inh, (230/21) 0.230mg-0.021mg/inh (120 inhalations)

CONTRAINDICATIONS: Status asthmaticus or other acute asthma.

WARNINGS/PRECAUTIONS: See Contraindications. Deaths due to adrenal insufficiency have occurred with transfer from systemic corticosteroids to inhaled corticosteroids. Resume oral corticosteroids during stress or severe asthma attack. Observe for adrenal insufficiency, systemic corticosteroid withdrawal effects, hypercorticism, reduction in growth velocity (pediatrics). More susceptible to infection. Not for acute bronchospasm. Discontinue if bronchospasm occurs after dosing. Caution with TB; untreated systemic fungal, bacterial, viral or parasitic infections; or ocular herpes simplex. Candida infection of mouth and pharynx, glaucoma, hypersensitivity reactions, increased IOP, cataracts reported. Monitor for increasing use of β_2 agonists. QTc interval prolongation reported with large doses. Discontinue if paradoxical bronchospasm occurs. Caution with cardiovascular disorders.

ADVERSE REACTIONS: Upper respiratory tract infection, throat irritation, upper respiratory tract inflammation, headaches, nausea, vomiting, musculoskeletal pain, menstruation symptoms.

INTERACTIONS: Extreme caution with TCAs or MAOIs during or within 14 days of use. Antagonized by β-blockers. Caution with non-potassium sparing diuretics; ECG changes, hypokalemia may develop. Potentiated by ketoconazole, other CYP3A4 inhibitors.

PREGNANCY: Category C, caution in nursing.

Aerobid
flunisolide (Forest)

RX

OTHER BRAND NAME: Aerobid-M (with menthol) (Forest)

THERAPEUTIC CLASS: Corticosteroid

INDICATIONS: Maintenance treatment of asthma as prophylactic therapy in patients ≥6 years and to reduce or eliminate the need for oral systemic corticosteroidal therapy.

DOSAGE: *Adults:* Initial: 2 inh bid. Max: 4 inh bid. Rinse mouth after use.
Pediatrics: 6-15 yrs: 2 inh bid. Rinse mouth after use.

HOW SUPPLIED: MDI: 0.25mg/inh (7g)

CONTRAINDICATIONS: Primary treatment of status asthmaticus or other acute asthma attacks.

WARNINGS/PRECAUTIONS: Deaths due to adrenal insufficiency have occurred with transfer from systemic corticosteroids to inhaled corticosteroids. Resume oral corticosteroids during stress or severe asthma attack. Observe for adrenal insufficiency, systemic corticosteroid withdrawal effects, and growth suppression (children). More susceptible to infections. Not for acute bronchospasm. D/C if bronchospasm occurs after dosing. Caution with tuberculosis of the respiratory tract; untreated systemic fungal, bacterial, viral or parasitic infections; or ocular herpes simplex. *Candida* infection of the mouth and pharynx reported.

ADVERSE REACTIONS: Upper respiratory infection, diarrhea, stomach upset, cold symptoms, nasal congestion, headache, nausea, vomiting, sore throat, unpleasant taste.

PREGNANCY: Category C, caution with nursing.

Agenerase
amprenavir (GlaxoSmithKline)

RX

> Oral solution contains propylene glycol; risk of toxicity in pediatrics <4 yrs, pregnant women, hepatic or renal failure, and concomitant disulfiram or metronidazole.

THERAPEUTIC CLASS: Protease inhibitor

AGRYLIN

INDICATIONS: Treatment of HIV infection in combination with other antiretrovirals.

DOSAGE: *Adults:* (Cap) 1200mg bid. Hepatic Impairment (Child-Pugh score 5-8): 450mg bid. (Child-Pugh score 9-12) 300mg bid. Avoid high-fat meals. (Sol): 1400mg bid
Pediatrics: (Cap) 13-16 yrs: 1200mg bid. 13-16 yrs and <50kg or 4-12yrs: 20mg/kg bid or 15mg/kg tid. Max: 2400mg/day. Hepatic Impairment (Child-Pugh score 5-8): 450mg bid. (Child-Pugh score 9-12) 300mg bid. Avoid high-fat meals. (Sol) >16 yrs or 13-16 yrs and ≥50kg: 1400mg bid. 4-12 yrs or 13-16 yrs and <50kg: 22.5mg/kg bid or 17mg/kg tid. Max: 2800mg/day.

HOW SUPPLIED: Cap: 50mg; Sol: 15mg/mL (240mL)

CONTRAINDICATIONS: (Cap, Sol) Drugs highly dependent on CYP450 3A4 for clearance (eg, dihydroergotamine, ergonovine, ergotamine, methylergonovine, cisapride, pimozide, midazolam, triazolam). (Sol) <4 yrs, pregnancy, hepatic or renal failure, concomitant disulfiram or metronidazole. (Cap) Flecanide and propafenone if coadministered with ritonavir.

WARNINGS/PRECAUTIONS: Caution with sulfonamide allergy. Spontaneous bleeding may occur with hemophilia A and B. Possible redistribution or accumulation of body fat. Caps and solution are not interchangeable on mg-mg basis. Severe life-threatening reactions including Stevens-Johnson syndrome reported. New onset and exacerbation of diabetes and hyperglycemia reported. May elevate LFTs; caution with hepatic impairment. May increase cholesterol and triglycerides; monitor before therapy and periodically thereafter.

ADVERSE REACTIONS: Severe skin reactions, rash, paresthesias, depression, nausea, vomiting, diarrhea, abdominal pain, hyperlipidemia.

INTERACTIONS: Serious/life-threatening interactions may occur with amiodarone, lidocaine (systemic), TCAs, and quinidine. Monitor INR with warfarin. Avoid supplemental vitamin E. Avoid astemizole, terfenadine, pimozide, ergonovine, methylergonovine, midazolam, triazolam, dihydroergotamine, ergotamine, and cisapride. Possible loss of virologic response and resistance with rifampin and St. John's wort. Give 50% of rifabutin dose. Increased risk of rhabdomyolysis with lovastatin, simvastatin. Increased sildenafil levels. Take 1 hr before or after antacids and didanosine. Increased levels of ketoconazole, itraconazole, alprazolam, clorazepate, diazepam, flurazepam, and calcium channel blockers. Oral contraceptives (ethinyl estradiol/norethindrone) may decrease efficacy and lead to resistance; use alternative non-hormonal contraception. Decreases methodone levels. Phenobarbital, phenytoin, and carbamazepine decrease levels. Increased bepridil levels; life-threatening reaction can occur. Decreased levels with dexamethasone. Monitor levels of cyclosporine, tacrolimus, rapamycin, and TCAs. Avoid solution administration with ritonavir solution. Reduce dose with ritonavir caps. Elevated LFTs, cholesterol, and TG with low-dose ritonavir. Use lowest possible dose of atorvastatin or consider other HMG-CoA reductase inhibitor.

PREGNANCY: (Cap) Category C, (Sol) Contraindicated in pregnancy; not for use in nursing.

AGRYLIN
anagrelide HCl (Shire US)

RX

THERAPEUTIC CLASS: Platelet-reducing agent

INDICATIONS: Treatment of thrombocythemia secondary to myeloproliferative disorders.

DOSAGE: *Adults:* Initial: 0.5mg qid or 1mg bid for at least 1 week. Moderate Hepatic Impairment: Initial: 0.5mg qd for at least 1 week. Titrate: Increase by no more than 0.5mg/day per week. Max: 10mg/day or 2.5mg/dose. Adjust lowest effective dose to reduce and maintain platelets <600,000/mcL. Monitor platelets every 2 days during first week, then weekly thereafter until reach maintenance dose.

Pediatrics: Initial: 0.5mg qd. Titrate: Increase by no more than 0.5mg/day per week. Max: 10mg/day or 2.5mg/dose. Adjust to lowest effective dose to reduce and maintain platelets <600,000/mcL. Monitor platelets every 2 days during first week, then weekly thereafter until reach maintenance dose.

HOW SUPPLIED: Cap: 0.5mg, 1mg

CONTRAINDICATIONS: Severe hepatic impairment.

WARNINGS/PRECAUTIONS: Caution with heart disease, renal or hepatic dysfunction. Perform pre-treatment cardiovascular exam and monitor during treatment; may cause cardiovascular effects (eg, vasodilation, tachycardia, palpitations, CHF). Monitor closely for renal toxicity if creatinine ≥2mg/dL or hepatic toxicity if bilirubin, SGOT, or LFTs >1.5X ULN). Monitor blood counts, renal and hepatic function while platelets are lowered. Increase in platelets after therapy interruption. Reduce dose in moderate hepatic impairment.

ADVERSE REACTIONS: Headache, palpitations, asthenia, edema, GI effects, dizziness, pain, dyspnea, fever, chest pain, rash, tachycardia, malaise, pharyngitis, cough, paresthesia.

INTERACTIONS: Sucralfate may interfere with absorption. Exacerbated effects of products that inhibit cyclic AMP PDE III (inotropes: milrinone, enoximone, amrinone, olparinone, cilostazol).

PREGNANCY: Category C, not for use in nursing.

AK-Fluor
fluorescein sodium (Akorn)

RX

THERAPEUTIC CLASS: Diagnostic dye

INDICATIONS: Indicated in diagnostic fluorescein angiography or angioscopy of the fundus and iris vasculature.

DOSAGE: *Adults:* Perform intradermal skin test before IV use if suspect potential allergy. Inject contents of ampule rapidly into antecubital vein. A syringe with fluorescein is attached to transparent tubing and a 25 gauge scalp vein needle for injection. Insert needle and draw patient's blood to hub of syringe so small air bubble separates patient's blood in tubing from fluorescein. With room lights on, inject blood back into vein while watching skin over needle tip. If needle extravasated, patient's blood will bulge skin; stop injection before injecting fluorescein. When certain there is no extravasation, turn room light off and complete fluorescein injection. Luminescence appears in retina and choroidal vessels in 9-14 seconds.

Pediatrics: Perform intradermal skin test before IV use if suspect potential allergy. Dose is 35mg/10lbs. Inject contents of ampule/vial rapidly into antecubital vein. A syringe with fluorescein is attached to transparent tubing and a 25 gauge scalp vein needle for injection. Insert needle and draw patient's blood to hub of syringe so small air bubble separates patient's blood in tubing from fluorescein. With room lights on, inject blood back into vein while watching skin over needle tip. If needle extravasated, patient's blood will bulge skin; stop injection before injecting fluorescein. When certain there is no extravasation, turn room light off and complete fluorescein injection. Luminescence appears in retina and choroidal vessels in 9-14 seconds.

HOW SUPPLIED: Inj: 10% (5mL), 25% (2mL)

WARNINGS/PRECAUTIONS: Avoid extravasation; severe local tissue damage can occur. Caution with history of allergy or bronchial asthma. Have emergency tray (eg, 0.1% epinephrine IV/IM, antihistamine, soluble steroid, IV aminophylline) and oxygen available. Avoid angiography in pregnancy, especially 1st trimester. Skin attains temporary yellowish discoloration and urine attains bright yellow color.

ADVERSE REACTIONS: Nausea, vomiting, headache, GI distress, syncope, hypotension, cardiac arrest, basilar artery ischemia, severe shock, convulsions, thrombophlebitis.

PREGNANCY: Safety in pregnancy not known, caution in nursing.

Alacol DM
phenylephrine HCl - dextromethorphan HBr - brompheniramine maleate
(Ballay)

RX

THERAPEUTIC CLASS: Antihistamine/antitussive/sympathomimetic

INDICATIONS: Relief of cough and upper respiratory symptoms including nasal congestion, associated with allergy or the common cold.

DOSAGE: *Adults:* 10mL q4h. Max: 6 doses/24 hrs.

Pediatrics: >12 yrs: 10mL q4h. 6-12 yrs: 5mL q4h. 2-6 yrs: 2.5mL q4h. Max: 6 doses/24 hrs.

HOW SUPPLIED: Syrup: (Brompheniramine-Dextromethorphan-Phenylephrine) 2mg-10mg-5mg/5mL

ALAMAST

CONTRAINDICATIONS: Newborns, premature infants, nursing, severe HTN or CAD, with MAOIs, lower respiratory tract conditions including asthma.

WARNINGS/PRECAUTIONS: Caution with persistent or chronic cough (eg, associated with asthma, emphysema, smoking, excessive phlegm). Persistent cough may be a sign of a serious condition. May diminish mental alertness. May produce excitation in children. Caution with asthma, narrow-angle glaucoma, GI obstruction, urinary bladder neck obstruction, DM, HTN, heart and thyroid disease.

ADVERSE REACTIONS: Sedation, thickening of bronchial secretions, dizziness, dryness of mouth, nose, and throat.

INTERACTIONS: Additive effects with alcohol, CNS depressants (eg, hypnotics, sedatives, tranquilizers, anxiolytics). MAOIs may prolong/intensify anticholinergic effects of antihistamines and phenylephrine. May reduce effects of antihypertensives.

PREGNANCY: Category C, contraindicated in nursing.

ALAMAST
pemirolast potassium (Vistakon)

RX

THERAPEUTIC CLASS: Mast cell stabilizer

INDICATIONS: Prevention of ocular itching due to allergic conjunctivitis.

DOSAGE: *Adults:* 1-2 drops in affected eye qid.
Pediatrics: ≥3 yrs: 1-2 drops in affected eye qid.

HOW SUPPLIED: Sol: 0.1% (10mL)

WARNINGS/PRECAUTIONS: May reinsert soft contact lens after 10 minutes, if eyes are not red. Contains lauralkonium chloride; may be absorbed by soft contact lens.

ADVERSE REACTIONS: Headache, rhinitis, cold/flu symptoms, ocular burning/discomfort, dry eye, foreign body sensation.

PREGNANCY: Category C, caution in nursing.

ALBENZA
albendazole (GlaxoSmithKline)

RX

THERAPEUTIC CLASS: Broad-spectrum anthelmintic

INDICATIONS: Treatment of parenchymal neurocysticercosis and cystic hydatid disease of the liver, lung, and peritoneum.

DOSAGE: *Adults:* Hydatid Disease: ≥60kg: 400mg bid. <60kg: 7.5mg/kg bid up to 800mg/day. Take with meals for 28 days, then 14 days drug-free, repeat for a total of 3 cycles. Neurocysticercosis: Same dose as Hydatid disease. Treat for 8-30 days.
Pediatrics: ≥6 yrs: Hydatid Disease: ≥60kg: 400mg bid. <60kg: 7.5mg/kg bid up to 800mg/day. Take with meals for 28 days, then 14 days drug-free, repeat for a total of 3 cycles. Neurocysticercosis: Same dose as Hydatid disease. Treat for 8-30 days.

HOW SUPPLIED: Tab: 200mg

WARNINGS/PRECAUTIONS: Monitor blood counts at the beginning of each 28-day cycle, and every 2 weeks during therapy. May continue if total WBC and absolute neutrophil count decrease are modest and do not progress. Not for use in pregnancy unless no other therapy is appropriate. Avoid pregnancy at least 1 month after discontinuing therapy. Discontinue immediately if become pregnant. Treatment for neurocysticercosis should include anticonvulsants and steroids. Examine for retinal lesions before therapy. Elevated LFTs reported.

ADVERSE REACTIONS: Abnormal LFTs, abdominal pain, nausea, vomiting, headache.

INTERACTIONS: Monitor theophylline levels after therapy. Increased levels with dexamethasone, praziquantel, and cimetidine.

PREGNANCY: Category C, caution in nursing.

ALBUTEROL
albuterol sulfate (Various)

RX

OTHER BRAND NAME: Proventil (Schering)

THERAPEUTIC CLASS: Beta$_2$ agonist

INDICATIONS: (Aerosol) Prevention and treatment of bronchospasm with reversible obstructive airway disease. Prevention of Exercise-Induced Bronchospasm (EIB). (Sol) Relief of bronchospasm with reversible obstructive airway disease and acute attacks of bronchospasm in patients ≥12 yrs. (Tab, Tab, Extended Release) Relief of bronchospasm with reversible obstructive airway disease in patients ≥6 yrs. (Syrup) Relief of bronchospasm in patients ≥2 yrs with reversible obstructive airway disease.

DOSAGE: *Adults:* Bronchospasm: (Aerosol) 2 inh q4-6h or 1 inh q4h. (Repetabs) Initial: 4-8mg q12h. Max: 32mg/day. (Sol) 2.5mg tid-qid by nebulizer. (Syrup, Tabs) 2-4mg tid-qid. Max: 32mg/day (8mg qid). Elderly/Beta-Adrenergic Sensitivity: (Syrup, Tabs) Initial: 2mg tid-qid. Max: (Tabs) 8mg tid-qid. EIB: (Aerosol) 2 inh 15 minutes before activity.

Pediatrics: Bronchospasm: >14 yrs: (Syrup) Initial: 2-4mg tid-qid. Max: 8mg qid. ≥12 yrs: (Aerosol) 2 inh q4-6h or 1 inh q4h. (Sol) 2.5mg tid-qid by nebulizer. (Tabs) Initial: 2-4mg tid-qid. Max: 8mg qid. >12 yrs: (Repetabs) Initial: 4-8mg q12h. Max: 32mg/day. 6-14 yrs: (Syrup) Initial: 2mg tid-qid. Max: 24mg/day. 6-12 yrs: (Repetabs) Initial: 4mg q12h. Max: 24mg/day. (Tabs) Initial: 2mg tid-qid. Max: 24mg/day. 2-5 yrs: (Syrup) Initial: 0.1mg/kg tid (not to exceed 2mg tid). Titrate: May increase to 0.2mg/kg/day. Max: 4mg tid. EIB: ≥12 yrs: (Aerosol) 2 inh 15 minutes before activity.

HOW SUPPLIED: Aerosol: 0.09mg/inh (17g); Sol (neb): 0.083% (3mL, 25's), 0.5% (20mL); Syrup: 2mg/5mL; Tab: 2mg*, 4mg*; Tab, Extended Release (Repetabs): 4mg *scored

WARNINGS/PRECAUTIONS: Hypersensitivity reactions reported. Monitor for worsening asthma. Fatalities reported with excessive use. Caution with cardiovascular disorders, especially coronary insufficiency, arrhythmias and HTN. May need concomitant corticosteroids. Can produce paradoxical bronchospasm. Caution with DM, hyperthyroidism, seizures. May cause transient hypokalemia.

ADVERSE REACTIONS: Tachycardia, increased BP, tremor, nervousness, dizziness, nausea/vomiting, palpitations, paradoxical bronchospasm, heartburn, rhinitis, respiratory tract infection.

INTERACTIONS: Avoid other sympathomimetic agents. Extreme caution with MAOIs and TCAs. Monitor digoxin. May worsen ECG changes and/or hypokalemia with nonpotassium-sparing diuretics. Antagonized by β-blockers.

PREGNANCY: Category C, not for use in nursing.

Alcortin
iodoquinol - hydrocortisone (Primus)   RX

THERAPEUTIC CLASS: Corticosteroid/Anti-infective

INDICATIONS: "Possibly" Effective: Contact or atopic dermatitis, impetiginized eczema, nummular eczema, endogenous chronic infectious dermatitis, stasis dermatitis, pyoderma, nuchal eczema and chronic eczematoid otitis externa, acne urticata, localized or disseminated neurodermatitis, lichen simplex chronicus, anogenital pruritus (vulvae, scroti, ani), folliculitis, bacterial dermatoses, mycotic dermatoses such as tinea (capitis, cruris, corporis, pedis), monliasis, intertrigo.

DOSAGE: *Adults:* Apply to affected area(s) tid-qid.

Pediatrics: ≥12 yrs: Apply to affected area(s) tid-qid.

HOW SUPPLIED: Gel: (Hydrocortisone-Iodoquinol) 2%-1% (2g)

WARNINGS/PRECAUTIONS: For external use only. Avoid eyes. Discontinue if irritation develops. May stain skin, hair, or fabrics. Risk of systemic absorption with treatment of extensive areas or use of occlusive dressings. Increased risk of systemic absorption in children. Iodoquinol may interfere with thyroid tests. False-positive phenylketonuria test reported.

ADVERSE REACTIONS: Burning, itching, irritation, dryness, folliculitis, hypertrichosis, acneiform eruptions, hypopigmentation, perioral dermatitis, allergic dermatitis, skin maceration, secondary infection, skin atrophy, striae, miliaria.

PREGNANCY: Category C, caution in nursing.

Aldara
imiquimod (Graceway)   RX

THERAPEUTIC CLASS: Immune response modifier

INDICATIONS: Actinic keratoses on face or scalp in immunocompetent adults. External genital and perianal warts/condyloma acuminata. Biopsy-confirmed, primary superfi-

ALEVE

cial basal cell carcinoma (sBCC) in immunocompetent adults, with a maximum tumor diameter of 2cm, located on the trunk (excluding anogenital skin), neck, or extremities (excluding hands and feet), only when surgical methods are medically less appropriate and patient follow-up can be assured.

DOSAGE: *Adults:* Use before bedtime. Actinic Keratosis: Usual: Apply 2x/week to defined area on face or scalp (but not both concurrently). Wash off after 8 hrs with soap and water. Max: 16 weeks. External Genital and Perianal Warts/Condyloma: Usual: Apply 3x/week. Wash off after 6-10 hrs with soap and water. Use until warts are clear. Max: 16 weeks. May suspend use for several days to manage local reactions. Do not occlude treatment area. sBCC: Apply 5x/week for 6 weeks. If tumor diameter is 0.5 to <1cm, use 4mm (10mg) of cream. If tumor is ≥1 to <1.5cm, use 5mm (25mg) of cream. If tumor is ≥1.5 to 2cm, use 7mm (40mg) of cream. Max diameter of tumor: ≤2cm. Treatment area should include a 1cm margin of skin around the tumor. Wash off after 8 hrs with soap and water.

Pediatrics: ≥12 yrs: External Genital and Perianal Warts/Condyloma: Usual: Apply 3x/week before bedtime. Wash off after 6-10 hrs with soap and water. Use until warts are clear. Max: 16 weeks. May suspend use for several days to manage local reactions. Do not occlude treatment area.

HOW SUPPLIED: Cre: 5% (12 pkt)

WARNINGS/PRECAUTIONS: Not for urethral, intra-vaginal, cervical, rectal, or intra-anal human papilloma viral disease. Avoid sexual contact while cream is on skin. May weaken condoms and diaphragms; avoid concurrent use. Avoid or minimize exposure to sunlight. May exacerbate inflammatory skin conditions. Avoid contact with eyes, lips, nostrils. Avoid after surgery or with sunburn until tissue is healed.

ADVERSE REACTIONS: Wart (erythema, erosion, flaking, edema) and application site reactions (bleeding, burning, itching, pain), flu-like symptoms, headache.

INTERACTIONS: Avoid topical drugs immediately after treatment of warts.

PREGNANCY: Category C, safety in nursing not known.

ALEVE OTC
naproxen sodium (Bayer Healthcare)

THERAPEUTIC CLASS: NSAID

INDICATIONS: Relief of minor aches and pains. Reduction of fever.

DOSAGE: *Adults:* Initial: 1 to 2 tabs, then 1 tab q8-12h. Max: 660mg/24hrs or 440mg/12hrs. Elderly: >65 yrs: 1 tab q12h.

Pediatrics: ≥12 yrs: Initial: 1 to 2 tabs, then 1 tab q8-12h. Max: 660mg/24hrs or 440mg/12hrs.

HOW SUPPLIED: Tab: 220mg

WARNINGS/PRECAUTIONS: Avoid during last trimester of pregnancy. Do not use >10 days for pain or >3 days for fever.

INTERACTIONS: Increased risk of GI bleeding with alcohol.

PREGNANCY: Safety in pregnancy or nursing not known.

ALINIA RX
nitazoxanide (Romark)

THERAPEUTIC CLASS: Antiprotozoal agent

INDICATIONS: Treatment of diarrhea caused by *Cryptosporidium parvum* and *Giardia lamblia*.

DOSAGE: *Adults:* ≥12 yrs: G.lamblia Diarhhea: 500mg q12h for 3 days. Take with food.
Pediatrics: C.parvum/G.lamblia Diarrhea: 1-3 yrs: 100mg (5mL) q12h for 3 days. 4-11yrs: 200mg (10mL) q12h for 3 days. G.lamblia Diarrhea: ≥12 yrs: 500mg (1 tab or 25mL) q12h for 3 days. Take with food.

HOW SUPPLIED: Sus: 100mg/5mL (60mL); Tab: 500mg (60^s, 3-Day Therapy Packs, 6^s)

ALLEGRA

WARNINGS/PRECAUTIONS: Caution with hepatic and biliary disease, renal disease. Contains 1.48g sucrose/5mL. Safety and effectiveness have not been established in HIV positive or immunodeficient patients.
ADVERSE REACTIONS: Abdominal pain, diarrhea, headache, nausea.
INTERACTIONS: Highly protein bound; caution with other highly plasma protein-bound drugs with narrow therapeutic indices.
PREGNANCY: Category B; caution in nursing.

All Clear
polyethylene glycol 300 - naphazoline HCl (Bausch & Lomb)   OTC

THERAPEUTIC CLASS: Decongestant/lubricant
INDICATIONS: To relieve eye redness due to minor eye irritations. Temporary relief of burning and irritation due to dryness of the eye and as a protectant against further irritation.
DOSAGE: *Adults:* 1-2 drops in affected eye up to qid.
Pediatrics: ≥6 yrs: 1-2 drops in affected eye up to qid.
HOW SUPPLIED: Sol: (Naphazoline-Polyethylene Glycol 300) 0.012%-0.2% (15mL)
WARNINGS/PRECAUTIONS: Overuse may cause more redness. Remove contact lenses before use. Do not touch container tip to any surface to avoid contamination. D/C if eye pain or vision changes occur, if redness or irritation continues, or if condition worsens or persists >72 hrs. Supervision required in patients with glaucoma.
PREGNANCY: Safety in pregnancy or nursing not known.

All Clear AR
hydroxypropyl methylcellulose - naphazoline HCl (Bausch & Lomb)   OTC

THERAPEUTIC CLASS: Decongestant/lubricant
INDICATIONS: Temporary relief of discomfort due to minor irritations of the eye or to exposure to wind or sun. To prevent further irritation or to relieve eye dryness. To relieve eye redness due to minor eye irritations.
DOSAGE: *Adults:* 1-2 drops in affected eye up to qid.
Pediatrics: ≥8 yrs: 1-2 drops in affected eye up to qid.
HOW SUPPLIED: Sol: (Naphazoline-Hydroxypropyl Methylcellulose) 0.03%-0.5% (15mL)
WARNINGS/PRECAUTIONS: Overuse may cause more redness. Remove contact lenses before use. Do not touch container tip to any surface to avoid contamination. D/C if eye pain or vision changes occur, if redness or irritation continues, or if condition worsens or persists >72 hrs. Supervision required in patients with glaucoma.
PREGNANCY: Safety in pregnancy or nursing not known.

Allegra
fexofenadine HCl (Sanofi-Aventis)   RX

THERAPEUTIC CLASS: H_1 antagonist
INDICATIONS: (Sus) Relief of symptoms associated with seasonal allergic rhinitis in children 2-11 yrs. Treatment of uncomplicated skin manifestations of chronic idiopathic urticaria in children 6 months to 11 yrs. (Tab) Relief of symptoms associated with seasonal allergic rhinitis and treatment of uncomplicated skin manifestations of chronic idiopathic urticaria in adults and children ≥6 yrs.
DOSAGE: *Adults:* Tab: Rhinitis/Urticaria: 60mg bid or 180mg qd. Renal Dysfunction: Initial: 60mg qd.
Pediatrics: Tab: ≥12 yrs: Rhinitis/Urticaria: 60mg bid or 180mg qd. Renal Dysfunction: Initial: 60mg qd. 6-11 yrs: Rhinitis/Urticaria: 30mg bid. Renal Dysfunction: Initial: 30mg qd. Sus: Rhinitis: 2-11 yrs: 30mg (5mL) bid. Renal Dysfunction: 30mg (5mL) qd. Urticaria: 2-11 yrs: 30mg (5mL) bid. Renal Dysfunction: 30mg (5mL) qd. 6 months to <2 yrs: 15mg (2.5mL) bid. Renal Dysfunction: 15mg (2.5mL) qd.
HOW SUPPLIED: Tab: 30mg, 60mg, 180mg; Sus: 30mg/5mL

Allegra-D

ADVERSE REACTIONS: Headache, cough, upper respiratory tract infection, back pain, fever, pain, otitis media, chronic idiopathic urticaria.

INTERACTIONS: Increased plasma levels with erythromycin or ketoconazole. Avoid concomitant aluminum- and magnesium-containing antacids. Fruit juices (eg, grapefruit, orange and apple) may decrease levels.

PREGNANCY: Category C, caution in nursing.

Allegra-D   RX
fexofenadine HCl - pseudoephedrine HCl (Sanofi-Aventis)

THERAPEUTIC CLASS: H_1 antagonist/sympathomimetic amine

INDICATIONS: Relief of symptoms of seasonal allergic rhinitis.

DOSAGE: *Adults:* 60-120mg tab bid or 180-240mg qd without food. Renal Dysfunction: Initial: 60-120mg tab qd; avoid 180-240mg tab. Do not crush or chew.

Pediatrics: ≥12 yrs: 60-120mg tab bid or 180-240mg qd without food. Renal Dysfunction: Initial: 60-120mg tab qd; avoid 180-240mg tab. Do not crush or chew.

HOW SUPPLIED: Tab, Extended Release: (Fexofenadine-Pseudoephedrine) (12 Hour) 60-120mg, (24 Hour) 180-240mg

CONTRAINDICATIONS: Narrow-angle glaucoma, urinary retention, severe HTN, severe CAD, within 14 days of MAOI therapy.

WARNINGS/PRECAUTIONS: Caution with HTN, DM, ischemic heart disease, increased IOP, hyperthyroidism, renal impairment, or prostatic hypertrophy. May produce CNS stimulation with convulsions or cardiovascular collapse with hypotension.

ADVERSE REACTIONS: Headache, insomnia, nausea, dry mouth, dyspepsia, throat irritation.

INTERACTIONS: Increased plasma levels with erythromycin or ketoconazole. Avoid MAOIs. Increased ectopic pacemaker activity can occur with digitalis. Caution with other sympathomimetic amines. Reduced effects of antihypertensive drugs which interfere with sympathetic activity (eg, methyldopa, mecamylamine, reserpine).

PREGNANCY: Category C, caution with nursing.

AlleRx   RX
pseudoephedrine HCl - methscopolamine nitrate - chlorpheniramine maleate
(Adams)

THERAPEUTIC CLASS: Antihistamine/anticholinergic/decongestant

INDICATIONS: Temporary relief of symptoms associated with allergic rhinitis, vasomotor rhinitis, sinusitis, and the common cold.

DOSAGE: *Adults:* 1 AM Dose tab in morning and 1 PM Dose tab in evening.

Pediatrics: ≥12 yrs: 1 AM Dose tab in morning and 1 PM Dose tab in evening.

HOW SUPPLIED: Tab, Extended Release: (AM Dose) (Methscopolamine-Pseudoephedrine) 2.5mg-120mg; (PM Dose) (Chlorpheniramine-Methscopolamine) 8mg-2.5mg

CONTRAINDICATIONS: Severe HTN or CAD, MAOI use or within 14 days of discontinuation, nursing mothers taking MAOIs, narrow-angle glaucoma, urinary retention, peptic ulcer, during asthma attack.

WARNINGS/PRECAUTIONS: Caution with elderly, HTN, DM, ischemic heart disease, hyperthyroidism, prostatic hypertrophy, cardiovascular disease, increased IOP. May produce CNS stimulation with convulsions or cardiovascular collapse with hypotension. Excitability reported especially in children.

ADVERSE REACTIONS: Drowsiness, lassitude, nausea, giddiness, dry mouth, blurred vision, cardiac palpitations, flushing, increased irritability.

INTERACTIONS: May enhance effects of TCAs, barbiturates, alcohol, other CNS depressants. May diminish antihypertensive effects of reserpine, veratrum alkaloids, methyldopa, mecamylamine. Increased sympathomimetic effect with β-blockers and MAOIs. Contraindicated with or within 14 days of discontinuing MAOIs. Hypotension potenti-

ated with sildenafil or other organic nitrates; avoid concomitant use. Caution with hyperactivity to sympathomimetics.
PREGNANCY: Category C, not for use in nursing.

ALOCRIL RX
nedocromil sodium (Allergan)

THERAPEUTIC CLASS: Mast cell stabilizer

INDICATIONS: Treatment of itching associated with allergic conjunctivitis.

DOSAGE: *Adults:* 1-2 drops bid. Continue throughout period of exposure.
Pediatrics: ≥3 yrs: 1-2 drops bid. Continue throughout period of exposure.

HOW SUPPLIED: Sol: 2% (5mL)

WARNINGS/PRECAUTIONS: Avoid wearing contacts while symptoms of allergic conjunctivitis persist.

ADVERSE REACTIONS: Headache, ocular burning, irritation, stinging, unpleasant taste, nasal congestion, asthma, conjunctivitis, eye redness, photophobia, rhinitis.

PREGNANCY: Category B, caution in nursing.

ALOMIDE RX
lodoxamide tromethamine (Alcon)

THERAPEUTIC CLASS: Mast cell stabilizer

INDICATIONS: Ocular disorders including vernal keratoconjunctivitis, vernal conjunctivitis, and vernal keratitis.

DOSAGE: *Adults:* 1-2 drops qid for up to 3 months.
Pediatrics: >2 yrs: 1-2 drops qid for up to 3 months.

HOW SUPPLIED: Sol: 0.1% (10mL)

WARNINGS/PRECAUTIONS: Do not wear soft contacts during treatment. Transient burning and stinging upon instillation.

ADVERSE REACTIONS: Ocular pruritus, blurred vision, dry eye, tearing, discharge, hyperemia, crystalline deposits, foreign body sensation.

PREGNANCY: Category B, caution in nursing.

ALOPRIM RX
allopurinol sodium (Nabi)

THERAPEUTIC CLASS: Xanthine oxidase inhibitor

INDICATIONS: Management of elevated serum and urinary uric acid levels in patients with leukemia, lymphoma, and solid tumor malignancies receiving cancer therapy when oral therapy is not tolerated.

DOSAGE: *Adults:* Initial: 200-400mg/m^2/day IV as qd or in divided doses every 6, 8, or 12 hrs. Max: 600mg/day. CrCl 10-20mL/min: 200mg/day. CrCl 3-10mL/min: 100mg/day. CrCl <3mL/min: 100mg/day at extended intervals.
Pediatrics: Initial: 200mg/m^2/day IV as qd or in divided doses every 6, 8, or 12 hrs.

HOW SUPPLIED: Inj: 500mg

CONTRAINDICATIONS: Previous severe reaction to therapy.

WARNINGS/PRECAUTIONS: D/C at first appearance of hypersensitivity; increased risk in decreased renal function. Monitor LFTs during early stages of therapy in liver disease. Monitor renal function and uric acid levels; adjust dose if needed. Maintain sufficient fluid intake to yield a daily urinary output ≥2 L. Drowsiness, hepatotoxicity, bone marrow suppression reported.

ADVERSE REACTIONS: Skin rash, eosinophilia, local injection site reaction, nausea, vomiting, diarrhea, renal failure/insufficiency.

INTERACTIONS: Decrease mercaptopurine and azathioprine dose to 1/3 to 1/4 of usual dose. Increased risk of skin rash with ampicillin, amoxicillin. Increased toxicity and risk of hypersensitivity with thiazide diuretics; monitor renal function. Caution with anticoagulants. Hypoglycemia reported with chlorpropamide. Enhanced myelosuppressive effects of cyclophosphamide, other cytotoxic agents. Increased cyclosporine levels. Increased urinary excretion of uric acid with uricosuric agents. Monitor PT with dicumarol.

PREGNANCY: Category C, caution with nursing.

ALPHAGAN P   RX
brimonidine tartrate (Allergan)

THERAPEUTIC CLASS: Selective alpha$_2$ agonist

INDICATIONS: Treatment of open-angle glaucoma and ocular hypertension.

DOSAGE: *Adults:* 1 drop tid, give q8h. Space dosing of other topical products that lower IOP by 5 minutes.

Pediatrics: ≥2 yrs: 1 drop tid, give q8h. Space dosing of other topical products that lower IOP by 5 minutes.

HOW SUPPLIED: Sol: 0.1% (5mL, 10mL, 15mL), 0.15% (5mL, 10mL, 15mL) (contains Purite®)

CONTRAINDICATIONS: Concomitant MAOI therapy.

WARNINGS/PRECAUTIONS: Caution with severe cardiovascular disease, hepatic or renal dysfunction, depression, cerebral or coronary insufficiency, Raynaud's phenomenon, orthostatic hypotension, thromboangiitis obliterans. Wait 15 minutes before reinserting contacts with 0.2% solution. Monitor IOP.

ADVERSE REACTIONS: Oral dryness, ocular hyperemia, ocular pruritus, burning, stinging, ocular allergic reaction, blurred vision, foreign body sensation, fatigue, drowsiness, headache, conjunctival follicles.

INTERACTIONS: May potentiate CNS depressants. May reduce BP; caution with β-blockers, antihypertensives, cardiac glycosides. Caution with TCAs. May be given with other topical products to lower IOP.

PREGNANCY: Category B, not for use in nursing.

ALTABAX   RX
retapamulin (GlaxoSmithKline)

THERAPEUTIC CLASS: Pleuromutilin antibacterial

INDICATIONS: Topical treatment of impetigo caused by susceptible strains of microorganisms, in patients ≥9 months.

DOSAGE: *Adults:* Apply thin layer (up to 100 cm^2 in total area) bid for 5 days. May cover with sterile bandage or gauze.

Pediatrics: ≥9 months: Apply thin layer (up to 2% total BSA) bid for 5 days. May cover with sterile bandage or gauze.

HOW SUPPLIED: Oint: 1% (5g, 10g, 15g)

WARNINGS/PRECAUTIONS: D/C if sensitization or irritation occurs. Not intended for oral, intranasal, ophthalmic or intravaginal use. May cause superinfection during therapy.

ADVERSE REACTIONS: Application site reactions.

INTERACTIONS: Co-administration with ketoconazole may increase levels.

PREGNANCY: Category B, caution in nursing.

AMBISOME   RX
amphotericin B (Astellas)

THERAPEUTIC CLASS: Polyene antifungal

INDICATIONS: Empiric therapy for presumed fungal infection in febrile, neutropenic patients. Treatment of *Aspergillus, Candida* or *Cryptococcus* infections refractory to amphotericin B deoxycholate or where renal impairment or unacceptable toxicity precludes its use. Treatment of visceral leishmaniasis and cryptococcal meningitis in HIV infected patients.

DOSAGE: *Adults:* Empiric Therapy: 3mg/kg/day IV. Systemic Infections (*Aspergillus, Candida, Cryptococcus*): 3-5mg/kg/day IV. Cryptococcal Meningitis in HIV: 6mg/kg/day IV. Visceral Leishmaniasis: Immunocompetent: 3mg/kg/day IV on days 1-5, 14, 21. May repeat course if needed. Immunocompromised: 4mg/kg/day IV on days 1-5, 10, 17, 24, 31, 38.

Pediatrics: 1 month-16 yrs: Empirical Therapy: 3mg/kg/day IV. Systemic Infections (*Aspergillus, Candida, Cryptococcus*): 3-5mg/kg/day IV. Cryptococcal Meningitis in HIV: 6mg/kg/day IV.Visceral Leishmaniasis: Immunocompetent: 3mg/kg/day IV on days 1-5, 14, 21. May repeat course if needed. Immunocompromised: 4mg/kg/day IV on days 1-5, 10, 17, 24, 31, 38.

HOW SUPPLIED: Inj: 50mg

WARNINGS/PRECAUTIONS: If anaphylaxis occurs, d/c all further infusions. Significantly less toxic than amphotericin B deoxycholate. Monitor renal, hepatic, hematopoietic function and electrolytes (especially K^+, Mg^{++}).

ADVERSE REACTIONS: Chills, asthenia, back pain, pain, infection, chest pain, HTN, hypotension, tachycardia, GI hemorrhage, diarrhea, nausea, vomiting, hyperglycemia, hypokalemia, dyspnea.

INTERACTIONS: Antineoplastic agents may potentiate renal toxicity, bronchospasm, hypotension. Corticosteroids and corticotropin may potentiate hypokalemia. May potentiate digitalis toxicity. May increase flucytosine toxicity. Acute pulmonary toxicity with leukocyte transfusions reported. Caution with imidazoles (eg, ketoconazole, clotrimazole, miconazole, fluconazole). Nephrotoxic drugs enhance potential for renal toxicity. May enhance curariform effect of skeletal muscle relaxants due to hypokalemia. Imidazoles (eg, ketocoazole, miconazole) may induce fungal resistance; caution with combination therapy in immunocompromised patients.

PREGNANCY: Category B, not for use in nursing.

AMIDATE
etomidate (Hospira)

RX

THERAPEUTIC CLASS: General anesthetic

INDICATIONS: For induction of general anesthesia. For supplementation of subpotent anesthetic agents, such as nitrous oxide in oxygen, during maintenance of anesthesia for short operative procedures.

DOSAGE: *Adults:* 0.2-0.6mg/kg IV. Usual: 0.3mg/kg IV, over 30 to 60 seconds.

Pediatrics: >10 yrs: 0.2-0.6mg/kg IV. Usual: 0.3mg/kg IV, over 30 to 60 seconds.

HOW SUPPLIED: Inj: 2mg/mL

WARNINGS/PRECAUTIONS: Not for prolonged infusion. Reduction of plasma cortisol and aldosterone concentrations have occurred; consider exogenous replacement during severely stressful conditions.

ADVERSE REACTIONS: Transient venous pain, transient skeletal muscle movements, including myoclonus, hyper/hypoventilation, apnea of short duration, hyper/hypotension, tachycardia, bradycardia.

PREGNANCY: Category C, caution in nursing.

AMIKIN
amikacin sulfate (Sandoz)

RX

> Potential for ototoxicity and nephrotoxicity. Neuromuscular blockade, respiratory blockade reported. Avoid potent diuretics, and other neurotoxic, nephrotoxic, and ototoxic drugs.

OTHER BRAND NAME: Amikin Pediatric (Sandoz)

THERAPEUTIC CLASS: Aminoglycoside

INDICATIONS: Short-term treatment of serious infections caused by gram-negative bacteria such as septicemia, and respiratory tract, bone/joint, CNS (including meningitis), skin and soft tissue, and intra-abdominal infections; burns and postoperative infections; complicated and recurrent urinary tract infections (UTI); and staphylococcal disease.

DOSAGE: *Adults:* (IM/IV)15mg/kg/day given q8h or q12h. Max: 15mg/kg/day. Heavier Weight Patients: Max: 1.5g/day. Recurrent Uncomplicated UTI: 250mg bid. Duration: 7-10 days. Stop therapy if no response after 3-5 days. Reduce dose if suspect renal dysfunction. Discontinue if azotemia increases or if a progressive decrease in urinary output occurs.

Pediatrics: 15mg/kg/day given bid-tid. Newborns: LD: 10mg/kg. MD: 7.5mg/kg q12h. Duration: 7-10 days.

HOW SUPPLIED: Inj: 50mg/mL, 250mg/mL

CONTRAINDICATIONS: History of serious toxic reactions to aminoglycosides.

WARNINGS/PRECAUTIONS: May aggravate muscle weakness; caution with muscular disorders (eg, myasthenia gravis, parkinsonism). May cause fetal harm in pregnancy. Contains sodium bisulfite, allergic reactions may occur especially in asthmatics. Maintain adequate hydration. Assess kidney function before therapy then daily.

ADVERSE REACTIONS: Ototoxicity, neuromuscular blockage, nephrotoxicity, skin rash, drug fever, headache, paresthesia, tremor, nausea, arthralgia, anemia, hypotension.

INTERACTIONS: Increased nephrotoxicity with cephalosporins. Significant mutual inactivation may occur with β-lactams (eg, penicillin, cephalosporins). Cross-allergenicity between aminoglycosides. Avoid diuretics, potent diuretics (eg, ethacrynic acid, furosemide), bacitracin, cisplatin, amphotericin B, paromomycin, polymyxin B, colistin, vancomycin, other aminoglycosides, and other neurotoxic, nephrotoxic and ototoxic drugs. Increased risk of neuromuscular blockade and respiratory paralysis with anesthetics, neuromuscular blockers, or massive transfusions of citrate-anticoagulated blood.

PREGNANCY: Category D, not for use in nursing.

Amoxil
amoxicillin (GlaxoSmithKline)

RX

THERAPEUTIC CLASS: Semisynthetic ampicillin derivative

INDICATIONS: Infections of the ear, nose, throat, genitourinary tract, skin and skin structure, lower respiratory tract due to susceptible (beta lactamase negative) organisms; gonorrhea (acute uncomplicated). *H. pylori* eradication to reduce the risk of duodenal ulcer recurrence.

DOSAGE: *Adults:* Ear/Nose/Throat/SSSI/GU: (Mild/Moderate) 500mg q12h or 250mg q8h. (Severe) 875mg q12h or 500mg q8h. LRTI: 875mg q12h or 500mg q8h. Gonorrhea 3g as single dose. H.pylori: (Dual Therapy) 1g + 30mg lansoprazole, both tid X 14 days. (Triple Therapy) 1g + 30mg lansoprazole + 500mg clarithromycin, all q12h X 14 days. CrCl 10-30mL/min: 250-500mg q12h. <10mL/min: 250-500mg q24h. Hemodialysis: 250-500mg or 250mg q24h, additional dose during and at the end.

Pediatrics: Neonates: ≤12 weeks: Max: 30mg/kg/day divided q12h. >3 months: Ear/Nose/Throat/SSSI/GU: (Mild/Moderate): 25mg/kg/day given q12h or 20mg/kg/day given q8h. (Severe): 45mg/kg/day given q12h or 40 mg/kg/day given q8h. LRTI: 45mg/kg/day given q12h or 40mg/kg/day given q8h. Gonorrhea: (Prepubertal) 50mg/kg with 25mg/kg probenecid as single dose. (Not for < 2yrs). >40kg: Dose as adult.

HOW SUPPLIED: Cap: 250mg, 500mg; Sus: 50mg/mL (15mL, 30mL), 125mg/5mL (80mL, 100mL, 150mL), 200mg/5mL (5mL, 50mL, 75mL, 100mL), 250mg/5mL (80mL, 100mL, 150mL), 400mg/5mL (5mL, 50mL, 75mL, 100mL); Tab: 500mg, 875mg; Tab, Chewable: 200mg, 400mg

WARNINGS/PRECAUTIONS: Monitor renal, hepatic, and blood with prolonged use. 200mg, 400mg chewable tabs contain phenylalanine.

ADVERSE REACTIONS: Nausea, vomiting, diarrhea, pseudomembranous colitis, hypersensitivity reactions, blood dyscrasias, superinfection (prolonged use).

INTERACTIONS: Increased levels with probenecid. Chloramphenicol, macrolides, sulfonamides, tetracyclines may interfere with bactericidal effects. False (+) for urine glucose with Clinitest®, Benedict's or Fehling's solution.

PREGNANCY: Category B, caution in nursing.

AMPHOTEC
amphotericin B cholesteryl sulfate (InterMune)

RX

THERAPEUTIC CLASS: Polyene antifungal

INDICATIONS: Treatment of invasive aspergillosis in patients with renal impairment, unacceptable toxicity, or previous failure to amphotericin deoxycholate.

DOSAGE: *Adults:* Test Dose: Infuse small amount over 15-30 minutes. Treatment: 3-4mg/kg/day IV at 1mg/kg/hr.
Pediatrics: Test Dose: Infuse small amount over 15-30 minutes. Treatment: 3-4mg/kg/day IV at 1mg/kg/hr.

HOW SUPPLIED: Inj: 50mg, 100mg

WARNINGS/PRECAUTIONS: Anaphylaxis may occur. Discontinue if severe respiratory distress occurs. Acute reactions (eg, fever, shaking chills, hypotension, nausea, tachypnea) 1-3 hrs after start infusion. Monitor renal/hepatic function, electrolytes, CBC, PT during therapy.

ADVERSE REACTIONS: Chills, fever, headache, hypotension, tachycardia, HTN, nausea, vomiting, thrombocytopenia, increased creatinine, hypokalemia, dyspnea, hypoxia.

INTERACTIONS: Antineoplastics may potentiate renal toxicity, bronchospasm, hypotension. Corticosteroids and corticotropin may potentiate hypokalemia. May increase flucytosine toxicity. Caution with imidazoles (eg, ketoconazole, clotrimazole, miconazole, fluconazole). Increased risk of renal toxicity with nephrotoxic drugs (eg, aminoglycosides, cyclosporine, pentamidine). May enhance curariform effect of skeletal muscle relaxants (eg, tubocurarine) or digitalis toxicity with hypokalemia.

PREGNANCY: Category B, not for use in nursing.

AMPICILLIN
ampicillin (Various)

RX

THERAPEUTIC CLASS: Semi-synthetic penicillin derivative

INDICATIONS: Genitourinary tract (GU) infections, including gonorrhea, respiratory and GI tract infections, and meningitis.

DOSAGE: *Adults:* GI/GU: 500mg qid. Use larger doses in chronic or severe infections. Gonorrhea: 3.5g single dose with 1g probenecid. Respiratory: 250mg qid. Treat minimum 48-72 hrs after eradication. Treat minimum 10 days for hemolytic strains of strep.
Pediatrics: >20kg: GI/GU: 500mg qid. Respiratory: 250mg qid. ≥20kg: GI/GU: 25mg/kg qid. Respiratory: 50mg/kg/day given tid-qid. Do not exceed adult doses. Use larger doses in chronic or severe infections. Treat minimum 48-72 hrs after eradication. Treat minimum 10 days for hemolytic strains of strep.

HOW SUPPLIED: Cap: 250mg, 500mg; Sus: 125mg/5mL, 250mg/5mL (100mL, 200mL)

CONTRAINDICATIONS: Infections caused by penicillinase-producing organisms.

WARNINGS/PRECAUTIONS: Possible cross-sensitivity with cephalosporins. Pseudomembranous colitis and anaphylatic reactions may occur.

ADVERSE REACTIONS: Stomatitis, nausea, vomiting, diarrhea, rash, SGOT elevation, blood dyscrasias, eosinophilia, thrombocytopenic purpura, hypersensitivity reactions, superinfection (prolonged use).

INTERACTIONS: Increased risk of rash with allopurinol. Bacteriostatic antibiotics (eg, chloramphenicol, erythromycins, sulfonamides or tetracyclines) may interfere with bactericidal activity. May decrease the effectiveness of oral contraceptives. Increased blood levels with probenecid.

PREGNANCY: Category B, not for use in nursing.

AMPICILLIN INJECTION
ampicillin sodium (Apothecon)

RX

THERAPEUTIC CLASS: Synthetic penicillin

INDICATIONS: Treatment of respiratory tract, urinary tract, and GI infections, bacterial meningitis, septicemia, endocarditis.

ANAFRANIL

DOSAGE: *Adults:* IM/IV: Respiratory Tract: ≥40kg: 250-500mg q8h. <40kg: 25-50mg/kg/day given q6-8h. GI/GU caused by N.gonorrhea females: ≥40kg: 500mg q6h. <40kg: 50mg/kg/day given q6-8h. Urethritis caused by N.gonorrhea (males): 500mg q8-12h for 2 doses; may retreat if needed. Bacterial Meningitis: 150-200mg/kg/day given q3-4h. Septicemia: 150-200mg/kg/day IV for 3 days, continue with IM q3-4h. Treat for minimum of 10 days and 48-72hrs after being asymptomatic.

Pediatrics: Bacterial Meningitis: 150-200mg/kg/day given q3-4h. Septicemia: 150-200mg/kg/day IV given q3-4h for 3 days, continue with IM q3-4h. Treat for minimum of 10 days and 48-72hrs after being asymptomatic.

HOW SUPPLIED: Inj: 125mg, 250mg, 500mg, 1g, 2g, 10g

WARNINGS/PRECAUTIONS: Caution with renal impairment. Cross-sensitivity with other β-lactams. May cause skin rash, especially in mononucleosis; avoid use. Pseudomembranous colitis reported. May result in overgrowth of nonsusceptible organisms.

ADVERSE REACTIONS: Headache, nausea, vomiting, oral and vaginal candidiasis, diarrhea, urticaria, allergic reactions, anaphylaxis, serum sickness-like reactions, exfoliative dermatitis.

INTERACTIONS: Potentiated by probenecid. Decreases effects of oral contraceptives. Allopurinol increases incidence of skin rash.

PREGNANCY: Category B, caution in nursing.

ANAFRANIL RX
clomipramine HCl (Mallinckrodt)

> Antidepressants increased the risk of suicidal thinking and behavior (suicidality) in short-term studies in children and adolescents with Major Depressive Disorder (MDD) and other psychiatric disorders. Clomipramine is not approved for use in pediatric patients except for patients with obsessive compulsive disorder.

THERAPEUTIC CLASS: Tricyclic antidepressant

INDICATIONS: Treatment of obsessive-compulsive disorder.

DOSAGE: *Adults:* Initial: 25mg/day with meals. Titrate: Increase within 2 weeks to 100mg/day. Increase further over several weeks. Max: 250mg/day. Maint: May give total daily dose at bedtime.

Pediatrics: >10 yrs: Initial: 25mg/day with meals. Titrate: Increase within 2 weeks to 3mg/kg or 100mg/day, whichever is smaller. Increase further over several weeks. Max: 3mg/kg/day or 200mg/day. Maint: May give total daily dose at bedtime.

HOW SUPPLIED: Cap: 25mg, 50mg, 75mg

CONTRAINDICATIONS: MAOI use within 14 days, acute recovery period following MI.

WARNINGS/PRECAUTIONS: Increased risks with electroconvulsive therapy. Discontinue prior to elective surgery. Avoid abrupt withdrawal. Caution with seizure disorder, conditions predisposing to seizures (eg, brain damage, alcoholism), urinary retention, narrow-angle glaucoma, adrenal medulla tumors, increased IOP, hyperthyroidism, cardiovascular disorders, liver dysfunction, significant renal dysfunction. Monitor hepatic enzymes with liver dysfunction. Weight changes, sexual dysfunction, blood dyscrasias, elevated liver enzymes reported. Hypomania/mania reported with affective disorder. Psychosis reported with schizophrenia.

ADVERSE REACTIONS: Dry mouth, constipation, nausea, dyspepsia, anorexia, weight gain, increased sweating, increased appetite, myoclonus, nervousness, libido change, dizziness, tremor, somnolence, impotence, visual changes.

INTERACTIONS: See Contraindications. Caution with anticholinergics, sympathomimetics, thyroid and CNS drugs. Blocks effects of clonidine, guanethidine. Increased levels with haloperidol, methylphenidate, highly protein bound drugs, CYP2D6 inhibitors (eg, quinidine, cimetidine, SSRIs) and enzyme substrates (eg, phenothiazines, propafenone, flecainide). At least 5 weeks must elapse before starting TCA therapy after fluoxetine discontinuation. Decreased levels with enzyme inducers (eg, barbiturates, phenytoin). Additive effects with CNS depressants, barbiturates, alcohol. NMS reported with neuroleptics. Increases phenobarbital and highly protein bound drugs (eg, warfarin, digoxin) plasma levels.

PREGNANCY: Category C, not for use in nursing.

ANALPRAM-HC
pramoxine HCl - hydrocortisone acetate (Ferndale)

RX

THERAPEUTIC CLASS: Corticosteroid/anesthetic

INDICATIONS: Corticosteroid responsive dermatoses of the anal region.

DOSAGE: *Adults:* Apply tid-qid. May use occlusive dressings in psoriasis or recalcitrant conditions. For cleansing anogenital area, spread lotion on cotton or tissue and wipe affected area.
Pediatrics: Apply tid-qid. May use occlusive dressings in psoriasis or recalcitrant conditions. For cleansing anogenital area, spread lotion on cotton or tissue and wipe affected area.

HOW SUPPLIED: Cre: (Hydrocortisone-Pramoxine) 1%-1%, 2.5%-1% (30g); Lot: 2.5%-1% (60mL)

WARNINGS/PRECAUTIONS: May produce reversible HPA axis suppression, manifestations of Cushing's syndrome, hyperglycemia, and glucosuria. D/C use if irritation occurs. Avoid eyes. Peds may be more susceptible to systemic toxicity. Use appropriate therapy with infections.

ADVERSE REACTIONS: Burning, itching, irritation, dryness, folliculitis, hypertrichosis, acneiform eruptions, hypopigmentation, perioral dermatitis, allergic contact dermatitis, secondary infection, skin maceration, skin atrophy, striae, miliaria.

PREGNANCY: Category C, caution in nursing.

ANCEF
cefazolin (GlaxoSmithKline)

RX

THERAPEUTIC CLASS: Cephalosporin (1st generation)

INDICATIONS: Treatment of serious respiratory tract, urinary tract (UTI), skin and skin structure, biliary tract, bone and joint, and genital infections, septicemia, endocarditis, and perioperative surgical prophylaxis.

DOSAGE: *Adults:* Moderate-Severe Infection: 500mg-1g q6-8h. Mild Gram-Positive Cocci Infection: 250-500mg q8h. Uncomplicated UTI: 1g q12h. Pneumococcal Pneumonia: 500mg q12h. Severe Life Threatening Infection (eg, Endocarditis, Septicemia): 1-1.5g q6h; Max: 12g/day (rare). Perioperative Surgical Prophylaxis: 1g IM/IV 0.5-1 hr before surgery. For Procedures ≥2 hrs: 500mg-1g IM/IV during surgery. Maint: 500mg-1g IM/IV q6-8h for 24 hrs post-op. Continue for 3-5 days for devastating procedures (eg, open-heart surgery and prosthetic arthroplasty). CrCl 35-54mL/min: Full dose q8h. CrCl 11-34mL/min: Half usual dose q12h. CrCl <10mL/min: Half usual dose q18-24h. Apply reduced dosage recommendations after initial LD is given.
Pediatrics: Mild-Moderately Severe Infection: 25-50mg/kg/day in 3-4 equal doses. Severe Infection: 100mg/kg/day in divided doses. CrCl 40-70mL/min: 60% of normal daily dose in equally divided doses q12h. CrCl 20-40mL/min: 25% of normal daily dose in equally divided doses q12h. CrCl 5-20mL/min: 10% of normal daily dose q24h. Apply reduced dosage recommendations after initial LD is given.

HOW SUPPLIED: Inj: 1g

WARNINGS/PRECAUTIONS: Prolonged use may result in overgrowth of nonsusceptible organisms. Possible cross-sensitivity between penicillins, cephalosporins, and other β-lactam antibiotics. Pseudomembranous colitis reported. Elevated levels with renal insufficiency can lead to seizures. Caution with colitis and other GI diseases. Safety in premature infants and neonates not established.

ADVERSE REACTIONS: Diarrhea, oral candidiasis, vomiting, nausea, stomach cramps, anorexia, allergic reactions, blood dyscrasias, renal failure, transient rise in SGOT/SGPT/BUN/SCr/alkaline phosphatase, local reactions.

INTERACTIONS: Decreased renal tubular secretion with probenecid.

PREGNANCY: Category B, caution in nursing.

ANDRODERM
testosterone (Watson)

CIII

THERAPEUTIC CLASS: Androgen

INDICATIONS: Testosterone replacement therapy in males due to primary or secondary hypogonadism.

ANECTINE

DOSAGE: *Adults:* Initial: 5mg/day. Maint: 2.5mg-7.5mg/day. Apply patch nightly to intact skin of the back, abdomen, upper arm or thigh. Rotate sites; avoid same site for 7 days. Do not apply to scrotum or oily, damaged, irritated areas. May apply 2 patches at same time.

Pediatrics: ≥15 yrs: Initial: 5mg/day. Maint: 2.5mg-7.5mg/day. Apply patch nightly to intact skin of the back, abdomen, upper arm or thigh. Rotate sites; avoid same site for 7 days. Do not apply to scrotum or oily, damaged, irritated areas. May apply 2 patches at same time.

HOW SUPPLIED: Patch: 2.5mg/24 hrs (60^s), 5mg/24 hrs (30^s)

CONTRAINDICATIONS: Breast or prostate cancer in men. Women.

WARNINGS/PRECAUTIONS: Prolonged use is associated with serious hepatic effects. Increased risk for prostatic hyperplasia/carcinoma in elderly. Risk of edema with pre-existing cardiac, renal, or hepatic disease; discontinue if edema occurs. Risk of virilization of female sex partner. Monitor LFTs, Hgb, Hct, PSA, cholesterol, lipids.

ADVERSE REACTIONS: Gynecomastia, pruritus/erythema/vesicles/blister at application site, prostate abnormalities, headache, depression.

INTERACTIONS: May potentiate effects of anticoagulants, oxyphenbutazone. May decrease blood glucose and insulin requirements in diabetics. Pretreatment with ointments may reduce testosterone absorption.

PREGNANCY: Category X, not for use in nursing.

ANECTINE
succinylcholine chloride (Sandoz)

RX

> Rare reports of acute rhabdomyolysis with hyperkalemia followed by ventricular dysrhythmias, cardiac arrest, and death in children with undiagnosed skeletal muscle myopathy. Reserve in children for emergency intubation where securing airway is necessary.

THERAPEUTIC CLASS: Skeletal muscle relaxant (depolarizing)

INDICATIONS: Adjunct to general anesthesia to facilitate tracheal intubation and to provide skeletal muscle relaxation during surgery or mechanical ventilation.

DOSAGE: *Adults:* Short Surgical Procedure: Average Dose: 0.6mg/kg IV. Range: 0.3-1.1mg/kg IV. Blockade develops in 1 minute, may persist up to 2 minutes. Long Surgical Procedure: 2.5-4.3mg/min IV; or 0.3-1.1mg/kg initial IV injection, then 0.04-0.07mg/kg IV at appropriate intervals. IM (if vein not accessible): Up to 3-4mg/kg IM. Max: 150mg/total dose. Effect observed in 2-3 minutes.

Pediatrics: Procedure to Secure Airway: Infants/Small Children: 2mg/kg IV. Older Children/Adolescents: 1mg/kg IV. IM (if vein not accessible): Infants/Older Children: Up to 3-4mg/kg IM. Max: 150mg/total dose. Effect observed in 2-3 minutes.

HOW SUPPLIED: Inj: 20mg/mL

CONTRAINDICATIONS: Personal or familial history of malignant hyperthermia, skeletal muscle myopathies. Acute phase of injury following major burns, multiple trauma, extensive skeletal muscle denervation, upper motor neuron injury.

WARNINGS/PRECAUTIONS: Avoid administration before unconsciousness has been induced. May induce arrhythmias or cardiac arrest in electrolyte abnormalities or massive digitalis toxicity. Caution with chronic abdominal infection, subarachnoid hemorrhage, conditions causing degeneration of central and peripheral nervous system, fractures, muscle spasms, reduced plasma cholinesterase activity, and acute phase of injury following major burns, multiple trauma, extensive skeletal muscle denervation, upper motor neuron injury. Malignant hyperthermia reported. Higher incidence of bradycardia progressing to asystole with 2nd dose. May increase IOP, intracranial or intragastric pressure. With prolonged therapy, Phase I block will progress to Phase II block associated with prolonged respiratory paralysis and weakness. Confirm Phase II block before therapy. Hypokalemia or hypocalcemia prolong neuromuscular blockade.

ADVERSE REACTIONS: Respiratory depression, cardiac arrest, malignant hyperthermia, arrhythmia, bradycardia, tachycardia, HTN, hypotension, hyperkalemia, increased IOP, muscle fasciculation, jaw rigidity, post-op muscle pains.

INTERACTIONS: Enhanced effects with promazine, oxytocin, certain non-penicillin antibiotics, β-blockers, procainamide, lidocaine, trimethaphan, lithium carbonate, magnesium salts, quinine, aprotinin, chloroquine, diethylether, isoflurane, desflurane, metoclopramide, terbutaline, and drugs that reduce plasma cholinesterase activity (eg, chronically administered oral contraceptives, glucocorticoids, certain MAOIs) or inhibit plasma cholinesterase. Increased risk of malignant hyperthermia with volatile anesthetics.
PREGNANCY: Category C, caution in nursing.

ANTIVERT
meclizine HCl (Pfizer)
RX

THERAPEUTIC CLASS: Antihistamine
INDICATIONS: Management of nausea, vomiting and dizziness associated with motion sickness. Management of vertigo associated with diseases affecting the vestibular system.
DOSAGE: *Adults:* Motion Sickness: 25-50mg 1 hr prior to trip/departure, repeat q24h prn. Vertigo: 25-100mg/day in divided doses.
Pediatrics: ≥12 yrs: Motion Sickness: 25-50mg 1 hr prior to trip/departure, repeat q24h prn. Vertigo: 25-100mg/day in divided doses.
HOW SUPPLIED: Tab: 12.5mg, 25mg, 50mg* *scored
WARNINGS/PRECAUTIONS: Caution with asthma, glaucoma, prostatic hypertrophy.
ADVERSE REACTIONS: Drowsiness, dry mouth, blurred vision (rare).
INTERACTIONS: Avoid alcoholic beverages.
PREGNANCY: Category B, safety in nursing is not known.

ANUSOL-HC CREAM
hydrocortisone (Salix)
RX

OTHER BRAND NAMES: Proctosol HC (NuCare) - Proctozone-HC (Rising) - Proctocream HC (Schwarz Pharma)
THERAPEUTIC CLASS: Corticosteroid
INDICATIONS: Corticosteroid responsive dermatoses.
DOSAGE: *Adults:* Apply bid-qid. May use occlusive dressings for psoriasis or recalcitrant conditions; d/c dressings if infection develops.
Pediatrics: Apply bid-qid. May use occlusive dressings for psoriasis or recalcitrant conditions; d/c dressings if infection develops.
HOW SUPPLIED: Cre: 2.5% (30g)
WARNINGS/PRECAUTIONS: May cause reversible adrenal suppression, manifestations of Cushing's syndrome, hyperglycemia, glucosuria. Caution when applied to large surface areas or under occlusive dressings. Use appropriate therapy with infections. Pediatrics may be more susceptible to systemic toxicity. D/C if irritation occurs. Avoid eyes.
ADVERSE REACTIONS: Burning, itching, irritation, dryness, folliculitis, hypertrichosis, acneiform eruptions, hypopigmentation, perioral dermatitis, allergic contact dermatitis, maceration skin, secondary infection, skin atrophy, striae, miliaria.
PREGNANCY: Category C, caution in nursing.

ANZEMET
dolasetron mesylate (Sanofi-Aventis)
RX

THERAPEUTIC CLASS: 5-HT$_3$ antagonist
INDICATIONS: (Inj) Prevention of nausea/vomiting associated with emetogenic cancer chemotherapy including high dose cisplatin. Prevention and treatment of post-op nausea/vomiting. (Tab) Prevention of nausea/vomiting associated with moderately emetogenic cancer chemotherapy and prevention of post-op nausea/vomiting.
DOSAGE: *Adults:* (Inj) Prevention of Chemotherapy Nausea/Vomiting: 1.8mg/kg IV single dose or 100mg IV 30 minutes before chemotherapy. Prevention/Treatment of

ARALEN

Post-op Nausea/Vomiting: 12.5mg IV single dose 15 minutes before cessation of anesthesia or as soon as nausea/vomiting presents. (Tab) Prevention of Chemotherapy Induced Nausea/Vomiting: 100mg PO within 1 hr before chemotherapy. Prevention of Postoperative Nausea/Vomiting: 100mg PO within 2 hrs before surgery.

Pediatrics: 2-16 yrs: (Inj) Prevention of Chemotherapy Nausea/Vomiting: 1.8mg/kg IV single dose 30 minutes before chemotherapy. Max: 100mg. May mix Inj in apple or grape juice and take orally within 1 hr before chemotherapy. Prevention/Treatment of Post-op Nausea/Vomiting: 0.35mg/kg IV single dose 15 minutes before cessation of anesthesia or as soon as nausea/vomiting presents. Max: 12.5mg single dose. May mix 1.2mg/kg Inj in apple or grape juice and take orally within 2 hrs before surgery. Max: 100mg/dose. (Tab) Prevention of Chemotherapy Induced Nausea/Vomiting: 1.8mg/kg PO within 1 hr before chemotherapy. Max: 100mg. Prevention of Postoperative Nausea/Vomiting: 1.2mg/kg PO within 2 hrs before surgery. Max: 100mg.

HOW SUPPLIED: Inj: 20mg/mL; Tab: 50mg, 100mg

WARNINGS/PRECAUTIONS: Caution in patients with or may develop cardiac conduction interval prolongation, especially those with congenital QT syndrome, hypokalemia and hypomagnesemia. Cross sensitivity may occur with other $5-HT_3$ antagonists. Can cause ECG interval changes.

ADVERSE REACTIONS: Headache, diarrhea, fever, fatigue, dizziness, abnormal hepatic function, chills/shivering, urinary retention, abdominal pain, HTN.

INTERACTIONS: Increased risk of prolongation of cardiac conduction intervals with diuretics, antiarrhythmics, drugs that prolong QT_c interval and cumulative high dose anthracycline therapy. Increased levels with cimetidine. Decreased levels with rifampin. Decreased clearance with IV atenolol.

PREGNANCY: Category B, caution in nursing.

ARALEN   RX
chloroquine (Sanofi-Aventis)

THERAPEUTIC CLASS: Aminoquinolone

INDICATIONS: Treatment of extraintestinal amebiasis and acute attacks of malaria. Suppression of malaria.

DOSAGE: *Adults:* Malaria: Initial: 1g, then 500mg 6-8 hrs later, then 500mg qd for 2 consecutive days (total of 2.5g in 3 days). Suppression: 500mg on the same day each week. Start 2 weeks before exposure (double initial dose if <2 weeks before exposure) and continue for 8 weeks after return. Extraintestinal Amebiasis: 1g qd for 2 days, then 500mg qd for at least 2-3 weeks. Treatment usually combined with intestinal amebicide.

Pediatrics: Malaria: Total dose of 25mg base/kg taken over 3 day, as follows: 1st Dose: 10mg base/kg (max 600mg base single dose). 2nd Dose: 5mg base/kg (300mg base single dose) 6 hrs after 1st dose. 3rd Dose: 5mg base/kg 18 hrs after 2nd dose. 4th Dose: 5mg base/kg 24 hrs after 3rd dose. Suppression: 5mg base/kg/week. Max: 300mg base/dose. Start 2 weeks before exposure (double initial dose if <2 weeks before exposure) and continue for 8 weeks after return.

HOW SUPPLIED: Tab: (Phosphate) 500mg (500mg tab=300mg base)

CONTRAINDICATIONS: Retinal or visual field changes.

WARNINGS/PRECAUTIONS: Caution with G6PD deficiency, pre-existing auditory damage, hepatic impairment, alcoholism, porphyria, psoriasis, elderly, and history of seizures. Monitor CBCs, vision, reflexes with prolonged use. D/C if visual or hematological disturbances, muscle weakness, hearing defects develop.

ADVERSE REACTIONS: Headache, pruritus, psychic stimulation, visual disturbances, pleomorphic skin eruptions, GI effects, convulsions.

INTERACTIONS: Caution with hepatotoxic drugs. Space dosing of antacids/kaolin by 4 hours. Increased levels with cimetidine; avoid concomitant use. Space dosing of ampicillin by at least 2 hours. May increase cyclosporine levels; monitor closely.

PREGNANCY: Avoid in pregnancy except for treatment of malaria if benefits outweigh risks. Not for use in nursing.

ARMOUR THYROID   RX
thyroid (Forest)

THERAPEUTIC CLASS: Thyroid replacement hormone

INDICATIONS: Treatment of hypothyroidism. As a pituitary TSH suppressant in the treatment or prevention of various types of euthyroid goiters. Diagnostic agent in suppression tests to differentiate suspected mild hyperthyroidism or thyroid gland autonomy. Management of thyroid cancer.

DOSAGE: *Adults:* Hypothyroidism: Initial: 30mg qd. Titrate: Increase by 15mg q2-3 weeks. Myxedema with Cardiovascular Disorder: 15mg qd. Maint: 60-120mg/day. Thyroid Cancer: Higher doses then replacement therapy is required. Myxedema Coma: Levothyroxine Sodium: Initial: 400mcg IV then 100-200mcg/day IV. Continue with oral therapy when stabilized. Thyroid Suppression: 1.56mg/kg/day for 7-10 days. Elderly: Initial: Use lower dose (eg, 15-30mg qd).

Pediatrics: Hypothyroidism: 0-6months: 4.8-6mg/kg/day; 6-12 months: 3.6-4.8mg/kg/day; 1-5 yrs: 3-3.6mg/kg/day; 6-12 yrs: 2.4-3mg/kg/day; >12 yrs: 1.2-1.8mg/kg/day.

HOW SUPPLIED: Tab: 15mg, 30mg, 60mg, 90mg, 120mg, 180mg, 240mg, 300mg

CONTRAINDICATIONS: Untreated thyrotoxicosis; uncorrected adrenal cortical insufficiency.

WARNINGS/PRECAUTIONS: Do not use in the treatment of obesity; larger doses in euthyroid patients can cause serious or even life threatening toxicity. Caution with cardiovascular disease, DM, diabetes insipidus, elderly, and adrenal cortical insufficiency.

INTERACTIONS: May increase insulin or oral hypoglycemic requirements. Reduced absorption with cholestyramine and colestipol; space dosing by 4-5 hours. Altered effect of oral anticoagulants; monitor PT/INR. Estrogens increase thyroxine-binding globulin; increase in thyroid dose may be needed. Serious or life-threatening side effects can occur with sympathomimetic amines. Androgens, corticosteroids, estrogens, iodine-containing preparations, and salicylates may interfere with thyroid lab tests.

PREGNANCY: Category A, caution in nursing.

Arranon RX
nelarabine (GlaxoSmithKline)

> Severe neurologic events reported; close monitoring is strongly recommended. Discontinue for neurologic events of NCI Common Toxicity Criteria ≥ grade 2.

THERAPEUTIC CLASS: Deoxyguanosine analogue

INDICATIONS: Treatment of T-cell acute lymphoblastic leukemia and T-cell lymphoblastic lymphoma in patients whose disease has not responded to or has relapsed following treatment with at least two chemotherapy regimens.

DOSAGE: *Adults:* 1500mg/m^2 IV over 2 hrs on days 1, 3, and 5 repeated every 21 days. CrCl <50ml/min: Insufficient data to support dose recommendation.

Pediatrics: 650mg/m^2/day IV over 1 hr daily for 5 consecutive days. Repeat every 21 days. CrCl <50ml/min: Insufficient data to support dose recommendation.

HOW SUPPLIED: Inj: 5mg/mL

WARNINGS/PRECAUTIONS: Leukopenia, thrombocytopenia, anemia, neutropenia/febrile neutropenia reported; regularly monitor CBC including platelets. Intravenous hydration recommended for management of hyperuricemia with risk of tumor lysis syndrome; may also consider allopurinol. Avoid administration of live vaccines. Closely monitor toxicities with severe renal impairment (eg, CrCl <30mL/min) and/or severe hepatic impairment (eg, bilirubin >3mg/dL); increased risk of adverse reactions.

ADVERSE REACTIONS: See Black Box Warning, Warnings/Precautions. Pediatrics: headache, increased transaminases, decreased blood potassium, decreased/increased blood albumin, vomiting. Adults: fatigue, nausea, diarrhea, vomiting, constipation, cough, dyspnea, dizziness, pyrexia, blurred vision.

PREGNANCY: Category D, not for use in nursing.

Asmanex RX
mometasone furoate (Schering)

THERAPEUTIC CLASS: Corticosteroid

INDICATIONS: Maintenance treatment of asthma as prophylactic therapy in patients ≥12 years; to reduce or eliminate the need for oral corticosteroidal therapy.

ASTELIN

DOSAGE: *Adults:* Previous Therapy with Bronchodilators Alone or Inhaled Corticosteroids: Initial: 220mcg qpm. Max: 440mcg qpm or 220mcg bid. Previous Therapy with Oral Corticosteroids: Initial: 440mcg bid. Max: 880mcg/day. Titrate to lowest effective dose once asthma stability is achieved.

Pediatrics: ≥12 yrs: Previous Therapy with Bronchodilators Alone or Inhaled Corticosteroids: Initial: 220mcg qpm. Max: 440mcg qpm or 220mcg bid. Previous Therapy with Oral Corticosteroids: Initial: 440mcg bid. Max: 880mcg/day. Titrate to lowest effective dose once asthma stability is achieved.

HOW SUPPLIED: Twisthaler: 220mcg/inh

CONTRAINDICATIONS: Primary treatment of status asthmaticus or other acute episodes of asthma where intensive measures are required.

WARNINGS/PRECAUTIONS: Deaths due to adrenal insufficiency have occurred with transfer from systemic corticosteroids to inhaled corticosteroids. Wean slowly from systemic corticosteroid therapy. Resume oral corticosteroids during stress or severe asthma attack. May unmask allergic conditions previously suppressed by systemic corticosteroid therapy. May increase susceptibility to infections. Not for rapid relief of bronchospasm or other acute episodes of asthma. Discontinue if bronchospasm occurs after dosing. Observe for systemic corticosteroid withdrawal effects, hypercorticism, reduced bone mineral density, and adrenal suppression; reduce dose slowly if needed. Decreased growth velocity may occur in pediatric patients. *Candida* infections in the mouth and pharynx reported. Caution with active or quiescent TB infection of the respiratory tract; untreated systemic fungal, bacterial, viral, or parasitic infections; or ocular herpes simplex. Glaucoma, increased IOP, and cataracts reported.

ADVERSE REACTIONS: Headache, allergic rhinitis, pharyngitis, upper respiratory tract infection, sinusitis, oral candidiasis, dysmenorrhea, musculoskeletal pain, back pain, dyspepsia, myalgia, abdominal pain, nausea.

INTERACTIONS: Ketoconazole may increase plasma levels.

PREGNANCY: Category C, caution in nursing.

ASTELIN   RX
azelastine HCl (MedPointe)

THERAPEUTIC CLASS: Antihistamine

INDICATIONS: Treatemnt of the symptoms of seasonal allergic rhinitis and vasomotor rhinitis.

DOSAGE: *Adults:* 2 sprays per nostril bid.
Pediatrics: Seasonal Allergic/Vasomotor Rhinitis: ≥12 yrs: 2 sprays per nostril bid. Seasonal Allergic Rhinitis: 5-11 yrs: 1 spray per nostril bid.

HOW SUPPLIED: Spray: 137mcg/spray (30mg)

ADVERSE REACTIONS: Bitter taste, somnolence, weight increase, headache, nasal burning, pharyngitis, paroxysmal sneezing, dry mouth, nausea.

INTERACTIONS: Avoid alcohol or other CNS depressants; additive CNS impairment may occur. Increased azelastine levels with cimetidine.

PREGNANCY: Category C, caution in nursing.

ATGAM   RX
lymphocyte immune globulin, anti-thymocyte globulin (equine) (Pharmacia & Upjohn)

> Administer in facility equipped and staffed with adequate lab and supportive medical resources.

THERAPEUTIC CLASS: Lymphocyte-selective immunosuppressant

INDICATIONS: Management of allograft rejection in renal transplantation. Treatment of moderate to severe aplastic anemia unsuitable for bone marrow transplantation.

DOSAGE: *Adults:* Renal Transplant: Delaying Rejection Onset: 15mg/kg/day for 14 days, then every other day for 14 days for total of 21 doses in 28 days. Give 1st dose 24 hrs before or after transplant. Rejection Treatment: 10-15mg/kg/day for 14 days. May give additional alternate day therapy up to a total of 21 doses. May delay 1st dose until diagnosis of 1st rejection episode. Aplastic Anemia: 10-20mg/kg/day for 8-14 days. May give additional alternate day therapy up to a total of 21 doses.

Pediatrics: Renal Transplant: Delaying Rejection Onset: 15mg/kg/day for 14 days, then every other day for 14 days for total of 21 doses in 28 days. Give 1st dose 24 hrs before or after transplant. Rejection Treatment: 10-15mg/kg/day for 14 days. May give additional alternate day therapy up to a total of 21 doses. May delay 1st dose until diagnosis of 1st rejection episode. Aplastic Anemia: 10-20mg/kg/day for 8-14 days. May give additional alternate day therapy up to a total of 21 doses.

HOW SUPPLIED: Inj: 50mg/mL

CONTRAINDICATIONS: History of severe systemic reaction to this product or other equine gamma globulin agents.

WARNINGS/PRECAUTIONS: Potency of agent may vary from lot to lot. Discontinue if anaphylaxis (eg, respiratory distress, hypotension) occurs, or if severe and unremitting thrombocytopenia or leukopenia occur in renal transplant patients. Risk of infectious transmission due to equine and human blood components. Monitor for leukopenia, thrombocytopenia, or infection (eg, CMV). Decide whether or not to continue therapy based on clinical circumstances (eg, infection).

ADVERSE REACTIONS: Fever, chills, leukopenia, thrombocytopenia, rash, pruritus, urticaria, wheal, flare, arthralgia, headache, phlebitis, chest/back pain, diarrhea, vomiting, nausea, dyspnea, hypotension, night sweats, stomatitis.

INTERACTIONS: Previously masked reactions may appear with corticosteroid or immunosuppressant dose reduction. Do not dilute with dextrose or use highly acidic infusions.

PREGNANCY: Category C, caution in nursing.

Ativan
lorazepam (Biovail)

CIV

THERAPEUTIC CLASS: Benzodiazepine

INDICATIONS: Management of anxiety.

DOSAGE: *Adults:* Initial: 2-3mg/day given bid-tid. Usual: 2-6mg/day in divided doses. Insomnia: 2-4mg qhs. Elderly/Debilitated: 1-2mg/day in divided doses.

Pediatrics: >12 yrs: Initial: 2-3mg/day given bid-tid. Usual: 2-6mg/day in divided doses. Insomnia: 2-4mg qhs.

HOW SUPPLIED: Tab: 0.5mg, 1mg*, 2mg* *scored

CONTRAINDICATIONS: Acute narrow-angle glaucoma.

WARNINGS/PRECAUTIONS: Avoid with primary depression or psychosis. Withdrawal symptoms with abrupt discontinuation. Careful supervision if addiction-prone. Caution with elderly, and renal or hepatic dysfunction. Monitor for GI disease with prolonged therapy. Periodic blood counts and LFTs with long-term therapy.

ADVERSE REACTIONS: Sedation, dizziness, weakness, unsteadiness, transient amnesia, memory impairment.

INTERACTIONS: CNS-depressant effects with barbiturates, alcohol. Diminished tolerance to alcohol and other CNS depressants.

PREGNANCY: Not for use in pregnancy or nursing.

Atropine Sulfate
atropine sulfate (Various)

RX

THERAPEUTIC CLASS: Anticholinergic

INDICATIONS: Antisialagogue for preanesthetic medication to prevent or reduce secretions of the respiratory tract. To restore cardiac rate and arterial pressure during anesthesia when vagal stimulation produced by intra-abdominal surgical traction causes a sudden decrease in pulse rate and cardiac action. To lessen degree of AV heart block when increased vagal tone is a major factor in the conduction defect (possibly due to digitalis). To overcome severe bradycardia and syncope due to hyperactive carotid sinus reflex, as an antidote (with external cardiac massage) for cardiovascular collapse from the injudicious use of choline ester (cholinergic) drug. In the treatment of anticho-

Atrovent

linesterase poisoning from organophosphorus insecticides, and as an antidote for the "rapid" type of mushroom poisoning due to presence of the alkaloid muscarine, in certain species of fungus such as *Amanita muscaria*.

DOSAGE: *Adults:* Usual: 0.5mg IM/IV/SC. Range: 0.4-0.6mg. If used as an antisialogogue, inject IM prior to anesthesia induction. Bradyarrhythmias: 0.4-1mg every 1-2 hrs prn. Max: 2mg/dose. May be used as an antidote for cardiovascular collapse resulting from injudicious administration of choline ester. When cardiac arrest has occurred, external cardiac massage or other method of resuscitation is required to distribute the drug after IV injection. Anticholinesterase Poisoning From Insecticide Poisoning: 2-3mg IV. Repeat until signs of atropine intoxication appear. Mushroom Poisoning: Administer sufficient doses to control parasympathomimetic signs before coma and cardiovascular collapse supervene.

Pediatrics: Range: 0.1mg (newborn) to 0.6mg (>12 yrs). Inject SC 30 minutes before surgery. Bradyarrhythmias: Range: 0.01-0.03mcg/kg IV.

HOW SUPPLIED: Inj: 0.05mg/mL, 0.1mg/mL, 0.4mg/mL, 0.5mg/mL, 1mg/mL

CONTRAINDICATIONS: Glaucoma, pyloric stenosis, or prostatic hypertrophy except in doses used for preanesthetic medication.

WARNINGS/PRECAUTIONS: Avoid overdose in IV administration. Increased susceptibility to toxic effects in children. Caution in patients >40 yrs. Conventional doses may precipitate glaucoma in susceptible patients, convert partial organic pyloric stenosis into complete obstruction, lead to complete urinary retention in patients with prostatic hypertrophy or cause inspissation of bronchial secretions and formation of dangerous viscid plugs in patients with chronic lung disease.

ADVERSE REACTIONS: Dryness of the mouth, blurred vision, photophobia, tachycardia, anhidrosis.

PREGNANCY: Category C, safety in nursing not known.

Atrovent   RX
ipratropium bromide (Boehringer Ingelheim)

OTHER BRAND NAME: Atrovent HFA (Boehringer Ingelheim)

THERAPEUTIC CLASS: Anticholinergic bronchodilator

INDICATIONS: Maintenance treatment of bronchospasm associated with COPD, including chronic bronchitis and emphysema.

DOSAGE: *Adults:* (MDI, HFA MDI) Initial: 2 inh qid. Max: 12 inh/24hrs. (Sol) 1 vial (500mcg/2.5mL) nebulized tid-qid; separate doses by 6-8 hrs.

Pediatrics: ≥12 yrs: (MDI) Initial: 2 inh qid. Max: 12 inh/24hrs. (Sol) 1 vial (500mcg/2.5mL) nebulized tid-qid; separate doses by 6-8 hrs.

HOW SUPPLIED: MDI: 0.018mg/inh (14g), (HFA) 0.017mg/inh (12.9g); Sol (neb): 0.02% (2.5mL, 25s)

CONTRAINDICATIONS: Hypersensitivity to atropine or its derivatives. (MDI) History of hypersensitivity to soya lecithin or related food products (eg, soybeans, peanuts).

WARNINGS/PRECAUTIONS: Not for acute episodes. Immediate hypersensitivity reaction reported. Caution with narrow-angle glaucoma, prostatic hypertrophy or bladder-neck obstruction.

ADVERSE REACTIONS: Nervousness, bronchitis, dyspnea, dizziness, headache, nausea, blurred vision, dry mouth, exacerbation of symptoms.

INTERACTIONS: Caution with anticholinergic-containing drugs.

PREGNANCY: Category B, caution in nursing.

Atrovent Nasal   RX
ipratropium bromide (Boehringer Ingelheim)

THERAPEUTIC CLASS: Anticholinergic agent

INDICATIONS: (0.03%) Relief of rhinorrhea associated with allergic and nonallergic perennial rhinitis. (0.06%) Relief of rhinorrhea associated with the common cold.

DOSAGE: *Adults:* (0.03%) 2 sprays per nostril bid-tid. (0.06%) 2 sprays per nostril tid-qid. Do not use >4 days with common cold.

Pediatrics: (0.03%) ≥6 yrs: 2 sprays per nostril bid-tid. (0.06%) ≥12 yrs: 2 sprays per nostril tid-qid. 5-11 yrs: 2 sprays per nostril tid. Do not use >4 days with common cold.

HOW SUPPLIED: Spray: (0.03%) 21mcg/spray (31g), (0.06%) 42mcg/spray (16.6g)

CONTRAINDICATIONS: Hypersensitivity to atropine or its derivatives.

WARNINGS/PRECAUTIONS: Immediate hypersensitivity reaction reported. Caution with narrow-angle glaucoma, prostatic hypertrophy or bladder-neck obstruction.

ADVERSE REACTIONS: Epistaxis, nasal dryness, dry mouth, dry throat, headache, upper respiratory infection, pharyngitis.

INTERACTIONS: May produce additive effects with other anticholinergic agents.

PREGNANCY: Category B, caution in nursing.

AUGMENTIN
amoxicillin - clavulanate potassium (GlaxoSmithKline)

RX

THERAPEUTIC CLASS: Aminopenicillin/beta lactamase inhibitor

INDICATIONS: Treatment of lower respiratory tract (LRTI), skin and skin structure (SSSI), and urinary tract infections (UTI), otitis media (OM), sinusitis.

DOSAGE: *Adults:* (Dose based on amoxicillin) 500mg q12h or 250mg q8h. Severe Infections/RTI: 875mg q12h or 500mg q8h. May use 125mg/5mL or 250mg/5mL sus in place of 500mg tab and 200mg/5mL sus or 400mg/5mL sus in place of 875mg tab. CrCl <30mL/min: Do not give 875mg tab. CrCl 10-30mL/min: 250-500mg q12h. CrCl <10mL/min: 250-500mg q24h. Hemodialysis: 250-500mg q24h, give additional dose during and at the end of dialysis.

Pediatrics: (Dose based on amoxicillin) ≥40kg: Use adult dose. ≥12 weeks: Sinusitis/OM/LRTI/Severe Infections: (Sus/Tab, Chewable) 45mg/kg/day given q12h or 40mg/kg/day given q8h. Less Severe Infections: 25mg/kg/day given q12h or 20mg/kg/day given q8h. <12 weeks:15mg/kg q12h (use 125mg/5mL sus).

HOW SUPPLIED: (Amoxicillin-Clavulanate) Sus: 125-31.25mg/5mL (75mL, 100mL, 150mL) 200-28.5mg/5mL (50mL, 75mL, 100mL), 250-62.5mg/5mL (75mL, 100mL, 150mL), 400-57mg/5mL (50mL, 75mL, 100mL); Tab: 250-125mg, 500-125mg, 875-125mg*; Tab, Chewable: 200-28.5mg, 250-62.5mg, 400-57mg *scored

CONTRAINDICATIONS: History of penicillin allergy or amoxicillin-clavulanate associated cholestatic jaundice/hepatic dysfunction.

WARNINGS/PRECAUTIONS: Pseudomembranous colitis reported. Possibility of superinfection. Caution with hepatic dysfunction. Monitor renal, hepatic, and hematopoietic functions with prolonged use. Avoid with mononucleosis. Fatal hypersensitivity reactions reported. Take with food to reduce GI upset. Chewable tabs and suspension contain phenylalanine. The 250mg tab and chewable tab are not interchangeable due to unequal clavulanic acid amounts. Only use 250mg tab in pediatrics ≥40kg. False (+) for urine glucose with Clinitest® and Benedict's or Fehling's solution.

ADVERSE REACTIONS: Diarrhea/loose stools, nausea, skin rashes, urticaria, vomiting, vaginitis.

INTERACTIONS: Increased and prolonged plasma levels with probenecid. May reduce effects of oral contraceptives. Allopurinol may increase incidence of rash. May increase PT with anticoagulant therapy.

PREGNANCY: Category B, caution in nursing.

AUGMENTIN ES-600
amoxicillin - clavulanate potassium (GlaxoSmithKline)

RX

THERAPEUTIC CLASS: Aminopenicillin/beta lactamase inhibitor

INDICATIONS: Treatment of recurrent or persistent acute otitis media.

DOSAGE: *Pediatrics:* (Dose based on amoxicillin) 3 months-12 yrs: <40kg: 45mg/kg q12h for 10 days.

Augmentin XR

HOW SUPPLIED: Sus: (Amoxicillin-Clavulanate) 600mg-42.9mg/5mL (50mL, 75mL, 100mL, 150mL)

CONTRAINDICATIONS: History of penicillin allergy or amoxicillin-clavulanate associated cholestatic jaundice/hepatic dysfunction.

WARNINGS/PRECAUTIONS: Pseudomembranous colitis reported. Possibility of superinfection. Caution with hepatic dysfunction. Monitor renal, hepatic, and hematopoietic functions with prolonged use. Avoid with mononucleosis. Fatal hypersensitivity reactions reported. Contains phenylalanine. False (+) for urine glucose with Clinitest® and Benedict's or Fehling's solution.

ADVERSE REACTIONS: Diaper rash, diarrhea, vomiting, moniliasis, rash.

INTERACTIONS: Increased and prolonged plasma levels with probenecid. May reduce effects of oral contraceptives. Allopurinol may increase incidence of rash. May increase PT with anticoagulant therapy.

PREGNANCY: Category B, caution in nursing.

Augmentin XR
amoxicillin - clavulanate potassium (GlaxoSmithKline)

RX

THERAPEUTIC CLASS: Aminopenicillin/beta lactamase inhibitor

INDICATIONS: Treatment of community acquired pneumonia (CAP) or acute bacterial sinusitis due to confirmed or suspected β-lactamase producing pathogens.

DOSAGE: *Adults:* Sinusitis: 2 tabs q12h for 10 days. CAP: 2 tabs q12h for 7-10 days. Take at the start of a meal.

Pediatrics: ≥16 yrs: Sinusitis: 2 tabs q12h for 10 days. CAP: 2 tabs q12h for 7-10 days. Take at the start of a meal.

HOW SUPPLIED: Tab, Extended Release: (Amoxicillin-Clavulanate) 1000mg-62.5mg

CONTRAINDICATIONS: History of penicillin allergy or amoxicillin-clavulanate associated cholestatic jaundice/hepatic dysfunction, severe renal impairment (CrCl <30mL/min), hemodialysis.

WARNINGS/PRECAUTIONS: Pseudomembranous colitis reported. Possibility of superinfection. Caution with hepatic dysfunction. Monitor renal, hepatic, and hematopoietic functions with prolonged use. Avoid with mononucleosis. Fatal hypersensitivity reactions reported. Not interchangeable with other Augmentin products due to unequal clavulanic acid amounts. False (+) for urine glucose with Clinitest® and Benedict's or Fehling's solution.

ADVERSE REACTIONS: Diarrhea, nausea, genital moniliasis, abdominal pain, vaginal mycosis.

INTERACTIONS: Increased and prolonged plasma levels with probenecid. May reduce effects of oral contraceptives. Allopurinol may increase incidence of rash. May increase PT with anticoagulant therapy.

PREGNANCY: Category B, caution in nursing.

Avapro
irbesartan (Bristol-Myers Squibb/Sanofi-Aventis)

RX

> Can cause death/injury to developing fetus during 2nd and 3rd trimesters. Stop therapy if pregnancy detected.

THERAPEUTIC CLASS: Angiotensin II receptor antagonist

INDICATIONS: Hypertension, alone or with other antihypertensives. Diabetic nephropathy with an elevated serum creatinine and proteinuria (>300mg/day) in patients with type 2 diabetes and hypertension.

DOSAGE: *Adults:* HTN: Initial: 150mg qd. Titrate: May increase to 300mg qd. Intravascular Volume/Salt Depletion: Initial: 75mg qd. Nephropathy: Maint: 300mg qd.

Pediatrics: HTN: ≥17 yrs: Initial: 150mg qd. Titrate: May increase to 300mg qd. Intravascular Volume/Salt Depletion: Initial: 75mg qd.

HOW SUPPLIED: Tab: 75mg, 150mg, 300mg

WARNINGS/PRECAUTIONS: Can cause fetal injury/death. Correct volume or salt depletion before therapy. Changes in renal function may occur; caution with renal artery stenosis, severe CHF. Angioedema reported.

ADVERSE REACTIONS: Diarrhea, dyspepsia/heartburn, musculoskeletal trauma, fatigue, upper respiratory infection.

PREGNANCY: Category C (1st trimester) and D (2nd and 3rd trimesters), not for use in nursing.

Axid
nizatidine (Reliant)
RX

OTHER BRAND NAME: Axid Oral Solution (Braintree)

THERAPEUTIC CLASS: H_2 blocker

INDICATIONS: Short term treatment of active duodenal ulcer (DU) and benign gastric ulcer (GU). Maintenance therapy for duodenal ulcers. Treatment of endoscopically diagnosed esophagitis, including erosive and ulcerative esophagitis, and heartburn due to GERD.

DOSAGE: *Adults:* Active DU/Active Benign GU: Usual: 300mg qhs or 150mg bid up to 8 weeks. Healed DU: Maint: 150mg qhs, up to 1 year. GERD: 150mg bid up to 12 weeks. Renal Impairment: Treatment: CrCl 20-50mL/min: 150mg/day. CrCl <20mL/min: 150mg every other day. Maint: CrCl 20-50mL/min: 150mg every other day. CrCl <20mL/min: 150mg every 3 days.

Pediatrics: ≥12 yrs: (Sol) Erosive Esophagitis/GERD: 150mg bid up to 8 weeks. Max: 300mg/day. Renal Impairment: Treatment: CrCl 20-50mL/min: 150mg/day. CrCl <20mL/min: 150mg every other day. Maint: CrCl 20-50mL/min: 150mg every other day. CrCl <20mL/min: 150mg every 3 days.

HOW SUPPLIED: Cap: 150mg, 300mg; Sol: 15mg/mL

WARNINGS/PRECAUTIONS: Caution with renal dysfunction; reduce dose. Symptomatic response does not preclude the presence of gastric malignancy. False positive tests for urobilinogen with Multistix®.

ADVERSE REACTIONS: Headache, abdominal pain, pain, asthenia, diarrhea, nausea, flatulence, vomiting, dyspepsia, rhinitis, pharyngitis, dizziness, headache.

INTERACTIONS: May elevate serum salicylate levels with high dose ASA.

PREGNANCY: Category B, not for use in nursing.

Azactam
aztreonam (Elan)
RX

THERAPEUTIC CLASS: Monobactam

INDICATIONS: Treatment of septicemia and lower respiratory tract (eg, pneumonia, bronchitis), skin and skin-structure, urinary tract (UTI), gynecologic (eg, endometritis), and intra-abdominal (eg, peritonitis) infections. Adjunct therapy to surgery for management of infections.

DOSAGE: *Adults:* UTI: 500mg-1g IM/IV q8-12h. Moderately Severe Systemic Infections: 1-2g IM/IV q8-12h. Severe Systemic/Life-Threatening Infections/*Pseudomonas aeruginosa*: 2g IV q6-8h. Max: 8g/day. CrCl 10-30mL/min: Initial: LD: 1 or 2g. Maint: 50% of usual dose. CrCl <10mL/min: Initial: LD: 500mg, 1g or 2g. Maint: 25% of initial dose at usual intervals. Serious/Life-Threatening Infections: In addition to maintenance dose, give 1/8 initial dose after each hemodialysis session. IV route is recommended for single dose >1g or for bacterial septicemia, localized parenchymal abscess (eg, intra-abdominal abscess), peritonitis, or other severe systemic or life-threatening infections. Continue for at least 48 hrs after patient is asymptomatic or bacterial eradication.

Pediatrics: 9 months-16 yrs: Mild-Moderate Infections: 30mg/kg IV q8h. Moderate-Severe Infections: 30mg/kg IV q6-8h. Max: 120mg/kg/day. IV route is recommended for single dose >1g or for bacterial septicemia, localized parenchymal abscess (eg, intra-abdominal abscess), peritonitis, or other severe systemic or life-threatening infections. Continue for at least 48 hrs after patient is asymptomatic or evidence of bacterial eradication.

AZASITE

HOW SUPPLIED: Inj: 500mg, 1g, 2g, 1g/50mL, 2g/50mL

WARNINGS/PRECAUTIONS: Caution with hypersensitivity to other beta-lactams or allergens. Pseudomembranous colitis reported. May promote overgrowth of nonsusceptible organisms. Monitor with renal or hepatic impairment. Toxic epidermal necrolysis reported (rarely) in bone marrow transplant with multiple risk factors including sepsis.

ADVERSE REACTIONS: Diarrhea, nausea, vomiting, rash, abdominal cramps, vaginal candidiasis, discomfort/swelling at injection site, hypersensitivity reaction.

INTERACTIONS: Monitor renal function with aminoglycosides; increased risk of nephrotoxicity, ototoxicity. Toxic epidermal necrolysis reported (rarely) in bone marrow transplant with radiation therapy and other drugs associated with toxic epidermal necrolysis.

PREGNANCY: Category B, not for use in nursing.

AZASITE   RX
azithromycin (Inspire)

THERAPEUTIC CLASS: Macrolide

INDICATIONS: Treatment of bacterial conjunctivitis caused by susceptible strains of microorganisms.

DOSAGE: *Adults:* Initial: 1 drop bid, 8 to 12 hrs apart, for first 2 days. Maint: 1 drop qd for next 5 days.
Pediatric: ≥1 yr: Initial: 1 drop bid, 8 to 12 hrs apart, for first 2 days. Maint: 1 drop qd for next 5 days.

HOW SUPPLIED: Sol: 1% (2.5mL)

WARNINGS/PRECAUTIONS: Not for injection; do not give systemically, inject subconjunctivally or into chamber of eye. Caution may cause hypersensitivity reactions. Growth of resistant organisms including fungi may occur with prolonged use. Avoid contact lens use.

ADVERSE REACTIONS: Eye irritation, burning, stinging and irritation upon instillation, contact dermatitis, corneal erosion, dry eye, dysgeusia, nasal congestion, ocular discharge, punctate keratitis, sinusitis.

PREGNANCY: Category B, caution in nursing.

AZELEX   RX
azelaic acid (Allergan)

THERAPEUTIC CLASS: Dicarboxylic acid antimicrobial

INDICATIONS: Mild-to-moderate inflammatory acne vulgaris.

DOSAGE: *Adults:* Wash and dry skin. Massage gently into affected area bid (am and pm).
Pediatrics: ≥12 yrs: Wash and dry skin. Massage gently into affected area bid (am and pm).

HOW SUPPLIED: Cre: 20% (30g, 50g)

WARNINGS/PRECAUTIONS: Avoid mouth, eyes, mucous membranes, and occlusive dressings.

ADVERSE REACTIONS: Pruritus, burning, stinging, tingling, hypopigmentation.

PREGNANCY: Category B, caution in nursing.

AZMACORT   RX
triamcinolone acetonide (Kos)

THERAPEUTIC CLASS: Corticosteroid

INDICATIONS: Maintenance treatment of asthma as prophylactic therapy in patients ≥6 yrs; to reduce or eliminate the need for oral corticosteroidal therapy.

DOSAGE: *Adults:* 2 inh tid-qid or 4 inh bid. Severe Asthma: Initial: 12-16 inh/day. Max: 16 inh/day. Rinse mouth after use.

Pediatrics: >12 yrs: 2 inh tid-qid or 4 inh bid. Severe Asthma: Initial: 12-16 inh/day. Max: 16 inh/day. 6-12 yrs: 1-2 inh tid-qid or 2-4 inh bid. Max: 12 inh/day. Rinse mouth after use.

HOW SUPPLIED: MDI: 100mcg/inh (20g)

CONTRAINDICATIONS: Primary treatment of status asthmaticus or other acute asthma attacks.

WARNINGS/PRECAUTIONS: Deaths due to adrenal insufficiency have occurred with transfer from systemic corticosteroids to inhaled corticosteroids. Resume oral corticosteroids during stress or severe asthma attack. Observe for adrenal insufficiency, systemic corticosteroid withdrawal effects, hypercorticism and growth suppression (children). More susceptible to infections. Not for acute bronchospasm. D/C if bronchospasm occurs after dosing. Caution with TB of respiratory tract; untreated systemic fungal, bacterial, viral or parasitic infections; or ocular herpes simplex. *Candida* infection of mouth and pharynx reported.

ADVERSE REACTIONS: Pharyngitis, sinusitis, headache, flu syndrome.

INTERACTIONS: Caution with prednisone.

PREGNANCY: Category C, caution in nursing.

AZULFIDINE
sulfasalazine (Pharmacia)

RX

THERAPEUTIC CLASS: 5-Aminosalicylic acid derivative/sulfapyridine

INDICATIONS: Treatment of mild to moderate ulcerative colitis. Adjunct therapy in severe ulcerative colitis. To prolong remission period between acute attacks of ulcerative colitis.

DOSAGE: *Adults:* Initial: 3-4g/day in divided doses. May initiate at 1-2g/day to reduce GI intolerance. Maint: 2g/day.
Pediatrics: ≥2 yrs: 40-60mg/kg/day divided into 3-6 doses. Maint: 7.5mg/kg qid.

HOW SUPPLIED: Tab: 500mg* *scored

CONTRAINDICATIONS: <2 yrs, intestinal or urinary obstruction, porphyria, hypersensitivity to sulfonamides, salicylates.

WARNINGS/PRECAUTIONS: Caution with hepatic/renal impairment, blood dyscrasias, severe allergy, bronchial asthma, G6PD deficiency. Monitor CBC, WBC, LFTs, at baseline, every 2nd week for 1st 3 months, monthly for next 3 months, and every 3 months thereafter. Monitor renal function periodically. Maintain adequate fluid intake to prevent crystalluria and stone formation. D/C if hypersensitivity or toxic reaction occurs.

ADVERSE REACTIONS: Anorexia, headache, nausea, vomiting, gastric distress, reversible oligospermia.

INTERACTIONS: Reduces absorption of folic acid, digoxin.

PREGNANCY: Category B, caution in nursing.

AZULFIDINE EN
sulfasalazine (Pharmacia & Upjohn)

RX

THERAPEUTIC CLASS: 5-Aminosalicylic acid derivative/sulfapyridine

INDICATIONS: Mild to moderate ulcerative colitis, as an adjunct treatment of severe ulcerative colitis, and for the prolongation of the remission period between acute attacks of ulcerative colitis. Rheumatoid arthritis and polyarticular-course juvenile rheumatoid arthritis that has responded inadequately to salicylates or other NSAIDs.

DOSAGE: *Adults:* Ulcerative Colitis: Initial: 1-4g/day in divided doses at intervals not exceeding 8 hrs. Maint: 2g/day. Rheumatoid Arthritis: Initial: 0.5-1g/day. Maint: 2g/day given bid. Swallow tabs whole after meals.
Pediatrics: ≥2 yrs: Ulcerative Colitis: Initial: 40-60mg/kg/24hrs in 3-6 divided doses. Maint: 7.5mg/kg qid. Juvenile Rheumatoid Arthritis: 30-50mg/kg/day given bid. To reduce GI effects give 1/4 to 1/3 initial dose; increase weekly for 1 month. Max: 2g/day. Swallow tabs whole after meals.

BACITRACIN INJECTION

HOW SUPPLIED: Tab, Delayed Release: 500mg

CONTRAINDICATIONS: Intestinal or urinary obstruction, porphyria, hypersensitivity to sulfonamides or salicylates.

WARNINGS/PRECAUTIONS: Caution with hepatic or renal impairment, blood dyscrasias, severe allergy, bronchial asthma or G6PD deficiency. Monitor CBC, WBC, and LFTs prior to therapy and every other week for the 1st 3 months, once monthly for next 3 months, then every 3 months. Monitor renal function periodically. Maintain adequate fluid intake. Fatal hypersensitivity reactions reported. D/C if tabs pass undisintegrated or if hypersensitivity reactions occur.

ADVERSE REACTIONS: Anorexia, headache, nausea, vomiting, gastric distress, oligospermia, rash, pruritus, urticaria, fever, orange-yellow urine or skin.

INTERACTIONS: Reduces absorption of folic acid and digoxin. Increased incidence of GI adverse events with combination of sulfasalazine (2g/day) and MTX (7.5mg/week).

PREGNANCY: Category B, caution in nursing.

BACITRACIN INJECTION
bacitracin (Pharmacia & Upjohn)

RX

> May cause renal failure due to tubular and glomerular necrosis. Monitor renal function prior to, and daily during therapy. Fluid intake and urinary output should be maintained at proper levels to avoid kidney toxicity. Discontinue if renal toxicity occurs. Avoid other nephrotoxic drugs.

THERAPEUTIC CLASS: Antibiotic

INDICATIONS: Treatment of pneumonia and empyema caused by staphylococci.

DOSAGE: Pediatrics: <2500g: 900U/kg/24h IM. >2500g: 1000U/kg/24h IM. Administer in 2-3 divided doses. Inject in upper outer quadrant of buttocks.

HOW SUPPLIED: Inj: 50,000U

WARNINGS/PRECAUTIONS: Use appropriate therapy if superinfection occurs.

ADVERSE REACTIONS: Albuminuria, cylindruria, azotemia, nausea, vomiting, pain at injection site, skin rashes, rising blood levels without increase in dosage.

INTERACTIONS: Avoid with other nephrotoxic drugs (eg, streptomycin, kanamycin, polymyxin B, polymyxin E, neomycin).

PREGNANCY: Safety in pregnancy or nursing not known.

BACLOFEN
baclofen (Various)

RX

OTHER BRAND NAME: Kemstro (Schwarz)

THERAPEUTIC CLASS: GABA analog

INDICATIONS: Treatment of spasticity associated with multiple sclerosis. May be effective in spinal cord injuries and other spinal cord diseases.

DOSAGE: *Adults:* Initial: 5mg tid for 3 days. Titrate: May increase dose by 5mg tid every 3 days. Usual: 40-80mg/day. Max: 80 mg/day (20mg qid). Renal Impairment: Reduce dose.

Pediatrics: ≥12 yrs: Initial: 5mg tid for 3 days. Titrate: May increase dose by 5mg tid every 3 days. Usual: 40-80mg/day. Max: 80 mg/day (20mg qid). Renal Impairment: Reduce dose.

HOW SUPPLIED: Tab: (Generic) 10mg, 20mg; Tab, Disintegrating (ODT): (Kemstro) 10mg, 20mg

WARNINGS/PRECAUTIONS: Caution with psychosis, schizophrenia, confusional states; may exacerbate conditions. Caution with bladder sphincter hypertonia, peptic ulceration, seizures, elderly, cerebrovascular disorder, respiratory failure, hepatic or renal failure. Abnormal AST, alkaline phosphatase and blood glucose reported. Caution when used to maintain locomotion or to obtain increased function. Decreased alertness with operating machinery. Has not significantly benefited stroke patients. Avoid abrupt discontinuation; reduce dose slowly over 1-2 weeks.

ADVERSE REACTIONS: Drowsiness, dizziness, weakness, fatigue, confusion, daytime sedation, headache, insomnia, hypotension, nausea, constipation, urinary frequency.

INTERACTIONS: May potentiate antihypertensives. May increase CNS depressant effects with MAO inhibitors. Potentiated by TCAs. Mental confusion, hallucinations and agitation with levodopa plus carbidopa therapy. May increase blood glucose and require dosage adjustment of antidiabetic agents. Synergistic effects with magnesium sulfate and other neuromuscular blockers. Additive CNS effects with alcohol and other CNS depressants.

PREGNANCY: Category C, caution in nursing.

Bactrim RX
trimethoprim - sulfamethoxazole (AR Scientific)

OTHER BRAND NAME: Bactrim DS (AR Scientific)
THERAPEUTIC CLASS: Sulfonamide/tetrahydrofolic acid inhibitor
INDICATIONS: Treatment of urinary tract infection (UTI), acute otitis media, acute exacerbation of chronic bronchitis (AECB), travelers' diarrhea, Shigellosis, and pneumocystitis carinii pneumonia (PCP).
DOSAGE: *Adults:* UTI: 800mg SMX-160mg TMP q12h for 10-14 days. Shigellosis: 800mg SMX-160mg TMP q12h for 5 days. AECB: 800mg SMX-160mg TMP q12h for 14 days. PCP Treatment: 15-20mg/kg TMP and 75-100mg/kg SMX per 24 hrs given q6h for 14-21 days. PCP Prophylaxis: 800mg SMX-160mg TMP qd. Traveler's Diarrhea: 800mg SMX-160mg TMP q12h for 5 days. CrCl: 15-30mL/min: 50% usual dose. CrCl: <15mL/min: Not recommended.
Pediatrics: ≥2 months: UTI/Otitis Media: 4mg/kg TMP and 20mg/kg SMX q12h for 10 days. Shigellosis: 8mg/kg TMP and 40mg/kg SMX per 24 hrs given q12h for 5 days. PCP Treatment: 15-20mg/kg TMP and 75-100mg/kg SMX per 24 hrs given q6h for 14-21 days. PCP Prophylaxis: 150mg/m^2/day TMP with 750mg/m^2/day SMX given bid, on 3 consecutive days/week. Max: 320mg TMP/1600mg SMX/day. CrCl: 15-30mL/min: 50% usual dose. CrCl: <15mL/min: Not recommended.
HOW SUPPLIED: (Sulfamethoxazole (SMX)-Trimethoprim (TMP)) Tab: 400mg-80mg*; Tab, DS: 800mg-160mg* *scored
CONTRAINDICATIONS: Megaloblastic anemia due to folate deficiency, pregnancy, nursing, infants <2 months, marked hepatic damage, severe renal insufficiency if cannot monitor renal status.
WARNINGS/PRECAUTIONS: Fatal hypersensitivity reactions (eg, Stevens-Johnson syndrome, toxic epidermal necrolysis, fulminant hepatic necrosis, agranulocytosis, aplastic anemia) may occur. Pseudomembranous colitis, cough, SOB, and pulmonary infiltrates reported. Avoid with group A β-hemolytic streptococcal infections. Caution with hepatic/renal impairment, elderly, folate deficiency (eg, chronic alcoholics, anticonvulsants, malabsorption, malnutrition), bronchial asthma, and other allergies. In G6PD deficiency, hemolysis may occur. Increased incidence of adverse events with AIDS. Ensure adequate fluid intake and urinary output. Caution with porphyria, thyroid dysfunction.
ADVERSE REACTIONS: Nausea, vomiting, anorexia, rash, urticaria.
INTERACTIONS: Diuretics (especially thiazides) may increase risk of thrombocytopenia with purpura in elderly patients. Caution with warfarin, may prolong PT. Increased effects of phenytoin, oral hypoglycemics. Increased plasma levels of methotrexate, digoxin (especially in elderly). Marked but reversible nephrotoxicity reported with cyclosporine. May develop megaloblastic anemia with pyrimethamine >25mg/week. Increased levels with indomethacin. May decrease effects of TCAs. Single case of toxic delirium with amantadine.
PREGNANCY: Category C, contraindicated in nursing.

Bactroban RX
mupirocin (GlaxoSmithKline)

THERAPEUTIC CLASS: Bacterial protein synthesis inhibitor
INDICATIONS: (Oint) Topical treatment of impetigo due to *S.aureus* and *S.pyogenes*. (Cre) Treatment of secondarily infected traumatic skin lesions (up to 10 cm in length or 100 cm^2) due to *S.aureus* and *S.pyogenes*.

BALAMINE DM

DOSAGE: *Adults:* (Oint) Apply tid. (Cre) Apply tid for 10 days. May cover with gauze. Re-evaluate if no response within 3-5 days.

Pediatrics: (Oint) 2-16 yrs: Apply tid. (Cre) 3 months-16 yrs: Apply tid for 10 days. May cover with gauze. Re-evaluate if no response within 3-5 days.

HOW SUPPLIED: Cre: 2% (15g, 30g); Oint: 2% (22g)

WARNINGS/PRECAUTIONS: Avoid eyes. Discontinue if sensitization or irritation occurs. May cause superinfection with prolonged use. Caution with ointment in renal dysfunction. Avoid mucosal surfaces. Avoid open wounds or damaged skin with ointment.

ADVERSE REACTIONS: Burning, pain, pruritus, headache, rash, nausea.

PREGNANCY: Category B, caution in nursing.

BALAMINE DM   RX
pseudoephedrine HCl - dextromethorphan HBr - carbinoxamine maleate
(Ballay)

THERAPEUTIC CLASS: Antihistamine/cough suppressant/decongestant

INDICATIONS: Relief of cough and upper respiratory symptoms, including nasal congestion associated with allergy or the common cold.

DOSAGE: *Adults:* (Syrup) 5mL qid.

Pediatrics: (Syrup) ≥6 yrs: 5mL qid. 18 months-6yrs: 2.5mL qid. (Drops) 9-18 months: 1mL qid. 6-9 months: 0.75mL qid. 3-6 months: 0.5mL qid. 1-3 months: 0.25mL qid.

HOW SUPPLIED: Drops: (Carbinoxamine-Dextromethorphan-Pseudoephedrine) 2mg-3.5mg-25mg/mL (30mL); Syrup: (Carbinoxamine-Dextromethorphan-Pseudoephedrine) 4mg-12.5mg-60mg/5mL

CONTRAINDICATIONS: Severe HTN or CAD, MAOI use or within 14 days of discontinuation, narrow-angle glaucoma, urinary retention, peptic ulcer, during asthma attack.

WARNINGS/PRECAUTIONS: Caution with elderly, atopic children, sedated/debilitated, patients confined to supine positions, HTN, DM, ischemic heart disease, hyperthyroidism, prostatic hypertrophy, asthma, and increased IOP. May produce CNS stimulation with convulsions or cardiovascular collapse with hypotension. Excitability reported especially in children. Caution while operating machinery.

ADVERSE REACTIONS: Sedation, dizziness, diplopia, vomiting, diarrhea, dry mouth, headache, arrhythmias, increased heart rate and BP, tremors, nervousness, insomnia.

INTERACTIONS: May enhance effects of TCAs, barbiturates, alcohol, other CNS depressants. May diminish antihypertensive effects of reserpine, veratrum alkaloids, methyldopa, mecamylamine. Increased sympathomimetic effect with beta-blockers and MAOIs. Additive cough-suppressant effect with narcotic antitussives. Contraindicated with or within 14 days of discontinuing MAOIs.

PREGNANCY: Category C, not for use in nursing.

BARACLUDE   RX
entecavir (Bristol-Myers Squibb)

> Lactic acidosis and severe, possibly fatal, hepatomegaly with steatosis reported. Reports of severe acute exacerbations of hepatitis B upon discontinuation of therapy. Follow-up liver function monitoring required.

THERAPEUTIC CLASS: Guanosine nucleoside analogue

INDICATIONS: Treatment of chronic hepatitis B virus (HBV) infection with active viral replication and persistent elevations in serum aminotransferases (ALT or AST) or histologically active disease.

DOSAGE: *Adults:* Nucleoside-Treatment-Naive: 0.5mg qd. CrCl 30 to <50mL/min: 0.25mg qd. CrCl 10 to <30mL/min: 0.15mg qd. CrCl <10mL/min: 0.05mg qd. Receiving Lamivudine or Known Lamivudine Resistance Mutation: 1mg qd. CrCl 30 to <50mL/min: 0.5mg qd. CrCl 10 to <30mL/min: 0.3mg qd. CrCl <10mL/min: 0.1mg qd. Take on empty stomach.

Pediatrics: ≥16 yrs: Nucleoside-Treatment-Naive: 0.5mg qd. CrCl 30 to <50mL/min: 0.25mg qd. CrCl 10 to <30mL/min: 0.15mg qd. CrCl <10mL/min: 0.05mg qd. Receiving Lamivudine or Known Lamivudine Resistance Mutation: 1mg qd. CrCl 30 to <50mL/min: 0.5mg qd. CrCl 10 to <30mL/min: 0.3mg qd. CrCl <10mL/min: 0.1mg qd. Take on empty stomach.

HOW SUPPLIED: Sol: 0.05mg/mL; Tab: 0.5mg, 1mg

WARNINGS/PRECAUTIONS: Reduce dose in renal dysfunction (CrCl <50mL/min) including patients on hemodialysis or CAPD (continuous ambulatory peritoneal dialysis).Exacerbations of hepatitis after discontinuation of treatment

ADVERSE REACTIONS: Headache, fatigue, dizziness, nausea, hyperglycemia, lipase > or equal to 2.1 X ULN, glycosuria, hematuria and increase in total bilirubin.

INTERACTIONS: May increase serum concentrations of entecavir or coadministered drug with drugs that reduce renal function or compete for active tubular secretion.

PREGNANCY: Category C, not for use in nursing.

BAYER ASPIRIN OTC
aspirin (Bayer Healthcare LLC)

OTHER BRAND NAMES: Bayer Extra Strength (Bayer Healthcare LLC) - Bayer Aspirin Regimen (Bayer Healthcare LLC) - Genuine Bayer Aspirin (Bayer Healthcare LLC) - Bayer Aspirin Children's (Bayer Healthcare LLC) - Bayer Aspirin Regimen with Calcium (Bayer Healthcare LLC)

THERAPEUTIC CLASS: Salicylate

INDICATIONS: To reduce the risk of death and nonfatal stroke with previous ischemic stroke or transient ischemia of the brain. To reduce risk of vascular mortality with suspected acute MI. To reduce risk of death and nonfatal MI with previous MI or unstable angina. To reduce risk of MI and sudden death in chronic stable angina pectoris. For patients who have undergone revascularization procedures with a pre-existing condition for which ASA is indicated. Relief of signs of rheumatoid arthritis (RA), juvenile rheumatoid arthritis (JRA), osteoarthritis (OA), spondyloarthropathies, arthritis, and pleurisy associated with SLE. For minor aches and pains.

DOSAGE: *Adults:* Ischemic Stroke/TIA: 50-325mg qd. Suspected Acute MI: Initial: 160-162.5mg qd as soon as suspect MI. Maint: 160-162.5mg qd for 30 days post-infarction, consider further therapy for prevention/recurrent MI. Prevention or Recurrent MI/Unstable Angina/Chronic Stable Angina: 75-325mg qd. CABG: 325mg qd, start 6 hrs post-surgery. Continue for 1 year. PTCA: Initial: 325mg, 2 hrs pre-surgery. Maint: 160-325mg qd. Carotid Endarterectomy: 80mg qd to 650mg bid, start pre-surgery. RA: Initial: 3g qd in divided doses. Increase for anti-inflammatory efficacy to 150-300mcg/mL plasma salicylate level. Spondyloarthropathies: Up to 4g/day in divided doses. OA: Up to 3g/day in divided doses. Arthritis/SLE Pleurisy: Initial: 3g/day in divided doses. Increase for anti-inflammatory efficacy to 150-300mcg/mL plasma salicylate level. Pain: 325-650mg q4-6h. Max: 4g/day.

Pediatrics: JRA: Initial: 90-130mg/kg/day in divided doses. Increase for anti-inflammatory efficacy to 150-300mcg/mL plasma salicylate level. Pain: ≥12 yrs: 325-650mg q4-6h. Max: 4g/day.

HOW SUPPLIED: Tab: (Genuine Bayer Aspirin) 325mg; Tab: (Bayer Extra Strength) 500mg; Tab: (Bayer Aspirin Regimen with Calcium) 81mg; Tab, Chewable: (Bayer Aspirin Children's) 81mg; Tab, Delayed Release: (Bayer Aspirin Regimen) 81mg, 325mg

CONTRAINDICATIONS: NSAID allergy, viral infections in children or teenagers, syndrome of asthma, rhinitis, and nasal polyps.

WARNINGS/PRECAUTIONS: Increased risk of bleeding with heavy alcohol use (≥3 drinks/day). May inhibit platelet function; can adversely affect inherited (hemophilia) or acquired (hepatic disease, vitamin K deficiency) bleeding disorders. Monitor for bleeding and ulceration. Avoid in history of active peptic ulcer, severe renal failure, severe hepatic insufficiency, and sodium restricted diets. Associated with elevated LFTs, BUN, and serum creatinine; hyperkalemia; proteinuria; and prolonged bleeding time. Avoid 1 week before and during labor.

ADVERSE REACTIONS: Fever, hypothermia, dysrhythmias, hypotension, agitation, cerebral edema, dehydration, hyperkalemia, dyspepsia, GI bleed, hearing loss, tinnitus, problems in pregnancy.

BAYER ASPIRIN EXTRA STRENGTH

INTERACTIONS: Diminished hypotensive and hyponatremic effects of ACE inhibitors. May increase levels of acetazolamide, valproic acid. Increased bleeding risk with heparin, warfarin. Decreased levels of phenytoin. Decreased hypotensive effects of γ-blockers. Decreased diuretic effects with renal or cardiovascular disease. Decreased methotrexate clearance; increased risk of bone marrow toxicity. Avoid NSAIDs. Increased effects of hypoglycemic agents. Antagonizes uricosuric agents.

PREGNANCY: Avoid in 3rd trimester of pregnancy and nursing.

BAYER ASPIRIN EXTRA STRENGTH   OTC
aspirin (Bayer Healthcare LLC)

THERAPEUTIC CLASS: Salicylate

INDICATIONS: For the temporary relief of headache, pain and fever of colds, muscle aches and pains, menstrual pain, toothache pain, minor aches and arthritis pain.

DOSAGE: *Adults:* 500-1000mg q4-6h prn. Max: 4g/24hrs.
Pediatrics: ≥12 yrs: 500-1000mg q4-6h prn. Max: 4g/24hrs.

HOW SUPPLIED: Tab: 500mg

WARNINGS/PRECAUTIONS: Avoid in children or teenagers for chickenpox or flu symptoms; Reye's syndrome may occur. Do not take >10 days for pain or >3 days for fever. Avoid in asthma, stomach problems that persist or recur, gastric ulcers, or bleeding problems. Stop therapy if ringing in the ears or loss of hearing occurs.

INTERACTIONS: Avoid with drugs for anticoagulation, diabetes, gout, or arthritis. Increased risk of stomach bleeding with alcohol use (≥3 drinks/day).

PREGNANCY: Avoid in 3rd trimester of pregnancy; safety in nursing not known.

BECONASE AQ   RX
beclomethasone dipropionate (GlaxoSmithKline)

OTHER BRAND NAME: Beconase (Various)

THERAPEUTIC CLASS: Corticosteroid

INDICATIONS: Relief of symptoms of seasonal or perennial allergic and nonallergic rhinitis. Prevention of nasal polyp recurrence following surgical removal.

DOSAGE: *Adults:* (Beconase): 1 spray per nostril bid-qid. (Beconase AQ) 1-2 sprays per nostril bid. Max: 2 sprays per nostril bid.
Pediatrics: (Beconase) ≥12 yrs: 1 spray per nostril bid-qid. 6-12 yrs: 1 spray per nostril tid. (Beconase AQ) ≥6 yrs: 1-2 sprays per nostril bid. Max: 2 sprays per nostril bid.

HOW SUPPLIED: Aerosol: (Beconase) 42mcg/spray (6.7g, 16.8g); Spray: (Beconase AQ) 42mcg/spray (25g)

WARNINGS/PRECAUTIONS: Risk of adrenal insufficiency and withdrawal symptoms when replacing systemic corticosteroids with a topical corticosteroids. Caution with active or quiescent TB, ocular herpes simplex, or untreated bacterial, fungal and systemic viral infections. Avoid with recent nasal trauma, surgery or septum ulcers. Risk for more severe/fatal course of infections (eg, chickenpox, measles) and for Candida infection of the nose and pharynx. Potential for growth velocity reduction in pediatrics.

ADVERSE REACTIONS: Nasopharyngeal irritation, sneezing, headache, nausea, lightheadedness, irritated/dry nose and throat, unpleasant taste/smell.

INTERACTIONS: Concomitant systemic corticosteroids increases risk of hypercorticism and/or HPA axis suppression.

PREGNANCY: Category C, caution in nursing.

BENADRYL ALLERGY   OTC
diphenhydramine HCl (McNeil)

THERAPEUTIC CLASS: Antihistamine

INDICATIONS: Relief of hay fever or upper respiratory allergies, and rhinorrhea/sneezing due to the common cold.

DOSAGE: *Adults:* 25-50mg q4-6h. Max: 300mg/24hrs.
Pediatrics: ≥12 yrs: 25-50mg q4-6h. Max: 300mg/24 hrs. 6-11 yrs: 12.5-25mg q4-6h. Max: 150mg/24hrs.
HOW SUPPLIED: Cap: 25mg; Sol: 12.5mg/5mL; Tab: 25mg; Tab, Chewable: 12.5mg
WARNINGS/PRECAUTIONS: Caution with emphysema, chronic bronchitis, glaucoma, or difficulty in urination due to prostate gland enlargement. May impair mental/physical abilities.
ADVERSE REACTIONS: Drowsiness, excitability (especially in children).
INTERACTIONS: Increased drowsiness with alcohol, sedatives, tranquilizers.
PREGNANCY: Safety in pregnancy and nursing not known.

BENZACLIN RX
clindamycin - benzoyl peroxide (Dermik)

THERAPEUTIC CLASS: Antibacterial/keratolytic
INDICATIONS: Topical treatment of acne vulgaris.
DOSAGE: *Adults:* Wash face and pat dry. Apply bid (am and pm).
Pediatrics: ≥12 yrs: Wash face and pat dry. Apply bid (am and pm).
HOW SUPPLIED: Gel: (Clindamycin-Benzoyl Peroxide) 1%-5% (25g, 50g)
CONTRAINDICATIONS: Hypersensitivity to lincomycin. History of regional enteritis, ulcerative colitis, and antibiotic-associated colitis.
WARNINGS/PRECAUTIONS: Severe colitis reported with oral and parenteral clindamycin. Discontinue if severe diarrhea occurs. Avoid contact with eyes and mucous membranes.
ADVERSE REACTIONS: Dry skin, pruritus, peeling, erythema, sunburn.
INTERACTIONS: Cumulative irritancy possible with other topical acne agents. Avoid erythromycin agents.
PREGNANCY: Category C, not for use in nursing.

BENZAGEL RX
benzoyl peroxide (Dermik)

OTHER BRAND NAME: Benzagel Wash (Dermik)
THERAPEUTIC CLASS: Antibacterial/keratolytic
INDICATIONS: Treatment of mild to moderate acne, used alone or as an adjunct.
DOSAGE: *Adults:* (Wash) Wash area qd-bid. Rinse and dry area. (Gel) Apply qd or more often to clean affected area. Very fair patients should start with single application qhs.
Pediatrics: ≥12 yrs: (Wash) Wash area qd-bid. Rinse and dry area. (Gel) Apply qd or more often to clean affected area. Very fair patients should start with single application qhs.
HOW SUPPLIED: Gel: 5%, 10% (42.5g), (Wash) 10% (60g)
WARNINGS/PRECAUTIONS: Discontinue if itching, redness, burning, swelling, or undue dryness occurs. Avoid contact with eyes and mucous membranes. May bleach colored fabrics or hair.
ADVERSE REACTIONS: Irritation, contact dermatitis.
PREGNANCY: Category C, caution in nursing.

BENZAMYCIN RX
erythromycin - benzoyl peroxide (Dermik)

THERAPEUTIC CLASS: Antibacterial/keratolytic
INDICATIONS: Topical treatment of acne vulgaris.

BETAMETHASONE DIPROPIONATE

DOSAGE: Adults: Wash skin and dry. Apply bid (am and pm).
Pediatrics: ≥12 yrs: Wash skin and dry. Apply bid (am and pm).
HOW SUPPLIED: Gel: (Benzoyl Peroxide-Erythromycin) 5%-3% (46.6g, 60^s)
WARNINGS/PRECAUTIONS: D/C if severe irritation occurs. Avoid eyes, mouth, and mucous membranes. Keep refrigerated after reconstitution and discard after 3 months.
ADVERSE REACTIONS: Dryness, urticaria, skin irritation, skin discoloration, oiliness, tenderness.
INTERACTIONS: Additive irritation with peeling, desquamating, or abrasive agents.
PREGNANCY: Category C, caution in nursing.

BETAMETHASONE DIPROPIONATE   RX
betamethasone dipropionate (Various)

THERAPEUTIC CLASS: Corticosteroid
INDICATIONS: Corticosteroid responsive dermatoses.
DOSAGE: *Adults:* (Cre, Oint) Apply qd-bid. (Lot) Apply a few drops bid, am and pm.
Pediatrics: (Cre, Oint) Apply qd-bid. (Lot) Apply a few drops bid, am and pm.
HOW SUPPLIED: Cre, Oint: 0.05% (15g, 45g); Lot: 0.05% (20mL, 60mL)
WARNINGS/PRECAUTIONS: May produce reversible HPA axis suppression, manifestations of Cushing's syndrome, hyperglycemia, and glucosuria. Avoid occlusive dressings. Pediatrics are more prone to systemic toxicity. Discontinue if irritation occurs. Avoid eyes.
ADVERSE REACTIONS: Burning, itching, irritation, dryness, folliculitis, hypertrichosis, acneiform eruptions, hypopigmentation, perioral dermatitis, allergic contact dermatitis, skin maceration, secondary infection, skin atrophy, striae, miliaria.
PREGNANCY: Category C, caution in nursing.

BETAPACE   RX
sotalol HCl (Berlex)

> To minimize risk of arrhythmia, place patients initiated or reinitiated on therapy for minimum of 3 days in a facility that can provide ECG monitoring and cardiac resuscitation. Perform CrCl before therapy. Do not substitute Betapace® for Betapace AF®.

THERAPEUTIC CLASS: Beta-blocker (group II/III antiarrhythmic)
INDICATIONS: Treatment of documented life-threatening ventricular arrhythmias.
DOSAGE: *Adults:* Initial: 80mg bid. Titrate: Increase to 120-160mg bid if needed. Allow 3 days between dose increments. Usual: 160-320mg/day given bid-tid. Refractory Patients: 480-640mg/day. CrCl 30-59mL/min: Dose q24h. CrCl 10-29mL/min: Dose q36-48h. CrCl <10mL/min: Individualize dose. May increase dose with renal impairment after at least 5-6 doses.
Pediatrics: ≥2 yrs: Initial: 30mg/m^2 tid. Titrate: Wait at least 36 hrs between dose increases. Guide dose by response, heart rate and QTc. Max: 60mg/m^2. <2 yrs: See dosing chart in labeling. Reduce dose or discontinue if QTc >550msec. Renal Impairment: Reduce dose or increase interval. Preparation of 5mg/mL Oral Solution: Add five 120mg tabs to 120mL simple syrup in a 6oz plastic, amber bottle. Shake bottle to wet all tabs. Allow tabs to hydrate for 2 hrs then shake bottle intermittently over 2 hrs until tabs are completely disintegrated. Shake before administration. Store at room temp for 3 months.
HOW SUPPLIED: Tab: 80mg*, 120mg*, 160mg*, 240mg* *scored
CONTRAINDICATIONS: Bronchial asthma, sinus bradycardia, 2nd- and 3rd-degree AV block (unless a functioning pacemaker is present), long QT syndromes, cardiogenic shock, uncontrolled CHF.
WARNINGS/PRECAUTIONS: Caution with heart failure controlled by digitalis and/or diuretics, DM, left ventricular dysfunction, non-allergic bronchospasm, sick sinus syndrome, renal impairment, 2-weeks post-MI. Avoid with hypokalemia, hypomagnesemia, excessive QT interval prolongation (>550msec). Correct electrolyte imbalances before

therapy. May provoke new or worsen ventricular arrhythmias. Avoid abrupt withdrawal. Use in surgery is controversial. May mask hypoglycemia, hyperthyroidism symptoms. Proarrhythmic events reported.

ADVERSE REACTIONS: Dyspnea, fatigue, dizziness, bradycardia, chest pain, palpitation, asthenia, abnormal ECG, hypotension, headache, lightheadedness, edema.

INTERACTIONS: May block epinephrine effects. Caution with drugs that prolong the QT interval (eg, Class I and III antiarrhythmics, phenothiazines, TCAs, bepridil, certain quinolones and oral macrolides, astemizole). Avoid within 2 hrs of aluminum- or magnesium-containing antacids. Potentiates rebound HTN with clonidine withdrawal. May potentiate bradycardia or hypotension with catecholamine-depleting drugs (eg, reserpine). Antidiabetic agents may need adjustment. Avoid Class IA and Class III antiarrhythmics; potential to prolong refractoriness. $β_2$-agonists (eg, terbutaline) may need dose increase. Additive Class II effects with β-blockers. Additive conduction abnormalities with digoxin and calcium channel blockers. Caution with diuretics.

PREGNANCY: Category B, not for use in nursing.

BETAPACE AF
sotalol HCl (Berlex)

RX

> To minimize risk of arrhythmia, place patients initiated or reinitiated on therapy for minimum of 3 days in a facility that can provide CrCl, ECG monitoring, and cardiac resuscitation. Do not substitute Betapace® for Betapace AF®.

THERAPEUTIC CLASS: Beta-blocker (group II/III antiarrhythmic)

INDICATIONS: Maintenance of normal sinus rhythm with symptomatic atrial fibrillation/ atrial flutter (AFIB/AFL) in patients who are currently in sinus rhythm.

DOSAGE: *Adults:* Initiate with continuous ECG monitoring. Give dose qd for CrCl 40-60mL/min and bid for CrCl >60mL/min. Initial: 80mg. Monitor QT 2-4hrs after each dose. Discontinue if QT ≥500msec. If QT <500msec after 3 days (after 5th or 6th dose if receiving qd dosing) discharge on current treatment. Alternately, may increase dose to 120mg during hospitalization, and follow for 3 days with bid dose and for 5 or 6 doses if receiving qd dose. Max: 160mg qd or bid depending on CrCl.

Pediatrics: ≥2 yrs: Initial: 30mg/m^2 tid. Titrate: Wait at least 36 hrs between dose increases. Guide dose by response, heart rate and QTc. Max: 60mg/m^2. <2 yrs: See dosing chart in labeling. Reduce dose or discontinue if QTc >550msec. Renal Impairment: Reduce dose or increase interval. Preparation of 5mg/mL Oral Solution: Add five 120mg tabs to 120mL simple syrup in a 6oz plastic, amber bottle. Shake bottle to wet all tabs. Allow tabs to hydrate for 2 hrs then shake bottle intermittently over 2 hrs until tabs are completely disintegrated. Shake before administration. Store at room temp for 3 months.

HOW SUPPLIED: Tab: 80mg*, 120mg*, 160mg* *scored

CONTRAINDICATIONS: Sinus bradycardia (<50bpm during waking hrs), sick sinus syndrome or 2nd- or 3rd-degree AV block (unless a functioning pacemaker is present), long QT syndromes, baseline QT interval >450msec, cardiogenic shock, uncontrolled heart failure, hypokalemia (<4meq/L), CrCl <40mL/min, bronchial asthma.

WARNINGS/PRECAUTIONS: Can cause serious ventricular arrhythmias. Avoid with hypokalemia, hypomagnesemia. Correct electrolyte imbalances before therapy. Bradycardia reported. Caution with heart failure controlled by digitalis and/or diuretics, non-allergic bronchospasm, sick sinus syndrome, left ventricular dysfunction, DM, renal dysfunction, post-MI. Avoid abrupt withdrawal. Use in surgery is controversial. May mask hypoglycemia, hyperthyroidism symptoms.

ADVERSE REACTIONS: Bradycardia, dyspnea, fatigue, dose-related QT interval prolongation, abnormal ECG, chest pain, diarrhea, nausea, vomiting, hyperhidrosis, dizziness.

INTERACTIONS: May block epinephrine effects. Avoid drugs that prolong the QT interval (eg, antiarrhythmics, phenothiazines, TCAs, bepridil, certain oral macrolides). Avoid within 2 hrs of aluminum- or magnesium-containing antacids. Potentiates rebound HTN with clonidine withdrawal. May potentiate bradycardia or hypotension with catecholamine-depleting drugs (eg, reserpine). Antidiabetic agents may need adjustment. $β_2$-agonists (eg, terbutaline) may need dose increase. Additive conduction abnormalities with digoxin and calcium channel blockers. Caution with diuretics.

PREGNANCY: Category B, not for use in nursing.

Biaxin   RX
clarithromycin (Abbott)

THERAPEUTIC CLASS: Macrolide antibiotic

INDICATIONS: Adults: Pharyngitis/tonsillitis, acute maxillary sinusitis, acute bacterial exacerbation of chronic bronchitis (ABECB), community aquired pneumonia (CAP), uncomplicated skin and skin structure infections (SSSI), disseminated mycobacterial infections, combination therapy for *H.pylori* infection with duodenal ulcers. MAC prophylaxis in advanced HIV. *Pediatrics:* Pharyngitis/tonsillitis, CAP, acute maxillary sinusitis, acute otitis media, uncomplicated SSSI, disseminated mycobacterial infections. MAC prophylaxis in advanced HIV.

DOSAGE: *Adults:* Pharyngitis/Tonsillitis: 250mg q12h for 10 days. Sinusitis: 500mg q12h for 14 days. ABECB: 250-500mg q12h for 7-14 days. SSSI/CAP: 250mg q12h for 7-14 days. MAC Prophylaxis/Treatment: 500mg bid. H.pylori: Triple Therapy: 500mg + amoxicillin 1g + omeprazole 20mg, all q12h for 10 days; or 500mg + amoxicillin 1g + lansoprazole 30mg, all q12h for 10-14 days. Give additional omeprazole 20mg qd for 18 days with active ulcer. Dual Therapy: 500mg q8h + omeprazole 40mg qd for 14 days (give additional omeprazole 20mg qd for 14 days with active ulcer); or 500mg q8h or q12h + ranitidine bismuth citrate 400mg q12h for 14 days (give additional ranitidine bismuth citrate 400mg bid for 14 days with active ulcer). Avoid Biaxin and ranitidine bismuth citrate combination with CrCl<25mL/min.

Pediatrics: ≥6 months: Usual: 7.5mg/kg q12h for 10 days. MAC Prophylaxis/Treatment: ≥20 months: 7.5mg/kg bid, up to 500mg bid. CrCl <30mL/min: Give 50% dose or double interval.

HOW SUPPLIED: Sus: 125mg/5mL, 250mg/5mL (50mL, 100mL); Tab: 250mg, 500mg

CONTRAINDICATIONS: Concomitant cisapride, pimozide, terfenadine, or other macrolide antibiotics.

WARNINGS/PRECAUTIONS: Avoid in pregnancy. Pseudomembranous colitis reported. Adjust dose with severe renal impairment. Colchicine toxicity reported, avoid concomitant use especially in elderly.

ADVERSE REACTIONS: Diarrhea, nausea, abnormal taste, dyspepsia, abdominal pain, headache, vomiting, rash.

INTERACTIONS: Increases serum levels of theophylline, digoxin, HMG-CoA reductase inhibitors, omeprazole, carbamazepine, drugs metabolized by CYP450. Decreases zidovudine plasma levels. Potentiates oral anticoagulant effects. Acute ergot toxicity with ergotamine or dihydroergotamine reported. Decreased clearance of triazolam. Avoid astemizole. Avoid ranitidine, bismuth citrate if CrCl <25mL/min or history of porphyria. Reduce dose with ritonavir if CrCl <60mL/min. Increased levels with fluconazole. Caution with concomitant colchicine use.

PREGNANCY: Category C, caution in nursing.

Bicillin C-R   RX
penicillin G procaine - penicillin G benzathine (King)

THERAPEUTIC CLASS: Penicillin

INDICATIONS: Treatment of moderately severe to severe upper-respiratory tract (URTI) and skin and soft-tissue infections (SSTI), scarlet fever and erysipelas due to streptococci. Treatment of moderately severe pneumonia and otitis media due to pneumococci.

DOSAGE: *Adults:* Group A Strep: URTI/SSTI/Scarlet Fever/Erysipelas: 2.4MU IM. Treat at a single session using multiple IM sites, or use an alternative schedule and give 1/2 of the total dose on Day 1 and 1/2 on Day 3. Pneumococcal Infections (Except Meningitis): 1.2MU IM, repeat every 2-3 days until temperature is normal for 48 hrs. Administer IM into upper, outer quadrant of buttock.

Pediatrics: Group A Strep: URTI/SSTI/Scarlet Fever/Erysipelas: >60 lbs: 2.4MU IM. 30-60 lbs: 900,000U-1.2MU IM. <30 lbs: 600,000U IM. Treat at a single session using multiple IM sites, or use an alternative schedule and give 1/2 of the total dose on Day 1 and 1/2 on Day

3. Pneumococcal Infections (Except Meningitis): 600,000U IM, repeat every 2-3 days until temperature is normal for 48 hrs. Administer IM into upper, outer quadrant of buttock. Use the midlateral aspect of thigh in neonates, infants, and small children.

HOW SUPPLIED: Inj: (Penicillin G Benzathine-Penicillin G Procaine) 300,000-300,000U/mL

CONTRAINDICATIONS: Do not inject into or near an artery or nerve.

WARNINGS/PRECAUTIONS: Serious, fatal anaphylactic reactions reported; increased risk with hypersensitivity to penicillin, cephalosporins, and other allergens. Pseudomembranous colitis reported. Avoid IV, intra-arterial administration, or injection into/near major peripheral nerves or blood vessels may cause severe neurovascular and neurological damage. IM administration into anterolateral thigh may cause quadriceps femoris fibrosis and atrophy. Caution with asthma. Avoid with procaine sensitivity. May result in overgrowth of nonsusceptible organisms. Monitor culture after therapy completion to determine eradication. Monitor renal and hematopoietic systems periodically with prolonged and high-dose therapy.

ADVERSE REACTIONS: Maculopapular/exfoliative dermatitis, urticaria, laryngeal edema, fever, pseudomembranous colitis, hemolytic anemia, leukopenia, thrombocytopenia, neuropathy, nephropathy.

INTERACTIONS: Increased and prolonged levels with probenecid. Tetracycline may antagonize bacterial effect; avoid concomitant use.

PREGNANCY: Category B, caution in nursing.

BICILLIN C-R 900/300 RX
penicillin G procaine - penicillin G benzathine (King)

THERAPEUTIC CLASS: Penicillin

INDICATIONS: Treatment of moderately severe to severe upper-respiratory tract (URTI) and skin and soft-tissue infections (SSTI), scarlet fever and erysipelas due to streptococci. Treatment of moderately severe pneumonia and otitis media due to pneumococci.

DOSAGE: *Pediatrics:* Group A Strep: URTI/SSTI/Scarlet Fever/Erysipelas: 1.2MU IM single dose. Pneumococcal Infections (Except Meningitis): 1.2MU IM every 2-3 days until temperature is normal for 48 hrs. Administer IM into upper, outer quadrant of buttock. Use midlateral aspect of thigh in neonates, infants, and small children.

HOW SUPPLIED: Inj: (Penicillin G Benzathine-Penicillin G Procaine) 900,000-300,000U/2mL

CONTRAINDICATIONS: Do not inject into or near an artery or nerve.

WARNINGS/PRECAUTIONS: Serious, fatal anaphylactic reactions reported; increased risk with hypersensitivity to penicillin, cephalosporins, and other allergens. Pseudomembranous colitis reported. Avoid IV, intra-arterial administration, or injection into/near major peripheral nerves or blood vessels may cause severe neurovascular and neurological damage. IM administration into anterolateral thigh may cause quadriceps femoris fibrosis and atrophy. Caution with asthma. Avoid with procaine sensitivity. May result in overgrowth of nonsusceptible organisms. Monitor culture after therapy completion to determine eradication. Monitor renal and hematopoietic systems periodically with prolonged and high-dose therapy.

ADVERSE REACTIONS: Maculopapular/exfoliative dermatitis, urticaria, laryngeal edema, fever, pseudomembranous colitis, hemolytic anemia, leukopenia, thrombocytopenia, neuropathy, nephropathy.

INTERACTIONS: Increased and prolonged levels with probenecid. Tetracycline may antagonize bactericidal effect.

PREGNANCY: Category B, caution in nursing.

BICILLIN L-A RX
penicillin G benzathine (King)

THERAPEUTIC CLASS: Penicillin

INDICATIONS: Treatment of mild to moderate upper respiratory tract infections (URTI) due to streptococci and venereal infections (eg, syphilis, yaws, bejel, pinta). Prophylaxis to prevent recurrence of rheumatic fever or chorea.

BILTRICIDE

DOSAGE: *Adults:* Group A Strep: URTI: 1.2MU IM single dose. Primary/Secondary/Latent Syphilis: 2.4MU IM single dose. Late Syphilis (Tertiary/Neurosyphilis): 2.4MU IM every 7 days for 3 doses. Yaws/Bejel/Pinta: 1.2MU IM single dose. Rheumatic Fever/Glomerulonephritis Prophylaxis: 1.2MU IM once a month or 600,000U IM every 2 weeks. Administer IM into upper, outer quadrant of buttock.

Pediatrics: Group A Strep: URTI: Older Pediatrics: 900,000U IM single dose. <60 lbs: 300,000-600,000U IM single dose. Congenital Syphilis: 2-12 yrs: Adjust dose based on adult schedule. <2 yrs: 50,000U/kg IM single dose. Rheumatic Fever/Glomerulonephritis Prophylaxis: 1.2MU IM once a month or 600,000U every 2 weeks. Administer IM into upper, outer quadrant of buttock. Use the midlateral aspect of thigh in neonates, infants, and small children.

HOW SUPPLIED: Inj: 600,000U/mL

CONTRAINDICATIONS: Do not inject into or near an artery or nerve.

WARNINGS/PRECAUTIONS: Serious, fatal anaphylactic reactions reported; increased risk with hypersensitivity to penicillin, cephalosporins, and other allergens. Pseudomembranous colitis reported. Avoid IV, intra-arterial administration, or injection into/near major peripheral nerves or blood vessels may cause severe neurovascular and neurological damage. IM administration into anterolateral thigh may cause quadriceps femoris fibrosis and atrophy. Caution with asthma. May result in overgrowth of nonsusceptible organisms. Monitor culture after therapy completion to determine eradication.

ADVERSE REACTIONS: Maculopapular/exfoliative dermatitis, urticaria, laryngeal edema, fever, pseudomembranous colitis, hemolytic anemia, leukopenia, thrombocytopenia, neuropathy, nephropathy.

INTERACTIONS: Increased and prolonged levels with probenecid. Tetracycline may antagonize bactericidal effect.

PREGNANCY: Category B, caution in nursing.

BILTRICIDE   RX
praziquantel (Schering)

THERAPEUTIC CLASS: Trematodicide

INDICATIONS: Treatment of infections due to all species of schistosoma and due to liver flukes.

DOSAGE: *Adults:* Schistosomiasis: 3x 20mg/kg for 1 day. Clonorchiasis/Opisthorchiasis: 3x 25mg/kg for 1 day. Take with fluids during meals; do not chew. Dosage interval should not be <4 hrs or >6 hrs.

Pediatrics: ≥4 yrs: Schistosomiasis: 3 X 20mg/kg for 1 day. Clonorchiasis/Opisthorchiasis: 3 X 25mg/kg for 1 day. Take with fluids during meals; do not chew. Dosage interval should not be <4 hrs or >6 hrs.

HOW SUPPLIED: Tab: 600mg (6^s)

CONTRAINDICATIONS: Ocular cysticercosis.

WARNINGS/PRECAUTIONS: Avoid driving or operating machinery until one day after treatment. Minimal increases in liver enzymes reported. Hospitalize if schistosomiasis or fluke infection is associated with cerebral cysticercosis.

ADVERSE REACTIONS: Malaise, headache, dizziness, abdominal discomfort, nausea.

PREGNANCY: Category B, not for use in nursing.

BLEPH-10   RX
sulfacetamide sodium (Allergan)

OTHER BRAND NAME: AK-Sulf (Akorn)

THERAPEUTIC CLASS: Sulfonamide

INDICATIONS: (Oint, Sol) Treatment of conjunctivitis and other superficial ocular infections. (Sol) Adjunct to systemic sulfonamide therapy of trachoma.

DOSAGE: *Adults:* Conjunctivitis/Superficial Infections: (Sol) 1-2 drops q2-3h initially. (Oint) Apply 1/2 inch q3-4h and hs. Taper dose by decreasing frequency with improvement. Treat for 7-10 days. Trachoma: (Sol) 2 drops q2h with systemic therapy.

Pediatrics: ≥2 months: Conjunctivitis/Superficial Infections: (Sol) 1-2 drops q2-3h initially. (Oint) Apply 1/2 inch q3-4h and hs. Taper dose by decreasing frequency with improvement. Treat for 7-10 days. Trachoma: (Sol) 2 drops q2h with systemic therapy.

HOW SUPPLIED: Oint: (AK-Sulf) 10% (3.5g); Sol: (Bleph-10) 10% (5mL, 15mL)

WARNINGS/PRECAUTIONS: Fatalities reported from severe reactions to sulfonamides. D/C if develop sign of hypersensitivity. Ointments may retard corneal wound healing.

ADVERSE REACTIONS: Local irritation, stinging, burning.

INTERACTIONS: Incompatible with silver preparations.

PREGNANCY: Category C, not for use in nursing.

BLEPHAMIDE   RX
prednisolone acetate - sulfacetamide sodium (Allergan)

OTHER BRAND NAME: Blephamide S.O.P. (Allergan)

THERAPEUTIC CLASS: Sulfonamide/corticosteroid

INDICATIONS: For steroid-responsive inflammatory ocular conditions associated with bacterial infection or risks of bacterial infection (eg, corneal injury).

DOSAGE: *Adults:* (Sus) 2 drops into conjunctival sac q4h and qhs. (Oint) Apply 1/2 inch into conjunctival sac tid-qid and qd-bid at night. Re-evaluate if no improvement after 2 days. Decrease dose as condition improves. Max: 20mL or 8g prescribed initially.
Pediatrics: ≥6 yrs: (Sus) 2 drops into conjunctival sac q4h and qhs. (Oint) Apply 1/2 inch into conjunctival sac tid-qid and qd-bid at night. Re-evaluate if no improvement after 2 days. Decrease dose as condition improves. Max: 20mL or 8g prescribed initially.

HOW SUPPLIED: (Sulfacetamide-Prednisolone) Oint: 10%-0.2% (3.5g); Sus: 10%-0.2% (5mL, 10mL)

CONTRAINDICATIONS: Most viral diseases of the cornea and conjunctiva (eg, epithelial herpes simplex keratitis, vaccinia, and varicella), mycobacterial infection of the eye, fungal diseases of ocular structures.

WARNINGS/PRECAUTIONS: Not for injection. Ocular HTN, glaucoma, secondary infections may occur with prolonged use. Acute anterior uveitis may occur. May mask or enhance infection with acute purulent conditions. Caution with glaucoma, treatment of herpes simplex. Monitor IOP. Staphylococcal isolates may be resistant to sulfonamides. Not effective in mustard gas keratitis and Sjogren's keratoconjunctivitis. Sensitization may recur with sulfonamides. May delay healing after cataract surgery. Fatalities reported due to adverse effects.

ADVERSE REACTIONS: Local irritation, intraocular pressure elevation, acute anterior uveitis, mydriasis, allergic sensitization (Stevens-Johnson syndrome, toxic epidermal necrolysis, fulminant hepatic necrosis, etc.).

INTERACTIONS: Incompatible with silver preparations. Local anesthetics related to p-amino benzoic acid may antagonize sulfonamides.

PREGNANCY: Category C, not for use in nursing.

BONTRIL SLOW-RELEASE   CIII
phendimetrazine tartrate (Amarin)

OTHER BRAND NAME: Bontril PDM (Amarin)

THERAPEUTIC CLASS: Anorectic sympathomimetic amine

INDICATIONS: Short term adjunct treatment of exogenous obesity.

DOSAGE: *Adults:* (Slow-Release) 105mg qam, 30-60 minutes before breakfast. (PDM) 35mg bid-tid, 1 hr before meals; may reduce to 17.5mg/dose. Max: 70mg tid.
Pediatrics: ≥12 yrs: (Slow-Release) 105mg qam, 30-60 minutes before breakfast. (PDM) 35mg bid-tid, 1 hr before meals; may reduce to 17.5mg/dose. Max: 70mg tabs tid.

HOW SUPPLIED: Cap, Extended Release: (Slow-Release) 105mg; Tab: (PDM) 35mg*
*scored

CONTRAINDICATIONS: Advanced arteriosclerosis, symptomatic cardiovascular disease, moderate and severe HTN, hyperthyroidism, glaucoma, agitated states, history of drug abuse, concomitant CNS stimulants including MAOIs.

BOOSTRIX

WARNINGS/PRECAUTIONS: Tolerance to anorectic effect develops within a few weeks, d/c if this occurs. Fatigue and depression with abrupt withdrawal after prolonged high dose therapy. Caution with mild HTN.

ADVERSE REACTIONS: Palpitation, tachycardia, BP elevation, overstimulation, restlessness, dizziness, dry mouth, diarrhea, constipation, nausea, libido changes, dysuria, insomnia.

INTERACTIONS: Hypertensive crisis if used within 14 days of MAOIs. May decrease hypotensive effects of guanethidine. May alter insulin requirements.

PREGNANCY: Not for use in pregnancy, safety in nursing not known.

BOOSTRIX   RX
tetanus toxoid - diphtheria toxoid - pertussis vaccine, acellular (GlaxoSmithKline)

THERAPEUTIC CLASS: Vaccine/toxoid combination

INDICATIONS: Active booster immunization against tetanus, diphtheria, and pertussis as a single dose in individuals 10-18 yrs of age.

DOSAGE: *Pediatrics:* 10-18 yrs: 0.5mL IM into the deltoid muscle.

HOW SUPPLIED: Inj: (Tetanus-Diphtheria-Pertussis) 5LF-2.5LF-8mcg/0.5mL.

CONTRAINDICATIONS: Hypersensitivity to any component; serious allergic reaction (eg, anaphylaxis) associated with previous dose. Encephalopathy not due to an identifiable cause within 7 days prior to pertussis immunization and progressive neurologic disorder, uncontrolled epilepsy, or progressive encephalopathy.

WARNINGS/PRECAUTIONS: May cause allergic reactions in latex sensitive patients. Caution if within 48 hrs of fever $\geq 105°F$ not due to another identifiable cause; collapse or shock-like state; persistent, inconsolable crying lasting ≥ 3 hrs. Caution if within 3 days of seizure with or without fever. Do not administer in patients with bleeding disorders such as hemophilia or thrombocytopenia, or patients on anticoagulant therapy unless potential benefit outweighs risk. Caution if Guillian Barre syndrome within 6 weeks of tetanus toxoid vaccine. Do not give Td, Tdap, or emergency dose of Td more frequently then every 10 yrs if patient has experienced Arthus-type reaction. Hypersensitivity reaction possible; epinephrine injection (1:1000) should be readily available.

ADVERSE REACTIONS: Local: pain, redness, swelling. Systemic: headache, fatigue, fever, nausea, vomiting, diarrhea, abdominal pain.

INTERACTIONS: Immunosuppressive therapies, including irradiation, antimetabolites, alkylating agents, cytotoxic drugs, and corticosteroids may reduce the immune response to vaccines.

PREGNANCY: Category C, caution in nursing.

BOTOX   RX
botulinum toxin type A (Allergan)

THERAPEUTIC CLASS: Purified neurotoxin complex

INDICATIONS: Treatment of strabismus and blepharospasm associated with dystonia, including benign essential blepharospasm or VII nerve disorders. Treatment of cervical dystonia to decrease severity of abnormal head position and neck pain. Treatment of severe primary axillary hyperhidrosis that is inadequately managed with topical agents

DOSAGE: *Adults:* Cervical Dystonia: Average Dose: 236U divided among affected muscles. Adjust to individual response. Max: 100U total dose in sternocleidomastoid muscles. Strabismus: Initial: Vertical Muscle and Horizontal Strabismus <20 Prism Diopters: 1.25-2.5U in any muscle. Horizontal Strabismus of 20-50 Prism Diopters: 2.5-5U in any one muscle. Persistent VI Nerve Palsy ≥ 1 Month: 1.25-2.5U into medial rectus muscle. Increase dose by 2-fold if previous dose results in incomplete paralysis. Max: 25U/muscle. Reassess 7-14 after each injection. Blepharospasm: Initial: 1.25-2.5U into medial and lateral pre-tarsal orbicularis oculi of the upper lid and into lateral pre-tarsal orbicularis oculi of the lower lid. Max: 200U/30 day. Primary Axillary Hyperhidrosis: 50 units per axilla.

Pediatrics: ≥ 16 yrs: Cervical Dystonia: 236U divided among affected muscles. Adjust dose to individual response. Max: 100U in sternocleidomastoid muscles. ≥ 12 yrs: Strabismus: Initial: Vertical Muscle and Horizontal Strabismus <20 Prism Diopters: 1.25-2.5U in any muscle. Horizontal Strabismus of 20-50 Prism Diopters: 2.5-5U in any one muscle. Persistent VI Nerve Palsy ≥1 Month: 1.25-2.5U into medial rectus muscle. Increase dose by 2-fold if previous dose results in incomplete paralysis. Max: 25U/muscle. Reassess 7-14 after each injection. Blepharospasm: Initial: 1.25-2.5U into medial and lateral pre-tarsal orbicularis oculi of the upper lid and into lateral pre-tarsal orbicularis oculi of the lower lid. Max: 200U/30 day.

HOW SUPPLIED: Inj: 100U

WARNINGS/PRECAUTIONS: Do not exceed dosing recommendations. Caution with peripheral motor neuropathic diseases (eg, amyotrophic lateral sclerosis, motor neuropathy), neuromuscular junctional disorders (eg, myasthenia gravis, Lambert-Eaton syndrome); increased risk of dysphagia and respiratory compromise. Contains albumin. Have epinephrine available if anaphylactic reaction occurs. Caution with inflammation at injection sites, excessive weakness or atrophy in target muscles. Injection of orbicularis muscle may reduce blinking. Caution to resume activities gradually. Retrobulbular hemorrhages compromising retinal circulation reported; have instruments to decompress orbit accessible. Increased risk of dysphagia in patients with smaller neck muscle mass and those with bilateral injections into sternocleidomastoid muscle; limit dose. Caution in elderly.

ADVERSE REACTIONS: (Cervical Dystonia) dysphagia, upper respiratory infection, neck pain, headache, (Blepharospasm) ptosis, keratitis, eye dryness, (Strabismus) ptosis, vertical deviation.

INTERACTIONS: May be potentiated with aminoglycosides, agents interfering with neuromuscular transmission (eg, curare-like compounds). Excessive neuromuscular weakness may be exacerbated if administer another botulinum toxin before effects resolve from the previous botulinum toxin injection.

PREGNANCY: Category C, caution in nursing.

BREVITAL
methohexital sodium (King)

CIV

> Should be used only in hospital or ambulatory care settings that provide for continuous monitoring of respiratory and cardiac function. Immediate availability of resuscitative drugs and age-and size-appropriate equipment for bag/valve/mask ventilation and intubation and personnel trained in their use and skilled in airway management should be assured. For deeply sedated patients, a designated individual other than the practitioner performing the procedure should be present to continuously monitor the patient.

THERAPEUTIC CLASS: Barbituate anesthetic

INDICATIONS: IV induction of anesthesia prior to the use of other general anesthetic agents. IV induction of anesthesia and as an adjunct to subpotent inhalational anesthetic agents (such as nitrous oxide in oxygen) for short surgical procedures. For use along with other parenteral agents, usually narcotic analgesics, to supplement subpotent inhalational anesthetic agents (such as nitrous oxide in oxygen) for longer surgical procedures. IV anesthesia for short surgical, diagnostic, or therapeutic procedures associated with minimal painful stimuli. Agent for inducing a hypnotic state. Pediatrics (older than 1 month): Rectal or intramuscular induction of anesthesia prior to the use of other general anesthetic agents; rectal or intramuscular induction of anesthesia and as an adjunct to subpotent inhalational anesthetic agents for surgical procedures; rectal or intramuscular anesthesia for short surgical, diagnostic, or therapeutic procedures associated with minimal painful stimuli.

DOSAGE: *Adults:* Individualize dose. Induction: 1% solution administered at a rate of 1mL/5 seconds. Range: 50-120mg or more (average: 70mg). Usual dose: 1-1.5mg/kg. Maint: Intermittent: 20-40mg (2 to 4mL of a 1% solution) q 4-7 minutes. Continuous drip: Average rate of administration is 3mL of a 0.2% solution/minute (1 drop/second).

Pediatrics: ≥1 month: Individualize dose: Induction: IM: 6.6 to 10mg/kg IM of the 5% concentration. Rectal: 25mg/kg rectally of the 1% solution.

HOW SUPPLIED: Inj: 500mg, 2.5g

CONTRAINDICATIONS: Patients with latent or manifest porphyria.

WARNINGS/PRECAUTIONS: Seizures may be elicited in patients with previous history of convulsive activity. Caution in severe hepatic dysfunction, severe cardiovascular insta-

BREVOXYL

bility, shock-like condition, asthma, COPD, severe HTN or hypotension, MI, CHF, severe anemia, status asthmaticus, extreme obesity, debilitated patients or those with impaired function of respiratory, circulatory, renal, hepatic, or endocrine system. Unintended intra-arterial injection may produce platelet aggregates and thrombosis at the site of injection.

ADVERSE REACTIONS: Circulatory depression, thrombophlebitis, hypotension, tachycardia, respiratory depression, skeletal muscle hypersensitivity (twitching), emergence delirium.

INTERACTIONS: May influence the metabolism of other concomitantly used drugs, such as phenytoin, halothane, anticoagulants, corticosteroids, ethyl alcohol, and propyleneglycol-containing solutions. Prior chronic administration of barbituates or phenytoin may reduce the effectiveness of methohexital. Additive CNS effects with other CNS depressants, including ethyl alcohol and propylene alcohol.

PREGNANCY: Category B, caution in nursing.

BREVOXYL   RX
benzoyl peroxide (Stiefel)

THERAPEUTIC CLASS: Antibacterial/keratolytic

INDICATIONS: Topical treatment of mild to moderate acne vulgaris.

DOSAGE: *Adults:* (Gel) Apply qd-bid to clean affected area. (Lotion) Shake well. Wet affected area and wash qd for 1st week, then bid thereafter if tolerated.
Pediatrics: ≥12 yrs: (Gel) Apply qd-bid to clean affected area. (Lotion) Shake well. Wet affected area and wash qd for 1st week, then bid thereafter if tolerated.

HOW SUPPLIED: Gel: 4%, 8% (42.5g, 90g); Lot: (Cleanser) 4%, 8% (297g); Lot: (Creamy Wash) 4%, 8% (170g)

WARNINGS/PRECAUTIONS: Avoid contact with hair, eyes, mucous membranes, carpeting, and fabrics.

ADVERSE REACTIONS: Erythema, peeling.

PREGNANCY: Category C, caution in nursing.

BROMFED   RX
pseudoephedrine HCl - brompheniramine maleate (Muro)

OTHER BRAND NAMES: Bromfed-PD (Muro) - Bromfenex (Ethex) - Bromfenex-PD (Ethex)

THERAPEUTIC CLASS: Antihistamine/decongestant

INDICATIONS: Treatment of symptoms of seasonal and perennial allergic rhinitis, and vasomotor rhinitis, including nasal congestion.

DOSAGE: *Adults:* (12mg-120mg) 1 cap q12h. (6mg-60mg) 1-2 caps q12h.
Pediatrics: ≥12 yrs: (12mg-120mg) 1 cap q12h. (6mg-60mg) 1-2 caps q12h. 6-11 yrs: (6mg-60mg) 1 cap q12h.

HOW SUPPLIED: (Brompheniramine-Pseudoephedrine) Cap, Extended Release: (PD) 6mg- 60mg, (Bromfed, Bromfenex) 12mg-120mg

CONTRAINDICATIONS: Severe HTN, CAD, narrow-angle glaucoma, MAOI therapy, urinary retention, peptic ulcer, during an asthmatic attack.

WARNINGS/PRECAUTIONS: Caution with HTN, DM, ischemic heart disease, hyperthyroidism, increased IOP, prostatic hypertrophy, and elderly. Caution while operating machinery.

ADVERSE REACTIONS: Drowsiness, lassitude, nausea, giddiness, dryness of the mouth, blurred vision, palpitations, flushing, increased irritability or excitement.

INTERACTIONS: Potentiated by MAOIs and β-blockers. Reduced antihypertensive effects of methyldopa, mecamylamine, reserpine, and veratrum alkaloids. Additive effects with alcohol and other CNS depressants.

PREGNANCY: Safety in pregnancy and nursing not known.

BUPRENEX   CV
buprenorphine HCl (Reckitt Benckiser)

THERAPEUTIC CLASS: Opioid analgesic

INDICATIONS: Relief of moderate to severe pain.

DOSAGE: *Adults:* 0.3mg IM/IV q6h prn. Repeat if needed, 30-60 minutes after initial dose and then prn. High Risk Patients/Concomitant CNS depressants: Reduce dose by approximately 50%. May use single doses ≤0.6mg IM if not at high-risk.

Pediatrics: ≥13 yrs: 0.3mg IM/IV q6h prn. Repeat if needed, 30-60 minutes after initial dose and then prn. High Risk Patients/Concomitant CNS depressants: Reduce dose by approximately 50%. May use single doses ≤0.6mg IM if not at high-risk. 2-12 yrs: 2-6mcg/kg IM/IV q4-6h.

HOW SUPPLIED: Inj: 0.3mg/mL

WARNINGS/PRECAUTIONS: Significant respiratory depression reported; caution with compromised respiratory function. May increase CSF pressure; caution with head injury, intracranial lesions. Caution with debilitated, BPH, biliary tract dysfunction, myxedema, hypothyroidism, urethral stricture, acute alcoholism, Addison's disease, CNS disease, coma, toxic psychoses, delirium tremens, elderly, pediatrics, kyphoscoliosis or hepatic/renal/pulmonary impairment. May impair mental or physical abilities. May precipitate withdrawal in narcotic-dependence. May lead to psychological dependence.

ADVERSE REACTIONS: Nausea, dizziness, sweating, hypotension, vomiting, headache, miosis, hypoventilation.

INTERACTIONS: Caution with MAOIs, CNS and respiratory depressants. Respiratory and cardiovascular collapse reported with diazepam. Increased CNS depression with other narcotic analgesics, general anesthetics, antihistamines, benzodiazepines, phenothiazines, other tranquilizers, sedative-hypnotics. Decreased clearance with CYP3A4 inhibitors (eg, macrolides, azole antifungals, protease inhibitors). Increased clearance with CYP3A4 inducers (eg, rifampin, carbamazepine, phenytoin).

PREGNANCY: Category C, not for use in nursing.

CADUET
amlodipine besylate - atorvastatin calcium (Pfizer)
RX

THERAPEUTIC CLASS: Calcium channel blocker/HMG-CoA reductase inhibitor

INDICATIONS: When treatment with both amlodipine and atorvastatin is appropriate. (Amlodipine) Treatment of hypertension, chronic stable or vasospastic angina (Prinzmetal's or Variant Angina). (Atorvastatin) Adjunct to diet to reduce total cholesterol (total-C), LDL-C, TG, and Apo B levels, and to increase HDL-C in primary hypercholesterolemia (heterozygous familial and nonfamilial) and mixed dyslipidemia (Types IIa and IIb). Adjunct to diet for elevated serum TG levels (Type IV). Treatment of primary dysbetalipoproteinemia (Type III) inadequately responding to diet. Adjunct to other lipid-lowering treatments or if treatments are unavailable, to reduce total-C and LDL-C in homozygous familial hypercholesterolemia. Adjunct to diet to lower total-C, LDL-C and Apo B in boys and postmenarchal girls with heterozygous familial hypercholesterolemia.

DOSAGE: *Adults:* Dosing should be individualized and based on the appropriate combination of recommendations for the monotherapies. (Amlodipine): HTN: Initial: 5mg qd. Titrate over 7-14 days. Max: 10mg qd. Small, Fragile, or Elderly/Hepatic Dysfunction/Concomitant Antihypertensive: Initial: 2.5mg qd. Angina: 5-10mg qd. Elderly/Hepatic Dysfunction: 5mg qd. (Atorvastatin): Hypercholesterolemia/Mixed Dyslipidemia: Initial: 10-20mg qd (or 40mg qd for LDL-C reduction >45%). Titrate: Adjust dose if needed at 2-4 week intervals. Usual: 10-80mg qd. Homozygous Familial Hypercholesterolemia: 10-80mg qd.

Pediatrics: ≥10 yrs (postmenarchal): (Amlodipine): HTN: 2.5-5mg qd. 10-17 yrs (postmenarchal): (Atorvastatin): Heterozygous Familial Hypercholesterolemia: Initial: 10mg/day. Titrate: Adjust dose if needed at intervals of ≥4 weeks. Max: 20mg/day.

HOW SUPPLIED: Tab: (Amlodipine-Atorvastatin) 2.5mg-10mg, 2.5mg-20mg, 2.5mg-40mg, 5mg-10mg, 5mg-20mg, 5mg-40mg, 5mg-80mg, 10mg-10mg, 10mg-20mg, 10mg-40mg, 10mg-80mg

CONTRAINDICATIONS: Active liver disease, unexplained persistent elevations of serum transaminases, pregnancy, nursing mothers.

WARNINGS/PRECAUTIONS: May, rarely, increase angina or MI with severe obstructive CAD. Monitor LFTs prior to therapy, at 12 weeks after initiation, with dose elevation, and periodically thereafter. Reduce dose or withdraw if AST or ALT >3x ULN persist. Caution

CAFCIT

with heavy alcohol use and/or history of hepatic disease, severe aortic stenosis, CHF. D/C if markedly elevated CPK levels occur, if myopathy is diagnosed or suspected, or if predisposition to renal failure secondary to rhabdomyolysis.

ADVERSE REACTIONS: Headache, edema, palpitation, dizziness, fatigue, constipation, flatulence, dyspepsia, abdominal pain.

INTERACTIONS: Increases levels with erythromycin. Increases levels of oral contraceptives (norethindrone, ethinyl estradiol), digoxin. Cyclosporine, fibric acid derivatives, niacin, erythromycin, azole antifungals may increase risk of myopathy. Caution with drugs that decrease levels or activity of endogenous steroid hormones (eg, ketoconazole, spironolactone, cimetidine). Decreased levels with Maalox® TC, but LDL-C reduction not altered. Colestipol decreases levels when coadministered, but greater LDL-C reduction with coadministration than when each given alone. Avoid fibrates.

PREGNANCY: Category X, not for use in nursing

CAFCIT RX
caffeine citrate (Mead Johnson)

THERAPEUTIC CLASS: Methylxanthine

INDICATIONS: Short-term treatment of apnea of prematurity in infants.

DOSAGE: *Pediatrics:* 28-<33 weeks: LD: 1mL/kg IV. Maint: 0.25mL/kg IV/PO q24h beginning 24 hrs after LD.

HOW SUPPLIED: Inj: 20mg/mL (3mL); Sol: 20mg/mL (3mL)

WARNINGS/PRECAUTIONS: Necrotizing enterocolitis, seizures reported. Rule out other possible causes of apnea before initiating therapy. Caution with cardiovascular disease, seizure disorder, renal/hepatic impairment. Monitor baseline caffeine levels if previously exposed to theophylline.

ADVERSE REACTIONS: Feeding intolerance, sepsis, hemorrhage, gastritis, GI hemorrhage, DIC, abnormal healing, dyspnea, cerebral hemorrhage, lung edema, dry skin, retinopathy of prematurity.

INTERACTIONS: Potential for interaction with CYP450 1A2 substrates, inducers, inhibitors. May need lower dose with cimetidine, ketoconazole. May need dose increase with phenobarbital, phenytoin.

PREGNANCY: Category C, safety in nursing not known.

CARBATROL RX
carbamazepine (Shire US)

> Aplastic anemia and agranulocytosis reported. Obtain complete pretreatment hematological testing as a baseline. Discontinue if develop evidence of bone marrow depression.

THERAPEUTIC CLASS: Carboxamide anticonvulsant

INDICATIONS: Treatment of partial seizures with complex symptomatology, generalized tonic-clonic seizures, and mixed seizure patterns of these or other partial or generalized seizures. Treatment of trigeminal neuralgia pain.

DOSAGE: *Adults:* Epilepsy: Initial: 200mg bid. Titrate: May increase weekly by 200mg/day. Maint: 800-1200mg/day. Max: 1200mg/day. Trigeminal Neuralgia: Initial (Day 1): 200mg qd. Titrate: May increase by 200mg/day q12h. Maint: 400-800mg/day. Max: 1200mg/day. Re-evaluate every 3 months.

Pediatrics: Epilepsy: >12 yrs: Initial: 200mg bid. Titrate: May increase weekly by 200mg/day. Max: 12-15 yrs: 1000mg/day. >15 yrs: 1200mg/day. 6 months-12 yrs: May convert immediate-release dose ≥400mg/day to equal daily dose using bid regimen. Usual/Max: ≤35mg/kg/day.

HOW SUPPLIED: Cap, Extended Release: 200mg, 300mg

CONTRAINDICATIONS: History of bone marrow depression, MAOI use within 14 days, sensitivity to TCAs.

WARNINGS/PRECAUTIONS: Lyell's syndrome and Stevens-Johnson syndrome, multi-organ hypersensitivity reactions reported. Caution with history of adverse hematologic reaction to any drug, increased IOP, the elderly, mixed seizure with atypical absence seizure. Fetal harm with pregnancy. May activate latent psychosis. Caution with cardiac, hepatic, or renal damage. Perform eye exam and monitor LFTs and renal function at baseline and periodically.

ADVERSE REACTIONS: Dizziness, drowsiness, unsteadiness, nausea, vomiting, bone marrow depression, rash, urticaria, hypersensitivity reactions, photosensitivity reactions, CHF, edema, HTN, hypotension.

INTERACTIONS: See Contraindications. Metabolism is inhibited by CYP3A4 inhibitors (eg, cimetidine, macrolides, etc.) and induced by CYP3A4 inducers (eg, rifampin, phenytoin, trazodone, etc.). Decreases oral contraceptive effectiveness. Increases plasma levels of clomipramine, phenytoin, and primidone. Decreases levels of APAP, alprazolam, clonazepam, clozapine, dicumarol, doxycycline, ethosuximide, haloperidol, methsuximide, phensuximide, phenytoin, theophylline, valproate, warfarin. Increased risk of neurotoxic side effects with lithium.

PREGNANCY: Category D, not for use in nursing.

Cathflo Activase
alteplase (Genentech)
RX

THERAPEUTIC CLASS: Thrombolytic agent

INDICATIONS: To restore function to central venous access devices as assessed by ability to withdraw blood.

DOSAGE: *Adults:* ≥30kg: 2mg in 2mL. <30kg: 110% of catheter internal lumen volume, not to exceed 2mg in 2mL. If function not restored after 120 minutes, may instill 2nd dose. Max: 2mg/dose. Reconstitute to final concentration of 1mg/mL.

Pediatrics: ≥2 yrs: ≥30kg: 2mg in 2mL. 10 to <30kg: 110% of catheter internal lumen volume, not to exceed 2mg in 2mL. If function not restored after 120 minutes, may instill 2nd dose. Max: 2mg/dose. Reconstitute to final concentration of 1mg/mL.

HOW SUPPLIED: Inj: 2mg

WARNINGS/PRECAUTIONS: Before therapy, consider catheter dysfunction due to causes other than thrombus formation. Avoid excessive pressure when instilling alteplase into catheter. Discontinue and withdraw drug from catheter if serious bleeding in critical location occurs. Caution if active internal bleeding, infection in the catheter, any bleeding condition that is difficult to manage, thrombocytopenia, hemostatic defects, or if high risk for emobolic complications. Caution if any of the following occurred within 48 hrs: sugery, OB delivery, percutaneous biopsy of viscera or deep tissues, or puncture of non-compressible vessels.

ADVERSE REACTIONS: Sepsis, GI bleeding, venous thrombosis.

PREGNANCY: Category C, caution in nursing.

Cedax
ceftibuten (Shionogi)
RX

THERAPEUTIC CLASS: Cephalosporin (3rd generation)

INDICATIONS: Acute bacterial exacerbations of chronic bronchitis (ABECB), acute bacterial otitis media, pharyngitis and tonsillitis.

DOSAGE: *Adults:* ABECB/Otitis Media/Pharyngitis/Tonsillitis: 400mg qd for 10 days. Max: 400mg/day. CrCl 30-49mL/min: 4.5mg/kg or 200mg qd. CrCl 5-29mL/min: 2.25mg/kg or 100mg qd. Take 2 hrs before or at least 1 hr after a meal.

Pediatrics: ≥6 months: Pharyngitis/Tonsillitis/Otitis Media: 9mg/kg qd for 10 days. Max: 400mg. ABECB/Otitis Media/Pharyngitis/Tonsillitis: ≥12 yrs: 400mg qd for 10 days. Max: 400mg/day. CrCl 30-49mL/min: 4.5mg/kg or 200mg qd. CrCl 5-29mL/min: 2.25mg/kg or 100mg qd. Take 2 hrs before or at least 1 hr after a meal.

HOW SUPPLIED: Cap: 400mg; Sus: 90mg/5mL (30mL, 60mL, 90mL, 120mL)

WARNINGS/PRECAUTIONS: Pseudomembranous colitis reported. Caution with history of GI disease. Cross-sensitivity with cephalosporins and penicillins.

ADVERSE REACTIONS: Diarrhea, vomiting, abdominal pain, anorexia, dizziness, dyspepsia, dry mouth, dyspnea, dysuria, fatigue, flatulence, loose stooles, headache, pruritus, rash, rigors, urticaria, superinfection (prolonged use).

PREGNANCY: Category B, caution in nursing.

CeeNU
lomustine (Bristol-Myers Squibb) — RX

> Bone marrow suppression (eg, thrombocytopenia, leukopenia) may contribute to bleeding and infections in compromised patients. Monitor blood counts weekly for 6 weeks after each dose. Adjust dose based on nadir blood counts from prior dose.

THERAPEUTIC CLASS: Nitrosourea alkylating agent

INDICATIONS: Single or adjunct treatment in primary/metastatic brain tumors in patients who already received surgical and/or radiation therapy. Secondary combination therapy of Hodgkin's disease in patients who relapse/fail primary therapy.

DOSAGE: *Adults:* Single Regimen/Previously Untreated: 130mg/m^2 PO single dose every 6 weeks. Compromised Bone Marrow: 100mg/m^2 PO single dose every 6 weeks. Subsequent Doses: Adjust according to hematologic response. Leukocytes 2000-2999, platelets 25,000-74,999: Give 70% of dose. Leukocytes <2000, platelets <25,000: Give 50% of dose.
Pediatrics: Single Regimen/Previously Untreated: 130mg/m^2 PO single dose every 6 weeks. Compromised Bone Marrow: 100mg/m^2 PO single dose every 6 weeks. Subsequent Doses: Adjust according to hematologic response. Leukocytes 2000-2999, platelets 25,000-74,999: Give 70% of dose. Leukocytes <2000, platelets <25,000: Give 50% of dose.

HOW SUPPLIED: Cap: 10mg, 40mg, 100mg

WARNINGS/PRECAUTIONS: Pulmonary toxicity is dose-related. May develop secondary malignancies with long-term use. Monitor hepatic and renal function. Caution in elderly.

ADVERSE REACTIONS: Delayed myleosuppression, pulmonary infiltrates/fibrosis, nausea, vomiting, hepatotoxicity, azotemia, renal failure, stomatitis, alopecia, optic atrophy, visual disturbances, lethargy, ataxia.

PREGNANCY: Category D, not for use in nursing.

Cefaclor
cefaclor (Various) — RX

THERAPEUTIC CLASS: Cephalosporin (2nd generation)

INDICATIONS: Treatment of otitis media, pharyngitis, tonsillitis, lower respiratory tract, urinary tract, and skin and skin structure infections caused by susceptible strains of microorganisms.

DOSAGE: *Adults:* Usual: 250mg q8h. Severe Infections/Pneumonia: 500mg q8h. Treat β-hemolytic strep for 10 days.
Pediatrics: ≥1 month: Usual: 20mg/kg/day given q8h. Otitis Media/Serious Infections: 40mg/kg/day. Max: 1g/day. May administer q12h for otitis media and pharyngitis. Treat β-hemolytic strep for 10 days.

HOW SUPPLIED: Cap: 250mg, 500mg; Sus: 125mg/5mL (75mL, 150mL), 187mg/5mL (50mL, 100mL), 250mg/5mL (75mL, 150mL), 375mg/5mL (50mL, 100mL)

WARNINGS/PRECAUTIONS: Cross sensitivity to penicillins and other cephalosporins may occur. Pseudomembranous colitis reported. Positive direct Coombs' tests reported. Caution with markedly impaired renal function, history of GI disease. False (+) for urine glucose with Benedict's, Fehling's solution, and Clinitest tablets.

ADVERSE REACTIONS: Hypersensitivity reactions, diarrhea, eosinophilia, genital pruritus and vaginitis, serum-sickness-like reactions, superinfection.

INTERACTIONS: Renal excretion inhibited by probenecid. May potentiate warfarin and other anticoagulants; monitor PT/INR.

PREGNANCY: Category B, caution in nursing.

Cefaclor ER
cefaclor (Various) — RX

THERAPEUTIC CLASS: Cephalosporin (2nd generation)

INDICATIONS: Acute bacterial exacerbation of chronic bronchitis (ABECB), secondary bacterial infections of acute bronchitis, pharyngitis, tonsillitis, and uncomplicated skin and skin structure infections (SSSI) caused by susceptible strains of microorganisms.

DOSAGE: *Adults:* ABECB/Acute Bronchitis: 500mg q12h for 7 days. Pharyngitis/Tonsillitis: 375mg q12h for 10 days. SSSI: 375mg q12h for 7-10 days. Take with meals. Do not crush, cut or chew tab.
Pediatrics: ≥16 yrs: ABECB/Acute Bronchitis: 500mg q12h for 7 days. Pharyngitis/Tonsillitis: 375mg q12h for 10 days. SSSI: 375mg q12h for 7-10 days. Take with meals. Do not crush, cut or chew tab.

HOW SUPPLIED: Tab, Extended Release: 375mg, 500mg

WARNINGS/PRECAUTIONS: Cross sensitivity to penicillins and other cephalosporins may occur. Pseudomembranous colitis reported. False (+) direct Coombs' tests reported. Caution with markedly impaired renal function, history of GI disease. False (+) for urine glucose with Benedict's, Fehling's solution, and Clinitest® tablets.

ADVERSE REACTIONS: Headache, rhinitis, diarrhea, nausea, vomiting, vaginitis, abdominal pain, pharyngitis, increased cough, pruritus, back pain, serum-sickness-like reactions, superinfection (prolonged use).

INTERACTIONS: Decreased absorption with antacids containing aluminum or magnesium hydroxide; space dose by 1 hr. Potentiated by probenecid. May potentiate warfarin, and other anticoagulants; monitor PT/INR.

PREGNANCY: Category B, caution in nursing.

CEFIZOX   RX
ceftizoxime (Astellas)

THERAPEUTIC CLASS: Cephalosporin (3rd generation)

INDICATIONS: Treatment of lower respiratory tract, skin and skin structure, intra-abdominal, bone and joint, and urinary tract infections (UTI), gonorrhea, pelvic inflammatory disease (PID), meningitis, and septicemia.

DOSAGE: *Adults:* Uncomplicated UTI: 500mg q12h IM/IV. Other Sites: 1g q8-12h IM/IV. Severe/Refractory Infections: 1-2g IM/IV q8-12h. PID: 2g IV q8h. Life Threatening Infections: 3-4g IV q8h. Uncomplicated Gonorrhea: 1g IM as single dose. Renal Impairment: LD: 500mg-1g IM/IV. Less Severe Infection: Maint: CrCl 50-79mL/min: 500mg q8h. CrCl 5-49mL/min: 250-500mg q12h. CrCl 0-4mL/min (Dialysis): 500mg q48h or 250mg q24h. Life Threatening Infection: Maint: CrCl 50-79mL/min: 0.75-1.5g q8h. CrCl 5-49mL/min: 0.5-1g q12h. CrCl 0-4mL/min (Dialysis): 0.5-1g q48h or 0.5g q24h.
Pediatrics: ≥6 months: 50mg/kg IM/IV q6-8h, up to 200mg/kg/day. Max: 6g/day for serious infections.

HOW SUPPLIED: Inj: 1g, 2g, 10g

WARNINGS/PRECAUTIONS: Pseudomembranous colitis reported. Caution with history of GI disease. Cross-sensitivity with cephalosporins and penicillins. Prolonged use may result in overgrowth of superinfection, positive Coombs test.

ADVERSE REACTIONS: Rash, pruritus, fever, BUN elevation, injection site reactions (eg, burning, cellulitis, phlebitis, pain, induration, tenderness), eosinophilia, thrombocytosis, elevated liver enzymes, GI effects.

INTERACTIONS: Risk of nephrotoxicity with aminoglycosides.

PREGNANCY: Category B, caution in nursing.

CEFOXITIN   RX
cefoxitin sodium (Various)

OTHER BRAND NAME: Mefoxin (Merck)

THERAPEUTIC CLASS: Cephalosporin (2nd generation)

INDICATIONS: Treatment of lower respiratory tract, urinary tract, intra-abdominal, gynecological, skin and skin structure, and bone and joint infections, and septicemia. For surgical prophylaxis.

DOSAGE: *Adults:* Usual: 1-2g IV q6-8h. Uncomplicated Infections: 1g IV q6-8h. Moderate-Severe: 1g IV q4h or 2g IV q6-8h. Gas Gangrene/Other Infections Requiring Higher Dose: 2g IV q4h or 3g IV q6h. Renal Insufficiency: LD: 1-2g IV. Maint: CrCl 30-50mL/min: 1-2g IV q8-12h. CrCl 10-29mL/min: 1-2g IV q12-24h. CrCl 5-9mL/min: 0.5-1g IV q12-24h. CrCl <5mL/min: 0.5-1g IV q24-48h. Hemodialysis: LD: 1-2g IV after dialysis.

CEFTIN

Maint: See renal insufficiency doses above. Prophylaxis: Uncontaminated GI Surgery/Hysterectomy: 2g IV 0.5-1 hr prior to surgery, then 2g IV q6h after first dose up to 24 hrs. C-Section: 2g IV single dose after umbilical cord is clamped, or 2g IV after umbilical cord is clamped followed by 2g IV 4 and 8 hrs after initial dose.

Pediatrics: ≥3 months: 80-160mg/kg/day divided into 4-6 equal doses. Max: 12g/day. Prophylaxis: Uncontaminated GI Surgery/Hysterectomy: 30-40mg/kg IV 0.5-1 hr prior to surgery, then 30-40mg/kg IV q6h after first dose up to 24 hrs.

HOW SUPPLIED: Inj: 1g, 1g/50mL, 2g, 2g/50mL, 10g

WARNINGS/PRECAUTIONS: Possible cross-sensitivity between penicillins and cephalosporins. Pseudomembranous colitis reported. Caution with allergies, GI disease, particularly colitis. Prolonged use may result in overgrowth of nonsusceptible organisms. Monitor renal, hepatic, hematopoietic functions, especially with prolonged therapy. False positive for urine glucose with Clinitest tablets.

ADVERSE REACTIONS: Thrombophlebitis, rash, pseudomembranous colitis, pruritus, fever, dyspnesa hypotension, diarrhea, blood dyscrasias, elevated LFTs, changes in renal function tests, exacerbation of myasthenia gravis.

INTERACTIONS: Increased nephrotoxicity with concomitant aminoglycosides.

PREGNANCY: Category B, caution use in nursing.

CEFTIN
cefuroxime axetil (GlaxoSmithKline)

RX

THERAPEUTIC CLASS: Cephalosporin (2nd generation)

INDICATIONS: (Sus/Tab) Pharyngitis/tonsillitis, acute otitis media, and impetigo. (Tab) Uncomplicated skin and skin structure (SSSI), and urinary tract infection (UTI), gonorrhea, early lyme disease, acute bacterial maxillary sinusitis, acute bacterial exacerbations of chronic bronchitis (ABECB) and secondary bacterial infections of acute bronchitis.

DOSAGE: *Adults:* (Tab) Pharyngitis/Tonsillitis/Sinusitis: 250mg bid for 10 days. ABECB/SSSI: 250-500mg bid for 10 days. Acute Bronchitis: 250-500mg bid for 5-10 days. UTI: 125-250mg bid for 7-10 days. Gonorrhea: 1000mg single dose. Lyme Disease: 500mg bid for 20 days.

Pediatrics: ≥13 yrs: (Tab) Pharyngitis/Tonsillitis/Sinusitis: 250mg bid for 10 days. ABECB/SSSI: 250-500mg bid for 10 days. Acute Bronchitis: 250-500mg bid for 5-10 days. UTI: 125-250mg bid for 7-10 days. Gonorrhea: 1000mg single dose. Lyme Disease: 500mg bid for 20 days. 3 months-12 yrs: (Sus) Pharyngitis/Tonsillitis: 10mg/kg bid for 10 days. Max: 500mg/day. Otitis Media/Sinusitis/Impetigo: 15mg/kg bid for 10 days. Max: 1000mg/day. (Tab-if can swallow whole) Pharyngitis/Tonsillitis: 125mg bid for 10 days. Otitis Media/Sinusitis: 250mg bid for 10 days.

HOW SUPPLIED: Sus: 125mg/5mL (100mL), 250mg/5mL (50mL, 100mL); Tab: 125mg, 250mg, 500mg

WARNINGS/PRECAUTIONS: Tablets are not bioequivalent to suspension. Caution with colitis, renal impairment. Cross-sensitivity with cephalosporins and penicillins. Pseudomembranous colitis reported. False (+) for urine glucose with Benedict's, Fehling's solution, and Clinitest® tablets. May cause fall in PT; risk in patients stable on anticoagulants, if receiving protracted course of antibiotics, renal/hepatic impairment, or a poor nutritional state; give vitamin K as needed.

ADVERSE REACTIONS: Diarrhea, nausea, vomiting, vaginitis, (suspension in peds) taste dislike, superinfection (prolonged use).

INTERACTIONS: Probenecid increases plasma levels. Lower bioavailability with drugs that lower gastric acidity. Caution with agents causing adverse effects on renal function (diuretics).

PREGNANCY: Category B, not for use in nursing.

CEFZIL
cefprozil (Bristol-Myers Squibb)

RX

THERAPEUTIC CLASS: Cephalosporin (2nd generation)

INDICATIONS: Mild to moderate pharyngitis/tonsillitis, otitis media, acute sinusitis, secondary bacterial infection of acute bronchitis, acute bacterial exacerbation of chronic bronchitis (ABECB), and uncomplicated skin and skin structure infections (SSSI).

DOSAGE: *Adults:* ≥13 yrs: Pharyngitis/Tonsillitis: 500mg q24h for 10 days. Acute Sinusitis: 250-500mg q12h for 10 days. ABECB/Acute Bronchitis: 500mg q12h for 10 days. SSSI: 250-500mg q12h or 500mg q24h. CrCl <30mL/min: 50% of standard dose.

Pediatrics: 2-12 yrs: Pharyngitis/Tonsillitis: 7.5mg/kg q12h for 10 days. SSSI: 20mg/kg q24h for 10 days. 6 months-12 yrs: Otitis Media: 15mg/kg q12h for 10 days. Acute Sinusitis: 7.5-15mg/kg q12h for 10 days. Do not exceed adult dose. CrCl <30mL/min: 50% of standard dose.

HOW SUPPLIED: Sus: 125mg/5mL, 250mg/5mL (50mL, 75mL, 100mL); Tab: 250mg, 500mg

WARNINGS/PRECAUTIONS: Cross-sensitivity with cephalosporins and penicillins. False (+) direct Coombs' tests reported. Pseudomembranous colitis reported. Caution with GI disease, renal impairment, elderly. False (+) for urine glucose with Benedict's, Fehling's solution, and Clinitest® tablets. Suspension contains phenylalanine.

ADVERSE REACTIONS: Diarrhea, nausea, hepatic enzyme elevations, eosinophilia, genital pruritus, genital vaginitis, superinfection (prolonged use).

INTERACTIONS: Nephrotoxicity with aminoglycosides reported. Probenecid may increase plasma levels. Caution with agents causing adverse effects on renal function (diuretics).

PREGNANCY: Category B, caution in nursing.

Celebrex
celecoxib (Searle)

RX

> NSAIDs may cause an increased risk of serious cardiovascular thrombotic events, MI, stroke and serious GI adverse events including bleeding, ulceration, and perforation of the stomach or intestines. Contraindicated for the treatment of peri-operative pain in the setting of coronary artery bypass graft (CABG) surgery.

THERAPEUTIC CLASS: COX-2 inhibitor

INDICATIONS: Relief of signs and symtoms of rheumatoid arthritis (RA) in adults, osteoarthritis (OA), and ankylosing spondylitis (AS). Management of acute pain in adults. Treatment of primary dysmenorrhea. To reduce the number of adematous colorectal polyps in familial adenomatous polyposis (FAP). Relief of signs and symptoms of juvenile rheumatoid arthitis (JRA) in patients ≥2 yrs.

DOSAGE: *Adults:* ≥18 yrs: OA: 200mg qd or 100mg bid. RA: 100-200mg bid. AS: 200mg qd or 100mg bid. Titrate: May increase to 400mg/day after 6 weeks. FAP: 400mg bid with food. Acute Pain/Primary Dysmenorrhea: Day 1: 400mg, then 200mg if needed. Maint: 200mg bid prn. Moderate Hepatic Insufficiency: Reduce daily dose by 50%.

Pediatrics: JRA: ≥2 yrs: 10-25 kg: 50mg bid. >25 kg: 100mg bid.

HOW SUPPLIED: Cap: 50mg, 100mg, 200mg, 400mg

CONTRAINDICATIONS: Sulfonamide hypersensitivity. Asthma, urticaria, or allergic type reactions after ASA or NSAID use. Treatment of peri-operative pain in the setting of CABG surgery.

WARNINGS/PRECAUTIONS: May lead to onset of new HTN or worsening of pre-existing HTN; monitor BP closely. Fluid retention and edema reported; caution with fluid retention or heart failure. Renal papillary necrosis and other renal injury reported after long-term use. Not recommended for use with advanced renal disease; if therapy must be initiated, monitor renal function. Anaphylactoid reactions may occur. May cause serious skin adverse events (eg, exfoliative dermatitis, Stevens-Johnson syndrome, and toxic epidermal necrolysis). Avoid in late pregnancy; may cause premature closure of ductus arteriosis. May cause elevations of LFTs; d/c if liver disease develops or systemic manifestations occur. Caution in elderly. Anemia may occur; with long-term use, monitor Hgb/Hct if signs or symptoms of anemia or blood loss develop. May inhibit platelet aggregation and prolong bleeding time (prolonged APTT); monitor with coagulation disorders. Caution with asthma and avoid with aspirin-sensitive asthma. Caution in pediatric patients with systemic onset JRA due to increased possibly of DIC.

ADVERSE REACTIONS: Dyspepsia, diarrhea, abdominal pain, nausea, dizziness, headache, sinusitis, upper respiratory infection, rash, fever, cough, arthralgia.

INTERACTIONS: Monitor oral anticoagulants; reports of serious bleeding, some fatal, with warfarin. Decrease effects of ACEIs, furosemide, and thiazides. Increased levels with

CELESTONE

fluconazole. Monitor lithium. Caution with CYP2C9 inhibitors and drugs metabolized by CYP2D6. Celecoxib is not a substitute for ASA for cardiovascular prophylaxis; may use with low-dose ASA but may increase GI complications.

PREGNANCY: Category C, not for use in nursing.

CELESTONE RX
betamethasone (Schering)

THERAPEUTIC CLASS: Glucocorticoid

INDICATIONS: Steroid responsive disorders.

DOSAGE: *Adults:* Initial: 0.6-7.2mg/day depending on disease. Maintain until sufficient response. Maint: Decrease dose by small amounts to lowest effective dose. Discontinue gradually.
Pediatrics: Initial: 0.6-7.2mg/day depending on disease. Maintain until sufficient response. Maint: Decrease dose by small amounts to lowest effective dose. Discontinue gradually.

HOW SUPPLIED: Syrup: 0.6mg/5mL (118mL)

CONTRAINDICATIONS: Systemic fungal infections.

WARNINGS/PRECAUTIONS: May need to increase dose before, during, and after stressful situations. May mask signs of infection or cause new infections. Prolonged use may produce posterior subcapsular cataracts, glaucoma, optic nerve damage, secondary ocular infections. Increases BP, salt/water retention, potassium and calcium excretion. More severe/fatal course of infections reported with chickenpox, measles. Caution with threadworm infestation, latent TB, hypothyroidism, cirrhosis, ocular herpes simplex, HTN, diverticulitis, fresh intestinal anastomosis, ulcerative colitis, osteoporosis, myasthenia gravis, renal insufficiency, peptic ulcer disease. Growth and development of children on prolonged therapy should be monitored. Monitor for psychic disturbances. Avoid abrupt withdrawal.

ADVERSE REACTIONS: Sodium retention, fluid retention, potassium loss, muscle weakness, myopathy, peptic ulcer, impaired wound healing, thin fragile skin, convulsions, menstrual irregularities, cataracts.

INTERACTIONS: Caution with ASA in hypoprothrombinemia. Increased susceptibility to infections with immunosuppressives. Avoid smallpox vaccines and other immunization procedures at high doses. Increased requirements of insulin or oral hypoglycemic agents.

PREGNANCY: Safety in pregnancy and nursing not known.

CELESTONE SOLUSPAN RX
betamethasone acetate - betamethasone sodium phosphate (Schering)

THERAPEUTIC CLASS: Glucocorticoid

INDICATIONS: When oral therapy is not feasible, use IM route for steroid responsive treatment of endocrine, rheumatic, collagen, dermatologic, respiratory, ophthalmic, neoplastic, hematologic, and GI disorders, allergic and edematous states and Tuberculous meningitis with subarachnoid block and trichinosis with neurologic/myocardial involvement. Intra-articular or soft tissue administration for short-term adjunct treatment of synovitis, osteoarthritis (OA), rheumatoid arthritis (RA), bursitis, acute gouty arthritis, epicondylitis, acute nonspecific tenosynovitis. Intralesional injection for keloids, discoid lupus erythematosus, necrobiosis lipoidica diabeticorum, alopecia areata, lesions of: lichen planus, psoriatic plaques, granuloma, annulare, lichen simplex chronicus.

DOSAGE: *Adults:* Initial: 0.5-9mg/day IM. Parenteral dose is usually 1/2-1/3 the oral dose given q12h. Maintain until sufficient response occurs. Maint: Decrease in small increments at appropriate time intervals until lowest effective dose. Discontinue gradually. Bursitis/Tenosynovitis/Peritendinitis: 1mL intrabursal injection. Tenosynovitis/Tendinitis: Give 3-4 injections every 1-2 weeks. Chronic Bursitis: Reduce initial dose. Ganglion Cysts: 0.5mL into cyst. RA/OA: 0.5-2mL intra-articularly. Dermatologic Conditions: 0.2mL/sq cm intradermally. Max: 1mL/week.

Pediatrics: Initial: 0.5-9mg/day IM. Parenteral dose is usually 1/2-1/3 the oral dose given q12h. Maintain until sufficient response. Maint: Decrease in small increments at appropriate time intervals until reach lowest dose that sustains response. Discontinue gradually.

HOW SUPPLIED: Inj: (Betamethasone Acetate-Betamethasone Sodium Phosphate) 3mg-3mg/mL

CONTRAINDICATIONS: Systemic fungal infections.

WARNINGS/PRECAUTIONS: May need to increase dose before, during, and after stressful situations. May mask signs of infection or cause new infections. Prolonged use may produce posterior subcapsular cataracts, glaucoma, optic nerve damage, secondary ocular infections. Increases BP, salt/water retention, potassium and calcium excretion. More severe/fatal course of infections reported with chickenpox, measles. Caution with threadworm infestation, latent TB, hypothyroidism, cirrhosis, ocular herpes simplex, HTN, diverticulitis, fresh intestinal anastomosis, ulcerative colitis, osteoporosis, myasthenia gravis, renal insufficiency, peptic ulcer disease. Growth and development of children on prolonged therapy should be monitored. Monitor for psychic disturbances. Avoid abrupt withdrawal. (Intra-articular) Examine joint fluid to rule out a septic process. Avoid injection into previously infected joint.

ADVERSE REACTIONS: Sodium retention, fluid retention, potassium loss, muscle weakness, myopathy, peptic ulcer, impaired wound healing, thin fragile skin, convulsions, menstrual irregularities, cataracts.

INTERACTIONS: Caution with ASA in hypoprothrombinemia. Increased susceptibility to infections with immunosuppressives. Avoid smallpox vaccines and other immunization procedures at high doses. Increased requirements of insulin or oral hypoglycemic agents. Avoid diluents containing methylparaben, phenol, propylparaben; may cause flocculation of steroid.

PREGNANCY: Safety in pregnancy and nursing not known.

Celontin
methsuximide (Parke-Davis)

RX

THERAPEUTIC CLASS: Succinimide

INDICATIONS: Management of absence (petit mal) seizures refractory to other drugs.

DOSAGE: *Adults:* Initial: 300mg qd for 7 days. Titrate: Increase weekly by 300mg/day for 3 weeks if needed. Max: 1.2g/day.
Pediatrics: Initial: 300mg qd for 7 days. Titrate: Increase weekly by 300mg/day 3 weeks if needed. Max: 1.2g/day. Use 150mg caps in small children.

HOW SUPPLIED: Cap: 150mg, 300mg

WARNINGS/PRECAUTIONS: Fatal blood dyscrasias reported; monitor blood counts periodically or if signs of infection. SLE reported. Withdraw slowly if altered behavior appears. May increase frequency of grand mal seizures if given alone in mixed type of seizures. Avoid abrupt withdrawal. Caution with renal/hepatic disease.

ADVERSE REACTIONS: GI effects, blood dyscrasias, dermatologic manifestations, drowsiness, ataxia, dizziness, hyperemia, proteinuria, periorbital edema.

INTERACTIONS: May interact with other anticonvulsants; monitor serum levels periodically.

PREGNANCY: Safety in pregnancy and nursing not known.

Ceptaz
ceftazidime (GlaxoSmithKline)

RX

THERAPEUTIC CLASS: Cephalosporin (3rd generation)

INDICATIONS: Treatment of lower respiratory tract (eg, pneumonia), skin and skin structure (SSSI), bone and joint, gynecologic, CNS (eg, meningitis), intra-abdominal, and urinary tract infections (UTI), and septicemia. For use in sepsis.

DOSAGE: *Adults:* Usual: 1g IM/IV q8-12h. Uncomplicated UTI: 250mg IM/IV q12h. Complicated UTI: 500mg IM/IV q8-12h. Bone and Joint Infection: 2g IV q12h. Uncomplicated Pneumonia/SSSI: 500mg-1g IM/IV q8h. Gynecological/Intra-Abdominal/Meningitis/

CEREZYME

Severe Life-Threatening Infection: 2g IV q8h. Lung Infection caused by Pseudomonas spp. in Cystic Fibrosis (normal renal function): 30-50mg/kg IV q8h. Max: 6g/day. CrCl 31-50mL/min: 1g q12h. CrCl 16-30mL/min: 1g q24h. CrCl 6-15mL/min: 500mg q24h. CrCl <5mL/min: 500mg q48h. For severe infections (6g/day), increase renal impairment dose by 50% or increase dosing interval. Apply reduced dosage recommendations after initial 1g LD is given. Hemodialysis: Give 1g before then 1g after each hemodialysis. Intra-Peritoneal Dialysis/Continuous Ambulatory Peritoneal Dialysis: Give 1g followed by 500mg q24h.

Pediatrics: ≥12 yrs: Usual: 1g IM/IV q8-12h. Uncomplicated UTI: 250mg IM/IV q12h. Complicated UTI: 500mg IM/IV q8-12h. Bone and Joint Infection: 2g IV q12h. Uncomplicated Pneumonia/SSSI: 500mg-1g IM/IV q8h. Gynecological/Intra-Abdominal/Meningitis/Severe Life-Threatening Infection: 2g IV q8h. Lung Infection caused by Pseudomonas spp. in Cystic Fibrosis (normal renal function): 30-50mg/kg IV q8h. Max: 6g/day. CrCl 31-50mL/min: 1g q12h. CrCl 16-30mL/min: 1g q24h. CrCl 6-15mL/min: 500mg q24h. CrCl <5mL/min: 500mg q48h. For severe infections (6g/day), increase renal impairment dose by 50% or increase dosing interval. Apply reduced dosage recommendations after initial 1g LD is given. Hemodialysis: Give 1g before then 1g after each hemodialysis. Intra-Peritoneal Dialysis/Continuous Ambulatory Peritoneal Dialysis: Give 1g followed by 500mg q24h.

HOW SUPPLIED: Inj: 10g

WARNINGS/PRECAUTIONS: Monitor renal function; potential for nephrotoxicity. Prolonged use may result in overgrowth of nonsusceptible organisms. Possible cross-sensitivity between penicillins, cephalosporins, and other beta-lactam antibiotics. Pseudomembranous colitis reported. Elevated levels with renal insufficiency can lead to seizures, encephalopathy, asterixis, coma, and neuromuscular excitability. Possible decrease in PT; caution with renal or hepatic impairment, poor nutritional state; monitor PT and give vitamin K if needed. Caution with colitis and other GI diseases. Distal necrosis can occur after inadvertent intra-arterial administration. Continue therapy for 2 days after the signs and symptoms of infection have disappeared, but in complicated infections longer therapy may be required. False positive for urine glucose with Benedict's, Fehling's solution, and Clinitest® tablets.

ADVERSE REACTIONS: Phlebitis and inflammation at injection site, pruritus, rash, fever, diarrhea.

INTERACTIONS: Nephrotoxicity reported with aminoglycosides or potent diuretics (eg, furosemide). Avoid with chloramphenicol; may decrease effect of beta-lactam antibiotics.

PREGNANCY: Category B, not for use in nursing.

CEREZYME RX
imiglucerase (Genzyme)

THERAPEUTIC CLASS: Beta-glucocerebrosidase

INDICATIONS: Long-term enzyme replacement therapy in Type 1 Gaucher disease.

DOSAGE: *Adults:* Initial: 2.5U/kg TIW to 60U/kg once every 2 weeks IV infusion over 1-2 hours. Adjust dose based on therapeutic goals.
Pediatrics: ≥2 yrs: Initial: 2.5U/kg TIW to 60U/kg once every 2 weeks IV infusion over 1-2 hours. Adjust dose based on therapeutic goals.

HOW SUPPLIED: Inj: 200U, 400U

WARNINGS/PRECAUTIONS: Monitor for IgG antibody formation during the 1st year of therapy. Reduce rate of infusion and pretreat with antihistamines and/or corticosteroids if anaphylactoid reactions occur. Caution in patients who developed antibodies or hypersensitivity reactions to alglucerase.

ADVERSE REACTIONS: Injection site reactions, pruritus, flushing, urticaria, angioedema, chest discomfort, dyspnea, coughing, cyanosis, hypotension, nausea, vomiting, rash, headache, fever.

PREGNANCY: Category C, caution in nursing.

CERUBIDINE RX
daunorubicin HCl (Bedford)

> Avoid IM/SQ route. Severe local tissue necrosis with extravasation. Myocardial toxicity may occur during or after terminate therapy; increased risk if cumulative dose >400-550mg/m² in adults, >300mg/m² in pediatrics >2 yrs, or >10mg/m² in pediatrics <2 yrs. Severe myelosuppression may occur. Reduce dose with impaired hepatic or renal function.

THERAPEUTIC CLASS: Anthracycline

INDICATIONS: In combination with other anticancer drugs, for remission induction in acute nonlymphocytic leukemia (ANLL) in adults, and for remission induction in acute lymphocytic leukemia (ALL) in children and adults.

DOSAGE: *Adults:* ANLL: Combination Therapy: <60 yrs: 45mg/m^2/day IV on days 1, 2, 3 of 1st course and on days 1, 2 of subsequent courses. ≥60 yrs: 30mg/m^2/day IV on days 1, 2, 3 of 1st course and on days 1, 2 of subsequent courses. ALL: Combination Therapy: 45mg/m^2/day IV on days 1, 2, 3. Renal Impairment: If SCr >3mg%, reduce dose by 50%. Hepatic Impairment: If serum bilirubin 1.2-3mg%, reduce dose by 25%. If >3mg%, reduce dose by 50%.
Pediatrics: ALL: Combination Therapy: 25mg/m^2 IV on day 1 every week. If complete remission not obtained after 4 courses, may give additional 1-2 courses. If <2 yrs or <0.5m^2 BSA, calculate dose based on weight (1mg/kg) instead of BSA.

HOW SUPPLIED: Inj: 20mg

WARNINGS/PRECAUTIONS: Avoid if pre-existing drug-induced bone marrow suppression occurs unless benefit warrants the risk. May cause fetal harm during pregnancy. May impart red color to urine. Monitor blood uric acid levels. Determine CBC frequently. Evaluate cardiac, renal, and hepatic function before each course.

ADVERSE REACTIONS: Cardiotoxicity, myelosuppression, alopecia, nausea, vomiting, diarrhea, abdominal pain, hyperuricemia, mucositis (3-7 days after therapy).

INTERACTIONS: Possible secondary leukemias with other antineoplastics or radiation therapy. Increased risk of cardiotoxicity with previous doxorubicin therapy or with concomitant cyclophosphamide. May need dose reduction with other myelosuppressants. Hepatotoxic agents (eg, high dose MTX) may increase risk of toxicity.

PREGNANCY: Category D, not for use in nursing.

CHERACOL W/CODEINE CV
guaifenesin - codeine phosphate (Lee Pharmaceuticals)

OTHER BRAND NAMES: Guaituss AC (Alpharma) - Halotussin AC (Watson) - Cheratussin AC (Vintage) - Mytussin AC (Morton Grove)

THERAPEUTIC CLASS: Cough suppressant/expectorant

INDICATIONS: Relief of cough due to minor throat and bronchial irritation from a cold or inhaled irritants. Loosens phlegm and thins bronchial secretions to make coughs more productive.

DOSAGE: *Adults:* 10mL q4h. Max: 60mL/24 hrs.
Pediatrics: ≥12 yrs: 10mL q4h. Max: 60mL/24 hrs. 6 to <12 yrs: 5mL q4h. Max: 30mL/24 hrs.

HOW SUPPLIED: Syrup: (Codeine-Guaifenesin) 10-100mg/5mL (120mL)

WARNINGS/PRECAUTIONS: Use caution with persistant/chronic cough, cough with excessive phlegm, chronic pulmonary disease, or shortness of breath. May cause or aggravate constipation.

ADVERSE REACTIONS: Constipation, sedation.

INTERACTIONS: Increased sedation with sedatives, tranquilizers and antidepressants, especially MAOIs.

PREGNANCY: Safety in pregnancy and nursing not known.

CHILDREN'S MYLANTA OTC
calcium carbonate (J&J -- Merck)

THERAPEUTIC CLASS: Antacid

INDICATIONS: For the relief of acid indigestion, sour stomach, and upset stomach due to these symptoms or overindulgence in food and drink.

DOSAGE: *Pediatrics:* 24-47 lbs or 2-5 yrs: 1 tab; 48-95 lbs or 6-11 yrs: 2 tabs. Max: 2-5 yrs: 3 tabs/24hrs; 6-11 yrs: 6 tabs/24hrs. Repeat as needed. Do not use for >2 weeks unless under supervision of a doctor.

HOW SUPPLIED: Tab, Chewable: 400mg

INTERACTIONS: Antacids may interact with other prescription drugs.

CHLORAL HYDRATE
chloral hydrate (Pharmaceutical Associations)

THERAPEUTIC CLASS: Trichloroacetaldehyde monohydrate

INDICATIONS: Short-term sedative/hypnotic (<2 weeks). To allay anxiety or induce sedation preoperatively or prior to EEG evaluations. Alone or with paraldehyde to prevent or suppress alcohol withdrawal syndrome. To reduce anxiety associated with withdrawal of other drugs such as narcotics or barbiturates.

DOSAGE: *Adults:* Dilute in half glass of water, fruit juice, or ginger ale. Hypnotic: Usual: 500mg-1g 15-30 min before bedtime. Sedative: Usual: 250mg tid pc. Alcohol Withdrawal: Usual: 500mg-1g q6h prn. Max: 2g/day.
Pediatrics: Hypnotic: 50mg/kg. Max: 1g/dose. Sedative: 8mg/kg tid. Max: 500mg tid. Prior to EEG: 20-25mg/kg.

HOW SUPPLIED: Syr: 500mg/5mL

CONTRAINDICATIONS: Marked hepatic or renal impairment.

WARNINGS/PRECAUTIONS: May be habit forming. Caution with depression, suicidal tendencies, history of drug abuse. Avoid with esophagitis, gastritis or gastric or duodenal ulcers, large doses with severe cardiac disease. May impair mental/physical abilities. Risk of gastritis, skin eruptions, parenchymatous renal damage with prolonged use. Withdraw gradually with chronic use.

ADVERSE REACTIONS: Nausea, vomiting, diarrhea, ataxia, dizziness.

INTERACTIONS: Reduces effectiveness of coumarin anticoagulants. May result in transient potentiation of warfarin-induced hypoprothrombinemia. Additive CNS effects with other CNS depressants (eg, paraldehyde, barbiturates, alcohol). Use with IV furosemide may cause diaphoresis, flushes, variable BP; use alternative hypnotic.

PREGNANCY: Category C, caution in nursing.

CHLORPROMAZINE RX
chlorpromazine (Various)

THERAPEUTIC CLASS: Phenothiazine

INDICATIONS: Treatment of schizophrenia. Control of nausea and vomiting. Relief of restlessness and apprehension before surgery. Treatment of acute intermittent porphyria. Adjunct treatment of tetanus. To control the manic type of manic-depressive illness. Relief of intractable hiccups. Treatment of severe behavioral problems in children. Short-term treatment of hyperactivity in children.

DOSAGE: *Adults:* Severe Behavioral Problems: Inpatient: Acute Schizophrenic/Manic State: 25mg IM, then 25-50mg IM in 1 hr if needed. Titrate: Increase over several days up to 400mg q4-6h until controlled then switch to PO. Usual: 500mg/day PO. Max: 1000mg/day PO. Less Acutely Disturbed: 25mg PO tid. Titrate: Increase gradually to 400mg/day. Outpatient: 10mg PO tid-qid or 25mg PO bid-tid. More Severe: 25mg PO tid. Titrate: After 1-2 days, increase by 20-50mg twice weekly until calm. Prompt Control of Severe Symptoms: 25mg IM, may repeat in 1 hr then 25-50mg PO tid. Nausea/Vomiting: Usual: 10-25mg PO q4-6h prn; 25mg IM then, if no hypotension, 25-50mg q3-4h prn until vomiting stops then switch to PO; 100mg rectally q6-8h prn. Nausea/Vomiting in Surgery: 12.5mg IM, may repeat in 1/2 hr; 2mg IV per fractional injection at 2 minute intervals. Max: 25mg. Presurgical Apprehension: 25-50mg PO 2-3 hrs pre-op; 12.5-25mg IM 1-2 hrs pre-op. Intractable Hiccups: 25-50mg PO tid-qid; if symptoms persist after 2-3 days, give 25-50mg IM; if symptoms still persist, give 25-50mg slow IV. Porphyria: 25-50mg PO tid-qid; 25mg IM tid-qid until PO therapy. Tetanus: 25-50mg IM tid-qid; 25-50mg IV. Elderly: Use lower doses, increase dose more gradually, monitor closely.
Pediatrics: 6 months-12 yrs: Severe Behavioral Problems: Outpatient: 0.25mg/lb PO q4-6h prn; 0.5mg/lb sup rectally q6-8h prn; 0.25mg/lb IM q6-8h prn. Inpatient: Start low and increase gradually to 50-100mg/day; ≥200mg/day in older children. Max: 500mg/day. <5 yrs (<50lbs): Max: ≤40mg/day IM; 5-12 yrs (50-100lbs): Max: ≤75mg/day IM. Nausea/Vomiting: 0.25mg/lb PO q4-6h; 0.5mg/lb sup rectally q6-8 prn. 0.25mg/lb IM q6-8h prn. Max: 6 months-5 yrs (or 50 lbs): <40mg/day. 5-12 yrs (or 50-100lbs): <75mg/day except in severe cases. During Surgery: 0.125mg/lb IM repeat in 1/2 hr if needed;

1mg IV per fractional injection at 2-minute intervals and not exceeding recommended IM dosage. Presurgical Apprehension: 0.25mg/lb PO 2-3 hrs (or IM 1-2 hrs) before operation. Tetanus: 0.25mg/lb IM/IV q6-8h. <50lbs: Max: ≤40mg/day; 50-100lbs: Max: ≤75mg/day.

HOW SUPPLIED: Cap, Extended Release: 30mg, 75mg, 150mg; Inj: 25mg/mL; Sup: 25mg, 100mg; Syrup: 10mg/5mL (120mL); Tab: 10mg, 25mg, 50mg, 100mg, 200mg

CONTRAINDICATIONS: Comatose states, or with large amounts of CNS depressants. Hypersensitivity to phenothiazines.

WARNINGS/PRECAUTIONS: Tardive dyskinesia, NMS may occur. Caution with chronic respiratory disorders, acute respiratory infections (especially in children), glaucoma, cardiovascular, hepatic, or renal disease, history of hepatic encephalopathy due to cirrhosis. Suppresses cough reflex; aspiration of vomitus possible. Caution if exposed to extreme heat or organophosphates. Avoid in children/adolescents with signs of Reye's syndrome. Lowers seizure threshold. Reduce dose gradually to prevent side effects. May mask signs of overdoses to other drugs and obscure diagnosis of other conditions (eg, intestinal obstruction, brain tumor, Reye's syndrome). May produce false-positive PKU test. May elevate prolactin levels. Injection contains sulfites.

ADVERSE REACTIONS: Drowsiness, jaundice, agranulocytosis, hypotensive effects, EKG changes, dystonias, motor restlessness, pseudo-parkinsonism, tardive dyskinesia, anticholinergic effects, NMS, ocular changes.

INTERACTIONS: See Contraindications. May decrease effects of oral anticoagulants, guanethidine. Propranolol increases plasma levels of both agents. Thiazide diuretics may potentiate orthostatic hypotension. Potentiates effects of CNS depressants (eg, anesthetic, barbiturates, narcotics); reduce doses of these drugs by 1/4 to 1/2. Anticonvulsants may need adjustment; phenytoin toxicity reported. Do not use with Amipaque®; discontinue at least 48 hrs before myelography and resume at least 24 hrs after. Can cause alpha-adrenergic blockade. Caution with atropine or related drugs. Encephalopathic syndrome reported with lithium.

PREGNANCY: Safety in pregnancy not known. Not for use in nursing.

Chlor-Trimeton   OTC
chlorpheniramine maleate (Schering)

THERAPEUTIC CLASS: Antihistamine

INDICATIONS: Allergic rhinitis and conjunctivitis.

DOSAGE: *Adults:* (Tab/Syrup) 4mg q4-6h. (Tab, ER) 8mg q8-12h or 12mg q12h. Max: 24mg/day.

Pediatrics: ≥12 yrs: (Tab/Syrup) 4mg q4-6h. Tab, ER: 8mg q8-12h or 12mg q12h. Max: 24mg/day. 6-12 yrs: (Tab/Syrup) 2mg q4-6h. Max: 12mg/24hrs.

HOW SUPPLIED: Syrup: 2mg/5mL; Tab: 4mg; Tab, Extended Release: 8mg, 12mg

WARNINGS/PRECAUTIONS: Avoid with emphysema, chronic bronchitis, glaucoma, and difficulty in urination due to prostate gland enlargement.

ADVERSE REACTIONS: Drowsiness, excitability.

INTERACTIONS: Alcohol, sedatives, hypnotics potentiate CNS depression.

PREGNANCY: Safety in pregnancy or nursing not known.

Ciloxan   RX
ciprofloxacin HCl (Alcon)

THERAPEUTIC CLASS: Fluoroquinolone

INDICATIONS: Bacterial conjunctivitis and corneal ulcers.

DOSAGE: *Adults:* Bacterial Conjunctivitis: Sol: 1-2 drops q2h while awake for 2 days, then 1-2 drops every 4 hrs while awake for 5 days. Oint: 1/2 inch tid for 2 days, then bid for 5 days. Corneal Ulcer: Sol: 2 drops every 15 minutes for the first 6 hrs, then 2 drops every 30 minutes for the rest of day 1, then 2 drops every hr on day 2, then 2 drops every 4 hrs on days 3-14. May continue if re-epithelialization has not occurred.

Pediatrics: Bacterial Conjunctivitis: ≥1 yr: Sol: 1-2 drops q2h while awake for 2 days, then 1-2 drops every 4 hrs while awake for 5 days. ≥2 yr: Oint: 1/2 inch tid for 2 days,

CIMETIDINE

then bid for 5 days. Corneal Ulcer: Sol: ≥1 yr: 2 drops every 15 minutes for the first 6 hrs, then 2 drops every 30 minutes for the rest of day 1, then 2 drops every hr on day 2, then 2 drops every 4 hrs on days 3-14. May continue if re-epithelialization has not occurred.

HOW SUPPLIED: Oint: 0.3% (3.5g); Sol: 0.3% (2.5mL, 5mL, 10mL)

WARNINGS/PRECAUTIONS: Not for injection into eye. Superinfection may result with prolonged use. Fatal hypersensitivity reactions reported after 1st dose of systemic quinolone therapy. Avoid allowing tip of container to contact eye or surrounding structures. Avoid contact lenses with conjunctivitis. Risk of crystalline precipitate in cornea. Ointment may slow corneal healing and cause visual blurring.

ADVERSE REACTIONS: Local burning, white crystalline precipitants, lid margin crusting, crystals/scales, foreign body sensation, itching, conjunctival hyperemia, bad taste.

INTERACTIONS: Systemic quinolone therapy may increase theophylline levels, interfere with caffeine metabolism, enhance warfarin effects, and elevate serum creatinine with cyclosporine.

PREGNANCY: Category C, caution in nursing.

CIMETIDINE
cimetidine (Various)
RX

OTHER BRAND NAME: Tagamet (GlaxoSmithKline)

THERAPEUTIC CLASS: H_2 blocker

INDICATIONS: Short-term treatment of active duodenal ulcer (DU), active benign gastric ulcer (GU). Maintenance of healed duodenal ulcer. Treatment of GERD and/or pathological hypersecretory conditions (eg, Zollinger-Ellison syndrome). Prevention of upper GI bleeding in critically ill patients.

DOSAGE: *Adults:* (PO) Active DU: 800mg qhs or 300mg qid or 400mg bid for 4-8 weeks. Maint: 400mg qhs. Active Benign GU: 800mg qhs or 300mg qid for 6 weeks. GERD: 800mg bid or 400mg qid for 12 weeks. Hypersecretory Conditions: 300mg qid. Max: 2400mg/day. (Inj) 300mg IM/IV q6-8h. Max: 2400mg/day. Rapid Gastric pH Elevation: LD: 150mg IV, then 37.5mg/hr IV. Upper GI Bleed Prevention: Continuous IV infusion of 50mg/hr for 7 days. CrCl <30mL/min: Give half the recommended dose.

Pediatrics: ≥16 yrs: (PO) Active DU: 800mg qhs or 300mg qid or 400mg bid for 4-8 weeks. Maint: 400mg qhs. Active Benign GU: 800mg qhs or 300mg qid for 6 weeks. GERD: 800mg bid or 400mg qid for 12 weeks. Hypersecretory Conditions: 300mg qid. Max: 2400mg/day. (Inj) 300mg IM/IV q6-8h. Max: 2400mg/day. Rapid Gastric pH Elevation: LD: 150mg IV, then 37.5mg/hr IV. Upper GI Bleed Prevention: Continuous IV infusion of 50mg/hr for 7 days. CrCl <30mL/min: Give half the recommended dose.

HOW SUPPLIED: Inj: (HCl) 150mg/mL, 300mg/50mL; Sol: (HCl) 300mg/5mL; Tab: 300mg, 400mg*, 800mg* *scored

WARNINGS/PRECAUTIONS: Cardiac arrhythmias and hypotension reported following rapid IV administration (rare). Symptomatic response does not preclude the presence of gastric malignancy. Reversible confusional states reported, especially in severely ill patients. Elderly, renal and/or hepatic impairment are risk factors for confusional states. Risk of hyperinfection of strongyloidiasis in immunocompromised patients.

ADVERSE REACTIONS: Diarrhea, headache, dizziness, somnolence, reversible confusional states, impotence, increased serum transaminases, rash, gynecomastia, blood dyscrasias.

INTERACTIONS: Reduces metabolism of warfarin-type anticoagulants, phenytoin, propranolol, nifedipine, chlordiazepoxide, diazepam, certain TCAs, lidocaine, theophylline and metronidazole. Monitor PT/INR. Adverse effects reported with phenytoin, lidocaine and theophylline; monitor levels. May affect absorption of drugs (eg, ketoconazole) affected by gastric pH; give 2 hrs before cimetidine. Antacids may interfer with absorption of cimetidine; space the dosing.

PREGNANCY: Category B, not for use in nursing.

CIPRO HC
hydrocortisone - ciprofloxacin HCl (Alcon)
RX

THERAPEUTIC CLASS: Antibacterial/corticosteroid combination

INDICATIONS: Acute otitis externa in adults and pediatric patients ≥1 year.

DOSAGE: *Adults:* 3 drops into affected ear bid for 7 days. Warm bottle in hand for 1-2 minutes to avoid dizziness. Shake well before use.
Pediatrics: ≥1 yr: 3 drops into affected ear bid for 7 days. Warm bottle in hand for 1-2 minutes to avoid dizziness. Shake well before use.
HOW SUPPLIED: Sus: (Ciprofloxacin-Hydrocortisone) 0.2%-1% (10mL)
CONTRAINDICATIONS: Perforated tympanic membrane, viral infections of external ear canal (eg, varicella and herpes simplex infections).
WARNINGS/PRECAUTIONS: D/C if hypersensitivity reaction occurs. Re-evaluate if no improvement after one week.
ADVERSE REACTIONS: Headache, pruritus.
PREGNANCY: Category C, not for use in nursing.

Cipro IV
ciprofloxacin (Schering)

RX

THERAPEUTIC CLASS: Fluoroquinolone
INDICATIONS: Treatment of skin and skin structure (SSSI), bone and joint, complicated intra-abdominal infections, lower respiratory (LRTI), and urinary tract infections (UTI), nosocomial pneumonia, acute sinusitis, chronic bacterial prostatitis, post-exposure inhalational anthrax, empirical therapy for febrile neutropenia, complicated UTI and pyelonephritis in pediatrics.
DOSAGE: *Adults:* ≥18 yrs: IV: UTI: Mild-Moderate: 200mg q12h for 7-14 days. Complicated/Severe: 400mg q12h for 7-14 days. LRTI/SSSI: Mild-Moderate: 400mg q12h for 7-14 days. Complicated/Severe: 400mg q8h for 7-14 days. Bone and Joint: Mild-Moderate: 400mg q12h for ≥4-6 weeks. Complicated/Severe: 400mg q8h for ≥4-6 weeks. Nosocomial Pneumonia: 400mg q8h for 10-14 days. Complicated Intra-Abdominal: 400mg q12h (w/metronidazole) for 7-14 days. Acute Sinusitis: 400mg q12h for 10 days. Chronic Bacterial Prostatitis: 400mg q12h for 28 days. Febrile Neutropenia: 400mg q8h (w/piperacillin 50mg/kg q4h) for 7-14 days. Max: 24g/day. Inhalational Anthrax: 400mg q12h for 60 days. Administer over 60 minutes. CrCl 5-29mL/min: 200-400mg q18-24h.
Pediatrics: <18 yrs: Inhalational Anthrax: 10mg/kg q12h for 60 days. Max: 400mg/dose; 800mg/day. 1-17 yrs: Complicated UTI/Pyelenophritis: 6-10mg/kg q8h for 10-21 days. Max: 400mg/dose.
HOW SUPPLIED: Inj: 10mg/mL, 200mg/100mL, 400mg/200mL
CONTRAINDICATIONS: Concomitant administration with tizanidine.
WARNINGS/PRECAUTIONS: Convulsions, increased intracranial pressure, and toxic psychosis reported. Caution with CNS disorders or if predisposed to seizures. Severe, fatal hypersensitivity reactions may occur. Pseudomembranous colitis, achilles and other tendon ruptures reported. D/C at first sign of rash/hypersensitivity or if pain, inflammation, or ruptured tendon occur. May permit overgrowth of clostridia. Maintain hydration; avoid alkaline urine. Avoid excessive sunlight and UV light. Do not give via feeding tube. Monitor renal, hepatic and hematopoietic function with prolonged use. Adust dose with renal dysfunction.
ADVERSE REACTIONS: Nausea, diarrhea, CNS disturbances, local IV site reactions, hepatic enzyme abnormalities, eosinophilia, headache, restlessness rash.
INTERACTIONS: See Contraindications. Increases theophylline and caffeine levels and prolongs effects. Altered serum levels of phenytoin. Severe hypoglycemia with glyburide (rare). Potentiated by probenecid. Transient serum creatinine elevations with cyclosporine. Enhances oral anticoagulant effects. Caution with drugs that lower seizure threshold.
PREGNANCY: Category C, not for use in nursing.

Cipro Oral
ciprofloxacin HCl (Schering)

RX

THERAPEUTIC CLASS: Fluoroquinolone
INDICATIONS: Treatment of lower respiratory tract (LRTI), complicated intra-abdominal, skin and skin structure (SSSI), bone and joint, and urinary tract infections (UTI), acute

CIPRODEX

exacerbations of chronic bronchitis, acute sinusitis, acute uncomplicated cystitis in females, chronic bacterial prostatitis, infectious diarrhea, typhoid fever, post-exposure inhalational anthrax, uncomplicated cervical and urethral gonorrhea, complicated UTI and pyelonephritis in pediatrics.

DOSAGE: *Adults:* ≥18 yrs: Acute Sinusitis/Typhoid Fever: 500mg q12h for 10 days. LRTI/SSSI: Mild-Moderate: 500mg q12h for 7-14 days. Severe/Complicated: 750mg q12h for 7-14 days. Cystitis/Acute Uncompilcated UTI: 250mg q12h for 3 days. Mild-Moderate UTI: 250mg q12h for 7-14 days. Severe/Complicated UTI: 500mg q12h for 7-14 days. Chronic Bacterial Prostatitis: 500mg q12h for 28 days. Intra-Abdominal: 500mg q12h (w/ metronidazole) for 7-14 days. Bone and Joint: Mild-Moderate: 500mg q12h for ≥4-6 weeks. Severe/Complicated: 750mg q12h for ≥4-6 weeks. Infectious Diarrhea: 500mg q12h for 5-7 days. Uncomplicated Urethral/Cervical Gonococcal: 250mg single dose. Inhalational Anthrax: 500mg q12h for 60 days. CrCl 30-50mL/min: 250-500mg q12h. CrCl 5-29mL/min: 250-500mg q18h. Hemodialysis/Peritoneal Dialysis: 250-500mg q24h (after dialysis). Administer at least 2 hrs before or 6 hrs after magnesium or aluminum containing antacids, sucralfate, Videx (didanosine) chewable/buffered tablets or pediatric powder, or other products containing calcium, iron or zinc.

Pediatrics: <18 yrs: Inhalational Anthrax: 15mg/kg q12h for 60 days. Max: 500mg/dose. 1-17 yrs: Complicated UTI/Pyelonephritis: 10-20mg/kg q12h for 10-21 days. Max: 750mg/dose.

HOW SUPPLIED: Sus: 250mg/5mL, 500mg/5mL (100mL); Tab: 250mg, 500mg, 750mg

CONTRAINDICATIONS: Concomitant administration with tizanidine.

WARNINGS/PRECAUTIONS: Convulsions, increased intracranial pressure, and toxic psychosis reported. Caution with CNS disorders or if predisposed to seizures. Severe, fatal hypersensitivity reactions may occur. Pseudomembranous colitis, achilles and other tendon ruptures reported. D/C at first sign of rash or if pain, inflammation, or ruptured tendon occurs. Maintain hydration; avoid alkaline urine. Avoid excessive sunlight and UV light. Do not give via feeding tube. Monitor renal, hepatic, and hematopoietic function with prolonged use. Adjust dose with renal dysfunction.

ADVERSE REACTIONS: Nausea, dizziness, headache, CNS disturbances, vomiting, diarrhea, rash, abdominal pain/discomfort.

INTERACTIONS: See Contraindications. Increases theophylline and caffeine levels and prolongs effects. Fatal reactions have occurred with theophylline. Magnesium or aluminum containing antacids, sucralfate, Videx (didanosine) chewable/buffered tablets or pediatric powder, and products containing calcium, iron, or zinc decrease serum and urine levels; space doses at least 2 hrs before or 6 hrs after administration. Altered serum levels of phenytoin. Severe hypoglycemia with glyburide (rare). Potentiated by probenecid. Transient serum creatinine elevations with cyclosporine. Enhances oral anticoagulant effects. Monitor PT. Caution with drugs that lower seizure threshold.

PREGNANCY: Category C, not for use in nursing.

CIPRODEX
ciprofloxacin - dexamethasone (Alcon)

RX

THERAPEUTIC CLASS: Antibacterial/corticosteroid combination

INDICATIONS: Acute otitis media in pediatric patients with tympanostomy tubes. Acute otitis externa.

DOSAGE: *Adults:* Acute Otitis Externa: 4 drops in affected ear(s) bid for 7 days. Warm bottle in hand for 1-2 minutes to avoid dizziness. Shake well before use.

Pediatrics: ≥6 months: 4 drops in affected ear(s) bid for 7 days. Warm bottle in hand for 1-2 minutes to avoid dizziness. Shake well before use.

HOW SUPPLIED: Sus: (Ciprofloxacin-Dexamethasone) 0.3%-0.1% (5mL, 7.5mL)

CONTRAINDICATIONS: Viral infections of external ecr canal including herpes simplex infections.

WARNINGS/PRECAUTIONS: Discontinue if hypersensitivity reaction occurs. Reevaluate if no improvement after one week.

ADVERSE REACTIONS: Ear pain/discomfort/pruritus.

PREGNANCY: Category C, not for use in nursing.

CLAFORAN
cefotaxime sodium (Sanofi-Aventis)

RX

THERAPEUTIC CLASS: Cephalosporin (3rd generation)

INDICATIONS: Treatment of lower respiratory tract, genitourinary, gynecologic, intra-abdominal, skin and skin structure, bone and joint, and CNS infections (eg, meningitis), bacteremia, and septicemia. For surgical prophylaxis.

DOSAGE: *Adults:* Gonococcal Urethritis/Cervicitis (males/females): 500mg single dose IM. Rectal Gonorrhea: 0.5g (females) or 1g (males) single dose IM. Uncomplicated Infections: 1g IM/IV q12h. Moderate-Severe Infections: 1-2g IM/IV q8h. Septicemia: 2g IV q6-8h. Life-Threatening Infections: 2g IV q4h. Max: 12g/day. Surgical Prophylaxis: 1g IM/IV 30-90 minutes before surgery. Cesarean Section: 1g IV when umbilical cord is clamped, then 1g IV at 6 and 12 hrs after 1st dose. CrCl <20mL/min/1.73 m^2: Give 1/2 of usual dose.
Pediatrics: ≥50kg: Use adult dose. Max: 12g/day. 1month-12 yrs and ≤50kg: 50-180mg/kg/day IM/IV divided in 4-6 doses. 1-4 weeks: 50mg/kg IV q8h. 0-1 week: 50mg/kg IV q12h. CrCl <20mL/min/1.73 m^2: Give 1/2 of usual dose.

HOW SUPPLIED: Inj: 500mg, 1g, 2g, 10g

WARNINGS/PRECAUTIONS: Cross sensitivity to penicillins and other cephalosporins may occur. Pseudomembranous colitis reported. May result in overgrowth of nonsusceptible organisms. Caution with history of GI disease. Reduce dose with renal dysfunction. Granulocytopenia may occur with long-term use. Monitor blood counts if therapy >10 days. Monitor injection site for tissue inflammation. False positive direct Coombs' tests reported.

ADVERSE REACTIONS: Injection site reactions, rash, pruritus, fever, eosinophilia, colitis, diarrhea.

INTERACTIONS: Increased nephrotoxicity with aminoglycosides.

PREGNANCY: Category B, caution in nursing.

CLARINEX
desloratadine (Schering)

RX

OTHER BRAND NAMES: Clarinex Syrup (Schering) - Clarinex RediTabs (Schering)

THERAPEUTIC CLASS: H_1 antagonist

INDICATIONS: Relief of perennial allergic rhinitis and chronic idiopathic urticaria in patients ≥6 months of age. Relief of seasonal allergic rhinitis in patients ≥2 yrs of age.

DOSAGE: *Adults:* 5mg qd. Hepatic/Renal Impairment: 5mg every other day. Dissolve RediTabs on tongue with or without water.
Pediatrics: Tabs: ≥12 yrs: 5mg qd. 6-11 yrs: 2.5mg qd. Syrup: ≥12 yrs: 10mL (5mg) qd. 6-11 yrs: 5mL (2.5mg) qd. 12 months-5 yrs: 2.5mL (1.25mg) qd. 6-11 months: 2mL (1mg) qd. Dissolve RediTabs on tongue with or without water.

HOW SUPPLIED: Tab: 5mg; Tab, Disintegrating: (RediTabs) 2.5mg, 5mg; Syrup: 0.5mg/mL

WARNINGS/PRECAUTIONS: Adjust dose with renal or hepatic impairment. Caution in elderly.

ADVERSE REACTIONS: Pharyngitis, dry mouth, headache, fever, diarrhea, cough, upper respiratory tract infection, cough, irritability, somnolence, bronchitis, otitis media, vomiting, nausea, fatigue.

INTERACTIONS: Erythromycin, ketoconazole increase plasma levels.

PREGNANCY: Category C, not for use in nursing.

CLARINEX-D 24 HOUR
desloratadine - pseudoephedrine sulfate (Schering)

RX

THERAPEUTIC CLASS: H_1 antagonist/sympathomimetic amine

INDICATIONS: Relief of nasal and non-nasal symptoms of seasonal allergic rhinitis including nasal congestion.

CLARIPEL

DOSAGE: *Adults:* 1 tab qd. Renal Impairment: 1 tab qod.
Pediatrics: ≥12 yrs: 1 tab qd. Renal Impairment: 1 tab qod.
HOW SUPPLIED: Tab, Extended Release: (Desloratadine-Pseudoephedrine) 5mg-240mg
CONTRAINDICATIONS: Narrow-angle glaucoma, urinary retention, MAOI therapy or within 14 days of discontinuation, severe HTN, severe CAD, hypersensitivity or idiosyncrasy to adrenergic agents, or to other drugs of similar chemical structures.
WARNINGS/PRECAUTIONS: Caution with HTN, DM, ischemic heart disease, increased intraocular pressure, hyperthyroidism, renal impairment, or prostatic hypertrophy. CNS stimulation with convulsions or cardiovascular collapse with accompanying hypotension may be produced by sympathomimetic amines. Avoid with hepatic insufficiency.
ADVERSE REACTIONS: Dry mouth, headache, insomnia, fatigue, pharyngitis, somnolence
INTERACTIONS: Do not use with MAOIs or within 14 days of discontinuation. Antihypertensive effects of β-adrenergic blocking agents, methyldopa, mecamylamine, reserpine, and veratrum alkaloids may be reduced by sympathomimetics (eg, pseudoephedrine). Increased ectopic pacemaker activity with digitalis.
PREGNANCY: Category C, not for use in nursing.

CLARIPEL   RX
hydroquinone (Stiefel)

THERAPEUTIC CLASS: Depigmenting agent
INDICATIONS: Gradual treatment of ultraviolet induced dyschromia and discoloration resulting from use of oral contraceptives, pregnancy, hormone replacement therapy, or skin trauma.
DOSAGE: *Adults:* Apply bid.
Pediatrics: ≥12 yrs: Apply bid.
HOW SUPPLIED: Cre: 4% (28g, 45g)
WARNINGS/PRECAUTIONS: Avoid sun exposure on bleached skin. Claripel contains sunscreen. May produce unwanted cosmetic effects if not used as directed. Test for skin sensitivity. Discontinue if no lightening effect after 2 months of therapy, if blue-black skin discoloration occurs, or if itching, vesicle formation, or excessive inflammatory reactions occur. Contains sodium metabisulfite; may cause serious allergic type reactions. Avoid contact with eyes.
ADVERSE REACTIONS: Cutaneous hypersensitivity (contact dermatitis).
PREGNANCY: Category C, caution in nursing.

CLARITIN OTC   OTC
loratadine (Schering)

OTHER BRAND NAME: Claritin Reditab OTC (Schering)
THERAPEUTIC CLASS: H_1 antagonist
INDICATIONS: Relief of symptoms due to hay fever or other upper respiratory allergies.
DOSAGE: *Adults:* (Reditab, Syrup, Tab) 10mg qd. Max: 10mg/d. Dissolve Reditab on tongue. Hepatic/Renal Impairment: May need to adjust dose.
Pediatrics: ≥6 yrs: (Reditab, Syr, Tab) 10mg qd. Max: 10mg/d. 2-5 yrs: (Syr) 5mg qd. Max: 5mg/d. Dissolve Reditab on tongue. Hepatic/Renal Impairment: May need to adjust dose.
HOW SUPPLIED: Syrup: 1mg/mL; Tab, Extended Release: (24 hr) 10mg; Tab, Disintegrating: (Reditab) 10mg
WARNINGS/PRECAUTIONS: Caution with hepatic or renal impairment.
PREGNANCY: Safety in pregnancy and nursing is not known.

CLARITIN-D OTC   OTC
loratadine - pseudoephedrine sulfate (Schering)

THERAPEUTIC CLASS: H_1 antagonist/sympathomimetic amine
INDICATIONS: Relief of symptoms due to hay fever or other upper respiratory allergies. Reduces swelling of nasal passages. Relief of sinus congestion and pressure.

DOSAGE: *Adults:* 5-120mg tab q12h or 10-240mg tab qd (with full glass of water). Max: 10-240mg/24 hrs. Hepatic/Renal Impairment: May need to adjust dose. Do not divide, crush, chew or dissolve tabs.
Pediatrics: ≥12 yrs: 5-120mg tab q12h, or 10-240mg tab qd (with full glass of water). Max: 10-240mg/24 hrs. Hepatic/Renal Impairment: May need to adjust dose. Do not divide, crush, chew or dissolve tabs.

HOW SUPPLIED: Tab, Extended Release: (Loratadine-Pseudoephedrine) (12 Hour) 5-120mg, (24 Hour) 10-240mg

WARNINGS/PRECAUTIONS: Caution with hepatic or renal impairment, heart disease, thyroid disease, high BP, diabetes, enlarged prostate.

ADVERSE REACTIONS: Dizziness, insomnia, nervousness.

INTERACTIONS: Avoid during or within 14 days MAOIs.

PREGNANCY: Safety in pregnancy and nursing is not known.

CLENIA
sulfur - sulfacetamide sodium (Upsher-Smith)
RX

THERAPEUTIC CLASS: Sulfonamide/sulfur combination

INDICATIONS: Topical treatment of acne vulgaris, acne rosacea, and seborrheic dermatitis.

DOSAGE: *Adults:* (Cleanser) Wash qd-bid. Massage into skin for 10-20 seconds, then rinse and dry. (Cream) Initial: Apply qd. Titrate: Increase up to bid-tid prn.
Pediatrics: ≥12 yrs: (Cleanser) Wash qd-bid. Massage into skin for 10-20 seconds, then rinse and dry. (Cream) Initial: Apply qd. Titrate: Increase up to bid-tid prn.

HOW SUPPLIED: Cleanser: (Sulfacetamide-Sulfur) 10%-5% (170g, 340g); Cre: 10%-5% (28g)

CONTRAINDICATIONS: Kidney disease.

WARNINGS/PRECAUTIONS: Discontinue if excessive irritation occurs. Avoid contact with eyes, eyelid, lips, or mucous membranes. Caution with denuded or abraded skin. Can cause reddening and scaling of epidermis.

ADVERSE REACTIONS: Dryness, erythema, itching, edema.

PREGNANCY: Category C, caution in nursing.

CLEOCIN
clindamycin HCl (Pharmacia & Upjohn)
RX

Pseudomembranous colitis reported; may range in severity from mild to life threatening.

THERAPEUTIC CLASS: Lincomycin derivative

INDICATIONS: Serious infections caused by anaerobes, streptococci, pneumococci and staphylococci.

DOSAGE: *Adults:* Serious Infection: 150-300mg PO q6h or 600-1200mg/day IM/IV given bid-qid. More Severe Infection: 300-450mg PO q6h or 1200-2700mg/day IM/IV given bid-qid. Life-threatening Infections: Up to 4800mg/day IV. Max: 600mg per IM injection. Take oral form with full glass of water. Treat β-hemolytic strep for at least 10 days.
Pediatrics: Birth-16 yrs: Serious Infection: 8-16mg/kg/day PO. More Severe Infection: 16-20mg/kg/day PO. 1 month-16 yrs: 20-40mg/kg/day IM/IV given tid-qid; use higher dose for more severe infection. <1 month: 15-20mg/kg/day IM/IV given tid-qid. Take oral form with full glass of water. Treat β-hemolytic strep for at least 10 days.

HOW SUPPLIED: Cap: (HCl) 75mg, 150mg, 300mg; Inj: (Phosphate) 150mg/mL, 300mg/50mL, 600mg/50mL, 900mg/50mL; Sus: (HCl) 75mg/5mL (100g)

WARNINGS/PRECAUTIONS: D/C if diarrhea occurs. May permit overgrowth of clostridia. Not for treatment of meningitis. Caution with atopic patients, GI disease (eg, colitis), hepatic disease and the elderly. Monitor blood, hepatic and renal function with long-term use. Do not give injection undiluted as a bolus. The 75mg and 100mg caps contain tartrazine.

CLEOCIN T

ADVERSE REACTIONS: Abdominal pain, pseudomembranous colitis, esophagitis, nausea, vomiting, diarrhea, hypersensitivity reactions, metallic taste (Inj), jaundice, blood dyscrasias, pruritus, vaginitis, superinfection (prolonged use).

INTERACTIONS: Antagonism may occur with erythromycin. May potentiate neuromuscular blockers.

PREGNANCY: Category B, not for use in nursing.

CLEOCIN T   RX
clindamycin phosphate (Pharmacia & Upjohn)

THERAPEUTIC CLASS: Lincomycin derivative

INDICATIONS: Acne vulgaris.

DOSAGE: *Adults:* Apply thin film bid.

Pediatrics: ≥12 yrs: Apply thin film bid. May use more than 1 pledget.

HOW SUPPLIED: Gel: 1% (30g, 60g); Lot: 1% (60mL); Sol: 1% (30mL, 60mL); Swab (Pledgets): 1% (60^s)

CONTRAINDICATIONS: Hypersensitivity to lincomycin. History of regional enteritis, ulcerative colitis, or antibiotic-associated colitis.

WARNINGS/PRECAUTIONS: Avoid eyes, abraded skin, mucous membranes, and mouth. Caution in atopic patients. D/C if significant diarrhea occurs.

ADVERSE REACTIONS: Dryness, oily skin, erythema, peeling, burning, itching, pseudomembranous colitis (rare).

INTERACTIONS: May potentiate neuromuscular blockers.

PREGNANCY: Category B, not for use in nursing.

CLEOCIN VAGINAL   RX
clindamycin phosphate (Pharmacia & Upjohn)

OTHER BRAND NAMES: Clindamax Vaginal (PharmaDerm) - Cleocin Vaginal Ovules (Pharmacia & Upjohn)

THERAPEUTIC CLASS: Lincomycin derivative

INDICATIONS: (Cream) Treatment of bacterial vaginosis in non-pregnant women and pregnant women during the 2nd and 3rd trimester. (Sup) Treatment of bacterial vaginosis in non-pregnant women.

DOSAGE: *Adults:* (Cream) 1 applicatorful intravaginally qhs. Treat non-pregnant females for 3 or 7 days. Treat pregnant females (2nd and 3rd trimester) for 7 days. (Sup) 1 suppository intravaginally qhs for 3 days.

Pediatrics: Post-Menarchal: (Sup) 1 suppository intravaginally qhs for 3 days.

HOW SUPPLIED: Cre: 2% (40g); Sup, Vaginal: (Ovules) 100mg (3^s)

CONTRAINDICATIONS: Hypersensitivity to lincomycin. History of regional enteritis, ulcerative colitis, or antibiotic-associated colitis.

WARNINGS/PRECAUTIONS: Do not use condoms or contraceptive diaphragms within 72 hrs following treatment. Monitor for pseudomembranous colitis. Avoid eye contact. Do not engage in vaginal intercourse or use other vaginal products (such as tampons or douches) during treatment. Monitor for pseudomembranous colitis.

ADVERSE REACTIONS: Vaginitis, vulvovaginal disorder, candidiasis, moniliasis, pruritus, abnormal labor.

INTERACTIONS: May potentiate neuromuscular blockers.

PREGNANCY: Category B, not for use in nursing.

CLINDAGEL   RX
clindamycin phosphate (Galderma)

THERAPEUTIC CLASS: Lincomycin derivative

INDICATIONS: Acne vulgaris.

DOSAGE: *Adults:* Apply thin film once daily.
Pediatrics: ≥12 yrs: Apply thin film once daily.
HOW SUPPLIED: Gel: 1% (40mL, 75mL)
CONTRAINDICATIONS: Hypersensitivity to lincomycin. History of regional enterative colitis, or antibiotic-associated colitis.
WARNINGS/PRECAUTIONS: Discontinue if significant diarrhea occurs. Caution in atopic individuals.
ADVERSE REACTIONS: Peeling, pruritus, pseudomembranous colitis (rare).
INTERACTIONS: May potentiate neuromuscular blockers.
PREGNANCY: Category B, not for use in nursing.

CLOBEVATE
clobetasol propionate (Stiefel)
RX

THERAPEUTIC CLASS: Corticosteroid
INDICATIONS: Inflammatory and pruritic manifestations of corticosteroid-responsive dermatoses.
DOSAGE: *Adults:* Apply thin layer bid. Limit treatment to 2 consecutive weeks. Max: 50g/week. Avoid with occlusive dressings.
Pediatrics: ≥12 yrs: Apply thin layer bid. Limit treatment to 2 consecutive weeks. Max: 50g/week. Avoid with occlusive dressings.
HOW SUPPLIED: Gel: 0.05% (45g)
WARNINGS/PRECAUTIONS: May produce reversible HPA axis suppression, Cushing's syndrome, hyperglycemia, and glucosuria. Pediatrics may be more susceptible to systemic toxicity. Discontinue if irritation occurs. Use appropriate antifungal or antibacterial with concomitant skin infections; discontinue if infection does not clear. Should not be used to treat rosacea or perioral dermatitis. Avoid use on face, groin, or axillae.
ADVERSE REACTIONS: Burning, stinging, irritation, pruritus, erythema, folliculitis, cracking and fissuring of the skin, numbness of fingers, skin atrophy, telangiectasia.
PREGNANCY: Category C, caution in nursing.

CLODERM
clocortolone pivalate (Healthpoint)
RX

THERAPEUTIC CLASS: Topical corticosteroid
INDICATIONS: Corticosteroid-responsive dermatoses.
DOSAGE: *Adults:* Apply tid. Use with occlusive dressing for management of psoriasis or recalcitrant conditions.
Pediatrics: Apply TID. Use with occlusive dressing for management of psoriasis or recalcitrant conditions.
HOW SUPPLIED: Cre: 0.1% (15g, 45g, 90g)
WARNINGS/PRECAUTIONS: May produce reversible HPA axis suppression, manifestations of Cushing's syndrome, hyperglycemia, glucosuria. Caution when applied to large surface areas or under occlusive dressings. Use appropriate antifungal or antibacterial agent with dermatological infections. D/C if infection is not adequately controlled or if irritation develops.
ADVERSE REACTIONS: Burning, itching, irritation, dryness, folliculitis, hypertrichosis, acneform eruptions, hypopigmentation, perioral/allergic contact dermatitis, secondary infection, skin atrophy.
PREGNANCY: Category C, caution in nursing.

CLOLAR
clofarabine (Genzyme)
RX

THERAPEUTIC CLASS: Antimetabolite
INDICATIONS: Treatment of pediatric patients 1-21 years old with relapsed or refractory acute lymphoblastic leukemia after at least two prior regimens.

COLACE

DOSAGE: *Pediatrics:* 1-21 yrs: 52mg/m^2 IV over 2 hours daily for 5 consecutive days. Treatment cycles are repeated following recovery or return to baseline organ function, approximately 2-6 weeks. Continuous IV fluids throughout 5 days of clofarabine therapy is recommended. The use of prophylactic steroids (eg, 100mg/m^2 hydrocortisone on Days 1-3) may be of benefit in preventing signs and symptoms of systemic inflammatory response syndrome (SIRS) or capillary leak. If patient develops signs and symptoms of SIRS or capillary leak, clofarabine therapy should be discontinued and appropriate supportive measures should be provided. Close monitoring of renal and hepatic function is required. If substantial increases in creatine or bilirubin occur, clofarabine therapy should be discontinued.

HOW SUPPLIED: Inj: 1mg/mL

WARNINGS/PRECAUTIONS: Suppression of bone marrow function should be anticipated. Increased risk of infection, including severe sepsis is possible. Monitor for signs and symptoms of tumor lysis syndrome, as well as cytokine release that could develop into SIRS/capillary leak syndrome and organ dysfunction. D/C immediately if SIRS or capillary leak syndrome develop. Severe bone marrow suppression, including neutropenia, anemia and thrombocytopenia have been observed. Dehydration may occur due to vomiting and diarrhea. Clofarabine should be discontinued if patient develops hypotension for any reason during the 5 days of administration. Since clofarabine is excreted primarily by the kidneys, drugs with known renal toxicity should be avoided during the 5 days of administration. Since the liver is a known target of clofarabine, concomitant use of medications known to induce hepatic toxicity should also be avoided. Patients taking medications known to affect BP or cardiac function should be closely monitored during administration.

ADVERSE REACTIONS: Vomiting, nausea, diarrhea, anemia, leukopenia, thrombocytopenia, neutropenia, febrile neutropenia, and infection.

PREGNANCY: Category D, not for use in nursing.

COLACE
docusate sodium (Purdue Products)
OTC

THERAPEUTIC CLASS: Stool softener

INDICATIONS: (PO) Stool softener for constipation, painful anorectal conditions and in cardiac conditions.

DOSAGE: *Adults:* 50-200mg/day. (Retention or Flushing Enema) Add 5-10mL of liquid to enema fluid. Mix Liq/Syr into 6-8 oz of milk or juice.

Pediatrics: ≥12 yrs: 50-200mg/day. 6-12 yrs: 40-120mg/day Liq. 3-6 yrs: 2mL Liq tid. Mix Liq/Syr into 6-8 oz of milk, juice or formula. (Retention/Flushing Enema) Add 5-10mL of liquid to enema fluid.

HOW SUPPLIED: Cap: 50mg, 100mg; Liq: 10mg/mL; Syrup: 20mg/5mL

WARNINGS/PRECAUTIONS: Avoid with abdominal pain, nausea, or vomiting. D/C enema if rectal bleeding occurs or fail to have a bowel movement.

ADVERSE REACTIONS: Bitter taste, throat irritation, nausea, rash.

PREGNANCY: Safety in pregnancy and nursing not known.

COLAZAL
balsalazide disodium (Salix)
RX

THERAPEUTIC CLASS: Anti-inflammatory Agent

INDICATIONS: Treatment of mild-to-moderate active ulcerative colitis in patients ≥5 yrs.

DOSAGE: *Adults:* 3 caps tid for up to 8 weeks (or 12 weeks if needed). May open capsule and sprinkle on applesauce.

Pediatrics: 5-17 yrs: 1 or 3 caps tid for 8 weeks. May open capsule and sprinkle on applesauce.

HOW SUPPLIED: Cap: 750mg

CONTRAINDICATIONS: Hypersensitivity to salicylates.

WARNINGS/PRECAUTIONS: May exacerbate symptoms of colitis. Prolonged gastric retention with pyloris stenosis. Caution with renal dysfunction or history of renal disease.

ADVERSE REACTIONS: Headache, abdominal pain, diarrhea, nausea, vomiting, respiratory problems, arthralgia, rhinitis, insomnia, fatigue, rectal bleeding, flatulence, fever, dyspepsia.

INTERACTIONS: Oral antibiotics may interfere with the release of mesalamine in the colon.

PREGNANCY: Category B, caution in nursing.

Coly-Mycin M
colistimethate sodium (King)

RX

THERAPEUTIC CLASS: Polypeptide antibiotic

INDICATIONS: Treatment of acute or chronic infections due to certain gram-negative bacilli (eg, *Pseudomonas aeruginosa, Enterobacter aerogenes, E. coli, Klebsiella pneumoniae*).

DOSAGE: *Adults:* Usual: 2.5-5mg/kg/day IV/IM in 2-4 divided doses. Max: 5mg/kg/day. SCr 1.3-1.5mg/dL: 2.5-3.8mg/kg/day IV/IM in 2 divided doses. SCr 1.6-2.5mg/dL: 2.5mg/kg/day IV/IM in 1-2 divided doses. SCr 2.6-4mg/dL: 1.5mg/kg/day IV/IM q36h. Obesity: Base dose on IBW.
Pediatrics: Usual: 2.5-5mg/kg/day IV/IM in 2-4 divided doses. Max: 5mg/kg/day. SCr 1.3-1.5mg/dL: 2.5-3.8mg/kg/day IV/IM in 2 divided doses. SCr 1.6-2.5mg/dL: 2.5mg/kg/day IV/IM in 1-2 divided doses. SCr 2.6-4mg/dL: 1.5mg/kg/day IV/IM q36h. Obesity: Base dose on IBW.

HOW SUPPLIED: Inj: 150mg

WARNINGS/PRECAUTIONS: Transient neurological disturbances may occur; dose reduction may alleviate symptoms. Respiratory arrest reported after IM administration. Increased risk of apnea and neuromuscular blockade with renal impairment. Reversible dose-dependent nephrotoxicity reported. Pseudomembranous colitis reported. May permit overgrowth of clostridia. Use extreme caution with renal impairment; d/c with further impairment.

ADVERSE REACTIONS: GI upset, tingling of extremities and tongue, slurred speech, dizziness, vertigo, paresthesia, itching, urticaria, rash, fever, increased BUN and creatinine, decreased creatinine clearance, respiratory distress, apnea, nephrotoxicity, decreased urine output.

INTERACTIONS: Avoid certain antibiotics (eg, aminoglycosides, polymyxin); may interfere with nerve transmission at neuromuscular junction. Extreme caution with curariform muscle relaxants (eg, tubocurarine), succinylcholine, gallamine, decamethonium and sodium citrate; may potentiate neuromuscular blocking effect. Avoid sodium cephalothin; may enhance nephrotoxicity.

PREGNANCY: Category C, caution in nursing.

Combivir
lamivudine - zidovudine (GlaxoSmithKline)

RX

> Zidovudine has been associated with hematologic toxicity (eg, granulocytopenia, severe anemia), especially with advanced HIV disease, and symptomatic myopathy reported with prolonged use. Lactic acidosis and severe, fatal hepatomegaly reported with nucleoside analogues.

THERAPEUTIC CLASS: Nucleoside analogue

INDICATIONS: Treatment of HIV infection in combination with other antiretrovirals.

DOSAGE: *Adults:* 1 tab bid. Do not give if CrCl ≤50mL/min or with dose-limiting adverse events.
Pediatrics: ≥12 yrs: 1 tab bid. Do not give if CrCl ≤50mL/min or with dose-limiting adverse events.

HOW SUPPLIED: Tab: (Lamivudine-Zidovudine) 150mg-300mg

WARNINGS/PRECAUTIONS: Caution with granulocyte count <1000cells/mm^3 or Hgb <9.5g/dL; monitor blood counts frequently with advanced HIV and periodically with asymptomatic or early HIV. Hepatic decompensation occured when used with interferon alfa w/ or w/o ribavirin. Avoid with CrCl ≤50mL/min, and hepatic impairment.

COMPAZINE

Myopathy, myositis may occur. Posttreatment exacerbation of hepatitis reported. Lamivudine-resistant hepatitis B virus reported. Caution in elderly. Possible redistribution or accumulation of body fat. Immune reconstitution syndrome reported.

ADVERSE REACTIONS: Headache, malaise, fatigue, fever, chills, nausea, diarrhea, anorexia, abdominal pain/cramps, neuropathy, insomnia, dizziness, neutropenia, musculoskeletal pain, myalgia, rash, cough, aplastic anemia, gynecomastia, oral mucosal pigmentation.

INTERACTIONS: Ganciclovir, interferon-alpha, other bone marrow suppressives and cytotoxic agents may increase the hematologic toxicity of zidovudine. Increased lamivudine exposure with trimethoprim 160mg/sulfamethoxazole 800mg. Avoid with zalcitabine, stavudine, doxorubicin, ribavirin, zidovudine, lamivudine, and fixed-dose combinations of abacavir, lamivudine, and zidovudine.

PREGNANCY: Category C, not for use in nursing.

COMPAZINE RX
prochlorperazine (GlaxoSmithKline)

OTHER BRAND NAME: Compro (Paddock)

THERAPEUTIC CLASS: Phenothiazine derivative

INDICATIONS: Control of severe nausea and vomiting. Management of psychotic disorders (eg, schizophrenia). Short-term treatment of generalized non-psychotic anxiety.

DOSAGE: *Adults:* Nausea/Vomiting: (Tab) Usual: 5-10mg tid-qid. Max: 40mg/day. (IM) 5-10mg IM q3-4h prn. Max: 40mg/day. (IV) 2.5-10mg IV (not bolus). Max: 10mg single dose and 40mg/day. Nausea/Vomiting with Surgery: 5-10mg IM 1-2 hrs or 5-10mg IV 15-30 minutes before anesthesia, or during or after surgery; repeat once if needed. Non-Psychotic Anxiety: (Tab) 5mg tid-qid; Psychosis: Mild/Outpatient: 5-10mg PO tid-qid. Moderate-Severe/Hospitalized: Initial: 10mg PO tid-qid. May increase in small increments every 2-3 days. Severe: (PO) 100-150mg/day. (IM) 10-20mg, may repeat q2-4 hrs if needed. Switch to oral after obtain control or if needed, 10-20mg IM q4-6h. Elderly: use lower dosing range and titrate more gradually.
Pediatrics: Nausea/Vomiting: >2 yrs and >20lbs: (PO/PR) 20-29 lbs: Usual: 2.5mg qd-bid. Max: 7.5mg/day. 30-39 lbs: 2.5mg bid-tid. Max: 10mg/day. 40-85 lbs: 2.5mg tid or 5mg bid. Max: 15mg/day. (IM) 0.06mg/lb, usually single dose for control. Psychosis: (PO/PR) 2-12 yrs: Initial: 2.5mg bid-tid, up to 10mg/day on 1st day. Max: 2-5 yrs: 20mg/day. 6-12 yrs: 25mg/day. (IM) <12 yrs: 0.06mg/lb single dose. Switch to oral after obtain control.

HOW SUPPLIED: Inj: (Comazine as edisylate) 5mg/mL; Sup: (Compazine as edisylate) 2.5mg, (Compro) 25mg; Tab: (Compazine as maleate) 5mg, 10mg

CONTRAINDICATIONS: Comatose states, concomitant large dose CNS depressants (alcohol, barbiturates, narcotics), pediatric surgery, pediatrics <2 yrs or <20 lbs.

WARNINGS/PRECAUTIONS: Secondary extrapyramidal symptoms can occur. Tardive dyskinesia, NMS may develop. Caution with activities requiring alertness. May mask symptoms of overdose of other drugs. May obscure diagnosis of intestinal obstruction, brain tumor, and Reye's syndrome. May interfere with thermoregulation. Caution with glaucoma, cardiac disorders. Caution in children with dehydration or acute illness and the elderly. Discontinue 48 hrs before myelography and may resume after 24 hrs postprocedure.

ADVERSE REACTIONS: Drowsiness, dizziness, amenorrhea, blurred vision, skin reactions, hypotension, NMS, cholestatic jaundice.

INTERACTIONS: Decreases oral anticoagulant effects. Potentiates α-adrenergic blockade. Thiazide diuretics potentiate orthostatic hypotension. Increased levels of both drugs with propranolol. Anticonvulsants may need adjustment. Risk of encephalopathic syndrome with lithium. Antagonizes antihypertensive effects of guanethidine and related compounds.

PREGNANCY: Safety in pregnancy is not known; caution in nursing.

CONCERTA CII
methylphenidate HCl (McNeil Consumer)

THERAPEUTIC CLASS: Sympathomimetic amine

INDICATIONS: Treatment of attention deficit hyperactivity disorder (ADHD) in patients ≥6 years old.

DOSAGE: Adults: Methylphenidate-Naive or Receiving Other Stimulant: Initial: 18mg qam. Titrate: Adjust dose at weekly intervals. Previous Methylphenidate Use: Initial: 18mg qam if previous dose 10-15mg/day; 36mg qam if previous dose 20-30mg/day; 54mg qam if previous dose 30-45mg/day. Initial conversion should not exceed 54mg/day. Titrate: Adjust dose at weekly intervals. Max: 72mg/day. Reduce dose or discontinue if paradoxical aggravation of symptoms occurs. Discontinue if no improvement after appropriate dosage adjustments over 1 month. Swallow whole with liquids. Do not crush, chew, or divide.

Pediatrics: ≥6 yrs: Methylphenidate-Naive or Receiving Other Stimulant: Initial: 18mg qam. Titrate: Adjust dose at weekly intervals. Max: 6-12 yrs: 54mg/day; 13-17 yrs: 72mg/day not to exceed 2mg/kg/day. Previous Methylphenidate Use: Initial: 18mg qam if previous dose 10-15mg/day; 36mg qam if previous dose 20-30mg/day; 54mg qam if previous dose 30-45mg/day. Initial conversion should not exceed 54mg/day. Titrate: Adjust dose at weekly intervals. Max: 72mg/day. Reduce dose or discontinue if paradoxical aggravation of symptoms occurs. Discontinue if no improvement after appropriate dosage adjustments over 1 month. Swallow whole with liquids. Do not crush, chew, or divide.

HOW SUPPLIED: Tab, Extended-Release: 18mg, 27mg, 36mg, 54mg

CONTRAINDICATIONS: Marked anxiety, tension, and agitation; glaucoma; motor tics or family history or diagnosis of Tourette's syndrome, during or within 14 days of MAOI use.

WARNINGS/PRECAUTIONS: Monitor growth during treatment in children. Not for severe depression or fatigue. May exacerbate symptoms of behavior disturbance and thought disorder in psychotic patients. Avoid with severe GI narrowing (eg, esophageal motility disorders, small bowel inflammatory disease, short-gut syndrome). May lower seizure threshold, especially in known EEG abnormalities. Caution with HTN, conditions affected by BP or HR elevation, history of drug abuse or alcoholism. Monitor during withdrawal from abusive use. Visual disturbances may occur (rare). Monitor CBC, differential, and platelets with prolonged use. Caution when using stimulants to treat patients with comorbid bipolar disorder because of concern for possible induction of mixed/manic episode in such patients. Stimulants at usual does can cause treatment emergent psychotic or manic symptoms (eg, hallucinations, delusional thinking, mania) in children and adolescents without prior history of psychotic illness. Aggressive behavior or hostility reported in clinical trials and postmarketing experience of some medications indicated for the treatment of ADHD. Avoid with known structural cardiac abnormalities or other serious cardiac problems.

ADVERSE REACTIONS: Headache, abdominal pain, anorexia, insomnia, upper respiratory tract infection.

INTERACTIONS: Avoid MAOIs. Potentiates anticoagulants, anticonvulsants (eg, phenobarbital, phenytoin, primidone), TCAs, and SSRIs. Caution with α_2-agonists (eg, clonidine) and pressor agents.

PREGNANCY: Category C, caution in nursing.

Cordran
flurandrenolide (Watson)

RX

OTHER BRAND NAME: Cordran SP (Watson)

THERAPEUTIC CLASS: Corticosteroid

INDICATIONS: Treatment of corticosteroid responsive dermatoses.

DOSAGE: *Adults:* (Cre, Lot) Apply qd-qid depending on severity. For moist lesions, apply cream bid-tid. Apply lotion bid-tid. (Tape) Clean and dry skin. Shave or clip hair. Apply tape q12-24h.

Pediatrics: (Cre, Lot) Apply qd-qid depending on severity. For moist lesions, apply cream bid-tid. Apply lotion bid-tid. (Tape) Clean and dry skin. Shave or clip hair. Apply tape q12-24h.

HOW SUPPLIED: Cre (SP): 0.05% (15g, 30g, 60g); Lot: 0.05% (15mL, 60mL); Tape: 4mcg/cm^2

CONTRAINDICATIONS: (Tape) Not for lesions exuding serum or in intertriginous areas.

WARNINGS/PRECAUTIONS: Systemic absorption may produce reversible HPA axis suppression, manifestations of Cushing's syndrome, hyperglycemia, and glucosuria. Appli-

CORMAX

cation of more potent steroids, use on large surfaces, prolonged use, or occlusive dressings may augment systemic absorption. Evaluate periodically for HPA suppression if large dose applied to large area or with occlusive dressings. Pediatrics are more susceptible to toxicity. D/C if irritation develops. May use occlusive dressing for psoriasis or recalcitrant conditions.

ADVERSE REACTIONS: Burning, itching, irritation, dryness, folliculitis, hypertrichosis, acneform eruptions, hypopigmentation, dermatitis. Occlusive dressing may cause skin maceration, secondary infection, skin atrophy, miliaria.

PREGNANCY: Category C, caution in nursing.

CORMAX   RX
clobetasol propionate (Watson)

OTHER BRAND NAME: Cormax Scalp (Watson)
THERAPEUTIC CLASS: Corticosteroid
INDICATIONS: Corticosteroid responsive dermatoses.
DOSAGE: *Adults:* Apply bid. Limit treatment to 2 consecutive weeks. Max: 50g/week or 50mL/week.
Pediatrics: ≥12 yrs: (Cre, Sol) Apply bid. Limit treatment to 2 consecutive weeks. Max: 50g/week or 50mL/week.
HOW SUPPLIED: Cre: 0.05% (15g, 30g, 45g); Sol (Scalp): 0.05% (25mL, 50mL)
CONTRAINDICATIONS: Primary infections of the scalp with solution.
WARNINGS/PRECAUTIONS: Not for treatment of rosacea or perioral dermatitis. May produce reversible HPA axis suppression, manifestations of Cushing's syndrome, hyperglycemia, and glucosuria. Reassess diagnosis if no improvement after 2 weeks. D/C if irritation occurs. Pediatrics may be more susceptible to systemic toxicity. Use appropriate antifungal or antibacterial agent with dermatological infections. Avoid occlusive dressings.
ADVERSE REACTIONS: Burning, stinging, pruritus, skin atrophy, cracking/fissuring of skin, irritation, (sol) tingling, (sol) folliculitis.
PREGNANCY: Category C, caution in nursing.

CORTANE-B   RX
chloroxylenol - hydrocortisone - pramoxine HCl (Blansett)

OTHER BRAND NAME: Zoto HC (Sciele)
THERAPEUTIC CLASS: Antimicrobial/Corticosteroid/Topical anesthetic
INDICATIONS: Treatment of superficial infections of the external ear and to control inflammation and itching.
DOSAGE: *Adults:* Instill 4-5 drops tid-qid. A gauze or wick may be inserted into ear canal after first administration. Add additional drops to saturate wick q4h. Remove wick after 24 hrs and continue to instill. Do not treat for >10 days.
Pediatrics: Instill 3 drops tid-qid. A gauze or wick may be inserted into ear canal after first administration. Add additional drops to saturate wick q4h. Remove wick after 24 hrs and continue to instill. Do not treat for >10 days.
HOW SUPPLIED: Sol: (Chloroxylenol-Hydrocortisone-Pramoxine) 1mg-10mg-10mg/mL (10mL)
CONTRAINDICATIONS: Varicella, vaccinia, perforated ear drum or when medication can reach the middle ear.
WARNINGS/PRECAUTIONS: Caution in long-standing otitis media. If local irritation or sensitization occurs, discontinue. Systemic absorption has produced HPA axis, manifestations of Cushing's syndrome, hyperglycemia, and glucosuria.
ADVERSE REACTIONS: Itching, burning, irritation, dryness, folliculitis, hypertrichosis, acneform eruptions, hypopigmentations.
PREGNANCY: Category C, caution in nursing.

CORTEF   RX
hydrocortisone (Pharmacia & Upjohn)

THERAPEUTIC CLASS: Corticosteroid
INDICATIONS: Steroid responsive disorders.

DOSAGE: *Adults:* Initial: 20-240mg/day depending on disease. Adjust until a satisfactory response. Maint: Decrease in small amounts to lowest effective dose. Acute Exacerbations of Multiple Sclerosis: Initial: (Tab) 200mg/day of prednisolone for 1 week, then 80mg every other day for 1 month (20mg hydrocortisone=5mg prednisolone).
Pediatrics: Initial: 20-240mg/day depending on disease. Adjust until a satisfactory response. Maint: After favorable response, decrease in small amounts to lowest effective dose. Acute Exacerbations of Multiple Sclerosis: Initial: (Tab) 200mg/day of prednisolone for 1 week, then 80mg every other day for 1 month (20mg hydrocortisone=5mg prednisolone).
HOW SUPPLIED: Sus: (Hydrocortisone Cypionate) 10mg/5mL (120mL); Tab: (Hydrocortisone) 5mg, 10mg, 20mg
CONTRAINDICATIONS: Systemic fungal infections.
WARNINGS/PRECAUTIONS: May need to increase dose before, during, and after stressful situations. May mask signs of infections. Avoid abrupt withdrawal. Prolonged use may produce glaucoma, optic nerve damage, secondary ocular infections. Increases BP, salt/water retention, potassium excretion. More severe/fatal course of infections reported with chickenpox, measles. Caution with TB, hypothyroidism, cirrhosis, ocular herpes simplex, HTN, diverticulitis, fresh intestinal anastomosis, ulcerative colitis, osteoporosis, myasthenia gravis, renal insufficiency, peptic ulcer disease. Growth and development of children on prolonged therapy should be monitored. Monitor for psychic disturbances. Kaposi's sarcoma reported.
ADVERSE REACTIONS: Fluid and electrolyte disturbances, HTN, osteoporosis, muscle weakness, cushingoid state, menstrual irregularities, nervousness, insomnia, impaired wound healing, DM, ulcerative esophagitis, excessive sweating, increases intracranial pressure, carbohydrate intolerance, glaucoma, cataracts.
INTERACTIONS: Reduced efficacy and increased clearance with hepatic enzyme inducers (eg, phenobarbital, phenytoin, and rifampin). Decreased clearance with ketoconazole and troleandomycin. Increases clearance of chronic high dose ASA; caution with hypoprothrombinemia. Effects on oral anticoagulants are variable; monitor PT. Increased insulin and oral hypoglycemic requirements in DM. Avoid live vaccines with immunosuppressive doses. Possible decreased vaccine response with killed or inactivated vaccines with immunosuppressive doses.
PREGNANCY: Safety in pregnancy and nursing not known.

Cortisporin Otic
neomycin - hydrocortisone - polymyxin B sulfate (King)

RX

THERAPEUTIC CLASS: Antibacterial/corticosteroid combination
INDICATIONS: (Sol/Sus) Treatment of superficial bacterial infections of the external auditory canal. (Sus) Treatment of infections of mastoidectomy and fenestration cavities.
DOSAGE: *Adults:* Clean and dry ear canal. Dropper: 4 drops tid-qid for up to 10 days. Alternate Regimen: Insert cotton wick into ear canal, then saturate cotton. Repeat q4h to keep cotton moist. Replace wick q24h.
Pediatrics: Clean and dry ear canal. Dropper: 3 drops tid-qid for up to 10 days. Alternate Regimen: Insert cotton wick into ear canal, then saturate cotton. Repeat q4h to keep cotton moist. Replace wick q24h.
HOW SUPPLIED: Sol, Sus: (Neomycin-Hydrocortisone-Polymyxin B) 0.35%-1%-10,000 U/mL (10mL)
CONTRAINDICATIONS: Herpes simplex, vaccinia, and varicella infections.
WARNINGS/PRECAUTIONS: Caution with perforated eardrum, chronic otitis media. Prolonged use may result in secondary infection. Re-evaluate if no improvement after 1 week. D/C after 10 days. Solution contains sulfites. May cause cutaneous sensitization.
ADVERSE REACTIONS: Skin sensitization, burning, itching, irritation, dryness, folliculitis, hypertrichosis, acneiform eruptions, secondary infection.
PREGNANCY: Category C, caution in nursing.

Cortisporin-TC Otic
colistin sulfate - neomycin sulfate - thonzonium bromide - hydrocortisone acetate (King)

RX

THERAPEUTIC CLASS: Antibacterial/corticosteroid combination
INDICATIONS: Treatment of infections of the external auditory canal, mastoidectomy and fenestration cavities.

CORTROSYN

DOSAGE: *Adults:* Clean and dry ear canal. Dropper: 5 drops (calibrated dropper) or 4 drops (dropper bottle) tid-qid. Alternate Regimen: Insert cotton wick into ear canal, then saturate cotton. Repeat q4h to keep cotton moist. Replace wick q24h.
Pediatrics: Clean and dry ear canal. Dropper: 4 drops (calibrated dropper) or 3 drops (dropper bottle) tid-qid. Alternate Regimen: Insert cotton wick into ear canal, then saturate cotton. Repeat q4h to keep cotton moist. Replace wick q24h.

HOW SUPPLIED: (Colistin-Hydrocortisone-Neomycin-Thonzonium) Sus: 3mg-10mg-3.3mg-0.5mg/mL (10mL)

CONTRAINDICATIONS: Herpes simplex, vaccinia, and varicella infections.

WARNINGS/PRECAUTIONS: Caution with perforated eardrum, chronic otitis media. Prolonged use may result in secondary infection. Re-evaluate if no improvement after 1 week. D/C after 10 days.

ADVERSE REACTIONS: Cutaneous sensitization.

PREGNANCY: Safety in pregnancy and nursing not known.

CORTROSYN   RX
cosyntropin (Amphastar)

THERAPEUTIC CLASS: Synthetic ACTH

INDICATIONS: Diagnostic agent used to screen for adrenocortical insufficiency.

DOSAGE: *Adults:* 0.25-0.75mg IM/IV injection or 0.25-0.75mg IV over 4-8 hrs. (See labeling for method details).
Pediatrics: >2 yrs: 0.25-0.75mg IM/IV injection or 0.25-0.75mg IV over 4-8 hrs. ≤2 yrs: 0.125mg IM/IV injection or IV over 4-8 hrs. (See labeling for method details).

HOW SUPPLIED: Inj: 0.25mg

WARNINGS/PRECAUTIONS: Exhibits slight immunologic activity. Patients known to be sensitized to natural ACTH with markedly positive skin tests will, with few exceptions, react negatively when tested intradermally. Falsely high fluorescence measurements with high plasma bilirubin or if plasma contains free Hgb.

ADVERSE REACTIONS: Hypersensitivity/anaphylactic reactions (rare), bradycardia, tachycardia, HTN, peripheral edema, rash.

INTERACTIONS: May potentiate electrolyte loss associated with diuretics.

PREGNANCY: Category C, caution in nursing.

COSMEGEN   RX
dactinomycin (Ovation)

> Drug is highly toxic; handle and administer with care. Avoid inhalation or contact with skin and mucous membranes. Extremely corrosive to soft tissue. Severe damage to soft tissue will occur with extravasation during IV use.

THERAPEUTIC CLASS: Actinomycin antibiotic

INDICATIONS: Concomitant treatment of Wilms' tumor, childhood rhabdomyosarcoma, Ewing's sarcoma, and metastatic nonseminomatous testicular carcinoma. Monotherapy for gestational trophoblastic neoplasia, and as palliative and/or adjunctive treatment of solid malignancies.

DOSAGE: *Adults:* Wilms' Tumor/Childhood Rhabdomyosarcoma/Ewing's Sarcoma: 15mcg/kg IV daily for 5 days. Testicular Cancer: 1000mcg/m^2 IV on day 1 of combination therapy. Gestational Trophoblastic Neoplasia: Monotherapy: 12mcg/kg IV daily for 5 days. Combination Therapy: 500mcg/m^2 IV on days 1 and 2. Solid Malignancies: 50mcg/kg IV for lower extremity or pelvis. 35mcg/kg IV for upper extremity. May need lower dose with obese patients, or with previous chemotherapy or radiation use. Dose intensity per 2-week cycle should not exceed 15mcg/kg/day or 400-600mcg/m^2 daily for 5 days. Calculate dose for obese or edematous patients based on BSA. Elderly: Start at low end of dosing range.
Pediatrics: >6-12 months: Wilms' Tumor, Childhood Rhabdomyosarcoma/Ewing's Sarcoma: 15mcg/kg IV daily for 5 days. Testicular Carcinoma: 1000mcg/m^2 IV on day 1 of combination therapy. Gestational Trophoblastic Neoplasia: Monotherapy: 12mcg/kg IV

daily for 5 days. Combination Therapy: 500mcg/m² IV on days 1 and 2. Solid Malignancies: 50mcg/kg IV for lower extremity or pelvis. 35mcg/kg IV for upper extremity. May need lower dose with obese patients, or with previous chemotherapy or radiation use. Dose intensity per 2-week cycle should not exceed 15mcg/kg/day or 400-600mcg/m² daily for 5 days. Calculate dose for obese or edematous patients based on BSA.

HOW SUPPLIED: Inj: 0.5mg

CONTRAINDICATIONS: At or about the time of infection with chickenpox or herpes zoster.

WARNINGS/PRECAUTIONS: Monitor renal, hepatic, and bone marrow functions frequently. Can cause fetal harm during pregnancy. Possible anaphylactoid reactions. If stomatitis, diarrhea, or severe hematopoietic depression occurs; d/c until recovery. Caution in elderly; increased risk of myelosuppression. Veno-occlusive disease (primarily hepatic) reported.

ADVERSE REACTIONS: Nausea, vomiting, fatigue, lethargy, fever, cheilitis, esophagitis, abdominal pain, liver toxicity, anemia, blood dyscrasias, skin eruptions, acne, alopecia.

INTERACTIONS: Increased GI toxicity, marrow suppression, and incidence of secondary tumors with radiation. May reactivate erythema from previous radiation therapy. Caution if used within 2 months of irradiation for treatment of right-sided Wilms' tumor; hepatomegaly and elevated AST levels reported. Only use with radiotherapy for Wilms' tumor if benefit outweighs risks.

PREGNANCY: Category D, not for use in nursing.

Cosopt
dorzolamide HCl - timolol maleate (Merck)

RX

THERAPEUTIC CLASS: Carbonic anhydrase inhibitor/nonselective beta-blocker

INDICATIONS: Treatment of ocular hypertension and open-angle glaucoma insufficiently responsive to β-blockers.

DOSAGE: *Adults:* 1 drop bid. Space dosing of other ophthalmic drugs by 10 minutes.
Pediatrics: ≥2 yrs: 1 drop bid. Space dosing of other ophthalmic drugs by 10 minutes.

HOW SUPPLIED: Sol: (Dorzolamide-Timolol) 2%-0.5% (5mL, 10mL)

CONTRAINDICATIONS: Bronchial asthma, history of bronchial asthma, severe COPD, sinus bradycardia, 2nd- or 3rd-degree AV block, overt cardiac failure, cardiogenic shock.

WARNINGS/PRECAUTIONS: Caution with sulfonamide allergy, cardiac failure, DM, COPD, bronchospastic disease, surgery and hepatic impairment. May mask symptoms of hypoglycemia and thyrotoxicosis. Bacterial keratitis reported with contaminated containers. Avoid in severe renal impairment. D/C if hypersensitivity or ocular reaction occur. Reinsert contact lenses 15 minutes after applying drops.

ADVERSE REACTIONS: Taste perversion, ocular burning, conjunctival hyperemia, blurred vision, superficial punctate keratitis, eye itching.

INTERACTIONS: Avoid oral carbonic anhydrase inhibitors, oral β-blockers, or topical β-blockers due to potential additive effects. Oral/IV calcium antagonists can cause AV-conduction disturbances, left ventricular failure or hypotension. Potentiated systemic β-blockade with concomitant CYP2D6 inhibitors. Reserpine can cause additive effects, hypotension and/or bradycardia. AV conduction time prolonged with digitalis. Quinidine may potentiate β-blockade. Increased risk of hypoglycemia with insulin or oral hypoglycemic agents. Wait 10 minutes before using another ophthalmic drug.

PREGNANCY: Category C, not for use in nursing.

Cotazym
lipase - amylase - protease (Organon)

RX

THERAPEUTIC CLASS: Pancreatic enzyme supplement

INDICATIONS: Treatment of steatorrhea due to exocrine pancreatic enzyme deficiency such conditions as cystic fibrosis and chronic pancreatitis.

CROFAB

DOSAGE: *Adults:* Individualize dose according to patient's remaining exocrine pancreatic function, gut lumen pH, and intake of fat and protein. Cystic Fibrosis: Usual: 2500 U lipase/kg/meal. Max: 6000 U lipase/kg/meal. Chronic Pancreatitis: Initial: 1-2 caps. Titrate: Adjust as needed.

Pediatrics: Infants: Usual: 2000-4000 U lipase/120mL of formula or each breast feeding. <4 yrs: Initial: 1000 U lipase/kg/meal. ≥4 yrs: Initial: 500 U lipase/kg/meal. For a snack, take 50% dose for a meal.

HOW SUPPLIED: Cap: (Amylase-Lipase-Protease) 30,000U-8000U-30,000U

CONTRAINDICATIONS: Hypersensitivity to antigens of porcine origin.

WARNINGS/PRECAUTIONS: Large doses of extended-release preparations associated with fibrosing colonopathy in cystic fibrosis. May interfere with folic acid absorption. Supplement with folic acid before and during pregnancy. Avoid inhalation or contact with hands when opening capsules; wear mask and gloves.

ADVERSE REACTIONS: Diarrhea, stool abnormalities, pharyngitis, vomiting, abdominal pain, gastric burning, syncope, mouth irritation/ulcers, anemia, abnormal smell and taste.

INTERACTIONS: Avoid calcium carbonate and magnesium hydroxide combination products (eg, antacids, supplements); may decrease fat absorption and increase steatorrhea. May interfere with folic acid and iron absorption.

PREGNANCY: Category C, caution in nursing.

CROFAB
crotalidae polyvalent immune fab (ovine) (Savage)

RX

THERAPEUTIC CLASS: Venom specific immunoglobulin Fab fragment

INDICATIONS: Management of minimal to moderate North American crotalid envenomation. Use within 6 hrs to prevent clinical deterioration and systemic coagulation abnormalities.

DOSAGE: *Adults:* Initial: 4-6 vials IV over 60 minutes. Observe patient for 1 hr following dose to determine if envenomation is controlled. If needed, administer additional 4-6 vials until envenomation controlled. Once control is achieved, give 2 vials q6h for up to 18 hrs (3 doses). Additional 2-vial doses may be given based on clinical course.

Pediatrics: Initial: 4-6 vials IV over 60 minutes. Observe patient for 1 hr following dose to determine if envenomation is controlled. If needed, administer additional 4-6 vials until envenomation controlled. Once control is achieved, give 2 vials q6h for up to 18 hrs (3 doses). Additional 2-vial doses may be given based on clinical course.

HOW SUPPLIED: Inj: 1g/vial

CONTRAINDICATIONS: Hypersensitivity to papaya or papain.

WARNINGS/PRECAUTIONS: Recurrent coagulopathy may persist for 1-2 weeks; monitor for symptoms. Risk of anaphylactic reaction. Sensitization may occur; caution with a repeat course of treatment for subsequent envenomation episode. Contains ethyl mercury; use with caution in children. Use caution with conditions that cause coagulation defects (eg, cancer, collagen disease, CHF, diarrhea, elevated temperature, hepatic disorders, hyperthyroidism, poor nutritional state, steatorrhea, vitamin K deficiency.

ADVERSE REACTIONS: Urticaria, rash.

PREGNANCY: Category C, caution in nursing.

CUPRIMINE
penicillamine (Aton)

RX

> Supervise closely due to toxicity, special dosage considerations, and therapeutic benefits.

OTHER BRAND NAME: Depen (Wallace)

THERAPEUTIC CLASS: Copper chelating agent

INDICATIONS: Treatment of Wilson's disease, cystinuria, and severe, active rheumatoid arthritis (RA) when conventional therapy has failed.

DOSAGE: *Adults:* Wilson's Disease: Determine dosage by 24-hr urinary copper excretion. Maint: 0.75-1.5g/day for 3 months. Max: Up to 2g/day, based on serum free copper. Cystinuria: Initial: 250mg qd. Usual: 250mg-1g qid. RA: Initial: 125-250mg/day. Titrate: May increase by 125-250mg/day every 1-3 months. If needed after 2-3 months, increase by 250mg/day every 2-3 months. D/C if no improvement after 3-4 months at dose of 1-1.5g/day. Maint: 500-750mg/day. Max: 1.5g/day. Give on empty stomach, 1 hr before or 2 hrs after meals, and 1 hr apart from any other drug, food or milk. Supplemental pyridoxine 25mg/day recommended.

Pediatrics: Cystinuria: 30mg/kg/day given qid.

HOW SUPPLIED: Cap: (Cuprimine): 250mg; Tab: (Depen) 250mg* *scored

CONTRAINDICATIONS: Pregnancy (except for treatment of Wilson's disease or certain cases of cystinuria), nursing, RA patients with renal insufficiency, history of penicillamine-related aplastic anemia or agranulocytosis.

WARNINGS/PRECAUTIONS: Aplastic anemia, agranulocytosis, drug fever, thrombocytopenia, Goodpasture's syndrome, myasthenia gravis, pemphigus foliaceus/vulgaris, obliterative bronchiolitis, proteinuria and hematuria reported. Routine urinalysis, CBC with differentials, Hgb and platelet count every 2 weeks for 6 months, then monthly.

ADVERSE REACTIONS: Rash, urticaria, anorexia, epigastric pain, nausea, vomiting, diarrhea, leukopenia, thrombocytopenia, proteinuria.

INTERACTIONS: Hematologic and renal adverse reactions increase with gold therapy, antimalarial or cytotoxic drugs, oxyphenbutazone and phenylbutazone. Systemic levels lowered by iron; separate doses by 2 hrs. Mineral supplements may block response to therapy.

PREGNANCY: Category D, not for use in nursing.

CUTIVATE RX
fluticasone propionate (GlaxoSmithKline)

THERAPEUTIC CLASS: Corticosteroid

INDICATIONS: Corticosteroid responsive dermatoses.

DOSAGE: *Adults:* (Cre) Atopic Dermatitis: Apply qd-bid. Other Dermatoses: Apply bid. Re-evaluate if no improvement after 2 weeks. (Oint) Apply bid. Avoid occlusive dressings.

Pediatrics: ≥3 months: (Cre) Atopic Dermatitis: Apply qd-bid. Other Dermatoses: Apply bid. Reassess if no improvement after 2 weeks. Avoid in diaper area. Oint not approved in peds. Avoid occlusive dressings.

HOW SUPPLIED: Cre: 0.05% (15g, 30g, 60g); Oint: 0.005% (15g, 30g, 60g)

WARNINGS/PRECAUTIONS: Caution with cre in peds. May produce reversible HPA axis suppression, manifestations of Cushing's syndrome, hyperglycemia, and glucosuria. D/C if irritation occurs. Use appropriate antifungal or antibacterial agent with dermatological infections. Peds may be more susceptible to systemic toxicity. Caution when applied to large surface areas. Avoid with pre-existing skin atrophy. Not for use in rosacea or perioral dermatitis.

ADVERSE REACTIONS: Stinging, burning, dryness, pruritus, erythema, irritation, hypertrichosis.

PREGNANCY: Category C, caution in nursing.

CYANIDE ANTIDOTE PACKAGE RX
amyl nitrite - sodium nitrite - sodium thiosulfate (Akorn)

THERAPEUTIC CLASS: Antidote

INDICATIONS: Treatment of cyanide poisoning.

DOSAGE: *Adults:* Apply 1 ampule of Amyl Nitrite to a handkerchief and hold in front of patient's mouth for 15 seconds followed by a rest for 15 seconds. Then reapply until

CYCLOCORT

Sodium Nitrite can be administered. Discontinue Amyl Nitrite and give Sodium Nitrite IV 300mg at the rate of 2.5-5mL/minute. Immediately after, inject 12.5g of Sodium Thiosulfate. If the poison was taken by mouth, gastric lavage should be performed as soon as possible. If signs of poisoning reappear, repeat Sodium Nitrite and Sodium Thiosulfate at one-half the original dose.

Pediatrics: Apply 1 ampule of Amyl Nitrite to a handkerchief and hold in front of patient's mouth for 15 seconds followed by a rest for 15 seconds. Then reapply until Sodium Nitrite can be administered. Discontinue Amyl Nitrite and give 6-8mL/m^2 of Sodium Nitrite IV; max: 10mL. Immediately after, inject 7g/m^2 of Sodium Thiosulfate; max: 12.5g. If the poison was taken by mouth, gastric lavage should be performed as soon as possible. If signs of poisoning reappear, repeat Sodium Nitrite and Sodium Thiosulfate at one-half the original dose.

HOW SUPPLIED: Sodium Nitrite: 300mg/10mL (2 ampules); Sodium Thiosulfate: 12.5mg/50mL (2 vials); Amyl Nitrite Inhalant: 0.3mL (12 ampules)

WARNINGS/PRECAUTIONS: Sodium Nitrite and Amyl Nitrite in high doses induce methemoglobinemia and can cause death.

PREGNANCY: Safety in pregnancy and nursing is not known.

CYCLOCORT RX
amcinonide (Astellas)

THERAPEUTIC CLASS: Corticosteroid

INDICATIONS: Corticosteroid responsive dermatoses.

DOSAGE: *Adults:* Apply bid-tid depending on severity.
Pediatrics: Apply bid-tid depending on severity.

HOW SUPPLIED: Cre, Oint: 0.1% (15g, 30g, 60g); Lot: 0.1% (20mL, 60mL)

WARNINGS/PRECAUTIONS: Systemic absorption may produce reversible HPA axis suppression, manifestations of Cushing's syndrome, hyperglycemia, and glucosuria. Discontinue if irritation occurs. Use appropriate antifungal or antibacterial agent with dermatological infections. Pediatrics may be more susceptible to systemic toxicity. Caution when applied to large surface areas or with occlusive dressings.

ADVERSE REACTIONS: Itching, stinging, soreness, burning, irritation, folliculitis, hypertrichosis, hypopigmentation, perioral dermatitis, skin maceration, striae, miliaria, skin atrophy, secondary infection, contact dermatitis.

PREGNANCY: Category C, not for use in nursing.

CYPROHEPTADINE RX
cyproheptadine HCl (Various)

THERAPEUTIC CLASS: Serotonin/histamine antagonist

INDICATIONS: Perennial and seasonal rhinitis, vasomotor rhinitis, allergic conjunctivitis, uncomplicated allergic skin manifestations, blood or plasma allergic reactions, cold urticaria, and dermatographism. Adjunct to anaphylaxis.

DOSAGE: *Adults:* Initial: 4mg tid. Usual: 4-20mg/day. Max: 0.5mg/kg/day.
Pediatrics: 7-14 yrs: Usual: 4mg bid-tid. Max: 16mg/day. 2-6 yrs: Usual: 2mg bid-tid or 0.25mg/kg/day. Max: 12mg/day.

HOW SUPPLIED: Syrup: 2mg/5mL; Tab: 4mg* *scored

CONTRAINDICATIONS: Newborn or premature infants, nursing mothers, concomitant MAOIs, angle-closure glaucoma, stenosing peptic ulcer, symptomatic prostatic hypertrophy, bladder neck obstruction, pyloroduodenal obstruction, elderly, debilitated.

WARNINGS/PRECAUTIONS: Caution with bronchial asthma, increased IOP, hyperthyroidism, CVD, HTN, and elderly. May impair mental/physical abilities.

ADVERSE REACTIONS: Drowsiness, somnolence, sedation, dizziness, confusion, restlessness, excitation, nervousness, insomnia, blurred vision, hypotension, palpitation, dry mouth, urinary frequency and retention.

INTERACTIONS: Avoid MAOIs. Additive effects with alcohol and other CNS depressants.

PREGNANCY: Category B, not for use in nursing.

Cytomel
liothyronine sodium (King)
RX

THERAPEUTIC CLASS: Thyroid replacement hormone

INDICATIONS: Hypothyroidism. As a pituitary TSH suppressant in the treatment and prevention of euthyroid goiters, including thyroid nodules, and Hashimoto's and multinodular goiter. Diagnostic agent in suppression tests to differentiate mild hyperthyroidism or thyroid gland autonomy.

DOSAGE: *Adults:* Mild Hypothyroidism: Initial: 25mcg qd. Titrate: May increase by up to 25mcg qd every 1-2 weeks. Maint: 25-75mcg qd. Myxedema: Initial: 5mcg qd. Titrate: May increase by 5-10mcg qd every 1-2 weeks up to 25mcg qd, then increase by 5-25mcg qd every 1-2 weeks. Maint: 50-100mcg/day. Goiter: Initial: 5mcg/day. Titrate: May increase by 5-10mcg qd every 1-2 weeks up to 25mcg qd, then by 12.5-25mcg qd every 1-2 weeks. Maint: 75mcg qd. Elderly/Coronary Artery Disease: Initial: 5mcg qd. Titrate: Increase by no more than 5mcg qd every 2 weeks. Thyroid Suppression Therapy: 75-100mcg qd for 7 days. Radioactive iodine uptake is determined before and after administration of hormone.

Pediatrics: Congenital Hypothyroidism: Initial: 5mcg qd. Titrate: Increase by 5mcg qd every 3-4 days until desired response. Maint: <1 yr: 20mcg qd. 1-3yrs: 50mcg qd. >3 yrs: 25-75mcg/day.

HOW SUPPLIED: Tab: 5mcg, 25mcg*, 50mcg* *scored

CONTRAINDICATIONS: Uncorrected adrenal cortical insufficiency and untreated thyrotoxicosis.

WARNINGS/PRECAUTIONS: Do not use in the treatment of obesity; larger doses in euthyroid patients can cause serious or even life threatening toxicity. Caution with angina pectoris and elderly; use lower doses. Rule out hypogonadism and nephrosis prior to therapy. With prolonged and severe hypothyroidism supplement with adrenocortical steroids. May aggravate diabetes mellitus or insipidus and adrenal cortical insufficiency. Add glucocorticoid with myxedema coma. Excessive doses may cause craniosynostosis in infants.

ADVERSE REACTIONS: Allergic skin reactions (rare).

INTERACTIONS: Hypothyroidism decreases and hyperthyroidism increases sensitivity to oral anticoagulants; monitor PT/INR. Monitor insulin and oral hypoglycemic requirements. Decreased absorption with cholestyramine; space dosing by 4-5 hrs. Large dose may cause life-threatening toxicities with sympathomimetic amines. Estrogens increase thyroxine-binding globulin; increase in thyroid dose may be needed. Additive effects of both agents with TCAs. HTN and tachycardia with ketamine. May potentiate digitalis toxicity. Increased adrenergic effects of catecholamines; caution with CAD.

PREGNANCY: Category A, caution in nursing.

Cytosar-U
cytarabine (Pharmacia & Upjohn)
RX

> Associated with bone marrow suppression, nausea, vomiting, oral ulceration, hepatic dysfunction, diarrhea, and abdominal pain. For induction therapy, treat in a facility able to monitor drug tolerance and toxicity.

THERAPEUTIC CLASS: Antimetabolite

INDICATIONS: Adjunct therapy for remission induction in acute non-lymphocytic leukemia (ANLL). Found useful in the treatment of acute lymphocytic leukemia (ALL) and blast phase of chronic myelocytic leukemia (CML). Prophylaxis and treatment of meningeal lymphoma.

DOSAGE: *Adults:* ANLL: Induction: 100mg/m^2/day continuous infusion or 100mg/m^2 IV q12h for days 1-7. Meningeal Leukemia: Give intrathecally. Range: 5-75mg/m^2 given qd to every 4 days. Usual: 30mg/m^2 every 4 days until CSF normal, followed by 1 additional treatment.

CYTOXAN

Pediatrics: ANLL: Induction: 100mg/m^2/day continuous infusion or 100mg/m^2 IV q12h for days 1-7. Meningeal Leukemia: Give intrathecally. Range: 5-75mg/m^2 given qd to every 4 days. Usual: 30mg/m^2 every 4 days until CSF normal, followed by 1 additional treatment.

HOW SUPPLIED: Inj: 100mg, 500mg, 1g, 2g

WARNINGS/PRECAUTIONS: Caution with pre-existing drug-induced bone marrow suppression, hepatic or renal dysfunction. Perform leukocyte and platelet counts daily during induction therapy. Monitor bone marrow, hepatic and renal functions, platelets, and leukocytes frequently. Sudden respiratory distress, cardiomyopathy, alopecia reported with high dose therapy. Severe and fatal CNS, GI, and pulmonary toxicity reported. Contains benzyl alcohol; fatal "Gasping Syndrome" in premature infants reported. Acute pancreatitis, hyperuricemia reported.

ADVERSE REACTIONS: Anorexia, nausea, vomiting, diarrhea, oral/anal inflammation or ulceration, hepatic dysfunction, fever, rash, thrombophlebitis, bleeding (all sites).

INTERACTIONS: Antagonizes susceptibility of gentamicin for K.pneumoniae. May inhibit efficacy of flucytosine. Monitor digoxin. Acute pancreatitis reported in patients receiving prior L-asparaginase treatment. Cardiomyopathy and death reported during high dose therapy with cyclophosphamide.

PREGNANCY: Category D, not for use in nursing.

CYTOXAN RX
cyclophosphamide (Bristol-Myers Squibb)

THERAPEUTIC CLASS: Nitrogen mustard alkylating agent

INDICATIONS: Treatment of malignant lymphomas, Hodgkin's disease, lymphocytic lymphoma, mixed-cell type or histiocytic lymphoma, Burkitt's lymphoma, multiple myeloma, chronic lymphocytic leukemia, chronic granulocytic leukemia, acute myelogenous and monocytic leukemia, acute lymphoblastic leukemia in children, mycosis fungoides, neuroblastoma, ovary adenocarcinoma, retinoblastoma, breast carcinoma. Treatment of biopsy proven "minimal change" nephrotic syndrome in children, but not as primary therapy.

DOSAGE: *Adults:* Malignant Diseases (Without Hematologic Deficiency): Monotherapy: Initial: 40-50mg/kg IV in divided doses over 2-5 days, or 10-15mg/kg IV given every 7-10 days, or 3-5mg/kg twice weekly. Oral Dosing: Initial/Maint: 1-5mg/kg/day PO. Adjust dose according to antitumor activity and/or leukopenia. May need to reduce dose when combined with other cytotoxic drugs.

Pediatrics: Malignant Diseases (Without Hematologic Deficiency): Monotherapy: Initial: 40-50mg/kg IV in divided doses over 2-5 days, or 10-15mg/kg IV given every 7-10 days, or 3-5mg/kg twice weekly. Oral Dosing: Initial/Maint: 1-5mg/kg/day PO. Adjust dose according to antitumor activity and/or leukopenia. May need to reduce dose when combined with other cytotoxic drugs. Nephrotic Syndrome: 2.5-3mg/kg/day PO for 60-90 days.

HOW SUPPLIED: Inj (Lyophilized): 500mg, 1g, 2g; Tab: 25mg, 50mg

CONTRAINDICATIONS: Severely depressed bone marrow function.

WARNINGS/PRECAUTIONS: Second malignancies, cardiac dysfunction, and hemorrhagic cystitis reported. May cause fetal harm in pregnancy. Serious, fatal infections may develop if severely immunosuppressed. Monitor for toxicity with leukopenia, thrombocytopenia, tumor cell infiltration of bone marrow, previous X-ray therapy or cytotoxic therapy, and impaired hepatic and/or renal function. Monitor hematologic profile for hematopoietic suppression. Examine urine for red blood cells. Anaphylactic reactions reported. Possible cross-sensitivity with other alkylating agents. May cause sterility. May interfere with normal wound healing. Consider dose adjustment with adrenalectomy.

ADVERSE REACTIONS: Impairment of fertility, amenorrhea, nausea, vomiting, anorexia, abdominal discomfort, diarrhea, alopecia, leukopenia, thrombocytopenia, hemorrhagic ureteritis, interstitial pneumonitis, malaise, asthenia, renal tubular necrosis.

INTERACTIONS: Chronic, high doses of phenobarbital increase metabolism and leukopenic activity. Potentiates succinylcholine chloride effects and doxorubicin-induced cardiotoxicity. Alert anesthesiologist if treated within 10 days of general anesthesia.

PREGNANCY: Category D, not for use in nursing.

DALLERGY   RX
phenylephrine HCl - methscopolamine nitrate - chlorpheniramine maleate (Laser)

THERAPEUTIC CLASS: Antihistamine/anticholinergic/ sympathomimetic

INDICATIONS: Relief of upper respiratory symptoms associated with allergies and the common cold.

DOSAGE: *Adults:* 1 tab or 10mL q4-6h. Max: 4 doses/24hrs.
Pediatrics: ≥12 yrs: 1 tab or 10mL q4-6h. 6-12 yrs: 1/2 tab or 5mL q4-6h. Max: 4 doses/24hrs.

HOW SUPPLIED: (Chlorpheniramine-Methscopolamine-Phenylephrine) Syrup: 2mg-0.625mg-10mg/5mL; Tab: 4mg-1.25mg-10mg*; Tab, Extended Release: 12mg-2.5mg-20mg *scored

CONTRAINDICATIONS: Severe HTN, severe CAD, MAOI therapy, narrow angle glaucoma, urinary retention, PUD, during asthma attack.

WARNINGS/PRECAUTIONS: Caution in HTN, DM, ischemic heart disease, hyperthyroidism, increased IOP, prostatic hypertrophy. Adverse events are more common in elderly. May cause excitability in children.

ADVERSE REACTIONS: Drowsiness, lassitude, nausea, giddiness, dry mouth, blurred vision, cardiac palpitations, flushing, increased irritability or excitement.

INTERACTIONS: Increased effect of sympathomimetic amines with MAOIs and β-blockers. May reduce antihypertensive effect of methyldopa, mecamylamine, reserpine, and veratrum alkaloids. Additive effect with alcohol, other CNS depressants.

PREGNANCY: Category C, caution in nursing.

DALLERGY JR   RX
phenylephrine HCl - chlorpheniramine maleate (Laser)

THERAPEUTIC CLASS: Antihistamine/sympathomimetic amine

INDICATIONS: Relief of upper respiratory symptoms associated with allergies and the common cold.

DOSAGE: *Adults:* 2 caps q12h. Max: 2 doses/24h.
Pediatrics: >12 yrs: 2 caps q12h. 6-12 yrs: 1 cap q12h. Max: 2 doses/24h.

HOW SUPPLIED: Cap: (Chlorpheniramine-Phenylephrine) 4mg-20mg

CONTRAINDICATIONS: Severe HTN, severe CAD, MAOI therapy, narrow angle glaucoma, urinary retention, PUD, during asthma attack.

WARNINGS/PRECAUTIONS: Caution with HTN, DM, ischemic heart disease, hyperthyroidism, increased IOP, prostatic hypertrophy, the elderly. May cause excitability especially in children.

ADVERSE REACTIONS: Drowsiness, lassitude, nausea, giddiness, dry mouth, blurred vision, cardiac palpitations, flushing, increased irritability or excitement.

INTERACTIONS: Increased sympathomimetic effect with MAOIs and β-blockers. May reduce antihypertensive effect of methyldopa, mecamylamine, reserpine, and veratum alkaloids. Additive effect with alcohol and other CNS depressants.

PREGNANCY: Category C, caution in nursing.

DALMANE   CIV
flurazepam HCl (Valeant)

THERAPEUTIC CLASS: Benzodiazepine

INDICATIONS: Treatment of insomnia.

DOSAGE: *Adults:* Usual: 15-30mg at bedtime. Elderly/Debilitated: Initial: 15mg at bedtime.
Pediatrics: ≥15 yrs: Usual: 15-30mg at bedtime.

HOW SUPPLIED: Cap: 15mg, 30mg

Dantrium

CONTRAINDICATIONS: Pregnancy.

WARNINGS/PRECAUTIONS: Caution in elderly, debilitated, severely depressed, those with suicidal tendencies, hepatic/renal impairment, respiratory disease. Ataxia and falls reported in elderly and debilitated. Withdrawal symptoms after discontinuation; avoid abrupt discontinuation.

ADVERSE REACTIONS: Confusion, dizziness, drowsiness, lightheadedness, ataxia.

INTERACTIONS: Additive effects with alcohol and other CNS depressants.

PREGNANCY: Not for use in pregnancy or nursing.

Dantrium   RX
dantrolene sodium (Procter & Gamble Pharmaceuticals)

> Associated with hepatotoxicity; monitor hepatic function. Discontinue if no benefit after 45 days.

THERAPEUTIC CLASS: Direct acting skeletal muscle relaxant

INDICATIONS: To control manifestations of clinical spasticity from upper motor neuron disorders (eg, spinal cord injury, stroke, cerebral palsy, multiple sclerosis). Preoperatively to prevent or attenuate development of malignant hyperthermia, and after a malignant hyperthermia crisis.

DOSAGE: *Adults:* Chronic Spasticity: Initial: 25mg qd for 7 days. Titrate: Increase to 25mg tid for 7 days, then 50mg tid for 7 days, then 100mg tid. Max: 100mg qid. If no further benefit at next higher dose, decrease to previous lower dose. Malignant Hyperthermia: Pre-Op: 4-8mg/kg/day given tid-qid for 1-2 days before surgery, with last dose given 3-4 hrs before surgery. Post-Op Following Malignant Hyperthermia Crisis: 4-8mg/kg/day given qid for 1-3 days.
Pediatrics: ≥5 yrs: Chronic Spasticity: Initial: 0.5mg/kg qd for 7 days. Titrate: Increase to 0.5mg/kg tid for 7 days, then 1mg/kg tid for 7 days, then 2mg/kg tid. Max: 100mg qid. If no further benefit at next higher dose, decrease to previous lower dose.

HOW SUPPLIED: Cap: 25mg, 50mg, 100mg

CONTRAINDICATIONS: Active hepatic disease, where spasticity is utilized to sustain upright posture and balance in locomotion, when spasticity is utilized to obtain or maintain increased function.

WARNINGS/PRECAUTIONS: Monitor LFTs at baseline, then periodically. Increased risk of hepatocellular disease in females and patients >35 yrs. Caution with pulmonary, cardiac, and liver dysfunction. Photosensitivity reaction may occur; limit sunlight exposure.

ADVERSE REACTIONS: Drowsiness, dizziness, weakness, malaise, fatigue, diarrhea, hepatitis, tachycardia, aplastic anemia, thrombocytopenia, depression, seizure.

INTERACTIONS: Increased drowsiness with CNS depressants. Caution with estrogens; risk of hepatotoxicity. Avoid with calcium channel blockers; risk of cardiovascular collapse. May potentiate vecuronium-induced neuromuscular block.

PREGNANCY: Safety in nursing not known. Not for use in nursing.

Dantrium IV   RX
dantrolene sodium (Procter & Gamble Pharmaceuticals)

THERAPEUTIC CLASS: Direct acting skeletal muscle relaxant

INDICATIONS: Adjunct management of fulminant hypermetabolism of skeletal muscle characteristic of malignant hyperthermia crises. For pre- and post-operative use to prevent or attenuate development of malignant hyperthermia.

DOSAGE: *Adults:* Malignant Hyperthermia: Initial: Minimum 1mg/kg IV push. Continue until symptoms subside or max cumulative dose 10mg/kg. Pre-Op Malignant Hyperthermia Prophylaxis: 2.5mg/kg 1.25 hrs before anesthesia and infuse over 1 hr. May need additional therapy during anesthesia/surgery if symptoms arise. Post-Op Prophylaxis: Initial: 1mg/kg or more as clinical situation dictates.
Pediatrics: Malignant Hyperthermia: Initial: Minimum 1mg/kg IV push. Continue until symptoms subside or max cumulative dose 10mg/kg.

HOW SUPPLIED: Inj: 20mg

WARNINGS/PRECAUTIONS: Use with supportive therapies to treat malignant hyperthermia. Take steps to prevent extravasation. Fatal and non-fatal hepatic disorders reported. Do not operate automobile or engage hazardous activity for 48 hrs after therapy. Caution at meals on day of administration because difficulty in swallowing/choking reported. Monitor vital signs if receive pre-operatively.

ADVERSE REACTIONS: Loss of grip strength, weakness in legs, drowsiness, dizziness, pulmonary edema, thrombophlebitis, urticaria, erythema.

INTERACTIONS: Plasma protein binding reduced by warfarin and clofibrate, and increased by tolbutamide. Avoid with calcium channel blockers; possible risk of cardiovascular collapse. Caution with tranquilizers. Possible increased metabolism by drugs known to induce hepatic microsomal enzymes. May potentiate vecuronium-induced neuromuscular block.

PREGNANCY: Category C, safety in nursing not known.

DAPSONE RX
dapsone (Jacobus)

THERAPEUTIC CLASS: Leprostatic agent

INDICATIONS: Treatment of dermatitis herpetiformis and leprosy.

DOSAGE: *Adults:* Dermatitis Herpetiformis: Initial: 50mg/day. Usual: 50-300mg/day, may increase dose if needed. Reduce to minimum maintenance dose. Leprosy: Give with 1 or more anti-leprosy drugs. Maint: 100mg/day.
Pediatrics: Same schedule as adults but with correspondingly smaller doses.

HOW SUPPLIED: Tab: 25mg*, 100mg* *scored

WARNINGS/PRECAUTIONS: Agranulocytosis, aplastic anemia and other blood dyscrasias reported. CBC weekly for the 1st month, monthly for 6 months and semi-annually thereafter. D/C if significant reduction in leukocytes, platelets or hemopoiesis occurs. Treat severe anemia prior to therapy. D/C if sensitivity occurs. Caution in those with G6PD deficiency, methemoglobin reductase deficiency, or hemoglobin M. Toxic hepatitis and cholestatic jaundice reported. Monitor LFT's.

ADVERSE REACTIONS: Hemolysis, peripheral neuropathy, nausea, vomiting, abdominal pain, pancreatitis, vertigo, blurred vision, tinnitus, insomnia, fever, headache, psychosis, phototoxicity, pulmonary eosinophilia, tachycardia, albuminuria, renal papillary necrosis, male infertility.

INTERACTIONS: Rifampin lowers plasma levels. Folic acid antagonists (eg, pyrimethamine) may increase hematologic reactions. Dapsone and trimethoprim each raise the level of the other.

PREGNANCY: Category C, not for use in nursing.

DAPTACEL RX
tetanus toxoid - diphtheria toxoid - pertussis vaccine acellular, adsorbed
(Aventis)

THERAPEUTIC CLASS: Vaccine

INDICATIONS: Active immunization against diphtheria, tetanus, and pertussis.

DOSAGE: *Pediatrics:* 6 weeks-up to 7 yrs: 0.5mL IM at intervals of 6-8 weeks, and at 17-20 months old. The interval between 3rd and 4th dose should be at least 6 months. May use to complete series in infants who received ≥1 dose of whole-cell pertussis (DTP). Usual age for 1st dose is 2 months old.

HOW SUPPLIED: Inj: (Diphtheria-Pertussis-Tetanus-) 15Lf U-23mcg-5Lf U/0.5mL

CONTRAINDICATIONS: Adults and pediatrics ≥7 yrs. Administration after immediate anaphylactic reaction, or encephalopathy not attributable to another identifiable cause within 7 days from initial vaccination. Moderate or serious illness. Outbreak of poliomyelitis.

WARNINGS/PRECAUTIONS: Stopper contains dry natural latex rubber. Evaluate risks/benefits of subsequent doses if temperature ≥105°F, or if collapse/shock occurs, or persistent crying for ≥3 hrs within 48 hrs, and convulsions with or without fever within 3 days of vaccine. Continue with DT vaccine if pertussis must be withheld. Avoid in coagulation disorder. Increased risk of neurological events with family history of convulsions; administer antipyretic at time of and for 24 hrs after immunization. Enhanced risk of manifestation of underlying neurological within 2-3 days following vaccine. May not achieve expected immune response in immunosuppressed patients. Avoid injection into blood vessel.

ADVERSE REACTIONS: Local tenderness, fever, fretfulness, anorexia, drowsiness, vomiting.

INTERACTIONS: Caution with anticoagulants. Immunosuppressives (eg, irradiation, antimetabolites, alkylating agents, cytotoxic drugs, corticosteroids) may reduce immune response to vaccine. Adequate immune response may not occur after recent immune globulin injection.

PREGNANCY: Category C, safety in nursing not known.

Daraprim
pyrimethamine (GlaxoSmithKline) — RX

THERAPEUTIC CLASS: Folic acid antagonist

INDICATIONS: Adjunct treatment of toxoplasmosis and acute malaria. Prophylaxis of malaria.

DOSAGE: *Adults:* Toxoplasmosis: Initial: 50-75mg qd with 1-4g/day of sulfonamide. After 1-3 weeks, reduce dose of each drug to 1/2 of previous dose for additional 4-5 weeks. Acute Malaria: 25mg qd for 2 days with sulfonamide. As monotherapy in semi-immune persons, 50mg for 2 days. Follow with prophylaxis dose through periods of early recrudescence and late relapse. Malaria Prophylaxis: 25mg once weekly.
Pediatrics: Toxoplasmosis: 0.5mg/kg bid. After 2-4 days, reduce to 0.25mg/kg bid for 1 month. Use with usual pediatric sulfonamide dose. Acute Malaria: 4-10 yrs: As monotherapy in semi-immune persons, 25mg for 2 days. Follow with prophylaxis dose through periods of early recrudescence and late relapse. Malaria Prophylaxis: >10 yrs: 25mg once weekly. 4-10 yrs: 12.5 once weekly. <4 yrs: 6.25mg once weekly.

HOW SUPPLIED: Tab: 25mg* *scored

CONTRAINDICATIONS: Megaloblastic anemia due to folate deficiency.

WARNINGS/PRECAUTIONS: Dose for toxoplasmosis approaches toxic levels; reduce dose or d/c if develop folate deficiency. Administer leucovorin 5-15mg qd (po, IV, or IM) until normal hematopoiesis. May be carcinogenic. Pediatric deaths reported with accidental ingestion. Use small initial dose with convulsive disorders to avoid nervous system toxicity. Caution with renal or hepatic dysfunction or if possible folate deficiency (eg, pregnancy, malabsorption syndrome, alcoholism). Perform semiweekly blood counts, including platelets with high doses.

ADVERSE REACTIONS: Hypersensitivity reactions (eg, Stevens-Johnson syndrome, toxic epidermal necrolysis) hyperphenylalinemia (with sulfonamides), anorexia, vomiting, blood dyscrasias, cardiac rhythm disorders.

INTERACTIONS: Concurrent phenytoin may affect folate levels. Increased risk of bone marrow suppression with antifolic drugs (eg, sulfonamides or trimethoprim-sulfamethoxazole). Mild hepatotoxicity reported with lorazepam.

PREGNANCY: Category C, not for use in nursing.

Daypro
oxaprozin (Pharmacia & Upjohn) — RX

> **NSAIDs may cause an increased risk of serious cardiovascular thrombotic events, MI, stroke and serious GI adverse events including bleeding, ulceration, and perforation of the stomach or intestines. Contraindicated for the treatment of peri-operative pain in the setting of coronary artery bypass graft (CABG) surgery.**

THERAPEUTIC CLASS: NSAID (propionic acid derivative)

INDICATIONS: Relief of signs and symptoms of osteoarthritis (OA), rheumatoid arthritis (RA), and juvenile rheumatoid arthritis (JRA).

DOSAGE: *Adults:* RA: 1200mg qd. Max: 1800mg/day in divided doses (not to exceed 26mg/kg/day). OA: 1200mg qd, give 600mg qd for low weight or milder disease. Max: 1800mg/day in divided doses (not to exceed 26mg/kg/day). Renal Dysfunction/Hemodialysis: Initial: 600mg qd.

Pediatrics: 6-16yrs: JRA: ≥55kg: 1200mg qd. 32-54kg: 900mg qd. 22-31kg: 600mg qd.

HOW SUPPLIED: Tab: 600mg* *scored

CONTRAINDICATIONS: Complete or partial syndrome of nasal polyps, angioedema and bronchospastic reactivity to ASA or other NSAIDs. Treatment of peri-operative pain in the setting of CABG surgery.

WARNINGS/PRECAUTIONS: May lead to onset of new HTN or worsening of pre-existing HTN; monitor BP closely. Fluid retention and edema reported; caution with fluid retention or heart failure. Renal papillary necrosis and other renal injury reported after long-term use. Not recommended for use with advanced renal disease; if therapy must be initiated, monitor renal function. Anaphylactoid reactions may occur. May cause serious skin adverse events (eg, exfoliative dermatitis, Stevens-Johnson syndrome, and toxic epidermal necrolysis). Avoid in late pregnancy; may cause premature closure of ductus arteriosis. May cause elevations of LFTs; d/c if liver disease develops or systemic manifestations occur. Caution in elderly. Anemia may occur; with long-term use, monitor Hgb/Hct if signs or symptoms of anemia develop. May inhibit platelet aggregation and prolong bleeding time; monitor with coagulation disorders. Caution with asthma and avoid with aspirin-sensitive asthma. Rash and/or mild photosensitivity reactions reported.

ADVERSE REACTIONS: Constipation, diarrhea, dyspepsia, flatulence, nausea, rash.

INTERACTIONS: Avoid with ASA. Caution with oral anticoagulants. Monitor BP with β-blockers.

PREGNANCY: Category C, not for use in nursing.

Daytrana   CII
methylphenidate (Shire)

THERAPEUTIC CLASS: Sympathomimetic amine

INDICATIONS: Treatment of attention deficit hyperactivity disorder (ADHD).

DOSAGE: *Adults:* Individualize dose. Apply to hip area 2 hrs before effect is needed and remove 9 hrs after application. Recommended Titration Schedule: Week 1: 10mg/9 hrs. Week 2: 15mg/9 hrs. Week 3: 20mg/9 hrs. Week 4: 30mg/9 hrs.

Pediatrics: ≥6 yrs: Individualize dose. Apply to hip area 2 hrs before effect is needed and remove 9 hrs after application. Recommended Titration Schedule: Week 1: 10mg/9 hrs. Week 2: 15mg/9 hrs. Week 3: 20mg/9 hrs. Week 4: 30mg/9 hrs.

HOW SUPPLIED: Patch: 10mg/9 hrs, 15mg/9 hrs, 20mg/9 hrs, 30mg/9 hrs (10^s, 30^s)

CONTRAINDICATIONS: Marked anxiety, tension, and agitation; glaucoma; motor tics or family history or diagnosis of Tourette's syndrome; treatment with MAOIs and within minimum of 14 days following discontinuation.

WARNINGS/PRECAUTIONS: Avoid use with known structural cardiac abnormalities; sudden death reported. D/C if contact sensitization is suspected. Monitor growth during treatment. May exacerbate symptoms of behavior disturbance and thought disorder in psychotic patients. Caution when using stimulants to treat patients with comorbid bipolar disorder because of concern for possible induction of mixed/manic episode in such patients. Stimulants at usual doses can cause treatment emergent psychotic or manic symptoms (eg, hallucinations, delusional thinking, mania) in children and adolescents without prior history of psychotic illness. Aggressive behavior or hostility reported in clinical trials and postmarketing experience of some medications indicated for the treatment of ADHD. May lower convulsive threshold; d/c in the presence of seizures. Caution with HTN; monitor BP. Caution when underlying medical conditions might be compromised by increases in BP or HR (eg, pre-existing HTN, heart failure, recent MI, or hyperthyroidism). Visual disturbances reported. Caution with history of drug dependence or alcoholism. Avoid exposing application site to external heat sources (eg, heating pads, electric blankets, heated water beds, etc). Monitor CBC, differential, and platelet counts during prolonged therapy.

DDAVP

ADVERSE REACTIONS: Nausea, vomiting, nasopharyngitis, weight decrease, anorexia, decreased appetite, affect lability, insomnia, tic, nasal congestion.

INTERACTIONS: See Contraindications. Caution with pressor agents. May decrease effectiveness of antihypertensive agents. May inhibit metabolism of coumarin anticoagulants, anticonvulsants (eg, phenobarbital, phenytoin, primidone), some tricyclic drugs (eg, imipramine, clomipramine, desipramine), and SSRIs. Monitor drug levels (or coagulation times with coumarin) and consider dose adjustments with concomitant use. Serious adverse events reported with concomitant clonidine use.

PREGNANCY: Category C, caution in nursing.

DDAVP   RX
desmopressin acetate (Sanofi-Aventis)

OTHER BRAND NAMES: DDAVP Nasal Spray (Sanofi-Aventis) - DDAVP Rhinal Tube (Sanofi-Aventis)

THERAPEUTIC CLASS: Synthetic vasopressin analog

INDICATIONS: (Spray/Tube/Tab) Primary nocturnal enuresis. (Inj/Spray/Tube/Tab) Central (cranial) diabetes insipidus. Temporary polyuria and polydipsia after head trauma or surgery in the pituitary region. (Inj) Hemophilia A and von Willebrand's disease (Type I).

DOSAGE: *Adults:* Nocturnal Enuresis: (Tab) Initial: 0.2mg PO qhs. Titrate: May increase up to 0.6mg. (Spray/Tube) Initial: 20mcg intranasally qhs. Titrate: Decrease to 10mcg or increase up to 40mcg if needed. Max: 4-8 weeks. Administer 1/2 dose in each nostril. Diabetes Insipidus: (Tab) Initial: 0.05mg bid. Titrate: Increase/decrease by 0.1-1.2mg/day given bid-tid. Maint: 0.1-0.8mg/day in divided doses. (Spray/Tube) Usual: 0.1-0.4mL/day given qd-tid. (Inj) 1-2mcg IV/SQ bid. Hemophilia A and von Willebrand's Disease: 0.3mcg/kg IV. Add 50mL diluent. Give 30 minutes preoperatively.

Pediatrics: Nocturnal Enuresis: ≥6 yrs: (Tab) Initial: 0.2mg PO hs. Titrate: May increase up to 0.6mg. (Spray/Tube) Initial: 20mcg intranasally qhs. Titrate: Decrease to 10mcg or increase up to 40mcg if needed. Max: 4-8 weeks. Administer 1/2 dose per nostril. Diabetes Insipidus: (Tab) ≥4 yrs: Initial: 0.05mg bid. Titrate: Increase/decrease by 0.1-1.2mg/day given bid-tid. Maint: 0.1-0.8mg/day in divided doses. (Spray/Tube) 3 months-12 yrs: Usual: 0.05-3mL/day given qd-bid. (Inj) ≥12 yrs: 1-2mcg IV/SQ bid. Hemophilia A and von Willebrand's Disease: ≥3 months: (Inj) 0.3mcg/kg IV. Add 50mL diluent if >10kg; add 10mL diluent if ≤10kg. Give 30 minutes preoperatively.

HOW SUPPLIED: Inj: 4mcg/mL; Nasal Spray: 10mcg/inh (5mL); Tab: 0.1mg*, 0.2mg*; Rhinal Tube: 0.01% (2.5mL) *scored

WARNINGS/PRECAUTIONS: Mucosal changes with nasal forms may occur; d/c until resolved. Decrease fluid intake in pediatrics and elderly to decrease risk of water intoxication and hyponatremia; monitor osmolality. Caution with coronary artery insufficiency, hypertensive cardiovascular disease, fluid and electrolyte imbalance (eg, cystic fibrosis). Anaphylaxis reported with IV use. Caution with IV use if history of thrombus formation. For diabetes insipidus, dosage must be adjusted according to diurnal pattern of response; estimate response by adequate duration of sleep and adequate, not excessive, water turnover.

ADVERSE REACTIONS: Inj: Headache, nausea, abdominal cramps, vulval pain, injection site reactions, facial flushing, BP changes. Spray: Headache, dizziness, rhinitis, nausea, nasal congestion, sore throat, cough, respiratory infection, epistaxis. Tab: Nausea, flushing, abdominal cramps, headache, increased SGOT, water intoxication, hyponatremia.

INTERACTIONS: Caution with other pressor agents.

PREGNANCY: Category B, caution in nursing.

DECLOMYCIN   RX
demeclocycline HCl (Wyeth)

THERAPEUTIC CLASS: Tetracycline derivative

INDICATIONS: Treatment of infections due to rickettsiae, *Mycoplasma pneumoniae*, *B.recurrentis*, agents of psittacosis, ornithosis, lymphomagranuloma venereum or granuloma inguinale. Treatment of gram-negative infections (eg, respiratory, urinary tract), gram-positive infections (eg, respiratory tract, skin and soft tissue), trachoma, inclusion conjunctivitis. When PCN is contraindicated, treatment of gonorrhea, syphilis, listeriosis, anthrax, *Clostridium* species, and others. Adjunct therapy for amebicides.

DOSAGE: *Adults:* Usual: 150mg qid or 300mg bid. Gonorrhea: Initial: 600mg, then 300mg q12h for 4 days. Gonorrhea: 600mg followed by 300mg q12h for 4 days to a total of 3g. Renal/Hepatic Impairment: Reduce dose and/or extend dose intervals. Continue therapy for at least 24-48 hrs after symptoms subside. Treat strep infections for at least 10 days. Take at least 1 hr before or 2 hrs after meals with plenty of fluids.

Pediatrics: >8 yrs: Usual: 3-6mg/lb/day given bid-qid. Gonorrhea: 600mg followed by 300mg q12h for 4 days to a total of 3g. Renal/Hepatic Impairment: Reduce dose and/or extend dose intervals. Continue therapy for at least 24-48 hrs after symptoms subside. Treat strep infections for at least 10 days. Take at least 1 hr before or 2 hrs after meals with plenty of fluids.

HOW SUPPLIED: Tab: 150mg, 300mg

CONTRAINDICATIONS: Hypersensitivity to any of the tetracyclines.

WARNINGS/PRECAUTIONS: May cause fetal harm during pregnancy. Use during tooth development (last half of pregnancy, infancy, <8 yrs), or long-term use, or repeated short-term use may cause permanent discoloration of the teeth. Pseudotumor cerebri (adults), bulging fontanels (infants) reported. Caution with renal or hepatic impairment. Long-term use may cause reversible, nephrogenic diabetes insipidus syndrome. May result in overgrowth of nonsusceptible organisms; d/c if superinfection develops. CNS symptoms may occur; caution when operating machinery. May decrease bone growth in premature infants. Monitor hematopoietic, renal, and hepatic function with long-term use. D/C at first evidence of skin erythema after sun/UV light exposure.

ADVERSE REACTIONS: GI problems, rash, esophageal ulceration, hypersensitivity reactions, dizziness, headache, tinnitus, blood dyscrasias, photosensitivity reactions, enamel hypoplasia, elevated BUN.

INTERACTIONS: Decreases PT; may need to decrease dose of anticoagulants. May interfere with bactericidal action of penicillin; avoid concomitant use. May decrease efficacy of oral contraceptives; use alternate method. Decreased absorption with antacids and iron-containing products. Fatal renal toxicity with methoxyflurane reported. Foods/dairy products interfere with absorption.

PREGNANCY: Category D, not for use in nursing.

DECONAMINE RX
pseudoephedrine HCl - chlorpheniramine maleate (Kenwood Therapeutics)

OTHER BRAND NAMES: Kronofed-A (Ferndale) - De-Congestine TR (Qualitest) - Deconamine SR (Kenwood Therapeutics)

THERAPEUTIC CLASS: Antihistamine/decongestant

INDICATIONS: Temporary relief of symptoms associated with rhinorrhea, sneezing, and nasal congestion.

DOSAGE: *Adults:* (Cap, SR) 1 cap q12h, (Tab) 1 tab tid-qid. (Syrup) 5-10mL tid-qid.
Pediatrics: ≥12 yrs: (Cap, SR) 1 cap q12h, (Tab) 1 tab tid-qid. (Syrup) 5-10mL tid-qid. 2-6 yrs: (Syrup) 2.5mL tid-qid. Max: 10mL/24hrs. 6-12 yrs: 2.5-5mL tid-qid. Max: 20mL/24hrs.

HOW SUPPLIED: (Chlorpheniramine-Pseudoephedrine) Cap, Sustained Release: 8mg-120mg; Syrup: 2mg-30mg/5mL; Tab: 4mg-60mg

CONTRAINDICATIONS: Severe HTN, severe CAD, concomitant MAOIs.

WARNINGS/PRECAUTIONS: Extreme caution in narrow angle glaucoma, stenosing peptic ulcer, pyloroduodenal obstruction, symptomatic prostatic hypertrophy, bladder neck obstruction. Caution in bronchial asthma, emphysema, chronic pulmonary disease, HTN, ischemic heart disease, DM, increased IOP, hyperthyroidism. May cause excitability in children. May produce CNS stimulation with convulsions or cardiovascular collapse with hypotension.

ADVERSE REACTIONS: Drowsiness, urticaria, drug rash, hypotension, hemolytic anemia, sedation, epigastric distress, urinary frequency, nervousness, dizziness.

DELATESTRYL

INTERACTIONS: Hypertensive crisis may occur with MAOIs. May reduce antihypertensive effect of methyldopa, reserpine, veratrum alkaloids, mecamylamine. Sedative effects potentiated by alcohol, other CNS depressants.

PREGNANCY: Category C, not for use in nursing.

Delatestryl   CIII
testosterone enanthate (Savient)

THERAPEUTIC CLASS: Androgen

INDICATIONS: Testosterone replacement in males with primary hypogonadism and hypogonadotropic hypogonadism. To stimulate puberty in males with delayed puberty. May also be used secondarily in females with advancing inoperable metastatic (skeletal) mammary cancer who are 1-5 years postmenopausal.

DOSAGE: *Adults:* Dose based on age, sex, and diagnosis. Adjust dose according to response and adverse reactions. Male Hypogonadism: 50-400mg IM every 2-4 weeks. Delayed Puberty: 50-200mg every 2-4 weeks for a limited duration (eg, 4-6 months). Breast Cancer: 200-400mg every 2-4 weeks.

Pediatrics: Dose based on age, sex, and diagnosis. Adjust dose according to response and adverse reactions. Male Hypogonadism: 50-400mg IM every 2-4 weeks. Delayed Puberty: 50-200mg every 2-4 weeks for a limited duration (eg, 4-6 months). Caution in children.

HOW SUPPLIED: Inj: 200mg/mL

CONTRAINDICATIONS: Breast or prostate carcinoma in men. Pregnancy.

WARNINGS/PRECAUTIONS: D/C if hypercalcemia occurs in breast cancer or immobilized patients; monitor calcium levels. Risk of hepatic adenomas, hepatocellular carcinoma, and peliosis hepatitis with prolonged high doses. D/C if jaundice, cholestatic hepatitis, or abnormal LFTs occur. Avoid use in elderly who has age related hypogonadism. D/C if edema occurs in patients with pre-existing cardiac, renal, or hepatic disease; restart at lower dose. Risk of compromised stature in children; monitor bone growth every 6 months. Monitor for virilization in females. Caution with a history of MI or CAD due to altered serum cholesterol levels. Monitor cholesterol, LFTs, Hct, Hgb periodically.

ADVERSE REACTIONS: Amenorrhea, virilization, menstrual irregularities, gynecomastia, excessive frequency/duration of penile erections, male pattern baldness, increased/decreased libido, oligospermia, hirsutism, acne, fluid and electrolyte disturbances, nausea, hypercholesterolemia, clotting factor suppression, polycythemia, altered LFTs, oligospermia, anxiety, depression.

INTERACTIONS: Potentiates oral anticoagulants and oxyphenbutazone. May decrease blood glucose and insulin requirements. ACTH and corticosteroids may enhance edema.

PREGNANCY: Category X, not for use in nursing.

Demerol Injection   CII
meperidine HCl (Hospira)

THERAPEUTIC CLASS: Opioid analgesic

INDICATIONS: For relief of moderate to severe pain. For preoperative medication, anesthesia support, and obstetrical analgesia.

DOSAGE: *Adults:* Pain: Usual: 50-150mg IM/SQ q3-4h prn. Preoperative: Usual: 50-100mg IM/SQ 30-90 minutes before anesthesia. Anesthesia Support: Use repeated slow IV injections of fractional doses (eg, 10mg/mL) or continuous IV infusion of a more dilute solution (eg, 1mg/mL). Titrate as needed. Obstetrical Analgesia: Usual: 50-100mg IM/SQ when pain is regular, may repeat at 1- to 3-hr intervals. Elderly: Start at lower end of dosage range and observe. With Phenothiazines/Other Tranquilizers: Reduce dose by 25 to 50%). IM method preferred with repeated use. For IV injection: Reduce dose and administer slowly, preferably using diluted solution.

Pediatrics: Pain: Usual: 0.5-0.8mg/lb IM/SQ, up to 50-150mg, q3-4h prn. Preoperative: Usual: 0.5-1mg/lb IM/SQ, up to 50-100mg, 30-90 minutes before anesthesia. With

Phenothiazines/Other Tranquilizers: Reduce dose by 25 to 50%). IM method preferred with repeated use. For IV injection: Reduce dose and administer slowly, using diluted solution.

HOW SUPPLIED: Inj: 25mg/mL, 50mg/mL, 75mg/mL, 100mg/mL
CONTRAINDICATIONS: MAOI during or within 14 days of use.
WARNINGS/PRECAUTIONS: May develop tolerance and dependence; abuse potential. Extreme caution with head injury, increased intracranial pressure, intracranial lesions, acute asthmatic attack, chronic COPD or cor pulmonale, decreased respiratory reserve, respiratory depression, hypoxia, and hypercapnia. Rapid IV infusion may result in increased adverse reactions. Caution with acute abdominal conditions, atrial flutter, supraventricular tachycardias. May aggravate convulsive disorders. Caution and reduce initial dose with elderly or debilitated, renal/hepatic impairment, hypothyroidism, Addison's disease, prostatic hypertrophy or urethral stricture. Severe hypotension may occur post-op or if depleted blood volume. Orthostatic hypotension may occur. May impair mental/physical abilities. Not for use in pregnancy prior to labor. May produce depression of respiration and psychophysiologic functions in the newborn when used as an obstetrical analgesic.
ADVERSE REACTIONS: Lightheadedness, dizziness, sedation, nausea, vomiting, sweating, respiratory/circulatory depression.
INTERACTIONS: See Contraindications. Caution and reduce dose with other CNS depressants (eg, narcotics, anesthetics, phenothiazines, tranquilizers, sedative-hypnotics, TCAs, alcohol).
PREGNANCY: Safety in pregnancy and nursing not known.

DEMEROL ORAL CII
meperidine HCl (Sanofi-Aventis)

THERAPEUTIC CLASS: Opioid analgesic
INDICATIONS: Moderate to severe pain.
DOSAGE: *Adults:* Usual: 50-150mg q3-4h prn. Concomitant Phenothiazines/Other Tranquilizers: Reduce dose by 25-50%. Dilute syrup in 1/2 glass of water.
Pediatrics: Usual: 1.1-1.8mg/kg up to 50-150mg q3-4h prn. Concomitant Phenothiazines/Other Tranquilizers: Reduce dose by 25-50%. Dilute syrup in 1/2 glass of water.
HOW SUPPLIED: Syrup: 50mg/5mL; Tab: 50mg*, 100mg *scored
CONTRAINDICATIONS: MAOI during or within 14 days of use.
WARNINGS/PRECAUTIONS: May develop tolerance and dependence; abuse potential. Extreme caution with head injury, increased intracranial pressure, intracranial lesions, acute asthma attack, chronic COPD, cor pulmonale, decreased respiratory reserve, respiratory depression, hypoxia, and hypercapnia. Caution with sickle cell anemia, pheochromocytoma, acute alcoholism, Addison's disease, CNS depression or coma, delirium tremens, elderly or debilitated, kyphoscoliosis associated with respiratory depression, myxedema, hypothyroidism, acute abdominal conditions, epilepsy, atrial flutter, other supraventricular tachycardias, renal or hepatic impairment, prostatic hypertrophy, urethral stricture, drug dependencies, neonates, and young infants. Severe hypotension may occur post-op or if depleted blood volume. Orthostatic hypotension may occur. Not for use in pregnancy prior to labor.
ADVERSE REACTIONS: Lightheadedness, dizziness, sedation, nausea, vomiting, sweating, respiratory depression.
INTERACTIONS: See Contraindications. Reduce dose with other CNS depressants (eg, narcotics, anesthetics, phenothiazines, tranquilizers, sedative-hypnotics, TCAs, alcohol). Mixed agonist/antagonist analgesics (eg, pentazocine, nalbuphine, butorphanol, buprenorphine) may reduce analgesic effects and/or precipitate withdrawal symptoms. Caution with acyclovir, cimetidine. Phenytoin may enhance hepatic metabolism. May enhance neuroblocking action of skeletal muscle relaxants. Increased levels with ritonavir; avoid concurrent administration.
PREGNANCY: Category C, not for use in nursing.

DEMSER RX
metyrosine (Merck)

THERAPEUTIC CLASS: Tyrosine hydroxylase inhibitor
INDICATIONS: Treatment of pheochromocytoma for preoperative preparation and when surgery is contraindicated. Chronic treatment with malignant pheochromocytoma.

DEPACON

DOSAGE: *Adults:* Initial: 250mg qid. Titrate: May increase by 250-500mg/day. Max: 4g/day. Titrate based on clinical symptoms and catecholamine excretion. Usual: 2-3g/day. Preoperative Preparation: Take 5-7 days before surgery.

Pediatrics: ≥12 yrs: Initial: 250mg qid. Titrate: May increase by 250-500mg/day. Max: 4g/day. Titrate based on clinical symptoms and catecholamine excretion. Usual: 2-3g/day. Preoperative Preparation: Take 5-7 days before surgery.

HOW SUPPLIED: Cap: 250mg

WARNINGS/PRECAUTIONS: When used preoperatively or with alpha-adrenergic blockers, maintain intravascular volume intra- and postoperatively to avoid hypotension and decreased perfusion. Maintain adequate water intake to achieve urine volume of ≥2000mL to prevent crystalluria. Risk of hypertensive crisis or arrhythmias during tumor manipulation. Monitor BP and ECG continuously during surgery.

ADVERSE REACTIONS: Sedation, EPS, anxiety, depression, hallucinations, disorientation, confusion, diarrhea.

INTERACTIONS: Additive sedative effects with alcohol and other CNS depressants (eg, hypnotics, sedatives, tranquilizers). May potentiate EPS with phenothiazines and haloperidol.

PREGNANCY: Category C, caution in nursing.

DEPACON
valproate sodium (Abbott)

RX

> Fatal hepatic failure (<2 yrs at considerable risk), teratogenic effects (eg, neural tube defects), and life-threatening pancreatitis reported.

THERAPEUTIC CLASS: Carboxylic acid derivative

INDICATIONS: Monotherapy and adjunctive therapy for treatment of simple and complex absence seizures, and complex partial seizures. Adjunct therapy for multiple seizure types.

DOSAGE: *Adults:* Simplex/Complex Absence Seizure: Initial: 15mg/kg/day. Titrate: Increase weekly by 5-10mg/kg/day until optimal response. Max: 60mg/kg/day. Complex Partial Seizure: Initial: 10-15mg/kg/day. Titrate: Increase weekly by 5-10mg/kg/day until optimal response. Max: 60mg/kg/day. Elderly: Reduce initial dose and titrate slowly. If dose >250mg/day, give in divided doses. Administer as 60 minute IV infusion, not >20mg/min. Not for use >14 days; switch to oral route as soon as clinically feasible. Decrease dose or discontinue if decreased food or fluid intake or if excessive somnolence occurs.

Pediatrics: ≥2 yrs: Simplex/Complex Absence Seizure: Initial: 15mg/kg/day. Titrate: Increase weekly by 5-10mg/kg/day until optimal response. Max: 60mg/kg/day. ≥10 yrs: Complex Partial Seizure: Initial: 10-15mg/kg/day. Titrate: Increase weekly by 5-10mg/kg/day until optimal response. Max: 60mg/kg/day. If dose >250mg/day, give in divided doses. Administer as 60 minute IV infusion, not >20mg/min. Not for use >14 days; switch to oral route as soon as clinically feasible. Decrease dose or discontinue with decreased food or fluid intake and if excessive somnolence.

HOW SUPPLIED: Inj: 100mg/mL

CONTRAINDICATIONS: Hepatic disease, significant hepatic dysfunction, known urea cycle disorders (UCD).

WARNINGS/PRECAUTIONS: Hyperammonemic encephalopathy in UCD patients; d/c if this occurs. Prior to therapy, evaluate for UCD in high risk patients (eg, history of unexplained encephalopathy, coma, etc). Measure ammonia levels if develop unexplained lethargy, vomiting, or mental status changes. Caution in elderly; monitor for fluid/nutritional intake, dehydration, somnolence. Monitor LFTs before therapy and during 1st 6 months. D/C if develop hepatic dysfunction, pancreatitis. Increased risk of hepatotoxicity with multiple anticonvulsants, congenital metabolic disorders, severe seizure disorder with mental retardation, organic brain disease, children <2 yrs. Avoid abrupt withdrawal. Monitor platelets and coagulation tests before therapy and periodically thereafter. Elevated liver enzymes and thrombocytopenia may be dose-related. Not for prophylaxis of post-traumatic seizures in acute head trauma. May interfere with urine ketone and thyroid function tests.

ADVERSE REACTIONS: Dizziness, headache, nausea, local reactions.

INTERACTIONS: Clonazepam may induce absence status in patients with absence seizures. Potentiates amitriptyline, nortriptyline, carbamazepine, diazepam, ethosuximide, lamotrigine, phenobarbital, primidone, phenytoin, tolbutamide, warfarin, zidovudine. Potentiated by ASA and felbamate. Antagonized by rifampin, carbamazepine, phenobarbital, phenytoin. Additive CNS depression with other CNS depressants (eg, alcohol).

PREGNANCY: Category D, not for use in nursing.

DEPAKENE
valproic acid (Abbott)
RX

> Fatal hepatic failure (<2 yrs at considerable risk), teratogenic effects (eg, neural tube defects), and life-threatening pancreatitis reported.

THERAPEUTIC CLASS: Carboxylic acid derivative

INDICATIONS: Monotherapy and adjunctive therapy for treatment of simple and complex absence seizures, and complex partial seizures. Adjunct therapy for multiple seizure types.

DOSAGE: *Adults:* Simplex/Complex Absence Seizure: Initial: 15mg/kg/day. Titrate: Increase weekly by 5-10mg/kg/day until optimal response. Max: 60mg/kg/day. Complex Partial Seizure: Initial: 10-15mg/kg/day. Titrate: Increase weekly by 5-10mg/kg/day until optimal response. Max: 60mg/kg/day. If dose >250mg/day, give in divided doses. Elderly: Reduce initial dose. Swallow caps whole, do not chew.
Pediatrics: ≥10 yrs: Complex Partial Seizure: Initial: 10-15mg/kg/day. Titrate: Increase weekly by 5-10mg/kg/day until optimal response. Max: 60mg/kg/day. If dose >250mg/day, give in divided doses. Swallow caps whole, do not chew.

HOW SUPPLIED: Cap: 250mg; Syrup: 250mg/5mL

CONTRAINDICATIONS: Hepatic disease, significant hepatic dysfunction, known urea cycle disorders (UCD).

WARNINGS/PRECAUTIONS: Hyperammonemic encephalopathy in UCD patients; d/c if this occurs. Prior to therapy, evaluate for UCD in high risk patients (eg, history of unexplained encephalopathy, coma, etc). Measure ammonia levels if develop unexplained lethargy, vomiting, or mental status changes. Caution in elderly; monitor for fluid/nutritional intake, dehydration, somnolence. Monitor LFTs before therapy and during 1st 6 months. D/C if develop hepatic dysfunction, pancreatitis. Increased risk of hepatotoxicity with multiple anticonvulsants, congenital metabolic disorders, severe seizure disorder with mental retardation, organic brain disease, children <2 yrs. Avoid abrupt withdrawal. Hyperammonemia reported. Monitor platelets and coagulation tests before therapy and periodically thereafter. Elevated liver enzymes and thrombocytopenia may be dose-related. May interfere with urine ketone and thyroid function tests.

ADVERSE REACTIONS: Headache, asthenia, nausea, vomiting, diarrhea, abdominal pain, somnolence, tremor, dizziness, thrombocytopenia, ecchymosis, nystagmus, alopecia.

INTERACTIONS: Clonazepam may induce absence status in patients with absence seizures. Potentiates amitriptyline, nortriptyline, carbamazepine, diazepam, ethosuximide, lamotrigine, phenobarbital, primidone, phenytoin, tolbutamide, warfarin, zidovudine. Potentiated by ASA and felbamate. Antagonized by rifampin, carbamazepine, phenobarbital, phenytoin. Additive CNS depression with other CNS depressants (eg, alcohol).

PREGNANCY: Category D, not for use in nursing.

DEPAKOTE
divalproex sodium (Abbott)
RX

> Fatal hepatic failure (<2 yrs at considerable risk), teratogenic effects (eg, neural tube defects), and life-threatening pancreatitis reported.

THERAPEUTIC CLASS: Valproate compound

DEPAKOTE ER

INDICATIONS: (Tab, Cap) Management of simple and complex absence seizures; complex partial seizures; and adjunctively with multiple seizure types including absence seizures. (Tab) Treatment of mania associated with bipolar disorder and migraine prophylaxis.

DOSAGE: *Adults:* (Cap/Tab) Complex Partial Seizures: Initial: 10-15mg/kg/day. Titrate: Increase by 5-10mg/kg/week. Max: 60mg/kg/day. Absence Seizures: Initial: 15mg/kg/day. Titrate: Increase weekly by 5-10mg/kg/day. Max: 60mg/kg/day. Give in divided doses if >250mg/day. (Tab) Migraine: Initial: ≥16 yrs: 250mg bid. Max: 1000mg/day. Mania: 750mg daily in divided doses. Titrate: Increase dose rapidly to clinical effect. Max: 60mg/kg/day. Elderly: Reduce initial dose and titrate slowly. Decrease dose or d/c if decreased food or fluid intake or if excessive somnolence occurs.

Pediatrics: ≥10 yrs: (Cap/Tab) Complex Partial Seizures: Initial: 10-15mg/kg/day. Titrate: Increase by 5-10mg/kg/week. Max: 60mg/kg/day. Absence Seizures: Initial: 15mg/kg/day. Titrate: Increase weekly by 5-10mg/kg/day. Max: 60mg/kg/day. Give in divided doses if >250mg/day.

HOW SUPPLIED: Cap, Delayed Release: (Sprinkle) 125mg; Tab, Delayed Release: 125mg, 250mg, 500mg

CONTRAINDICATIONS: Hepatic disease, significant hepatic dysfunction, known urea cycle disorders (UCD).

WARNINGS/PRECAUTIONS: Hyperammonemic encephalopathy in UCD patients; d/c if this occurs. Prior to therapy, evaluate for UCD in high risk patients (eg, history of unexplained encephalopathy, coma, etc). Measure ammonia levels if develop unexplained lethargy, vomiting, or mental status changes. Caution with hepatic disease. Check LFTs prior to therapy, then frequently during first 6 months. Dose-related thrombocytopenia and elevated liver enzymes reported. Monitor platelet and coagulation tests prior to therapy, then periodically. Altered thyroid function tests and urine ketone test. May stimulate replication of HIV and CMV viruses. Avoid abrupt discontinuation.

ADVERSE REACTIONS: Nausea, vomiting, diarrhea, somnolence, dyspepsia, thrombocytopenia, asthenia, abdominal pain, tremor, headache, anorexia, diplopia, blurred vision, weight gain, ataxia, nystagmus.

INTERACTIONS: Potentiates carbamazepine, amitriptyline, nortriptyline, diazepam, ethosuximide, primidone, lamotrigine, phenobarbital, phenytoin, tolbutamide, zidovudine, lorazepam. Efficacy potentiated by ASA, felbamate. Efficacy reduced by rifampin, carbamazepine, phenobarbital, phenytoin, primidone. Clonazepam may induce absence status in patients with absence type seizures. CNS depression with alcohol and other CNS depressants. Monitor PT/INR with warfarin.

PREGNANCY: Category D, not for use in nursing.

DEPAKOTE ER
divalproex sodium (Abbott)

RX

> Fatal hepatic failure (<2 yrs at considerable risk), teratogenic effects (eg, neural tube defects), and life-threatening pancreatitis reported.

THERAPEUTIC CLASS: Valproate compound

INDICATIONS: Migraine prophylaxis. Monotherapy and adjunct therapy for treatment of complex partial seizures, and simple and complex absence seizures. Adjunct for multiple seizure types that include absence seizures. Acute manic or mixed episodes associated with bipolar disorder.

DOSAGE: *Adults:* For qd dosing. Migraine: Initial: 500mg qd for 1 week. Titrate: Increase to 1000mg qd. Max: 1000mg/day. Complex Partial Seizures: Monotherapy/Adjunct Therapy: Initial: 10-15mg/kg/day. Titrate: Increase by 5-10mg/kg/week to optimal response. Usual: Less than 60mg/kg/day (accepted therapeutic range 50-100mcg/mL). When converting to monotherapy, reduce concomitant antiepilepsy drug by 25% every 2 weeks starting at initiation or delay 1-2 weeks after start of therapy. Simple and Complex Absence Seizures: Initial: 15mg/kg/day. Titrate: Increase weekly by 5-10mg/kg/day to optimal response. Max: 60mg/kg/day. Mania: Initial: 25mg/kg/day given once daily. Titrate: Increase dose rapidly to clinical effect. Max: 60mg/kg/day. Conversion from Depakote: Administer Depakote ER qd using a dose 8-20% higher than the total daily dose of Depakote. If cannot directly convert to Depakote ER, consider increasing to next higher Depakote total daily dose before converting to appropriate total daily Depakote ER dose. Elderly: Give lower initial dose and titrate slowly. Decrease dose or d/c if decreased food or fluid intake or if excessive somnolence occurs. Swallow whole; do not crush or chew.

Pediatrics: ≥10yrs: For qd dosing. Complex Partial Seizures: Monotherapy/Adjunct Therapy: Initial: 10-15mg/kg/day. Titrate: Increase by 5-10mg/kg/week to optimal response. Usual: Less than 60mg/kg/day (accepted therapeutic range 50-100mcg/mL). When converting to monotherapy, reduce concomitant antiepilepsy drug by 25% every 2 weeks starting at initiation or delay 1-2 weeks after start of therapy. Simple and Complex Absence Seizures: Initial: 15mg/kg/day. Titrate: Increase weekly by 5-10mg/kg/day to optimal response. Max: 60mg/kg/day. Conversion from Depakote: Administer Depakote ER qd using a dose 8-20% higher than the total daily dose of Depakote. If cannot directly convert to Depakote ER, consider increasing to next higher Depakote total daily dose before converting to appropriate total daily Depakote ER dose. Swallow whole; do not crush or chew.

HOW SUPPLIED: Tab, Extended Release: 250mg, 500mg

CONTRAINDICATIONS: Hepatic disease, significant hepatic dysfunction, known urea cycle disorders (UCD).

WARNINGS/PRECAUTIONS: Hyperammonemic encephalopathy in UCD patients; d/c if this occurs. Prior to therapy, evaluate for UCD in high risk patients (eg, history of unexplained encephalopathy, coma, etc). If unexplained lethargy, vomiting, or mental status changes occur measure ammonia levels. Caution with hepatic disease and elderly. Check LFTs prior to therapy, then frequently during 1st 6 months. Dose-related thrombocytopenia and elevated liver enzymes reported. Thrombocytopenia significantly increases with plasma trough levels >110mcg/mL in females and >135mcg/mL in males. Monitor platelet and coagulation tests prior to therapy, then periodically. Altered thyroid function tests and urine ketone test. May stimulate replication of HIV and CMV viruses. Avoid abrupt discontinuation.

ADVERSE REACTIONS: Nausea, dyspepsia, diarrhea, vomiting, abdominal pain, increased appetite, asthenia, somnolence, infection, dizziness, tremor, weight gain, back pain, alopecia.

INTERACTIONS: Potentiates carbamazepine, amitriptyline, nortriptyline, diazepam, ethosuximide, primidone, lamotrigine, phenobarbital, phenytoin, tolbutamide, zidovudine, lorazepam. Efficacy potentiated by ASA, felbamate. Efficacy reduced by rifampin, carbamazepine, phenobarbital, phenytoin, primidone. Clonazepam may induce absence status in patients with history of absence type seizures. CNS depression with alcohol and other CNS depressants. Monitor PT/INR with warfarin.

PREGNANCY: Category D, not for use in nursing.

DEPO-MEDROL RX
methylprednisolone acetate (Pharmacia & Upjohn)

THERAPEUTIC CLASS: Glucocorticoid

INDICATIONS: Steroid responsive disorders.

DOSAGE: *Adults:* Local Effect: Rheumatoid/Osteoarthritis: Large Joint: 20-80mg. Medium Joint: 10-40mg. Small Joint: 4-10mg. Administer intra-articularly into synovial space every 1-5 weeks or more depending on relief. Ganglion/Tendinitis/Epicondylitis: 4-30mg into cyst/area of greatest tenderness. May repeat if necessary. Dermatologic Conditions: Inject 20-60mg into lesion. Distribute 20-40mg doses by repeated injections into large lesions. Usual: 1-4 injections. Systemic Effect: Substitute for Oral Therapy: IM dose should equal total daily PO methylprednisolone dose q24h. Prolonged Therapy: Administer weekly PO dose as single IM injection. Androgenital Syndrome: 40mg IM every 2 weeks. Rheumatoid Arthritis: 40-120mg IM weekly. Dermatologic Lesions: 40-120mg IM weekly for 1-4 weeks. Acute Severe Dermatitis (Poison Ivy): 80-120mg IM single dose. Chronic Contact Dermatitis: May repeat injections every 5-10 days. Seborrheic Dermatitis: 80mg IM weekly. Multiple Sclerosis: 200mg/day prednisolone for 1 week, then 80mg every other day for 1 month (4mg methylprednisolone=5mg prednisolone). Asthma/Allergic Rhinitis: 80-120mg IM.

Pediatrics: Use lower adult doses. Determine dose by severity of condition and response.

Depo-Testosterone

HOW SUPPLIED: Inj: 20mg/mL, 40mg/mL, 80mg/mL

CONTRAINDICATIONS: Intrathecal administration, systemic fungal infections.

WARNINGS/PRECAUTIONS: Dermal and subdermal atrophy reported; do not exceed recommended doses. May need to increase dose before, during, and after stressful situations. May mask signs of infection or cause new infections. Prolonged use may produce cataracts, glaucoma, secondary ocular infections. Increases BP, salt/water retention, potassium and calcium excretion. More severe/fatal course of infections reported with chickenpox, measles. Caution with Strongyloides, latent TB, hypothyroidism, cirrhosis, ocular herpes simplex, HTN, diverticulitis, fresh intestinal anastomoses, ulcerative colitis, osteoporosis, myasthenia gravis, renal insufficiency, peptic ulcer disease. Kaposi's sarcoma reported. Growth and development of children on prolonged therapy should be monitored. Monitor for psychic disturbances. Avoid abrupt withdrawal. Do not use intra-articularly, intrabursally, or for intratendinous administration in acute infection. Avoid injection into unstable and previously infected joints. Monitor urinalysis, blood sugar, BP, weight, chest x-ray, and upper GI x-ray (if ulcer history) regularly during prolonged therapy.

ADVERSE REACTIONS: Fluid and electrolyte disturbances, HTN, osteoporosis, muscle weakness, cushingoid state, menstrual irregularities, impaired wound healing, DM, ulcerative esophagitis, excessive sweating, increases intracranial pressure, carbohydrate intolerance, glaucoma, cataracts, urticaria, subcutaneous/cutaneous atrophy.

INTERACTIONS: Reduced efficacy with hepatic enzyme inducers (eg, phenobarbital, phenytoin, and rifampin). Increases clearance of chronic high dose ASA. Caution with ASA in hypoprothrombinemia. Effects on oral anticoagulants are variable; monitor PT. Increased insulin and oral hypoglycemic requirements in DM. Avoid live vaccines with immunosuppressive doses. Possible decreased vaccine response with killed or inactivated vaccines with immunosuppressive doses. Mutual inhibition of metabolism with cyclosporine; convulsions reported. Potentiated by ketoconazole and troleandomycin. Do not dilute or mix with other solutions.

PREGNANCY: Safety in pregnancy and nursing not known.

Depo-Testosterone `CIII`
testosterone cypionate (Pharmacia & Upjohn)

THERAPEUTIC CLASS: Androgen

INDICATIONS: Testosterone replacement in males with primary hypogonadism and hypogonadotropic hypogonadism.

DOSAGE: *Adults:* Male Hypogonadism: 50-400mg IM every 2-4 weeks. Dose based on age, sex, and diagnosis. Adjust dose according to response and adverse reactions.
Pediatrics: ≥12 yrs: Male Hypogonadism: 50-400mg IM every 2-4 weeks. Dose based on age, sex, and diagnosis. Adjust dose according to response and adverse reactions.

HOW SUPPLIED: Inj: 100mg/mL, 200mg/mL

CONTRAINDICATIONS: Severe renal, hepatic and cardiac disease. Males with carcinoma of the breast or prostate gland. Pregnancy.

WARNINGS/PRECAUTIONS: May accelerate bone maturation without linear growth; monitor bone growth every 6 months. Risk of hepatic damage with long-term use. Discontinue if hypercalcemia occurs in immobilized patients. Discontinue with acute urethral obstruction, priapism, excessive sexual stimulation, or oligospermia; restart at lower doses. Risk of edema; caution with pre-existing cardiac, renal or hepatic disease. Caution in the elderly; increased risk of prostatic hypertrophy and prostatic carcinoma. Caution with BPH. Should not be used for enhancement of athletic performance. Do not administer IV. Monitor Hct, Hgb, cholesterol periodically.

ADVERSE REACTIONS: Gynecomastia, excessive frequency/duration of penile erections, male pattern baldness, increased/decreased libido, oligospermia, hirsutism, acne, fluid and electrolyte disturbances, nausea, hypercholesterolemia, clotting factor suppression, polycythemia, altered LFTs, priapism, anxiety, depression.

INTERACTIONS: Potentiates oral anticoagulants (eg, warfarin) and oxyphenbutazone. May decrease blood glucose and insulin requirements in diabetics.

PREGNANCY: Category X, not for use in nursing.

DERMA-SMOOTHE/FS
fluocinolone acetonide (Hill Dermaceuticals)

RX

THERAPEUTIC CLASS: Corticosteroid

INDICATIONS: Treatment of atopic dermatitis and scalp psoriasis.

DOSAGE: *Adults:* Atopic Dermatitis: Apply tid. Scalp Psoriasis: Wet/dampen hair and scalp thoroughly. Massage into scalp and cover with shower cap. Wash hair with regular shampoo after minimum of 4 hrs and rinse thoroughly.

Pediatrics: Atopic Dermatitis: ≥2 yrs: Moisten skin and apply bid up to 4 weeks.

HOW SUPPLIED: Oil: 0.01% (120mL)

WARNINGS/PRECAUTIONS: May produce reversible HPA axis suppression, manifestations of Cushing's syndrome, hyperglycemia, and glucosuria. Pediatrics may be more susceptible to systemic toxicity. Use appropriate antifungal or antibacterial agent with dermatological infections. Contains refined peanut oil NF. Discontinue if develop hypersensitivity. Avoid face, diaper area, and intertriginous areas with pediatrics.

ADVERSE REACTIONS: Dryness, folliculitis, acneiform eruptions, perioral dermatitis, allergic contact dermatitis, secondary infections, skin atrophy, striae, miliaria, burning, itching, irritation, hypopigmentation.

PREGNANCY: Category C, caution in nursing.

DERMATOP
prednicarbate (Dermik)

RX

THERAPEUTIC CLASS: Corticosteroid (medium-potency)

INDICATIONS: Corticosteroid responsive dermatoses.

DOSAGE: *Adults:* (Cre, Oint) Apply bid.

Pediatrics: ≥1 yr: (Cre) Apply bid. Max: 3 weeks of therapy. ≥10 yrs: (Oint) Apply bid.

HOW SUPPLIED: Cre, Oint: 0.1% (15g, 60g)

WARNINGS/PRECAUTIONS: May produce reversible HPA axis suppression, manifestations of Cushing's syndrome, hyperglycemia, and glucosuria. D/C if irritation occurs. Use appropriate antifungal or antibacterial agent with dermatological infections. Pediatrics may be more susceptible to systemic toxicity. Re-evaluate if no improvement after 2 weeks. Avoid eyes, occlusive dressings. Not for treatment of diaper dermatitis.

ADVERSE REACTIONS: Stinging, burning, dry skin, pruritus, urticaria, allergic contact dermatitis, edema, paresthesia, rash, skin atrophy.

PREGNANCY: Category C, caution in nursing.

DESFERAL
deferoxamine mesylate (Novartis)

RX

THERAPEUTIC CLASS: Iron-chelating agent

INDICATIONS: Treatment of acute iron intoxication and of chronic iron overload due to transfusion-dependent anemias.

DOSAGE: *Adults:* See labeling for solution preparation. Iron Intoxication: IM preferred for all patients not in shock. Only use IV slow infusion with cardiovascular collapse, and do not exceed 15mg/kg/hr for the 1st 1g. Subsequent IV dosing should not exceed 125mg/hr. IM: Initial: 1g, then 500mg q4h for 2 doses. Give subsequent 500mg doses q4-12h depending upon clinical response. Max: 6g/24 hrs. IV: 1g, then 500mg over 4 hrs for 2 doses. Give subsequent 500mg doses over 4-12 hrs depending upon clinical response. Max: 6g/24 hrs. Iron Overload: IM: 500mg-1g/day IM. In addition, 2g IV per unit of blood transfused; not to exceed 15mg/kg/hr. Max: 1g without transfusion or 6g even with ≥3 units of blood or PRBC. SQ: 1-2g (20-40mg/kg/day) SQ over 8-24 hrs using small pump for continuous infusion. Individualize duration.

DESMOPRESSIN ACETATE

Pediatrics: ≥3 yrs: See labeling for solution preparation. Iron Intoxication: IM preferred for all patients not in shock. Only use IV slow infusion with cardiovascular collapse, and do not exceed 15mg/kg/hr for the 1st 1g. Subsequent IV dosing should not exceed 125mg/hr. IM: Initial: 1g, then 500mg q4h for 2 doses. Give subsequent 500mg doses q4-12h depending upon clinical response. Max: 6g/24 hrs. IV: 1g, then 500mg over 4 hrs for 2 doses. Give subsequent 500mg doses over 4-12 hrs depending upon clinical response. Max: 6g/24 hrs. Iron Overload: IM: 500mg-1g/day IM. In addition, 2g IV per unit of blood transfused; not to exceed 15mg/kg/hr. Max: 1g without transfusion or 6g even with ≥3 units of blood or PRBC. SQ: 1-2g (20-40mg/kg/day) SQ over 8-24 hrs using small pump for continuous infusion. Individualize duration.

HOW SUPPLIED: Inj: 500mg, 2g

CONTRAINDICATIONS: Severe renal disease, anuria.

WARNINGS/PRECAUTIONS: Ocular and auditory disturbances reported with prolonged use, high doses, or low ferritin levels. Periodic visual acuity tests, slit-lamp exams, funduscopy, and audiometry with prolonged treatment. High doses with low ferritin levels associated with growth retardation. Adult respiratory distress syndrome, also in children, reported after high IV doses in acute iron intoxication or thalassemia. Give IM, slow SQ, or IV infusion; skin flushing, urticaria, hypotension, and shock reported with rapid IV injection. High dose may exacerbate neurological dysfunction in aluminum-related encephalopathy. May precipitate onset of dialysis dementia. Aluminum overload with deferoxamine may decrease serum calcium and aggravate hyperparathyroidism. D/C with mucormycosis, *Yersinia enterocolitica* or *Yersinia pseudotuberculosis* infections. Monitor pediatrics body weight and growth every 3 months. Caution in elderly patients.

ADVERSE REACTIONS: Injection site reactions, hypersensitivity reactions, tachycardia, hypotension, shock, abdominal discomfort, diarrhea, nausea, vomiting, blood dyscrasia, leg cramps, growth retardation, bone changes, reddish urine.

INTERACTIONS: Cardiac dysfunction reported with high dose vitamin C (>500mg/day in adults) in patients with severe chronic iron overload; avoid vitamin C supplements in cardiac failure patients. Only give vitamin C after 1 month of deferoxamine therapy and monitor cardiac function. Do not exceed vitamin C 200mg/day in adults; 50mg/day for pediatrics <10 yrs and 100mg/day for older children usually suffices. Concurrent prochlorperazine may lead to temporary impairment of consciousness. May distort imaging results with gallium-67; discontinue deferoxamine 48 hrs before scintigraphy.

PREGNANCY: Category C, caution in nursing.

DESMOPRESSIN ACETATE RX
desmopressin acetate (Ferring)

THERAPEUTIC CLASS: Synthetic vasopressin analog

INDICATIONS: Management of primary nocturnal enuresis, central cranial diabetes insipidus and temporary polyuria and polydipsia following head trauma or surgery.

DOSAGE: *Adults:* Central Cranial Diabetes Insipidus: 0.1-0.4mL/day as single dose or divided into 2-3 doses.

Pediatrics: Primary Nocturnal Enuresis: ≥6 yrs: 20mcg intranasally hs. Administer 1/2 the dose into each nostril. Max: 40mcg/day. Central Cranial Diabetes Insipidus: >12 yrs: 0.1-0.4mL/day as single dose or divided into 2-3 doses. 3 months-12 yrs: 0.05-0.3mL/day as single dose or divided into 2-3 doses.

HOW SUPPLIED: Sol: 0.01% (5mL)

WARNINGS/PRECAUTIONS: For intranasal use only. Adjust fluid intake downward in order to decrease the potential for water intoxication and hyponatremia. May increase BP, caution in coronary insufficiency and cardiovascular disease. Caution in fluid and electrolyte imbalance. Anaphylaxis reported. Changes in the nasal mucosa may cause erratic absorption, use IV administration in these cases.

ADVERSE REACTIONS: Transient headache, nausea, nasal congestion, rhinitis, flushing, abdominal cramps, nosebleed, sore throat, cough, upper respiratory tract infection, water intoxication, hyponatremia, asthenia, dizziness, epistaxis, GI disorder, conjunctivitis, edema lachrymation disorder.

INTERACTIONS: Caution with pressor agents.

PREGNANCY: Category B, caution in nursing.

Desonate
desonide (SkinMedica)

RX

THERAPEUTIC CLASS: Corticosteroid

INDICATIONS: Mild to moderate atopic dermatitis.

DOSAGE: *Adults:* Apply thin layer bid to affected area and rub in gently. Not recommended beyond 4 consecutive weeks.

Pediatrics: ≥3 months: Apply a thin layer bid to the affected area and rub in gently. Not recommended beyond 4 consecutive weeks.

HOW SUPPLIED: Gel: 0.05% (15g, 30g, 60g)

WARNINGS/PRECAUTIONS: May produce reversible HPA axis suppression, manifestations of Cushing's syndrome, hyperglycemia, and glucosuria. Discontinue if irritation occurs. Pediatrics may be more susceptible to systemic toxicity. Caution when applied to large surface areas. Avoid occlusive dressings. Avoid use beyond 4 wks.

ADVERSE REACTIONS: Burning, rash, application site pruritus.

PREGNANCY: Category C, caution in nursing.

Desoxyn
methamphetamine HCl (Ovation)

CII

> High potential for abuse. Avoid prolonged therapy in obesity.

THERAPEUTIC CLASS: Sympathomimetic amine

INDICATIONS: Attention deficit disorder with hyperactivity. Short term adjunct to treat exogenous obesity.

DOSAGE: *Adults:* Obesity: 5mg, 1/2 hr before each meal. Do not exceed a few weeks of treatment.

Pediatrics: ADHD: ≥6 yrs: Initial: 5mg qd-bid. Titrate: Increase weekly by 5mg/day until optimum response. Usual: 20-25mg/day given bid. Obesity: ≥12 yrs: 5mg, 1/2 hr before each meal. Do not exceed a few weeks of treatment.

HOW SUPPLIED: Tab: 5mg

CONTRAINDICATIONS: Advanced arteriosclerosis, symptomatic cardiovascular disease, moderate to severe HTN, hyperthyroidism, glaucoma, agitated states, history of drug abuse, during or within 14 days of MAOI use.

WARNINGS/PRECAUTIONS: Tolerance to anorectic effect develops within a few weeks, do not exceed recommended dose to increase effect. Monitor growth in children. Caution with HTN. Do not use to combat fatigue or replace rest. Exacerbation of motor and phonic tics and Tourette's syndrome. May exacerbate behavior disturbance and thought disorder in psychotic pediatrics. Interrupt occasionally to determine if patient requires continued therapy.

ADVERSE REACTIONS: BP elevation, tachycardia, palpitation, dizziness, insomnia, tremor, diarrhea, constipation, dry mouth, urticaria, impotence, changes in libido.

INTERACTIONS: May alter insulin requirements. May decrease hypotensive effect of guanethidine. Avoid MAOIs. Caution with TCAs and indirect acting sympathomimetic amines. Antagonized by phenothiazines.

PREGNANCY: Category C, not for use in nursing.

Dexamethasone
dexamethasone (Various)

RX

OTHER BRAND NAME: Decadron (Merck)

THERAPEUTIC CLASS: Glucocorticoid

INDICATIONS: Treatment of steroid responsive disorders.

DOSAGE: *Adults:* Individualize for disease and patient response. Withdraw gradually. (Tab) Initial: 0.75-9mg/day PO. Maint: Decrease in small amounts to lowest effective dose. Cushing's Syndrome Test: 1mg PO at 11pm; draw blood at 8am next morning. Or,

DEXEDRINE

0.5mg PO q6h for 48 hrs; or 2mg (to distinguish if excess pituitary ACTH or other causes) PO q6h for 48 hrs; obtain 24 hr urine collections. (Inj) Initial: 0.5-9mg/day IV/IM. Cerebral Edema: Initial: 10mg IV, then 4mg IM q6h until edema subsides. Reduce dose after 2-4 days and gradually discontinue over 5-7 days. Palliative Management of Recurrent/Inoperable Brain Tumors: Maint: 2mg IV/PO bid-tid. Acute Allergic Disorders: 4-8mg IM on 1st day, then 1.5mg PO bid for 2 days, then 0.75mg PO bid for 1 day, then 0.75mg PO qd for 2 days. (Inj) Usual: 0.2-9mg. Maint: Decrease in small amounts to lowest effective dose. Intra-Articular/Intralesional/Soft Tissue Injection: Usual: 0.2-6mg once every 3-5 days to once every 2-3 weeks. See labeling for Shock Treatment. Take with meals and antacids to prevent peptic ulcer.

Pediatrics: Individualize for disease and patient response. Withdraw gradually. (Tab) Initial: 0.75-9mg/day PO. Maint: Decrease in small amounts to lowest effective dose. Cushing's Syndrome Test: 1mg PO at 11pm; draw blood at 8am next morning. Or, 0.5mg PO q6h for 48 hrs; or 2mg (to distinguish if excess pituitary ATCH or other causes) PO q6h for 48 hrs; obtain 24 hr urine collections. (Inj) Initial: 0.5-9mg/day IV/IM. Cerebral Edema: Initial: 10mg IV, then 4mg IM q6h until edema subsides. Reduce dose after 2-4 days and gradually discontinue over 5-7 days. Palliative Management of Recurrent/Inoperable Brain Tumors: Maint: 2mg IV/PO bid-tid. Acute Allergic Disorders: 4-8mg IM on 1st day, then 1.5mg PO bid for 2 days, then 0.75mg PO bid for 1 day, then 0.75mg PO qd for 2 days. (Inj) Usual: 0.2-9mg. Maint: Decrease in small amounts to lowest effective dose. Intra-Articular/Intralesional/Soft Tissue Injection: Usual: 0.2-6mg once every 3-5 days to once every 2-3 weeks. See labeling for shock treatment. Take with meals and antacids to prevent peptic ulcer.

HOW SUPPLIED: Inj: (Dexamethasone Sodium Phosphate) 4mg/mL, 10mg/mL; Sol: (Dexamethasone) 0.5mg/5mL, 1mg/mL; Tab: (Dexamethasone) 0.5mg*, 0.75mg*, 1mg*, 1.5mg*, 2mg*, 4mg*, 6mg* *scored

CONTRAINDICATIONS: Systemic fungal infections.

WARNINGS/PRECAUTIONS: Increase dose before, during, and after stressful situations. Avoid abrupt withdrawal. May mask signs of infection, activate latent amebiasis, elevate BP, cause salt/water retention, increase excretion of potassium and calcium. Prolonged use may produce cataracts, glaucoma, secondary ocular infections. Caution with recent MI, ocular herpes simplex, emotional instability, nonspecific ulcerative colitis, diverticulitis, peptic ulcer, renal insufficiency, HTN, osteoporosis, myasthenia gravis, threadworm infection, active tuberculosis. Enhanced effect with hypothyroidism, cirrhosis. Consider prophylactic therapy if exposed to measles or chickenpox. Risk of glaucoma, cataracts and eye infections. False negative dexamethasone suppression test with indomethacin.

ADVERSE REACTIONS: Fluid/electrolyte disturbances, muscle weakness, osteoporosis, peptic ulcer, pancreatitis, ulcerative esophagitis, impaired wound healing, headache, psychic disturbances, growth suppression (children), glaucoma, hyperglycemia, weight gain, nausea, malaise.

INTERACTIONS: Caution with ASA. Inducers of CYP3A4 (eg, phenytoin, phenobarbital, carbamazepine, rifampin) and ephedrine enhance clearance; increase steroid dose. Inhibitors of CYP3A4 (ketoconazole, macrolides) may increase plasma levels. Drugs that affect metabolism may interfere with dexamethasone suppression tests. Increased clearance of drugs metabolized by CYP3A4 (eg, indinavir, erythromycin). May increase or decrease phenytoin levels. Ketoconazole may inhibit adrenal corticosteroid synthesis and cause adrenal insufficiency during corticosteroid withdrawal. Antagonizes or potentiates coumarins. Hypokalemia with potassium-depleting diuretics. Live virus vaccines are contraindicated with immunosuppressive doses.

PREGNANCY: Safety in pregnancy not known, not for use in nursing.

DEXEDRINE
dextroamphetamine sulfate (GlaxoSmithKline)

`CII`

> High potential for abuse. Avoid prolonged use. Misuse may cause sudden death and serious CV adverse events.

OTHER BRAND NAME: Dexedrine Spansules (GlaxoSmithKline)
THERAPEUTIC CLASS: Sympathomimetic amine

DextroStat

INDICATIONS: Treatment of attention deficit disorder with hyperactivity (ADHD) and narcolepsy.

DOSAGE: *Adults:* Narcolepsy: Initial: 10mg/day. Titrate: May increase by 10mg/day every week. Usual: 5-60mg/day. For tabs, give 1st dose upon awakening and additional every 4-6 hrs. May give caps once daily.
Pediatrics: Narcolepsy: 6-12 yrs: Initial: 5mg qd. Titrate: Increase weekly by 5mg/day. ≥12 yrs: Initial: 10mg qd. Titrate: Increase weekly by 10mg/day. Usual: 5-60mg/day in divided doses. ADHD: Initial: 3-5 yrs: 2.5mg qd. Titrate: Increase weekly by 2.5mg/day. ≥6 yrs: 5mg qd-bid. Titrate: Increase weekly by 5mg/day. Max: 40mg/day. For tabs, give 1st dose upon awakening and additional every 4-6 hrs. May give caps once daily.

HOW SUPPLIED: Cap, Extended-Release: (Spansules) 5mg, 10mg, 15mg; Tab: 5mg*
*scored

CONTRAINDICATIONS: Advanced arteriosclerosis, symptomatic cardiovascular disease, moderate to severe HTN, hyperthyroidism, glaucoma, agitated states, history of drug abuse, during or within 14 days of MAOI use.

WARNINGS/PRECAUTIONS: May exacerbate symptoms of behavior disturbance and thought disorder in psychotic patients. Caution when using stimulants to treat patients with comorbid bipolar disorder because of concern for possible induction of mixed/manic episode in such patients. Stimulants at usual doses can cause treatment emergent psychotic or manic symptoms (eg, hallucinations, delusional thinking, mania) in children and adolescents without prior history of psychotic illness. Aggressive behavior or hostility reported in clinical trials and the postmarketing experience of some medications indicated for the treatment of ADHD. Caution with HTN. Tablets contain tartrazine; may cause allergy reactions. Exacerbation of motor and phonic tics and Tourette's syndrome. Monitor growth in children. Avoid with serious structural cardiac abnormalities, cardiomyopathy, serious heart rhythm abnormalities, CAD, or other serious cardiac problems. Avoid use in the presence of seizure. Visual disturbances reported with stimulant treatment.

ADVERSE REACTIONS: Palpitations, tachycardia, BP elevation, CNS overstimulation, restlessness, insomnia, dry mouth, GI disturbances, anorexia, urticaria, impotence.

INTERACTIONS: GI acidifying agents (guanethidine, reserpine, glutamic acid, etc.) and urinary acidifying agents (ammonium chloride, etc) decrease efficacy. MAOIs may cause hypertensive crisis. Potentiated by GI and urinary alkalinizers, propoxyphene overdose. Potentiated effects of both agents with TCAs. May delay absorption of phenytoin, ethosuximide, phenobarbital. Potentiates meperidine, norepinephrine, phenobarbital, phenytoin. Antagonized by haloperidol, chlorpromazine, lithium. Antagonizes adrenergic blockers, antihistamines, antihypertensives, veratrum alkaloids (antihypertensive).

PREGNANCY: Category C, not for use in nursing.

DextroStat   CII
dextroamphetamine sulfate (Shire US)

> High potential for abuse. Avoid prolonged use.

THERAPEUTIC CLASS: Sympathomimetic amine

INDICATIONS: Treatment of narcolepsy and attention deficit disorder with hyperactivity (ADHD).

DOSAGE: *Adults:* Narcolepsy: Initial: 10mg/day. Titrate: May increase by 10mg/day every week. Usual: 5-60mg/day. Give 1st dose upon awakening, and additional doses every 4-6 hrs.
Pediatrics: Narcolepsy: 6-12 yrs: Initial: 5mg/day. Titrate: Increase weekly by 5mg/day. ≥12 yrs: Initial: 10mg/day. Titrate: Increase weekly by 10mg/day. Usual: 5-60mg/day in divided doses. ADHD: 3-5 yrs: Initial: 2.5mg/day. Titrate: Increase weekly by 2.5mg/day until optimum response. 6-16 yrs: Initial 5mg qd-bid. Titrate: Increase weekly by 5mg/day optimum response. Give 1st dose upon awakening, and additional doses q4-6h.

HOW SUPPLIED: Tab: 5mg*, 10mg* *scored

CONTRAINDICATIONS: Advanced arteriosclerosis, symptomatic cardiovascular disease, moderate to severe HTN, hyperthyroidism, glaucoma, agitated states, history of drug abuse, during or within 14 days of MAOI use.

DIASTAT

WARNINGS/PRECAUTIONS: Caution in HTN. Contains tartrazine, may cause allergic reactions. Exacerbation of motor and phonic tics and Tourette's syndrome. May exacerbate behavior disturbance and thought disorder in psychotic pediatrics. Interrupt occasionally to determine if patient requires continued therapy. Monitor growth in children.

ADVERSE REACTIONS: BP elevation, tachycardia, palpitation, dizziness, insomnia, tremor, diarrhea, constipation, dry mouth, urticaria, impotence, changes in libido.

INTERACTIONS: GI acidifying agents (guanethidine, reserpine, glutamic acid, etc.) and urinary acidifying agents (ammonium chloride, etc.) decrease efficacy. MAOIs may cause hypertensive crisis. Potentiated by GI and urinary alkalinizers, propoxyphene overdose. Potentiated effects of both agents with TCAs. May delay absorption of phenytoin, ethosuximide, phenobarbital. Potentiates meperidine, norepinephrine, phenobarbital, phenytoin. Antagonized by haloperidol, chlorpromazine, lithium. Antagonizes adrenergic blockers, antihistamines, antihypertensives, veratrum alkaloids (antihypertensive).

PREGNANCY: Category C, not for use in nursing.

Diastat
diazepam (Valeant) — CIV

THERAPEUTIC CLASS: Benzodiazepine

INDICATIONS: Management of refractory patients with epilepsy, on stable regimens of anti-epileptic drugs, who require intermittent use to control bouts of increased seizure activity.

DOSAGE: *Adults:* 0.2mg/kg rectally. Calculate amount and round upwards to next available dose. May give 2nd dose 4-12 hrs later. Max: 5 episodes/month or 1 episode every 5 days.

Pediatrics: ≥12 yrs: 0.2mg/kg. 6-11yrs: 0.3mg/kg. 2-5 yrs: 0.5mg/kg. Calculate amount and round upwards to next available dose. May give 2nd dose 4-12 hrs later. For rectal administration. Max: 5 episodes/month and 1 episode every 5 days.

HOW SUPPLIED: Kit: 2.5mg, 5mg, 10mg, 15mg, 20mg

CONTRAINDICATIONS: Acute narrow angle glaucoma, untreated open angle glaucoma.

WARNINGS/PRECAUTIONS: Produces CNS depression. Avoid abrupt withdrawal. Caution with elderly, hepatic/renal dysfunction, compromised respiratory function, neurologic damage. Not for daily chronic use. Withdrawal symptoms reported with discontinuation.

ADVERSE REACTIONS: Somnolence, dizziness, headache, pain, abdominal pain, nervousness, vasodilation, diarrhea, ataxia, euphoria, incoordination, asthma, rhinitis, rash.

INTERACTIONS: Potentiated by phenothiazines, narcotics, barbiturates, valproate, MAOIs, and other antidepressants. Potential inhibitors of CYP450 2C19 (eg, cimetidine, quinidine, tranylcypromine) and CYP450 3A4 (eg, ketoconazole, troleandomycin, clotrimazole) may decrease elimination. CYP450 2C19 (eg, rifampin) and CYP450 3A4 (eg, carbamazepine, phenytoin, dexamethasone, phenobarbital) inducers could increase elimination. May interfere with metabolism of substrates for CYP450 2C19 (eg, omeprazole, propranolol, imipramine) and CYP450 3A4 (eg, cyclosporine, paclitaxel, terfenadine, theophylline, warfarin).

PREGNANCY: Category D, not for use in nursing.

Diazepam Injection
diazepam (Various) — CIV

THERAPEUTIC CLASS: Benzodiazepine

INDICATIONS: Management of anxiety disorders and short-term relief of anxiety symptoms. Symptomatic relief of acute alcohol withdrawal. Adjunct prior to endoscopic procedures, surgical procedures and cardioversion. Adjunct therapy in skeletal muscle spasm (eg, tetanus, etc), status epilepticus and severe recurrent convulsive disorders.

DOSAGE: *Adults:* Anxiety (moderate): 2-5mg IM/IV, may repeat in 3-4 hrs. Anxiety (severe): 5-10mg IM/IV, may repeat in 3-4 hrs. Alcohol Withdrawal (acute): 10mg IM/IV, then 5-10mg in 3-4 hrs if needed. Endoscopic Procedures: Usual: ≤10mg IV (up to 20mg) or 5-10mg IM 30 minutes prior to procedure. Muscle Spasm: 5-10mg IM/IV, then 5-10mg in 3-4 hrs if needed. Status Epilepticus/Severe Seizures: Initial: 5-10mg IV. Maint: May repeat at 10-15 minute intervals. Max: 30mg. Preoperative: 10mg IM. Cardioversion: 5-15mg IV, 5-10 minutes prior to procedure. Elderly/Debilitated: Usual: 2-5mg.

Pediatrics: Tetanus: 30 days-5 yrs: 1-2mg IM/IV (slowly), may repeat every 3-4 hrs prn. ≥5 yrs: 5-10mg IM/IV, may repeat every 3-4 hrs. Status Epilepticus/Severe Seizures: 30 days-5 yrs: 0.2-0.5mg IV (slowly) every 2-5 minutes up to 5mg. ≥5 yrs: 1mg IV (slowly) every 2-5 minutes up to 10mg, may repeat in 2-4 hrs.

HOW SUPPLIED: Inj: 5mg/mL

CONTRAINDICATIONS: Acute narrow angle glaucoma, untreated open angle glaucoma.

WARNINGS/PRECAUTIONS: Inject slowly and avoid small veins with IV. Do not mix or dilute with other products in syringe or infusion flask. Extreme caution in elderly, severely ill and those with limited pulmonary reserve. Avoid if in shock, coma or acute alcohol intoxication with depressed vital signs. May impair mental/physical abilities. Increase in grand mal seizures reported. Caution with kidney or hepatic dysfunction. Not for obstetrical use. Withdrawal symptoms may occur. Hypotension and muscular weakness reported. Monitor blood counts and LFT's. Not for maintenance of seizures once controlled.

ADVERSE REACTIONS: Drowsiness, fatigue, ataxia, venous thrombosis and phlebitis (injection site).

INTERACTIONS: Phenothiazines, narcotics, barbiturates, MAOIs, and other antidepressants may potentiate effects. Delayed clearance with cimetidine. Reduce narcotic dose by at least one-third. Risk of apnea with concomitant barbiturates, alcohol, or other CNS depressants.

PREGNANCY: Not for use during pregnancy, safety in nursing unknown.

DICLOXACILLIN   RX
dicloxacillin sodium (Various)

THERAPEUTIC CLASS: Penicillin (penicillinase-resistant)

INDICATIONS: Infections caused by penicillinase-producing staphylococci.

DOSAGE: *Adults:* Mild-Moderate Infection: 125mg q6h. Severe Infection: 250mg q6h for at least 14 days.

Pediatrics: <40kg: Mild-Moderate Infection: 12.5mg/kg/day in divided doses q6h. Severe Infection: 25mg/kg/day in divided doses q6h for at least 14 days.

HOW SUPPLIED: Cap: 250mg, 500mg; Sus: 62.5mg/5mL (100mL)

WARNINGS/PRECAUTIONS: Serious, fatal hypersensitivity reactions reported. Caution with history of allergy and/or asthma. Monitor renal, hepatic, and hematopoietic function with prolonged use. Not for use as initial therapy with serious, life-threatening infections, or with nausea, vomiting, gastric dilation, cardiospasm, or intestinal hypermotility.

ADVERSE REACTIONS: Allergic reactions, nausea, vomiting, diarrhea, stomatitis, black or hairy tongue, superinfection (prolonged use).

INTERACTIONS: Tetracycline may antagonize the bactericidal effects. Potentiated by probenecid.

PREGNANCY: Category B, caution in nursing.

DIDREX   CIII
benzphetamine HCl (Pharmacia & Upjohn)

THERAPEUTIC CLASS: Anorectic sympathomimetic amine

INDICATIONS: Short term adjunct treatment of exogenous obesity.

DIFFERIN

DOSAGE: *Adults:* Initial: 25-50mg qd. Usual: 25-50mg qd-tid.

Pediatrics: ≥12 yrs: Initial: 25-50mg qd. Usual: 25-50mg qd-tid.

HOW SUPPLIED: Tab: 50mg* *scored

CONTRAINDICATIONS: Advanced arteriosclerosis, symptomatic cardiovascular disease, moderate to severe HTN, agitated states, hyperthyroidism, glaucoma, history of drug abuse, concomitant CNS stimulants, MAOI use within 14 days, pregnancy.

WARNINGS/PRECAUTIONS: Caution with mild HTN. Discontinue if tolerance develops. Psychological disturbances reported when used with restrictive dietary regimen.

ADVERSE REACTIONS: Palpitations, tachycardia, BP elevation, restlessness, dizziness, insomnia, headache, tremor, sweating, dry mouth, nausea, diarrhea, unpleasant tastes, urticaria, altered libido.

INTERACTIONS: Hypertensive crisis risk if used within 14 days of MAOIs. Potentiates TCAs. Avoid with other CNS stimulants. Decreases effects of antihypertensives. Potentiated by urinary alkalinizing agents and reduced effect with urinary acidifying agents. May alter insulin requirements.

PREGNANCY: Category X, not for use in nursing.

DIFFERIN   RX
adapalene (Galderma)

THERAPEUTIC CLASS: Naphthoic acid derivative (retinoid-like)

INDICATIONS: Topical treatment of acne vulgaris.

DOSAGE: *Adults:* Apply qhs after washing.

Pediatrics: ≥12 yrs: Apply qhs after washing.

HOW SUPPLIED: Cre: 0.1% (45g); Gel: 0.1%, 0.3% (45g)

WARNINGS/PRECAUTIONS: Avoid contact with eyes, lips, paranasal creases, mucous membranes, cuts, abrasions, eczematous or sunburned skin. Minimize sun exposure. Extreme weather may increase skin irritation.

ADVERSE REACTIONS: Erythema, scaling, dryness, pruritus, burning, sunburn, acne flares.

INTERACTIONS: Caution with other topicals with strong drying effects, high concentration of alcohol, astringents, spices, or lime. Allow effects of sulfur, resorcinol, or salicylic acid to subside before use.

PREGNANCY: Category C, caution in nursing.

DIFLUCAN   RX
fluconazole (Pfizer)

THERAPEUTIC CLASS: Triazole antifungal

INDICATIONS: Treatment of vaginal, oropharyngeal, esophageal, and systemic candidiasis. Treatment of peritonitis and UTI caused by Candida. Treatment of cryptococcal meningitis. Prophylaxis in patients undergoing BMT.

DOSAGE: *Adults:* Vaginal Candidiasis: 150mg PO single dose. IV/PO: Oropharyngeal Candidiasis: 200mg 1st day then 100mg qd for minimum 2 weeks. Esophageal Candidiasis: 200mg 1st day then 100mg qd for minimum 3 weeks then treat 2 weeks following resolution of symptoms. Max: 400mg/day. Systemic Infections: 400mg/day. UTI/Peritonitis: 50-200mg/day. Cryptococcal Meningitis: 400mg 1st day then 200mg qd for 10-12 weeks after negative CSF culture. Suppression of relapse in AIDS: 200mg/day. Prophylaxis in BMT: 400mg/day. CrCl <50mL/min: Initial: LD 50-400mg. Maint: Give 50% of recommended dose.

Pediatrics: IV/PO: Oropharyngeal Candidiasis: 6mg/kg 1st day then 3mg/kg/day for minimum of 2 weeks. Esophageal Candidiasis: 6mg/kg 1st day then 3mg/kg/day for minimum 3 weeks and 2 weeks following resolution of symptoms. Max: 12mg/kg/day. Systemic Infections: 6-12mg/kg/day. Cryptococcal Meningitis: 12mg/kg 1st day then 6mg/kg/day for 10-12 weeks after negative CSF culture. Suppression of relapse in AIDS: 6mg/kg/day. CrCl <50mL/min: Initial: 50-400mg. Maint: Give 50% of recommended dose.

DILANTIN

HOW SUPPLIED: Inj: 200mg/100mL, 400mg/200mL; Sus: 50mg/5mL, 200mg/5mL (35mL); Tab: 50mg, 100mg, 150mg, 200mg

CONTRAINDICATIONS: Coadministration with cisapride or terfenadine (with multiple diflucan doses of ≥400mg). Caution if hypersensitive to other azoles.

WARNINGS/PRECAUTIONS: Monitor LFTs. D/C if hepatic dysfunction develops or exfoliative skin disorder progresses. Anaphylaxis reported.

ADVERSE REACTIONS: Headache, nausea, abdominal pain, diarrhea, skin rash, vomiting.

INTERACTIONS: Severe hypoglycemia with oral hypoglycemics. May increase PT with coumarin-type drugs. Increases levels of phenytoin, cyclosporine, cisapride, astemizole, zidovudine and theophylline. Rifampin enhances metabolism of fluconazole. Cimetidine may decrease levels. HCTZ may increase levels. Contraindicated with terfenadine and cisapride due to prolongation of QTc interval. Cardiac events (torsade de pointes) reported with cisapride. Uveitis reported with rifabutin. Nephrotoxicity reported with tacrolimus. May increase or decrease levels of ethinyl estradiol- and levonorgestrel-containing oral contraceptives.

PREGNANCY: Category C, not for use in nursing.

DIGIBIND   RX
digoxin immune fab (ovine) (GlaxoSmithKline)

THERAPEUTIC CLASS: Antidote, digoxin toxicity

INDICATIONS: Treatment of life-threatening digoxin intoxication.

DOSAGE: *Adults:* Acute Ingestion of Unknown Amount: Usual: Administer 10 vials, observe response, then additional 10 vials if clinically indicated. Calculation: # vials = total digitalis body load (mg)/0.5mg of digitalis bound per vial. 1 vial will bind approximately 0.5mg of digoxin (or digitoxin). Digoxin Concentrations At Steady State: # of vials = (serum dig conc in ng/mL) x (wt in kg)/100. Digitoxin Concentrations At Steady State: # of vials = (serum digitoxin conc in ng/mL) x (wt in kg)/1000. If toxicity not adequately reversed after several hrs or appears to recur, may need readministration. See labeling for details.

Pediatrics: Acute Ingestion of Unknown Amount: Usual: Administer 10 vials, observe response, then additional 10 vials if clinically indicated. Calculation: # vials = total digitalis body load (mg)/0.5mg of digitalis bound per vial. 1 vial will bind approximately 0.5mg of digoxin (or digitoxin). Digoxin Concentrations At Steady State: Dose (mg) = (# vials) (38mg/vial). Digitoxin Concentrations At Steady State: # of vials = (serum digitoxin conc in ng/mL) x (wt in kg)/1000. If toxicity not adequately reversed after several hrs or appears to recur, may need readministration. See labeling for details.

HOW SUPPLIED: Inj: 38mg

WARNINGS/PRECAUTIONS: Obtain digoxin level before initiation. Do not overlook possibility of multiple drug overdose. Risk of hypersensitivity is greater with allergies to papain, chymopapain, or other papaya extracts; skin testing may be appropriate for high risk individuals. K+ levels may drop rapidly after administration; monitor closely. Digitalis toxicity may recur with renal dysfunction. Caution with cardiac dysfunction, further deterioration may occur from digoxin withdrawal. Can provide additional support with inotropes or vasodilators. Monitor for volume overload in children.

ADVERSE REACTIONS: Allergic reactions, exacerbation of low cardiac output, CHF.

PREGNANCY: Category C, caution in nursing.

DILANTIN   RX
phenytoin (Parke-Davis)

THERAPEUTIC CLASS: Hydantoin

INDICATIONS: (CER, CTB) Control of generalized tonic-clonic (grand mal) and complex partial (psychomotor, temporal lobe) seizures. Prevention and treatment of neurosurgically induced seizures. (Sus) Control of tonic-clonic (grand mal) and psychomotor (temporal lobe) seizures.

Diphenhydramine HCl Injection

DOSAGE: *Adults:* (CER) Initial: 100mg tid. Titrate: May increase at 7-10 day intervals. Max: 200mg tid. May give once daily with extended release if controlled on 300mg daily. LD (clinic/hospital): 1g in 3 divided doses (400mg, 300mg, 300mg) given 2 hrs apart. Start maintenance 24 hrs later. (CTB) Initial: 100mg tid. Titrate: May increase at 7-10 day intervals. Usual: 300-400mg/day. Max: 600mg/day. May chew or swallow tab whole. Not for once daily dosing. (Sus) Initial: 125mg tid. Titrate: May increase at 7-10 day intervals. Max: 625mg/day.

Pediatrics: (CER, CTB, Sus) Initial: 5mg/kg/day given bid-tid. Titrate: May increase at 7-10 day intervals. Maint: 4-8mg/kg/day. Max: 300mg/day. >6 yrs: May require the minimum adult dose (300mg/day).

HOW SUPPLIED: Cap, Extended Release (CER): 30mg, 100mg; Sus: 125mg/5mL (237mL); Tab, Chewable (CTB): 50mg* *scored

WARNINGS/PRECAUTIONS: Avoid abrupt discontinuation. Caution with porphyria, hepatic dysfunction, elderly, diabetes, debilitated. D/C if rash occurs. Lymphadenopathy reported. Serum sickness may occur with lymph node involvement. Gingival hyperplasia reported; maintain proper dental hygiene. Hyperglycemia, birth defects and osteomalacia reported. Monitor levels. Confusional states reported with increased levels. Increased seizure frequency during pregnancy. Neonatal coagulation defects reported within first 24 hrs of birth. Give Vitamin K to mother before delivery and to neonate after birth. Avoid use with seizures due to hypoglycemia or other metabolic causes.

ADVERSE REACTIONS: Nystagmus, ataxia, slurred speech, decreased coordination, confusion, dizziness, insomnia, transient nervousness, motor twitchings, headaches, nausea, vomiting, constipation, rash, hypersensitivity reactions.

INTERACTIONS: Increased levels with acute alcohol intake, amiodarone, chloramphenicol, chlordiazepoxide, diazepam, dicumarol, disulfiram, estrogens, H_2-antagonists, halothane, isoniazid, methylphenidate, phenothiazines, phenylbutazone, salicylates, succinamides, sulfonamides, tolbutamide, trazodone. Decreased levels with chronic alcohol abuse, carbamazepine, reserpine, sucralfate. Decreases effects of corticosteroids, coumarin anticoagulants, digitoxin, doxycycline, estrogens, furosemide, oral contraceptives, quinidine, rifampin, theophylline, vitamin D. Phenobarbital, sodium valproate, valproic acid may increase or decrease levels. May increase or decrease levels of phenobarbital, sodium valproate, valproic acid. Calcium antacids decrease absorption; space dosing. Moban® contains calcium ions which interfere with absorption. TCAs may precipitate seizures. Increased risk of phenytoin hypersensitivity with barbiturates, succinamides, oxazolidinediones.

PREGNANCY: Possibly teratogenic, weigh benefits versus risk; not for use in nursing.

DIPHENHYDRAMINE HCl INJECTION RX
diphenhydramine HCl (Various)

THERAPEUTIC CLASS: Antihistamine

INDICATIONS: Amelioration of allergic reactions to blood or plasma. Adjunct to epinephrine in anaphylaxis. For other uncomplicated immediate type allergic conditions when oral therapy is contraindicated. Treatment of motion sickness. For parkinsonism when oral therapy is not possible or contraindicated.

DOSAGE: *Adults:* Usual: 10-50mg IV or up to 100mg IM if needed. Max: 400mg/day.
Pediatrics: Usual: 5mg/kg/24hrs or 150mg/m^2/24hrs IV/IM in 4 divided doses. Max: 300mg/day.

HOW SUPPLIED: Inj: 50mg/mL

CONTRAINDICATIONS: Neonates, premature infants, nursing, as a local anesthetic.

WARNINGS/PRECAUTIONS: Caution with narrow-angle glaucoma, stenosing peptic ulcer, pyloroduodenal obstruction, symptomatic prostatic hypertrophy, or bladder-neck obstruction. May cause excitation in pediatrics. Increased risk of dizziness, sedation, and hypotension in elderly. Caution with lower respiratory diseases, bronchial asthma, increased IOP, hyperthyroidism, cardiovascular disease, or HTN. Local necrosis with SQ or intradermal use.

ADVERSE REACTIONS: Sedation, drowsiness, dizziness, disturbed coordination, epigastric distress, thickening of bronchial secretions.

INTERACTIONS: Additive effects with alcohol, CNS depressants. MAOIs prolong and intensify anticholinergic effects.

PREGNANCY: Category B, contraindicated in nursing.

Diprivan
propofol (Various)

RX

THERAPEUTIC CLASS: General anesthetic

INDICATIONS: Sedative-hypnotic agent used for both induction and maintenance of anesthesia. For initiation and maintenance of monitored anesthesia care (MAC) sedation during diagnostic procedures and in conjunction with local/regional anesthesia in patients undergoing surgical procedures. To provide continuous sedation and control of stress responses in intubated, mechanically ventilated adult patients in ICU.

DOSAGE: Adults: General Anesthesia: <55 yrs: 40mg IV every 10 seconds until induction onset. Maint: 100-200mcg/kg/min IV or 20-50mg intermittently byIV bolus prn. Elderly/Debilitated/ASA III & IV: 20mg IV every 10 seconds until induction onset. Maint: 50-100mcg/kg/min IV. Cardiac Anesthesia: 20mg IV every 10 seconds until induction onset. Maint: 100-150mcg/kg/min IV with secondary opioid or 50-100mcg/kg/min IV with primary opioid. Neurosurgical Patients: 20mg IV every 10 seconds until induction onset. Maint: 100-200mcg/kg/min IV. MAC Sedation: 100-150mcg/kg/min IV infusion or 0.5mg/kg slow IV injection over 3-5 min followed immediately by maintenance infusion. Maint: 25-75mcg/kg/min IV infusion or 10-20mg incremental IV boluses. Elderly/Debilitated/ASA III & IV: Use doses similar to healthy adults. Avoid rapid boluses. Maint: 80% of the usual adult dose. ICU Sedation: Initial: 5mcg/kg/min IV infusion for 5 min. Increase 5-10mcg/kg/min IV over 5-10 min. Maint: 5-50mcg/kg/min IV or higher may be required.

Pediatrics: 3-16 yrs: General Anesthesia: 2.5-3.5mg/kg IV over 20-30 seconds. Maint: 2 months-16 yrs: 125-300mcg/kg/min IV.

HOW SUPPLIED: Inj: 10mg/mL

WARNINGS/PRECAUTIONS: Avoid rapid bolus administration in elderly, debilitated or ASA III/IV patients. Monitor oxygen saturation and for signs of significant hypotension, bradycardia, cardiovascular depression, apnea or airway obstruction. Caution with hyperlipoproteinemia, diabetic hyperlipemia, pancreatitis, epilepsy. Rare reports of anaphylaxis reactions, pulmonary edema, perioperative myoclonia, postoperative pancreatitis, bradycardia, asystole, cardiac arrest, rhabdomyolysis. Minimize transient local pain by using larger veins of forearm or antecubital fossa and/or prior lidocaine injection. May elevate serum TG. Do not infuse for >5 days without drug holiday to replace zinc losses; consider supplemental zinc with chronic use in those predisposed to zinc deficiency. In renal impairment, perform baseline urinalysis/urinary sediment then monitor on alternate days during sedation. (Neurosurgical Anesthesia) Use infusion or slow bolus to avoid significant hypotension and decreases in cerebral perfusion pressure. (Cardiac Anesthesia) Use slower rates of administration in premedicated and geriatric patients, patients with recent fluid shifts or those hemodynamically unstable. Correct fluid deficits prior to use.

ADVERSE REACTIONS: Bradycardia, arrhythmia, hypotension, HTN, tachycardia nodal, decreased cardiac output, CNS movement, injection site burning/stinging/pain, hyperlipemia, apnea, rash, pruritus, respiratory acidosis during weaning.

INTERACTIONS: Increased effects with narcotics (eg, morphine, meperidine, fentanyl), combinations of opioids and sedatives (eg, benzodiazepines, barbiturates, chloral hydrate, droperidol) and potent inhalational agents (eg, isoflurane, enflurane, halothane). Concomitant fentanyl may cause bradycardia in pediatrics.

PREGNANCY: Category B, not for use in nursing.

Diprolene
betamethasone (augmented) dipropionate (Schering)

RX

OTHER BRAND NAME: Diprolene AF (Schering)

THERAPEUTIC CLASS: Corticosteroid

DisperMox

INDICATIONS: Relief of inflammatory and pruritic manifestations of corticosteroid responsive dermatoses.

DOSAGE: *Adults:* (Gel, Lot) Apply qd-bid for no more than 2 weeks. Limit to (Gel) 50g/week, (Lot) 50mL/week. (Cre, Oint) Apply qd-bid, up to 45g/week.
Pediatrics: ≥13 yrs: (Cre) Apply qd-bid for no more than 2 weeks. Limit to 45g/week. ≥12 yrs: (Gel, Lot) Apply qd-bid for no more than 2 weeks. Limit to (Gel) 50g/week, (Lot) 50mL/week. (Oint) Apply qd-bid, up to 45g/week.

HOW SUPPLIED: Cre (AF), Gel, Oint: 0.05% (15g, 50g); Lot: 0.05% (30mL, 60mL)

WARNINGS/PRECAUTIONS: May produce reversible HPA axis suppression, manifestations of Cushing's syndrome, hyperglycemia and glucosuria. Discontinue if irritation occurs. Use appropriate antifungal or antibacterial agent with dermatological infections. Pediatrics may be more susceptible to systemic toxicity. Caution when applied to large surface areas. Not for use with occlusive dressings. Gel is not for use in rosacea or perioral dermatitis or on the face, groin, or in the axillae.

ADVERSE REACTIONS: Stinging, burning, dry skin, pruritus, folliculitis, acneiform papules, irritation, hypopigmentation, skin maceration, secondary infection, skin atrophy, striae, miliaria.

PREGNANCY: Category C, (Cre, Lot) not for use in nursing; (Gel, Oint) caution in nursing.

DisperMox RX
amoxicillin (Ranbaxy)

THERAPEUTIC CLASS: Semisynthetic ampicillin derivative

INDICATIONS: Infections of the ear, nose, throat, genitourinary tract, skin and skin structure, lower respiratory tract due to susceptible (beta lactamase negative) organisms; gonorrhea (acute uncomplicated).

DOSAGE: *Adults:* ENT/SSSI/GU: (Mild/Moderate): 500mg q12h or 250mg q8h. (Severe): 875mg q12h or 500mg q8h. LRTI: 875mg q12h or 500mg q8h. Gonorrhea: 3g as single oral dose. Do not chew or swallow dispersible tabs.
Pediatrics: Neonates: ≤12 weeks: Max: 30mg/kg/day divided q12h. >3 months: ENT/SSSI/GU: (Mild/Moderate): 25mg/kg/day given q12h or 20mg/kg/day given q8h. (Severe): 45mg/kg/day given q12h or 40 mg/kg/day given q8h. LRTI: 45mg/kg/day given q12h or 40mg/kg/day given q8h. Gonorrhea: (Prepubertal) 50mg/kg with 25mg/kg probenecid as single dose (regimen not for use if <2 yrs). >40kg: Dose as adult. Do not chew or swallow dispersible tabs.

HOW SUPPLIED: Tab, Dispersible: 200mg, 400mg, 600mg

WARNINGS/PRECAUTIONS: Monitor renal, hepatic, and blood with prolonged use. Dispersible tabs contain phenylalanine.

ADVERSE REACTIONS: Nausea, vomiting, diarrhea, pseudomembranous colitis, hypersensitivity reactions, blood dyscrasias, superinfection (prolonged use).

INTERACTIONS: Increased levels with probenecid. Chloramphenicol, macrolides, sulfonamides, tetracyclines may interfere with bactericidal effects. False (+) for urine glucose with Clinitest, Benedict's or Fehling's solution.

PREGNANCY: Category B, caution in nursing.

Ditropan XL RX
oxybutynin chloride (Ortho-McNeil)

OTHER BRAND NAME: Ditropan (Ortho-McNeil)

THERAPEUTIC CLASS: Anticholinergic agent

INDICATIONS: (All) Overactive bladder/bladder instability with symptoms of urge urinary incontinence, urgency, and frequency. (Tab, Extended Release) Detrusor overactivity associated with a neurological condition in pediatrics ≥6 years old.

DOSAGE: *Adults:* (Tab, Syrup) Usual: 5mg bid-tid. Max: 5mg qid. (Tab, Extended Release) Initial: 5 or 10mg qd. Titrate: May increase by 5mg weekly. Max: 30mg/day. Swallow XL whole with liquid; do not chew, divide or crush tab.

Pediatrics: >5 yrs: (Tab, Syrup) Usual: 5mg bid. Max: 5mg tid. ≥6 yrs: (Tab, Extended Release) Initial: 5mg qd. Titrate: May increase by 5mg weekly. Max: 20mg/day. Swallow XL whole with liquid; do not chew, divide, or crush tab.

HOW SUPPLIED: Syrup: 5mg/5mL; Tab: 5mg*; Tab, Extended Release: 5mg, 10mg, 15mg *scored

CONTRAINDICATIONS: (Tab/Syrup) Untreated angle closure glaucoma and narrow anterior chamber angles, GI tract obstruction, paralytic ileus, intestinal atony, megacolon, toxic megacolon complicating ulcerative colitis, severe colitis, myasthenia gravis, obstructive uropathy, unstable cardiovascular status in acute hemorrhage. (Tab, Extended-Release) Urinary retention, gastric retention, uncontrolled narrow-angle glaucoma, and in patients at risk for these conditions.

WARNINGS/PRECAUTIONS: Caution with hepatic or renal impairment, bladder outflow obstruction, GI obstruction/narrowing, ulcerative colitis, intestinal atony, myasthenia gravis, autonomic neuropathy, hyperthyroidism, CHD, CHF, arrhythmias, HTN, tachycardia, prostatic hypertrophy, and GERD. Heat prostration can occur with high environmental temperatures. D/C if diarrhea develops. Tab, Extended-Release shell may be excreted in the stool.

ADVERSE REACTIONS: Dry mouth, constipation, somnolence, headache, diarrhea, nausea, blurred vision, dyspepsia, asthenia, pain, dizziness, rhinitis, dry eyes, UTI.

INTERACTIONS: Increased adverse effects with other anticholinergics. Increased drowsiness with alcohol or other sedatives. May alter GI absorption of other drugs due to GI motility effects. Increased levels with ketoconazole; caution with CYP3A4 inhibitors (eg, antimycotics, macrolides). Caution with bisphosphonates or other drugs that may exacerbate esophagitis.

PREGNANCY: Category B, caution in nursing.

DIURIL RX
chlorothiazide (Salix)

THERAPEUTIC CLASS: Thiazide diuretic

INDICATIONS: (PO/IV) Adjunct therapy in edema associated with CHF, hepatic cirrhosis, corticosteroid and estrogen therapy, renal dysfunction. (PO) Management of hypertension.

DOSAGE: *Adults:* (PO/IV) Edema: 0.5-1g qd-bid. May give every other day or 3-5 days/week. Substitute IV for oral using same dosage. (PO) HTN: 0.5-1g qd or in divided doses. Max: 2g/day.
Pediatrics: (PO) Diuresis/HTN: Usual: 10-20mg/kg/day given qd-bid. Max: Infants up to 2 yrs: 375mg/day. 2-12 yrs: 1g/day. <6 months: Up to 15mg/kg bid may be required.

HOW SUPPLIED: Inj: 0.5g; Sus: 250mg/5mL (237mL); Tab: 250mg*, 500mg* *scored

CONTRAINDICATIONS: Anuria, sulfonamide hypersensitivity.

WARNINGS/PRECAUTIONS: Caution in severe renal disease, liver dysfunction, electrolyte/fluid imbalance. Monitor electrolytes. Hyperuricemia, hyperglycemia, hypokalemia, hyponatremia, hypomagnesemia, hypercalcemia may occur. Increases in cholesterol and triglyceride levels reported. May exacerbate SLE. Sensitivity reactions reported. D/C prior to parathyroid test. Enhanced effects in post-sympathectomy patient. IV use not recommended in infants or children.

ADVERSE REACTIONS: Weakness, hypotension, pancreatitis, jaundice, diarrhea, vomiting, blood dyscrasias, rash, photosensitivity, electrolyte imbalance, impotence.

INTERACTIONS: May potentiate orthostatic hypotension with alcohol, barbiturates, narcotics. Adjust antidiabetic drugs. Possible decreased response to pressor amines. Corticosteroids, ACTH increase electrolyte depletion. May potentiate nondepolarizing skeletal muscle relaxants, antihypertensives. Lithium toxicity. NSAIDs decrease effects. Decreased PO absorption with cholestyramine, colestipol.

PREGNANCY: Category C, not for use in nursing.

DOLOBID RX
diflunisal (Merck)

> NSAIDs may cause an increased risk of serious cardiovascular thrombotic events, MI, stroke and serious GI adverse events including bleeding, ulceration, and perforation of the stomach or intestines. Contraindicated for the treatment of peri-operative pain in the setting of coronary artery bypass graft (CABG) surgery.

THERAPEUTIC CLASS: NSAID

DONNATAL

INDICATIONS: Acute or long-term symptomatic treatment of mild to moderate pain, osteoarthritis (OA), rheumatoid arthritis (RA).

DOSAGE: *Adults:* Pain: Initial: 1g, then 500mg q8-12h. OA/RA: 250-500mg bid. Max: 1500mg/day.

Pediatrics: ≥12 yrs: Pain: Initial: 1g, then 500mg q12h or 500mg q8h. OA/RA: 250-500mg bid. Max: 1500mg/day.

HOW SUPPLIED: Tab: 250mg, 500mg

CONTRAINDICATIONS: ASA or other NSAID allergy that precipitates acute asthmatic attack, urticaria, or rhinitis. Treatment of peri-operative pain in the setting of CABG surgery.

WARNINGS/PRECAUTIONS: May lead to onset of new HTN or worsening of pre-existing HTN; monitor BP closely. Fluid retention and edema reported; caution with fluid retention or heart failure. Renal papillary necrosis and other renal injury reported after long-term use. Not recommended for use with advanced renal disease; if therapy must be initiated, monitor renal function. Anaphylactoid reactions may occur. May cause serious skin adverse events (eg, exfoliative dermatitis, Stevens-Johnson syndrome, and toxic epidermal necrolysis). Avoid in late pregnancy; may cause premature closure of ductus arteriosis. May cause elevations of LFTs; d/c if liver disease develops or systemic manifestations occur. Caution in elderly. Anemia may occur; with long-term use, monitor Hgb/Hct if signs or symptoms of anemia develop. May inhibit platelet aggregation and prolong bleeding time; monitor with coagulation disorders. Caution with asthma and avoid with aspirin-sensitive asthma. Adverse eye findings reported. Hypersensitivity syndrome reported; d/c if hypersensitivity occurs. Reye's syndrome may develop.

ADVERSE REACTIONS: Nausea, dyspepsia, GI pain, diarrhea, rash, headache, insomnia, dizziness, tinnitus, fatigue.

INTERACTIONS: May prolong PT with oral anticoagulants. Decreases hyperuricemic effect of HCTZ, furosemide. Antacids may reduce plasma levels. Avoid other NSAIDs. May potentiate methotrexate, cyclosporine toxicities. Increased plasma levels of APAP. Decreased plasma levels with ASA. Caution with nephrotoxic or hepatotoxic drugs.

PREGNANCY: Category C, not for use in nursing.

DONNATAL RX
phenobarbital - atropine sulfate - hyoscyamine sulfate - scopolamine hydrobromide (PBM Pharmaceuticals)

OTHER BRAND NAME: Donnatal Extentabs (PBM Pharmaceuticals)

THERAPEUTIC CLASS: Anticholinergic/barbiturate

INDICATIONS: Adjunct therapy for irritable bowel syndrome, acute enterocolitis, duodenal ulcers.

DOSAGE: *Adults:* (Elixir/Tab) 1-2 tabs or 5-10mL tid-qid. (Extentabs) 1 tab q8-12h. Hepatic Disease: Use lower doses.

Pediatrics: (Elixir) 4.5kg: 0.5mL q4h or 0.75mL q6h. 9.1kg: 1mL q4h or 1.5mL q6h. 13.6kg: 1.5mL q4h or 2mL q6h. 22.7kg: 2.5mL q4h or 3.75mL q6h. 34kg: 3.75mL q4h or 5mL q6h. 45.4kg: 5mL q4h or 7.5mL q6h. Hepatic Disease: Use lower doses.

HOW SUPPLIED: (Atropine-Hyoscyamine-Phenobarbital-Scopolamine) Elixir: 0.0194mg-0.1037mg-16.2mg-0.0065mg/5mL; Tab: 0.0194mg-0.1037mg-16.2mg-0.0065mg; Tab, Extended Release: (Extentabs) 0.0582mg-0.3111mg-48.6mg-0.0195mg

CONTRAINDICATIONS: Glaucoma, obstructive uropathy, obstructive GI disease, paralytic ileus, intestinal atony in elderly or debilitated, unstable cardiovascular status in acute hemorrhage, severe ulcerative colitis, myasthenia gravis, hiatal hernia with reflux esophagitis, intermittent porphyria, and for patients in whom phenobarbital produces restlessness and/or excitement.

WARNINGS/PRECAUTIONS: Inconclusive whether anticholinergic/antispasmodic drugs aid in duodenal ulcer healing, decrease recurrence rate, or prevent complications. Heat prostration can occur with high environmental temperatures. Avoid with intestinal obstruction. May be habit forming; caution with history of physical and/or psychological drug dependence. Caution with hepatic disease, renal disease, autonomic neuropathy, hyperthyroidism, coronary heart disease, CHF, arrhythmias, tachycardia, HTN.

May delay gastric emptying. Diarrhea may be an early symptom of incomplete intestinal obstruction, especially with ileostomy or colostomy; treatment would be inappropriate.

ADVERSE REACTIONS: Xerostomia, urinary hesitancy/retention, blurred vision, tachycardia/palpitation, mydriasis, cycloplegia, increased ocular tension, loss of taste, headache, nervousness, drowsiness, weakness, dizziness, insomnia, nausea, vomiting, impotence, suppression of lactation, constipation, bloated feeling, musculoskeletal pain, allergic reaction/drug idiosyncrasies, decreased sweating.

INTERACTIONS: Phenobarbital may decrease anticoagulant effects; adjust dose.

PREGNANCY: Category C, caution in nursing.

Doryx
doxycycline hyclate (Warner Chilcott)

RX

THERAPEUTIC CLASS: Tetracycline derivative

INDICATIONS: Treatment of susceptible infections including respiratory, urinary, skin and skin structure, lymphogranuloma, psittacosis, trachoma, uncomplicated urethral/endocervical/rectal, nongonococcal urethritis, rickettsiae, chancroid, plague, cholera, brucellosis, anthrax. When penicillin is contraindicated, treatment of syphilis, listeriosis, *Clostridium* species, and others. Adjunct therapy for amebiasis and severe acne.

DOSAGE: *Adults:* Usual: 100mg q12h on 1st day, followed by 100mg qd. Severe Infections/Chronic UTI: 100mg q12h. Uncomplicated Gonococcal Infections (Men, except anorectal infections): 100mg bid for 7 days, or 300mg followed in 1 hr by another 300mg dose. Acute Epididymo-Orchitis: 100mg bid for at least 10 days. Primary/Secondary Syphilis: 300mg/day in divided doses for at least 10 days. Nongonococcal Urethritis, Uncomplicated Urethral/Endocervical/Rectal Infection: 100mg bid for at least 7 days. Inhalational Anthrax (post-exposure): 100mg bid for 60 days. Treat Strep infections for 10 days.

Pediatrics: >8 yrs: >100lbs: 100mg q12h on 1st day, followed by 100mg qd. Severe Infections/Chronic UTI: 100mg q12h. ≤100lbs: 2mg/lb given bid on day 1, followed by 1mg/lb given qd-bid thereafter. Severe Infections: Up to 2mg/lb. Inhalational Anthrax (post-exposure): <100lbs: 1mg/lb bid for 60 days. ≥100lbs: 100mg bid for 60 days.

HOW SUPPLIED: Cap: 75mg, 100mg

WARNINGS/PRECAUTIONS: May cause fetal harm during pregnancy. Use during tooth development (last half of pregnancy, infancy, <8 yrs) may cause permanent discoloration of the teeth or enamel hypoplasia. Photosensitivity, increased BUN, superinfection may occur. Monitor hematopoietic, renal and hepatic values periodically with long term therapy. Bulging fontanels in infants and benign intracranial HTN in adults reported. May decrease bone growth in premature infants.

ADVERSE REACTIONS: Anorexia, nausea, vomiting, diarrhea, dysphagia, enterocolitis, rash, exfoliative dermatitis, renal toxicity, hypersensitivity reactions, blood dyscrasias.

INTERACTIONS: May require downward adjustments of anticoagulant dosage. May interfere with bactericidal action of penicillin; avoid concurrent use when possible. Avoid antacids containing aluminum, calcium, or magnesium, sodium bicarbonate, and iron-containing preparations.

PREGNANCY: Category D, not for use in nursing.

Dryvax
smallpox vaccine, dried (Wyeth)

RX

> Acute myopericarditis has been observed after administration. Encephalitis and progressive vaccinia have occured following smallpox immunization, almost always in immunocompromised patients. Severe vaccinal skin infections have occured among persons with eczema. Do not administer in persons with eczema, cardiac disease and immunocompromised.

THERAPEUTIC CLASS: Vaccine

INDICATIONS: For active immunization against smallpox disease.

DOSAGE: *Adults:* Give IM into deltoid muscle or posterior aspect of arm over triceps muscle. Use 2 or 3 needle punctures for primary vaccination and 15 punctures for revaccination. May cover vaccination site with a porous bandage, until scab separates and underlying skin has healed. Inspect vaccination site 6-8 days later to interpret response.

Pediatrics: ≥12 months: Give IM into deltoid muscle or posterior aspect of arm over triceps muscle. Use 2 or 3 needle punctures for primary vaccination and 15 punctures for revaccination. May cover vaccination site with a porous bandage, until scab separates and underlying skin has healed. Inspect vaccination site 6-8 days later to interpret response.

HOW SUPPLIED: Inj: 100 million PFU

CONTRAINDICATIONS: (Routine non-emergency use) Hypersensitivity to polymyxin B sulfate, dihydrostreptomycin sulfate, chlortetracycline HCl, and neomycin sulfate; infants <12 months of age; eczema, history of eczema, or other acute, chronic, or exfoliative skin conditions (including household contacts of such persons); systemic corticosteroid use at doses ≥2mg/kg or ≥20mg/day of prednisone for ≥2 weeks, or immunosuppressive use (eg, alkylating agents, antimetabolites), or radiation (including household contacts of such persons); congenital or acquired immune deficiencies (including household contacts of such persons); immunosuppressed individuals (including household contacts of such persons); pregnancy (including household contacts of such persons).

WARNINGS/PRECAUTIONS: Vial stopper contains dry natural rubber; caution with latex sensitivity. Patients susceptible to adverse effects of caccinia virus should avoid contact with persons with active vaccination lesions. Vaccinia virus may be cultured from site of primary vaccine from time of papule development until scab separates from skin lesion. Not recommended for elderly in non-emergency conditions.

ADVERSE REACTIONS: Fever, rash, secondary pyogenic infections at vaccination site, inadvertent inoculation at other sites, regional lymphadenopathy, malaise.

INTERACTIONS: Avoid salves or ointments on vaccination site.

PREGNANCY: Category C, not for use in nursing in non-emergency conditions.

Duac   RX
clindamycin - benzoyl peroxide (Stiefel)

THERAPEUTIC CLASS: Antibacterial/keratolytic

INDICATIONS: Topical treatment of inflammatory acne vulgaris.

DOSAGE: *Adults:* Wash face and pat dry. Apply qd in the evening.

Pediatrics: ≥12 yrs: Wash face and pat dry. Apply qd in the evening.

HOW SUPPLIED: Gel: (Clindamycin-Benzoyl Peroxide) 1%-5% (45g)

CONTRAINDICATIONS: Hypersensitivity to lincomycin. History of regional enteritis, ulcerative colitis, pseudomembranous colitis, or antibiotic-associated colitis.

WARNINGS/PRECAUTIONS: Severe colitis reported with oral and parenteral clindamycin. Discontinue if severe diarrhea occurs. Avoid contact with eyes and mucous membranes. May bleach hair or colored fabric. Limit sunlight exposure.

ADVERSE REACTIONS: Dry skin, erythema, peeling, burning.

INTERACTIONS: Cumulative irritancy possible with other topical acne agents. Avoid erythromycin agents.

PREGNANCY: Category C, not for use in nursing.

Dulcolax   OTC
bisacodyl (Boehringer Ingelheim)

THERAPEUTIC CLASS: Stimulant laxative

INDICATIONS: Relief of occasional constipation and irregularity. For bowel cleansing regimen for surgery or endoscopic exam.

DOSAGE: *Adults:* (Tab) Take 2-3 tabs qd. Do not crush/chew. (Sup) Insert 1 sup rectally; retain for 15-20 minutes. May coat tip with petroleum jelly with anal fissures or hemorrhoids. X-Ray Endoscopy For Barium Enema: Avoid food after tab administration. Insert 1 sup rectally 1-2 hrs before exam.

Pediatrics ≥12 yrs: (Tab) 2-3 tabs qd. 6-12 yrs: 1 tab qd. Do not crush/chew. (Sup) ≥12 yrs: Insert 1 sup rectally; retain for 15-20 minutes. 6-12 yrs: Insert 1/2 sup rectally qd. May coat tip with petroleum jelly with anal fissures or hemorrhoids. X-Ray Endoscopy For Barium Enema: ≥6 yrs: Avoid food after tab administration. Insert 1 sup 1-2 hrs before exam. <6 yrs: Avoid tab. Insert 1/2 sup rectally 1-2 hrs before exam.

HOW SUPPLIED: Sup: 10mg; Tab, Delayed Release: 5mg

CONTRAINDICATIONS: Acute abdominal surgery, appendicitis, rectal bleeding, gastroenteritis, intestinal obstruction.

WARNINGS/PRECAUTIONS: Avoid with abdominal pain, nausea, or vomiting. Not for long-term use (>7 days). D/C with rectal bleeding or fail to have bowel movement.

ADVERSE REACTIONS: Abdominal discomfort.

INTERACTIONS: Avoid tabs within 1 hr after antacids or milk.

PREGNANCY: Safety in pregnancy and nursing not known.

DURAGESIC
fentanyl (Ortho-McNeil)

CII

> Life-threatening hypoventilation can occur. Contraindicated for acute or post-op pain, mild/intermittent pain responsive to PRN or non-opioids, or in doses >25mcg/hr at initiation of opioid therapy. Avoid in patients <12 yrs or if <18 yrs and weigh <50kg. Only for use in opioid tolerant patients. Concomitant use with potent CYP450 3A4 inhibitors may result in an increase in fentanyl plasma concentrations which may cause potentially fatal respiratory depression. Monitor patients receiving potent CYP450 3A4 inhibitors.

THERAPEUTIC CLASS: Opioid analgesic

INDICATIONS: Management of chronic pain when continuous opioid analgesia is required and cannot be managed by lesser means.

DOSAGE: *Adults:* Individualize dose. Determine dose based on opioid tolerance. Initial: 25mcg/hr for 72 hr.

Pediatrics: >12 yrs: Individualize dose. Determine dose based on opioid tolerance. Initial: 25mcg/hr for 72 hr.

HOW SUPPLIED: Patch: 12.5mcg/hr, 25mcg/hr, 50mcg/hr, 75mcg/hr, 100mcg/hr (5^s)

CONTRAINDICATIONS: Management of acute/post-op pain, mild/intermittent pain responsive to PRN or non-opioid therapy. Doses >25mcg/hr at initiation. Hypersensitivity to adhesives. Diagnosis or suspicion of paralytic ileus.

WARNINGS/PRECAUTIONS: Monitor patients with adverse events for at least 12 hrs after removal. Avoid exposing application site to direct external heat. Hypoventilation may occur; caution with chronic pulmonary diseases. Caution with brain tumors, bradyarrhythmias, renal/hepatic impairment. Avoid with increased intracranial pressure, impaired consciousness, or coma. May obscure clinical course of head injury. Tolerance and physical dependence can occur.

ADVERSE REACTIONS: Hypoventilation, hypotension, HTN, nausea, vomiting, constipation, dry mouth, somnolence, confusion, asthenia, sweating.

INTERACTIONS: See Black Box Warning. Concomitant use with CNS depressants (opioids, sedatives, hypnotics, tranquilizers, general anesthetics, phenothiazines, skeletal muscle relaxants, alcohol) may cause respiratory depression, hypotension, profound sedation, or potentially coma or death. May increase clearance with CYP3A4 inducers (eg, rifampin, carbamazepine, phenytoin). Avoid use within 14 days of MAOI.

PREGNANCY: Category C, not for use in nursing.

DURATUSS
guaifenesin - pseudoephedrine HCl (Victory)

RX

THERAPEUTIC CLASS: Expectorant/decongestant

INDICATIONS: Relief of nasal congestion due to the common cold, hay fever, sinusitis, or other upper respiratory allergies. Relief of eustachian tube congestion and cough. Adjunct therapy in serious otitis media.

DOSAGE: *Adults:* 1 tab q12h.

Duratuss DM

Pediatrics: ≥12 yrs: 1 tab q12h. 6-12 yrs: 1/2 tab q12h.

HOW SUPPLIED: Tab, Extended Release: (Guaifenesin-Pseudoephedrine) 600mg-120mg* *scored

CONTRAINDICATIONS: Hypersensitivity to sympathomimetics, severe HTN, with MAOIs.

WARNINGS/PRECAUTIONS: Do not crush or chew tabs. Caution with HTN, hyperthyroidism, DM, heart disease, peripheral vascular disease, glaucoma, prostatic hypertrophy.

ADVERSE REACTIONS: Nervousness, insomnia, restlessness, headache.

INTERACTIONS: Avoid MAOIs. May reduce effects of antihypertensive drugs which interfere with sympathetic activity (eg, methyldopa, mecamylamine, reserpine). Increased ectopic pacemaker activity with digitalis. Caution with concomitant sympathomimetic amines.

PREGNANCY: Category C, not for use in nursing.

Duratuss DM
guaifenesin - dextromethorphan hydrobromide (Victory)

RX

THERAPEUTIC CLASS: Cough suppressant/expectorant

INDICATIONS: Relief of cough due to minor throat and bronchial irritation complicated by viscous mucus.

DOSAGE: *Adults:* 5mL q4h. Max: 30mL/24 hrs.

Pediatrics: >12 yrs: 5mL q4h. Max: 30mL/24 hrs. 6-12 yrs: 2.5mL q4h. Max: 15mL/24 hrs. 2-6 yrs: 1.25mL q4h. Max: 7.5mL/24 hrs.

HOW SUPPLIED: Elixir: (Dextromethorphan-Guaifenesin) 25mg-225mg/5mL

CONTRAINDICATIONS: Within 14 days of MAOI therapy.

WARNINGS/PRECAUTIONS: Re-evaluate if cough persists >1 week or recurs.

ADVERSE REACTIONS: Nausea, GI disturbances, dizziness, drowsiness, vomiting, headache, rash.

INTERACTIONS: Avoid use within 14 days of MAOI therapy; may cause serotonin syndrome. Additive CNS depressant effects with alcohol, antihistamines, psychotropics, other CNS depressants.

PREGNANCY: Category C, caution in nursing.

Duratuss G
guaifenesin (Victory)

RX

OTHER BRAND NAMES: Guaifenex G (Ethex) - Muco-Fen 1200 (Ivax) - Liquibid-D (Capellon) - Guaifenesin ER (Amide)

THERAPEUTIC CLASS: Expectorant

INDICATIONS: Temporary relief of symptoms associated with respiratory tract infections and related conditions. Loosens phlegm and thins bronchial secretions

DOSAGE: *Adults:* 1 tab q12h. Max: 2 tabs/24 hrs. May break tabs in half; do not crush or chew.

Pediatrics: >12 yrs: 1 tab q12h. Max: 2 tabs/24 hrs. 6-12 yrs: 1/2 tab q12h. Max: 1 tab/24 hrs. May break tabs in half; do not crush or chew.

HOW SUPPLIED: Tab, Extended Release: 1200mg* *scored

ADVERSE REACTIONS: Nausea, vomiting.

PREGNANCY: Category C, caution in nursing.

Duricef
cefadroxil monohydrate (Warner Chilcott)

RX

THERAPEUTIC CLASS: Cephalosporin (1st generation)

INDICATIONS: Skin and skin structure (SSSI) and urinary tract infection (UTI), pharyngitis, and tonsillitis.

DOSAGE: *Adults:* Uncomplicated Lower UTI: 1-2g/day given qd or bid. Other UTI: 1gm bid. SSSI: 1g qd or 500mg bid. Group A β-hemolytic Strep Pharyngitis/Tonsillitis: 1g qd or 500mg bid for 10 days. CrCl ≤50mL/min: Initial: 1g. Maint: CrCl 25-50mL/min: 500mg q12h; CrCl 10-25mL/min: 500mg q24h; CrCl 0-10mL/min: 500mg q36h.
Pediatrics: UTI/SSSI: 15mg/kg q12h. Pharyngitis/Tonsillitis/Impetigo: 30mg/kg qd or 15mg/kg q12h. Treat β-hemolytic strep infections for at least 10 days.

HOW SUPPLIED: Cap: 500mg; Sus: 250mg/5mL (50mL, 100mL), 500mg/5mL (50mL, 75mL, 100mL); Tab: 1g* *scored

WARNINGS/PRECAUTIONS: Caution with markedly impaired renal function, history of GI disease. Cross-sensitivity with cephalosporins and penicillins. False (+) direct Coombs' tests, pseudomembranous colitis reported.

ADVERSE REACTIONS: Diarrhea, rash, hypersensitivity reactions, pruritus, hepatic dysfunction, genital moniliasis, vaginitis, fever, superinfection (prolonged use).

PREGNANCY: Category B, caution in nursing.

DYNACIN
minocycline HCl (Medicis)

RX

THERAPEUTIC CLASS: Tetracycline derivative

INDICATIONS: Treatment of inclusion conjunctivitis, nongonococcal urethritis, and other infections (eg, respiratory tract, endocervical, rectal, urinary tract, skin and skin structure) caused by susceptible strains of microorganisms. Alternative treatment in certain other infections (eg, urethritis, gonococcal, syphilis, anthrax). Adjunctive therapy in acute intestinal amebiasis and severe acne. Treatment of *Mycobacterium marinum* and asymptomatic carriers of *Neisseria meningitidis*.

DOSAGE: *Adults:* Usual: 200mg initially, then 100mg q12h; alternative is 100-200mg initially, then 50mg qid. Uncomplicated Gonococcal Infection (Men, other than urethritis and anorectal infections): 200mg initially, then 100mg q12h for minimum 4 days. Uncomplicated Gonococcal Urethritis (Men): 100mg q12h for 5 days. Syphilis: Administer usual dose for 10-15 days. Meningococcal Carrier State: 100mg q12h for 5 days. *Mycobacterium marinum:* 100mg q12h for 6-8 weeks. Uncomplicated urethral, endocervical, or rectal infection: 100mg q12h for at least 7 days. Renal Dysfunction: Reduce dose and/or extend dose intervals.
Pediatrics: >8 yrs: 4mg/kg initially followed by 2mg/kg q12h. Take with plenty of fluids.

HOW SUPPLIED: Cap: 50mg, 75mg, 100mg; Tab: 50mg, 75mg, 100mg

WARNINGS/PRECAUTIONS: May cause fetal harm during pregnancy. Use during tooth development (last half of pregnancy, infancy, <8yrs) may cause permanent discoloration of the teeth or enamel hypoplasia; avoid use during this period. Renal toxicity, hepatotoxicity, photosensitivity, increased BUN, superinfection, pseudotumor cerebri may occur; perform hematopoietic, renal, and hepatic monitoring. May impair mental/physical abilities. Use alternate form of contraception other than oral contraceptives. May decrease bone growth in premature infants.

ADVERSE REACTIONS: Anorexia, nausea, vomiting, diarrhea, dysphagia, enterocolitis, pancreatitis, increased LFTs, hepatitis, liver failure, renal toxicity, rash, exfoliative dermatitis, Stevens-Johnson syndrome, skin and mucous membrane pigmentation, blood dyscrasias, headache, tooth discoloration.

INTERACTIONS: May require downward adjustments of anticoagulant dosage. May interfere with bactericidal action of penicillin; avoid concurrent use when possible. May decrease efficacy of oral contraceptives. Impaired absorption with antacids containing aluminum, calcium, or magnesium and iron-containing products. Fatal renal toxicity with methoxyflurane has been reported.

PREGNANCY: Category D, not for use in nursing.

E.E.S.
erythromycin ethylsuccinate (Abbott)

RX

THERAPEUTIC CLASS: Macrolide antibiotic

INDICATIONS: Mild to moderate upper and lower respiratory tract and skin and skin structure infections, listeriosis, pertussis, diphtheria, erythrasma, intestinal amebiasis,

Ecotrin

acute pelvic inflammatory disease (PID) (*N.gonorrhea*), primary syphilis in PCN allergy, Legionnaires' disease, chlamydial infections (eg, newborn conjunctivitis urethral, endocervical, or rectal, etc), and nongonococcal urethritis. Prophylaxis of endocarditis or rheumatic fever.

DOSAGE: *Adults:* Usual: 1600mg/day given q6h, q8h or q12h. Max: 4g/day. Treat strep infections for 10 days. Streptococcal Infection Prophylaxis with Rheumatic Heart Disease: 400mg bid. Urethritis (*C.trachomatis* or *U.urealyticum*): 800mg tid for 7 days. Primary Syphilis: 48-64g in divided doses over 10-15 days. Intestinal Amebiasis: 400mg qid for 10-14 days. Pertussis: 40-50mg/kg/day in divided doses for 5-14 days. Legionnaires' Disease: 1.6-4g/day in divided doses.

Pediatrics: Usual: 30-50mg/kg/day in divided doses q6h, q8h or q12h. Double dose for more severe infections. Treat strep infections for 10 days. Intestinal Amebiasis: 30-50mg/kg/day in divided doses for 10-14 days. Pertussis: 40-50mg/kg/day in divided doses for 5-14 days.

HOW SUPPLIED: Sus: 200mg/5mL, 400mg/5mL (100mL, 480mL), Tab: 400mg

CONTRAINDICATIONS: Concomitant terfenadine, astemizole, cisapride, pimozide.

WARNINGS/PRECAUTIONS: Pseudomembranous colitis, hepatic dysfunction reported. May aggravate myasthenia gravis.

ADVERSE REACTIONS: Nausea, vomiting, abdominal pain, diarrhea, anorexia, hepatic dysfunction, abnormal LFTs, allergic reactions, superinfection (prolonged use).

INTERACTIONS: Rhabdomyolysis reported with lovastatin. May increase levels of theophylline, digoxin, drugs metabolized by CYP450 (eg, carbamazepine, cyclosporine, tacrolimus, phenytoin, alfentanil, disopyramide, lovastatin, bromocriptine, valproate, etc). Increases effects of oral anticoagulants, triazolam, midazolam. Risk of acute ergot toxicity with ergotamine or dihydroergotamine. May potentiate sildenafil. Avoid terfenadine, astemizole, cisapride, pimozide.

PREGNANCY: Category B, caution in nursing.

Ecotrin   OTC
aspirin (GlaxoSmithKline Consumer)

THERAPEUTIC CLASS: Salicylate

INDICATIONS: To reduce the risk of death and nonfatal stroke with previous ischemic stroke or transient ischemia of the brain. To reduce risk of vascular mortality with suspected acute MI. To reduce risk of death and nonfatal MI with previous MI or unstable angina. To reduce risk of MI and sudden death in chronic stable angina. Indicated for patients who have undergone revascularization procedures with a pre-existing condition for which ASA is indicated. Relief of signs of rheumatoid arthritis (RA), juvenile rheumatoid arthritis (JRA), osteoarthritis (OA), spondyloarthropathies, arthritis, and pleurisy associated with SLE.

DOSAGE: *Adults:* Ischemic Stroke/TIA: 50-325mg qd. Suspected Acute MI: Initial: 160-162.5mg qd as soon as suspect MI. Maint: 160-162.5mg for 30 days post-infarction, consider further therapy for prevention/recurrent MI. Prevention or Recurrent MI/Unstable Angina/Chronic Stable Angina: 75-325mg qd. CABG: 325mg qd, start 6 hrs post-surgery. Continue for 1 year. PTCA: Initial: 325mg, 2 hrs pre-surgery. Maint: 160-325mg qd. Carotid Endarterectomy: 80mg qd to 650mg bid, start pre-surgery. RA/Arthritis/SLE Pleurisy: Initial: 3g qd in divided doses. Increase for anti-inflammatory efficacy to 150-300 mcg/mL plasma salicylate level. Spondyloarthropathies: Up to 4g/day in divided doses. OA: Up to 3g/day in divided doses.

Pediatrics: JRA: Initial: 90-130 mg/kg/day in divided doses. Increase for anti-inflammatory efficacy to 150-300 mcg/mL plasma salicylate level.

HOW SUPPLIED: Tab, Delayed Release: 81mg, 325mg, 500mg

CONTRAINDICATIONS: NSAID allergy, children or teenagers for viral infections with or without fever, syndrome of asthma, rhinitis, and nasal polyps.

WARNINGS/PRECAUTIONS: Increased risk of bleeding with heavy alcohol use (≥3 drinks/day). May inhibit platelet function; can adversely affect inherited (hemophilia) or acquired (hepatic disease, vitamin K deficiency) bleeding disorders. Monitor for bleeding and ulceration. Avoid in history of active peptic ulcer, severe renal failure, severe hepatic insufficiency, and sodium restricted diets. Associated with elevated LFTs, BUN, and serum creatinine; hyperkalemia; proteinuria; and prolonged bleeding time. Avoid one week before and during labor.

ADVERSE REACTIONS: Fever, hypothermia, dysrhythmias, hypotension, agitation, cerebral edema, dehydration, hyperkalemia, dyspepsia, GI bleed, hearing loss, tinnitus, problems in pregnancy.

INTERACTIONS: Diminished hypotensive and hyponatremic effects of ACE inhibitors. May increase levels of acetazolamide, valproic acid. Increased risk of bleeds with heparin, warfarin. Decreased levels of phenytoin. Decreased hypotensive effects of β-blockers. Decreased diuretic effects with renal or cardiovascular disease. Decreased methotrexate clearance; increased risk of bone marrow toxicity. Avoid NSAIDs. Increased effects of hypoglycemic agents. Antagonizes uricosuric agents.

PREGNANCY: Avoid in 3rd trimester of pregnancy and nursing.

EDECRIN
ethacrynic acid (Merck)
RX

THERAPEUTIC CLASS: Aryloxyacetic acid derivative

INDICATIONS: Treatment of edema when agent of greater diuretic potential is required. Treatment of edema in CHF, hepatic cirrhosis, and renal disease. Short term management of ascites due to malignancy, idiopathic edema, lymphedema; congenital heart disease and nephrotic syndrome in hospitalized pediatrics.

DOSAGE: *Adults:* Initial: 50-100mg qd. Titrate: 25-50mg increments. Usual: 50-200mg/day. After diuresis achieved, give smallest effective dose continuously or intermittently.
Pediatrics: Initial: 25mg. Titrate: Increase by 25mg increments. Maint: Reduce dose and frequency once dry weight achieved; may give intermittently.

HOW SUPPLIED: Tab: 25mg*, 50mg* *scored

CONTRAINDICATIONS: Anuria, infants. Discontinue if increasing electrolyte imbalance, azotemia, or oliguria develops during treatment of severe, progressive renal disease. Discontinue if severe, watery diarrhea occurs.

WARNINGS/PRECAUTIONS: Caution in advanced liver cirrhosis. Monitor serum electrolytes, CO2, BUN early in therapy and periodically during active diuresis. Vigorous diuresis may induce acute hypotensive episode and in elderly cardiac patients, hemoconcentration resulting in thromboembolic disorders. Ototoxicity reported with severe renal dysfunction. Hypomagnesemia and transient increase in serum urea nitrogen may occur. Reduce dose or withdraw if excessive electrolyte loss occurs. Initiate therapy in the hospital for cirrhotic patients with ascites. Liberalize salt intake and supplement with K^+ if needed. Reduced responsiveness in renal edema with hypoproteinemia; use salt poor albumin.

ADVERSE REACTIONS: Anorexia, malaise, abdominal discomfort, gout, deafness, tinnitus, vertigo, headache, fatigue, rash, chills.

INTERACTIONS: Risk of lithium toxicity. May increase ototoxic potential of aminoglycosides and some cephalosporins. Displaces warfarin from plasma protein; may need dose reduction. NSAIDs may decrease effects. Orthostatic hypotension may occur with antihypertensives. Increased risk of gastric hemorrhage with corticosteroids. Excessive K^+ loss may precipitate digitalis toxicity. Caution with K^+-depleting steroids.

PREGNANCY: Category B, not for use in nursing.

ELDOPAQUE FORTE
hydroquinone (Valeant)
RX

OTHER BRAND NAME: Eldoquin Forte (Valeant)

THERAPEUTIC CLASS: Depigmenting agent

INDICATIONS: For the gradual bleaching of hyperpigmented skin conditions (eg, chloasma, melasma, freckles, senile lentigines).

DOSAGE: *Adults:* Apply bid. Do not rub in Eldopaque Forte. Use sunscreen with Eldoquin Forte.

ELESTAT

Pediatrics: ≥12 yrs: Apply bid. Do not rub in Eldopaque Forte. Use sunscreen with Eldoquin Forte.

HOW SUPPLIED: Cre: 4% (28.4g)

WARNINGS/PRECAUTIONS: Avoid sun exposure on bleached skin. Eldopaque Forte contains sunblock; use sunscreen. May produce unwanted cosmetic effects if not used as directed. Test for skin sensitivity. D/C if no lightening effect after 2 months. Contains sodium metabisulfite; may cause serious allergic type reactions. Limit treatment to small areas of body at one time. Avoid contact with eyes.

ADVERSE REACTIONS: Cutaneous hypersensitivity (contact dermatitis).

PREGNANCY: Category C, caution in nursing.

ELESTAT RX
epinastine HCl (Allergan)

THERAPEUTIC CLASS: H_1 antagonist

INDICATIONS: For the prevention of itching associated with allergic conjunctivitis.

DOSAGE: *Adults:* 1 drop in each eye bid.

Pediatrics: ≥3 yrs: 1 drop in each eye bid.

HOW SUPPLIED: Sol: 0.05% (5mL)

WARNINGS/PRECAUTIONS: Not for contact lens related irritation. May reinsert contact lens 10 minutes after dosing if eye is not red.

ADVERSE REACTIONS: Burning sensation in the eye, folliculosis, hyperemia, pruritus.

PREGNANCY: Category C, caution in nursing.

ELIDEL RX
pimecrolimus (Novartis)

THERAPEUTIC CLASS: Macrolactam ascomycin derivative

INDICATIONS: Short-term and intermittent long-term therapy of moderate to severe atopic dermatitis in non-immunocompromised patients intolerant to or unresponsive to conventional therapy.

DOSAGE: *Adults:* Apply bid. Re-evaluate if symptoms persist after 6 weeks.

Pediatrics: ≥2 yrs: Apply bid. Re-evaluate if symptoms persist after 6 weeks.

HOW SUPPLIED: Cre: 1% (30g, 60g, 100g)

WARNINGS/PRECAUTIONS: Increased risk of varicella zoster infection, herpes simplex virus infection or eczema herpeticum. Lymphadenopathy reported; discontinue if unknown etiology of lymphadenopathy or acute mononucleosis presents. Skin papilloma or warts reported; consider discontinuation if worsening or unresponsive skin papilloma. Minimize or avoid natural or artificial sunlight exposure. Avoid with Netherton's syndrome, areas of active cutaneous viral infections, or occlusive dressings. Long-term safety has not been established. Rare cases of malignancy (eg, skin and lymphoma) have been reported with topical calcineurin inhibitors; therefore, continuous long-term use should be avoided and application limited to areas of involvement. Not indicated for use in children <2 yrs.

ADVERSE REACTIONS: Application site burning, headache, nasopharyngitis, influenza, pharyngitis, viral infection, pyrexia, cough.

INTERACTIONS: Caution with CYP3A4 inhibitors (eg, erythromycin, itraconazole, ketoconazole, fluconazole, calcium channel blockers, cimetidine) in widespread and/or erythrodermic disease.

PREGNANCY: Category C, not for use in nursing.

ELIMITE RX
permethrin (Allergan)

THERAPEUTIC CLASS: Pyrethroid scabicidal agent

INDICATIONS: Treatment of scabies.

DOSAGE: *Adults:* Massage into skin from head to soles of feet. Wash off after 8-14 hrs. One treatment should be adequate. Retreat if living mites present after 14 days.

Pediatrics: ≥2 months: Massage into skin from head (scalp, temples and forehead) to soles of feet. Wash off after 8-14 hrs. One treatment should be adequate. Retreat if living mites present after 14 days.

HOW SUPPLIED: Cre: 5% (60g)

CONTRAINDICATIONS: Allergy to synthetic pyrethroid or pyrethrin.

WARNINGS/PRECAUTIONS: May temporarily exacerbate infection (eg, pruritus, edema, erythema). Avoid eyes. D/C if hypersensitivity occurs.

ADVERSE REACTIONS: Burning, stinging, pruritus, erythema, numbness, tingling, rash.

PREGNANCY: Category B, not for use in nursing.

ELITEK
rasburicase (Sanofi-Aventis)

RX

> May cause serious hypersensitivity reactions including anaphylaxis; discontinue if this occurs. Hemolysis may occur in G6PD deficiency; discontinue with hemolysis. Before initiate, screen patients at high risk for G6PD deficiency. Discontinue if develop methemoglobinemia. Causes enzymatic degradation of uric acid within blood samples left at room temperature. Collect blood in pre-chilled tubes containing heparin; immediately immerse and maintain in ice water bath and assay sample within 4 hrs of collection.

THERAPEUTIC CLASS: Recombinant urate-oxidase enzyme

INDICATIONS: Initial management of plasma uric acid levels in pediatrics with leukemia, lymphoma, and solid tumor malignancies who are receiving anti-cancer therapy expected to result in tumor lysis and subsequent elevation of plasma uric acid.

DOSAGE: *Pediatrics:* 1 month-17 yrs: 0.15 or 0.2mg/kg IV as a single daily dose for 5 days. Administer over 30 minutes, not as a bolus infusion. Dosing >5 days or >1 course is not recommended. Initiate chemotherapy 4-24 hrs after 1st dose.

HOW SUPPLIED: Inj: 1.5mg

CONTRAINDICATIONS: G6PD deficiency, history of anaphylaxis or hypersensitivity reactions, hemolytic or methemoglobinemia reactions to rasburicase or any of the excipients.

WARNINGS/PRECAUTIONS: Screen patients at high risk for G6PD deficiency (eg, African or Mediterranean ancestry) prior to initiation. Administer IV hydration.

ADVERSE REACTIONS: Vomiting, fever, nausea, headache, abdominal pain, constipation, diarrhea, mucositis, rash, respiratory distress, sepsis, neutropenia with or without fever.

PREGNANCY: Category C, not for use in nursing.

ELMIRON
pentosan sodium (Ortho-McNeil)

RX

THERAPEUTIC CLASS: Analgesic, urinary

INDICATIONS: Relief of bladder pain/discomfort associated with interstitial cystitis.

DOSAGE: *Adults:* Take 1 hr before or 2 hrs after meals with water. 100mg tid for 3 months. Re-evaluate after 3 months; may continue for another 3 months.

Pediatrics: ≥16 yrs: Take 1 hr before or 2 hrs after meals with water. 100mg tid for 3 months. Re-evaluate after 3 months; may continue for another 3 months.

HOW SUPPLIED: Cap: 100mg

WARNINGS/PRECAUTIONS: Bleeding complications (eg, ecchymosis, epistaxis, gum hemorrhage), alopecia, increased PT/PTT reported. Caution with invasive procedures, coagulopathy, aneurysms, thrombocytopenia, hemophilia, GI ulcers, polyps, diverticula, history of heparin-induced thrombocytopenia, and hepatic impairment. Transient liver enzyme elevation reported.

ADVERSE REACTIONS: Nausea, diarrhea, alopecia, headache, rash, dyspepsia, abdominal pain.

ELOCON

INTERACTIONS: Increased risk of bleeding with anticoagulants, heparin, t-PA streptokinase, or high dose aspirin.

PREGNANCY: Category B, caution in nursing.

ELOCON RX
mometasone furoate (Schering)

THERAPEUTIC CLASS: Corticosteroid

INDICATIONS: Corticosteroid responsive dermatoses.

DOSAGE: *Adults:* (Cre, Oint) Apply qd. (Lot) Apply a few drops qd. Reassess if no improvement within 2 weeks.

Pediatrics: (Cre, Oint) ≥2 yrs: Apply qd for up to 3 weeks if needed. Avoid in diaper area. Reassess if no improvement within 2 weeks.

HOW SUPPLIED: Cre, Oint: 0.1% (15g, 45g); Lot: 0.1% (30mL, 60mL)

WARNINGS/PRECAUTIONS: May produce reversible HPA axis suppression, manifestations of Cushing's syndrome, hyperglycemia and glucosuria. Discontinue if irritation occurs. Use appropriate antifungal or antibacterial agent with dermatological infections. Pediatrics may be more susceptible to systemic toxicity. Caution when applied to large surface areas or with occlusive dressings.

ADVERSE REACTIONS: Burning, pruritus, skin atrophy, rosacea, acneiform reaction, tingling, stinging, furunculosis, folliculitis.

PREGNANCY: Category C, caution (Cre, Oint) or not for use (Lot) in nursing.

EMADINE RX
emedastine difumarate (Alcon)

THERAPEUTIC CLASS: H_1 receptor antagonist

INDICATIONS: Temporary relief of signs and symptoms of allergic conjunctivitis.

DOSAGE: *Adults:* 1 drop in affected eye up to qid.

Pediatrics: ≥3 yrs: 1 drop in affected eye up to qid.

HOW SUPPLIED: Sol: 0.05% (5mL)

WARNINGS/PRECAUTIONS: Wait at least 10 minutes after application to insert contact lens (if eye is not red). Not for irritation due to contact lens.

ADVERSE REACTIONS: Headache, abnormal dreams, asthenia, bad taste, blurred vision, burning, stinging, corneal infiltrates, corneal staining, dermatitis, discomfort, dry eye, foreign body sensation, hyperemia, keratitis, pruritus, rhinitis, sinusitis, tearing.

PREGNANCY: Category B, caution in nursing.

EMBELINE E RX
clobetasol propionate (Healthpoint)

THERAPEUTIC CLASS: Corticosteroid

INDICATIONS: Corticosteroid responsive dermatoses.

DOSAGE: *Adults:* Apply bid. Limit to 2 consecutive weeks. Max: 50g/week. Moderate-Severe Psoriasis: Apply to 5%-10% BSA up to 4 weeks. Max: 50g/week.

Pediatrics: ≥12 yrs: Apply bid. Limit to 2 consecutive weeks. Max: 50g/week. Moderate-Severe Psoriasis: ≥16 yrs: Apply to 5%-10% BSA up to 4 weeks. Max: 50g/week.

HOW SUPPLIED: Cre: 0.05% (15g, 30g, 60g)

WARNINGS/PRECAUTIONS: Not for use on the face, groin, or axillae, or for treatment of rosacea or perioral dermatitis. May produce reversible HPA axis suppression, manifestations of Cushing's syndrome, hyperglycemia, and glucosuria. Reassess if no improvement after 2 weeks. D/C if irritation occurs. Peds may be more susceptible to systemic toxicity. Avoid occlusive dressings.

ADVERSE REACTIONS: Burning/stinging, pruritus, irritation, erythema, folliculitis, cracking/fissuring of skin, numbness of fingers, tenderness in elbows, telangiectasia, skin atrophy.

PREGNANCY: Category C, caution in nursing.

EMLA
lidocaine - prilocaine (AstraZeneca LP)

RX

OTHER BRAND NAME: EMLA Anesthetic Disc (AstraZeneca LP)

THERAPEUTIC CLASS: Acetamide local anesthetic

INDICATIONS: Topical anesthetic for use on normal intact skin or on genital mucous membranes for minor surgery. Pretreatment for infiltration anesthesia.

DOSAGE: *Adults:* Apply 1 disc or thick layer of cream to intact skin and cover with occlusive dressing. Minor Dermal Procedure: Apply 2.5g (1/2 tube) over 20-25cm^2 of skin surface or 1 disc for 1 hr. Major Dermal Procedure: Apply 2g/10cm^2 of skin for 2 hrs. Adult Male Genital Skin: Apply 1g/10cm^2 of skin surface for 15 minutes. Female External Genitalia: Apply 5-10g for 5-10 minutes.

Pediatrics: All following doses are Max: 0-3 months or <5kg: 1g/10cm^2 for up to 1 hr. 3-12 months and ≥5 kg: 2g/20 cm^2 for up to 4 hrs. 1-6 yrs and >10 kg: 10g/100cm^2 for up to 4 hrs. 7-12 yrs and >20kg: 20g/200cm^2 for up to 4 hrs.

HOW SUPPLIED: (Lidocaine-Prilocaine) Cre: 2.5%-2.5%; Disc: 2.5%-2.5%

WARNINGS/PRECAUTIONS: Avoid application for longer than recommended times or large areas. Avoid with methemoglobinemia. Risk of methemoglobinemia in very young or with G6P deficiency. Avoid eye contact, use in ear. Caution with severe hepatic disease, acutely ill, debilitated, elderly, history of drug sensitivities. Avoid in neonates with a gestational age <37 weeks and infants <12 months receiving treatment with methemoglobin-inducing agents.

ADVERSE REACTIONS: Local reactions such as: erythema, edema, abnormal sensations, paleness (pallor or blanching), altered temperature sensations, itching, rash.

INTERACTIONS: Caution with Class I antiarrhythmics (eg, tocainide, mexiletine). Avoid drugs associated with drug-induced methemoglobinemia (eg, sulfonamides, APAP, nitrates/nitrites, nitrofurantoin, phenobarbital, phenytoin, quinine). Caution with other products containing local anesthetics; consider the amount absorbed from all formulations.

PREGNANCY: Category B, caution in nursing.

Emtriva
emtricitabine (Gilead)

RX

> Lactic acidosis and severe hepatomegaly with steatosis, including fatal cases, reported with nucleoside analogs alone or with concomitant antiretrovirals. Not indicated for the treatment of chronic HBV infection; severe acute exacerbations of hepatitis B reported in patients co-infected with HBV and HIV upon discontinuation of emtricitabine.

THERAPEUTIC CLASS: Nucleoside analogue

INDICATIONS: Treatment of HIV-1 infection in combination with other antivirals.

DOSAGE: *Adults:* ≥18 yrs: Cap: 200mg qd. CrCl 30-49mL/min: 200mg q48h. CrCl 15-29mL/min: 200mg q72h. CrCl <15mL/min (including hemodialysis): 200mg q96h. Sol: 240mg (24mL) qd. CrCl 30-49mL/min: 120mg (12mL) qd. CrCl 15-29mL/min: 80mg (8mL) qd. CrCl <15mL/min (including hemodialysis): 60mg (6mL) qd.

Pediatrics: 0-3 months: Sol: 3mg/kg qd. 3 months-17 yrs: Cap: >33kg: 200mg qd. Sol: 6mg/kg qd. Max: 240mg (24mL).

HOW SUPPLIED: Cap: 200mg; Sol: 10mg/mL

WARNINGS/PRECAUTIONS: Test for chronic hepatitis B prior to initiation; post-treatment exacerbations reported. Monitor hepatic function for several months in patients who discontinue the drug and are co-infected with HIV and HBV. Reduce dose with renal dysfunction. Monitor changes in fasting cholesterol, serum amylase, creatinine kinase, and neutrophil count. Redistribution/accumulation of body fat reported. Immune reconstitution syndrome reported.

ADVERSE REACTIONS: Headache, diarrhea, nausea, rash, vomiting, dyspepsia, asthenia, abdominal pain, dizziness, insomnia, neuropathy, paresthesia, increased cough, rhinitis.

INTERACTIONS: Avoid co-administration with Atripla, Truvada, or lamivudine-containing products.

PREGNANCY: Category B, not for use in nursing.

ENBREL
etanercept (Amgen)

RX

THERAPEUTIC CLASS: TNF receptor blocker

INDICATIONS: To reduce signs/symptoms, induce major clinical response, improve physical function, and inhibit progression of structural damage in moderate to severe rheumatoid arthritis (RA) (may be initiated in combination with methotrexate (MTX) or alone). To reduce signs/symptoms, inhibit progression of structural damage of active arthritis, and improve physical function in psoriatic arthritis (may be used with MTX in patients not responding to MTX alone). To reduce signs/symptoms of moderate to severe polyarticular-course juvenile rheumatoid arthritis (JRA) unresponsive to one or more DMARDs. To reduce signs/symptoms of active ankylosing spondylitis (AS). Chronic moderate to severe plaque psoriasis for candidates of systemic therapy or phototherapy.

DOSAGE: *Adults:* ≥18 yrs: RA/Psoriatic Arthritis/AS: 50mg SQ per week, given as one SQ injection. May continue MTX, glucocorticoids, salicylates, NSAIDs, or analgesics. Psoriasis: Initial: 50mg SQ twice weekly given 3 or 4 days apart for 3 months. May begin with 25-50mg/week. Maint: 50mg/week.

Pediatrics: 4-17 yrs: JRA: 0.8mg/kg SQ per week. Max: 50mg/week. Max per injection site: 25mg. ≤31kg: One SQ injection once weekly. >31kg: Two SQ injections on same day or 3 or 4 days apart. May continue glucocorticoids, NSAIDs, or analgesics.

HOW SUPPLIED: Inj: 25mg (vial), 50mg/mL (syringe)

CONTRAINDICATIONS: Sepsis.

WARNINGS/PRECAUTIONS: D/C if severe allergic reaction or infection (eg, sepsis) occurs. May cause autoimmune antibodies. Serious, fatal infections including sepsis reported. Avoid with active infections. Monitor closely if develop new infection. JRA patients should be brought up to date with current immunization guidelines prior to initiating therapy. D/C temporarily with significant varicella virus exposure and consider prophylaxis. Avoid with Wegener's granulomatosis.

ADVERSE REACTIONS: (Adults/Pediatrics) Injection site reactions, infections, headache. (Pediatrics) Varicella, gastroenteritis, depression, cutaneous ulcer, esophagitis.

INTERACTIONS: Do not give live vaccines. Avoid with cyclophosphamide.

PREGNANCY: Category B, not for use in nursing.

ENTEX HC
guaifenesin - phenylephrine HCl - hydrocodone bitartrate (Andrx)

THERAPEUTIC CLASS: Opioid antitussive

INDICATIONS: Temporary relief of nonproductive cough.

DOSAGE: *Adults:* 5-10mL q4-6h. Max 40mL/24 hrs.

Pediatrics: ≥12 yrs: 5-10mL q4-6h. Max 40mL/24 hrs. 6-12 yrs: 5mL q4-6h. Max 20mL/24 hrs. 2-6 yrs: 2.5mL q4-6h. Max 10mL/24 hrs.

HOW SUPPLIED: Liq: (Guaifenesin-Hydrocodone-Phenylephrine) 100mg-5mg-7.5mg/5mL (473mL)

CONTRAINDICATIONS: Infants, newborns, severe HTN or CAD, hyperthyroidism, or MAOI therapy.

WARNINGS/PRECAUTIONS: May be habit-forming. May cause respiratory depression or increase CSF pressure in the presence of other intracranial pathology. May obscure head injuries or acute abdominal conditions. Caution in elderly, debilitated, hepatic/renal dysfunction, Addison's disease, hypothyroidism, postoperative use, prostatic hypertrophy, pulmonary disease, and urethral stricture. Suppresses cough reflex.

ADVERSE REACTIONS: CNS stimulation, constipation, drowsiness, dizziness, excitability, headache, insomnia, lightheadedness, nausea, vomiting, nervousness, respiratory depression, restlessness, tachycardia, tremors, urinary retention, weakness, arrhythmias, and cardiovascular.

INTERACTIONS: Additive CNS effects with alcohol, antianxiety agents, antihistamines, antipsychotics, narcotics, tranquilizers, or other CNS depressants. Increased sympathomimetic effects with MAOIs or beta blockers. Sympathomimetics may reduce antihypertensive effects of methyldopa, mecamylamine, reserpine, veratrum alkaloids. May enhance the effects of TCAs, barbiturates, alcohol, other CNS depressants.

PREGNANCY: Category C, not for use in nursing.

Entex LA
guaifenesin - phenylephrine HCl (Andrx)

RX

THERAPEUTIC CLASS: Expectorant/sympathomimetic

INDICATIONS: Temporary relief of symptoms associated with upper respiratory tract disorders and cough associated with respiratory tract infections and related disorders when complicated by tenacious mucous or mucous plugs and congestion.

DOSAGE: *Adults:* 1 tab q12h. Max: 2 tabs/24hrs.

Pediatrics: ≥12 yrs: 1 tab q12h. Max: 2 tabs/24hrs. 6-12 yrs: 1/2 tab q12h. Max: 1 tab/24hrs.

HOW SUPPLIED: Tab, Extended Release: (Guaifenesin-Phenylephrine) 400mg-30mg* *scored

CONTRAINDICATIONS: HTN, ventricular tachycardia, MAOI use within 14 days. Extreme caution in elderly, hyperthyroidism, bradycardia, partial heart block, myocardial disease, severe arteriosclerosis.

WARNINGS/PRECAUTIONS: Caution in HTN, DM, ischemic heart disease, increase IOP, hyperthyroidism, or prostatic hypertrophy. May produce CNS stimulation with convulsions or cadiovascular collapse with hypotension. Adverse effects occur more often in elderly.

ADVERSE REACTIONS: Palpitations, headache, dizziness, nausea, anxiety, restlessness, tremor, weakness, pallor, dysuria, respiratory difficulty.

INTERACTIONS: β-blockers and MAOIs may potentiate pressor response. Increased risk of arrhythmias with digitalis glycosides and halothane anesthesia. May reduce hypotensive effects of guanethidine, mecamylamine, methyldopa, reserpine, and veratrum alkaloids. TCAs may antagonize effects.

PREGNANCY: Category C, not for use in nursing.

Entex PSE
guaifenesin - pseudoephedrine HCl (Andrx)

RX

OTHER BRAND NAMES: Ami-Tex PSE (Amide) - Guaifenex PSE 120 (Ethex)

THERAPEUTIC CLASS: Expectorant/decongestant

INDICATIONS: Relief of nasal congestion due to common cold, hay fever, upper respiratory allergies, and nasal congestion associated with sinusitis. To promote nasal or sinus drainage. For symptomatic relief of respiratory conditions characterized by dry nonproductive cough and in the presence of tenacious mucous plugs in the respiratory tract.

DOSAGE: *Adults:* 1 tab q12h.

Pediatrics: ≥12 yrs: 1 tab q12h. 6 to <12 yrs: 1/2 tab q12h.

HOW SUPPLIED: Tab, Extended Release: (Guaifenesin-Pseudoephedrine) 400mg-120mg* *scored

CONTRAINDICATIONS: Nursing, severe HTN, severe CAD, prostatic hypertrophy, concomitant MAOIs.

WARNINGS/PRECAUTIONS: Caution in HTN, DM, heart disease, peripheral vascular disease, increased IOP, hyperthyroidism, or prostatic hypertrophy.

ADVERSE REACTIONS: Nausea, vomiting, nervousness, dizziness, sleeplessness, lightheadedness, tremor, palpitations, tachycardia, weakness, respiratory difficulties.

EPIFOAM
pramoxine HCl - hydrocortisone acetate (Schwarz) — RX

INTERACTIONS: MAOI and β-blockers increase sympathomimetic effects. May reduce antihypertensive effects of methyldopa, guanethidine, mecamylamine, reserpine, and veratrum alkaloids.

PREGNANCY: Category C, contraindicated in nursing.

EPIFOAM
pramoxine HCl - hydrocortisone acetate (Schwarz) — RX

THERAPEUTIC CLASS: Corticosteroid

INDICATIONS: Corticosteroid responsive dermatoses.

DOSAGE: *Adults:* Apply tid-qid. Use occlusive dressings for management of psoriasis or recalcitrant conditions.

Pediatrics: Use least amount necessary for effective regimen. Use occlusive dressings for management of psoriasis or recalcitrant conditions.

HOW SUPPLIED: Foam: (Hydrocortisone-Pramoxine) 1%-1% (10g)

WARNINGS/PRECAUTIONS: Avoid prolonged use. Discontinue use if irritation persists. May produce reversible HPA axis suppression, manifestations of Cushing's syndrome, hyperglycemia, glucosuria. Pediatrics more susceptible to systemic toxicity.

ADVERSE REACTIONS: Burning, itching, irritation, dryness, folliculitis, hypertrichosis, acneiform eruptions, hypopigmentation, perioral dermatitis, maceration, secondary infection, skin atrophy, striae, miliaria.

PREGNANCY: Category C, caution in nursing.

EPIPEN
epinephrine (Dey) — RX

OTHER BRAND NAME: EpiPen Jr. (Dey)

THERAPEUTIC CLASS: Sympathomimetic catecholamine

INDICATIONS: Emergency treatment of allergic reactions (anaphylaxis) to insect stings or bites, foods, drugs, other allergens, and idiopathic or exercise-induced anaphylaxis.

DOSAGE: *Adults:* 0.3mg IM in thigh. May repeat with severe anaphylaxis.

Pediatrics: 0.15mg or 0.3mg (0.01mg/kg) IM in thigh. May repeat with severe anaphylaxis.

HOW SUPPLIED: Inj: (Epipen Jr) 0.5mg/mL, (Epipen) 1mg/mL

WARNINGS/PRECAUTIONS: Not for IV use. Contains sulfites. Extreme caution with heart disease. Anginal pain may be induced with coronary insufficiency. Increased risk of adverse reactions with hyperthyroidism, CVD, HTN, DM, elderly, pregnancy, pediatrics <30kg with Epipen and <15kg with Epipen, Jr.

ADVERSE REACTIONS: Palpitations, tachycardia, sweating, nausea, vomiting, respiratory difficulty, pallor, dizziness, weakness, tremor, headache, apprehension, anxiety.

INTERACTIONS: Potentiated by TCAs and MAOIs. Increased risk of arrhythmias with digitalis, mercurial diuretics, or quinidine. Pressor effects may be counteracted by rapidly acting vasodilators.

PREGNANCY: Category C, safety in nursing not known.

EPIQUIN MICRO
hydroquinone (SkinMedica) — RX

THERAPEUTIC CLASS: Depigmenting agent

INDICATIONS: Gradual treatment of ultraviolet induced dyschromia and discoloration resulting from the use of oral contraceptives, pregnancy, hormone replacement therapy, or skin trauma.

DOSAGE: *Adults:* Apply bid (am and hs). Use sunscreen.

Pediatrics: ≥12yrs: Apply bid (am and hs). Use sunscreen.

HOW SUPPLIED: Cre: 4% (30g)

WARNINGS/PRECAUTIONS: Avoid sun exposure on bleached skin. Use sunscreen. May produce unwanted cosmetic effects if not used as directed. Test for skin sensitivity. Discontinue if no lightening effect after 2 months of therapy, if blue-black darkening of the skin occurs, or if itching, vesicle formation, or excessive inflammatory reactions occur. Contains sodium metabisulfite, may cause serious allergic type reactions. Avoid contact with eyes.

ADVERSE REACTIONS: Cutaneous hypersensitivity (contact dermititis).

PREGNANCY: Category C, caution in nursing.

Epivir
lamivudine (GlaxoSmithKline)

RX

> Lactic acidosis and severe, possibly fatal hepatomegaly reported. Tablets and solution have higher dose of active ingredient than Epivir-HBV; only dose with appropriate forms for HIV.

THERAPEUTIC CLASS: Nucleoside analogue

INDICATIONS: Treatment of HIV infection in combination with other antiretrovirals.

DOSAGE: *Adults:* 150mg bid or 300mg qd, concomitantly with other antiretrovirals. CrCl 30-49mL/min: 150mg qd. CrCl 15-29mL/min: 150mg first dose, then 100mg qd. CrCl 5-14mL/min: 150mg first dose, then 50mg qd. CrCl <5mL/min: 50mg first dose, then 25mg qd.

Pediatrics: 3 months-16 yrs: 4mg/kg bid, concomitantly with other antiretrovirals. Max: 150mg bid. Adolescents: CrCl 30-49mL/min: 150mg qd. CrCl 15-29mL/min: 150mg first dose, then 100mg qd. CrCl 5-14mL/min: 150mg first dose, then 50mg qd. CrCl <5mL/min: 50mg first dose, then 25mg qd.

HOW SUPPLIED: Sol: 10mg/mL (240mL); Tab: 150mg, 300mg

WARNINGS/PRECAUTIONS: Caution in peds with history of prior antiretroviral nucleoside exposure, history of pancreatitis, or other significant risk factors for developing pancreatitis. D/C if pancreatitis develops. Post-treatment exacerbations of hepatitis reported. Lactic acidosis and severe, fatal hepatomegaly reported. Hepatic decompensation occured when used with interferon alfa w/ or w/o ribavirin. Reduce dose in renal dysfunction. Possible redistribution or accumulation of body fat. Suspend therapy if develop lactic acidosis or pronounced hepatotoxicity. Immune reconstitution syndrome reported.

ADVERSE REACTIONS: Headache, malaise, fatigue, fever, chills, nausea, diarrhea, vomiting, anorexia, abdominal pain, neuropathy, dizziness, skin rash, musculoskeletal pain, cough, pancreatitis.

INTERACTIONS: TMP/SMX increases levels of lamivudine. Avoid with zalcitabine, zidovudine, lamivudine, and fixed-dose combinations of abacavir, lamivudine, and zidovudine.

PREGNANCY: Category C, not for use in nursing.

Epivir-HBV
lamivudine (GlaxoSmithKline)

RX

> Lactic acidosis and severe, possibly fatal, hepatomegaly reported. If prescribed for patients with unrecognized or untreated HIV infection, rapid emergence of HIV resistance is likely. Reports of severe acute exacerbations of hepatitis B upon discontinuation of therapy. Follow up liver function monitoring required.

THERAPEUTIC CLASS: Nucleoside analogue

INDICATIONS: Treatment of chronic hepatitis B associated with viral replication and active liver inflammation.

DOSAGE: *Adults:* 100mg qd. CrCl 30-49mL/min: 100mg day 1, then 50mg qd. CrCl: 15-29mL/min: 100mg day 1, then 25mg qd. CrCl 5-14mL/min: 35mg day 1, then 15mg qd. CrCl <5mL/min: 35mg day 1, then 10mg qd.

Pediatrics: 2-17 yrs: 3mg/kg qd. Max: 100mg/day.

HOW SUPPLIED: Sol: 5mg/mL (240mL); Tab: 100mg

EPOGEN

WARNINGS/PRECAUTIONS: Reduce dose in renal dysfunction. Caution in elderly. This formulation is not appropriate in both HBV and HIV infections. Posttreatment exacerbations of hepatitis reported. Pancreatitis reported, especially in HIV-infected pediatrics with prior nucleoside exposure. Monitor patient regularly during treatment. Safety and efficacy with treatment after 1 yr is not known. Suspend therapy if develop lactic acidosis or pronounced hepatotoxicity.

ADVERSE REACTIONS: Pancreatitis, lactic acidosis, severe hepatomegaly, GI complaints, sore throat, infections, elevated LFTs, arthralgia.

INTERACTIONS: TMP/SMX may increase lamivudine levels. Avoid with zalcitabine.

PREGNANCY: Category C, not for use in nursing.

EPOGEN   RX
epoetin alfa (Amgen)

> Erythropoiesis-stimulating agents (ESAs) may increase risk for death and/or serious cardiovascular events when administered to a target Hgb >12g/dL. Use lowest dose that will gradually increase Hgb concentration to lowest level sufficient to avoid need for RBC transfusion. When ESAs are used preoperatively for reduction of allogenic RBC transfusions, a higher incidence of DVT was reported in patients not receiving prophylactic anticoagulation. Antithrombotic prophylaxis should be strongly considered when ESAs are used to reduce allogenic RBC transfusions.

THERAPEUTIC CLASS: Erythropoiesis stimulator

INDICATIONS: Treatment of anemia of chronic renal failure (CRF), anemia related to zidovudine in HIV, chemotherapy-induced anemia in patients with non-myeloid malignancies (serum erythropoietin ≤200mU/mL), and reduction of allogeneic blood transfusions in anemic (≤13 to >10 g/dL) patients scheduled for elective, noncardiac, nonvascular surgery.

DOSAGE: *Adults:* CRF: Initial: 50-100 U/kg IV/SQ 3x/week. IV is preferred route in dialysis patients. Reduce dose when Hct approaches 36% or increase by >4 points in any 2 week period. Increase dose if Hct does not increase by 5-6 points after 8 weeks of therapy and Hct is below target range. Maint: Individually titrate. Zidovudine-Treated HIV Patients: Serum erythropoietin ≤500 mU/mL and zidovudine dose ≤4200mg/week: 100 U/kg IV/SQ 3x/week for 8 weeks. Max: 300 U/kg 3x/week. Maint: Individualize dose to maintain Hct within 30%-36%. Chemotherapy-Induced Anemia: Initial: 150 U/kg SQ 3x/week. Titrate: May increase to 300U/kg 3x/week after 8 weeks of therapy. Surgery: 300 U/kg/day SQ for 10 days before, on day of, and 4 days after surgery; or 600 U/kg SQ once weekly on 21, 14, and 7 days before surgery, and a 4th dose on day of surgery.
Pediatrics: CRF: Initial: 50 U/kg 3x/week IV/SQ. Reduce dose when Hct approaches 36% or increase by >4 points in any 2 week period. Increase dose if Hct does not increase by 5-6 points after 8 weeks of therapy and Hct is below target range. Maint: Individually titrate.

HOW SUPPLIED: Inj: 2000 U/mL, 3000 U/mL, 4000 U/mL, 10,000 U/mL, 20,000 U/mL, 40,000 U/mL

CONTRAINDICATIONS: Uncontrolled HTN. Hypersensitivity to mammalian cell-derived products and Albumin (human).

WARNINGS/PRECAUTIONS: Pure red cell aplasia and severe anemia (with or without other cytopenias) may occur. Caution with porphyria, HTN or a history of seizures. Evaluate iron stores prior to and during therapy. Most patients need iron supplementation. Monitor Hct, BP, iron levels, serum chemistry, and CBC. Menses may resume. Multidose formulation contains benzyl alcohol.

ADVERSE REACTIONS: HTN, headache, fatigue, arthralgias, nausea, vomiting, diarrhea, edema, rash, pyrexia, clotted vascular access, respiratory congestion, dyspnea, asthenia, dizziness, seizures, thrombotic events.

INTERACTIONS: Adjust anticoagulant dose in dialysis patients.

PREGNANCY: Category C, caution in nursing.

EQUAGESIC
aspirin - meprobamate (Wyeth/Women First)

THERAPEUTIC CLASS: Carbamate derivative/salicylate

INDICATIONS: Adjunct in short-term treatment of pain accompanied by tension and/or anxiety in patients with musculoskeletal disease.

DOSAGE: *Adults:* 1-2 tabs tid-qid prn. Elderly/Debilitated: Use lowest effective dose. *Pediatrics:* ≥12 yrs: 1-2 tabs tid-qid prn.

HOW SUPPLIED: Tab: (Meprobamate-ASA) 200mg-325mg* *scored

CONTRAINDICATIONS: Acute intermittent porphyria.

WARNINGS/PRECAUTIONS: Extreme caution with peptic ulcer, asthma, coagulation abnormalities, hypoprothrombinemia, or vitamin K deficiency. Abuse, physical and psychological dependence reported. Abrupt withdrawal after prolonged and excessive use may precipitate recurrence of pre-existing symptoms. May impair mental and physical abilities. Caution with hepatic or kidney dysfunction. May precipitate seizures in epileptic patients. Prescribe cautiously and in small amounts to suicidal patients.

ADVERSE REACTIONS: Epigastric discomfort, nausea, vomiting, drowsiness, ataxia, dizziness, slurred speech, headache, vertigo, weakness.

INTERACTIONS: Additive CNS suppression with alcohol or other psychotropic drugs. May antagonize uricosuric activity of probenecid and sulfinpyrazone. Extreme caution with anticoagulants. May enhance hypoglycemic effects of sulfonylureas.

PREGNANCY: Safety in pregnancy or nursing not known.

ERTACZO
sertaconazole nitrate (Ortho Neutrogena)   RX

THERAPEUTIC CLASS: Azole antifungal

INDICATIONS: Treatment of interdigital tinea pedis in immunocompetent patients caused by *Trichophyton rubrum*, *Trichophyton mentagrophytes*, and *Epidermophyton floccosum*.

DOSAGE: *Adults:* Apply bid to affected areas between toes and adjacent areas for 4 weeks. Re-evaluate if no clinical improvement after 2 weeks.
Pediatrics: ≥12 yrs: Apply bid to affected areas between toes and adjacent areas for 4 weeks. Re-evaluate if no clinical improvement after 2 weeks.

HOW SUPPLIED: Cre: 2% (30g)

WARNINGS/PRECAUTIONS: Not for ophthalmic, oral, or intravaginal use. Discontinue if irritation or sensitivity occurs.

ADVERSE REACTIONS: Contact dermatitis, dry skin, burning skin, application site reaction, skin tenderness.

PREGNANCY: Category C, caution in nursing.

ERYC
erythromycin (Warner Chilcott)   RX

THERAPEUTIC CLASS: Macrolide antibiotic

INDICATIONS: Mild-to-moderate upper and lower respiratory tract and skin and soft tissue infections, pertussis, diphtheria, erythrasma, intestinal amebiasis, acute pelvic inflammatory disease (PID) (*N. gonorrhea*), Listeria monocytogenes infections, primary syphilis in PCN allergy, Legionnaires' disease, chlamydial infections (eg, newborn conjunctivitis, urethral, endocervical, or rectal, etc), and nongonococcal urethritis. Prophylaxis of endocarditis or rheumatic fever in PCN allergy.

DOSAGE: *Adults:* Usual: 250mg q6h or 500mg q12h. Max: 4g/day. Treat strep infections for 10 days. Chlamydial Urogenital Infection During Pregnancy: 500mg qid for at least 7 days or 250mg qid for 14 days. Urethral/Endocervical/Rectal Chlamydial Infections: 500mg qid for 7 days. Primary Syphilis: 30-40g in divided doses for 10-15 days. Acute PID: 500mg (erythromycin lactobionate) IV q6h for 3 days, then 250mg PO q6h for 7 days. Streptococcal Infection Long-Term Prophylaxis of Rheumatic Fever: 250mg bid. Intestinal Amebiasis: 250mg qid for 10-14 days. Pertussis: 40-50mg/kg/day in divided doses for 5-14 days. Legionnaires' Disease: 1-4g/day in divided doses. Bacterial Endocarditis Prophylaxis: 1g 1 hr before procedure, then 500mg 6 hrs later.
Pediatrics: Usual: 30-50mg/kg/day in divided doses without food. Max: 4g/day. Severe Infections: Double dose up to 4g/day. Treat strep infections for 10 days. Intestinal Amebiasis: 30-50mg/kg/day in divided doses for 10-14 days. Bacterial Endocarditis Prophylaxis: 20mg/kg 1 hr before procedure, then 10mg/kg 6 hrs later.

ERYPED

HOW SUPPLIED: Cap, Delayed Release: 250mg

CONTRAINDICATIONS: Concomitant terfenadine or cisapride.

WARNINGS/PRECAUTIONS: Pseudomembranous colitis, hepatic dysfunction reported.

ADVERSE REACTIONS: Nausea, vomiting, abdominal pain, diarrhea, anorexia, abnormal LFTs, allergic reaction, superinfection (prolonged use).

INTERACTIONS: May increase levels of theophylline, digoxin, drugs metabolized by CYP450 (eg, carbamazepine, cyclosporine, phenytoin, tacrolimus, hexobarbital). Increases effects of oral anticoagulants and triazolam. Risk of acute ergot toxicity with ergotamine or dihydroergotamine. Avoid terfenadine and cisapride.

PREGNANCY: Category B, caution in nursing.

ERYPED
erythromycin ethylsuccinate (Abbott)

RX

THERAPEUTIC CLASS: Macrolide antibiotic

INDICATIONS: Treatment of mild to moderate upper and lower respiratory tract and skin and skin structure infections, listeriosis, pertussis, diphtheria, erythrasma, intestinal amebiasis, acute pelvic inflammatory disease (PID) (*N.gonorrhea*), primary syphilis in PCN allergy, Legionnaires' disease, chlamydial infections (eg, newborn conjunctivitis, urethral, endocervical, or rectal, etc.), and nongonococcal urethritis. Prophylaxis of endocarditis or rheumatic fever.

DOSAGE: *Adults:* Usual: 1600mg/day given q6h, q8h or q12h. Max: 4g/day. Treat strep infections for 10 days. Streptococcal Infection Prophylaxis with Rheumatic Heart Disease: 400mg bid. Urethritis (*C.trachomatis* or *U.urealyticum*): 800mg tid for 7 days. Primary Syphilis: 48-64g in divided doses over 10-15 days. Intestinal Amebiasis: 400mg qid for 10-14 days. Pertussis: 40-50mg/kg/day in divided doses for 5-14 days. Legionnaires' Disease: 1.6-4g/day in divided doses.
Pediatrics: Usual: 30-50mg/kg/day in divided doses q6h, q8h or q12h. Double dose for more severe infections. Treat strep infections for 10 days. Intestinal Amebiasis: 30-50mg/kg/day in divided doses for 10-14 days. Pertussis: 40-50mg/kg/day in divided doses for 5-14 days.

HOW SUPPLIED: Sus: 100mg/2.5mL (50mL), 200mg/5mL, 400mg/5mL (5mL, 100mL, 200mL); Tab, Chewable: 200mg* *scored

CONTRAINDICATIONS: Concomitant terfenadine, astemizole, cisapride, pimozide.

WARNINGS/PRECAUTIONS: Pseudomembranous colitis, hepatic dysfunction reported. May aggravate myasthenia gravis.

ADVERSE REACTIONS: Nausea, vomiting, abdominal pain, diarrhea, anorexia, hepatic dysfunction, abnormal LFTs, allergic reactions, superinfection (prolonged use).

INTERACTIONS: Rhabdomyolysis reported with lovastatin. May increase levels of theophylline, digoxin, drugs metabolized by CYP450 (eg, carbamazepine, cyclosporine, tacrolimus, phenytoin, alfentanil, disopyramide, lovastatin, bromocriptine, valproate, etc). Increases effects of oral anticoagulants, triazolam, midazolam. Risk of acute ergot toxicity with ergotamine or dihydroergotamine. May potentiate sildenafil. Avoid terfenadine, astemizole, cisapride, pimozide.

PREGNANCY: Category B, caution in nursing.

ERY-TAB
erythromycin (Abbott)

RX

THERAPEUTIC CLASS: Macrolide antibiotic

INDICATIONS: Mild-to-moderate upper and lower respiratory tract and skin and skin structure infections, listeriosis, pertussis, diphtheria, erythrasma, intestinal amebiasis, acute pelvic inflammatory disease (PID) (*N.gonorrhea*), primary syphilis in PCN allergy, Legionnaires' disease, chlamydial infections (eg, newborn conjunctivitis urethral, endocervical, and rectal, etc), and nongonococcal urethritis. Prophylaxis of rheumatic fever.

DOSAGE: *Adults:* Usual: 250mg qid, 333mg q8h or 500mg q12h without food. Max: 4g/day. Do not take bid when dose is ≥1g/day. Treat strep infections for 10 days. Chlamydial Urogenital Infection During Pregnancy: 500mg qid or 666mg q8h for 7 days, or 500mg q12h, 333mg q8h or 250mg qid for 14 days. Urethral/Endocervical/Rectal Chlamydial Infections and Nongonococcal Urethritis: 500mg qid or 666mg q8h for at least 7 days. Primary Syphilis: 30-40g in divided doses for 10-15 days. Acute PID: 500mg (erythromycin lactobionate) IV q6h for 3 days, then 500mg PO q12h or 333mg q8h for 7 days. Streptococcal Infection Long-Term Prophylaxis of Rheumatic Fever: 250mg bid. Intestinal Amebiasis: 500mg q12h, 333mg q8h or 250mg q6h for 10-14 days. Pertussis: 40-50mg/kg/day in divided doses for 5-14 days. Legionnaires' Disease: 1-4g/day in divided doses.

Pediatrics: Usual: 30-50mg/kg/day in divided doses without food. Max: 4g/day. Severe Infections: Double dose up to 4g/day. Treat strep infections for 10 days. Chlamydial Conjunctivitis of Newborns and Chlamydial Pneumonia in Infancy: 12.5mg/kg qid for 2 weeks and 3 weeks, respectively. Intestinal Amebiasis: 30-50mg/kg/day in divided doses for 10-14 days. Long-Term Prophylaxis of Rheumatic Fever: 250mg bid. Intestinal Amebiasis: 30-50mg/kg/day in divided doses for 10-14 days. Pertussis: 40-50mg/kg/day in divided doses for 5-14 days. Legionnaire's Disease: 1-4g/day in divided doses.

HOW SUPPLIED: Tab, Delayed Release: 250mg, 333mg, 500mg

CONTRAINDICATIONS: Concomitant terfenadine, astemizole, or cisapride.

WARNINGS/PRECAUTIONS: Pseudomembranous colitis, hepatic dysfunction reported. May aggravate myasthenia gravis. Erythromycin does not reach adequate concentrations in fetus to prevent congenital syphilis.

ADVERSE REACTIONS: Nausea, vomiting, abdominal pain, diarrhea, anorexia, abnormal LFTs, allergic reactions, superinfection (prolonged use).

INTERACTIONS: Rhabdomyolysis reported with lovastatin. May increase levels of theophylline, digoxin, drugs metabolized by CYP450 (eg, carbamazepine, cyclosporine, phenytoin, alfentanil, disopyramide, lovastatin, bromocriptine, valproate, etc). Increases effects of oral anticoagulants, triazolam, midazolam. Risk of acute ergot toxicity with ergotamine or dihydroergotamine. Avoid terfenadine, astemizole, or cisapride.

PREGNANCY: Category B, caution in nursing.

Erythrocin RX
erythromycin stearate (Abbott)

THERAPEUTIC CLASS: Macrolide antibiotic

INDICATIONS: Mild-to-moderate upper and lower respiratory tract, and skin and skin structure infections, listeriosis, pertussis, diphtheria, erythrasma, intestinal amebiasis, acute pelvic inflammatory disease (PID) (*N.gonorrhea*), primary syphilis in PCN allergy, Legionnaires' disease, chlamydial infections (eg, newborn conjunctivitis urethral, endocervical, or rectal, etc), and nongonococcal urethritis. Prophylaxis of rheumatic fever.

DOSAGE: *Adults:* Usual: 250mg q6h or 500mg q12h without food. Max: 4g/day. Treat strep infections for 10 days. Streptococcal Infection Prophylaxis of Rheumatic Fever: 250mg bid. Chlamydial Urogenital Infection During Pregnancy: 500mg qid for 7 days or 250mg qid for 14 days. Urethral/Endocervical/Rectal Chlamydial Infections and Nongonococcal Urethritis: 500mg qid for at least 7 days. Primary Syphilis: 30-40g in divided doses over 10-15 days. Acute PID: 500mg (erythromycin lactobionate) IV q6h for 3 days, then 500mg PO q12h for 7 days. Intestinal Amebiasis: 250mg qid for 10-14 days. Pertussis: 40-50mg/kg/day in divided doses for 5-14 days. Legionnaires' Disease: 1-4g/day in divided doses.

Pediatrics: Usual: 30-50mg/kg/day in divided doses without food. Severe Infections: Double dose up to 4g/day. Treat strep infections for 10 days. Streptococcal Infection Prophylaxis of Rheumatic Fever: 250mg bid. Chlamydial Conjunctivitis of Newborns/Chlamydial Pneumonia in Infancy: 12.5mg/kg qid for 2 weeks and 3 weeks, respectively. Intestinal Amebiasis: 30-50mg/kg/day in divided doses for 10-14 days. Pertussis: 40-50mg/kg/day in divided doses for 5-14 days.

HOW SUPPLIED: Tab: 250mg, 500mg

WARNINGS/PRECAUTIONS: Hepatic dysfunction, pseudomembranous colitis reported.

ADVERSE REACTIONS: Nausea, vomiting, abdominal pain, diarrhea, anorexia, abnormal LFTs, superinfection (prolonged use).

ERYTHROMYCIN

INTERACTIONS: Rhabdomyolysis reported with lovastatin. May increase levels of theophylline, digoxin, drugs metabolized by CYP450 (eg, carbamazepine, cyclosporine, phenytoin, etc). Increases effects of oral anticoagulants, triazolam. Risk of acute ergot toxicity with ergotamine or dihydroergotamine.

PREGNANCY: Category B, caution in nursing.

ERYTHROMYCIN RX
erythromycin (Abbott)

THERAPEUTIC CLASS: Macrolide antibiotic

INDICATIONS: Mild to moderate upper and lower respiratory tract and skin and skin structure infections, listeriosis, pertussis, diphtheria, erythrasma, intestinal amebiasis, primary syphilis in PCN allergy, Legionnaires' disease, chlamydial infections (eg, newborn conjunctivitis urethral, endocervical, rectal, etc), and nongonococcal urethritis. Prophylaxis of endocarditis or rheumatic fever.

DOSAGE: *Adults:* Usual: 250mg q6h or 500mg q12h without food. Max: 4g/day. Treat strep infections for 10 days. Streptococcal Infection Prophylaxis of Rheumatic Fever: 250mg bid. Chlamydial Urogenital Infection During Pregnancy: 500mg qid for 7 days or 250mg qid for 14 days. Urethral/Endocervical/Rectal Chlamydial Infections: 500mg qid for at least 7 days. Primary Syphilis: 30-40g in divided doses over 10-15 days. Intestinal Amebiasis: 250mg q6h for 10-14 days. Pertussis: 40-50mg/kg/day in divided doses for 5-14 days. Legionnaires' Disease: 1-4g/day in divided doses. Bacterial Endocarditis Prophylaxis: 1g 1 hr before procedure, then 500mg 6 hrs later.

Pediatrics: Usual: 30-50mg/kg/day in divided doses without food. Severe Infections: Double dose up to 4g/day. Treat strep infections for 10 days. Streptococcal Infection Prophylaxis of Rheumatic Fever: 250mg bid. Intestinal Amebiasis: 30-50mg/kg/day in divided doses for 10-14 days. Pertussis: 40-50mg/kg/day in divided doses for 5-14 days. Bacterial Endocarditis Prophylaxis: 20mg/kg 1 hr before procedure, then 10mg/kg 6 hrs later.

HOW SUPPLIED: Cap, Delayed Release: 250mg

WARNINGS/PRECAUTIONS: Caution with hepatic dysfunction.

ADVERSE REACTIONS: Nausea, vomiting, abdominal pain, diarrhea, anorexia, hepatic dysfunction, abnormal LFTs, superinfection (prolonged use).

INTERACTIONS: Rhabdomyolysis reported with lovastatin. May increase levels of theophylline, digoxin, drugs metabolized by CYP450 (eg, carbamazepine, cyclosporine, phenytoin, etc). Increases effects of oral anticoagulants, triazolam. Risk of acute ergot toxicity with ergotamine or dihydroergotamine. Extreme caution with terfenadine.

PREGNANCY: Category B, caution in nursing.

ERYTHROMYCIN BASE RX
erythromycin (Abbott)

THERAPEUTIC CLASS: Macrolide antibiotic

INDICATIONS: Mild to moderate upper and lower respiratory tract and skin and skin structure infections, listeriosis, pertussis, diphtheria, erythrasma, intestinal amebiasis, acute pelvic inflammatory disease (PID) (*N.gonorrhea*), primary syphilis in PCN allergy, Legionnaires' disease, chlamydial infections (eg, newborn conjunctivitis urethral, endocervical, rectal, etc), and nongonococcal urethritis. Prophylaxis of rheumatic fever.

DOSAGE: *Adults:* Usual: 250mg q6h or 500mg q12h without food. Max: 4g/day. Treat strep infections for 10 days. Streptococcal Infection Prophylaxis of Rheumatic Fever: 250mg bid. Chlamydial Urogenital Infection During Pregnancy: 500mg qid for 7 days or 250mg qid for 14 days. Urethral/Endocervical/Rectal Chlamydial Infections and Nongonococcal Urethritis: 500mg qid for at least 7 days. Primary Syphilis: 30-40g in divided doses over 10-15 days. Acute PID: 500mg (erythromycin lactobionate) IV q6h for 3 days, then 500mg PO q12h for 7 days. Intestinal Amebiasis: 250mg qid for 10-14 days. Pertussis: 40-50mg/kg/day in divided doses for 5-14 days. Legionnaires' Disease: 1-4g/day in divided doses.

Pediatrics: Usual: 30-50mg/kg/day in divided doses without food. Severe Infections: Double dose up to 4g/day. Treat strep infections for 10 days. Streptococcal Infection

Prophylaxis of Rheumatic Fever: 250mg bid. Chlamydial Conjunctivitis of Newborns and Chlamydial Pneumonia in Infancy: 12.5mg/kg qid for 2 weeks and 3 weeks, respectively. Intestinal Amebiasis: 30-50mg/kg/day in divided doses for 10-14 days. Pertussis: 40-50mg/kg/day in divided doses for 5-14 days.

HOW SUPPLIED: Tab: 250mg

CONTRAINDICATIONS: Concomitant terfenadine, astemizole, or cisapride.

WARNINGS/PRECAUTIONS: Pseudomembranous colitis, hepatic dysfunction reported. May aggravate myasthenia gravis.

ADVERSE REACTIONS: Nausea, vomiting, abdominal pain, diarrhea, anorexia, abnormal LFTs, allergic reactions, superinfection (prolonged use).

INTERACTIONS: Rhabdomyolysis reported with lovastatin. May increase levels of theophylline, digoxin, drugs metabolized by CYP450 (eg, carbamazepine, cyclosporine, phenytoin, etc). Increases effects of oral anticoagulants, triazolam. Risk of acute ergot toxicity with ergotamine or dihydroergotamine. Extreme caution with terfenadine.

PREGNANCY: Category B, caution in nursing.

ERYTHROMYCIN OPHTHALMIC   RX
erythromycin (Various)

THERAPEUTIC CLASS: Macrolide

INDICATIONS: Superficial ocular infections of the conjunctiva and/or cornea. Prophylaxis of ophthalmia neonatorum due to N.gonorrhoeae or C.trachomatis.

DOSAGE: *Adults:* Superficial Ocular Infections: Apply 1 cm to eye up to 6 times/day, depending on severity. Do not flush ointment from eye.

Pediatrics: Superficial Ocular Infections: Apply 1 cm to eye up to 6 times/day, depending on severity. Neonatal Gonococcal or Chlamydial Ophthalmia Prophylaxis: Apply 1 cm into lower conjunctival sac. Do not flush ointment from eye.

HOW SUPPLIED: Oint: 5mg/g (1g, 3.5g)

ADVERSE REACTIONS: Minor ocular irritations, redness, hypersensitivity reactions, superinfection (prolonged use).

PREGNANCY: Category B, caution in nursing.

ESGIC   RX
caffeine - butalbital - acetaminophen (Forest)

THERAPEUTIC CLASS: Barbiturate/analgesic

INDICATIONS: Tension or muscle contraction headaches.

DOSAGE: *Adults:* 1-2 caps/tabs q4h prn. Max: 6 caps/tabs/day.

Pediatrics: ≥12 yrs: 1-2 caps/tabs q4h prn. Max: 6 caps/tabs/day.

HOW SUPPLIED: Cap/Tab: (Butalbital-APAP-Caffeine) 50mg-325mg-40mg* *scored

CONTRAINDICATIONS: Porphyria.

WARNINGS/PRECAUTIONS: May be habit-forming; potential for abuse. Not for long-term use. Caution in elderly, debilitated, severe renal or hepatic impairment, acute abdominal conditions, suicidal tendencies, history of drug abuse.

ADVERSE REACTIONS: Drowsiness, lightheadedness, dizziness, sedation, shortness of breath, nausea, vomiting, abdominal pain, intoxicated feeling.

INTERACTIONS: Enhanced CNS effects with MAOIs. May enhance CNS depressant effects of other narcotic analgesics, alcohol, general anesthetics, tranquilizers, sedative hypnotics, or other CNS depressants.

PREGNANCY: Category C, not for use in nursing.

ESGIC-PLUS   RX
caffeine - butalbital - acetaminophen (Forest)

THERAPEUTIC CLASS: Barbiturate/analgesic

INDICATIONS: Tension or muscle contraction headaches.

ESKALITH

DOSAGE: *Adults:* 1 cap/tab q4h prn. Max: 6 caps/tabs/day.
Pediatrics: ≥12 yrs: 1 cap/tab q4h prn. Max: 6 caps/tabs/day.
HOW SUPPLIED: Cap/Tab: (Butalbital-APAP-Caffeine) 50mg-500mg-40mg* *scored
CONTRAINDICATIONS: Porphyria.
WARNINGS/PRECAUTIONS: May be habit-forming; potential for abuse. Not for long-term use. Caution in elderly, debilitated, severe renal or hepatic impairment, acute abdominal conditions, suicidal tendencies, history of drug abuse.
ADVERSE REACTIONS: Drowsiness, lightheadedness, dizziness, sedation, shortness of breath, nausea, vomiting, abdominal pain, intoxicated feeling.
INTERACTIONS: Enhanced CNS effects with MAOIs. May enhance CNS depressant effects of other narcotic analgesics, alcohol, general anesthetics, tranquilizers, sedative hypnotics, or other CNS depressants.
PREGNANCY: Category C, not for use in nursing.

ESKALITH   RX
lithium carbonate (GlaxoSmithKline)

> Lithium toxicity is related to serum levels, and can occur at doses close to therapeutic levels.

OTHER BRAND NAME: Eskalith CR (GlaxoSmithKline)
THERAPEUTIC CLASS: Antimanic agents
INDICATIONS: Treatment of manic episodes of manic-depressive illness.
DOSAGE: *Adults:* (Cap) 300mg tid-qid. (Tab, Extended-Release) 450mg q12h. Monitor every 1-2 weeks and adjust dose if needed. When stable, monitor every 2 months to achieve levels of 0.6-1.2mEq/L. Maint: 900-1200mg/day. Acute Mania: 1800mg/day in divided doses. Monitor levels twice weekly to achieve 1-1.5mEq/L. When switching to extended-release tabs, give same total daily dose when possible.
Pediatrics: ≥12 yrs: (Cap) 300mg tid-qid. (Tab, Extended-Release) 450mg q12h. Monitor every 1-2 weeks and adjust dose if needed. When stable, monitor every 2 months to achieve levels of 0.6-1.2 mEq/L. Maint: 900-1200mg/day. Acute Mania: 1800mg/day in divided doses. Monitor levels twice weekly to achieve 1-1.5mEq/L. When switching to extended-release tabs, give same total daily dose when possible.
HOW SUPPLIED: Cap: (Eskalith) 300mg; Tab, Extended Release: (Eskalith CR) 450mg* *scored
WARNINGS/PRECAUTIONS: Avoid with significant renal or cardiovascular disease, severe debilitation, dehydration, or sodium depletion. Risk of encephalopathic syndrome (eg, weakness, lethargy, fever, tremulousness, confusion, EPS); discontinue therapy. Maintain normal diet, adequate salt/fluid intake. Reduce dose or discontinue with sweating, diarrhea, infection with elevated temperatures. Caution with hypothyroidism; may need supplemental therapy. Chronic therapy associated with diminution of renal concentrating ability, glomerular and interstitial fibrosis, and nephron atrophy.
ADVERSE REACTIONS: Fine hand tremor, polyuria, mild thirst, nausea, general discomfort, diarrhea, vomiting, drowsiness, muscular weakness.
INTERACTIONS: Increased risk of neurotoxicity with calcium channel blockers. Increased risk of toxicity with diuretics, metronidazole. Increased plasma levels with indomethacin, piroxicam, other NSAIDs, COX-2 inhibitors, ACE inhibitors, angiotensin II receptor antagonists. Caution with SSRIs. Decreased levels with acetazolamide, urea, xanthine agents, alkalinizing agents. Interacts with methyldopa, phenytoin, carbamazepine. May prolong effects of neuromuscular blockers.
PREGNANCY: Safety in pregnancy not known, not for use in nursing.

ESTROSTEP FE   RX
ethinyl estradiol - norethindrone acetate (Warner Chilcott)

THERAPEUTIC CLASS: Estrogen/progestogen combination
INDICATIONS: Prevention of pregnancy. Treatment of acne vulgaris in females ≥15 yrs who want contraception (for at least 6 months), have achieved menarche and are unresponsive to topical acne agents.

DOSAGE: *Adults:* Contraception/Acne: 1 tab qd for 28 days, then repeat. Start 1st Sunday after menses begin or the 1st day of menses.

Pediatrics: ≥15 yrs: Contraception (Postpubertal Adolescents)/Acne: 1 tab qd for 28 days, then repeat. Start 1st Sunday after menses begin or the 1st day of menses.

HOW SUPPLIED: Tab: (Ethinyl Estradiol-Norethindrone) 0.035mg-1mg, 0.030mg-1mg, 0.020mg-1mg and 75mg ferrous fumarate

CONTRAINDICATIONS: Thrombophlebitis, history of DVT, active or history of thromboembolic disorders, pregnancy, cerebrovascular disease, CAD, undiagnosed abnormal genital bleeding, cholestatic jaundice of pregnancy, jaundice with prior pill use, hepatic adenoma or carcinoma, breast carcinoma, endometrium or other estrogen-dependent neoplasia.

WARNINGS/PRECAUTIONS: Cigarette smoking increases risk of serious cardiovascular side effects. This risk increases with age (especially >35 yrs) and heavy smoking. Increased risk of MI, vascular disease, thromboembolism, stroke, and gallbladder disease. Retinal thrombosis, hepatic neoplasia reported. May cause glucose intolerance. May increase BP, elevate LDL levels or cause other lipid changes, fluid retention, breakthrough bleeding, and spotting. May cause or exacerbate migraine. May develop visual changes with contact lens. Increased risk of MI with HTN, hyperlipidemia, obesity, and diabetes. D/C if jaundice, significant depression or ophthalmic irregularities develop. Perform annual physical exam. Use before menarche is not indicated. May affect certain endocrine, LFTs and blood components.

ADVERSE REACTIONS: Nausea, vomiting, breakthrough bleeding, spotting, amenorrhea, migraine, depression, vaginal candidiasis, edema, weight changes.

INTERACTIONS: Reduced effects, increased breakthrough bleeding, and menstrual irregularities with rifampin, barbiturates, phenylbutazone, phenytoin, carbamazepine, St. John's wort, and possibly with griseofulvin, ampicillin, and tetracyclines. Increased plasma levels with atorvastatin. Ascorbic acid and APAP may increase plasma levels. Decreased plasma levels of APAP. Increased clearance of temazepam, salicylic acid, morphine, and clofibric acid. Increased plasma levels of cyclosporine, prednisolone, and theophylline.

PREGNANCY: Category X, not for use in nursing.

Evoclin RX
clindamycin phosphate (Stiefel)

THERAPEUTIC CLASS: Lincomycin derivative

INDICATIONS: Treatment of acne vulgaris.

DOSAGE: *Adults:* Apply to affected area once daily.

Pediatrics: ≥12 yrs: Apply to affected area once daily.

HOW SUPPLIED: Foam: 1% (50g, 100g)

CONTRAINDICATIONS: History of regional enteritis, ulcerative colitis, or antibiotic-associated colitis.

WARNINGS/PRECAUTIONS: Diarrhea, bloody diarrhea, and colitis (including pseudomembranous colitis) reported with the use of topical and systemic clindamycin. Discontinue if significant diarrhea occurs. Caution in atopic individuals. Avoid eye contact.

ADVERSE REACTIONS: Headache, application site burning/pruritus/dryness, pseudomembranous colitis (rare).

INTERACTIONS: May potentiate neuromuscular blockers; caution with concomitant use.

PREGNANCY: Category B, caution in nursing.

Exjade RX
deferasirox (Novartis)

THERAPEUTIC CLASS: Iron Chelating Agent

INDICATIONS: Treatment of chronic iron overload due to blood transfusions (transfusional hemosiderosis).

Felbatol

DOSAGE: *Adults:* Initial: 20mg/kg/day. Titrate: May increase 5-10mg/kg q 3-6 months. Max: 30mg/kg/day. Take on empty stomach at least 30 minutes before food at same time each day. Tablets should be completely dispersed in 3.5oz of liquid if dose <1g or in 7oz if dose >1g. If serum ferritin falls below 500μg/L, consider interrupting therapy.

Pediatrics: ≥2 yrs: Initial: 20mg/kg/day. Titrate: May increase 5-10mg/kg q 3-6 months. Max: 30mg/kg/day. Take on empty stomach at least 30 minutes before food at same time each day. Tablets should be completely dispersed in 3.5oz of liquid if dose <1g or in 7oz if dose >1g. If serum ferritin falls below 500μg/L, consider interrupting therapy.

HOW SUPPLIED: Tab: 125mg, 250mg, 500mg

WARNINGS/PRECAUTIONS: Assess SCr before therapy and monitor monthly therafter; reduce dose, interrupt or d/c therapy if necessary. Intermittent proteinuria reported; monitor closely. Acute renal failure and cytopenias reported. Use caution and monitor SCr in those at risk of complications, having preexisting renal or comorbid conditions, receiving medicinal products that depress renal function, or elderly. Caution with pre-existing hematologic disorders; monitor CBC regularly. Hepatic abnormalities, increased transaminases reported; monitor LFTs monthly; modify dose for severe or persistent elevations. Reports of auditory (high frequency hearing loss, decreased hearing) and ocular distrubances (lens opacities, cataracts, elevated IOP, retinal disorders); initial and yearly auditory and ophthalmic testing recommended. Reports of skin rashes; d/c if severe, may reinitiate with short period of oral steriod.

ADVERSE REACTIONS: Diarrhea, vomiting, nausea, headache, abdominal pain, pyrexia, cough, increased SCr, rash, b-thalassemia, rare anemias, sicke cell disease.

INTERACTIONS: Avoid with aluminum-containing antacids or other iron chelator therapies.

PREGNANCY: Category B, caution in nursing.

Felbatol RX
felbamate (MedPointe)

> Associated with aplastic anemia and fatal hepatic failure. Monitor blood, LFTs. Avoid in history of hepatic dysfunction.

THERAPEUTIC CLASS: Dicarbamate anticonvulsant

INDICATIONS: Not for 1st line therapy. Monotherapy or adjunct therapy in partial seizures with and without generalization in adults. Adjunct therapy for partial and generalized seizures with Lennox-Gastaut syndrome in children.

DOSAGE: *Adults:* Initial Monotherapy: 300mg qid or 400mg tid. Titrate: Increase by 600mg every 2 weeks to 2.4g/day. Max: 3.6g/day. Initial Monotherapy Conversion/Adjunct Therapy: 300mg qid or 400mg tid while reducing present AED (see literature). Titrate: For conversion, increase at week 2 to 2.4g/day, at week 3 up to 3.6g/day. Adjunct Therapy: Increase by 1.2g/day every week up to 3.6mg/day. Renal Dysfunction: May need to reduce dose with concomitant AEDs.

Pediatrics: ≥14 yrs: Initial Monotherapy: 300mg qid or 400mg tid. Titrate: Increase by 600mg every 2 weeks to 2.4g/day. Max: 3.6g/day. Initial Monotherapy Conversion/Adjunct Therapy: 300mg qid or 400mg tid while reducing present AED (see literature). Titrate: For conversion, increase at week 2 to 2.4g/day, at week 3 up to 3.6g/day. Adjunct Therapy: Increase by 1.2g/day every week up to 3.6mg/day. 2-14 yrs: Lennox-Gastaut Adjunct Therapy: Initial: 15mg/kg/day in 3-4 divided doses. Titrate: Increase by 15mg/kg/day every week to 45mg/kg/day. Renal Dysfunction: May need to reduce dose with concomitant AEDs.

HOW SUPPLIED: Sus: 600mg/5mL (240mL, 960mL); Tab: 400mg*, 600mg* *scored

CONTRAINDICATIONS: History of blood dyscrasias, hepatic dysfunction.

WARNINGS/PRECAUTIONS: Avoid abrupt discontinuation. Caution with renal dysfunction. Obtain written, informed consent. Obtain full hematologic evaluations and LFTs before, during and after discontinuation. Discontinue if bone marrow depression or liver abnormalities occur.

ADVERSE REACTIONS: Anorexia, vomiting, insomnia, nausea, headache, anemias, hepatic failure.

INTERACTIONS: Increases plasma levels of phenytoin, valproate, active carbamazepine metabolite and phenobarbital. Decreases carbamazepine levels. Decreased felbamate levels with phenytoin, carbamazepine, and phenobarbital. Caution with OCs.
PREGNANCY: Category C, safety in nursing not known.

Feosol
iron carbonyl - ferrous sulfate (GlaxoSmithKline Consumer)
OTC

THERAPEUTIC CLASS: Iron supplement
INDICATIONS: Treatment of iron deficiency and iron deficiency anemia.
DOSAGE: *Adults:* 1 tab qd with food.
Pediatrics: ≥12 yrs: 1 tab qd with food.
HOW SUPPLIED: Tab: Feosol Caplet (Iron Carbonyl) 50mg (45mg elemental iron), Feosol Tablet (Ferrous Sulfate) 200mg (65mg elemental iron)
WARNINGS/PRECAUTIONS: Keep product out of reach of children. Accidental overdose of iron-containing products is a leading cause of fatal poisoning in children <6 yrs.
ADVERSE REACTIONS: Nausea, GI disturbance, constipation, diarrhea.
INTERACTIONS: Decreases absorption of tetracycline; space dose by 2 hrs.
PREGNANCY: Safety in pregnancy and nursing not known.

Fero-Grad-500
vitamin C - ferrous sulfate (Abbott)
OTC

THERAPEUTIC CLASS: Iron/vitamin
INDICATIONS: Iron supplementation.
DOSAGE: *Adults:* 1 tab qd.
Pediatrics: ≥4 yrs: 1 tab qd.
HOW SUPPLIED: Tab, Extended Release: Ferrous Sulfate 105mg-Vitamin C 500mg

Ferrlecit
sodium ferric gluconate complex (Watson)
RX

THERAPEUTIC CLASS: Hematinic
INDICATIONS: Treatment of iron deficiency anemia in patients ≥6 yrs old undergoing chronic hemodialysis and receiving supplemental epoetin therapy.
DOSAGE: *Adults:* 10mL (125mg) as IV infusion (diluted) or as slow IV injection (undiluted). Minimum Cumulative Dose: 1g elemental iron over 8 sequential dialysis sessions.
Pediatrics: ≥6 yrs: 0.12mL/kg (1.5mg/kg) as IV infusion over 1 hr at 8 sequential dialysis sessions. Max: 125mg/dose.
HOW SUPPLIED: Inj: 62.5mg elemental iron/5mL
CONTRAINDICATIONS: Anemia not associated with iron deficiency. Iron overload.
WARNINGS/PRECAUTIONS: Hypersensitivity reactions and hypotension reported. Iron overload is more common in patients with hemoglobinopathies and other refractory anemia. Should not be administered to patients with iron overload.
ADVERSE REACTIONS: Injection site reactions, nausea, vomiting, diarrhea, hypotension, cramps, HTN, dizziness, dyspnea, abnormal erythrocytes, leg cramps, pain, chest pain, hypoesthesia, dysgeusia.
PREGNANCY: Category B, caution in nursing.

Feverall
acetaminophen (Alpharma)
OTC

THERAPEUTIC CLASS: Analgesic
INDICATIONS: Treatment of pain and fever in patients who cannot tolerate oral meds due to nausea and vomiting.

FINEVIN

DOSAGE: *Pediatrics:* Insert sup rectally. 3-11 months: 80mg q6h. Max: 480mg/24hrs. 12-36 months: 80mg q4h. Max: 480mg/24hrs. 3-6 yrs: 120mg q4-6h. Max: 720mg/24hrs. 6-12 yrs: 325mg q4-6h. Max: 2600mg/24hrs.
HOW SUPPLIED: Sup: 80mg, 120mg, 325mg, 650mg
PREGNANCY: Safety in pregnancy or nursing not known.

FINEVIN RX
azelaic acid (Berlex)

THERAPEUTIC CLASS: Dicarboxylic acid antimicrobial
INDICATIONS: Mild-to-moderate inflammatory acne vulgaris.
DOSAGE: *Adults:* Wash and dry skin. Massage gently into affected area bid (am and pm).
Pediatrics: ≥12 yrs: Wash and dry skin. Massage gently into affected area bid (am and pm).
HOW SUPPLIED: Cre: 20% (30g, 50g)
WARNINGS/PRECAUTIONS: Hypopigmentation reported after use. Avoid the mouth, eyes, mucous membranes, occlusive dressings, or wrappings.
ADVERSE REACTIONS: Pruritus, burning, stinging, tingling.
PREGNANCY: Category B, caution in nursing.

FIORICET RX
caffeine - butalbital - acetaminophen (Watson)

THERAPEUTIC CLASS: Barbiturate/analgesic
INDICATIONS: Tension or muscle contraction headaches.
DOSAGE: *Adults:* 1-2 tabs q4h prn. Max: 6 tabs/day. Not for extended use.
Pediatrics: ≥12 yrs: 1-2 tabs q4h prn. Max: 6 tabs/day. Not for extended use.
HOW SUPPLIED: Tab: (Butalbital-APAP-Caffeine) 50mg-325mg-40mg
CONTRAINDICATIONS: Porphyria.
WARNINGS/PRECAUTIONS: May be habit forming. Not for extended use. Caution in elderly, debilitated, severe renal or hepatic impairment, acute abdominal conditions. Caution in mentally depressed and suicidal tendencies, history of drug abuse.
ADVERSE REACTIONS: Drowsiness, lightheadedness, dizziness, sedation, shortness of breath, nausea, vomiting, abdominal pain, intoxicated feeling.
INTERACTIONS: Enhanced CNS effects with MAOIs. May enhance CNS depressant effects of other narcotic analgesics, alcohol, general anesthetics, tranquilizers, sedative hypnotics, or other CNS depressants.
PREGNANCY: Category C, not for use in nursing.

FLAGYL RX
metronidazole (Pharmacia & Upjohn)

THERAPEUTIC CLASS: Nitroimidazole
INDICATIONS: Treatment of symptomatic/asymptomatic trichomoniasis, amebic dysentery, amebic liver abscess, and anaerobic infections. Following IV metronidazole therapy, treatment of intra-abdominal, skin and skin structure, bone and joint, CNS, lower respiratory tract, and gynecologic infections, septicemia, and endocarditis.
DOSAGE: *Adults:* Trichomoniasis (Female and Male Sex Partner): (Cap/Tab) 375mg bid or 250mg tid for 7 days. One-day Therapy: (Tab) 2gm as single or divided doses. If repeat course needed, reconfirm diagnosis and allow 4-6 weeks between courses. Abscess: 500mg or 750mg tid for 5-10 days. Dysentery: 750mg tid for 5-10 days. Anaerobic Bacterial Infection: Usually IV therapy initially if serious, 7.5mg/kg q6h for 7-10 days or longer. Max: 4g/24 hrs. Elderly: Adjust dose based on serum levels. Hepatic Disease: Give lower dose cautiously; monitor levels.

Pediatrics: Amebiasis: 35-50mg/kg/24hrs given tid for 10 days.

HOW SUPPLIED: Cap: 375mg; Tab: 250mg, 500mg

CONTRAINDICATIONS: Treatment during 1st trimester of pregnancy.

WARNINGS/PRECAUTIONS: Seizures and peripheral neuropathy reported. Discontinue if abnormal neurological signs occur. Caution with severe hepatic impairment, blood dyscrasias, or CNS diseases. Monitor leukocytes before and after therapy.

ADVERSE REACTIONS: Seizures, peripheral neuropathy, nausea, vomiting, headache, anorexia, urticaria, rash, metallic taste, dysuria, vaginal candidiasis, vaginitis, dizziness, leukopenia.

INTERACTIONS: Avoid alcohol during and for 3 days after use. Avoid within 2 weeks of disulfiram use; increased possibility of psychotic reactions. Potentiates anticoagulant effects of warfarin; monitor PT. Increased elimination with phenytoin, phenobarbital and other hepatic enzyme inducers. May impair phenytoin clearance. Potentiated by cimetidine and other hepatic enzyme inhibitors. Increased lithium levels.

PREGNANCY: Category B, not for use in nursing.

Fleet Bisacodyl OTC
bisacodyl (Fleet)

THERAPEUTIC CLASS: Stimulant laxative

INDICATIONS: Relief of occasional constipation. For bowel cleansing for X-ray and endoscopic exam. Laxative in postoperative, antepartum, or postpartum care.

DOSAGE: *Adults:* (Enema) Use 1 rectally single dose qd. (Sup) Insert 1 rectally qd. Retain for 15-20 minutes. (Tab) 2-3 tabs single dose qd. Swallow tabs whole; do not chew or crush.

Pediatrics: ≥12 yrs: (Enema) Use 1 rectally single dose qd. (Sup) Insert 1 rectally qd. Retain for 15-20 minutes. (Tab) 2-3 tabs single dose qd. 6-11 yrs: (Sup) Insert 1/2 suppository rectally qd. Retain for 15-20 minutes. (Tab) 1 tab qd. Swallow tabs whole; do not chew or crush.

HOW SUPPLIED: Enema: 10mg; Sup: 10mg; Tab, Delayed Release: 5mg

WARNINGS/PRECAUTIONS: Do not use with nausea, vomiting, or abdominal pain. Rectal bleeding or failure to have a bowel movement after use may indicate a serious condition. Should not be used longer than 1 week.

ADVERSE REACTIONS: Abdominal discomfort, faintness, cramps.

INTERACTIONS: Do not administer tabs within 1 hr after taking an antacid, milk, or milk products.

PREGNANCY: Safety in pregnancy and nursing is not known.

Fleet Glycerin Laxatives OTC
glycerin (Fleet)

THERAPEUTIC CLASS: Laxative

INDICATIONS: Relief of constipation.

DOSAGE: *Adults:* 1 enema (5.6g) or 1 suppository (2g or 3g) rectally.

Pediatrics: 2-5 yrs: 1 enema (2.3g) or 1 suppository (1g) rectally. ≥ 6 yrs: 1 enema (5.6g) or 1 suppository (2g or 3g) rectally.

HOW SUPPLIED: Enema: (Babylax) 2.3g, (Liquid Glycerin) 5.6g; Sup: 1g, 2g, 3g

WARNINGS/PRECAUTIONS: Rectal irritation may occur. Do not use with nausea, vomiting, or abdominal pain. Rectal bleeding or failure to have a bowel movement after use may indicate a serious condition. Do not use longer than 1 week.

ADVERSE REACTIONS: Rectal discomfort, burning sensation.

PREGNANCY: Safety in pregnancy and nursing in not known.

Flexeril RX
cyclobenzaprine HCl (McNeil Consumer)

THERAPEUTIC CLASS: Skeletal muscle relaxant (central-acting)

INDICATIONS: Relief of muscle spasm associated with acute, painful musculoskeletal conditions.

Flonase

DOSAGE: *Adults:* Usual: 5mg tid. Titrate: May increase to 10mg tid. Mild Hepatic Dysfunction/Elderly: Initial: 5mg qd, then slowly increase. Moderate/Severe Hepatic Dysfunction: Avoid use. Treatment should not exceed 2-3 weeks.

Pediatrics: ≥15 yrs: Usual: 5mg tid. Titrate: May increase to 10mg tid. Mild Hepatic Dysfunction/Elderly: Initial: 5mg qd, then slowly increase. Moderate/Severe Hepatic Dysfunction: Avoid use. Treatment should not exceed 2-3 weeks.

HOW SUPPLIED: Tab: 5mg, 10mg

CONTRAINDICATIONS: Acute recovery phase of MI, arrhythmias, heart block or conduction disturbances, CHF, hyperthyroidism, MAOI use during or within 14 days.

WARNINGS/PRECAUTIONS: Caution with history of urinary retention, angle-closure glaucoma, increased IOP, hepatic dysfunction. Caution in elderly due to increased risk of CNS effects. May produce arrhythmias, sinus tachycardia and conduction time prolongation. May impair ability to drive.

ADVERSE REACTIONS: Drowsiness, dry mouth, headache, fatigue.

INTERACTIONS: Enhances effects of alcohol, barbiturates, and other CNS depressants. May block antihypertensive action of guanethidine and similar compounds. May enhance seizure risk with tramadol. Contraindicated with MAOIs. Caution with anticholinergic medication.

PREGNANCY: Category B, caution in nursing.

Flonase RX
fluticasone propionate (GlaxoSmithKline)

THERAPEUTIC CLASS: Corticosteroid

INDICATIONS: Management of the nasal symptoms of seasonal and perennial allergic rhinitis, and nonallergic rhinitis.

DOSAGE: *Adults:* Initial: 2 sprays per nostril qd or 1 spray per nostril bid. Maint: 1 spray per nostril qd. May dose as 2 sprays per nostril qd as needed for seasonal allergic rhinitis.

Pediatrics: ≥4 yrs: Initial: 1 sprays per nostril qd. If inadequate response, may increase to 2 sprays per nostril. Maint: 1 spray per nostril qd. Max: 2 sprays per nostril/day. ≥12 yrs: May dose as 2 sprays per nostril qd as needed for seasonal allergic rhinitis.

HOW SUPPLIED: Spray: 50mcg/spray (16g)

WARNINGS/PRECAUTIONS: Risk of adrenal insufficiency and withdrawal symptoms when replacing systemic corticosteroids with a topical corticosteroids. Caution with active or quiescent TB, ocular herpes simplex, or untreated bacterial, fungal and systemic viral infections. Avoid with recent nasal trauma, surgery or septum ulcers. Risk for more severe/fatal course of infections (eg, chickenpox, measles); avoid exposure in patients who have not had disease or been properly immunized. Candida infection of nose and pharynx reported (rare). Potential for growth velocity reduction in pediatrics. Excessive use may cause signs of hypercorticism or HPA suppression.

ADVERSE REACTIONS: Headache, pharyngitis, epistaxis, nasal burning/irritation, asthma symptoms, nausea/vomiting, cough.

INTERACTIONS: Caution with ketoconazole or other potent CYP3A4 inhibitors, may increase serum fluticasone levels. Concomitant inhaled corticosteroids increases risk of hypercorticism and/or HPA axis suppression. Increased levels with ritonavir; avoid use.

PREGNANCY: Category C, caution in nursing.

Flovent HFA RX
fluticasone propionate (GlaxoSmithKline)

THERAPEUTIC CLASS: Corticosteroid

INDICATIONS: Maintenance treatment of asthma as prophylactic therapy in patients ≥4 years; to reduce or eliminate the need for oral corticosteroidal therapy.

DOSAGE: *Adults:* Previous Bronchodilator Only: Initial: 88mcg bid. Max: 440mcg bid. Previous Inhaled Corticosteroids: Initial: 88-220mcg bid. Max: 440mcg bid. Previous Oral

Corticosteroids: Initial: 440mcg bid. Max: 880mcg bid. Reduce PO prednisone no faster than 2.5 to 5mg/day weekly, beginning at least 1 week after starting fluticasone. Rinse mouth after use.

Pediatrics: ≥12 yrs: Previous Bronchodilator Only: Initial: 88mcg bid. Max: 440mcg bid. Previous Inhaled Corticosteroids: Initial: 88-220mcg bid. Max: 440mcg bid. Previous Oral Corticosteroids: Initial: 440mcg bid. Max: 880mcg bid. 4-11 yrs: Initial/Max: 88mcg bid. Reduce PO prednisone no faster than 2.5 to 5mg/day weekly, beginning at least 1 week after starting fluticasone. Rinse mouth after use.

HOW SUPPLIED: MDI: 44mcg/inh (10.6g), 110mcg/inh (12g), 220mcg/inh (12g)

CONTRAINDICATIONS: Primary treatment of status asthmaticus or other acute asthma attacks.

WARNINGS/PRECAUTIONS: Deaths due to adrenal insufficiency have occurred with transfer from systemic corticosteroids to inhaled corticosteroids. Resume oral corticosteroids during stress or severe asthma attack. Wean slowly from systemic corticosteroid therapy. Observe for adrenal insufficiency, systemic corticosteroid withdrawal effects, hypercorticism, adrenal suppression (including adrenal crisis), reduction in growth velocity (children and adolescents). May increase susceptibility to infections. Not for acute bronchospasm. D/C if bronchospasm occurs after dosing. Caution with TB of respiratory tract; untreated systemic fungal, bacterial, viral or parasitic infections; or ocular herpes simplex. *Candida* infection of mouth and pharynx reported. Glaucoma, increased IOP and cataracts reported. Rare cases of eosinophilic conditions.

ADVERSE REACTIONS: Pharyngitis, cough, bronchitis, nasal congestion, sinusitis, dysphonia, oral candidiasis, upper respiratory infection, influenza, headache, nasal discharge, allergic rhinitis, fever, paradoxical bronchospasm..

INTERACTIONS: Increased levels with ritonavir; avoid use. Caution with ketoconazole and other potent CYP3A4 inhibitors; may increase serum fluticasone levels.

PREGNANCY: Category C, caution in nursing.

Floxin Otic
ofloxacin (Daiichi)

RX

OTHER BRAND NAME: Floxin Otic Singles (Daiichi)

THERAPEUTIC CLASS: Fluoroquinolone

INDICATIONS: Otitis externa in patients ≥6 mos. Chronic suppurative otitis media in patients ≥12 yrs with perforated tympanic membranes. Acute otitis media in patients ≥1 yr with tympanostomy tubes.

DOSAGE: *Adults:* Otitis Externa: 10 drops or 2 single-dispensing containers (SDCs) once daily for 7 days. Chronic Suppurative Otitis Media with Perforated Tympanic Membrane: 10 drops or 2 SDCs bid for 14 days.

Pediatrics: Otitis Externa: 6 mos-13 yrs: 5 drops or 1 single-dispensing container (SDC) once daily for 7 days. ≥13 yrs: 10 drops or 2 SDCs once daily for 7 days. Chronic Suppurative Otitis Media with Perforated Tympanic Membrane: ≥12 yrs: 10 drops or 2 SDCs bid for 14 days. Acute Otitis Media with Tympanostomy Tubes: 1-12 yrs: 5 drops or 1 SDC bid for 10 days.

HOW SUPPLIED: Sol: 0.3% (5mL, 10mL), (Singles) 0.3% (20^s)

WARNINGS/PRECAUTIONS: D/C if hypersensitivity reaction occurs. Re-evaluate if no improvement after one week.

ADVERSE REACTIONS: Pruritus, application site reaction, taste perversion.

PREGNANCY: Category C, not for use in nursing.

Flumadine
rimantadine HCl (Forest)

RX

THERAPEUTIC CLASS: Adamantane class antiviral

INDICATIONS: Prophylaxis and treatment of influenza A virus.

DOSAGE: *Adults:* Prophylaxis/Treatment: 100mg bid. Elderly/Severe Hepatic Dysfunction/CrCl ≤10mL/min: 100mg qd. Initiate treatment within 48 hrs of onset of symptoms. Treat for 7 days from initial onset of symptoms.

FluMist

Pediatrics: Prophylaxis: 1-9 yrs: 5mg/kg qd. Max: 150mg qd. ≥10 yrs: 100mg bid.
HOW SUPPLIED: Syrup: 50mg/5mL (240mL); Tab: 100mg
WARNINGS/PRECAUTIONS: Caution with a history of epilepsy. D/C if seizures develop. Caution with renal or hepatic dysfunction.
ADVERSE REACTIONS: Insomnia, dizziness, nervousness, nausea, vomiting, anorexia, dry mouth, abdominal pain, asthenia.
INTERACTIONS: May be potentiated by cimetidine. APAP and ASA may decrease levels of rimantadine. Avoid use of Live Influenza Virus Vaccine within 2 weeks before or 48 hrs after use.
PREGNANCY: Category C, not for use in nursing.

FluMist   RX
influenza virus vaccine Live (MedImmune)

THERAPEUTIC CLASS: Vaccine
INDICATIONS: Active immunization for the prevention of disease caused by influenza A and B viruses in healthy children and adolescents, 5-17 years of age, and healthy adults, 18-49 years of age.
DOSAGE: *Adults:* 0.25mL per nostril.
Pediatrics: ≥9 yrs: 0.25mL per nostril. 5-8 yrs: Not Previously Vaccinated With FluMist: 0.25mL per nostril for 2 doses 60 days (+/- 14 days) apart. Previously Vaccinated With FluMist: 0.25mL per nostril.
HOW SUPPLIED: Nasal Spray: 0.5mL (10s)
CONTRAINDICATIONS: Parenteral use. Hypersensitivity to eggs or egg products. Children and adolescents 5-17 years of age receiving aspirin or aspirin-containing therapy. History of Guillain-Barre syndrome. Immune deficiency diseases such as combined immuno immunodeficiency, agammaglobulinemia, and thymic abnormalities, and conditions such as HIV infection, malignancy, leukemia, or lymphoma. Immunosuppressed or altered/compromised immune status due to treatment with systemic corticosteroids, alkylating drugs, antimetabolites, radiation, or other immunosuppressive therapies.
WARNINGS/PRECAUTIONS: Avoid with history of asthma or reactive airways disease, chronic disorders of the cardiovascular and pulmonary systems, second or third trimester of pregnancy, chronic metabolic diseases (including diabetes), renal dysfunction, hemoglobinopathies, congenital or acquired immunosuppression. Avoid close contact with immunocompromised individuals for at least 21 days. Have epinephrine available. Delay administration until after the acute phase (at least 72 hrs) of febrile and/or respiratory illnesses.
ADVERSE REACTIONS: Runny nose, congestion, cough, irritability, headache, sore throat, fever, chills, muscle aches, vomiting, tiredness/weakness.
INTERACTIONS: Avoid concurrent use with other vaccines and within 48 hrs after cessation of antiviral therapy; antiviral agents until 2 weeks after vaccination unless medically indicated; aspirin or aspirin-containing products in children and adolescents 5-17 yrs.
PREGNANCY: Category C, caution in nursing.

Flunisolide Nasal Spray   RX
flunisolide (Various)

THERAPEUTIC CLASS: Corticosteroid
INDICATIONS: Relief of seasonal or perennial rhinitis.
DOSAGE: *Adults:* Initial: 2 sprays per nostril bid. Titrate: May increase to 2 sprays per nostril tid. Max: 8 sprays per nostril/day.
Pediatrics: 6-14 yrs: Initial: 1 spray per nostril tid or 2 sprays per nostril bid. Max: 4 sprays per nostril/day.
HOW SUPPLIED: Spray: 25mcg/spray (25mL)
CONTRAINDICATIONS: Untreated localized infection of the nasal mucosa.

WARNINGS/PRECAUTIONS: Risk of adrenal insufficiency and withdrawal symptoms when replacing systemic corticosteroids with a topical corticosteroids. Caution with active or quiescent TB, ocular herpes simplex, or untreated bacterial, fungal and systemic viral infections. Avoid with recent nasal trauma, surgery or septum ulcers. Risk for more severe/fatal course of infections (eg, chickenpox, measles) and for *Candida* infections of the nose and pharynx.

ADVERSE REACTIONS: Nasal congestion, sneezing, epistaxis, bloody mucous, nasal irritation, watery eyes, sore throat, nausea, vomiting, headache.

INTERACTIONS: Concomitant systemic corticosteroids increases risk of hypercorticism and/or HPA axis suppression.

PREGNANCY: Category C, caution in nursing.

FLUVIRIN
influenza virus vaccine (Chiron)

RX

THERAPEUTIC CLASS: Vaccine

INDICATIONS: Immunization against influenza viruses containing antigens related to those in the vaccine.

DOSAGE: *Adults:* 0.5mL IM in deltoid or thigh single dose. Shake well.

Pediatrics: ≥4 yrs: 0.5mL IM. <9 yrs (Not Previously Vaccinated): Repeat dose minimum 1 month apart. Administer in deltoid muscle to older children and thigh muscle in infants and young children.

HOW SUPPLIED: Inj: 45mcg/0.5mL

CONTRAINDICATIONS: Allergy to chicken eggs, chicken, chicken feathers, chicken dander, or thimerosal (a mercury derivative). Delay administration to patients with an active neurological disorder or an acute febrile illness until disease stabilizes or symptoms subside. History of any neurological signs or symptoms following administration of any vaccine is contraindicated to further use.

WARNINGS/PRECAUTIONS: Do not administer in children younger than 6 months. Caution in children between the ages of 6 months through 4 years. Caution with thrombocytopenia, coagulation disorders, and impaired immune responses.

ADVERSE REACTIONS: Soreness at the injection site, fever, malaise, myalgia.

INTERACTIONS: Immunosuppressive therapies (eg, irradiation, corticosteroids, antimetabolites, alkylating and cytotoxic agents) may reduce effectiveness. May inhibit clearance of warfarin and theophylline.

PREGNANCY: Category C, safe for use in nursing.

FLUVOXAMINE MALEATE
fluvoxamine maleate (Various)

RX

> Antidepressants increased the risk of suicidal thinking and behavior (suicidality) in short-term studies in children and adolescents with Major Depressive Disorder (MDD) and other psychiatric disorders. Fluvoxamine is not approved for use in pediatric patients except for pateints with Obsessive Compulsive Disorder (OCD).

THERAPEUTIC CLASS: Selective serotonin reuptake inhibitor

INDICATIONS: Treatment of OCD.

DOSAGE: *Adults:* Initial: 50mg qhs. Titrate: Increase by 50mg every 4-7 days. Maint: 100-300mg/day. Give bid if total dose >100mg daily. Max: 300mg/day. Elderly/Hepatic Impairment: Modify initial dose and titration.

Pediatrics: 8-17 yrs: Initial: 25mg qhs. Titrate: Increase by 25mg every 4-7 days. Maint: 50-200mg/day. Max: 8-11 yrs: 200mg/day. Adolescents: 300mg/day. Give bid if total dose >50mg daily.

HOW SUPPLIED: Tab: 25mg, 50mg*, 100mg* *scored

CONTRAINDICATIONS: Co-administration of thioridazine, terfenadine, astemizole, cisapride, pimozide, alosetron, tizanidine.

FLUZONE

WARNINGS/PRECAUTIONS: Activation of mania/hypomania, SIADH, and hyponatremia reported. Close supervision with high risk suicide patients. Caution with history of seizures, hepatic dysfunction, with conditions altering metabolism or hemodynamic responses. Smoking increases metabolism.

ADVERSE REACTIONS: Headache, asthenia, nausea, diarrhea, vomiting, anorexia, dyspepsia, insomnia, somnolence, nervousness, agitation, dizziness, anxiety, dry mouth, sweating, tremor, abnormal ejaculation.

INTERACTIONS: See Contraindications. May potentiate metoprolol, propranolol. Avoid alcohol, diazepam, terfenadine, astemizole, cisapride, primozide. Increases serum levels of theophylline, warfarin, clozapine, carbamazepine, methadone. Bradycardia with diltiazem. Potential for serious, fatal interactions with MAOIs. Lithium may increase serotonergic effects. Reduces clearance of mexiletine and benzodiazepines metabolized by hepatic oxidation (eg, alprazolam, midazolam, triazolam). Caution with sumatriptan, TCAs, tryptophan. Avoid thioridazine; produces dose-related QTc interval prolongation. Increases tacrine serum levels.

PREGNANCY: Category C, not for use in nursing.

FLUZONE   RX
influenza virus vaccine (Sanofi Pasteur)

THERAPEUTIC CLASS: Vaccine

INDICATIONS: Active immunization against influenza disease caused by influenza virus types A and B contained in vaccine in subjects from 6 months of age and older.

DOSAGE: *Adults:* 0.5mL IM in the deltoid muscle.
Pediatrics: ≥9 yrs: 0.5mL IM. 3-8 yrs: 0.5mL IM. 6-35 months: 0.25mL IM. Children <9 yrs who have not previously been vaccinated should recevie two doses of vaccine ≥1 month apart. Older children should be given the IM injection in deltoid muscle, infants and young children should receive the IM injection in the anterolateral aspect of the thigh.

HOW SUPPLIED: Inj: 0.25mL, 0.5mL

CONTRAINDICATIONS: Hypersensitivity reactions to egg proteins or to chicken proteins. Vaccination may be postponed in case of febrile or acute disease. Immunization should be delayed in patients with an active neurologic disorder.

WARNINGS/PRECAUTIONS: Avoid in individuals who have a prior history of Guillain-Barre syndrome and in patients with bleeding disorders, such as hemophilia or thrombocytopenia or if patients is on anticoagulant therapy. Immunosuppressed patients may not obtain expected antibody response. Have epinephrine injection (1:1000) available.

ADVERSE REACTIONS: Local: soreness, pain, swelling. Systemic: fever, malaise, myalgia.

PREGNANCY: Category C, safety in nursing not known.

FML   RX
fluorometholone (Allergan)

OTHER BRAND NAME: FML Forte (Allergan)

THERAPEUTIC CLASS: Corticosteroid

INDICATIONS: Treatment of inflammation of the palpebral and bulbar conjunctiva, cornea, and anterior segment of the globe.

DOSAGE: *Adults:* (Sus) 1 drop bid-qid or (Oint) apply 1/2 inch qd-tid. May give 0.1% q4h during initial 24-48 hrs. Re-evaluate after 2 days if no improvement.
Pediatrics: ≥2 yrs: (Sus) 1 drop bid-qid or (Oint) apply 1/2 inch qd-tid. May give 0.1% q4h during initial 24-48 hrs. Re-evaluate after 2 days if no improvement.

HOW SUPPLIED: Oint: (S.O.P.) 0.1% (3.5g); Sus: 0.1% (5mL, 10mL, 15mL); (Forte) 0.25% (2mL, 5mL, 10mL, 15mL)

CONTRAINDICATIONS: Viral diseases of the cornea and conjunctiva including epithelial herpes simplex keratitis, vaccinia, and varicella. Mycobacterial infection and fungal diseases of the eye.

WARNINGS/PRECAUTIONS: Caution with glaucoma, herpes simplex, diseases causing thinning of cornea/sclera and other ocular viral infections. Prolonged use can cause glaucoma or secondary ocular infections (eg, fungal). Monitor IOP after 10 days of therapy. Re-evaluate if no response after 2 days. Ointment may retard corneal healing. May delay healing and increase incidence of bleb formation after cataract surgery. Avoid abrupt withdrawal with chronic use.

ADVERSE REACTIONS: Elevation of IOP, glaucoma, infrequent optic nerve damage, posterior subcapsular cataract formation, delayed wound healing, burning/stinging upon instillation, ocular irritation, taste perversion, visual disturbance.

PREGNANCY: Category C, not for use in nursing.

Focalin
dexmethylphenidate HCl (Novartis)   CII

THERAPEUTIC CLASS: Sympathomimetic amine

INDICATIONS: Treatment of attention deficit hyperactivity disorder (ADHD).

DOSAGE: *Adults:* Take bid at least 4 hrs apart. Methylphenidate Naive: Initial: 2.5mg bid. Titrate: Increase weekly by 2.5-5mg/day. Max: 20mg/day. Currently on Methylphenidate: Initial: Take 1/2 of methylphenidate dose. Max: 20mg/day. Reduce or discontinue if paradoxical aggravation of symptoms. Discontinue if no improvement after appropriate dosage adjustments over 1 month.

Pediatrics: ≥6 yrs: Take bid at least 4 hrs apart. Methylphenidate Naive: Initial: 2.5mg bid. Titrate: Increase weekly by 2.5-5mg/day. Max: 20mg/day. Currently on Methylphenidate: Initial: Take 1/2 of methylphenidate dose. Max: 20mg/day. Reduce or discontinue if paradoxical aggravation of symptoms. Discontinue if no improvement after appropriate dosage adjustments over 1 month.

HOW SUPPLIED: Tab: 2.5mg, 5mg, 10mg

CONTRAINDICATIONS: Marked anxiety, tension, and agitation; glaucoma; motor tics or family history or diagnosis of Tourette's syndrome; during or within 14 days of MAOI use.

WARNINGS/PRECAUTIONS: Caution in drug dependence or alcoholism. Avoid with known serious structural cardiac abnormalities, cardiomyopathy, serious heart rhythm abnormalities, CAD, or other serious cardiac problems. May cause modest increase in BP; caution with HTN, heart failure, recent MI, or ventricular arrhythmia. May exacerbate symptoms of behavior disturbance and thought disorder with pre-existing psychotic disorder. Caution when using stimulants to treat patients with comorbid bipolar disorder becuase of concern for possible induction of mixed/manic episodes in such patients. Stimulants at usual doses may cause treatment-emergent psychotic or manic symptoms (eg, hallucinations, delusional thinking, mania) in children and adolescents without prior history of psychotic illness or mania. Aggressive behavior or hostility reported in clinical trials and the postmarketing experience of some medications indicated for the treatment of ADHD. Suppression of growth reported with long-term use; monitor growth. May lower convulsive threshold; d/c in the presence of seizures. Visual disturbances reported. Monitor CBC, differential, and platelets with prolonged therapy.

ADVERSE REACTIONS: Abdominal pain, fever, anorexia, nausea, nervousness, insomnia. (Pediatrics) Loss of appetite, weight loss, tachycardia.

INTERACTIONS: See Contraindications. May decrease the effectiveness of antihypertensives. Caution with pressor agents. May inhibit metabolism of coumarin anticoagulants, anticonvulsants, and some antidepressants; adjust dose. Adverse events reported with clonidine.

PREGNANCY: Category C, caution in nursing.

Focalin XR
dexmethylphenidate HCl (Novartis)   CII

THERAPEUTIC CLASS: Sympathomimetic amine

INDICATIONS: Treatment of attention deficit hyperactivity disorder (ADHD) in patients aged 6 yrs and older.

FOLIC ACID

DOSAGE: *Adults:* Methylphenidate Naive: Initial: 10mg/day. Titrate: May adjust weekly by 10mg/day. Max: 20mg/day. Currently on Methylphenidate: Initial: Take 1/2 of methylphenidate dose. Max: 20mg/day. Reduce or discontinue if paradoxical aggravation of symptoms. Swallow capsule whole or sprinkle contents on applesauce. Contents should not be crushed, chewed or divided. Discontinue if no improvement after appropriate dosage adjustments over 1 month.

Pediatrics: ≥6 yrs: Methylphenidate Naive: Initial: 5mg/day. Titrate: May adjust weekly by 5mg/day. Max: 20mg/day. Currently on Methylphenidate: Initial: Take 1/2 of methylphenidate dose. Max: 20mg/day. Reduce or discontinue if paradoxical aggravation of symptoms. Swallow capsule whole or sprinkle contents on applesauce: contents should not be crushed, chewed or divided. Discontinue if no improvement after appropriate dosage adjustments over 1 month.

HOW SUPPLIED: Cap, Extended Release: 5mg, 10mg, 15mg, 20mg

CONTRAINDICATIONS: Marked anxiety, tension, and agitation; glaucoma; motor tics or family history or diagnosis of Tourette's syndrome; during or within 14 days of MAOI use.

WARNINGS/PRECAUTIONS: Caution in drug dependence or alcoholism. Avoid with known serious structural cardiac abnormalities, cardiomyopathy, serious heart rhythm abnormalities, CAD, or other serious cardiac problems. May cause modest increase in BP; caution with HTN, heart failure, recent MI, or ventricular arrhythmia. May exacerbate symptoms of behavior disturbance and thought disorder with pre-existing psychotic disorder. Caution when using stimulants to treat patients with comorbid bipolar disorder becuase of concern for possible induction of mixed/manic episodes in such patients. Stimulants at usual doses may cause treatment-emergent psychotic or manic symptoms (eg, hallucinations, delusional thinking, mania) in children and adolescents without prior history of psychotic illness or mania. Aggressive behavior or hostility reported in clinical trials and the postmarketing experience of some medications indicated for the treatment of ADHD. Suppression of growth reported with long-term use; monitor growth. May lower convulsive threshold; d/c in the presence of seizures. Visual disturbances reported. Monitor CBC, differential, and platelets with prolonged therapy.

ADVERSE REACTIONS: Dyspepsia, headache, anxiety. (Adults) dry mouth, pharyngolaryngeal pain, feeling jittery, dizziness. (Pediatrics) decreased appetite, nausea.

INTERACTIONS: See Contraindications. May decrease the effectiveness of antihypertensives. Caution with pressor agents. May inhibit metabolism of coumarin anticoagulants, anticonvulsants, and tricyclic drugs; adjust dose. Adverse events reported with clonidine. Antacids or acid supressants could alter the release of dexmethylphenidate.

PREGNANCY: Category C, caution in nursing.

Folic Acid
folic acid (Various)
RX

THERAPEUTIC CLASS: Erythropoiesis agent

INDICATIONS: Treatment of megaloblastic anemia due to folic acid deficiency and in anemias of nutritional origin, pregnancy, infancy or childhood.

DOSAGE: *Adults:* Usual: Up to 1mg/day. Maint: 0.4mg qd. Pregnancy/Nursing: Maint: 0.8mg qd. Max: 1mg/day. Increase maintenance dose with alcoholism, hemolytic anemia, anticonvulsant therapy, chronic infection.

Pediatrics: Usual: Up to 1mg/day. Maint: Infants: 0.1mg qd. <4 yrs: 0.3mg qd. ≥4 yrs: 0.4mg qd.

HOW SUPPLIED: Inj: 5mg/mL; Tab: (OTC) 0.4mg, 0.8mg, (RX) 1mg

WARNINGS/PRECAUTIONS: Not for monotherapy in pernicious anemia and other megaloblastic anemias with B_{12} deficiency. May obscure pernicious anemia in dosage >0.1 mg/day. Decreased B_{12} serum levels with prolonged therapy.

ADVERSE REACTIONS: Allergic sensitization.

INTERACTIONS: Antagonizes phenytoin effects. Methotrexate, phenytoin, primidone, barbiturates, alcohol, alcoholic cirrhosis, nitrofurantoin, and pyrimethamine increase loss of folate. Increased seizures with phenytoin, primidone and phenobarbital reported. Tetracycline may cause false low serum and red cell folate due to suppression of Lactobacillus casei.

PREGNANCY: Category A, requirement increases during nursing.

FORADIL
formoterol fumarate (Schering) — RX

> Long-acting β₂-agonists may increase the risk of asthma-related death.

THERAPEUTIC CLASS: Beta$_2$ agonist

INDICATIONS: Long-term maintenance treatment of asthma and prevention of bronchospasm with reversible obstructive airway disease (including nocturnal asthma) in patients who require regular treatment with inhaled short acting β$_2$-agonists. Maintenance treatment of bronchoconstriction in chronic obstructive pulmonary disease (COPD). Acute prevention of excercise-induced bronchospasm (EIB).

DOSAGE: *Adults:* Do not swallow cap; give only by inhalation with Aerolizer Inhaler. Asthma/COPD: 12mcg q12h. Max: 24mcg/day. EIB: 12mcg 15 minutes before exercise (do not give added dose if already on q12h dose).

Pediatrics: ≥5 yrs: Do not swallow cap; give only by inhalation with Aerolizer™ Inhaler. Asthma/COPD: 12mcg q12h. Max: 24mcg/day. ≥12 yrs: EIB: 12mcg 15 minutes before exercise (do not give added dose if already on q12h dose).

HOW SUPPLIED: Cap (Inhalation): 12mcg (12^s, 60^s)

WARNINGS/PRECAUTIONS: Do not discontinue inhaled corticosteroids. Only use short-acting β$_2$-agonist inhaler for acute symptoms. Discontinue if paradoxical bronchospasm occurs. Discontinue if ECG changes, QT interval increases, or ST depression occurs. Caution with cardiovascular disorders (eg, HTN, arrhythmias), thyrotoxicosis and convulsive disorders. Anaphylactic and other allergic reactions reported. Not for use in acute asthmatic conditions. Should not be used with other long-acting β$_2$-agonist medications. May cause hypokalemia.

ADVERSE REACTIONS: Viral infection, dyspnea, chest pain, tremor, HTN, hypotension, tachycardia, arrhythmias, headache, nausea, vomiting, fatigue, hypokalemia, hyperglycemia, exacerbation of asthma.

INTERACTIONS: Potentiates other sympathomimetics. Hypokalemia potentiated by xanthine derivatives (eg, theophylline), steroids and non-potassium sparing diuretics. Extreme caution with MAOIs, TCAs, and drugs known to prolong QT interval. Antagonized effect with β-blockers.

PREGNANCY: Category C, caution in nursing.

FORTAZ
ceftazidime (GlaxoSmithKline) — RX

THERAPEUTIC CLASS: Cephalosporin (3rd generation)

INDICATIONS: Treatment of lower respiratory tract (eg, pneumonia), skin and skin structure (SSSI), bone and joint, gynecologic, CNS (eg, meningitis), intra-abdominal, and urinary tract infections (UTI), and septicemia. For use in sepsis.

DOSAGE: *Adults:* Usual: 1g IM/IV q8-12h. Uncomplicated UTI: 250mg IM/IV q12h. Complicated UTI: 500mg IM/IV q8-12h. Bone and Joint Infection: 2g IV q12h. Uncomplicated Pneumonia/SSSI: 500mg-1g IM/IV q8h. Gynecological/Intra-Abdominal/Meningitis/Severe Life-Threatening Infection: 2g IV q8h. Lung Infection Caused by *Pseudomonas* spp. in Cystic Fibrosis (normal renal function): 30-50mg/kg IV q8h. Max: 6g/day. CrCl 31-50mL/min: 1g q12h. CrCl 16-30mL/min: 1g q24h. CrCl 6-15mL/min: 500mg q24h. CrCl <5mL/min: 500mg q48h. For severe infections (6g/day), increase renal impairment dose by 50% or increase dosing interval. Apply reduced dosage recommendations after initial 1g LD is given. Hemodialysis: Give 1g before then 1g after each hemodialysis. Intra-Peritoneal Dialysis/Continuous Ambulatory Peritoneal Dialysis: Give 1g followed by 500mg q24h, or add to fluid at 250mg/2L.

Pediatrics: 1 month-12 yrs: 30-50mg/kg IV q8h. Max: 6g/day. Neonates (0-4 weeks): 30mg/kg IV q12h. Higher doses for cystic fibrosis or meningitis. CrCl 31-50mL/min: 1g q12h. CrCl 16-30mL/min: 1g q24h. CrCl 6-15mL/min: 500mg q24h. CrCl <5mL/min: 500mg q48h. For severe infections (6g/day), increase renal impairment dose by 50% or increase dosing interval. Apply reduced dosage recommendations after initial 1g LD is

Fortovase

given. Hemodialysis: Give 1g before then 1g after each hemodialysis. Intra-Peritoneal Dialysis/Continuous Ambulatory Peritoneal Dialysis: Give 1g followed by 500mg q24h, or add to fluid at 250mg/2L.

HOW SUPPLIED: Inj: 500mg, 1g, 1g/50mL, 2g, 2g/50mL, 6g

WARNINGS/PRECAUTIONS: Monitor renal function; potential for nephrotoxicity. Prolonged use may result in overgrowth of nonsusceptible organisms. Possible cross-sensitivity between penicillins, cephalosporins, and other β-lactam antibiotics. Pseudomembranous colitis reported. Elevated levels with renal insufficiency can lead to seizures, encephalopathy, coma, asterixis and neuromuscular excitability. Possible decrease in PT; caution with renal or hepatic impairment, poor nutritional state; monitor PT and give vitamin K if needed. Caution with colitis, other GI diseases, and the elderly. Distal necrosis can occur after inadvertent intra-arterial administration. Continue therapy for 2 days after the signs and symptoms of infection have disappeared, but in complicated infections longer therapy may be required. False positive for urine glucose with Benedict's solution, Fehling's solution, and Clinitest tablets.

ADVERSE REACTIONS: Phlebitis and inflammation at injection site, pruritus, rash, fever, diarrhea.

INTERACTIONS: Nephrotoxicity reported with cephalosporins or potent diuretics (eg, furosemide). Avoid with chloramphenicol; may decrease effect of β-lactam antibiotics. Possible decrease in PT; caution with a protracted course of antimicrobial therapy; monitor PT and give vitamin K if needed. May reduced efficacy of oral contraceptives.

PREGNANCY: Category B, caution in nursing.

Fortovase RX
saquinavir (Roche Labs)

THERAPEUTIC CLASS: Protease inhibitor

INDICATIONS: Treatment of HIV infection in combination with other antiretrovirals.

DOSAGE: *Adults:* 1200mg tid with meals or up to 2 hrs after meals.
Pediatrics: >16 yrs: 1200mg tid with meals or up to 2 hrs after meals.

HOW SUPPLIED: Cap: 200mg

CONTRAINDICATIONS: Concomitant terfenadine, cisapride, astemizole, triazolam, midazolam, or ergot derivatives.

WARNINGS/PRECAUTIONS: Not interchangeable with saquinavir mesylate formulation. New onset DM, exacerbation of pre-existing DM, and hyperglycemia may occur. Exacerbation of chronic liver dysfunction reported with hepatitis or cirrhosis. Spontaneous bleeding may occur with hemophilia A and B. Possible redistribution or accumulation of body fat. Caution with hepatic dysfunction. Interrupt therapy if serious toxicity occurs.

ADVERSE REACTIONS: Nausea, diarrhea, abdominal discomfort, dyspepsia, flatulence, headache, fatigue.

INTERACTIONS: Avoid terfenadine, cisapride, astemizole, triazolam, midazolam, ergot derivatives, lovastatin, St. John's wort, and simvastatin. Decreased plasma levels with nevirapine. Consider alternatives to rifampin, rifabutin. Ritonavir increases adverse effects. Delavirdine increases plasma levels; monitor LFTs frequently. Ketoconazole, nelfinavir, indinavir increase plasma levels. Increased plasma levels of both clarithromycin and saquinavir. Increased sildenafil plasma levels; consider 25mg as initial sildenafil dose. Carbamazepine, phenobarbital, phenytoin, dexamethasone may decrease plasma levels.

PREGNANCY: Category B, not for use in nursing.

Furadantin RX
nitrofurantoin (Sciele)

THERAPEUTIC CLASS: Imidazolidinedione antibacterial

INDICATIONS: Treatment of urinary tract infection (UTI).

DOSAGE: *Adults:* Usual: 50-100mg qid with food for 1 week or at least 3 days after sterility of urine. Use lower doses for uncomplicated UTI. Long-Term Suppressive Therapy: 50-100mg qhs.
Pediatrics: >1 month: Usual: 5-7mg/kg/day given qid with food for 1 week or at least 3 days after sterility of urine. Long-Term Suppressive Therapy: 1mg/kg/day qd or bid.
HOW SUPPLIED: Sus: 25mg/5mL
CONTRAINDICATIONS: Anuria, oliguria, CrCl <60 mL/min, pregnancy at term (38-42 weeks gestation), during labor and delivery, neonates <1 month of age.
WARNINGS/PRECAUTIONS: Acute, subacute or chronic pulmonary reactions have occurred. Enhanced occurrence of peripheral neuropathy with anemia, DM, renal dysfunction, electrolyte imbalance, vitamin B deficiency, and debilitating disease. D/C therapy with acute and chronic pulmonary reactions, hepatic disorders, hemolysis, or peripheral neuropathy. Monitor renal function, LFTs and pulmonary function periodically during long-term therapy. Pseudomembranous colitis reported.
ADVERSE REACTIONS: Pulmonary disorders, hepatic damage, peripheral neuropathy, nausea, emesis, anorexia, dizziness, exfoliative dermatitis, Stevens-Johnson syndrome, anaphylaxis, blood dyscrasias.
INTERACTIONS: Antacids, especially magnesium trisilicate, decrease rate and extent of absorption. Probenecid and sulfinpyrazone increase nitrofurantoin levels.
PREGNANCY: Category B, not for use in nursing.

FUROSEMIDE RX
furosemide (Various)

> Can lead to profound water and electrolyte depletion with excessive use.

OTHER BRAND NAMES: Lasix (Aventis)
THERAPEUTIC CLASS: Loop diuretic
INDICATIONS: (Inj, PO) Treatment of edema associated with CHF, liver cirrhosis, and renal disease including nephrotic syndrome. (PO) Treatment of hypertension. (Inj) Adjunct therapy for acute pulmonary edema.
DOSAGE: *Adults:* (PO) HTN: Initial: 40mg bid. Edema: Initial: 20-80mg PO. May repeat or increase by 20-40mg after 6-8 hrs. Max: 600mg/day. Alternative Regimen: Dose on 2-4 consecutive days each week. Closely monitor if on >80mg/day. (Inj) Edema: Initial: 20-40mg IV/IM. May repeat or increase by 20mg after 2 hrs. Acute Pulmonary Edema: Initial: 40mg IV. May increase to 80mg IV after 1 hr.
Pediatrics: Edema: (PO) Initial: 2mg/kg single dose. May increase by 1-2mg/kg after 6-8 hrs. Max: 6mg/kg. (Inj) Initial: 1mg/kg IV/IM single dose. May increase by 1mg/kg IV/IM after 2 hrs. Max: 6mg/kg.
HOW SUPPLIED: Inj: 10mg/mL; Sol: 10mg/mL, 40mg/5mL; Tab: 20mg, 40mg*, 80mg
*scored
CONTRAINDICATIONS: Anuria.
WARNINGS/PRECAUTIONS: Monitor for fluid/electrolyte imbalance (eg, hypokalemia), renal or hepatic dysfunction. Initiate in hospital with hepatic cirrhosis and ascites. Tinnitus, hearing impairment, hyperglycemia, hyperuricemia reported. May activate SLE. Cross-sensitivity with sulfonamide allergy. Avoid excessive diuresis, especially in elderly.
ADVERSE REACTIONS: Pancreatitis, jaundice, anorexia, paresthesias, ototoxicity, blood dyscrasias, dizziness, rash, urticaria, photosensitivity, fever, thrombophlebitis, restlessness.
INTERACTIONS: Ototoxicity with aminoglycosides, ethacrynic acid. Caution with high dose salicylates. Lithium toxicity. Antagonizes tubocurarine. Potentiates antihypertensives, succinylcholine, ganglionic or peripheral adrenergic blockers. Decreases arterial response to norepinephrine. Separate sucralfate dose by 2 hrs. Indomethacin may decrease effects. Hypokalemia with ACTH, corticosteroids. Renal changes with NSAIDs. Orthostatic hypotension may be aggravated by alcohol, barbiturates, or narcotics.
PREGNANCY: Category C, caution in nursing.

FUZEON RX
enfuvirtide (Roche Labs)

THERAPEUTIC CLASS: Fusion inhibitor
INDICATIONS: Treatment of HIV-1 infection in combination with other antiretroviral agents in treatment-experienced patients with evidence of HIV-1 replication despite ongoing antiretroviral therapy.

GABITRIL

DOSAGE: *Adults:* 90mg SQ bid. Inject SQ into the upper arm, anterior thigh, or abdomen. Do not inject into moles, scar tissue, bruises, the navel, or near any blood vessels. Rotate sites; do not give if injection site reaction occurred from an earlier dose.

Pediatrics: 6-16 yrs: 2mg/kg SQ bid. Max: 90mg bid. 11-15.5kg: 27mg bid. 15.6-20.0kg: 36mg bid. 20.1-24.5kg: 45mg bid. 24.6-29.0kg: 54mg bid. 29.1-33.5kg: 63mg bid. 33.6-38.0kg: 72mg bid. 38.1-42.5kg: 81mg bid. ≥ 42.6kg: 90mg bid. Inject SQ into the upper arm, anterior thigh, or abdomen. Do not inject into moles, scar tissue, bruises, or the navel. Rotate sites; do not give if injection site reaction occurred from an earlier dose.

HOW SUPPLIED: Inj: 90mg (60^s)

WARNINGS/PRECAUTIONS: Monitor for signs and symptoms of pneumonia, cellulitis, or local infection. Discontinue if hypersensitivity reactions occur. Theoretically may lead to production of anti-enfuvirtide antibodies; may result in false positive HIV test with an ELISA assay. Immune reconstitution syndrome reported. Increased risk of bleeding or bruising in patients with coagulation disorders.

ADVERSE REACTIONS: Diarrhea, nausea, fatigue, local injection site reactions, peripheral neuropathy, insomnia, depression, anxiety, cough, sinusitis, herpes simplex, decreased weight/appetite, pancreatitis, asthenia, pruritus, myalgia, nerve pain, bruising, hematomas.

PREGNANCY: Category B, not for use in nursing.

GABITRIL
tiagabine HCl (Cephalon)
RX

THERAPEUTIC CLASS: Nipecotic acid derivative

INDICATIONS: Adjunctive therapy in the treatment of partial seizures.

DOSAGE: *Adults:* Initial: 4mg qd. Titrate: May increase weekly by 4-8mg until clinical response. Max: 56mg/day given bid-qid. Take with food.

Pediatrics: ≥12 yo: Initial: 4mg qd. Titrate: May increase to 8mg qd at beginning of Week 2, then increase weekly by 4-8mg until clinical response. Max: 32mg/day. Take with food.

HOW SUPPLIED: Tab: 2mg, 4mg, 6mg, 8mg, 10mg, 12mg, 16mg

WARNINGS/PRECAUTIONS: Reports of new onset seizure or status epilepticus in patients without epilepsy. D/C and evaluate for underlying seizure disorder. Avoid abrupt withdrawal. Monitor during initial titration for impaired concentration, speech problem, somnolence, fatigue; may require hospitalization if reaction is severe. May exacerbate EEG abnormalities; adjust dose. Status epilepticus and sudden death reported. Reduce dose or d/c if generalized weakness occurs. Reduce dose with hepatic impairment. Serious skin rash reported.

ADVERSE REACTIONS: Dizziness, asthenia, somnolence, nausea, vomiting, nervousness, tremor, abdominal pain, abnormal thinking, depression, confusion, pharyngitis, rash.

INTERACTIONS: May reduce valproate levels. Diminished effects with carbamazepine, phenytoin. Additive CNS depression with alcohol, triazolam, CNS depressants.

PREGNANCY: Category C, caution in nursing.

GAMMAR-P
immune globulin (ZLB Behring)
RX

THERAPEUTIC CLASS: Immunoglobulin

INDICATIONS: Patients with primary defective antibody synthesis (eg, agammaglobulinemia or hypogammaglobulinemia), who are at increased risk of infection.

DOSAGE: *Adults:* 200-400mg/kg IV every 3-4 weeks. Adjust dose to maintain desired IgG levels and clinical response.

Pediatrics/Adolescents: 200mg/kg IV every 3-4 weeks. Adjust dose to maintain desired IgG levels and clinical response.

HOW SUPPLIED: Inj: 5g, 10g

CONTRAINDICATIONS: History of allergic reactions to human albumin, anaphylactic or severe systemic response to IM/IV immune globulin, isolated IgA deficiency.

WARNINGS/PRECAUTIONS: Make sure patient is not volume depleted before administration. Caution if predisposed to acute renal failure (eg, any degree of pre-existing renal insufficiency, DM, >65 yrs, volume depletion, sepsis, paraproteinemia, with nephrotoxic drugs). Monitor renal function and infusion rate. Aseptic meningitis syndrome reported. Made from human blood; risk of transmitting infection.

ADVERSE REACTIONS: Acute renal failure, acute tubular necrosis, proximal tubular nephropathy, osmotic nephrosis, chills, headache, backache, neck pain.

INTERACTIONS: May interfere with response to live viral vaccines (eg, measles, mumps, rubella).

PREGNANCY: Category C, safety in nursing not known.

Gantrisin Pediatric   RX
sulfisoxazole (Roche Labs)

THERAPEUTIC CLASS: Sulfonamide

INDICATIONS: Treatment of acute, recurrent or chronic urinary tract infection. Treatment and prophylaxis in meningococcal meningitis. Adjunct treatment of Haemophilus influenzae meningitis, acute otitis media, malaria, and toxoplasmosis. Treatment of trachoma, inclusion conjunctivitis, nocardiosis, chancroid.

DOSAGE: Pediatrics: >2 months: Initial: 1/2 of 24hr dose. Maint: 150mg/kg/24hr or 4g/m^2/24hr given q4-6h. Max: 6g/24hr.

HOW SUPPLIED: Sus: 500mg/5mL

CONTRAINDICATIONS: Infants <2 months (except in congenital toxoplasmosis treatment), pregnancy at term, mothers nursing infants <2 months old.

WARNINGS/PRECAUTIONS: Fatalities reported due to Stevens-Johnson syndrome, toxic epidermal necrolysis, fulminant hepatic necrosis, agranulocytosis, aplastic anemia and other blood dyscrasias. Discontinue if develop skin rash or sign of an adverse reaction. Hypersensitivity reactions of the respiratory tract reported. Do not use in group A β-hemolytic streptococcal infections. Pseudomembranous colitis reported. Caution with renal/hepatic impairment, severe allergy or bronchial asthma. Hemolysis may occur in G6PD-deficient patients.

ADVERSE REACTIONS: Anaphylaxis, erythema multiforme, toxic epidermal necrolysis, tachycardia, hepatitis, nausea, anorexia, hematuria, crystalluria, BUN and creatinine elevations, blood dyscrasias, dizziness, psychosis, cough.

INTERACTIONS: May prolong PT with anticoagulants. May require less thiopental for anesthesia. May potentiate hypoglycemia effects of sulfonylureas. May displace methotrexate from plasma proteins.

PREGNANCY: Category C, not for use in nursing.

Gardasil   RX
human papillomavirus recombinant vaccine, quadrivalent (Merck)

THERAPEUTIC CLASS: Vaccine

INDICATIONS: Vaccination of girls and women ages 9-26 yrs for the prevention of cervical cancer, genital warts, cervical adenocarcinoma *in situ*, cervical intraepithelial neoplasia grades 2 and 3, vulvar intraepithelial neoplasia grades 2 and 3, vaginal intraepithelial neoplasia grades 2 and 3, and cervical intraepithelial neoplasia grade 1 caused by Human Papillomavirus types 6, 11, 16, and 18.

DOSAGE: *Adults:* Give 3 separate 0.5mL IM doses in the deltoid region of upper arm or higher anterolateral area of the thigh. First dose: At elected date; Second dose: 2 months after first dose; Third dose: 6 months after first dose.
Pediatrics: ≥9 yrs: Give 3 separate 0.5mL IM doses in the deltoid region of upper arm or higher anterolateral area of the thigh. First dose: At elected date; Second dose: 2 months after first dose; Third dose: 6 months after first dose.

HOW SUPPLIED: Inj: Vial/Syringe: 0.5mL

WARNINGS/PRECAUTIONS: Should not be administered with bleeding disorders or anticoagulant therapy unless the potential benefits outweigh the risk. Patients with impaired immune responsiveness may have reduced antibody response to active immunization. Medical treatment should be readily available in case of rare anaphylactic reactions.

ADVERSE REACTIONS: Local site reactions, fever, pyrexia, nausea, nasopharyngitis, dizziness, diarrhea.

INTERACTIONS: Immunosuppressive therapies, including irradiation, antimetabolites, alkylating agents, cytotoxic drugs, and corticosteroids (used in greater than physiologic doses) may reduce the immune responses to vaccines.

PREGNANCY: Category B, caution in nursing.

Genotropin RX
somatropin (Pharmacia & Upjohn)

OTHER BRAND NAME: Genotropin MiniQuick (Pharmacia & Upjohn)

THERAPEUTIC CLASS: Human growth hormone

INDICATIONS: Long-term treatment of pediatrics with growth failure due to growth hormone deficiency (GHD) or Prader-Willi syndrome (PWS) or who are born small for gestational age (SGA) and fail to catch-up by age 2. Long-term replacement therapy in adults with GHD of either childhood- or adult-onset etiology. Long-term treatment of growth failure associated with Turner Syndrome (TS) in patients who have open epiphyses.

DOSAGE: *Adults:* Individualize dose: GHD: Initial: Up to 0.04mg/kg/week. May increase at 4-8 week intervals. Max: 0.08mg/kg/week. Divide dose into 6-7 SQ injections. Elderly patients should receive a lower starting dose.
Pediatrics: Individualize dose. GHD: 0.16-0.24mg/kg/week. PWS: 0.24mg/kg/week. SGA: 0.48mg/kg/week. TS: 0.33mg/kg/week. Divide doses into 6-7 SQ injections.

HOW SUPPLIED: Inj: 1.5mg, 5.8mg, 13.8mg; Inj; MiniQuick: 0.2mg, 0.4mg, 0.6mg, 0.8mg, 1mg, 1.2mg, 1.4mg, 1.6mg, 1.8mg, 2mg

CONTRAINDICATIONS: Evidence of neoplastic activity. Pediatrics with closed epiphyses. Patients with diabetic retinopathy or active malignancy. Acute critical illness due to complications after open heart or abdominal surgery, multiple accidental trauma, or with acute respiratory failure. Patients with PWS who are severely obese or have severe respiratory impairment.

WARNINGS/PRECAUTIONS: In PWS, evaluate for upper airway obstruction prior to initiation; monitor weight, for sleep apnea, signs of upper airway obstruction (eg, suspend therapy with onset of or increased snoring), respiratory infections (treat early and aggressively if occur). Monitor GHD secondary to intracranial lesion for progression/recurrence. Monitor gait, glucose intolerance because insulin sensitivity is decreased, for malignant transformation of skin lesions, scoliosis progression, intracranial HTN (perform fundoscopic exam at start and periodically). Caution with DM, endocrine disorders, hypopituitarism, and Turner syndrome. Tissue atrophy may occur (rotate injection site).

ADVERSE REACTIONS: Peripheral swelling/edema, arthralgia, pain/stiffness in extremities, myalgia, upper respiratory infection, paresthesia.

INTERACTIONS: Antagonized by glucocorticoids. May alter clearance of CYP450 substrates (eg, corticosteroids, sex steroids, anticonvulsants, cyclosporine). May need dose adjustment if taking oral estrogen replacement. May need insulin dose adjustment.

PREGNANCY: Category B, caution in nursing.

Gentamicin Ophthalmic RX
gentamicin sulfate (Various)

THERAPEUTIC CLASS: Aminoglycoside

INDICATIONS: Treatment of ocular bacterial infections including conjunctivitis, keratitis, keratoconjunctivitis, corneal ulcers, blepharitis, blepharoconjunctivitis, acute meibomianitis and dacryocystitis.

DOSAGE: *Adults:* Usual: 1-2 drops q4h or apply 1/2 inch of ointment bid-tid. Severe Infection: 2 drops every hour.

Pediatrics: Usual: 1-2 drops q4h or apply half-inch of ointment bid-tid. Severe Infection: 2 drops every hour.

HOW SUPPLIED: Oint: 0.3% (3.5g); Sol: 0.3% (5mL)

WARNINGS/PRECAUTIONS: Discontinue if develop irritation, hypersensitivity, purulent discharge, inflammation or pain. Prolonged use may result in superinfection. Ointment may retard corneal healing.

ADVERSE REACTIONS: Bacterial and fungal corneal ulcers, burning, irritation, conjunctivitis, conjunctival epithelial defects, conjunctival hyperemia.

PREGNANCY: Category C. Safety in nursing is not known.

GENTAMICIN SULFATE INJECTION RX
gentamicin sulfate (Various)

> Potential nephrotoxicity, neurotoxicity, ototoxicity. Risk of toxicity is greater with impaired renal function, high dosage, or prolonged therapy. Monitor serum concentrations closely. Avoid prolonged peak levels >12mcg/mL and trough levels >2mcg/mL. Monitor renal and eight cranial nerve function, urine, BUN, serum creatinine, and CrCl. Obtain serial audiograms. Advanced age and dehydration increase risk of toxicity. Adjust dose or discontinue use with evidence of ototoxicity or nephrotoxicity. May cause fetal harm during pregnancy. Avoid concurrent and/or sequential systemic or topical use of other potentially neurotoxic and/or nephrotoxic drugs, such as cisplatin, cephaloridine, kanamycin, amikacin, neomycin, polymyxin B, colistin, paromomycin, streptomycin, tobramycin, vancomycin, and viomycin. Avoid concurrent use with potent diuretics, such as ethacrynic acid or furosemide.

THERAPEUTIC CLASS: Aminoglycoside

INDICATIONS: Treatment of bacterial neonatal sepsis, bacterial septicemia, and serious bacterial infections of the CNS (meningitis), urinary tract, respiratory tract, gastrointestinal tract (including peritonitis), skin, bone and soft tissue (including burns) caused by susceptible strains of microorganisms.

DOSAGE: *Adults:* IM/IV: Serious Infections: 3mg/kg/day given q8h. Life-Threatening Infections: 5mg/kg/day tid-qid; reduce to 3mg/kg/day as soon as clinically indicated. Treat for 7-10 days; may need longer course in difficult and complicated infections. Renal Impairment: Reduced dose given q8h or usual dose given at prolonged intervals based on either CrCl or serum creatinine. Dialysis: 1-1.7mg/kg, depending on severity of infection, at end of each dialysis period. Obese Patients: Calculate dose based on estimated lean body mass.

Pediatrics: Children: 6-7.5mg/kg/day (2-2.5mg/kg given q8h). Infants and Neonates: 7.5mg/kg/day (2.5mg/kg given q8h). Premature and Full-Term Neonates ≤1 week: 5mg/kg/day (2.5mg/kg given q12h). Treat for 7-10 days; may need longer course in difficult and complicated infections. Renal Impairment: Reduced dose given q8h or usual dose given at prolonged intervals based on either CrCl or serum creatinine. Dialysis: 2mg/kg at end of each dialysis period. Obese Patients: Calculate dose based on estimated lean body mass.

HOW SUPPLIED: Inj: 10mg/mL, 40mg/mL

WARNINGS/PRECAUTIONS: Contains metabisulfite. Neuromuscular blockade, respiratory paralysis, ototoxicity, and nephrotoxicity may occur after local irrigation or topical application during surgical procedures. Caution with neuromuscular disorders (eg, myasthenia gravis, parkinsonism). Caution in elderly; monitor renal function. Keep patients well-hydrated during treatment. May cause fetal harm when administered to pregnant women.

ADVERSE REACTIONS: Nephrotoxicity, neurotoxicity, rash, fever, urticaria, nausea, vomiting, headache, lethargy, confusion, depression, decreased appetite, weight loss, BP changes, blood dyscrasias, elevated LFTs.

INTERACTIONS: Increased nephrotoxicity with cephalosporins. Do not premix with other drugs; administer separately. Neuromuscular blockade and respiratory paralysis may occur in anesthetized patients or those receiving neuromuscular blockers (eg, succinylcholine, tubocurarine, decamethonium). See Black Box Warning.

PREGNANCY: Category D, safety not known in nursing.

GENTAMICIN TOPICAL RX
gentamicin sulfate (Various)

THERAPEUTIC CLASS: Aminoglycoside

INDICATIONS: Treatment of primary skin infections such as impetigo contagiosa, folliculitis, ecthyma, furunculosis, sycosis barbae, and pyoderma gangrenosum; and second-

GLEEVEC

ary skin infections such as infectious eczematoid dermatitis, pustular acne, pustular psoriasis, infected seborrheic dermatitis, infected contact dermatitis, infected excoriations, and bacterial superinfections.

DOSAGE: *Adults:* Apply gently tid-qid. May apply gauze dressing.

Pediatrics: >1 yr: Apply gently tid-qid. May apply gauze dressing.

HOW SUPPLIED: Cre, Oint: 0.1% (15g, 30g)

WARNINGS/PRECAUTIONS: Discontinue if irritation, sensitization, or superinfection develops.

ADVERSE REACTIONS: Irritation (erythema and pruritus).

PREGNANCY: Unknown use in pregnancy and nursing.

GLEEVEC RX
imatinib mesylate (Novartis)

THERAPEUTIC CLASS: Protein-tyrosine kinase inhibitor

INDICATIONS: Treatment of Philadelphia chromosome positive chronic myeloid leukemia (CML) in blast crisis, accelerated phase, or in chronic phase after failure of interferon-alpha therapy or in newly adult diagnosed patients. Treatment of pediatric patients with Ph+ chronic phase CML whose disease has recurred after stem cell transplant or who are resistant to interferon-alpha therapy. Treatment of Kit (CD117) positive unresectable and/or metastatic malignant gastrointestinal stromal tumors (GIST).

DOSAGE: *Adults:* ≥18 yrs: CML: Chronic Phase: 400mg qd, may increase to 600 mg qd. Accelerated Phase/Blast Crisis: 600mg qd, may increase to 400 mg bid. See labeling for dose increase with CML. GIST: 400mg qd or 600mg qd. Hepatotoxicity/Non-Hematologic Adverse Reaction: If bilirubin >3X ULN or transaminases >5X ULN, hold drug until bilirubin <1.5X ULN and transaminases <2.5X ULN. Continue at reduced dose. Neutropenia/Thrombocytopenia: See labeling for dose adjustment. Take with food and water.

Pediatrics: ≥3 yrs: CML: Chronic Phase: 260mg/m^2/day given qd or split into 2 doses (morning and evening). Neutropenia/Thrombocytopenia: See labeling for dose adjustment. Take with food and water.

HOW SUPPLIED: Tab: 100mg, 400mg

WARNINGS/PRECAUTIONS: Fluid retention/edema reported; monitor weight. Neutropenia/thrombocytopenia reported; monitor CBC weekly during 1st month, biweekly during 2nd month, and periodically thereafter. May be hepatotoxic; monitor LFTs at baseline, then monthly or as needed. Avoid becoming pregnant. Interrupt treatment if severe non-hematologic adverse reaction develops (eg, severe hepatotoxicity or severe fluid retention); resume if appropriate. GI bleeds reported. Severe congestive heart failure and left ventricular dysfunction. Hypereosinophilic cardiac toxicity.

ADVERSE REACTIONS: Nausea, vomiting, fluid retention, neutropenia, thrombocytopenia, diarrhea, hemorrhage, pyrexia, rash, headache, fatigue, abdominal pain, elevated transaminases or bilirubin, edema, muscle cramps, musculoskeletal pain, flatulence, nasopharyngitis, insomnia, anemia, anorexia, rhinitis.

INTERACTIONS: Increased levels with CYP3A4 inhibitors (eg, ketoconazole, erythromycin, clarithromycin, itraconazole). Decreased levels with CYP3A4 inducers (eg, dexamethasone, phenytoin, carbamazepine, rifampin, phenobarbital, St. John's Wort). Caution with CYP3A4 substrates with narrow therapeutic windows (eg, cyclosporine, pimozide). Increases levels of drugs metabolized by CYP3A4 (eg, dihydropyridines, triazolobenzodiazepines, HMG-CoA reductase inhibitors). Switch patients on warfarin to low molecular weight or standard heparin.

PREGNANCY: Category D, not for nursing.

GLUCAGON RX
glucagon (Lilly)

THERAPEUTIC CLASS: Glucagon

INDICATIONS: Treatment for severe hypoglycemia. Diagnostic aid for radiologic examination of the stomach, duodenum, small bowel, and colon.

GLUCOPHAGE XR

DOSAGE: *Adults:* Severe Hypoglycemia: 1mg (1U) SQ/IM/IV. May give another dose after 15 minutes if patient does not respond, but IV glucose would be a better alternative. Use immediately after reconstitution; discard unused portion. Diagnostic Aid: Stomach/Duodenum/Small Bowel: 0.5mg (0.5U) IV or 2mg (2U) IM before procedure. Colon: 2mg (2U) IM 10 minutes before procedure.

Pediatrics: Severe Hypoglycemia: ≥20kg: 1mg (1U) SQ/IM/IV. <20kg: 0.5mg (0.5U) or 20-30mcg/kg. May give another dose after 15 minutes if patient does not respond, but IV glucose would be a better alternative. Use immediately after reconstitution; discard unused portion.

HOW SUPPLIED: Inj: 1mg

CONTRAINDICATIONS: Pheochromocytoma.

WARNINGS/PRECAUTIONS: Caution with history suggestive of insulinoma and/or pheochromocytoma. Glucagon can cause pheochromocytoma tumor to release catecholamines, which may result in a sudden and marked increase in BP. Effective in treating hypoglycemia only if sufficient liver glycogen is present. Glucagon is not effective in states of starvation, adrenal insufficiency, or chronic hypoglycemia; use glucose to treat instead.

ADVERSE REACTIONS: Nausea, vomiting, allergic reactions, urticaria, respiratory distress, hypotension.

PREGNANCY: Category B, caution in nursing.

GLUCOPHAGE XR   RX
metformin HCl (Bristol-Myers Squibb)

OTHER BRAND NAMES: Riomet (Ranbaxy) - Glucophage (Bristol-Myers Squibb)

THERAPEUTIC CLASS: Biguanide

INDICATIONS: Adjunct to diet or with a sulfonylurea or insulin, to improve glycemic control in type 2 diabetes mellitus.

DOSAGE: *Adults:* (Sol, Tab) Initial: 500mg bid or 850mg qd with meals. Titrate: Increase by 500mg/week, or 850mg every 2 weeks, or may increase from 500mg bid to 850mg bid after 2 weeks. Max: 2550mg/day. Give in 3 divided doses with meals if dose is >2g/day. (Tab, Extended Release) Initial: ≥17 yrs: 500mg qd with evening meal. Titrate: Increase by 500mg/week. Max: 2000mg/day. With Insulin: Initial: 500mg qd. Titrate: Increase by 500mg/week. Max: 2500mg/day and 2000mg/day (XR). Decrease insulin dose by 10-25% when FPG <120mg/dL. Swallow whole; do not crush or chew. Elderly/Debilitated/Malnourished: Conservative dosing; do not titrate to Max.

Pediatrics: 10-16 yrs: (Sol, Tab) Initial: 500mg bid with meals. Titrate: Increase by 500mg/week. Max: 2000mg/day.

HOW SUPPLIED: Sol: (Riomet) 500mg/5mL; Tab: 500mg, 850mg, 1000mg*; Tab, Extended Release: 500mg, 750mg *scored

CONTRAINDICATIONS: Renal disease/dysfunction (SrCr ≥1.5mg/dL (males), ≥1.4mg/dL (females), abnormal CrCl), CHF, metabolic acidosis, diabetic ketoacidosis. Discontinue temporarily (48 hrs) for radiologic studies with intravascular iodinated contrast materials.

WARNINGS/PRECAUTIONS: Lactic acidosis reported (rare); increased risk with renal dysfunction, increased age, DM, CHF, and other conditions with risk of hypoperfusion and hypoxemia. Avoid use in patients ≥80 yrs unless renal function is normal. Monitor renal function and for ketoacidosis and metabolic acidosis. Avoid in renal/hepatic impairment. D/C in hypoxic states (eg, CHF, shock, acute MI), loss of blood glucose control due to stress (give insulin), acidosis, dehydration, sepsis. Temporarily d/c prior to surgery (due to restricted food intake) and procedures requiring intravascular iodinated contrast materials. May decrease serum vitamin B_{12} levels. Increased risk of hypoglycemia in elderly, debilitated/malnourished, adrenal or pituitary insufficiency, or alcohol intoxication. Monitor renal function.

ADVERSE REACTIONS: Lactic acidosis, diarrhea, nausea, vomiting, flatulence, abdominal discomfort, abnormal stools, hypoglycemia, myalgia, dizziness, dyspnea, nail disorder, rash, sweating, taste disorder, chest discomfort, chills, flu syndrome, palpitations, asthenia, indigestion, headache.

INTERACTIONS: Furosemide, nifedipine, cimetidine, cationic drugs (eg, digoxin, amiloride, procainamide, quinidine, quinine, ranitidine, trimethoprim, vancomycin, triamterene, morphine) may increase metformin levels. Thiazides, other diuretics, corticosteroids, phenothiazines, thyroid products, estrogens, oral contraceptives, phenytoin, nicotinic acid, sympathomimetics, calcium channel blockers, isoniazid may cause hyperglycemia. Risk of hypoglycemia with alcohol. Excess alcohol may increase potential for lactic acidosis. May decrease furosemide levels.

PREGNANCY: Category B, not for use in nursing.

GRANULEX RX
trypsin - castor oil - peruvian balsam (Mylan Bertek)

THERAPEUTIC CLASS: Debriding agent

INDICATIONS: Treatment of decubitus ulcers, varicose ulcers, debridement of eschar, dehiscent wounds and sunburn.

DOSAGE: *Adults:* Spray wound at least bid or more often prn.
Pediatrics: Spray wound at least bid or more often prn.

HOW SUPPLIED: Spray: (Castor Oil-Peruvian Balsam-Trypsin) 650mg-72.5mg-0.1mg/0.82mL (60mL, 120mL)

WARNINGS/PRECAUTIONS: Do not spray on fresh arterial clots. Avoid spraying in eyes. Wound may be left open or a wet bandage may be applied.

PREGNANCY: Safety in pregnancy and nursing is not known.

GRIFULVIN V RX
griseofulvin (Ortho Neutrogena)

THERAPEUTIC CLASS: *Penicillium*-derived antifungal

INDICATIONS: Management of tinea capitis, tinea corporis, tinea pedis, tinea unguium, tinea barbae, and tinea cruris.

DOSAGE: *Adults:* Tinea Capitis: 500mg qd for 4-6 weeks. Tinea Corporis: 500mg qd for 2-4 weeks. Tinea Pedis: 1g qd for 4-8 weeks. Tinea Cruris: 500mg qd. Tinea Unguium: 1g qd for at least 4 months (fingernail) or at least 6 months (toenails).
Pediatrics: Usual: 5mg/lb/day. 30-50lb: 125-250mg qd. >50lb: 250-500mg qd. Tinea Capitis: Treat for 4-6 weeks. Tinea Corporis: Treat for 2-4 weeks. Tinea Pedis: Treat for 4-8 weeks. Tinea Unguium: Treat for at least 4 months (fingernail) or at least 6 months (toenails).

HOW SUPPLIED: Sus: 125mg/5mL (120mL); Tab: 500mg

CONTRAINDICATIONS: Porphyria, hepatocellular failure, pregnancy.

WARNINGS/PRECAUTIONS: Confirm diagnosis. Not for prophylactic use. Monitor renal, hepatic, and hematopoietic functions periodically with prolonged therapy. Cross-sensitivity with penicillin may exist. Photosensitivity reported. D/C if granulocytopenia occurs.

ADVERSE REACTIONS: Rash, urticaria, oral thrush, nausea, vomiting, epigastric distress, diarrhea, headache, dizziness, insomnia, mental confusion.

INTERACTIONS: Oral anticoagulants may need adjustment. Barbiturates decrease effects. Decreases effects of oral contraceptives; may increase incidence of breakthrough bleeding.

PREGNANCY: Not for use in pregnancy and in nursing.

GRIS-PEG RX
griseofulvin (Pedinol)

THERAPEUTIC CLASS: *Penicillium*-derived antifungal

INDICATIONS: Treatment of tinea capitis, t.corporis, t.pedis, t.unguium, t.barbae and t.cruris.

DOSAGE: *Adults:* T.capitis: 375mg qd in single or divided doses for 4-6 weeks. T.corporis: 375mg qd in single or divided doses for 2-4 weeks. T.pedis: 375mg bid for 4-8 weeks. T.cruris: 375mg qd in single or divided doses. T.unguium: 375mg bid for at least 4 months (fingernail) or at least 6 months (toenails).

Pediatrics: Usual: 3.3mg/lb/day. 35-60lb: 125-187.5mg qd. >60lb: 187.5-375mg qd. T.capitis: Treat for 4-6 weeks. T.corporis: Treat for 2-4 weeks. T.pedis: Treat for 4-8 weeks. T.unguium: Treat for at least 4 months (fingernail) or at least 6 months (toenails).

HOW SUPPLIED: Tab: 125mg*, 250mg* *scored

CONTRAINDICATIONS: Porphyria, hepatocellular failure, pregnancy.

WARNINGS/PRECAUTIONS: Not for prophylactic use. Periodically monitor renal, hepatic, and hematopoietic functions in prolonged therapy. Cross-sensitivity with penicillin may exist. Photosensitivity reported. D/C if granulocytopenia occurs.

ADVERSE REACTIONS: Rash, urticaria, oral thrush, nausea, vomiting, epigastric distress, diarrhea, headache, dizziness, insomnia, mental confusion.

INTERACTIONS: Oral anticoagulants may need dose adjustments. Decreased effects with barbiturates. Decreased effects of oral contraceptives. Increased alcohol effects.

PREGNANCY: Not for use in pregnancy and in nursing.

GUAIFED-PD   RX
guaifenesin - phenylephrine HCl (Victory)

THERAPEUTIC CLASS: Nasal decongestant and expectorant

INDICATIONS: Temporary relief of nasal congestion and dry nonproductive cough associated with the common cold and other respiratory allergies.

DOSAGE: *Adults:* 1-2 caps q12h.
Pediatrics: ≥12 yrs: 1-2 caps q12h. 6 to <12yrs: 1 cap q12h.

HOW SUPPLIED: Cap: (Guaifenesin-Phenylephrine) 200mg-7.5mg

CONTRAINDICATIONS: Severe HTN, severe CAD, concomitant MAOIs, pregnancy, nursing mothers.

WARNINGS/PRECAUTIONS: Caution with HTN, DM, ischemic heart disease, hyperthyroidism, increased IOP, prostatic hypertrophy, and the elderly. Not for persistent or chronic cough such as occurs with smoking, asthma, emphysema, or where cough is accompanied by excessive secretions.

ADVERSE REACTIONS: Nausea, cardiac palpitations, increased irritability, headache, dizziness, tachycardia, diarrhea, drowsiness, stomach pain, seizures, slowed heart rate, shortness of breath.

INTERACTIONS: MAOIs and β-adrenergic blockers may increase the effect of sympathomimetics. Sympathomimetics may reduce the antihypertensive effects of methyldopa, mecamylamine, reserpine and veratrum alkaloids. Pseudoephedrine may increase the possibility of cardiac arrhythmias with digitalis glycosides.

PREGNANCY: Category B, not for use in nursing.

GUAIFENESIN-HYDROCODONE BITARTRATE   CIII
guaifenesin - hydrocodone bitartrate (Various)

OTHER BRAND NAME: Codiclear DH (Victory)

THERAPEUTIC CLASS: Opioid antitussive

INDICATIONS: Nonproductive cough.

DOSAGE: *Adults:* Initial: 5mL pc and qhs (at least 4 hrs apart). Max: 30mL/day, and 15mL/single dose.

Pediatrics: >12 yrs: Initial: 5mL pc and qhs (at least 4 hrs apart); up to 10mL/single dose. 6-12 yrs: Initial: 2.5mL pc and qhs (at least 4 hrs apart); up to 5mL/single dose.

HOW SUPPLIED: Syrup: (Hydrocodone-Guaifenesin) 5mg-100mg/5mL

WARNINGS/PRECAUTIONS: May obscure diagnosis or clinical course of acute abdominal conditions or head injuries. May produce dose-related respiratory depression. Monitor for tolerance.

GUIATUSS DAC

ADVERSE REACTIONS: Respiratory depression, nausea, vomiting, HTN, postural hypotension, palpitations, ureteral spasm, vesical sphincter spasms, urinary retention, sedation, drowsiness, nausea, vomiting.

INTERACTIONS: Additive CNS depression with other narcotic analgesics, general anesthetics, phenothiazines, tranquilizers, sedative hypnotics, alcohol, CNS depressants.

PREGNANCY: Category C, not for use in nursing.

GUIATUSS DAC CV
guaifenesin - codeine phosphate - pseudoephedrine HCl (Scientific Labs)

THERAPEUTIC CLASS: Cough suppressant/expectorant/ decongestant

INDICATIONS: Relief of nasal congestion and cough due to throat and bronchial irritation from a cold or inhaled irritants. Loosens phlegm and thins bronchial secretions to make coughs more productive.

DOSAGE: *Adults:* 10mL q4h. Max: 40mL/24 hrs.

Pediatrics: ≥12 yrs: 10mL q4h. Max: 40mL/24 hrs. 6 to <12 yrs: 5mL q4h. Max: 20mL/24 hrs.

HOW SUPPLIED: Syrup: (Codeine-Guaifenesin-Pseudoephedrine) 10mg-100mg-30mg/5mL

WARNINGS/PRECAUTIONS: Use caution with persistent/chronic cough, cough with excessive phlegm, chronic pulmonary disease, high BP, heart disease, DM, thyroid disease, or shortness of breath. May cause or aggravate constipation.

ADVERSE REACTIONS: Constipation, sedation.

INTERACTIONS: Caution with antidepressants, especially MAOIs.

PREGNANCY: Safety in pregnancy and nursing not known.

GYNE-LOTRIMIN OTC
clotrimazole (Schering)

OTHER BRAND NAMES: Gyne-Lotrimin 3 (Schering) - Gyne-Lotrimin Combination Pack (Schering) - Gyne-Lotrimin 3 Combination Pack (Schering)

THERAPEUTIC CLASS: Azole antifungal

INDICATIONS: Treatment of vaginal candidiasis.

DOSAGE: *Adults:* 200mg sup or 2% cream intravaginally qhs for 3 days, or 100mg sup or 1% cream intravaginally qhs for 7 days. Apply 1% cream externally qd-bid prn.

Pediatrics: ≥12 yrs: 200mg sup or 2% cream intravaginally qhs for 3 days, or 100mg sup or 1% cream intravaginally qhs for 7 days. Apply 1% cream externally qd-bid prn.

HOW SUPPLIED: (Gyne-Lotrimin) Cre: 1% (5g, 45g); Sup: 100mg (7^s); (Combination Pack) Cre: 1% (7g); Sup: 100mg (7^s); (Gyne-Lotrimin 3) Sup: 200mg (3^s); (3 Combination Pack) Cre: 1% (7g); Sup: 200mg (3^s)

WARNINGS/PRECAUTIONS: Do not use if fever (>100°F), foul smelling vaginal discharge or abdominal, back or shoulder pain. Do not use with douches, spermicide or tampons. Do not rely on condoms or diaphragm to prevent STDs or pregnancy while using these products.

HALOG RX
halcinonide (Westwood-Squibb)

OTHER BRAND NAME: Halog-E (Westwood-Squibb)

THERAPEUTIC CLASS: Corticosteroid

INDICATIONS: Corticosteroid responsive dermatoses.

DOSAGE: *Adults:* (Cre, Oint, Sol) Apply bid-tid. (Cre in hydrophilic base) Apply qd-tid. May use occlusive dressings for psoriasis and recalcitrant conditions.

Pediatrics: Limit to least amount compatible with an effective therapeutic regimen.

HOW SUPPLIED: (Halog) Cre, Oint: 0.1% (15g, 30g, 60g, 240g); Sol: 0.1% (20mL, 60mL); (Halog-E) Cre: 0.1% in a hydrophilic vanishing cream (30g, 60g)

WARNINGS/PRECAUTIONS: May produce reversible HPA axis suppression, manifestations of Cushing's syndrome, hyperglycemia and glucosuria. Occlusive dressings and application to large surface areas may augment systemic absorption. Pediatrics may be more susceptible to systemic toxicity. Discontinue if irritation occurs.

ADVERSE REACTIONS: Burning, itching, irritation, dryness, folliculitis, hypertrichosis, acneiform eruptions, hypopigmentation, perioral dermatitis, contact dermatitis, skin maceration, secondary infection.

PREGNANCY: Category C, caution in nursing.

Haloperidol
haloperidol (Various)

RX

OTHER BRAND NAMES: Haldol (Ortho-McNeil) - Haldol Decanoate (Ortho-McNeil)

THERAPEUTIC CLASS: Butyrophenone

INDICATIONS: (Immediate-Release) Treatment of psychosis, Tourette's disorder, severe childhood behavioral problems. Short-term treatment of hyperactivity in children. (Decanoate) Prolonged management of psychosis.

DOSAGE: *Adults:* Psychosis: (Immediate Release) PO: Moderate Symptoms/Elderly/Debilitated: 0.5-2mg bid-tid. Severe Symptoms/Resistant Patients: 3-5mg bid-tid. Max: 100mg/day. IM: Acute Agitation: 2-5mg every 4-8 hrs or hourly as needed for moderately severe to very severe symptoms. Max: 100mg/day. (Decanoate) Give every 4 weeks or monthly. Initial: 10-20 times daily oral dose up to 100mg. Give remainder of dose 3-7 days later if initial dose >100mg. Usual: 10-15 times daily oral dose. Max: 450mg/month. Elderly/Debilitated: Initial: 10-15 times daily oral dose.

Pediatrics: 3-12 yrs (15-40 kg): PO: Psychosis: 0.05-0.15mg/kg/day given bid-tid. Nonpsychotic Disorder/Tourette's: 0.05-0.075mg/kg/day given bid-tid. Max: 6mg/day.

HOW SUPPLIED: Inj: 5mg/mL; Inj: (Decanoate) 50mg/mL, 100mg/mL; Sol: 2mg/mL; Tab: 0.5mg*, 1mg*, 2mg*, 5mg*, 10mg*, 20mg* *scored

CONTRAINDICATIONS: Comatose states, severe toxic CNS depression, Parkinson's disease.

WARNINGS/PRECAUTIONS: Risk of tardive dyskinesia, especially in elderly. NMS, hyperpyrexia, heat stroke, bronchopneumonia reported. Decreased cholesterol, cutaneous and/or ocular changes may occur. Neurotoxicity may occur with thyrotoxicosis. Caution with cardiovascular disease, seizures, EEG abnormalities, elderly.

ADVERSE REACTIONS: Extrapyramidal symptoms, tardive dyskinesia, tardive dystonia, ECG changes, gynecomastia, insomnia, drowsiness, skin reactions, anorexia, anticholinergic effects, laryngospasm, cataracts.

INTERACTIONS: Caution with rifampin, anticonvulsants, anticoagulants, anticholinergics, antiparkinson agents. May potentiate CNS depression with alcohol, opiates, anesthetics and other CNS depressants. Antagonizes epinephrine. Monitor for neurological toxicity with lithium.

PREGNANCY: Category C, not for use in nursing.

Halotestin
fluoxymesterone (Pharmacia & Upjohn)

CIII

THERAPEUTIC CLASS: Androgen

INDICATIONS: Testosterone replacement therapy in males with primary hypogonadism or hypogonadotrophic hypogonadism. To stimulate puberty in males with delayed puberty. Palliation of androgen-responsive recurrent mammary cancer in females who are >1 to <5yrs postmenopausal or who have a hormone-dependent tumor as shown by previous beneficial response to castration.

DOSAGE: *Adults:* Male Replacement Therapy: 5-20mg/day, qd or in divided doses tid-qid. Breast Cancer: 10-40mg/day in divided doses tid-qid. Continue therapy for at least 1 month for a satisfactory subjective response, and for 2-3 months for an objective response.

Pediatrics: Male Replacement Therapy: 5-20mg/day, qd or in divided doses tid-qid. Delayed Puberty: Initial: Use low dose, titrate carefully; use for 4-6 months. Caution in children.

HOW SUPPLIED: Tab: 2mg*, 5mg*, 10mg* *scored

CONTRAINDICATIONS: Males with breast or prostate cancer, pregnancy, serious cardiac, hepatic or renal disease.

WARNINGS/PRECAUTIONS: Discontinue if hypercalcemia occurs in breast cancer or immobilized patients; monitor calcium levels. Risk of hepatic adenomas, hepatocellular carcinoma, and peliosis hepatitis with prolonged high doses. Discontinue if jaundice, cholestatic hepatitis occurs. Caution in the elderly; increased risk of prostatic hypertrophy and prostatic carcinoma. Risk of edema; caution with pre-existing cardiac, renal, or hepatic disease. Risk of compromised stature in children; monitor bone growth every 6 months. Should not be used for enhancement of athletic performance. Monitor for virilization in females. Patients with BPH may develop acute urethral obstruction. If priapism occurs, discontinue and if restarted use lower dose. Contains tartrazine; may cause allergic type reactions especially in those with aspirin hypersensitivity. Monitor LFTs, Hct, Hgb periodically.

ADVERSE REACTIONS: Amenorrhea, virilization, menstrual irregularities, gynecomastia, excessive frequency/duration of penile erections, male pattern baldness, increased/decreased libido, oligospermia, hirsutism, acne, fluid and electrolyte disturbances, nausea, hypercholesterolemia, clotting factor suppression, polycythemia, altered LFTs, oligospermia, priapism, anxiety, depression.

INTERACTIONS: Potentiates oral anticoagulants and oxyphenbutazone. May decrease blood glucose and insulin requirements.

PREGNANCY: Category X, not for use in nursing.

Havrix   RX
hepatitis A vaccine (Inactivated) (GlaxoSmithKline)

THERAPEUTIC CLASS: Vaccine

INDICATIONS: Active immunization in persons ≥12 months against hepatitis A virus.

DOSAGE: *Adults:* ≥18 yrs: 1440 EL U IM (deltoid), then booster after 6-12 months. *Pediatrics:* 1-18 yrs: 720 EL U IM (deltoid), then booster after 6-12 months.

HOW SUPPLIED: Inj: 720 EL U/0.5mL, 1440 EL U/mL

CONTRAINDICATIONS: Hypersensitivity to any component, including neomycin.

WARNINGS/PRECAUTIONS: Have epinephrine available for anaphylaxis. Delay with febrile illness. Caution with thrombocytopenia or bleeding disorders. Immunosuppressed may show suboptimal response. May not prevent hepatitis A in patients already infected.

ADVERSE REACTIONS: Injection site soreness, induration, redness, swelling, fever, fatigue, malaise, anorexia, nausea, headache.

INTERACTIONS: Caution with anticoagulant therapy and IM injection. Give immunoglobulins and other vaccines in different syringe and injection site.

PREGNANCY: Category C, caution in nursing.

Heparin Sodium   RX
heparin sodium (Wyeth)

THERAPEUTIC CLASS: Glycosaminoglycan

INDICATIONS: Prophylaxis and treatment of venous thrombosis and its extension, PE in atrial fibrillation, and peripheral arterial embolism. Prevention of postoperative DVT and PE. Diagnosis and treatment of acute and chronic consumptive coagulopathies, for prevention of clotting in arterial and cardiac surgery.

DOSAGE: *Adults:* Based on 68kg: Initial: 5000U IV, then 10,000-20,000U SQ. Maint: 8000-10,000U q8h or 15,000-20,000U q12h. Intermittent IV Injection: Initial: 10,000U. Maint: 5000-10,000U q4-6h. Continuous IV Infusion: Initial: 5000U. Maint: 20,000-40,000U/24 hours. Adjust to coagulation test results. See labeling for details in specific disease states.

Pediatrics: Initial: 50U/kg IV drip. Maint: 100U/kg IV drip q4h or 20,000U/m^2/24 hrs continuously.

HOW SUPPLIED: Inj: 1000U/mL, 2500U/mL, 5000U/mL, 7500U/mL, 10,000U/mL

CONTRAINDICATIONS: Severe thrombocytopenia, if cannot perform appropriate blood-coagulation tests (with full-dose heparin), uncontrollable active bleeding state (except in DIC).

WARNINGS/PRECAUTIONS: Not for IM use. Hemorrhage can occur at any site; caution with increased danger of hemorrhage (severe HTN, bacterial endocarditis, surgery, etc.). Monitor blood coagulation tests frequently. Thrombocytopenia reported; discontinue if platelets <100,000mm^3 or if recurrent thrombosis develops. Contains benzyl alcohol. "White-clot syndrome" reported. Monitor platelets, Hct, and occult blood in the stool. Increased heparin resistance with fever, thrombosis, thrombophlebitis, infections with thrombosing tendencies, MI, cancer, and post-op. Higher bleeding incidence in women >60 yrs.

ADVERSE REACTIONS: Hemorrhage, local irritation, erythema, mild pain, hematoma, chills, fever, urticaria.

INTERACTIONS: Wait ≥5 hrs after last IV dose or 24 hrs after last SQ dose before measure PT for dicumarol or warfarin. Platelet inhibitors (eg, acetylsalicylic acid, dextran, phenylbutazone, ibuprofen, indomethacin, dipyridamole, hydroxychloroquine) may induce bleeding. Digitalis, tetracyclines, nicotine, or antihistamines may counteract anticoagulant action.

PREGNANCY: Category C, safe in nursing.

HIPREX
methenamine hippurate (Sanofi-Aventis)

RX

THERAPEUTIC CLASS: Hippuric acid salt

INDICATIONS: Prophylaxis or suppression of recurrent urinary tract infections when long-term therapy is necessary. For use only after infection is eradicated by other appropriate antimicrobials.

DOSAGE: *Adults:* 1g bid.

Pediatrics: >12 yrs: 1g bid. 6 to 12 yrs: 0.5g-1g bid.

HOW SUPPLIED: Tab: 1g* *scored

CONTRAINDICATIONS: Renal insufficiency, severe hepatic insufficiency, severe dehydration, concomitant sulfonamides.

WARNINGS/PRECAUTIONS: Maintain acid urine. Doses of 8g/day may cause bladder irritation, painful and frequent micturition, albuminuria, gross hematuria. Monitor LFTs and repeated urine cultures. Contains tartrazine.

ADVERSE REACTIONS: Nausea, upset stomach, dysuria, rash.

INTERACTIONS: Avoid alkalinizing agents or foods. Sulfonamides may precipitate in the urine; avoid concomitant use.

PREGNANCY: Safety in pregnancy and nursing unknown.

HISTA-VENT DA
phenylephrine HCl - methscopolamine nitrate - chlorpheniramine maleate
(Ethex)

RX

THERAPEUTIC CLASS: Antihistamine/anticholinergic/sympathomimetic

INDICATIONS: Temporary relief of symptoms of allergic rhinitis, vasomotor rhinitis, sinusitis, and the common cold.

DOSAGE: *Adults:* 1 tab q12h. Do not crush or chew.

Pediatrics: ≥12 yrs: 1 tab q12h. 6 to <12 yrs: 1/2 tab q12h. May cut in 1/2; do not crush or chew.

HOW SUPPLIED: Tab, Extended Release: (Chlorpheniramine-Methscopolamine-Phenylephrine) 8mg-2.5mg-20mg* *scored

Histussin D

CONTRAINDICATIONS: Severe HTN, severe CAD, MAOI therapy, narrow angle glaucoma, urinary retention, PUD, during asthma attack.

WARNINGS/PRECAUTIONS: Caution in HTN, DM, ischemic heart disease, hyperthyroidism, increased IOP, prostatic hypertrophy. May produce CNS stimulation, convulsions, or cardiovascular collapse with accompanying hypotension; more common in the elderly. May cause excitability in children. May impair ability to operate machinery.

ADVERSE REACTIONS: Tachycardia, palpitations, nervousness, insomnia, restlessness, headache, gastric irritation, irritability, fear, anxiety, tenseness, restlessness, tremor.

INTERACTIONS: Increased effect of sympathomimetic amines with MAOI and β-blockers. May reduce antihypertensive effect of methyldopa, mecamylamine, and reserpine. Additive effect with alcohol, TCAs, barbiturates, other CNS depressants.

PREGNANCY: Category C, not for use in nursing.

Histussin D
pseudoephedrine HCl - hydrocodone bitartrate (Victory) — CIII

THERAPEUTIC CLASS: Opioid antitussive

INDICATIONS: Relief of cough with upper respiratory tract congestion associated with the common cold, influenza, bronchitis and sinusitis.

DOSAGE: *Adults:* 5mL qid prn. May be taken with meals.
Pediatrics: >90 lbs: 5mL qid prn. 50-90 lbs: 2.5mL qid prn. 25-50 lbs: 1.25mL qid prn. May be taken with meals.

HOW SUPPLIED: Sol: (Hydrocodone-Pseudoephedrine) 5mg-60mg/5mL

CONTRAINDICATIONS: Severe HTN, severe CAD, MAOIs. Hypersensitivity to sympathomimetic amines and phenanthrene derivatives.

WARNINGS/PRECAUTIONS: Caution with DM, HTN, CVD, decreased respiration, and hypersensitivity to ephedrine. Decreases mental alertness/physical coordination.

ADVERSE REACTIONS: Nausea, GI upset, drowsiness, constipation.

INTERACTIONS: Potentiate effects of other narcotics, general anesthetics, tranquilizers, sedatives, hypnotics, β-adrenergic blockers, alcohol, and other CNS depressants. Increased effect of antidepressant or hydrocodone with MAOIs or TCAs. Reduced antihypertensive effects of methyldopa, mecamylamine, reserpine alkaloids.

PREGNANCY: Safety in pregnancy and nursing are unknown.

Hivid
zalcitabine (Roche Labs) — RX

> Severe peripheral neuropathy, pancreatitis (rare), hepatic failure (rare), lactic acidosis, and severe hepatomegaly with steatosis, reported. Extreme caution with pre-existing neuropathy.

THERAPEUTIC CLASS: Reverse transcriptase inhibitor

INDICATIONS: Treatment of HIV infection in combination with other antiretrovirals.

DOSAGE: *Adults:* 0.75mg q8h. CrCl 10-40mL/min: 0.75mg q12h. CrCl <10mL/min: 0.75mg q24h.
Pediatrics: ≥13 yrs: 0.75mg q8h.

HOW SUPPLIED: Tab: 0.375mg, 0.75mg

WARNINGS/PRECAUTIONS: Decreased CD4 counts increase risk of adverse effects including peripheral neuropathy, pancreatitis, lactic acidosis, severe hepatomegaly with steatosis, hepatic toxicity, oral/esophageal ulcers, cardiomyopathy and CHF. Caution in elderly. Reduce dose in renal impairment. Increased risk of lymphoma with high doses. D/C if moderate peripheral neuropathy develops; may reintroduce at 50% of dose if improve to mild symptoms. Interrupt or reduce dose if serious toxicities occur (eg, peripheral neuropathy, severe oral ulcers, pancreatitis, elevated LFTs). Monitor CBC and clinical chemistry tests before therapy and at appropriate intervals thereafter. Monitor hematologic indices frequently with poor bone marrow reserve. Interrupt therapy if severe anemia or granulocytopenia occurs; reduce dose if less severe. Possible redistribution or accumulation of body fat.

ADVERSE REACTIONS: Peripheral neuropathy, oral lesions/stomatitis, headache, elevated amylase, fatigue, abdominal pain, nausea, vomiting, hepatic dysfunction, blood dyscrasias, rash, urticaria, redistribution/accumulation of body fat.

INTERACTIONS: Avoid drugs associated with peripheral neuropathy. Monitor renal function and neuropathy development with amphotericin, foscarnet, aminoglycosides. Cimetidine and probenecid decrease clearance. Metoclopramide, aluminum- and magnesium-containing antacids reduce absorption. Interrupt therapy with pancreatitis causing agents (eg, intravenous pentamidine).

PREGNANCY: Category C, not for use in nursing.

HUMALOG
insulin lispro (Lilly)

RX

THERAPEUTIC CLASS: Insulin

INDICATIONS: To control hyperglycemia in diabetes.

DOSAGE: *Adults:* Individualize dose. Inject SQ within 15 minutes before or immediately after a meal. May use with external insulin pump; do not dilute or mix with other insulin when used with pump.

Pediatrics: ≥3 yrs: Individualize dose. Inject SQ within 15 minutes before or immediately after a meal. May use with external insulin pump; do not dilute or mix with other insulin when used with pump.

HOW SUPPLIED: Cartridge: 100 U/mL; Inj: 100 U/mL; Pen: 100 U/mL

CONTRAINDICATIONS: Hypoglycemia.

WARNINGS/PRECAUTIONS: Any change of insulin should be made cautiously. Changes in strength, manufacturer, type or method of manufacture may result in the need for a change in dosage. Hypoglycemia may occur with taking too much insulin, missing or delaying meals, exercising or working more than usual. An infection or illness (especially with diarrhea or vomiting) may change insulin requirements. With type 1 DM a longer-acting insulin is usually required to maintain glucose control; not required with type 2 DM if regimen includes sulfonylureas. May be diluted with sterile diluent.

ADVERSE REACTIONS: Hypoglycemia, hypokalemia, allergic reaction, injection site reaction, lipodystrophy, pruritus, rash.

INTERACTIONS: Increased insulin requirements with corticosteroids, isoniazid, niacin, estrogens, oral contraceptives, phenothiazines, thyroid replacement therapy. Decreased insulin requirements with oral hypoglycemics, salicylates, sulfa antibiotics, MAOIs, ACEIs, β-blockers, octreotide and alcohol. β-blockers may mask symptoms of hypoglycemia. Caution with potassium-lowering drugs or drugs sensitive to serum potassium levels.

PREGNANCY: Category B, caution in nursing.

HUMATROPE
somatropin (Lilly)

RX

THERAPEUTIC CLASS: Human growth hormone

INDICATIONS: Long-term treatment of pediatrics with growth failure due to growth hormone deficiency (GHD). For short stature associated with Turner syndrome if epiphyses are not closed. Long-term treatment of idiopathic short stature in pediatrics. Replacement therapy in adults.

DOSAGE: *Adults:* GHD: Up to 0.006mg/kg SQ qd. Titrate: Increase by individual requirements. Max: 0.0125mg/kg/day.

Pediatrics: GHD: 0.18mg/kg weekly SQ/IM. Max: 0.3mg/kg weekly in equally divided doses given either on 3 alternate days, 6 times per week or daily. Turner Syndrome: Up to 0.375mg/kg SQ weekly equally divided given either daily or on 3 alternate days. Idiopathic Short Stature: Up to 0.37mg/kg SQ weekly given 6 to 7 times per week equally divided.

HOW SUPPLIED: Inj: 5mg, 6mg, 12mg, 24mg

HUMIBID

CONTRAINDICATIONS: Pediatrics with closed epiphyses. Active malignancy. Hypersensitivity to Metacresol or glycerin. Acute critical illness due to complications after open heart or abdominal surgery, multiple accidental trauma. Acute respiratory failure.

WARNINGS/PRECAUTIONS: If sensitivity to diluent occurs reconstitute with bacteriostatic (contains benzyl alcohol; avoid in newborns) or sterile water for injection. Monitor GHD secondary to intracranial lesion for progression/recurrence. Monitor gait, glucose intolerance, for malignant transformation of skin lesions, scoliosis progression, intracranial HTN (perform fundoscopic exam at start and periodically). Caution with DM, endocrine disorders, hypopituitarism. With Turner syndrome monitor for otic or cardiovascular disorders, autoimmune thyroid disease. Caution with endocrine disorders, monitor for otic and cardiovascular disorder.

ADVERSE REACTIONS: Injection site pain, headache, edema, myalgia, pain, rhinitis. (Adults) arthralgia, paresthesia, HTN, back pain. (Pediatrics) flu-syndrome, AST/ALT increases, pharyngitis, gastritis, respiratory disorder.

INTERACTIONS: Antagonized by glucocorticoids. May alter clearance of CYP450 substrates (eg, corticosteroids, sex steroids, anticonvulsants, antipyrine, cyclosporine).

PREGNANCY: Category C, caution in nursing.

HUMIBID
guaifenesin (Adams)

OTC

THERAPEUTIC CLASS: Expectorant

INDICATIONS: Help loosen phlegm and thin bronchial secretions to rid the bronchial passageways of bothersome mucus and make coughs more productive.

DOSAGE: *Adults*: 1200mg q12h. Max: 2400mg/24hrs. Do not crush, chew, or break tablet. Take with full glass of water.

Pediatrics: ≥12 yrs: 1200mg q12h. Max: 2400mg/24hrs. Do not crush, chew, or break tablet. Take with full glass of water.

HOW SUPPLIED: Tab, Extended-Release: 1200mg

WARNINGS/PRECAUTIONS: Stop use if cough lasts >7 days, comes back, or occurs with fever, rash, or persistent headache.

PREGNANCY: Safety in pregnancy and nursing is not known.

HUMULIN
insulin, human regular - insulin, human isophane - insulin human, rDNA origin (Lilly)

OTC

OTHER BRAND NAMES: Humulin N (Lilly) - Humulin R (Lilly)

THERAPEUTIC CLASS: Insulin

INDICATIONS: To control hyperglycemia in diabetes.

DOSAGE: *Adults:* Individualize dose.

Pediatrics: Individualize dose.

HOW SUPPLIED: Inj: 100U/mL (Humulin N, Humulin R), 500U/mL (Humulin R U-500); Pen: 100U/mL (Humulin N).

WARNINGS/PRECAUTIONS: Human insulin differs from animal source insulin. Any change of insulin should be made cautiously. Changes in strength, manufacturer, type or method of manufacture may result in the need for a change in dosage. Hypoglycemia may occur with taking too much insulin, missing or delaying meals, exercising or working more than usual. An infection or illness (especially with diarrhea or vomiting) may change insulin requirements. Administration of insulin SQ can result in lipoatrophy.

ADVERSE REACTIONS: Hypoglycemia, sweating, dizziness, palpitation, tremor, hunger, restlessness, lightheadedness, inability to concentrate, headache, injection site reaction, allergic reaction.

INTERACTIONS: Increased insulin requirements with oral contraceptives, corticosteroids, or thyroid replacement therapy. Reduced insulin requirements with oral hypoglycemics, salicylates, sulfa antibiotics, and certain antidepressants. Alcoholic beverages may change insulin requirements. β-blockers may mask symptoms of hypoglycemia.

PREGNANCY: Pregnancy category is not known.

Humulin 70/30 OTC
insulin human, rDNA origin - insulin, human (isophane/regular) (Lilly)

OTHER BRAND NAME: Humulin 50/50 (Lilly)
THERAPEUTIC CLASS: Insulin
INDICATIONS: To control hyperglycemia in diabetes.
DOSAGE: *Adults:* Individualize dose. Administer SQ.
Pediatrics: Individualize dose. Administer SQ.
HOW SUPPLIED: (Isophane-Regular) Inj: (Humulin 70/30) 70U-30U/mL, (Humulin 50/50) 50U-50U/mL

WARNINGS/PRECAUTIONS: Human insulin differs from animal source insulin. Make any change of insulin cautiously. Changes in strength, manufacturer, type, or method of manufacture may result in the need for a change in dosage. Hypoglycemia may occur with too much insulin, missing or delaying meals, exercising, or working more than usual. Infection or illness (especially with diarrhea or vomiting) may change insulin requirements. Administration of insulin SQ can result in lipoatrophy.

ADVERSE REACTIONS: Hypoglycemia, sweating, dizziness, palpitation, tremor, hunger, restlessness, lightheadedness, inability to concentrate, headache, injection site reaction, allergic reaction.

INTERACTIONS: Increased insulin requirements with oral contraceptives, corticosteroids, or thyroid replacement therapy. Reduced insulin requirements with oral hypoglycemics, salicylates, sulfa antibiotics, and certain antidepressants. Alcoholic beverages may change insulin requirements. β-blockers may mask symptoms of hypoglycemia.

PREGNANCY: Pregnancy category is not known.

Hycotuss CIII
guaifenesin - hydrocodone bitartrate (Endo)

OTHER BRAND NAME: Vi-Q-Tuss (Vintage)
THERAPEUTIC CLASS: Cough suppressant/expectorant
INDICATIONS: Symptomatic relief of irritating nonproductive cough associated with upper and lower respiratory tract congestion.
DOSAGE: *Adults:* Initial: 5mL after meals and hs, not less than 4 hrs apart. Titrate: May increase up to 15mL after meals and hs. Max: 30mL/24 hrs.
Pediatrics: >12 yrs: Initial: 5mL after meals and hs, not less than 4 hrs apart. Max Single Dose: 10mL. 6-12 yrs: Initial: 2.5mL after meals and hs, not less than 4 hrs apart. Max Single Dose: 5mL.
HOW SUPPLIED: Syrup: (Hydrocodone-Guaifenesin) 5mg-100mg/5mL
CONTRAINDICATIONS: Cross sensitivity to other opioids. Intracranial lesion associated with increased intracranial pressure and whenever ventilatory function is depressed.
WARNINGS/PRECAUTIONS: May be habit forming. Risk of psychic dependence, physical dependence, tolerance, and potential for abuse. Dose-related respiratory depression. Caution with head injury, other intracranial lesions or a pre-existing increase in intracranial pressure. May obscure the clinical course head injuries, acute abdominal conditions.
ADVERSE REACTIONS: Respiratory depression, HTN, postural hypotension, palpitations, urinary retention, sedation, drowsiness, mental clouding, lethargy.
INTERACTIONS: Additive CNS depression with other narcotics, analgesics, general anesthetics, phenothiazines, other tranquilizers, sedative hypnotics or other CNS depressants (including alcohol).
PREGNANCY: Category C, not for use in nursing.

HYDRALAZINE
hydralazine HCl (Various)
RX

THERAPEUTIC CLASS: Vasodilator

INDICATIONS: Management of hypertension.

DOSAGE: *Adults:* Initial: 10mg qid for 2-4 days. Titrate: Increase to 25mg qid for the rest of the week, then increase to 50mg qid. Maint: Use lowest effective dose. Resistant Patients: 300mg/day or titrate to lower dose combined with thiazide diuretic and/or reserpine, or β-blocker.
Pediatrics: Initial: 0.75mg/kg/day given qid. Titrate: Increase gradually over 3-4 weeks to a max of 7.5mg/kg/day or 200mg/day.

HOW SUPPLIED: Inj: 20mg/mL; Tab: 10mg, 25mg, 50mg, 100mg

CONTRAINDICATIONS: CAD and mitral valvular rheumatic heart disease.

WARNINGS/PRECAUTIONS: Discontinue if SLE symptoms occur. May cause angina and ECG changes of MI. Caution with suspected CAD, CVA, advanced renal impairment. May increase pulmonary artery pressure in mitral valvular disease. Postural hypotension reported. Add pyridoxine if develop peripheral neuritis. Monitor CBC and ANA titer before and periodically during therapy.

ADVERSE REACTIONS: Headache, anorexia, nausea, vomiting, diarrhea, tachycardia, angina.

INTERACTIONS: Caution with MAOIs. Profound hypotension with potent parenteral antihypertensives (eg, diazoxide). May reduce pressor response to epinephrine.

PREGNANCY: Category C, safety in nursing not known.

HYDROCHLOROTHIAZIDE
hydrochlorothiazide (Various)
RX

THERAPEUTIC CLASS: Thiazide diuretic

INDICATIONS: Adjunct therapy in edema associated with CHF, hepatic cirrhosis, corticosteroid and estrogen therapy, renal dysfunction. Management of hypertension.

DOSAGE: *Adults:* Edema: 25-100mg qd or in divided doses. May give every other day or 3-5 days/week. HTN: Initial: 25mg qd. Titrate: May increase to 50mg/day.
Pediatrics: Diuresis/HTN: 1-2mg/kg/day given qd-bid. Max: Infants up to 2 yrs: 37.5mg/day. 2-12 yrs: 100mg/day. <6 months: Up to 1.5mg/kg bid may be required.

HOW SUPPLIED: Tab: 25mg*, 50mg* *scored

CONTRAINDICATIONS: Anuria, sulfonamide hypersensitivity.

WARNINGS/PRECAUTIONS: Caution in severe renal disease, liver dysfunction, electrolyte/fluid imbalance. Monitor electrolytes. Hyperuricemia, hyperglycemia, hypokalemia, hyponatremia, hypomagnesemia, hypercalcemia may occur. Increases in cholesterol and triglyceride levels reported. May exacerbate SLE. Sensitivity reactions reported. D/C prior to parathyroid test. Enhanced effects in post-sympathectomy patients.

ADVERSE REACTIONS: Weakness, hypotension, pancreatitis, jaundice, diarrhea, vomiting, blood dyscrasias, rash, photosensitivity, electrolyte imbalance, impotence.

INTERACTIONS: May potentiate orthostatic hypotension with alcohol, barbiturates, narcotics. Adjust antidiabetic drugs. Possible decreased response to pressor amines. Corticosteroids, ACTH increase electrolyte depletion. May potentiate nondepolarizing skeletal muscle relaxants, antihypertensives. Lithium toxicity. NSAIDs decrease effects. Decreased PO absorption with cholestyramine, colestipol.

PREGNANCY: Category B, not for use in nursing.

HYDROCORTISONE ACETATE
hydrocortisone acetate (Truxton)
RX

THERAPEUTIC CLASS: Corticosteroid

INDICATIONS: By intra-articular or soft tissue injection as adjunctive therapy for short-term administration in: synovitis of osteoarthritis, rheumatoid arthritis, bursitis, gouty arthritis, epicondylitis, nonspecific tenosynovitis, and post-traumatic osteoarthritis. By intralesional injection in: keloids, localized inflammatory lesions, discoid lupus erythematosus, necrobiosis lipoidica diabeticorum, alopecia areata, and cystic tumors of an aponeurosis or tendon.

DOSAGE: *Adults:* Usual: Large joints: 25-37.5mg. Max: 50mg. Small joints: 10-25mg. Bursae: 25-37.5mg. Tendon Sheaths: 5-12.5mg. Soft Tissue Infiltration: 25-50mg, occasionally 75mg. Ganglia: 12.5-25mg. For intra-articular, intralesional, and soft tissue injection only. Injection given once every 2-3 weeks; once a week for more severe conditions.
Pediatrics: Usual: Large joints: 25-37.5mg. Max: 50mg. Small joints: 10-25mg. Bursae: 25-37.5mg. Tendon Sheaths: 5-12.5mg. Soft Tissue Infiltration: 25-50mg, occasionally 75mg. Ganglia: 12.5-25mg. For intra-articular, intralesional, and soft tissue injection only. Injection given once every 2-3 weeks; once a week for more severe conditions.

HOW SUPPLIED: Inj: 25mg/mL.

CONTRAINDICATIONS: Systemic fungal infections.

WARNINGS/PRECAUTIONS: May need to increase dose before, during, and after stressful situations. May mask signs of infection or cause new infections. Avoid with cerebral malaria. May activate latent amebiasis. Prolonged use may produce glaucoma, optic nerve damage, secondary ocular infections. Increases BP, salt/water retention, potassium excretion. More severe/fatal course of infections reported with chickenpox, measles. Caution with Strongyloides, latent TB, recent MI, hypothyroidism, cirrhosis, ocular herpes simplex, HTN, diverticulitis, fresh intestinal anastomosis, ulcerative colitis, osteoporosis, myasthenia gravis, renal insufficiency, peptic ulcer disease. May increase or decrease sperm count. Growth and development of children on prolonged therapy should be monitored. Monitor for psychic disturbances. Avoid abrupt withdrawal. Avoid injection into an infected site or unstable joint. Frequent intra-articular injections may cause joint tissue damage.

ADVERSE REACTIONS: Fluid and electrolyte disturbances, HTN, osteoporosis, muscle weakness, cushingoid state, menstrual irregularities, nervousness, insomnia, impaired wound healing, DM, ulcerative esophagitis, excessive sweating, increases intracranial pressure, carbohydrate intolerance, glaucoma, cataracts, weight gain, nausea, malaise.

INTERACTIONS: Reduced efficacy and increased clearance with hepatic enzyme inducers (eg, phenobarbital, phenytoin, ephedrine, and rifampin). Caution with ASA in hypoprothrombinemia. Effects on oral anticoagulants are variable; monitor PT. Increased insulin and oral hypoglycemic requirements in DM. Avoid live vaccines with immunosuppressive doses. Possible decreased vaccine response with killed or inactivated vaccines with immunosuppressive doses. Monitor for hypokalemia with potassium-depleting diuretics.

PREGNANCY: Safety in pregnancy not known, not for use in nursing.

HYDROXYZINE HCL
hydroxyzine HCl (Various)

RX

OTHER BRAND NAME: Atarax (Pfizer)

THERAPEUTIC CLASS: Piperazine antihistamine

INDICATIONS: (PO) Relief of anxiety associated with psychoneurosis and as adjunct in organic disease states with anxiety. As a sedative when used as premedication and following general anesthesia. Management of allergic pruritus. (Inj) Management of anxiety, tension, and psycomotor agitation in conditions of emotional stress. As pre-/postoperative and pre-/postpartum adjunctive medication to permit reduction in narcotic dosage, allay anxiety, and control emesis. To control nausea and vomiting, excluding pregnancy.

DOSAGE: *Adults:* PO: Anxiety: 50-100mg qid. Pruritus: 25mg tid-qid. Sedation: 50-100mg. IM: Nausea/Vomiting: 25-100mg. Pre-/Postoperative and Pre-/Postpartum Adjunct: 25-100mg. Psychiatric/Emotional Emergencies: 50-100mg q4-6h prn.
Pediatrics: PO: Anxiety/Pruritus: <6 yrs: 50mg/day in divided doses. ≥6 yrs: 50-100mg in divided doses. Sedation: 0.6mg/kg. IM: Nausea/Vomiting: 0.5mg/lb. Pre-/Postoperative Adjunct: 0.5mg/lb.

HOW SUPPLIED: Inj: 25mg/mL, 50mg/mL; Syrup: 10mg/5mL; Tab: 10mg, 25mg, 50mg, 100mg

HYDROXYZINE PAMOATE

CONTRAINDICATIONS: Early pregnancy. Inj is intended only for IM administration and should not, under any circumstances, be injected subcutaneously, intra-arterially, or IV.
WARNINGS/PRECAUTIONS: Caution in elderly. May impair mental/physical abilities. Effectiveness as an antianxiety agent for long term use (>4 months) has not been established.
ADVERSE REACTIONS: Dry mouth, drowsiness, involuntary motor activity.
INTERACTIONS: Potentiates CNS depression with other CNS depressants (eg, narcotics, non-narcotic analgesics, barbiturates, alcohol). May increase alcohol effects.
PREGNANCY: Not for use in pregnancy or nursing.

HYDROXYZINE PAMOATE RX
hydroxyzine pamoate (Various)

OTHER BRAND NAME: Vistaril (Pfizer)
THERAPEUTIC CLASS: Piperazine antihistamine
INDICATIONS: Relief of anxiety. Allergic pruritus. For sedation as premedication and following anesthesia.
DOSAGE: *Adults:* Anxiety: 50-100mg qid. Pruritus: 25mg tid-qid. Sedation: 50-100mg.
Pediatrics: Anxiety/Pruritus: >6 yrs: 50-100mg/day in divided doses. <6 yrs: 50mg/day in divided doses. Sedation: 0.6mg/kg.
HOW SUPPLIED: Cap: 25mg, 50mg, 100mg; Sus: 25mg/5mL (120mL, 480mL)
CONTRAINDICATIONS: Early pregnancy.
WARNINGS/PRECAUTIONS: Caution in elderly. May impair mental/physical abilities. Effectiveness as an antianxiety agent for long term use (>4 months) has not been established.
ADVERSE REACTIONS: Dry mouth, drowsiness, involuntary motor activity.
INTERACTIONS: Potentiated by CNS depressants(eg, narcotics, non-narcotic analgesics, barbiturates); reduce dose.
PREGNANCY: Safety unknown in pregnancy and is contraindicated in early pregnancy, not for use in nursing.

HYTONE RX
hydrocortisone (Dermik)

THERAPEUTIC CLASS: Corticosteroid
INDICATIONS: Corticosteroid responsive dermatoses.
DOSAGE: *Adults:* Apply bid-qid depending on the severity. May use occlusive dressings for psoriasis or recalcitrant conditions. Discontinue dressings if infection develops.
Pediatrics: Apply bid-qid depending on the severity. May use occlusive dressings for psoriasis or recalcitrant conditions. Discontinue dressings if infection develops.
HOW SUPPLIED: Cre: 2.5% (30g, 60g); Lot: 2.5% (60mL); Oint: 2.5% (30g)
WARNINGS/PRECAUTIONS: May produce reversible HPA axis suppression, manifestations of Cushing's syndrome, hyperglycemia, and glucosuria. Caution when applied to large surface areas or under occlusive dressings. Use appropriate antifungal or antibacterial agent with dermatological infections; discontinue if infection does not clear. Pediatrics may be more susceptible to systemic toxicity. Avoid eyes. Discontinue if irritation occurs.
ADVERSE REACTIONS: Burning, itching, irritation, dryness, folliculitis, hypertrichosis, acneiform eruptions, hypopigmentation, perioral dermatitis, allergic contact dermatitis, skin maceration, secondary infection, skin atrophy, striae, miliaria.
PREGNANCY: Category C, caution in nursing.

HYTONE 1% OTC
hydrocortisone (Dermik)

THERAPEUTIC CLASS: Corticosteroid
INDICATIONS: Relief of itching associated with minor skin irritation, inflammation and rashes due to eczema, insect bites, poison ivy/oak/sumac, soaps/detergents, cosmet-

ics, jewelry, seborrheic dermatitis, psoriasis, and/or external feminine and external anal itching.

DOSAGE: *Adults:* Apply up to tid-qid. External Anal Itching: Clean and dry area before applying.

Pediatrics: ≥2 yrs: Apply up to tid-qid. External Anal Itching: ≥12 yrs: Clean and dry area before applying.

HOW SUPPLIED: Lot: 1% (30mL, 120mL)

WARNINGS/PRECAUTIONS: Avoid eyes. Discontinue use if condition worsens, if symptoms persist for more than 7 days, or if symptoms recur after clearing up. Not for diaper rash. For external feminine itching, avoid use with vaginal discharge. For external anal itching, do not insert into rectum with fingers or applicator.

PREGNANCY: Safety in pregnancy and nursing is not known.

IB-STAT RX
hyoscyamine sulfate (InKine)

THERAPEUTIC CLASS: Anticholinergic

INDICATIONS: Adjunct treatment of peptic ulcer, irritable bowel syndrome, functional GI disorders, neurogenic bladder, neurogenic bowel disturbances. Management of functional intestinal disorders (eg, mild dysenteries, diverticulitis). To control gastric secretion, visceral spasm, and hypermotility in spastic colitis, spastic bladder, cystitis, pylorospasm, and associated abdominal cramps. Symptomatic relief of biliary and renal colic with concomitant morphine or other narcotics. "Drying agent" for symptomatic relief of acute rhinitis. To reduce rigidity and tremors of Parkinson's disease and control associated sialorrhea and hyperhidrosis. For anticholinesterase poisoning.

DOSAGE: *Adults:* 1-2 sprays q4h or prn. Max: 12 sprays/24hrs.

Pediatrics: ≥12 yrs: 1-2 sprays q4h or prn. Max: 12 sprays/24hrs.

HOW SUPPLIED: Sol: 0.125mg/mL (30mL)

CONTRAINDICATIONS: Glaucoma, obstructive uropathy, GI tract obstructive disease, paralytic ileus, intestinal atony of elderly/debilitated, unstable cardiovascular status in acute hemorrhage, severe ulcerative colitis, toxic megacolon, myasthenia gravis.

WARNINGS/PRECAUTIONS: Risk of heat prostration with high environmental temperature. May impair mental/physical abilities. Psychosis has been reported. Caution with diarrhea, autonomic neuropathy, hyperthyroidism, coronary heart disease, CHF, arrhythmias/tachycardia, HTN, renal disease, hiatal hernia with reflux esophagitis.

ADVERSE REACTIONS: Drowsiness, dizziness, blurred vision, mouth dryness, urinary hesitancy and retention, tachycardia, palpitations.

INTERACTIONS: Additive effects with other antimuscarinics, amantadine, haloperidol, phenothiazines, MAOIs, TCAs, or some antihistamines. Antacids interfere with absorption; take ac and antacids pc.

PREGNANCY: Category C, caution in nursing.

IC-GREEN RX
indocyanine green (Akorn)

THERAPEUTIC CLASS: Diagnostic dye

INDICATIONS: To determine cardiac output, hepatic function and liver blood flow, and for ophthalmic angiography.

DOSAGE: *Adults:* For Dilution Curves: 5mg. Max: 2 mg/kg. Refer to prescribing information for further instructions for dilution curves and administration depending on study being conducted.

Pediatrics: For Dilution Curves: 2.5mg. Infants: 1.25mg. Max: 2 mg/kg. Refer to prescribing information for further instructions for dilution curves and administration depending on study being conducted.

HOW SUPPLIED: Inj: 25mg

CONTRAINDICATIONS: Caution with allergy to iodides.

Imodium A-D

WARNINGS/PRECAUTIONS: Use solvent provided for dissolution. Use aqueous solution within 6 hrs.

ADVERSE REACTIONS: Anaphylactic or urticarial reactions.

INTERACTIONS: Do not use with heparin preparations containing sodium bisulfate; may reduce absorption. Do not perform radioactive iodine uptake studies for at least 1 week following use.

PREGNANCY: Category C, caution in nursing.

Imodium A-D OTC
loperamide HCl (McNeil Consumer)

THERAPEUTIC CLASS: Anti-peristalsis agent

INDICATIONS: Management of diarrhea and traveler's diarrhea.

DOSAGE: *Adults:* ≥12 yrs: Initial: 4mg after the first loose bowel movement then 2mg after each additional loose bowel with plenty of liquid. Max: 8mg/day for no more than 2 days.

Pediatrics: 9-11 yrs (60-95 lbs): 2mg after the first loose bowel movement then 1mg after each additional loose bowel with plenty of liquid. Max: 6mg/day for no more than 2 days. 6-8 yrs (48-59 lbs): 2mg after the first loose bowel movement then 1mg after each additional loose bowel. Max: 4mg/day for no more than 2 days. 2-5 yrs (24-47 lbs): 1mg after the first loose bowel movement then 1mg after each additional loose bowel. Max: 3mg/day

HOW SUPPLIED: Sol: 1mg/5mL; Tab: 2mg

WARNINGS/PRECAUTIONS: Do not use if diarrhea is accompanied with high fever, blood, or mucus in stool. Caution with history of liver disease.

PREGNANCY: Safety in pregnancy and nursing is not known.

Imogam Rabies-HT RX
rabies immune globulin (Sanofi Pasteur)

THERAPEUTIC CLASS: Immunoglobulin

INDICATIONS: Suspected exposure to rabies, particularly severe exposure, except persons previously immunized with HDCV Rabies Vaccine in a pre- or post-exposure.

DOSAGE: *Adults:* 20IU/kg IM. Infiltrate as much of dose around wound, if feasible, with remaining portion given IM in gluteal region.

Pediatrics: 20IU/kg IM. Infiltrate as much of dose around wound, if feasible, with remaining portion given IM in gluteal region.

HOW SUPPLIED: Inj: 150IU/mL

CONTRAINDICATIONS: Do not repeat dose once vaccine treatment has started.

WARNINGS/PRECAUTIONS: Do not give in same syringe or into same site as vaccine. Made from human plasma, risk of infection. Patients with IgA deficiency could have anaphylactic reaction to IgA containing blood products. Have epinephrine (1:1000) available.

ADVERSE REACTIONS: Local reactions: tenderness, pain, soreness, stiffness. Systemic reactions: headache, malaise.

INTERACTIONS: Wait 3 months before giving live vaccines.

PREGNANCY: Category C, safety in nursing not known.

Imovax Rabies Vaccine RX
rabies vaccine (Sanofi Pasteur)

THERAPEUTIC CLASS: Vaccine

INDICATIONS: Pre-exposure immunization and postexposure treatment of rabies.

DOSAGE: *Adults:* Pre-exposure: 3 doses of 1mL IM on days 0, 7, and either 21 or 28. 1mL booster every 2 yrs (see labeling for details). Post-exposure: 1mL IM on days 0, 3, 7, 14, 30 (ACIP recommendations; 5 doses) and 90 (WHO recommendations; 6 doses). Give 1st dose with rabies immune globulin (RIG) or antirabies serum (ARS). If possible, infiltrate half of RIG or ARS into wound. Previously Immunized: 2 doses; immediately after exposure and 3 days later (no RIG needed).

Pediatrics: Pre-exposure: 3 doses of 1mL IM on days 0, 7, and either 21 or 28. 1mL booster every 2 yrs (see labeling for details). Post-exposure: 1mL IM on days 0, 3, 7, 14, 30 (ACIP recommendations; 5 doses), and 90 (WHO recommendations; 6 doses). Give 1st dose with rabies immune globulin (RIG) or antirabies serum (ARS). If possible, infiltrate half of the RIG or ARS into the wound. Previously Immunized: 2 doses; immediately after exposure and 3 days later (no RIG needed).

HOW SUPPLIED: Inj: 2.5IU

WARNINGS/PRECAUTIONS: Postpone preexposure immunization during acute febrile illness. Neurologic illness resembling Guillain-Barre syndrome reported. May give antihistamines with history of hypersensitivity. Have epinepherine (1:1000) available. Suboptimal response may occur in immunocompromised patients.

ADVERSE REACTIONS: Local reactions: pain, erythema, swelling, itching. Systemic reactions: headache, nausea, abdominal pain, muscle aches, dizziness.

INTERACTIONS: Immunosuppressants can interfere with development of active immunity.

PREGNANCY: Category C, safety in nursing not known.

INAPSINE   RX
droperidol (Akorn)

> QT prolongation, torsade de pointes, arrhythmias reported. Use in patients resistant or intolerant to other therapies. Monitor ECG before and 2-3 hrs after treatment. Extreme caution if at risk for developing prolonged QT syndrome.

THERAPEUTIC CLASS: Neuroleptic butyrophenone

INDICATIONS: To reduce incidence of nausea and vomiting associated with surgical and diagnostic procedures.

DOSAGE: *Adults:* Initial (Max): 2.5mg IM/IV. May give additional 1.25mg cautiously to achieve desired effect. Lower initial doses in elderly, debilitated, poor-risk patients.

Pediatrics: 2-12 yrs: Initial (Max): 0.1 mg/kg IM/IV. May give additional dose cautiously. Lower initial doses in debilitated, poor-risk patients.

HOW SUPPLIED: Inj: 2.5mg/mL

CONTRAINDICATIONS: Known or suspected QT prolongation, including congenital long QT syndrome.

WARNINGS/PRECAUTIONS: Caution with renal/hepatic impairment. HTN, tachycardia reported with pheochromocytoma. Risk of prolonged QT syndrome with CHF, cardiac disease, bradycardia, cardiac hypertrophy, electrolyte imbalances (eg, hypokalemia, hypomagnesemia), >65 yrs, alcohol abuse. NMS reported; give dantrolene with increased temperature, HR, or carbon dioxide production. May decrease pulmonary arterial pressure.

ADVERSE REACTIONS: QT interval prolongation, torsade de pointes, cardiac arrest, hypotension, tachycardia, dysphoria, post-op drowsiness, restlessness, hyperactivity, anxiety, depression, syncope, irregular cardiac rhythm.

INTERACTIONS: Avoid drugs that prolong the QT interval (eg, antimalarials, calcium channel blockers, antidepressants, Class I and III antiarrhythmics, certain antihistamines, neuroleptics). Caution with MAOIs, alcohol, diuretics and drugs that induce hypokalemia, hypomagnesemia. May potentiate and be potentiated by CNS depressants (eg, barbiturates, benzodiazepines, tranquilizers, opioids, general anesthetics); use lower doses. Caution with conduction anesthesia (eg, spinal, peridural). Increased BP with fentanyl citrate or other parenteral analgesics. Epinephrine may paradoxically decrease BP.

PREGNANCY: Category C, caution in nursing.

INDERAL
propranolol HCl (Wyeth)
RX

THERAPEUTIC CLASS: Nonselective beta-blocker

INDICATIONS: (Tab) Management of hypertension, angina pectoris, hypertrophic subaortic stenosis. Migraine prophylaxis. (Inj/Tab) For cardiac arrhythmias (supraventricular, ventricular tachycardia, tachyarrhythmia of digitalis intoxication, resistant tachyarrhythmia), reduction of cardiovascular mortality post-MI, essential tremor, and pheochromocytoma.

DOSAGE: *Adults:* HTN: (Tab) Initial: 40mg bid. Titrate: Increase gradually. Maint: 120-240mg/day. Angina: (Tab) 80-320mg/day, given bid-qid. Arrhythmia: (Inj) 1-3mg IV at 1 mg/min. (Tab) 10-30mg tid-qid ac and qhs. MI: (Tab) 180-240mg/day, given bid-tid. Migraine: (Tab) Initial: 80mg/day in divided doses. Usual: 160-240mg/day in divided doses. Tremor: (Tab) Initial: 40mg bid. Maint: 120mg/day. Max: 320mg/day. Hypertrophic Subaortic Stenosis: (Tab) 20-40mg tid-qid, ac and qhs. Pheochromocytoma: (Tab) 60mg/day in divided doses for 3 days before surgery with alpha-blocker. Inoperable Tumor: (Tab) 30mg/day in divided doses.
Pediatrics: HTN (Tab): Initial: 1mg/kg/day PO. Usual: 1-2mg/kg bid. Max: 16mg/kg/day.

HOW SUPPLIED: Inj: 1mg/mL; Tab: 10mg*, 20mg*, 40mg*, 60mg*, 80mg* *scored

CONTRAINDICATIONS: Cardiogenic shock, sinus bradycardia and >1st-degree block, bronchial asthma, CHF (unless failure is secondary to tachyarrhythmia treatable with propranolol).

WARNINGS/PRECAUTIONS: Caution with well-compensated cardiac failure, nonallergic bronchospasm, Wolff-Parkinson-White syndrome, hepatic or renal dysfunction. Withdrawal before surgery is controversial. May mask hypoglycemia or hyperthyroidism symptoms. Avoid abrupt discontinuation. May reduce IOP. Can cause cardiac failure.

ADVERSE REACTIONS: Bradycardia, CHF, hypotension, lightheadedness, mental depression, nausea, vomiting, allergic reactions, agranulocytosis.

INTERACTIONS: Bradycardia/hypotension with catecholamine-depleting drugs. Potentiated by chlorpromazine, cimetidine. Antagonized by NSAIDs, phenytoin, phenobarbital, rifampin. May increase cardiac effects of calcium channel blockers. Reduces clearance of antipyrine, lidocaine, and theophylline. Aluminum hydroxide gel reduces intestinal absorption. Alcohol decreases absorption rate. May block epinephrine, thyroxine effects. Hypotension and cardiac arrest reported with haloperidol. May increase warfarin concentration; monitor prothrombin time. Concomitant use with alcohol may increase plasma levels of propranolol.

PREGNANCY: Category C, caution in nursing. Intrauterine growth retardation, small placenta, and congenital abnormalities have been reported in neonates whose mothers received propranolol during pregnancy. Neonates whose mothers received propranolol at parturition have exhibited bradycardia, hypoglycemia, and/or respiratory depression.

INDOCIN I.V.
indomethacin sodium trihydrate (Merck)
RX

THERAPEUTIC CLASS: NSAID (indole derivative)

INDICATIONS: To close hemodynamically significant patent ductus arteriosus in premature infants weighing between 500-1750g after 48 hrs of ineffective medical management.

DOSAGE: *Pediatrics:* Neonates 500-1750g: Therapy includes 3 doses at 12-24 hr intervals. <48 hrs old: 0.2mg/kg IV followed by 0.1mg/kg IV then 0.1mg/kg IV. 2-7 days old: 0.2mg/kg IV for 3 doses. >7 days old: 0.2mg/kg IV followed by 0.25mg/kg IV then 0.25mg/kg IV. If anuria or marked oliguria (urinary output <0.6mL/kg/hr) occurs at scheduled time of second or third dose, hold doses until renal function normalizes. May repeat course if ductus arteriosus reopens. Surgery may be needed if unresponsive after 2 courses.

HOW SUPPLIED: Inj: 1mg

CONTRAINDICATIONS: Untreated infection, bleeding, thrombocytopenia, coagulation defects, necrotizing enterocolitis, significant renal impairment, congenital heart disease when patency of ductus arteriosus is necessary for pulmonary or systemic blood flow.

WARNINGS/PRECAUTIONS: Risk of minor GI bleeding, intraventricular bleeding. May reduce urine output, CrCl, glomerular filtration rate and may increase serum creatinine, BUN. May cause renal insufficiency, including acute renal failure; caution with extracellular volume depletion, CHF, sepsis, hepatic dysfunction. Monitor renal function and serum electrolytes. May mask signs of infection. D/C if liver disease develops. Avoid extravascular injection or leakage.

ADVERSE REACTIONS: Intracranial bleeding, GI bleeding, hyponatremia, elevated serum potassium, retrolental fibroplasia.

INTERACTIONS: May prolong half-life of digitalis; monitor ECG and serum digitalis levels. May elevate gentamicin and amikacin levels. May decrease natriuretic effect of furosemide. May reduce renal function; consider reducing dosage of medications that rely on adequate renal function for elimination. Increased risk of renal insufficiency with nephrotoxic drugs. Increased risk of bleeding with anticoagulants.

PREGNANCY: Safety in pregnancy or nursing not known.

Indomethacin RX
indomethacin (Various)

> NSAIDs may cause an increased risk of serious cardiovascular thrombotic events, MI, stroke and serious GI adverse events including bleeding, ulceration, and perforation of the stomach or intestines. Contraindicated for the treatment of perioperative pain in the setting of coronary artery bypass graft (CABG) surgery.

OTHER BRAND NAME: Indocin (Merck)

THERAPEUTIC CLASS: NSAID (indole derivative)

INDICATIONS: Management of moderate to severe rheumatoid arthritis (RA), ankylosing spondylitis, osteoarthritis (OA), acute painful shoulder (bursitis and/or tendinitis) and/or acute gouty arthritis.

DOSAGE: *Adults:* RA/Ankylosing Spondylitis/OA: Initial: 25mg PO bid-tid. Titrate: May increase by 25-50mg/day at weekly intervals. Max: 200mg/day. Bursitis/Tendinitis: 75-150mg/day given tid-qid for 7-14 days. Acute Gouty Arthritis: 50mg PO tid until pain is tolerable, then d/c. Take with food.
Pediatrics: ≥14 yrs: RA/Ankylosing Spondylitis/OA: Initial: 25mg PO bid-tid. Titrate: May increase by 25-50mg/day at weekly intervals. Max: 200mg/day. Bursitis/Tendinitis: 75-150mg/day given tid-qid for 7-14 days. Acute Gouty Arthritis: 50mg PO tid until pain is tolerable, then d/c. 2-14 yrs (safety and effectiveness not established): Initial: 1-2mg/kg/day in divided doses. Max: 3mg/kg/day or 150-200mg/day. Take with food.

HOW SUPPLIED: Cap: 25mg, 50mg; Sus: 25mg/5mL (237mL)

CONTRAINDICATIONS: ASA or other NSAID allergy that precipitates acute asthmatic attack, urticaria or rhinitis. Do not give suppositories with history of proctitis or recent rectal bleeding. Treatment of perioperative pain in the setting of CABG surgery.

WARNINGS/PRECAUTIONS: May lead to onset of new HTN or worsening of pre-existing HTN; monitor BP closely. Fluid retention and edema reported; caution with fluid retention or heart failure. Renal papillary necrosis and other renal injury reported after long-term use. Not recommended for use with advanced renal disease; if therapy must be initiated, monitor renal function. Anaphylactoid reactions may occur. May cause serious skin adverse events (eg, exfoliative dermatitis, Stevens-Johnson syndrome, and toxic epidermal necrolysis). Avoid in late pregnancy; may cause premature closure of ductus arteriosis. May cause elevations of LFTs; d/c if liver disease develops or systemic manifestations occur. Caution in elderly. Anemia may occur; with long-term use, monitor Hgb/Hct if signs or symptoms of anemia develop. May inhibit platelet aggregation and prolong bleeding time; monitor with coagulation disorders. Caution with asthma and avoid with aspirin-sensitive asthma. Corneal deposits and retinal disturbances reported with prolonged therapy; monitor eye exams at periodic intervals during prolonged therapy. May aggravate depression or other psychiatric disturbances, epilepsy, and parkinsonism; use with caution. D/C if severe CNS adverse reactions develop. May impair mental/physical abilities.

ADVERSE REACTIONS: Headache, dizziness, nausea, vomiting, dyspepsia, diarrhea, abdominal pain, constipation, vertigo, somnolence, depression, fatigue.

INTERACTIONS: Avoid salicylates, diflunisal, other NSAIDs and triamterene. Potassium sparing diuretics may cause hyperkalemia. Increase toxicity of methotrexate, cyclosporine, lithium and digoxin. Probenecid increases levels. Caution with antihypertensives and anticoagulants. May decrease effects of diuretics, β-blockers, captopril.

PREGNANCY: Category C, not for use in nursing.

INFANRIX
RX
tetanus toxoid - diphtheria toxoid - pertussis vaccine, acellular (GlaxoSmithKline)

THERAPEUTIC CLASS: Vaccine/toxoid combination

INDICATIONS: Active immunization against diphtheria, tetanus, and pertussis as a 5-dose series in infants and children 6wks-7yrs old.

DOSAGE: *Pediatrics:* ≥6 weeks up to 7 yrs: 3 doses of 0.5mL IM at 4-8 week intervals. Start at 2 months or as early as 6 weeks if necessary. 2 Booster doses: Give at 15-20 months and at 4 to 6 years. Do not start series over again, regardless of time elapsed between doses. May use to complete primary series in infants who received 1-2 doses of whole-cell DTP vaccine.

HOW SUPPLIED: Inj: (Diphtheria-Tetanus-Pertussis) 25Lf-10Lf-25mcg/0.5mL

CONTRAINDICATIONS: Hypersensitivity to any component; serious allergic (eg, anaphylaxis) associated with previous dose. Encephalopathy not due to an identifiable cause within 7 days prior to pertussis immunization and progressive neurologic disorder, uncontrolled epilepsy, or progressive encephalopathy. Not contraindicated in individuals with HIV infection.

WARNINGS/PRECAUTIONS: Caution if within 48 hrs of previous whole-cell DTP or acellular DTP vaccine, fever ≥105°F not due to another identifiable cause, collapse or shock-like state, or inconsolable crying lasting ≥3 hrs occurs, or if convulsions occur within 3 days. For high seizure risk, give APAP at time of vaccination and q4-6h for 24 hrs. Caution with neurologic or CNS disorders. Avoid with coagulation disorders. Have epinephrine available. Suboptimal response may occur in immunocompromised patients.

ADVERSE REACTIONS: Local reactions, fever, irritability, drowsiness, anorexia, vomiting, diarrhea, crying.

INTERACTIONS: Avoid with anticoagulants. Immunosuppressive therapy (eg, irradiation, antimetabolites, alkylating agents, cytotoxic drugs, corticosteroids) may decrease response. Administer tetanus immune globulin, diphtheria antitoxin, hepatitis B vaccine, and *Haemophilus influenzae* type b vaccine at separate site.

PREGNANCY: Category C, safety in nursing not known.

INFeD
RX
iron dextran (Watson)

> Anaphylactic-type reactions and death possible. Only use when indication clearly established and lab investigations confirm iron deficient state not amenable to oral therapy.

THERAPEUTIC CLASS: Iron supplement

INDICATIONS: Treatment of iron deficiency when oral administration is not possible.

DOSAGE: *Adults:* Iron Deficiency Anemia: Dose (mL)=0.0442 (desired Hgb-observed Hgb) x LBW + (0.26 x LBW); LBW=lean body weight (kg). See labeling for more details. Blood Loss: Replace equivalent amount of iron in blood loss.

Pediatrics: ≥4 months: >15kg: Iron Deficiency Anemia: Dose (mL)=0.0442 (desired Hgb-observed Hgb) x LBW + (0.26 x LBW); LBW=lean body weight (kg). 5-15kg: Dose (mL)=0.0442 (desired Hgb-observed Hgb) x weight + (0.26 x weight). See labeling for more details. Blood Loss: Replace equivalent amount of iron in blood loss.

HOW SUPPLIED: Inj: 50mg/mL

CONTRAINDICATIONS: Anemia not associated with iron deficiency.

WARNINGS/PRECAUTIONS: Large IV doses associated with increased incidence of adverse effects. Caution with serious hepatic impairment, significant allergies, asthma.

Avoid during acute phase of infectious kidney disease. May exacerbate cardiovascular complications in pre-existing cardiovascular disease and joint pain or swelling in rheumatoid arthritis. Hypersensitivity reactions reported after uneventful test doses. Unwarranted therapy can cause exogenous hemosiderosis. Have epinephrine (1:1000) available. Risk of carcinogenesis with IM use. Give 0.5mL test dose before IM/IV administration.

ADVERSE REACTIONS: Anaphylactic reactions, chest pain/tightness, urticaria, pruritus, abdominal pain, nausea, arthralgia, convulsions, respiratory arrest, hematuria, febrile episodes.

INTERACTIONS: Discontinue oral iron before use.

PREGNANCY: Category C, caution in nursing.

INTAL RX
cromolyn sodium (King)

THERAPEUTIC CLASS: Mast cell stabilizer

INDICATIONS: Prophylactic treatment of bronchial asthma and of acute bronchoconstriction due to exercise, environmental agents, and known antigens.

DOSAGE: *Adults:* Asthma: (Inhaler) Usual/Max: 2 inh qid. (Sol) 20mg nebulized qid. Acute Bonchospasm Prevention: (Inhaler) Usual: 2 inh 10-60 minutes before exposure to precipitant. (Sol) 20mg nebulized shortly before exposure to precipitant. Renal/Hepatic Dysfunction: Decrease inhaler dose.

Pediatrics: Asthma: (Inhaler) ≥5 yrs: Usual/Max: 2 inh qid. (Sol) ≥2 yrs: 20mg nebulized qid. Acute Bronchospasm Prevention: (Inhaler) ≥5 yrs: Usual: 2 inh 10-60 minutes before exposure to precipitant. (Sol) ≥2 yrs: 20mg nebulized shortly before exposure to precipitant. Renal/Hepatic Dysfunction: Decrease inhaler dose.

HOW SUPPLIED: MDI: 0.8mg/inh (8.1g, 14.2g); Sol (neb): 10mg/mL (2mL, 10s 60s)

WARNINGS/PRECAUTIONS: Not for treatment of acute attack. Severe anaphylaxis may occur. D/C if eosinophilic pneumonia or pulmonary infiltrates with eosinophilia develop. May experience cough and/or bronchospasm. Caution with inhaler in CAD or history of cardiac arrhythmias. Decrease dose or d/c with renal/hepatic dysfunction.

ADVERSE REACTIONS: Throat irritation/dryness, bad taste, cough, nausea, bronchospasm, sneezing, wheezing.

INTERACTIONS: Avoid with isoproterenol during pregnancy.

PREGNANCY: Category B, caution in nursing.

INTRON A RX
interferon alfa-2b (Schering)

> May cause or aggravate fatal or life-threatening neuropsychiatric, autoimmune, ischemic, and infectious disorders. Monitor closely with periodic clinical and laboratory evaluations.

THERAPEUTIC CLASS: Biological response modifier

INDICATIONS: Treatment of hairy cell leukemia, malignant melanoma, follicular lymphoma, condylomata acuminata, AIDS-related Kaposi's sarcoma, chronic hepatitis C and B.

DOSAGE: *Adults:* ≥18 yrs: Hairy Cell Leukemia: 2MIU/m^2 IM/SQ 3x/week up to 6 months. Reduce dose by 50% or stop therapy with severe reactions. Malignant Melanoma: Initial: 20MIU/m^2 IV for 5 consecutive days/week for 4 weeks. Maint: 10MIU/m^2 SQ 3x/week for 48 weeks. Follicular Lymphoma: 5MIU SQ 3x/week up to 18 months. Condylomata Acuminata: 1MIU into lesion 3x/week alternating days for 3 weeks. Kaposi's Sarcoma: 30MIU/m^2 3x/week IM/SQ. Hepatitis C: 3MIU IM/SQ 3x/week for 18-24 months. Hepatitis B: IM/SC: 5MIU qd or 10MIU IM/SQ 3x/week for 16 weeks.

Pediatrics: ≥1 yr: Hepatitis B: 3MIU/m^2 SQ 3x/week for 1 week, then 6MIU/m^2 3x/week for total therapy of 16-24 weeks. Max: 10MIU/m^2 3x/week. Reduce dose by 50% or stop therapy with severe reactions. Adjust based on WBC, granulocyte, and/or platelet counts.

INVANZ

HOW SUPPLIED: Inj: 10MIU, 18MIU, 50MIU, 10MIU/mL, 3MIU/0.2mL, 5MIU/0.2mL, 10MIU/0.2mL

WARNINGS/PRECAUTIONS: Do not give IM if platelet count is less than 50,000/mm^3. Hepatotoxicity, retinal hemorrhages, autoimmune diseases, pulmonary infiltrates, pneumonitis, thyroid abnormalities and pneumonia reported. Avoid with immunosuppressed transplant, autoimmune disorders, decompensated liver disease. Caution with cardiac disease, coagulation disorders, severe myelosuppression, pulmonary disease, thyroid disorders, or DM prone to ketoacidosis. Avoid with pre-existing psychiatric condition; depression and suicidal behavior reported. May exacerbate psoriasis or sarcoidosis. Do not interchange brands.

ADVERSE REACTIONS: Fever, headache, chills, fatigue, myalgia, GI disturbances, alopecia, dyspnea, depression.

INTERACTIONS: Increases theophylline levels by 100%. Caution with myelosuppressive agents (eg, zidovudine). Antidiabetics and thyroid agents may need adjustments. Increased risk of hemolytic anemia when coadministered with ribavirin.

PREGNANCY: Category C, Category X when used with ribavirn, not for use in nursing.

INVANZ RX
ertapenem sodium (Merck)

THERAPEUTIC CLASS: Carbapenem

INDICATIONS: Treatment of complicated intra-abdominal infections; skin and skin structure infections (SSSI), including diabetic foot infections without osteomyelitits; community acquired pneumonia (CAP); complicated urinary tract infections (UTI) including pyelonephritis; acute pelvic infections including postpartum endomyometritis, septic abortion, and post surgical gynecologic infections; prophylaxis of surgical site infection following elective colorectal surgery.

DOSAGE: *Adults:* Treatment: 1g IM/IV qd. Duration: Intra-Abdominal Infections: 5-14 days. SSSI: 7-14 days. CAP/UTI: 10-14 days. Pelvic Infection: 3-10 days. May administer IV for up to 14 days and IM for up to 7 days. CrCl ≤30mL/min/1.73m^2: 500mg IM/IV qd. Hemodialysis: Give 150mg IM/IV after dialysis only if 500mg dose was given within 6 hrs prior to dialysis. Prophylaxis: 1g IV as single dose given 1 hr prior to surgical incision.
Pediatrics: ≥13 years: 1g IM/IV qd. 3 mo-12 yrs: 15mg/kg IM/IV bid (not to exceed 1g/day). Treatment Duration: Intra-Abdominal Infections: 5-14 days. SSSI: 7-14 days. CAP/UTI: 10-14 days. Pelvic Infections: 3-10 days. May administer IV for up to 14 days and IM for up to 7 days. CrCl ≤30mL/min/1.73 m^2: 500mg IM/IV qd.

HOW SUPPLIED: Inj: 1g

CONTRAINDICATIONS: Hypersensitivity to drugs in same class, anaphylactic reactions to beta-lactams, hypersensitivity to local anesthetics of the amide type (due to lidocaine diluent).

WARNINGS/PRECAUTIONS: Anaphylactic reactions reported with beta-lactam therapy; increased incidence with sensitivity to multiple allergens. Seizures, CNS adverse experiences, pseudomembranous colitis reported. Increased risk of seizures with CNS disorders and/or compromised renal function. Use lidocaine HCl as the diluent; avoid dextrose-containing diluents. Monitor renal, hepatic, hematopoietic functions during prolonged therapy. Do not inject into blood vessel.

ADVERSE REACTIONS: Diarrhea, infused vein complication, nausea, headache, vaginitis, edema/swelling, fever, abdominal pain, constipation, altered mental status, headache, insomnia, phlebitis/thrombophlebitis, vomiting.

INTERACTIONS: Decreased clearance with probenecid. Do not mix or co-infuse with other drugs.

PREGNANCY: Category B, caution in nursing.

INVIRASE RX
saquinavir mesylate (Roche Labs)

> Not interchangeable with Fortovase®.

THERAPEUTIC CLASS: Protease inhibitor

INDICATIONS: Treatment of HIV infection in combination with other antiretrovirals.

DOSAGE: *Adults:* 1000mg bid with ritonavir 100mg bid. Take within 2 hrs after a full meal.

Pediatrics: >16 yrs: 1000mg bid with ritonavir 100mg bid. Take within 2 hrs after a full meal.

HOW SUPPLIED: Cap: 200mg; Tab: 500mg

CONTRAINDICATIONS: Concomitant amiodarone, bepridil, flecainide, propafenone, quinidine, rifampin, pimozide, terfenadine, cisapride, astemizole, triazolam, midazolam, ergot derivatives.

WARNINGS/PRECAUTIONS: New onset DM, exacerbation of pre-existing DM, hyperglycemia may occur. Exacerbation of chronic liver dysfunction reported with hepatitis or cirrhosis. Spontaneous bleeding may occur with hemophilia A, B. Possible redistribution or accumulation of body fat. Caution with hepatic dysfunction. Interrupt therapy if serious toxicity occurs.

ADVERSE REACTIONS: Diarrhea, abdominal discomfort, nausea, dyspepsia, mucosa damage, headache, paresthesia, extremity numbness, asthenia, myalgia.

INTERACTIONS: See contraindications. Avoid lovastatin, simvastatin, St. John's wort. Decreased plasma levels with nevirapine. Consider alternatives to CYP3A4 inducers (eg, phenobarbital, phenytoin, dexamethasone, carbamazepine). Ritonavir increases adverse effects. Risk of toxicity with substrates of CYP3A4 substrates (eg, calcium channel blockers, clindamycin, dapsone, quinidine, triazolam). Delavirdine increases plasma levels; monitor LFTs frequently.

PREGNANCY: Category B, not for use in nursing.

Ionamin
phentermine (Celltech)   CIV

THERAPEUTIC CLASS: Anorectic sympathomimetic amine

INDICATIONS: Short term adjunct for exogenous obesity if initial BMI ≥30kg/m^2 or ≥27kg/m^2 with other risk factors (eg, HTN, diabetes hyperlipidemia).

DOSAGE: *Adults:* 15-30mg before breakfast or 10-14 hrs before bedtime. Swallow caps whole.

Pediatrics: ≥16 yrs: 15-30mg prior to breakfast or 10-14 hrs before bedtime. Swallow caps whole.

HOW SUPPLIED: Cap: 15mg, 30mg

CONTRAINDICATIONS: Advanced arteriosclerosis, CVD, moderate to severe HTN, hyperthyroidism, glaucoma, agitated states, history of drug abuse, within 14 days of MAOI use.

WARNINGS/PRECAUTIONS: Primary pulmonary HTN and valvular heart disease reported. D/C if tolerance occurs. Abuse potential. Caution with mild HTN.

ADVERSE REACTIONS: Primary pulmonary HTN, palpitations, tachycardia, BP elevation, restlessness, dizziness, insomnia, headache, diarrhea, constipation, impotence.

INTERACTIONS: See Contraindications. May alter insulin requirements. Avoid with weight loss products including SSRIs. Valvular heart disease and primary pulmonary hypertension reported with fenfluramine and dexfenfluramine. May decrease effects of adrenergic neuron blocking agents.

PREGNANCY: Safety in pregnancy and nursing not known.

Iquix
levofloxacin (Vistakon)   RX

THERAPEUTIC CLASS: Fluoroquinolone

INDICATIONS: Bacterial corneal ulcer.

DOSAGE: *Adults:* Days 1-3: 1-2 drops q30min-2h while awake and 4-6 hrs after retiring. Days 4-completion: 1-2 drops q1-4h while awake.

Pediatrics: ≥6 yrs: Days 1-3: 1-2 drops q30min-2h while awake and 4-6 hrs after retiring. Days 4-completion: 1-2 drops q1-4h while awake.

HOW SUPPLIED: Sol: 1.5% (5mL)

IROFOL

WARNINGS/PRECAUTIONS: Discontinue if hypersensitivity or superinfection occurs. Avoid contact lenses with corneal ulcer.

ADVERSE REACTIONS: Headache, taste disturbance.

INTERACTIONS: Systemic quinolone therapy increases theophylline levels, interferes with caffeine metabolism, enhances warfarin effects, and elevates SCr with cyclosporine.

PREGNANCY: Category C, caution in nursing.

IROFOL   RX
folic acid - polysaccharide iron complex (Dayton)

THERAPEUTIC CLASS: Iron/vitamin

INDICATIONS: Prevention and treatment of iron and folic acid deficiencies.

DOSAGE: *Adults:* 1-2 tabs or 5-10mL qd.
Pediatrics: >12 yrs: 1-2 tabs or 5-10mL qd.

HOW SUPPLIED: (Folic Acid-Polysaccharide Iron Complex) Liquid: 1mg-100mg/5mL; Tab: 1mg-150mg

WARNINGS/PRECAUTIONS: Not for the treatment of pernicious anemia and other megaloblastic anemias. Folic acid >0.1mg/day may obscure pernicious anemia.

ADVERSE REACTIONS: Gastric intolerance, allergic sensitization.

INTERACTIONS: Absorption may be inhibited by eggs, milk, magnesium trisilicate or antacids containing carbonates.

PREGNANCY: Safety in pregnancy and nursing not known.

ISONIAZID   RX
isoniazid (Various)

> Severe, fatal hepatitis may develop. Monitor LFTs monthly.

OTHER BRAND NAME: Nydrazid (Sandoz)

THERAPEUTIC CLASS: Isonicotinic acid hydrazide

INDICATIONS: Prevention and treatment of tuberculosis (TB).

DOSAGE: *Adults:* Active TB: 5mg/kg single dose. Max: 300mg/day. Use with other antituberculosis agents. Prevention: 300mg qd single dose.
Pediatrics: Active TB: 10-20mg/kg single dose. Max: 300mg qd. Use with other antituberculosis agents. Prevention: 10mg/kg qd single dose. Max: 300mg qd.

HOW SUPPLIED: Inj: 100mg/mL; Syrup: 50mg/5mL; Tab: 100mg, 300mg

CONTRAINDICATIONS: Severe hypersensitivity reactions including drug-induced hepatitis, previous INH-associated hepatic injury, severe adverse effects to INH (eg, drug fever, chills, arthritis), acute liver disease.

WARNINGS/PRECAUTIONS: Discontinue if hypersensitivity occurs. Monitor closely with liver or renal disease. Take with vitamin B_6 in malnourished and those predisposed to neuropathy.

ADVERSE REACTIONS: Peripheral neuropathy, nausea, vomiting, epigastric distress, elevated serum transaminases, bilirubinemia, jaundice, hepatitis, skin eruptions, pyridoxine deficiency.

INTERACTIONS: Alcohol is associated with hepatitis. May increase phenytoin, theophylline, and valproate serum levels. Do not take with food. Severe acetaminophen toxicity reported. Decreases carbamazepine metabolism and AUC of ketoconazole.

PREGNANCY: Safety in pregnancy and nursing is not known.

KALETRA   RX
lopinavir - ritonavir (Abbott)

THERAPEUTIC CLASS: Protease inhibitor

INDICATIONS: Treatment of HIV infection in combination with other antiretrovirals.

DOSAGE: *Adults:* Therapy-Naive: 400/100mg (2 tabs or 5mL) bid or 800/200mg qd (4 tabs or 10mL). Therapy-Experienced: 400/100mg (2 tabs or 5mL) bid. Once daily administration not recommended. Concomitant Efavirenz, Nevirapine, Fosamprenavir, Nelfinavir: Therapy-Naive: 400/100mg (2 tabs) bid. Concomitant Efavirenz, Nevirapine, Amprenavir or Nelfinavir: 533/133mg (6.5mL) bid. Concomitant Efavirenz, Nevirapine, Fosamprenavir without Ritonavir, or Nelfinavir: Treatment-Experienced with Decreased Susceptibility to Lopinavir: 600/150mg (3 tabs) bid. Tablets can be taken with or without food. Oral solution must be taken with food.

Pediatrics: >12 yrs: Therapy-Naive: 400/100mg (2 tabs or 5mL) bid or 800/200mg qd (4 tabs or 10mL). Therapy-Experienced: 400/100mg (2 tabs or 5mL) bid. Once daily administration not recommended. Concomitant Efavirenz, Nevirapine, Fosamprenavir, Nelfinavir: Therapy-Naive: 400/100mg (2 tabs) bid. Concomitant Efavirenz, Nevirapine, Amprenavir or Nelfinavir: 533/133mg (6.5mL) bid. Concomitant Efavirenz, Nevirapine, Fosamprenavir without Ritonavir, or Nelfinavir: Treatment-Experienced with Decreased Susceptibility to Lopinavir: 600/150mg (3 tabs) bid. 6 months-12 yrs: >40kg: 400/100mg (2 tabs or 5 mL) bid. 15-40kg: (Sol) 10/2.5mg/kg bid. 7-<15kg: (Sol) 12/3mg/kg bid. Concomitant Efavirenz, Nevirapine, Amprenavir: >45kg: 533/133mg (2 tabs or 6.5mL) bid. 15-45kg: (Sol) 11/2.75mg/kg bid. 7-<15kg: (Sol) 13/3.25mg/kg bid. Tablets can be taken with or without food. Oral solution must be taken with food.

HOW SUPPLIED: Tab: (Lopinavir-Ritonavir) 200mg-50mg; Sol: (Lopinavir-Ritonavir) 80mg-20mg/mL (160mL)

CONTRAINDICATIONS: Concomitant drugs dependent on CYP3A or CYP2D6 for clearance (eg, flecainide, propafenone, astemizole, terfenadine, dihydroergotamine, ergonovine, ergotamine, methylergonovine, cisapride, pimozide, midazolam, triazolam).

WARNINGS/PRECAUTIONS: May elevate triglyceride and total cholesterol levels; monitor levels at baseline then periodically. Possible redistribution or accumulation of body fat. Discontinue if symptoms of pancreatitis occur. May exacerbate DM or cause hyperglycemia. Caution in hepatic impairment. Increased bleeding may occur with hemophilia A and B. Risk of further transaminase elevation or hepatic decompensation in patients with underlying hepatitis B or C or marked transaminase elevation prior to treatment; monitor ALT/AST more frequently during first several months of therapy.

ADVERSE REACTIONS: Abdominal pain, asthenia, headache, diarrhea, nausea, vomiting, dyspepsia, flatulence.

INTERACTIONS: See Contraindications. Avoid use with rifampin, St. John's wort; may cause loss of virologic response and resistance. Avoid use with lovastatin and simvastatin; risk of myopathy and rhabdomyolysis. May increase levels of antiarrhythmics (eg, amiodarone, bepridil, systemic lidocaine, quinidine), dihydropyridine calcium channel blockers (eg, felodipine, nifedipine, nicardipine), immunosuppressants (eg, cyclosporine, tacrolimus, rapamycin); monitoring recommended. May increase levels of trazodone; use with caution and consider lower trazodone dose. May increase levels of fluticasone; coadministration not recommended. CYP3A inducers may decrease lopinavir levels. CYP3A inhibitors may increase lopinavir levels. May increase levels of drugs primarily metabolized by CYP3A. May increase levels of amprenavir, indinavir, saquinavir. May increase levels of clarithromycin with renal impairment; reduce clarithromycin dose by 50% if CrCl 30-60mL/min and by 75% if CrCl <30mL/min. Decreased effect with dexamethasone, carbamazepine, phenobarbital, phenytoin. Monitor PT/INR with warfarin. Space dosing with didanosine; give 1 hr before or 2 hrs after lopinavir/ritonavir. Increased levels with delavirdine. Efavirenz and nevirapine may decrease levels; adjust dose. May increase levels of ketoconazole or itraconazole; avoid ketoconazole or itraconazole doses >200mg/day. May increase rifabutin levels; reduce usual rifabutin dose by 75%. Decreases atovaquone levels. Oral solution contains alcohol; disulfiram reaction may occur with disulfiram or metronidazole. May increase sildenafil, tadalafil, vardenafil levels; reduce dose of sildenafil (eg, 25mg q48h); reduce dose of tadalafil (eg, 10mg q72h); reduce dose of vardenafil (eg, 2.5mg q72h). May decrease methadone levels; may need to increase methadone dose. May decrease ethinyl estradiol levels; use alternate/additional contraception. Increased atorvastatin levels; use lowest atorvastatin dose or consider alternate HMG-CoA reductase inhibitors (eg, pravastatin, fluvastatin). Increases tenofovir levels. May increase nelfinavir levels; dosage adjustments needed. Increased levels with ritonavir.

PREGNANCY: Category C, not for use in nursing.

KAYEXALATE
sodium polystyrene sulfonate (Sanofi-Aventis)

RX

THERAPEUTIC CLASS: Cation-exchange resin
INDICATIONS: Treatment of hyperkalemia.

KEFLEX

DOSAGE: *Adults:* Oral: 15g qd-qid. Rectal Enema: 30-50g q6h.

Pediatrics: Oral: Use 1g per 1mEq of potassium as basis of calculation.

HOW SUPPLIED: Sus: 15g/60mL

CONTRAINDICATIONS: Hypokalemia.

WARNINGS/PRECAUTIONS: May be insufficient for emergency correction of hyperkalemia. Monitor for electrolyte disturbances. Caution in those intolerant to sodium increases (eg, severe CHF or HTN, or marked edema). Treat constipation with sorbital.

ADVERSE REACTIONS: Anorexia, nausea, vomiting, constipation, hypokalemia, hypocalcemia, sodium retention, diarrhea, (elderly) fecal impaction.

INTERACTIONS: Avoid nonabsorbable cation-donating antacids and laxatives; systemic alkalosis may occur (eg, magnesium hydroxide, aluminum carbonate). Hypokalemia exaggerates toxic effects of digitalis. Intestinal obstruction reported with aluminum hydroxide.

PREGNANCY: Category C, caution in nursing.

KEFLEX RX
cephalexin (Advancis)

THERAPEUTIC CLASS: Cephalosporin (1st generation)

INDICATIONS: Treatment of otitis media and skin and skin structure (SSSI), bone, genitourinary tract, and respiratory tract infections.

DOSAGE: *Adults:* Usual: 25-50mg/kg/day in divided doses. Streptococcal Pharyngitis/SSSI/Uncomplicated Cystitis (>15 yrs): 500mg q12h. Treat cystitis for 7-14 days. Max: 4g/day.

Pediatrics: Usual: 25-50mg/kg/day in divided doses. Streptococcal Pharyngitis (>1 yr)/SSSI: May divide dose and give q12h. Otitis Media: 75-100mg/kg/day in divided doses. Administer for ≥10 days in β-hemolytic streptococcal infections.

HOW SUPPLIED: Cap: 250mg, 333mg, 500mg, 750mg; Sus: 125mg/5ml, 250mg/5ml (100ml, 200ml)

WARNINGS/PRECAUTIONS: Caution with markedly impaired renal function, history of GI disease. Cross-sensitivity with cephalosporins and penicillins. Pseudomembranous colitis reported. False (+) direct Coombs' tests reported. False (+) for urine glucose with Benedict's, Fehling's solution, and Clinitest tablets.

ADVERSE REACTIONS: Diarrhea, allergic reactions, dyspepsia, gastritis, abdominal pain, superinfection (prolonged use).

INTERACTIONS: Probenecid inhibits excretion.

PREGNANCY: Category B, caution in nursing.

KEPPRA RX
levetiracetam (UCB Pharma)

THERAPEUTIC CLASS: Pyrrolidine derivative

INDICATIONS: (PO) Adjunctive therapy for partial onset seizures in adults and children ≥4 yrs of age. Adjunctive therapy in the treatment of myoclonic seizures in adults and children ≥12 yrs with juvenile myoclonic epilepsy (JME). Adjunctive therapy in the treatment of primary generalized tonic-clonic (PGTC) seizures in adults and children ≥6 yrs with idiopathic generalized epilepsy. (Inj) Adjunctive therapy for partial onset seizures in adults and as alternative when oral administration is temporarily not feasible.

DOSAGE: *Adults:* Inj/PO: Initial: 500mg bid. Titrate: Increase by 1000mg/day every 2 weeks. Max: 3000mg/day. Inj: Replacement Therapy: Initial total daily dosage and frequency should equal total daily dosage and frequency of oral therapy. Dilute injection in 100mL of compatible diluent and give as 15-min IV infusion. CrCl 50-80mL/min: 500-1000mg q12h. CrCl 30-50mL/min: 250-750mg q12h. CrCl <30mL/min: 250-500mg q12h. ESRD with Dialysis: 500-1000mg q24h; supplemental 250-500mg after dialysis.

Pediatrics: PO: Partial Onset Seizures/PGTC: ≥16 yrs or JME: ≥ 12 yrs: Initial: 500mg bid. Titrate: Increase by 1000mg/day every 2 weeks. Max: 3000mg/day. Partial Onset Seizures: 4 to <16 yrs or PGTC: 6-16 yrs: Initial: 10mg/kg bid: Titrate: Increase by 20mg/kg/

day every 2 weeks. Max: 60mg/kg/day. Inj: Partial Onset Seizures: Initial: 500mg bid. Titrate: Increase by 1000mg/day every 2 weeks. Max: 3000mg/day. Replacement Therapy: Initial total daily dosage and frequency should equal total daily dosage and frequency of oral therapy. Dilute injection in 100mL of compatible diluent and give as 15-min IV infusion. CrCl 50-80mL/min: 500-1000mg q12h. CrCl 30-50mL/min: 250-750mg q12h. CrCl <30mL/min: 250-500mg q12h. ESRD with Dialysis: 500-1000mg q24h; supplemental 250-500mg after dialysis.

HOW SUPPLIED: Inj: 500mg/5mL; Sol: 100mg/mL; Tab: 250mg*, 500mg*, 750mg*, 1000mg* *scored

WARNINGS/PRECAUTIONS: Associated with somnolence, fatigue, coordination difficulties, and behavioral abnormalities. Avoid abrupt withdrawal. Hematologic abnormalities reported. Caution in renal dysfunction.

ADVERSE REACTIONS: Somnolence, asthenia, headache, infection, pain, anorexia, dizziness, nervousness, vertigo, ataxia, vertigo, pharyngitis, rhinitis, irritability.

PREGNANCY: Category C, caution in nursing.

KETAMINE
ketamine HCl (Various)   CIII

THERAPEUTIC CLASS: Nonbarbiturate anesthetic

INDICATIONS: Sole anesthetic agent for diagnostic and surgical procedures that do not require skeletal muscle relaxation. Induction of anesthesia prior to the administration of other general anesthetic agents. To supplement low-potency agents (eg, nitrous oxide).

DOSAGE: *Adults:* Initial: IV: 1-4.5mg/kg. Infuse slowly over 60 seconds. May administer with 2-5mg doses of diazepam over 60 seconds. IM: 6.5-13mg/kg. Maint: Adjust according to anesthetic needs. May increase in increments of one-half to full induction dose.
Pediatrics: Initial: IV: 1-4.5mg/kg. Infuse slowly over 60 seconds. IM: 6.5-13mg/kg. Maint: Adjust according to anesthetic needs. May increase in increments of one-half to full induction dose.

HOW SUPPLIED: Inj: 50mg/mL

CONTRAINDICATIONS: Patients in whom a significant elevation in blood pressure would constitute a serious hazard.

WARNINGS/PRECAUTIONS: Monitor cardiac function in patients with hypertension or cardiac dysfunction. Postoperative confusional states may occur during recovery. Respiratory depression may occur; maintain airway and respiration. Do not use alone in pharynx, larynx, or bronchial tree procedures. Use with caution in chronic alcoholics and acutely intoxicated patients. May increase cerebrospinal fluid pressure, use with extreme caution in patients with preanesthetic cerebrospinal fluid pressure. Use with agent that obtunds visceral pain when surgical procedure involving visceral pain.

ADVERSE REACTIONS: Nausea, vomiting, anorexia, elevated blood pressure and pulse, hypotension, bradycardia, arrhythmia, respiratory depression, apnea, airway obstruction, diplopia, nystagmus, slight elevation of IOP, enhanced skeletal muscle tone.

INTERACTIONS: Prolonged recovery time with barbiturates and/or narcotics.

PREGNANCY: Not recommended with pregnancy, use in nursing unknown.

KETOROLAC
ketorolac tromethamine (Various)   RX

For short-term use only (≤5 days). Contraindicated with peptic ulcer disease, GI bleeding/perforation, perioperative pain in coronary artery bypass graft (CABG) surgery, advanced renal impairment, risk of renal failure due to volume depletion, CV bleeding, hemorrhagic diathesis, incomplete hemostasis, high-risk of bleeding, intraoperatively when hemostasis is critical, intrathecal/epidural use, L&D, nursing, and with ASA, NSAIDs, or probenecid. Caution greater risk of GI events with elderly patients. NSAIDs may cause an increased risk of CV thrombotic events (MI, stroke).

OTHER BRAND NAME: Toradol (Roche Labs)

THERAPEUTIC CLASS: NSAID (pyrrolo-pyrrole derivative)

KLARON

INDICATIONS: Short-term (≤5 days) management of moderately severe, acute pain.

DOSAGE: Adults: >16 to <65 yrs: Single-Dose: 60mg IM or 30mg IV. Multiple-Dose: 30mg IM/IV q6h. Max: 120mg/day. Transition from IM/IV to PO: 20mg PO single dose, then 10mg PO q4-6h. Max: 40mg/24 hrs. ≥65 yrs/Renal Impairment/<50kg: Single-Dose: 30mg IM or 15mg IV. Multiple-Dose: 15mg IM/IV q6h. Max: 60mg/day. Transition from IM/IV to PO: 10mg PO q4-6h. Max: 40mg/24 hrs.

Pediatrics: 2-16 yrs: Single-Dose: IM: 1mg/kg. Max: 30mg. IV: 0.5mg/kg. Max: 15mg.

HOW SUPPLIED: Inj: 15mg/mL, 30mg/mL; Tab: 10mg

CONTRAINDICATIONS: Active or history of peptic ulcer, GI bleeding, perioperative pain in CABG surgery, advanced renal impairment or risk of renal failure due to volume depletion, labor/delivery, nursing mothers, ASA or NSAID allergy, preoperatively or intraoperatively when hemostasis is critical, cerebrovascular bleeding, hemorrhagic diathesis, incomplete hemostasis, if high risk of bleeding, neuraxial (epidural or intrathecal) administration, and concomitant ASA, NSAIDs, probenecid, or pentoxifylline.

WARNINGS/PRECAUTIONS: Do not exceed 5 days of therapy. Risk of GI ulcerations, bleeding and perforation. Caution with renal or liver dysfunction, dehydration, HTN, congestive heart failure, coagulation disorders, debilitated and elderly, pre-existing asthma. Preoperative use prolongs bleeding. CV thrombotic events, fluid retention, edema, NaCl retention, oliguria, anaphylactic reactions, elevated BUN and serum creatinine, anemia reported. Correct hypovolemia before therapy.

ADVERSE REACTIONS: Nausea, dyspepsia, GI pain, diarrhea, edema, headache, drowsiness, dizziness.

INTERACTIONS: May increase risk of bleeding with anticoagulants. May reduce diuretic response to furosemide. Increased serum levels with salicylates. Avoid ASA, NSAIDs and probenecid. Increased lithium and methotrexate levels. May increase risk of renal impairment with ACE inhibitors. May increase seizures with phenytoin and carbamazepine. Hallucinations reported with fluoxetine, thiothixene and alprazolam. Do not mix in the same syringe as morphine. May have adverse effects with nondepolarizing muscle relaxants.

PREGNANCY: Category C, not for use in nursing.

KLARON
sulfacetamide sodium (Dermik)

RX

THERAPEUTIC CLASS: Sulfonamide

INDICATIONS: Topical treatment of acne vulgaris.

DOSAGE: *Adults:* Apply thin film bid.

Pediatrics: ≥12 yrs: Apply thin film bid.

HOW SUPPLIED: Lot: 10% (118mL)

WARNINGS/PRECAUTIONS: D/C if irritation, rash, or hypersensitivity reaction occurs. Avoid eyes. Contains sulfites. Caution with denuded or abraded skin.

ADVERSE REACTIONS: Erythema, itching, edema, stinging, burning, local irritation.

PREGNANCY: Category C, caution in nursing.

KLONOPIN
clonazepam (Roche Labs)

OTHER BRAND NAME: Klonopin Wafers (Roche Labs)

THERAPEUTIC CLASS: Benzodiazepine

INDICATIONS: Adjunct or monotherapy in Lennox-Gastaut syndrome, akinetic and myoclonic seizures. Absence seizures refractory to succinimides. Panic disorder with or without agoraphobia.

DOSAGE: *Adults:* Seizure Disorders: Initial: Not to exceed 1.5mg/day given tid. Titrate: May increase by 0.5-1mg every 3 days. Max: 20mg qd. Panic Disorder: Initial: 0.25mg bid. Titrate: Increase to 1mg/day after 3 days, then may increase by 0.125-0.25mg bid every 3 days. Max: 4mg/day. Wafer: Dissolve in mouth with or without water.

Pediatrics: <10 yrs or 30kg: Seizure Disorders: Initial: 0.01-0.03mg/kg/day up to 0.05mg/kg/day given bid-tid. Titrate: Increase by no more than 0.25-0.5mg every 3 days. Maint: 0.1-0.2mg/kg/day given tid. Wafer: Dissolve in mouth with or without water.

HOW SUPPLIED: Tab: 0.5mg*, 1mg, 2mg; Tab, Disintegrating (Wafer): 0.125mg, 0.25mg, 0.5mg, 1mg, 2mg *scored

CONTRAINDICATIONS: Significant liver disease, acute narrow angle glaucoma, untreated open angle glaucoma.

WARNINGS/PRECAUTIONS: May increase incidence of generalized tonic-clonic seizures. Monitor blood counts and LFT's periodically with long-term therapy. Caution with renal dysfunction, chronic respiratory depression. Increased fetal risks during pregnancy. Avoid abrupt withdrawal. Hypersalivation reported.

ADVERSE REACTIONS: Somnolence, depression, ataxia, CNS depression, upper respiratory tract infection, fatigue, dizziness, sinusitis, colpitis.

INTERACTIONS: Decreased serum levels with CYP450 inducers (eg, phenytoin, carbamazepine, phenobarbital). Caution with CYP3A inhibitors (eg, oral antifungals). Alcohol, narcotics, barbiturates, nonbarbiturate hypnotics, antianxiety agents, phenothiazines, thioxanthene and butyrophenone antipsychotics, MAOIs, TCAs and other anticonvulsant drugs potentiate CNS-depressant effects.

PREGNANCY: Category D, not for use in nursing.

KOGENATE FS RX
antihemophilic factor (Bayer)

THERAPEUTIC CLASS: Antihemophilic Factor (Recombinant)

INDICATIONS: Treatment of hemophilia A in which there is a deficiency of activity of clotting factor FVIII.

DOSAGE: *Adults:* Minor hemorrhage: 10-20 IU/kg IV; repeat if evidence of further bleeding. Moderate to major hemorrhage/surgery (minor): 15-30 IU/kg IV; repeat one dose at 12-24 hrs if needed. Major to life-threatening hemorrhage/fractures/head trauma: Initial: 40-50 IU/kg IV; repeat dose 20-25 IU/kg IV q 8-12 hrs. Surgery (major): Preoperative dose: 50 IU/kg IV (verify 100% FVIII activity prior to surgery); repeat as necessary after 6-12 hrs initially, and for 10-14 days until healing is complete.

Pediatrics: Minor hemorrhage: 10-20 IU/kg IV; repeat if evidence of further bleeding. Moderate to major hemorrhage/surgery (minor): 15-30 IU/kg IV; repeat one dose at 12-24 hrs if needed. Major to life-threatening hemorrhage/fractures/head trauma: Initial: 40-50 IU/kg IV; repeat dose 20-25 IU/kg IV q 8-12 hrs. Surgery (major): Preoperative dose: 50 IU/kg IV (verify 100% FVIII activity prior to surgery); repeat as necessary after 6-12 hrs initially, and for 10-14 days until healing is complete.

HOW SUPPLIED: Inj: 250 IU, 500 IU, 1000 IU

CONTRAINDICATIONS: Known hypersensitivity to mouse or hamster protein.

WARNINGS/PRECAUTIONS: Development of circulating neutralizing antibodies to FVIII may occur; monitor by appropriate clinical observation and laboratory tests. Hypotension, urticaria, and chest tightness in association with hypersensitivity reported.

ADVERSE REACTIONS: Local injection site reactions, dizziness, rash, unusual taste, mild increase in BP, pruritus, depersonalization, nausea, rhinitis.

PREGNANCY: Category C, safety not known in nursing.

KYTRIL RX
granisetron HCl (Roche Labs)

THERAPEUTIC CLASS: 5-HT$_3$ antagonist

INDICATIONS: (Inj, Sol, Tab) Prevention of nausea and vomiting associated with chemotherapy. (Sol, Tab) Prevention of nausea and vomiting associated with radiation. (Inj) Prevention and treatment of post-op nausea and vomiting.

DOSAGE: *Adults:* Prevention with Chemotherapy: (PO) 2mg qd up to 1 hr before chemotherapy or 1mg bid (up to 1 hr before chemotherapy and 12 hrs later). (IV) 10mcg/kg within 30 minutes before chemotherapy. Prevention with Radiation: (PO)

LAC-HYDRIN

2mg within 1 hr of radiation. Post-Op Prevention: (IV) Administer 1 mg over 30 seconds before induction of anesthesia or immediately before anesthesia reversal. Post-Op Treatment: (IV) Administer 1mg over 30 seconds.

Pediatrics: 2-16 yrs: Prevention with Chemotherapy: 10mcg/kg IV within 30 minutes before chemotherapy.

HOW SUPPLIED: Inj: 0.1mg/ml, 1mg/mL; Sol: 2mg/10mL; Tab: 1mg

WARNINGS/PRECAUTIONS: (Inj) Does not stimulate gastric or intestinal peristalsis. Do not use instead of nasogastric suction. May mask progressive ileus or gastric distension.

ADVERSE REACTIONS: Headache, asthenia, somnolence, diarrhea, constipation, abdominal pain, dizziness, insomnia, decreased appetite, fever.

INTERACTIONS: Hepatic CYP450 enzyme inducers or inhibitors may alter clearance.

PREGNANCY: Category B, caution in nursing.

LAC-HYDRIN   RX
ammonium lactate (Westwood-Squibb)

THERAPEUTIC CLASS: Emollient

INDICATIONS: Treatment of ichthyosis vulgaris and xerosis.

DOSAGE: *Adults:* Apply bid and rub thoroughly.

Pediatrics: (Lot) Infants/Children: (Cre) ≥2 yrs: Apply bid and rub in thoroughly.

HOW SUPPLIED: Cre: 12% (140g, 385g); Lot: 12% (225g, 400g)

WARNINGS/PRECAUTIONS: Avoid sun exposure to treated skin. Avoid eyes, lips, mucous membranes, intravaginal use and oral use. Caution if used on face; potential for irritation Stinging, burning may occur if applied to fissures, erosions, or abrasions. Discontinue if skin condition worsens.

ADVERSE REACTIONS: Burning, stinging, itching, erythema.

PREGNANCY: Category B, caution in nursing.

LAMICTAL   RX
lamotrigine (GlaxoSmithKline)

> Serious life threatening rash including Stevens-Johnson syndrome and toxic epidermal necrolysis reported. Occurs more often in peds than adults. D/C at 1st sign of rash.

OTHER BRAND NAME: Lamictal CD (GlaxoSmithKline)

THERAPEUTIC CLASS: Phenyltriazine

INDICATIONS: Adjunctive therapy in patients (≥2 yrs) with partial seizures and for generalized seizures of Lennox-Gastaut syndrome. For conversion to monotherapy in adults (≥16 yrs) with partial seizures receiving a single enzyme-inducing antiepileptic drug (EIAED) or valproate (VPA). Maintenance treatment of Bipolar I Disorder to delay the time to occurrence of mood episodes (depression, mania, hypomania, mixed episodes) in patients treated for acute mood episodes with standard therapy.

DOSAGE: *Adults:* Epilepsy: Concomitant AEDs with valproate (VPA): Weeks 1 and 2: 25mg every other day. Weeks 3 and 4: 25mg qd. Titrate: Increase every 1-2 weeks by 25-50mg/day. Maint: 100-400mg/day, given qd or bid; 100-200mg/day when added to VPA alone. Concomitant EIAEDs without VPA: Weeks 1 and 2: 50mg qd. Weeks 3 and 4: 50mg bid. Titrate: Increase every 1-2 weeks by 100mg/day. Maint: 150-250mg bid. Conversion to Monotherapy From Single EIAED: ≥16 yrs: Weeks 1 and 2: 50mg qd. Weeks 3 and 4: 50mg bid. Titrate: Increase every 1-2 weeks by 100mg/day. Maint: 250mg bid. Withdraw EIAED over 4 weeks. Conversion to Monotherapy From VPA: ≥16 yrs: Step 1: Follow Concomitant AEDs with VPA dosing regimen to achieve Lamictal dose of 200mg/day. Maintain previous VPA dose. Step 2: Maintain Lamictal 200mg/day. Decrease VPA to 500mg/day by decrements of ≤500mg/day per week. Maintain VPA 500mg/day for 1 week. Step 3: Increase to Lamictal 300mg/day for 1 week. Decrease VPA simultaneously to 250mg/day for 1 week. Step 4: D/C VPA. Increase Lamictal 100mg/day every week to maint dose of 500mg/day. Bipolar Disorder: Patients not taking carbamazepine, other enzyme-inducing drugs (EIDs) or VPA: Weeks 1 and 2: 25mg qd. Weeks 3 and 4: 50mg qd. Week 5: 100mg qd. Weeks 6 and 7: 200mg qd. Patients taking VPA: Weeks 1 and 2: 25mg every other day. Weeks 3 and 4: 25mg qd. Week 5: 50mg qd. Weeks 6 and 7: 100mg qd. Patients taking carbamazepine (or other EIDs) and not taking VPA: Weeks 1 and 2: 50mg qd. Weeks 3 and 4: 100mg qd (divided doses). Week 5: 200mg qd (divided doses). Week 6: 300mg qd (divided doses). Week 7: up to 400mg qd (divided doses). After d/c of psychotropic drugs excluding VPA, carbamazepine, or other EIDs: Maintain current dose. After d/c of VPA and current lamotrigine dose of 100mg qd: Week 1: 150mg qd. Week 2 and onward: 200mg qd. After d/c of carbamazepine or other EIDs and current lamotrigine dose of 400mg qd: Week 1: 400mg qd. Week 2: 300mg qd. Week 3 and Onward: 200mg qd. Concomitant or starting estrogen-containing oral contraceptives: not taking carbamazepine, phenytoin, phenobarbital, primidone, or rifampin, lamictal should be increased by as much as 2-fold over the recommended target maintenance dose; the dose increase should start at the same time as the initiation and continuation of contraceptives. Stopping estrogen-containing oral contraceptives: may decrease lamictal by as much as 50%. Hepatic Impairment: Initial/Titrate/Maint: Reduce by 50% for moderate (Child-Pugh Grade B) and 75% for severe (Child-Pugh Grade C) impairment. Significant Renal Impairment: Maint: Reduce dose. Elderly: Start at low end of dosing range.

Pediatrics: Round dose down to nearest whole tab. 2-12 yrs: ≥6.7kg: Lennox-Gastaut/Partial Seizures: Concomitant AEDs with VPA: Weeks 1 and 2: 0.15mg/kg/day given qd-bid. Weeks 3 and 4: 0.3mg/kg/day given qd or bid. Titrate: Increase every 1-2 weeks by 0.3mg/kg/day. Maint: 1-5mg/kg/day given qd or bid; 1-3mg/kg/day when added to VPA alone. Max: 200mg/day. Concomitant EIAEDs without VPA: Weeks 1 and 2: 0.3mg/kg bid. Weeks 3 and 4: 0.6mg/kg bid. Titrate: Increase every 1-2 weeks by 1.2mg/kg/day. Maint: 2.5-7.5mg/kg bid. Max: 400mg/day. >12 yrs: Concomitant AEDs with VPA: Weeks 1 and 2: 25mg every other day. Weeks 3 and 4: 25mg qd. Titrate: Increase every 1-2 weeks by 25-50mg/day. Maint: 100-400mg/day, given qd or bid; 100-200mg/day when added to VPA alone. Concomitant EIAEDs without VPA: Weeks 1 and 2: 50mg qd. Weeks 3 and 4: 50mg bid. Titrate: Increase every 1-2 weeks by 100mg/day. Maint: 150-250mg bid. Hepatic Impairment: Initial/Titrate/Maint: Reduce by 50% for moderate (Child-Pugh Grade B) and 75% for severe (Child-Pugh Grade C) impairment. Significant Renal Impairment: Maint: Reduce dose.

HOW SUPPLIED: Tab: 25mg*, 100mg*, 150mg*, 200mg*; Tab, Chewable: (Lamictal CD) 2mg, 5mg, 25mg *scored

WARNINGS/PRECAUTIONS: Risk of serious life-threatening rash; d/c if rash occurs. Multiorgan failure, sudden unexplained death, hypersensitivity reactions, and pure red cell aplasia reported. Avoid abrupt withdrawal. Caution with renal, hepatic, or cardiac functional impairment. May cause ophthalmic toxicity. Do not exceed recommended initial dose and dose escalations. Caution in elderly. Chewable tabs may be swallowed whole, chewed (with water/diluted fruit juice) or dispersed in water/diluted fruit juice; do administer partial quantities.

ADVERSE REACTIONS: Serious rash, dizziness, ataxia, somnolence, headache, diplopia, blurred vision, nausea, vomiting, insomnia, back/abdominal pain, fatigue, xerostomia, rhinitis.

INTERACTIONS: Decreased levels with phenytoin, carbamazepine, phenobarbital, primidone, rifampin, estrogen-containing oral contraceptives. Risk of life-threatening rash with valproic acid. Lamotrigine decreases valproic acid levels; valproic acid increases lamotrigine levels. Inhibits dihydrofolate reductase; may potentiate folate inhibitors.

PREGNANCY: Category C, not for use in nursing.

Lamisil AT
terbinafine HCl (Novartis Consumer) OTC

THERAPEUTIC CLASS: Allylamine antifungal

INDICATIONS: Treatment of tinea pedis, tinea cruris, tinea corporis.

DOSAGE: *Adults:* Wash and dry area. Tinea pedis: Apply bid for 1 week (interdigital) or for 2 weeks (bottom or sides of foot). Tinea cruris/corporis: Apply qd for 1 week.

Pediatrics: ≥12 yrs: Wash and dry area. Tinea pedis: Apply bid for 1 week (interdigital) or for 2 weeks (bottom or sides of foot). Tinea cruris/corporis: Apply qd for 1 week.

HOW SUPPLIED: Cre: 1% (12g, 24g); Spray: 1% (30mL)

LANOXIN

WARNINGS/PRECAUTIONS: Do not use on nails, scalp, in or near the mouth or eyes, or for vaginal yeast infections.

PREGNANCY: Not rated in pregnancy or nursing.

LANOXIN RX
digoxin (GlaxoSmithKline)

OTHER BRAND NAMES: Digitek (Mylan Bertek) - Lanoxicaps (GlaxoSmithKline)

THERAPEUTIC CLASS: Cardiac glycoside

INDICATIONS: Treatment of mild to moderate heart failure and to control ventricular response rate with chronic atrial fibrillation.

DOSAGE: *Adults:* Rapid Digitalization: LD: (Cap/Inj) 0.4-0.6mg PO/IV or (Tab) 0.5-0.75mg PO, may give additional (Cap/Inj) 0.1-0.3mg or (Tab) 0.125-0.375mg at 6-8 hr intervals until clinical effect. Maint: (Tab) 0.125-0.5mg qd. Elderly (>70 yrs)/Renal Dysfunction: Initial: 0.125mg qd. Marked Renal Dysfunction: Initial: 0.0625mg qd. Titrate: Increase every 2 weeks based on response. A-Fib: Titrate to minimum effective dose for desired response.

Pediatrics: (Ped Sol) Oral Digitalizing Dose: Premature Infants: 20-30mcg/kg. Full-Term Infants: 25-35mcg/kg. 1-24 months: 35-60mcg/kg. 2-5 yrs: 30-40mcg/kg. 5-10 yrs: 20-35mcg/kg. >10 yrs: 10-15mcg/kg. Maint: Premature Infants: 20-30% of PO digitalizing dose/day. Full-Term Infants to >10 yrs: 25-35% of PO digitalizing dose. (Ped Inj) IV Digitalizing Dose: Premature Infants: 15-25mcg/kg. Full-Term Infants: 20-30mcg/kg. 1-24 months: 30-50mcg/kg. 2-5 yrs: 25-35mcg/kg. 5-10 yrs: 15-30mcg/kg. >10 yrs: 8-12mcg/kg. Maint: Premature Infants: 20-30% of IV digitalizing dose. Full-Term Infants to >10 yrs: 25-35% of IV digitalizing dose/day. (Cap) Oral Digitalizing Dose: 2-5 yrs: 25-35mcg/kg. 5-10 yrs: 15-30mcg/kg. >10 yrs: 8-12mcg/kg. Maint: ≥2 yrs: 25-25% of PO or IV digitalizing dose. (Tab) Maint: 2-5 yrs: 10-15mcg/kg. 5-10 yrs: 7-10mcg/kg. >10 yrs: 3-5mcg/kg. A-Fib: Titrate to minimum effective dose for desired response.

HOW SUPPLIED: Cap: (Lanoxicaps) 0.1mg, 0.2mg; Inj: (Pediatric Inj) 0.1mg/mL, 0.25mg/mL; Sol: (Pediatric Sol) 0.05mg/mL (60mL); Tab: 0.125mg*, 0.25mg* *scored

CONTRAINDICATIONS: Ventricular fibrillation, digitalis hypersensitivity.

WARNINGS/PRECAUTIONS: May cause severe sinus bradycardia or sinoatrial block with pre-existing sinus node disease. May cause advanced or complete heart block with pre-existing incomplete AV block. May cause very rapid ventricular response or ventricular fibrillation. Caution with thyroid disorders, AMI, hypermetabolic states, restrictive cardiomyopathy, constrictive pericarditis, amyloid heart disease, elderly, acute cor pulmonale, and idiopathic hypertrophic subaortic stenosis. Caution with renal dysfunction; high risk for toxicity. Caution with hypokalemia, hypomagnesemia, or hypercalcemia; toxicity may occur. Hypocalcemia can nullify effects of digoxin. Monitor electrolytes and renal function periodically. Risk of ventricular arrhythmia with electrical cardioversion. Bioavailability is different between dosage forms.

ADVERSE REACTIONS: Heart block, rhythm disturbances, anorexia, nausea, vomiting, diarrhea, visual disturbances, headache, weakness, dizziness, mental disturbances.

INTERACTIONS: Risk of toxicity with K^+-depleting diuretics. Increased risk of arrhythmias with calcium, sympathomimetics, and succinylcholine. Increased serum levels with quinidine, verapamil, amiodarone, propafenone, indomethacin, itraconazole, alprazolam, and spironolactone; monitor for toxicity. Increased absorption with propantheline, diphenoxylate, macrolides, and tetracycline; monitor for toxicity. Decreased intestinal absorption with antacids, kaolin-pectin, sulfasalazine, neomycin, cholestyramine, certain anticancer drugs, and metoclopramide. Decreased serum levels with rifampin. Increased digoxin dose requirement with thyroid supplements. Additive effects on AV node conduction with β-blockers or calcium channel blockers. Caution with drugs that deteriorate renal function.

PREGNANCY: Category C, caution in nursing.

LANTUS RX
insulin glargine, human (Sanofi-Aventis)

THERAPEUTIC CLASS: Insulin

INDICATIONS: Treatment of adults and pediatrics with type 1 diabetes mellitus. Treatment of adults with type 2 diabetes mellitus who require basal (long-acting) insulin.

DOSAGE: *Adults:* Individualize dose. For SQ injection only. Administer qd at same time each day. Insulin naive patients on oral antidiabetic drugs, start with 10U qd. Switching from once-daily NPH or Ultralente does not require initial dose change. Switching from bid NPH, reduce initial dose by 20%. Maint: 2-100U/day.

Pediatrics: ≥6 yrs: Individualize dose. For SQ injection only. Administer qd at same time each day. Insulin naive patients on oral antidiabetic drugs, start with 10U qd. Switching from once-daily NPH or Ultralente does not require initial dose change. Switching from bid NPH, reduce initial dose by 20%. Maint: 2-100U/day.

HOW SUPPLIED: Inj: 100U/mL; OptiPen: 100U/mL

WARNINGS/PRECAUTIONS: Human insulin differs from animal source insulin. Any change of insulin should be made cautiously. Changes in strength, manufacturer, type or method of manufacture may result in the need for a change in dosage. Hypoglycemia may occur with taking too much insulin, missing or delaying meals, exercising or working more than usual. An infection or illness (especially with diarrhea or vomiting) may change insulin requirements. Administration of insulin SQ can result in lipodystrophy. Not for IV use. Do not mix with other insulins. May cause sodium retention and edema.

ADVERSE REACTIONS: Hypoglycemia, allergic reactions, injection site reactions, lipodystrophy, pruritus, rash.

INTERACTIONS: Increased glucose lowering effects with ACE inhibitors, disopyramide, fibrates, fluoxetine, MAOIs, propoxyphene, salicylates, somatostatin analog, sulfonamide antibiotics, and other antidiabetic agents. Decreased blood glucose lowering effects with corticosteroids, danazol, diuretics, sympathomimetic amines, isoniazid, phenothiazine derivatives, somatropin, thyroid hormones, estrogens, progestogens. Pentamidine may cause hypoglycemia, followed by hyperglycemia. β-blockers, clonidine, lithium salts, and alcohol may potentiate or weaken glucose lowering effect. β-blockers, clonidine, guanethidine, and reserpine may reduce or mask signs of hypoglycemia.

PREGNANCY: Category C, caution in nursing.

Lariam
mefloquine HCl (Roche Labs)

RX

THERAPEUTIC CLASS: Quinolinemethanol derivative

INDICATIONS: Treatment and prophylaxis of mild to moderate acute malaria caused by P.falciparum or P.vivax.

DOSAGE: *Adults:* Treatment: 1250mg single dose. Prophylaxis: 250mg/week. Start 1 week before arrival in endemic area and continue weekly (same day of week) while in area. Continue for 4 weeks after leaving the area. Take with food and 8 oz of water.

Pediatrics: ≥6 months: Treatment: Usual: 20-25mg/kg, split in 2 doses. Take 6-8 hrs apart. If vomiting occurs <30 minutes after dose, give a 2nd full dose. If vomiting occurs 30-60 minutes after dose, give additional half-dose. Prophylaxis: ≥3 months: 3-5mg/kg/week. >45kg: 250mg/week. 31-45kg: 3/4 tab/week. 21-30kg: 125mg/week. 5-20kg: 1/4 tab/week. Take with food and water. May crush and mix with water.

HOW SUPPLIED: Tab: 250mg* *scored

CONTRAINDICATIONS: Hypersensitivity to related compounds (eg, quinine, quinidine). Use as prophylaxis with active or recent history of depression, generalized anxiety disorder, psychosis or schizophrenia, or other major psychiatric disorder, or with a history of convulsions.

WARNINGS/PRECAUTIONS: In life-threatening malaria infection due to P.falciparum, use IV antimalarials. High risk of relapse seen with acute P.vivax; after initial treatment, subsequently treat with 8-aminoquinoline (eg, primaquine). May cause psychiatric symptoms. During prophylaxis, d/c if symptoms of acute anxiety, depression, restlessness, or confusion occur. In long-term therapy, monitor LFTs and perform ophthalmic exams. May impair mental/physical abilities. Increase risk of convulsions in epileptic patients. Caution with cardiac disease, hepatic dysfunction and elderly.

ADVERSE REACTIONS: Nausea, vomiting, myalgia, fever, dizziness, headache, somnolence, sleep disorders, loss of balance, chills, diarrhea, abdominal pain, fatigue, tinnitus, pruritus, skin rash.

Lescol XL

INTERACTIONS: Avoid halofantrine; may prolong QTc interval. Concomitant administration with other related compounds (eg, quinine, quinidine, chloroquine) may cause ECG abnormalities and increased risk of convulsions; delay mefloquine dose for 12 hrs after last dose of these drugs. Avoid propranolol; cardiopulmonary arrest reported. Drugs that may alter cardiac conduction (eg, anti-arrhythmic or β-blockers, calcium channel blockers, antihistamines, H_1-blockers, TCAs, and phenothiazines) may prolong QT_c interval. May lower plasma levels of anticonvulsants (eg, valproic acid, carbamazepine, phenobarbital, phenytoin); monitor blood levels and adjust dosage accordingly. Complete vaccinations with live, attenuated vaccines (eg, typhoid vaccine) at least 3 days before mefloquine therapy. Caution with anticoagulants, antidiabetic agents.
PREGNANCY: Category C, not for use in nursing.

Lescol XL RX
fluvastatin sodium (Novartis)

OTHER BRAND NAME: Lescol (Novartis)
THERAPEUTIC CLASS: HMG-CoA reductase inhibitor
INDICATIONS: Adjunct to diet, to reduce total cholesterol (Total-C), LDL-C, TG, and Apo B levels, and to increase HDL-C in primary hypercholesterolemia and mixed dyslipidemia (Types IIa and IIb) when response to nonpharmacological measures is inadequate. To slow coronary atherosclerosis progression in coronary heart disease by lowering Total-C and LDL-C. To reduce risk of undergoing coronary revascularization procedures in patients with coronary heart disease. Adjunct to diet to reduce Total-C, LDL-C, and Apo B levels in adolescent boys and girls who are at least one year post-menarche, 10-16 years of age, with heterozygous familial hypercholesterolemia when response to dietary restriction is inadequate and LDL-C remains ≥190mg/dL or if LDL-C remains ≥160mg/dL and there is positive family history of premature CV disease or 2 or more other CV disease risk factors are present.
DOSAGE: *Adults:* ≥18 yrs: (For LDL-C reduction of ≥25%) Initial: 40mg cap qpm or 80mg XL tab at anytime of day (or 40mg cap bid). (For LDL-C reduction of <25%) Initial: 20mg cap qpm. Usual: 20-80mg/day. Severe Renal Impairment: Caution with dose >40mg/day. Take 2 hrs after bile-acid resins qhs.
Pediatrics: Heterozygous Familial Hypercholesterolemia: 10-16 yrs (≥1 yr postmenarche): Individualize dose: Initial: 20mg cap. Titrate: Adjust dose at 6 week intervals. Max: 40mg cap bid or 80mg XL tab qd.
HOW SUPPLIED: Cap: (Lescol) 20mg, 40mg; Tab, Extended-Release: (Lescol XL) 80mg
CONTRAINDICATIONS: Active liver disease, unexplained persistent elevations of serum transaminases, pregnancy, nursing mothers.
WARNINGS/PRECAUTIONS: Monitor LFTs prior to therapy, at 12 weeks or with dose elevation. D/C if AST or ALT ≥3X ULN on 2 consecutive occasions. Risk of myopathy and/or rhabdomyolysis reported. D/C if markedly elevated CPK levels occur, if myopathy is diagnosed or suspected, or if predisposition to renal failure secondary to rhabdomyolysis. Less effective with homozygous familial hypercholesterolemia. Caution with heavy alcohol use and/or history of hepatic disease. Evaluate if endocrine dysfunction develops.
ADVERSE REACTIONS: Dyspepsia, abdominal pain, headache, nausea, diarrhea, abnormal LFTs, myalgia, flu-like symptoms.
INTERACTIONS: Rifampicin significantly decreases serum levels. Increases levels of glyburide, diclofenac, and phenytoin. Increase serum levels with glyburide, phenytoin, cimetidine, ranitidine, and omeprazole. Caution with drugs that decrease levels of endogenous steroid hormones (eg, ketoconazole, spironolactone, cimetidine). Avoid fibrates. Cyclosporine, gemfibrozil, erythromycin, or niacin may increase risk of myopathy/rhabdomyolysis. Cholestyramine given within 4 hrs decreases serum levels but has additive effects when given 4 hrs after fluvastatin (immediate-release). Monitor digoxin, anticoagulants.
PREGNANCY: Category X, not for use in nursing.

Levbid RX
hyoscyamine sulfate (Schwarz)

OTHER BRAND NAMES: Levsin (Schwarz) - Levsinex (Schwarz)
THERAPEUTIC CLASS: Anticholinergic

INDICATIONS: Adjunct treatment of peptic ulcer, irritable bowel syndrome, neurogenic bladder, and neurogenic bowel disturbances. Management of functional intestinal disorders (eg, mild dysenteries, diverticulitis). To control gastric secretion, visceral spasm, and hypermotility in spastic colitis, spastic bladder, cystitis, pylorospasm, and associated abdominal cramps. Symptomatic relief of biliary and renal colic with concomitant morphine or other narcotics. "Drying agent" for symptomatic relief of acute rhinitis. To reduce rigidity and tremors of Parkinson's disease and control associated sialorrhea and hyperhidrosis. For anticholinesterase poisoning. To reduce pain and hypersecretion in pancreatitis. For certain cases of partial heart block associated with vagal activity. (Elixir, Drops) Treatment of infant colic. (Inj) Facilitates GI diagnostic procedures. In anesthesia as a pre-op antimuscarinic. In urology to improve radiologic visibility of kidneys.

DOSAGE: *Adults:* May also chew or swallow SL tab. (Drops, Eli, Tab, and Tab, SL) 0.125-0.25mg q4h or prn. Max: 1.5mg/24hrs. (Cap and Tab, Extended Release) 0.375-0.75mg q12h; or 1 cap q8h. Max: 1.5mg/24hrs. Do not crush or chew. (Inj) GI Disorders: 0.25-0.5mg IM/IV/SQ as single dose or up to qid at 4 hr intervals. Diagnostic Procedures: 0.25-0.5mg IV 5-10 minutes before procedure. Anesthesia: 5mcg/kg IM/IV/SQ 30-60 minutes before anesthesia or with narcotic/sedative administration. Drug-Induced Bradycardia (Surgery): Increments of 0.25mL IV; repeat prn. Neuromuscular Blockade Reversal: 0.2mg for every 1mg neostigmine or equal dose of physostigmine or pyridostigmine.

Pediatrics: May also chew or swallow SL tab. ≥12 yrs: (Drops, Eli, Tab, and Tab, SL) 0.125-0.25mg q4h or prn. Max: 1.5mg/24hrs. (Cap and Tab, Extended Release) 0.375-0.75mg q12h; or 1 cap may be given q8h. Max: 1.5mg/24hrs. Do not crush or chew. 2 to <12 yrs: (Tab and Tab, SL) 0.0625-0.125mg q4h or prn. Max: 0.75mg/24hrs. (Eli) Give q4h or prn. 10kg: 1.25mL. 20kg: 2.5mL. 40kg: 3.75mL. 50kg: 5mL. Max: 30mL/24hrs. (Drops) 0.25-1mL q4h or prn. Max: 6mL/24 hrs. <2 yrs: (Drops) Give q4h or prn. 3.4kg: 4 drops. Max: 24 drops/24hrs. 5kg: 5 drops. Max: 30 drops/24hrs. 7kg: 6 drops. Max: 36 drops/24hrs. 10kg: 8 drops. Max: 48 drops/24hrs. >2 yrs: Anesthesia: (Inj) 5mcg/kg IM/IV/SQ 30-60 minutes before anesthesia or with narcotic/sedative administration.

HOW SUPPLIED: (Levbid) Tab, Extended Release: 0.375mg*. (Levsin) Drops: 0.125mg/mL (15mL); Elixir: 0.125mg/5mL (473mL); Inj: 0.5mg/mL; Tab: 0.125mg*; Tab, SL: 0.125mg*. (Levsinex) Cap, Extended Release: 0.375mg *scored

CONTRAINDICATIONS: Glaucoma, obstructive uropathy, GI tract obstruction, paralytic ileus; intestinal atony of elderly/debilitated, unstable cardiovascular status in acute hemorrhage, toxic megacolon complicating ulcerative colitis, myasthenia gravis.

WARNINGS/PRECAUTIONS: Risk of heat prostration with high environmental temperature. Avoid activities requiring mental alertness. Psychosis has been reported. Caution with diarrhea, autonomic neuropathy, hyperthyroidism, coronary heart disease, CHF, arrhythmias/tachycardia, HTN, renal disease, and hiatal hernia associated with reflux esophagitis.

ADVERSE REACTIONS: Anticholinergic effects, drowsiness, headache, nervousness.

INTERACTIONS: Additive effects with other antimuscarinics, amantadine, haloperidol, phenothiazines, MAOIs, TCAs, and some antihistamines. Antacids interfere with absorption; take ac and antacids pc.

PREGNANCY: Category C, caution in nursing.

LEVEMIR
RX
insulin detemir, rDNA origin (Novo Nordisk)

THERAPEUTIC CLASS: Insulin

INDICATIONS: Treatment of adults and pediatrics with type 1 diabetes or adults with type 2 diabetes who require basal (long acting) insulin for the control of hyperglycemia.

DOSAGE: *Adults:* Individualize dose. Administer SQ qd or bid. Once-Daily Dosing: Administer with evening meal or bedtime. Twice-Daily Dosing: Administer evening dose with evening meal, at bedtime, or 12 hrs after morning dose. Type 1/Type 2 Diabetes on Basal-Bolus Treatment or Patients Only on Basal Insulin: Change on a unit-to-unit basis. Insulin-Naive with Type 2 Diabetes Inadequately Controlled on Oral Antidiabetics: Initial: 0.1-0.2 U/kg in evening or 10 U qd or bid.

LEVOTHROID

Pediatrics: Individualize dose. Administer SQ qd or bid. Once-Daily Dosing: Administer with evening meal or bedtime. Twice-Daily Dosing: Administer evening dose with evening meal, at bedtime, or 12 hrs after morning dose. Type 1 Diabetes on Basal-Bolus Treatment or Patients Only on Basal Insulin: Change on a unit-to-unit basis.

HOW SUPPLIED: Inj: 100 U/mL (3mL, 10mL)

WARNINGS/PRECAUTIONS: Monitor glucose; may cause hypoglycemia. Not for use in an insulin infusion pump. Should not be diluted or mixed with any other insulin preparations. May cause lipodystrophy or hypersensitivity. Dose adjustment may be needed in renal or hepatic impairment and during intercurrent conditions such as illness, emotional distrubances, or other stresses.

ADVERSE REACTIONS: Allergic reactions, injection site reactions, lipodystrophy, pruritus, rash, hypoglycemia, weight gain.

INTERACTIONS: Avoid mixing with other insulins. Increased glucose lowering effects with ACE inhibitors, disopyramide, fibrates, fluoxetine, MAOIs, propoxyphene, salicylates, somatostatin analog, sulfonamide antibiotics, and other antidiabetic agents. Decreased blood glucose lowering effects with corticosteroids, danazol, diuretics, sympathomimetic agents, isoniazid, phenothiazine derivates, somatotropin, thyroid hormones, estrogens, progestogens. Pentamidine may cause hypoglycemia, followed by hyperglycemia. β-blockers, clonidine, lithium salts, and alcohol may potentiate or weaken glucose lowering effect. β-blockers, clonidine, guanethidine, and reserpine may reduce or mask signs of hypoglycemia.

PREGNANCY: Category C, caution in nursing.

LEVOTHROID
levothyroxine sodium (Forest)

RX

THERAPEUTIC CLASS: Thyroid replacement hormone

INDICATIONS: Hypothyroidism. As a pituitary TSH suppressant for nonendemic goiter and for chronic lymphocytic thyroiditis. Diagnostic agent in suppression tests to differentiate mild hyperthyroidism or thyroid gland autonomy. Adjunct therapy with antithyroid drugs to treat thyrotoxicosis. Adjunct to surgery and radioiodine therapy for TSH-dependent thyroid cancer.

DOSAGE: *Adults:* Hypothyroidism: Usual: 100-200mcg/day. Endocrine/Cardiovascular Complications: Initial: 50mcg/day. Titrate: Increase by 50mcg/day every 2-4 weeks until euthyroid. Hypothyroid with Angina: Initial: 25mcg/day. Titrate: Increase by 25-50mcg every 2-4 weeks until euthyroid.
Pediatrics: Hypothyroidism: >12 yrs: Usual: 100-200mcg/day. 6-12 yrs: 4-5mcg/kg/day. 1-5 yrs: 5-6mcg/kg/day. 6-12 months: 6-8mcg/kg/day. 0-6 months: 10-15mcg/kg/day. May crush tab and sprinkle over food (applesauce) or mix with 5-10mL water, formula (non-soy), or breast milk.

HOW SUPPLIED: Tab: 25mcg*, 50mcg*, 75mcg*, 88mcg*, 100mcg*, 112mcg*, 125mcg*, 137mcg*, 150mcg*, 175mcg*, 200mcg*, 300mcg* *scored

CONTRAINDICATIONS: Untreated thyrotoxicosis, acute MI, and uncorrected adrenal insufficiency.

WARNINGS/PRECAUTIONS: Do not use in the treatment of obesity; larger doses in euthyroid patients can cause serious or even life threatening toxicity. Caution with cardiovascular disease, HTN. May aggravate diabetes mellitus or insipidus and adrenal cortical insufficiency. Excessive doses in infants may produce craniosynostosis. Add glucocorticoid with myxedema coma.

ADVERSE REACTIONS: Lactose hypersensitivity, transient partial hair loss in children.

INTERACTIONS: Monitor insulin and oral hypoglycemic requirements. May potentiate anticoagulant effects of warfarin; adjust warfarin dose and monitor PT/INR. Increased adrenergic effects of catecholamines; caution with CAD. Decreased absorption with cholestyramine and colestipol; space dosing by 4-5 hrs. Estrogens increase thyroxine-binding globulin; increase in thyroid dose may be needed. Large dose may cause life-threatening toxicities with sympathomimetic amines. Avoid mixing crushed tabs with foods/formula with large amounts of iron, soybean or fiber.

PREGNANCY: Category A, caution in nursing.

LEVOXYL
levothyroxine sodium (King)

RX

THERAPEUTIC CLASS: Thyroid replacement hormone

INDICATIONS: Hypothyroidism. As a pituitary TSH suppressant in the treatment and prevention of euthyroid goiters, including thyroid nodules, lymphocytic thyroiditis, and multinodular goiter. Adjunct to surgery and radioiodine therapy for thyrotropin-dependent well-differentiated thyroid cancer.

DOSAGE: *Adults:* Take in the AM at least one-half hour before food. Hypothyroid: Usual: 1.7mcg/kg/day. >200mcg/day (seldom). >50 yrs/<50 yrs with Cardiac Disease: Initial: 25-50mcg/day. Titrate: Increase by 12.5-25mcg/day every 6-8 weeks until euthyroid. Elderly with Cardiac Disease: Initial: 12.5-25mcg/day. Titrate: Increase by 12.5-25mcg/day every 4-6 weeks until euthyroid. Severe Hypothyroidism: Initial: 12.5-25mcg/day. Titrate: Increase by 25mcg/day every 2-4 weeks until euthyroid. Pregnancy: May increase dose requirements. Subclinical Hypothyroidism: Lower doses required.

Pediatrics: Take in the AM at least one-half hour before food. Hypothyroidism: 0-3 months: 10-15mcg/kg/day. 3-6 months: 8-10mcg/kg/day. 6-12 months: 6-8mcg/kg/day. 1-5 yrs: 5-6mcg/kg/day. 6-12 yrs: 4-5mcg/kg/day. >12 yrs: 2-3mcg/kg/day. Growth/Puberty Complete: 1.7mcg/kg/day. Cardiac Risk: Initial: Use lower dose. Titrate: Increase dose every 4-6 weeks until euthyroid. Infants with Serum T_4 <5mcg/dL: Initial: 50mcg/day. Chronic/Severe Hypothyroidism: Children: Initial: 25mcg/day. Titrate: Increase by 25mcg/day every 2-4 weeks until desired effect. Minimize Hyperactivity in Older Children: Initial: Give 1/4 of full replacement dose. Titrate: Increase by same amount weekly until full dose achieved. May crush tab and mix with 5-10mL water.

HOW SUPPLIED: Tab: 25mcg*, 50mcg*, 75mcg*, 88mcg*, 100mcg*, 112mcg*, 125mcg*, 137mcg*, 150mcg*, 175mcg*, 200mcg*, 300mcg* *scored

CONTRAINDICATIONS: Untreated thyrotoxicosis, acute MI, and uncorrected adrenal insufficiency.

WARNINGS/PRECAUTIONS: Do not use in the treatment of obesity; larger doses in euthyroid patients can cause serious or even life threatening toxicity. Caution with cardiovascular disease, CAD, adrenal insufficiency, and the elderly with risk of occult cardiac disease. Carefully titrate dose to avoid over or under treatment. Decreased bone mineral density with long term use. Caution with nontoxic diffuse goiter or nodular thyroid disease. With adrenal insufficiency supplement with glucocorticoids before therapy.

ADVERSE REACTIONS: Pseudotumor cerebri in children reported. Seizures (rare), hypersensitivity reactions, dysphagia, choking, gagging, hyperthyroidism (increased appetite, weight loss, heat intolerance, hyperactivity, tremors, palpitations, tachycardia, diarrhea, vomiting, hair loss).

INTERACTIONS: Sympathomimetics may increase risk of coronary insufficiency with CAD. Upward dose adjustments needed for insulin and oral hypoglycemic agents. Decreased absorption with soybean flour (infant formula), cottonseed meal, walnuts, and fiber. May potentiate oral anticoagulant effects; adjust dose and monitor PT/INR. May decrease levels and effects of digitalis glycosides. Cholestyramine, colestipol, ferrous sulfate, aluminum hydroxide, sodium polystyrene, soybean flour, sucralfate may decrease absorption. Reduced TSH secretion with dopamine/dopamine agonists, glucocorticoids, octreotide. Decreased thyroid hormone secretion with aminoglutethimide, amiodarone, iodine (including iodine-containing radiographic contrast agents), lithium, methimazole, PTU, sulfonamides, tolbutamide. Increased thyroid hormone secretion with amiodarone, iodide (including iodine-containing radiographic contrast agents). Decreased T_4 absorption with antacids (aluminum & magnesium hydroxides), simethicone, bile acid sequestrants (cholestyramine, colestipol), calcium carbonate, cation exchange resins (kayexalate), ferrous sulfate, sucralfate. Increased serum TBG concentration with clofibrate, estrogens, heroin/methadone, 5-FU, mitotane, tamoxifen. Decreased serum TBG concentration with androgens/anabolic steroids, asparaginase, glucocorticoids, nicotinic acid (slow-release). Protein-binding site displacement with furosemide, heparin, hydantoins, NSAIDs, salicylates. Increased hepatic metabolism with carbamazepine, hydantoins, phenobarbital, rifampin. Decreased conversion of T_4 to T_3 levels with amiodarone, β-adrenergic antagonists (propranolol >160mg/day), glucocorticoids (dexamethasone >4mg/day), PTU. Additive effects of both agents with antidepressants. Interferon-(alpha) may cause development of antithyroid microsomal antibodies causing transient hypothyroidism, hyperthyroidism, or both. Interleukin-2 has been associated with transient painless thyroiditis. Excessive use with growth hormones may accelerate epiphyseal closure. Ketamine use may produce marked HTN and tachycardia. May reduce uptake of iodine-containing radiographic contrast agents. Altered levels of thyroid hormone and/or TSH level with choral hydrate, diazepam, ethionamide, lovastatin, metoclopramide, 6-mercaptopurine, nitroprusside, para-aminosalicylate sodium, perphenazine, resorcinol (excessive topical use), thiazide diuretics.

PREGNANCY: Category A, caution in nursing.

LIBRIUM
chlordiazepoxide HCl (Valeant)

CIV

THERAPEUTIC CLASS: Benzodiazepine

INDICATIONS: Management of anxiety disorders and short-term relief of anxiety symptoms, withdrawal symptoms of acute alcoholism, and preoperative apprehension and anxiety.

DOSAGE: *Adults:* Mild-Moderate Anxiety: 5-10mg tid-qid. Severe Anxiety: 20-25mg tid-qid. Alcohol Withdrawal: 50-100mg; repeat until agitation controlled. Max: 300mg/day. Preoperative Anxiety: 5-10mg PO tid-qid on days prior to surgery. Elderly/Debilitated: 5mg bid-qid.
Pediatrics: ≥ 6 yrs: 5mg bid-qid. May increase to 10mg bid-tid.

HOW SUPPLIED: Cap: 5mg, 10mg, 25mg

WARNINGS/PRECAUTIONS: Avoid in pregnancy. Paradoxical reactions reported in psychiatric patients and in hyperactive aggressive pediatrics. Caution with porphyria, renal or hepatic dysfunction. Reduce dose in elderly, debilitated. Avoid abrupt withdrawal after extended therapy.

ADVERSE REACTIONS: Drowsiness, ataxia, confusion, skin eruptions, edema, nausea, constipation, extrapyramidal symptoms, libido changes, EEG changes.

INTERACTIONS: Additive effects with CNS depressants and alcohol. Avoid other psychotropic agents.

PREGNANCY: Not for use in pregnancy, safety in nursing not known.

LIDEX
fluocinonide (Medicis)

RX

OTHER BRAND NAME: Lidex-E (Medicis)

THERAPEUTIC CLASS: Corticosteroid

INDICATIONS: Corticosteroid responsive dermatoses.

DOSAGE: *Adults:* Apply bid-qid. May use occlusive dressing for psoriasis or recalcitrant conditions; discontinue dressings if infection develops.
Pediatrics: Apply bid-qid. May use occlusive dressing for psoriasis or recalcitrant conditions; discontinue dressings if infection develops.

HOW SUPPLIED: (Lidex) Cre, Gel, Oint: 0.05% (15g, 30g, 60g); Sol: 0.05% (60mL); (Lidex-E) Cre: 0.05% (15g, 30g, 60g)

WARNINGS/PRECAUTIONS: May produce reversible HPA axis suppression, manifestations of Cushing's syndrome, hyperglycemia, and glucosuria. Caution when applied to large surface areas or under occlusive dressings. Use appropriate antifungal or antibacterial agent with dermatological infections; discontinue if infection does not clear. Pediatrics may be more susceptible to systemic toxicity. Avoid eyes. Discontinue if irritation occurs.

ADVERSE REACTIONS: Burning, itching, irritation, dryness, folliculitis, hypertrichosis, acneiform eruptions, hypopigmentation, perioral dermatitis, allergic contact dermatitis, skin maceration, secondary infection, skin atrophy, striae, miliaria.

PREGNANCY: Category C, caution in nursing.

LIDOCAINE OINTMENT
lidocaine (Fougera)

RX

THERAPEUTIC CLASS: Acetamide local anesthetic

INDICATIONS: Topical anesthesia of the oropharynx. Anesthetic lubricant for intubation. Temporary relief of pain associated with minor burns, abrasions, and insect bites.

DOSAGE: *Adults:* Apply up to 5g (6 inches)/application. Max: 17-20g/day.
Pediatrics: Determine dose by age and weight. Max: 4.5mg/kg.

HOW SUPPLIED: Oint: 5% (35g)

WARNINGS/PRECAUTIONS: Reduce dose in elderly, debilitated, acutely ill, and children. Avoid excessive dosage or too frequent administration; may result in serious adverse effects requiring resuscitative measures. Caution with heart block and severe shock. Extreme caution if mucosa is traumatized or sepsis is present in the area of application; risk of rapid systemic absorption.

ADVERSE REACTIONS: Lightheadedness, nervousness, confusion, euphoria, dizziness, drowsiness, blurred vision, tremors, convulsions, respiratory depression, bradycardia, hypotension, urticaria, edema, anaphylactoid reactions.

PREGNANCY: Category B, caution in nursing.

LINCOCIN   RX
lincomycin HCl (Pharmacia & Upjohn)

> Diarrhea, colitis, pseudomembranous colitis reported; may begin up to several weeks after discontinuation. Reserve for serious infections where less toxic antimicrobials are inappropriate.

THERAPEUTIC CLASS: *Streptomyces lincolnensis* derivative

INDICATIONS: Treatment of serious infections due to streptococci, pneumococci, and staphylococci. Reserve for PCN allergy or if PCN is inappropriate.

DOSAGE: *Adults:* IM: Serious Infection: 600mg q24h. More Severe Infection: 600mg q12h or more often. IV: Dose depends on severity. Serious Infection: 600mg-1g q8-12h. More Severe Infection: Increase dose. Infuse over ≥1 hr. Life-Threatening Situation: Up to 8g/day has been given. Max: 8g/day. Severe Renal Dysfunction: 25-30% of normal dose.
Pediatrics: >1 month: IM: Serious Infection: 10mg/kg q24h. More Severe Infection: 10mg/kg q12h or more often. IV: 10-20mg/kg/day, depending on severity infused in divided doses as described for adults. Severe Renal Dysfunction: 25-30% of normal dose.

HOW SUPPLIED: Inj: 300mg/mL

CONTRAINDICATIONS: Clindamycin hypersensitivity.

WARNINGS/PRECAUTIONS: May be inadequate for meningitis treatment. Contains benzyl alcohol. Monitor elderly for change in bowel frequency. Caution with severe renal/hepatic dysfunction, or with history of GI disease (eg, colitis), asthma, significant allergies. Superinfections may occur. Perform periodic CBC, LFTs, and renal function tests with prolonged therapy. Do not administer undiluted as IV bolus. Cardiopulmonary arrest and hypotension with too rapid IV administration.

ADVERSE REACTIONS: Glossitis, stomatitis, nausea, vomiting, diarrhea, colitis, pruritus, blood dyscrasias, hypersensitivity reactions, rash, urticaria, vaginitis, tinnitus, vertigo.

INTERACTIONS: Caution with neuromuscular blockers; may enhance effects. Possible antagonism with erythromycin; avoid concomitant use. Kaolin-pectin inhibits oral lincomycin.

PREGNANCY: Category C, not for use in nursing.

LINDANE   RX
lindane (Alpharma)

> Only for patients who are intolerant or have failed 1st-line therapy with safer agents. Seizures and deaths reported with repeat or prolonged use. Caution in infants, children, elderly, those with other skin conditions, and those <50kg due to increased risk of neurotoxicity. Contraindicated in premature infants or those with uncontrolled seizure disorders. Instruct patients on proper use and inform that itching occurs after successful killing of scabies or lice.

THERAPEUTIC CLASS: Ectoparasiticide/ovicide

INDICATIONS: (Lot) Treatment of *Sarcoptes scabiei* (scabies) resistant to other therapies. (Shampoo) Treatment of head and pubic lice resistant to or if intolerant to other therapies.

LIPITOR

DOSAGE: *Adults:* (Lot) Apply 1-2oz to dry skin; rub in thoroughly. Apply to whole body from neck down. Wash off after 8-12 hrs. Apply only once. (Shampoo) Wash and dry hair with regular shampoo. Apply Lindane to hair without water. Add water after 4 minutes; lather then rinse immediately. Towel briskly. Remove nits with comb or tweezers. Use 1oz for short hair, 1.5oz for medium length hair, and 2oz for long hair. Max: 2oz/application. Retreat if lice remain after 7 days.

Pediatrics: (Lot) Apply (≥6 yrs) 1-2oz or 1oz (<6 yrs) to dry skin; rub in thoroughly. Apply to whole body from neck down. Wash off after 8-12 hrs. Apply only once. (Shampoo) Wash and dry hair with regular shampoo. Apply Lindane to hair without water. Add water after 4 minutes; lather then rinse immediately. Towel briskly. Remove nits with comb or tweezers. Use 1oz for short hair, 1.5oz for medium length hair, and 2oz for long hair. Max: 2oz/application. Retreat if lice remain after 7 days.

HOW SUPPLIED: Lot, Shampoo: 1% (60mL, 480mL)

CONTRAINDICATIONS: Premature infants, Norwegian (crusted) scabies, skin conditions (eg, atopic dermatitis, psoriasis) that increase systemic absorption of the drug, uncontrolled seizure disorders.

WARNINGS/PRECAUTIONS: Adverse events with serious outcomes reported. Caution in those at increased risk of seizure (eg, HIV, head trauma, prior seizure, CNS tumor, severe hepatic cirrhosis, excessive alcohol use, abrupt alchol or sedative withdrawal). Give Medication Guide to each patient when dispensing. Avoid eyes and mouth. Do not use with open wounds, cuts, or scores. Use rubber gloves to apply.

ADVERSE REACTIONS: CNS stimulation, dizziness, convulsions.

INTERACTIONS: Avoid creams, ointments, oils, oil based hair dressings or conditioners; may enhance absorption. Caution with drugs that may lower seizure threshold (eg, antipsychotics, antidepressants, theophylline, cyclosporine, mycophenolate, tacrolimus, penicillins, imipenem, quinolones, chloroquine sulfate, pyrimethamine, isoniazid, meperidine, radiographic contrast agents, centrally active anticholinesterases, methocarbamol).

PREGNANCY: Category C, not for use in nursing.

LIPITOR RX
atorvastatin calcium (Parke-Davis/Pfizer)

THERAPEUTIC CLASS: HMG-CoA reductase inhibitor

INDICATIONS: Adjunct to diet, to reduce total cholesterol (total-C), LDL-C, TG, and Apo B levels, and to increase HDL-C in primary hypercholesterolemia (heterozygous familial and nonfamilial) and mixed dyslipidemia (Types IIa and IIb). Adjunct to diet for elevated serum TG levels (Type IV). Treatment of primary dysbetalipoproteinemia (Type III) inadequately responding to diet. Adjunct to other lipid-lowering treatments or if treatments are unavailable, to reduce total-C and LDL-C in homozygous familial hypercholesterolemia. Adjunct to diet to lower total-C, LDL-C and apolipoprotein B in postmenarchal adolescents with heterozygous familial hypercholesterolemia. To reduce the risk of MI, revascularization procedures, and angina in adults without clinically evident CHD but with multiple risk factors for CHD. To reduce the risk of MI and stroke in patients with Type II DM, and without clinically evident CHD, but with multiple risk factors for CHD. In patients with clinically evident CHD to reduce the risk of non-fatal MI, fatal and non-fatal stroke, revascularization procedures, hospitalization for CHF, and angina.

DOSAGE: *Adults:* Hypercholesterolemia/Mixed Dyslipidemia: Initial: 10-20mg qd (or 40mg qd for LDL-C reduction >45%). Titrate: Adjust dose if needed at 2-4 week intervals. Usual: 10-80mg qd. Homozygous Familial Hypercholesterolemia: 10-80mg qd.

Pediatrics: Heterozygous Familial Hypercholesterolemia: 10-17 yrs (postmenarchal): Initial: 10mg/day. Titrate: Adjust dose if needed at intervals of ≥4 weeks. Max: 20mg/day.

HOW SUPPLIED: Tab: 10mg, 20mg, 40mg, 80mg

CONTRAINDICATIONS: Active liver disease, unexplained persistent elevations of serum transaminases, pregnancy, nursing mothers.

WARNINGS/PRECAUTIONS: Monitor LFTs prior to therapy, at 12 weeks or with dose elevation, and periodically thereafter. Reduce dose or withdraw if AST or ALT ≥3x ULN persist. Caution with heavy alcohol use and/or history of hepatic disease. D/C if markedly elevated CPK levels occur, if myopathy is diagnosed or suspected, or if predisposition to renal failure secondary to rhabdomyolysis. Caution in patients with recent stroke or TIA.

ADVERSE REACTIONS: Constipation, flatulence, dyspepsia, abdominal pain, transaminase and CK elevation in higher doses.

INTERACTIONS: Increases levels with erythromycin. Increases levels of oral contraceptives (norethindrone, ethinyl estradiol), digoxin. Monitor digoxin. Cyclosporine, fibric acid derivatives, niacin, erythromycin, and azole antifungals may increase risk of myopathy. Caution with drugs that decrease levels or activity of endogenous steroid hormones (eg, ketoconazole, spironolactone, cimetidine). Decreases levels with Maalox TC, but LDL-C reduction not altered. Colestipol decreases levels when coadministered, but greater LDL-C reduction with coadministration than when each given alone. Avoid fibrates.

PREGNANCY: Category X, not for use in nursing.

Lithium Carbonate RX
lithium carbonate (Roxane)

> Lithium toxicity is related to serum lithium levels and can occur at doses close to therapeutic levels.

THERAPEUTIC CLASS: Antimanic agents

INDICATIONS: Treatment of manic episodes of bipolar disorder and maintenance treatment of bipolar disorder.

DOSAGE: *Adults:* Acute Mania: 600mg tid to achieve effective serum levels of 1-1.5mEq/L; monitor levels twice a week until stabilized. Maint: 300mg tid-qid to maintain serum levels of 0.6-1.2 mEq/L; monitor levels every 2 months. Elderly: Reduce dose.
Pediatrics: ≥12 yrs: Acute Mania: 600mg tid. Effective serum levels are 1-1.5mEq/L; monitor levels twice a week until stabilized. Maint: 300mg tid-qid to maintain serum levels of 0.6-1.2mEq/L; monitor levels every 2 months.

HOW SUPPLIED: Cap: 150mg, 300mg, 600mg; Tab: 300mg

CONTRAINDICATIONS: Renal or cardiovascular disease, severe debilitation or dehydration, sodium depletion, and diuretic use.

WARNINGS/PRECAUTIONS: May cause fetal harm; if possible withdraw for at least the 1st trimester of pregnancy. Caution in the elderly. Maintain normal diet, adequate salt/fluid intake. Assess kidney function prior to and during therapy. May impair mental/physical abilities. Reduce dose or d/c with sweating, diarrhea, infection with elevated temperatures. Caution with thyroid disorders; monitor thyroid function. Chronic therapy associated with diminution of renal concentrating ability (eg, diabetes insipidus), glomerular and interstitial fibrosis, and nephron atrophy.

ADVERSE REACTIONS: Fine hand tremor, polyuria, mild thirst, nausea, incoordination, diarrhea, vomiting, drowsiness, muscular weakness.

INTERACTIONS: Risk of encephalopathic syndrome (eg, weakness, lethargy, fever, tremulousness, confusion, EPS) with haloperidol and other antipsychotics; discontinue therapy if such signs occur. May prolong effects of neuromuscular blockers. Increased levels with indomethacin, piroxicam and other NSAIDs. Increased risk of toxicity due to decreased clearance with diuretics and ACE inhibitors; contraindicated with diuretics.

PREGNANCY: Category D, not for use in nursing.

Lithobid RX
lithium carbonate (JDS)

> Lithium toxicity is related to serum levels, and can occur at doses close to therapeutic levels.

THERAPEUTIC CLASS: Antimanic agent

INDICATIONS: Treatment of manic episodes of manic-depressive illness.

DOSAGE: *Adults:* Acute Mania: Initial: 900mg bid or 600mg tid to achieve effective serum levels of 1-1.5mEq/L; monitor levels twice weekly until stabilized. Maint: 900-1200mg/day, given bid-tid to maintain serum levels of 0.6-1.2mEq/L; monitor levels every 2 months.

LIVOSTIN

Pediatrics: ≥12 yrs: Acute Mania: Initial: 900mg bid or 600mg tid to achieve effective serum levels of 1-1.5mEq/L; monitor levels twice weekly until stabilized. Maint: 900-1200mg/day, given bid-tid to maintain serum levels of 0.6-1.2 mEq/L; monitor levels every 2 months.

HOW SUPPLIED: Tab, Extended Release: 300mg

WARNINGS/PRECAUTIONS: Avoid with significant renal or cardiovascular disease, severe debilitation, dehydration, or sodium depletion. Assess kidney function prior to and during therapy. Risk of encephalopathic syndrome (eg, weakness, lethargy, fever, tremulousness, confusion, EPS); discontinue therapy. May impair mental/physical abilities. Reduce dose or discontinue with sweating, diarrhea, infection with elevated temperatures. Caution with hypothyroidism; may need supplemental therapy. Chronic therapy associated with diminution of renal concentrating ability, glomerular and interstitial fibrosis, and nephron atrophy.

ADVERSE REACTIONS: Fine hand tremor, polyuria, mild thirst, nausea, general discomfort, diarrhea, vomiting, drowsiness, muscular weakness.

INTERACTIONS: Avoid diuretics and ACE inhibitors; risk of lithium toxicity due to reduced renal clearance. May prolong effects of neuromuscular blockers. Decreased levels with acetazolamide, urea, xanthine preparations, and alkalinizing agents. May produce hypothyroidism with iodide preparations. Increased plasma levels with indomethacin, piroxicam, other NSAIDs. Increased risk of neurotoxic effects with carbamazepine and calcium channel blockers. Reduced renal clearance with metronidazole. Fluoxetine may increase and/or decrease lithium levels.

PREGNANCY: Category D, not for use in nursing.

LIVOSTIN   RX
levocabastine HCl (Novartis Ophthalmics)

THERAPEUTIC CLASS: H_1 antagonist

INDICATIONS: Relief of signs and symptoms of seasonal allergic conjunctivitis.

DOSAGE: *Adults:* 1 drop qid.

Pediatrics: ≥12 yrs: 1 drop qid.

HOW SUPPLIED: Sus: 0.05% (5mL, 10mL)

CONTRAINDICATIONS: Do not use while wearing soft contact lenses.

WARNINGS/PRECAUTIONS: For topical use only.

ADVERSE REACTIONS: Transient stinging/burning, headache.

PREGNANCY: Category C, safety in nursing not known.

LOCOID   RX
hydrocortisone butyrate (Ferndale)

THERAPEUTIC CLASS: Corticosteroid

INDICATIONS: (Cre, Oint) Corticosteroid responsive dermatoses. (Sol) Seborrheic dermatitis.

DOSAGE: *Adults:* (Cre, Oint) Apply bid-tid. May use occlusive dressings for psoriasis or recalcitrant conditions. D/C dressings if infection develops. (Sol) Apply bid-tid.

Pediatrics: (Cre, Oint) Apply bid-tid. May use occlusive dressings for psoriasis or recalcitrant conditions. D/C dressings if infection develops. (Sol) Apply bid-tid.

HOW SUPPLIED: Cre, Oint: 0.1% (15g, 45g); Sol: 0.1% (20mL, 60mL)

WARNINGS/PRECAUTIONS: May produce reversible HPA axis suppression, manifestations of Cushing's syndrome, hyperglycemia, and glucosuria. D/C if irritation occurs. Use appropriate antifungal or antibacterial agent with dermatological infections. Peds may be more susceptible to systemic toxicity. Caution when applied to large surface areas. Avoid contact with eyes. Limit to least amount compatible with an effective therapeutic regimen. Chronic corticosteroid therapy may interfere with the growth and development of children.

ADVERSE REACTIONS: Burning, itching, irritation, dryness, folliculitis, hypertrichosis, acneiform eruptions, hypopigmentation, perioral dermatitis, allergic dermatitis, skin maceration, secondary infection, skin atrophy, striae, miliaria.

PREGNANCY: Category C, caution in nursing.

LODINE XL
etodolac (Wyeth)

RX

> NSAIDs may cause an increased risk of serious cardiovascular thrombotic events, MI, stroke and serious GI adverse events including bleeding, ulceration, and perforation of the stomach or intestines. Contraindicated for the treatment of peri-operative pain in the setting of coronary artery bypass graft (CABG) surgery.

THERAPEUTIC CLASS: NSAID (pyranocarboxylic acid derivative)

INDICATIONS: Relief of signs and symptoms of osteoarthritis (OA), rheumatoid arthritis (RA), and juvenile rheumatoid arthritis (JRA).

DOSAGE: *Adults:* Usual: 400-1000mg qd. Max: 1200mg/day.

Pediatrics: 6-16 yrs: JRA: >60kg: 1000mg. 46-60kg: 800mg. 31-45kg: 600mg. 20-30kg: 400mg.

HOW SUPPLIED: Tab, Extended Release: 400mg, 500mg, 600mg

CONTRAINDICATIONS: ASA or other NSAID allergy that precipitates asthma, urticaria or allergic reaction. Treatment of peri-operative pain in the setting of CABG surgery.

WARNINGS/PRECAUTIONS: May lead to onset of new HTN or worsening of pre-existing HTN; monitor BP closely. Fluid retention and edema reported; caution with fluid retention or heart failure. Renal papillary necrosis and other renal injury reported after long-term use. Not recommended for use with advanced renal disease; if therapy must be initiated, monitor renal function. Anaphylactoid reactions may occur. May cause serious skin adverse events (eg, exfoliative dermatitis, Stevens-Johnson syndrome, and toxic epidermal necrolysis). Avoid in late pregnancy; may cause premature closure of ductus arteriosis. May cause elevations of LFTs; d/c if liver disease develops or systemic manifestations occur. Caution in elderly. Anemia may occur; with long-term use, monitor Hgb/Hct if signs or symptoms of anemia develop. May inhibit platelet aggregation and prolong bleeding time; monitor with coagulation disorders. Caution with asthma and avoid with aspirin-sensitive asthma.

ADVERSE REACTIONS: Dyspepsia, abdominal pain, diarrhea, flatulence, nausea, constipation, vomiting, GI ulcers, gross bleeding/perforation.

INTERACTIONS: May elevate digoxin, lithium, and methotrexate serum levels. May enhance nephrotoxicity associated with cyclosporine. Avoid with phenylbutazone. Increased adverse effect potential with ASA. Caution with warfarin. May decrease antihypertensive effects with ACE inhibitors. May reduce natriuretic effect of furosemide and thiazides.

PREGNANCY: Category C, not for use in nursing.

LODRANE 24
brompheniramine maleate (ECR)

RX

THERAPEUTIC CLASS: Alkylamine Antihistamine

INDICATIONS: Temporary relief of seasonal and perennial allergic rhinitis and vasomotor rhinitis.

DOSAGE: *Adults:* 12-24mg qd.

Pediatrics: ≥12 yrs: 12-24mg qd. 6-12 yrs: 12mg qd.

HOW SUPPLIED: Cap, Extended Release: 12mg

CONTRAINDICATIONS: Nursing mothers, patients taking MAOIs, narrow angle glaucoma, urinary retention, peptic ulcer, and during an asthmatic attack.

WARNINGS/PRECAUTIONS: Caution with HTN, DM, ischemic heart disease, hyperthyroidism, bronchial asthma, increased IOP, prostatic hypertrophy, CVD, and elderly. May impair mental/physical abilities.

LOMOTIL

ADVERSE REACTIONS: Drowsiness, confusion, restlessness, nausea, vomiting, rash, vertigo, palpitation, anorexia, dizziness, headache, insomnia, anxiety, tension, excitability.

INTERACTIONS: See Contraindications. MAOIs and TCA's may prolong and intensify the anticholinergic effects of antihistamines. Concomitant use of antihistamines with alcohol, TCA's, barbiturates, other CNS depressants may have an additive effect.

PREGNANCY: Category C, not for use in nursing.

LOMOTIL
atropine sulfate - diphenoxylate HCl (Pharmacia & Upjohn)

OTHER BRAND NAME: Lonox (Sandoz)
THERAPEUTIC CLASS: Opioid/anticholinergic
INDICATIONS: Adjunctive therapy for management of diarrhea.
DOSAGE: *Adults:* Initial: 2 tabs or 10mL qid. Titrate: Reduce dose after symptoms are controlled. Maint: 2 tabs or 10mL qd. Max: 20mg/day diphenoxylate. Discontinue if symptoms are not controlled after 10 days of max dose 20mg/day (diphenoxylate).
Pediatrics: 2-12 yrs: Initial: 0.3-0.4mg/kg/day of solution given qid. 13-16 yrs: Initial: 2 tabs or 10mL tid. Titrate: Reduce dose after symptoms are controlled. Maint: 25% of initial dose. Discontinue if no improvement within 48 hrs.
HOW SUPPLIED: (Diphenoxylate-Atropine) Sol: 2.5mg-0.025/5mL (60mL); Tab: 2.5mg-0.025mg
CONTRAINDICATIONS: Obstructive jaundice, diarrhea associated with pseudomembranous enterocolitis or enterotoxin-producing bacteria.
WARNINGS/PRECAUTIONS: May induce toxic megacolon in ulcerative colitis; discontinue if abdominal distention occurs. May cause intestinal fluid retention. Avoid use with diarrhea associated with organisms that penetrate the intestinal mucosa, and with pseudomembranous enterocolitis. Caution in pediatrics, especially with Down's syndrome. Extreme caution advanced hepatorenal disease and liver dysfunction. Do not use with severe dehydration or electrolyte imbalance until corrective therapy is initiated.
ADVERSE REACTIONS: Numbness of extremities, dizziness, anaphylaxis, hyperthermia, tachycardia, urinary retention, flushing, drowsiness, toxic megacolon, nausea, vomiting.
INTERACTIONS: May potentiate barbiturates, tranquilizers and alcohol. MAOIs may precipitate hypertensive crisis.
PREGNANCY: Category C, caution in nursing.

LOPROX
ciclopirox (Medicis)

RX

OTHER BRAND NAME: Loprox TS (Medicis)
THERAPEUTIC CLASS: Broad-spectrum antifungal
INDICATIONS: (Cre/Sus) Treatment of dermal infections of tinea pedis, tinea cruris, tinea corporis, cutaneous candidiasis and tinea versicolor. (Gel) Treatment of interdigital tinea pedis and tinea corporis. (Gel/Shampoo) Treatment of seborrheic dermatitis of the scalp.
DOSAGE: *Adults:* (Cre/Gel/Sus) Massage affected and surrounding areas bid (am and pm) up to 4 weeks. (Shampoo) Apply about 5mL (up to 10mL for long hair) to wet scalp. Lather and rinse off after 3 minutes. Repeat twice weekly for 4 weeks, at least 3 days apart.
Pediatrics: ≥10 yrs: (Cre/Sus) Massage affected and surrounding areas bid (am and pm) up to 4 weeks. Gel or Shampoo not recommended in pediatrics <16 yrs.
HOW SUPPLIED: Cre: 0.77% (15g, 30g, 90g); Gel: 0.77% (30g, 45g, 100g); Shampoo: 1% (120mL); Sus: Loprox TS 0.77% (30mL, 60mL)

LOTENSIN

WARNINGS/PRECAUTIONS: Avoid eyes, mucous membranes, occlusive wrappings or dressings. D/C if sensitization or chemical irritation occurs. Hair discoloration reported in patients with lighter hair color.

ADVERSE REACTIONS: Contact dermatitis, pruritus, burning.

PREGNANCY: Pregnancy B, caution in nursing.

LORTAB
acetaminophen - hydrocodone bitartrate (UCB Pharma)

CIII

THERAPEUTIC CLASS: Opioid analgesic

INDICATIONS: Relief of moderate-to-moderately severe pain.

DOSAGE: *Adults:* (2.5/500, 5/500) 1-2 tabs q4-6h prn. Max: 8 tabs/day. (7.5/500, 10/500) 1 tab q4-6h prn. Max: 6 tabs/day. (Sol) 15mL q4-6h prn. Max: 90mL/day.

Pediatrics: ≥2 yrs: (Sol) 12-15kg: 3.75mL. 16-22kg: 5mL. 23-31kg: 7.5mL. 32-45kg: 10mL. ≥46kg: 15mL. May repeat q4-6h prn.

HOW SUPPLIED: (Hydrocodone-APAP) Sol: 7.5mg-500mg/15mL; Tab: 2.5mg-500mg*, 5mg-500mg*, 7.5mg-500mg*, 10mg-500mg* *scored

WARNINGS/PRECAUTIONS: May produce dose-related respiratory depression. May obscure acute abdominal conditions or head injuries. Caution in elderly, debilitated, severe hepatic or renal dysfunction, hypothyroidism, Addison's disease, prostatic hypertrophy, urethral stricture, pulmonary disease, postoperative use. May be habit-forming. Suppresses cough reflex.

ADVERSE REACTIONS: Lightheadedness, dizziness, sedation, nausea, vomiting.

INTERACTIONS: Additive CNS depression with other narcotics, antihistamines, antipsychotics, antianxiety agents, alcohol, CNS depressants. Increased effect of antidepressant or hydrocodone with MAOIs or TCAs.

PREGNANCY: Category C, not for use in nursing.

LOTENSIN
benazepril HCl (Novartis)

RX

> Avoid use in pregnancy, ACE inhibitors can cause injury and even death to the developing fetus. Discontinue when pregnancy is detected.

THERAPEUTIC CLASS: ACE inhibitor

INDICATIONS: Treatment of hypertension.

DOSAGE: *Adults:* If possible, discontinue diuretic 2-3 days prior to therapy. Initial: 10mg qd, 5mg with concomitant diuretic. Maint: 20-40mg/day given qd-bid. Resume diuretic if BP not controlled. Max: 80mg/day. CrCl <30mL/min: Initial: 5mg qd. Max: 40mg/day.

Pediatrics: ≥6 yrs: Initial: 0.2mg/kg qd. Max: 0.6mg/kg.

HOW SUPPLIED: Tab: 5mg, 10mg, 20mg, 40mg

WARNINGS/PRECAUTIONS: Discontinue if angioedema, jaundice, or if marked LFT elevation occurs. Risk of hyperkalemia with DM, renal dysfunction. Persistent nonproductive cough reported. Monitor WBCs in renal and collagen vascular disease. Anaphylactoid reactions reported. Fetal/neonatal morbidity and death reported. Monitor for hypotension in high risk patients (eg, surgery/anesthesia, prolonged diuretic therapy, heart failure, volume and/or salt depletion, etc). Caution with CHF, renal dysfunction, and renal artery stenosis. Less effective on BP in blacks and more reports of angioedema than nonblacks.

ADVERSE REACTIONS: Cough, dizziness, headache, fatigue, somnolence, postural dizziness, nausea.

INTERACTIONS: May increase lithium levels. Hypotension risk with diuretics. Increase risk of hyperkalemia with K^+-sparing diuretics, K^+-containing salt substitutes, or K^+ supplements.

PREGNANCY: Category C (1st trimester) and D (2nd and 3rd trimesters), not for use in nursing.

LOTRIMIN
clotrimazole (Schering) — RX

THERAPEUTIC CLASS: Azole antifungal
INDICATIONS: Topical treatment of candidiasis caused by *Candida albicans* and tinea versicolor caused by *Malassezia furfur*.
DOSAGE: *Adults:* Apply bid (am and pm). Re-evaluate if no improvement after 4 weeks.
Pediatrics: Apply bid (am and pm). Re-evaluate if no mprovement after 4 weeks.
HOW SUPPLIED: Cre: 1% (15g, 30g, 45g); Lot: 1% (30mL); Sol: 1% (10mL, 30mL)
WARNINGS/PRECAUTIONS: Discontinue if irritation or sensitivity occurs. Not for opthalmic use.
ADVERSE REACTIONS: Erythema, stinging, blistering, peeling, edema, pruritus, urticaria, burning, irritation.
PREGNANCY: Category B, caution in nursing.

LOTRIMIN AF
clotrimazole (Schering) — OTC

THERAPEUTIC CLASS: Azole antifungal
INDICATIONS: Tinea pedis, t.cruris, t.corporis.
DOSAGE: *Adults:* Cleanse skin with soap and water and dry thoroughly. Apply to affected area am and pm. Athlete's Foot and Ringworm: Treat for 4 weeks. Jock Itch: Treat for 2 weeks.
Pediatrics: ≥2 yrs: Cleanse skin with soap and water and dry thoroughly. Apply to affected area am and pm. Athlete's Foot and Ringworm: Treat for 4 weeks. Jock Itch: Treat for 2 weeks.
HOW SUPPLIED: Cre: 1% (24g); Lot: 1% (20mL); Sol: 1% (10mL)
WARNINGS/PRECAUTIONS: Discontinue if irritation occurs or no improvement in 4 weeks (t.pedis or t. corporis) or 2 weeks (t. cruris). Avoid eye contact. Not effective on scalp or nails.
PREGNANCY: Safety in pregnancy and nursing not known.

LOTRIMIN AF SPRAY & POWDER
miconazole nitrate (Schering) — OTC

THERAPEUTIC CLASS: Azole antifungal
INDICATIONS: To treat and relieve the itching, cracking, burning, and scaling of athlete's foot (tinea pedis), jock itch, (tinea cruris), and ringworm (tinea corporis). Powder aids in the drying of moist areas.
DOSAGE: *Adults:* Cleanse skin with soap and water anc dry thoroughly. (Powder) Sprinkle a thin layer over affected area am and pm. (Spray) Spray a thin layer over affected area am and pm. Athlete's Foot and Ringworm: Treat for 4 weeks. Jock Itch: Treat for 2 weeks.
Pediatrics: ≥2 yrs: Cleanse skin with soap and water and dry thoroughly. (Powder) Sprinkle a thin layer over affected area am and pm. (Spray) Spray a thin layer over affected area am and pm. Athlete's Foot and Ringworm: Treat for 4 weeks. Jock Itch: Treat for 2 weeks.
HOW SUPPLIED: Powder: 2% (90g); Spray, Powder: 2% (100g); Spray: 2% (113g)
WARNINGS/PRECAUTIONS: Avoid eye contact. Discontinue if irritation occurs or no improvement in 4 weeks (athlete's foot or ringworm) or 2 weeks (jock itch). Avoid while smoking or near heat/flame.
PREGNANCY: Safety in pregnancy and nursing not known.

LOTRIMIN ULTRA
butenafine HCl (Schering) — OTC

THERAPEUTIC CLASS: Benzylamine antifungal
INDICATIONS: To cure and relieve itching, cracking, burring, and scaling of athlete's foot (tinea pedis), jock itch, (tinea cruris), and ringworm (tinea corporis).

DOSAGE: *Adults:* Wash and dry area. Tinea Pedis: Apply between toes bid (am and pm) for 1 week, or qd for 4 weeks. Tinea Cruris/Corporis: Apply qd for 2 weeks.
Pediatrics: ≥12 yrs: Wash and dry area. Tinea Pedis: Apply between toes bid (am and pm) for 1 week, or qd for 4 weeks. Tinea Cruris/Corporis: Apply qd for 2 weeks.

HOW SUPPLIED: Cre: 1% (12g)

WARNINGS/PRECAUTIONS: Avoid nails, scalp, mouth, and eyes. Discontinue if too much irritation occurs. Not for vaginal yeast infections. Effectiveness on bottom of foot is unknown.

PREGNANCY: Safety in pregnancy and nursing not known.

LUPRON PEDIATRIC   RX
leuprolide acetate (TAP)

OTHER BRAND NAME: Lupron Depot-Ped (TAP)

THERAPEUTIC CLASS: Synthetic gonadotropin releasing hormone analog

INDICATIONS: Treatment of central precocious puberty.

DOSAGE: *Pediatrics:* Initial: 50mcg/kg/d as single SQ dose or (depot) 0.3mg/kg every 4 weeks (minimum 7.5mg) as single IM dose. Depot Start Dose: ≤25kg: 7.5mg; >25-37.5kg: 11.25mg; >37.5kg: 15mg. Titrate: Increase by 10 mcg/kg/day SQ or (depot) 3.75mg IM every 4 weeks if downregulation not achieved. Maint: Dose that produces adequate downregulation. Verify adequate downregulation with significant weight increase.

HOW SUPPLIED: Inj: 5mg/mL, (Depot) 7.5mg, 11.25mg, 15mg

CONTRAINDICATIONS: Pregnancy.

WARNINGS/PRECAUTIONS: Monitor hormonal effects after 1-2 months of therapy. Measure bone age every 6-12 months. Increase in clinical signs and symptoms may occur in early phase of therapy due to rise in gonadotropins and sex steroids. Discontinue before age 11 in females and age 12 in males.

ADVERSE REACTIONS: Initial exacerbation of signs and symptoms, injection site reactions, pain, acne/seborrhea, rash, urogenital bleeding/discharge, vaginitis.

PREGNANCY: Category X, not for use in nursing.

LURIDE   RX
sodium fluoride (Colgate Oral)

THERAPEUTIC CLASS: Fluoride supplement

INDICATIONS: To prevent dental caries in areas where drinking water fluoride content is <0.6ppm.

DOSAGE: *Pediatrics:* (Drops) <0.3ppm: 6 months-3 yrs: 0.5mL qd. 3-6 yrs: 1mL qd. 6-16 yrs: 2mL qd. 0.3-0.6ppm: 3-6 yrs: 0.5mL qd. 6-16 yrs: 1mL qd. (Tab) <0.3ppm: 6 months-<3 yrs: 0.25mg qd. 3-6 yrs: 0.5mg qd. 6-16 yrs: 1mg qd. 0.3-0.6ppm: 3-6 yrs: 0.25mg qd. 6-16 yrs: 0.5mg qd. Dissolve tab in mouth or chew tab before swallowing. Take at bedtime after brushing teeth.

HOW SUPPLIED: Drops: 0.5mg/mL (50mL); Tab, Chewable: 0.25mg, 0.5mg, 1mg

CONTRAINDICATIONS: (Drips) Areas where drinking water fluoride is >0.6 ppm, pediatrics <6 months. (Tab) 1mg: Water fluoride is >0.3ppm, pediatrics <6 yrs. 0.5mg: Water fluoride is >0.6ppm, pediatrics <6 yrs. 0.25mg: Water fluoride is >0.6ppm.

WARNINGS/PRECAUTIONS: Dental fluorosis may result from daily ingestion of excessive fluoride in pediatrics <6 yrs especially if water fluoride is >0.6ppm.

ADVERSE REACTIONS: Allergic rash.

INTERACTIONS: Do not eat or drink dairy products within 1 hour of administration.

PREGNANCY: Safety in pregnancy not known. Caution in nursing.

LUSTRA   RX
hydroquinone (Taro)

OTHER BRAND NAME: Lustra-AF (Taro)

THERAPEUTIC CLASS: Depigmenting agent

MACROBID

INDICATIONS: Gradual treatment of ultraviolet induced dyschromia and discoloration resulting from use of oral contraceptive, pregnancy, hormone replacement therapy, or skin trauma.

DOSAGE: *Adults:* Apply bid (am and hs). Use sunscreen with Lustra.

Pediatrics: ≥12 yrs: Apply bid (am and hs). Use sunscreen with Lustra.

HOW SUPPLIED: Cre: 4% (56.8g)

WARNINGS/PRECAUTIONS: Avoid sun exposure on bleached skin. Lustra-AF contains sunscreen; use sunscreen with Lustra. May produce unwanted cosmetic effects if not used as directed. Test for skin sensitivity. D/C if no lightening effect after 2 months of therapy, if blue-black darkening of the skin occurs, or if itching, vesicle formation, or excessive inflammatory reactions occur. Contains sodium metabisulfite, may cause serious allergic type reactions. Avoid contact wtih eyes.

ADVERSE REACTIONS: Cutaneous hypersensitivity (contact dermatitis).

PREGNANCY: Category C, caution in nursing.

MACROBID   RX
nitrofurantoin monohydrate (Procter & Gamble)

THERAPEUTIC CLASS: Imidazolidinedione antibacterial

INDICATIONS: Treatment of acute uncomplicated urinary tract infections (acute cystitis).

DOSAGE: *Adults:* 100mg every 12 hrs for 7 days. Take with food.

Pediatrics: >12 yrs: 100mg every 12 hrs for 7 days. Take with food.

HOW SUPPLIED: Cap: 100mg

CONTRAINDICATIONS: Anuria, oliguria, CrCl <60mL/min, pregnancy at term (38-42 weeks gestation), labor and delivery, and neonates <1 month of age.

WARNINGS/PRECAUTIONS: Acute, subacute, or chronic pulmonary reactions have occurred. Anemia, diabetes mellitus, renal dysfunction, electrolyte imbalance, vitamin B deficiency, and debilitating disease enhance occurrence of peripheral neuropathy. Stop therapy with acute and chronic pulmonary reactions, hepatic disorders, hemolysis, or peripheral neuropathy. Monitor renal function, LFTs and pulmonary function periodically during long-term therapy. Optic neuritis and hepatic reactions reported.

ADVERSE REACTIONS: Pulmonary disorders, hepatic damage, peripheral neuropathy, nausea, headache, flatulence, anorexia, diarrhea, dizziness, alopecia, exfoliative dermatitis, Stevens-Johnson syndrome, anaphylaxis, blood dyscrasias, aplastic anemia.

INTERACTIONS: Antacids, especially magnesium trisilicate, decrease rate and extent of absorption. Uricosuric drugs (eg, probenecid and sulfinpyrazone) increase nitrofurantoin levels.

PREGNANCY: Category B, not for use in nursing.

MACRODANTIN   RX
nitrofurantoin macrocrystals (Procter & Gamble)

THERAPEUTIC CLASS: Imidazolidinedione antibacterial

INDICATIONS: Treatment of urinary tract infection.

DOSAGE: *Adults:* 50-100mg qid for at least 7 days. Take with food. Long-term Suppressive Use: 50-100mg at bedtime.

Pediatrics: ≥1 month: 5-7mg/kg/day given qid for at least 7 days. Take with food. Long-term Suppressive Use: 1mg/kg/day given qd-bid.

HOW SUPPLIED: Cap: 25mg, 50mg, 100mg

CONTRAINDICATIONS: Anuria, oliguria, CrCl <60mL/min, pregnancy at term (38-42 weeks gestation), labor and delivery, neonates <1 month of age.

WARNINGS/PRECAUTIONS: Acute, subacute or chronic pulmonary reactions have occurred. Anemia, diabetes mellitus, renal dysfunction, electrolyte imbalance, vitamin B deficiency, and debilitating disease enhance occurrence of peripheral neuropathy.

Stop therapy with acute and chronic pulmonary reactions, hepatic disorders, hemolysis, or peripheral neuropathy. Monitor renal function, LFT's and pulmonary function periodically during long-term therapy. Optic neuritis and hepatic reactions reported.

ADVERSE REACTIONS: Pulmonary disorders, hepatic damage, peripheral neuropathy, nausea, emesis, anorexia, dizziness, alopecia, exfoliative dermatitis, Stevens-Johnson syndrome, anaphylaxis, blood dyscrasias, aplastic anemia.

INTERACTIONS: Antacids, especially magnesium trisilicate, decrease rate and extent of absorption. Uricosuric drugs (eg, probenecid and sulfinpyrazone) increase nitrofurantoin levels.

PREGNANCY: Category B, not for use in nursing

Malarone
atovaquone - proguanil HCl (GlaxoSmithKline)

RX

OTHER BRAND NAME: Malarone Pediatric (GlaxoSmithKline)

THERAPEUTIC CLASS: Pyrimidine synthesis inhibitor

INDICATIONS: Prophylaxis or treatment of malaria caused by P.falciparum.

DOSAGE: *Adults:* Prevention: Begin 1-2 days before entering endemic area, continue during stay and for 7 days after return. 1 tab qd. Treatment: 4 tabs qd for 3 days. Repeat dose if vomiting occurs within 1 hr after dosing. Take as single dose with food or milky drink.

Pediatrics: Prevention: Begin 1-2 days before entering endemic area, continue during stay and for 7 days after return. 11-20kg: 1 pediatric tab qd. 21-30kg: 2 pediatric tabs qd. 31-40kg: 3 pediatric tabs qd. >40kg: Dose as adult. Treatment: Treat for 2 consecutive days. 5-8kg: 2 pediatric tabs qd. 9-10kg: 3 pediatric tabs. 11-20kg: 1 tab qd. 21-30kg: 2 tabs qd. 31-40kg: 3 tabs. >40kg: Dose as adult. Repeat dose if vomiting occurs within 1 hr after dosing. Take as single dose with food or milky drink.

HOW SUPPLIED: (Atovaquone-Proguanil) Tab: 250mg-100mg; Tab, Pediatric: 62.5mg-25mg

CONTRAINDICATIONS: For prophylaxis in severe renal impairment (CrCl <30mL/min).

WARNINGS/PRECAUTIONS: Not for cerebral malaria. Patients with severe malaria are not candidates for oral therapy. Rare cases of anaphylaxis have been reported.

ADVERSE REACTIONS: Vomiting, pruritus, elevation of LFTs.

INTERACTIONS: Rifampin, rifabutin may decrease levels; concomitant use is not recommended. Reduced bioavailability with metoclopramide and tetracycline.

PREGNANCY: Category C, caution in nursing.

Marcaine
bupivacaine HCl (Hospira)

RX

THERAPEUTIC CLASS: Local anesthetic

INDICATIONS: Production of local or regional anesthesia for surgery, dental, or oral surgery procedures, diagnostic and therapeutic procedures, and for obstetrical procedures. Only 0.25% and 0.5% are indicated for obstetrical anesthesia.

DOSAGE: *Adults:* Individualize dose. Dosage varies depending on procedure, area to be anesthetized, vascularity of tissues, number of neural segments to be blocked, depth and duration of anesthesia, degree of muscle relaxation required, and patient tolerance and physical condition. Single Dose Max: 175mg. May repeat once every 3 hrs. Total Daily Dose Max: 400mg. Epidural Anesthesia: 0.5% or 0.75% in 3-5mL increments. In obstetrics, use only 0.25% or 0.5%. Use 3-5mL increments of 0.5% solution not to exceed 50-100mg at any dosing interval. Test dose using 0.5% with 1:200,000 epinephrine recommended prior to caudal and lumbar epidural blocks. Elderly/Debilitated/Cardiac or Liver Disease: Reduce dose.

Pediatrics: ≥12 yrs: Individualize dose. Dosage varies depending on procedure, area to be anesthetized, vascularity of tissues, number of neural segments to be blocked, depth and duration of anesthesia, degree of muscle relaxation required, and patient tolerance and physical condition. Single Dose Max: 175mg. May repeat once every 3 hrs. Total Daily Dose Max: 400mg. Epidural Anesthesia: 0.5% or 0.75% in 3-5mL incre-

MARCAINE WITH EPINEPHRINE

ments. In obstetrics, use only 0.25% or 0.5%. Use 3-5mL increments of 0.5% solution not to exceed 50-100mg at any dosing interval. Test dose using 0.5% with 1:200,000 epinephrine recommended prior to caudal and lumbar epidural blocks.

HOW SUPPLIED: Inj: 0.25%, 0.5%, 0.75%

CONTRAINDICATIONS: Obstetrical paracervical block anesthesia.

WARNINGS/PRECAUTIONS: The 0.75% strength is not recommended for obstetrical anesthesia. Acidosis, cardiac arrest, death reported from delay in toxicity management. Local anesthetic solutions containing antimicrobial preservatives should not be used for epidural or caudal anesthesia. Not recommended for IV regional anesthesia. Monitor cardiovascular and respiratory vital signs and state of consciousness after each injection. Caution with hepatic disease and impaired cardiovascular function. Monitor circulation and respiration with injections into head and neck area. Respiratory arrest following local anesthetic injection during retrobulbar blocks has been reported.

ADVERSE REACTIONS: Restlessness, anxiety, dizziness, tinnitus, blurred vision, tremors, convulsions, nausea, vomiting, chills, hypotension, bradycardia, ventricular arrhythmias, urticaria, pruritus, erythema, edema.

INTERACTIONS: Avoid use with any other local anesthetics.

PREGNANCY: Category C, not for use in nursing.

MARCAINE WITH EPINEPHRINE RX
epinephrine - bupivacaine HCl (Hospira)

THERAPEUTIC CLASS: Local anesthetic

INDICATIONS: Production of local or regional anesthesia for surgery, dental, or oral surgery procedures, diagnostic and therapeutic procedures, and for obstetrical procedures. Only 0.25% and 0.5% are indicated for obstetrical anesthesia.

DOSAGE: *Adults:* Individualize dose. Dosage varies depending on procedure, area to be anesthetized, vascularity of tissues, number of neural segments to be blocked, depth and duration of anesthesia, degree of muscle relaxation required, and patient tolerance and physical condition. Single Dose Max: 225mg. May repeat once every 3 hrs. Total Daily Dose Max: 400mg. Epidural Anesthesia: 0.5% or 0.75% in 3-5mL increments. In obstetrics, use only 0.25% or 0.5%. Use 3-5mL increments of 0.5% solution not to exceed 50-100mg at any dosing interval. Test dose using 0.5% with 1:200,000 epinephrine recommended prior to caudal and lumbar epidural blocks. Dentistry: 0.5% with epinephrine. Average Dose: 1.8mL (9mg) per injection site. May repeat after 2-10 minutes if necessary. Max: 90mg total dose for all sites. Elderly/Debilitated/Cardiac or Liver Disease: Reduce dose.

Pediatrics: ≥12 yrs: Individualize dose. Dosage varies depending on procedure, area to be anesthetized, vascularity of tissues, number of neural segments to be blocked, depth and duration of anesthesia, degree of muscle relaxation required, and patient tolerance and physical condition. Single Dose Max: 225mg. May repeat once every 3 hrs. Total Daily Dose Max: 400mg. Epidural Anesthesia: 0.5% or 0.75% in 3-5mL increments. In obstetrics, use only 0.25% or 0.5%. Use 3-5mL increments of 0.5% solution not to exceed 50-100mg at any dosing interval. Test dose using 0.5% with 1:200,000 epinephrine recommended prior to caudal and lumbar epidural blocks. Dentistry: 0.5% with epinephrine. Average Dose: 1.8mL (9mg) per injection site. May repeat after 2-10 minutes if necessary. Max: 90mg total dose for all sites.

HOW SUPPLIED: Inj: (Bupivacaine-Epinephrine) 0.25%/1:200,000, 0.5%/1:200,000

CONTRAINDICATIONS: Obstetrical paracervical block anesthesia.

WARNINGS/PRECAUTIONS: The 0.75% strength is not recommended for obstetrical anesthesia. Acidosis, cardiac arrest, death reported from delay in toxicity management. Local anesthetic solutions containing antimicrobial preservatives should not be used for epidural or caudal anesthesia. Not recommended for IV regional anesthesia. Bupivacaine with epinephrine solutions contain sodium metabisulfite which may cause allergic-type reactions in susceptible people. Monitor cardiovascular and respiratory vital signs and state of consciousness after each injection. Caution when local anesthetic solutions containing a vasoconstrictor are used in areas of the body supplied by end arteries or having otherwise compromised blood supply; ischemic injury or necrosis may result with hypertensive vascular disease. Caution with hepatic disease and impaired cardiovascular function. Monitor circulation and respiration with injections into head and neck area. Respiratory arrest following local anesthetic injection during retrobulbar blocks has been reported.

ADVERSE REACTIONS: Restlessness, anxiety, dizziness, tinnitus, blurred vision, tremors, convulsions, nausea, vomiting, chills, hypotension, bradycardia, ventricular arrhythmias, urticaria, pruritus, erythema, edema.

INTERACTIONS: Avoid use with any other local anesthetics. Anesthetic solutions containing epinephrine or norepinephrine with MAOIs or TCAs may produce severe, prolonged HTN; avoid concurrent use or monitor closely if concurrent use is necessary. Concurrent administration of vasopressors and ergot-type oxytocic drugs may cause severe, persistent HTN or CVA. Phenothiazines and butyrophenones may reduce or reverse the pressor effect of epinephrine. Serious dose-related cardiac arrhythmias may occur with use during or following administration of potent inhalation anesthetics.

PREGNANCY: Category C, not for use in nursing.

MATULANE
procarbazine HCl (Sigma-Tau)

RX

THERAPEUTIC CLASS: Hydrazine derivative

INDICATIONS: In combination with other antineoplastics for the treatment of Stage III/IV Hodgkin's disease.

DOSAGE: *Adults:* 2-4mg/kg/day as single or divided doses for first week then increase to 4-6mg/kg/day until maximum response or WBC <4000mm^3 or platelets <100,000/mm^3. Maint: 1-2mg/kg/day. In MOPP: 100mg/m^2 qd for 14 days. Adjust dose for combination regimens.

Pediatrics: 50mg/m^2/day for first week then increase to 100mg/m^2/day until response is obtained or leukopenia or thrombocytopenia occurs. Maint: 50mg/m^2/day. Adjust dose for combination regimens.

HOW SUPPLIED: Cap: 50mg

CONTRAINDICATIONS: Inadequate marrow reserve.

WARNINGS/PRECAUTIONS: Toxicity may occur in renal or hepatic impairment. Wait one month or longer with prior use of bone marrow suppressing radiation or chemotherapy. Discontinue if CNS symptoms (paresthesias, neuropathies, confusion), leukopenia, thrombocytopenia, hypersensitivity, stomatitis, diarrhea, hemorrhage or bleeding tendencies occur. Bone marrow depression often occurs 2-8 weeks after initiation. Monitor urinalysis, transaminases, LFTs weekly, hematologic status every 3-4 days.

ADVERSE REACTIONS: Leukopenia, anemia, thrombopenia, nausea, vomiting.

INTERACTIONS: Avoid sympathomimetics, TCAs, tyramine-containing drugs/foods, alcohol (may cause disulfiram-type reaction), tobacco. Caution with barbiturates, antihistamines, narcotics, hypotensives, phenothiazines.

PREGNANCY: Category D, not for use in nursing.

MAXAIR
pirbuterol acetate (Graceway)

RX

OTHER BRAND NAME: Maxair Autohaler (Graceway)

THERAPEUTIC CLASS: Beta$_2$ agonist

INDICATIONS: Prevention and reversal of bronchospasm in reversible bronchospasm (eg, asthma).

DOSAGE: *Adults:* 1-2 inh q4-6h. Max: 12 inh/day.
Pediatrics: ≥12 yrs: 1-2 inh q4-6h. Max: 12 inh/day.

HOW SUPPLIED: Autohaler: 0.2mg/inh (14g, 25.6g); MDI: 0.2mg/inh (14g)

WARNINGS/PRECAUTIONS: Caution with cardiovascular disorders, (eg, ischemic heart disease, HTN, arrhythmias), hyperthyroidism, diabetes, convulsive disorders. Fatalities reported with excessive use. Can produce paradoxical bronchospasm. Monitor BP.

ADVERSE REACTIONS: Nervousness, tremor, headache, dizziness, palpitations, tachycardia, cough, nausea.

INTERACTIONS: Avoid other aerosol β₂ agonists. Vascular effects may be potentiated by MAOIs, TCAs, and sympathomimetics. ECG changes and/or hypokalemia may occur with non-potassium sparing diuretics. Decreased effect with β-blockers.

PREGNANCY: Category C, caution in nursing.

MAXIPIME
cefepime HCl (Elan)

RX

THERAPEUTIC CLASS: Cephalosporin (4th generation)

INDICATIONS: Treatment of uncomplicated/complicated urinary tract (UTI), uncomplicated skin and skin structure (SSSI), and complicated intra-abdominal infections, and pneumonia. Emperic therapy for febrile neutropenia.

DOSAGE: *Adults:* Moderate-Severe Pneumonia: 1-2g IV q12h for 10 days. Febrile Neutropenia Emperic Therapy: 2g IV q8h for 7 days or until neutropenia resolved. Mild-Moderate UTI: 0.5-1g IM/IV q12h for 7-10 days. Severe UTI/Moderate-Severe SSSI: 2g IV q12h for 10 days. Complicated Intra-Abdominal Infections: 2g IV q12h for 7-10 days. CrCl ≤60mL/min: Initial: Same dose as normal renal function. Maint: Refer to prescribing information for dose-adjustment.

Pediatrics: 2 months-16 yrs: ≤40kg: UTI/SSSI/Pneumonia: 50mg/kg IV q12h. Febrile Neutropenia: 50mg/kg IV q8h. Max: Do not exceed adult dose. CrCl ≤60mL/min: Initial: Same dose as normal renal function. Maint: Refer to prescribing information for dose-adjustment.

HOW SUPPLIED: Inj: 500mg, 1g, 2g

WARNINGS/PRECAUTIONS: Caution with penicillin sensitivity; cross hypersensitivity may occur. Pseudomembranous colitis reported. Treatment may result in overgrowth of nonsusceptible organisms. Caution with renal impairment or history of GI disease especially colitis. Encephalopathy, myoclonus, seizures, and/or renal failure reported. D/C if seizure occurs. Associated with a fall in PT; monitor PT with renal or hepatic impairment, poor nutritional state, and protracted course of antimicrobials; give vitamin K as indicated.

ADVERSE REACTIONS: Local reactions (eg, phlebitis) rash, diarrhea.

INTERACTIONS: Increased risk of nephrotoxicity and ototoxicity with aminoglycosides. Risk of nephrotoxicity with potent diuretics (eg, furosemide).

PREGNANCY: Category B, caution in nursing.

MEBARAL
mephobarbital (Ovation)

CIV

THERAPEUTIC CLASS: Barbiturate

INDICATIONS: As a sedative for relief of anxiety, tension, and apprehension. Treatment of grand mal and petit mal epilepsy.

DOSAGE: *Adults:* Epilepsy: 400-600mg/day. Start with small dose, gradually increase over 4-5 days until optimum dose. Elderly/Debilitated/Renal or Hepatic Dysfunction: Reduce dose. Concomitant Phenobarbital: Give 50% of each drug. Concomitant Phenytoin: Reduce phenytoin dose. Sedation: 32-100mg tid-qid. Optimum Dose: 50mg tid-qid.

Pediatrics: Epilepsy: >5 yrs: 32-64mg tid-qid. <5 yrs: 16-32mg tid-qid. Start with small dose, gradually increase over 4-5 days until optimum dose. Sedation: 16-32mg tid-qid.

HOW SUPPLIED: Tab: 32mg, 50mg, 100mg

CONTRAINDICATIONS: Manifest or latent porphyria.

WARNINGS/PRECAUTIONS: May be habit forming; tolerance and dependence may occur with continued use. Avoid abrupt withdrawal. Caution in acute/chronic pain; paradoxal excitement may occur or symptoms masked. Can cause fetal damage. May cause marked excitement, depression and confusion in elderly or debilitated. Reduce initial dose with hepatic damage. Careful adjustment in impaired renal, cardiac, or respiratory function, myasthenia gravis, and myxedema. May increase vitamin D requirements. Caution with depression, suicidal tendencies and history of drug abuse.

ADVERSE REACTIONS: Somnolence, agitation, confusion, hyperkinesia, ataxia, CNS depression, hypoventilation, apnea, bradycardia, hypotension, syncope, nausea, vomiting, headache.

INTERACTIONS: MAOIs may prolong effects. Additive CNS depression with alcohol and other CNS depressants. Decreases effects of oral anticoagulants, oral contraceptives. Increases corticosteroid metabolism. Interferes with griseofulvin absorption. Decreases half-life of doxycycline. May alter phenytoin metabolism. Sodium valproate and valproic acid decrease metabolism.

PREGNANCY: Category D, caution with nursing.

Mebendazole
mebendazole (Various)
RX

THERAPEUTIC CLASS: Broad-spectrum anthelmintic

INDICATIONS: Treatment of Enterobiasis (pinworm), Trichuriasis (whipworm), Ascariasis (common roundworm), *Ancylostoma duodenale* (common hookworm), *Necator americanus* (American hookworm).

DOSAGE: *Adults:* Pinworm: 100mg single dose. Other Parasites: 100mg bid for 3 days. May repeat in 3 weeks if needed. Chew, swallow, crush or mix tab with food.
Pediatrics: ≥2 yrs: Pinworm: 100mg single dose. Other Parasites: 100mg bid for 3 days. May repeat in 3 weeks if needed. Chew, swallow, crush or mix tab with food.

HOW SUPPLIED: Tab, Chewable: 100mg

WARNINGS/PRECAUTIONS: Neutropenia, agranulocytosis reported with prolonged use. Periodically assess organ system functions with prolonged use.

ADVERSE REACTIONS: Abdominal pain, diarrhea.

INTERACTIONS: Cimetidine may increase plasma levels.

PREGNANCY: Category C, caution in nursing.

Meclofenamate
meclofenamate sodium (Various)
RX

THERAPEUTIC CLASS: NSAID

INDICATIONS: Relief of mild to moderate pain, primary dysmenorrhea, and idiopathic heavy menstrual blood loss. Symptomatic treatment of acute and chronic rheumatoid arthritis (RA) and osteoarthritis (OA).

DOSAGE: *Adults:* Mild to Moderate Pain: 50mg q4-6h. Max: 400mg/day. Excessive Menstrual Blood Loss/Primary Dysmenorrhea: 100mg tid for up to 6 days starting at onset of menstrual flow. RA/OA: 200-400mg/day in 3-4 divided doses. Max: 400mg/day.
Pediatrics: ≥14 yrs: Mild to Moderate Pain: 50mg q4-6h. Max: 400mg/day. Excessive Menstrual Blood Loss/Primary Dysmenorrhea: 100mg tid for up to 6 days starting at onset of menstrual flow. RA/OA: 200-400mg/day in 3-4 divided doses. Max: 400mg/day.

HOW SUPPLIED: Cap: 50mg, 100mg

CONTRAINDICATIONS: ASA or other NSAID allergy that precipitates bronchospasm, allergic rhinitis or urticaria.

WARNINGS/PRECAUTIONS: Risk of GI ulcerations, bleeding, and perforation. Borderline LFT elevations may occur. Renal and hepatic toxicity. Extreme caution in the elderly. If visual symptoms occur, discontinue.

ADVERSE REACTIONS: Diarrhea, nausea, vomiting, abdominal pain, edema, urticaria, pruritis, headache, dizziness, tinnitus, pyrosis, flatulence, anorexia, constipation, peptic ulcer.

INTERACTIONS: Enhanced effects of warfarin. ASA may lower levels.

PREGNANCY: Safety in pregnancy is not known. Not for use in nursing.

Medrol
methylprednisolone (Pharmacia & Upjohn)
RX

OTHER BRAND NAME: Medrol Dose Pack (Pharmacia & Upjohn)
THERAPEUTIC CLASS: Glucocorticoid
INDICATIONS: Steroid responsive disorders.

MENACTRA

DOSAGE: *Adults:* Initial: 4-48mg/day depending on disease and response. Maint: Decrease dose by small amounts to lowest effective dose. MS: Initial: 160mg/day for 1 week. Maint: 64mg every other day for 1 month. Alternate Day Therapy: Twice the usual dose every other day for long-term therapy.
Pediatrics: Initial: 4-48mg/day depending on disease and response. Maint: Decrease dose by small amounts to lowest effective dose. MS: Initial: 160mg/day for 1 week. Maint: 64mg every other day for 1 month. Alternate Day Therapy: Twice the usual dose every other day for long-term therapy.

HOW SUPPLIED: Tab: 2mg*, 4mg*, 8mg*, 16mg*, 32mg*; (Dose-Pak) 4mg* (21^s) *scored

CONTRAINDICATIONS: Systemic fungal infections.

WARNINGS/PRECAUTIONS: May need to increase dose before, during, and after stressful situations. May mask signs of infection or or cause new infections. Prolonged use may produce glaucoma, optic nerve damage, secondary ocular infections. Increases BP, salt/water retention, potassium excretion. More severe/fatal course of infections reported with chickenpox, measles. Caution with Strongyloides, latent TB, hypothyroidism, cirrhosis, ocular herpes simplex, HTN, diverticulitis, fresh intestinal anastomoses, ulcerative colitis, osteoporosis, myasthenia gravis, renal insufficiency, peptic ulcer disease. Kaposi's sarcoma reported. Growth and development of children on prolonged therapy should be monitored. Monitor for psychic disturbances. Avoid abrupt withdrawal. The 24mg tabs contain tartrazine; caution with tartrazine sensitivity.

ADVERSE REACTIONS: Fluid and electrolyte disturbances, HTN, osteoporosis, muscle weakness, cushingoid state, menstrual irregularities, nervousness, insomnia, impaired wound healing, DM, ulcerative esophagitis, excessive sweating, increases intracranial pressure, carbohydrate intolerance, glaucoma, cataracts, weight gain, nausea, malaise.

INTERACTIONS: Reduced efficacy with hepatic enzyme inducers (eg, phenobarbital, phenytoin, and rifampin). Increases clearance of chronic high dose ASA. Caution with ASA in hypoprothrombinemia. Effects on oral anticoagulants are variable; monitor PT. Increased insulin and oral hypoglycemic requirements in DM. Avoid live vaccines with immunosuppressive doses. Possible decreased vaccine response with killed or inactivated vaccines with immunosuppressive doses. Mutual inhibition of metabolism with cyclosporine; convulsions reported. Potentiated by ketoconazole and troleandomycin.

PREGNANCY: Safety in pregnancy and nursing not known.

MENACTRA RX
meningococcal polysaccharide diptheria toxoid conjugate vaccine (Sanofi Pasteur)

THERAPEUTIC CLASS: Vaccine

INDICATIONS: Active immunization of adolescents and adults 11-55 yrs of age for the prevention of invasive menigococcal disease caused by N.meningitidis serogroups A, C, Y and W-135.

DOSAGE: *Adults:* ≤55 yo: 0.5 mL IM into the deltoid region.
Pediatrics: ≥11 yo: 0.5mL IM into the deltoid region.

HOW SUPPLIED: Inj: 0.5mL

CONTRAINDICATIONS: Life-threatening reaction after previous administration of vaccine with similar contents. Known hypersensitivity to dry natural rubber latex.

WARNINGS/PRECAUTIONS: Guillain-Barre syndrome (GBS) has been reported. Avoid with bleeding disorders (eg. hemophilia, thrombocytopenia, anticoagulant therapy). Do not administer IV, SC, or intradermally. Have epinephrine injection (1:1000) available, in case of anaphylatic reaction.

ADVERSE REACTIONS: Redness, swelling, induration, pain, headache, fatigue, malaise, arthralgia, anorexia, chills, fever.

INTERACTIONS: Caution with anticoagulants. Immunosuppressive therapies may reduce immune response to vaccines.

PREGNANCY: Category C, caution in nursing.

MENTAX RX
butenafine HCl (Mylan Bertek)

THERAPEUTIC CLASS: Benzylamine antifungal

INDICATIONS: Interdigital tinea pedis, tinea corporis, tinea cruris, and tinea versicolor.

DOSAGE: *Adults:* T.pedis: Apply bid for 7 days or qd for 4 weeks. T.corporis/T.cruris/T.versicolor: Apply qd for 2 weeks.

Pediatrics: ≥12 yrs: T.pedis: Apply bid for 7 days or qd for 4 weeks. T.corporis/T.cruris/T.versicolor: Apply qd for 2 weeks.

HOW SUPPLIED: Cre: 1% (15g, 30g)

WARNINGS/PRECAUTIONS: Avoid eyes, nose, mouth, and other mucous membranes. D/C if irritation or sensitivity develops. Confirm diagnosis. Caution if sensitive to other allylamine antifungals.

ADVERSE REACTIONS: Burning, stinging, itching, contact dermatitis, irritation, erythema, worsening of condition.

PREGNANCY: Category B, caution in nursing.

Mepron
atovaquone (GlaxoSmithKline) — RX

THERAPEUTIC CLASS: Napthoquinone antiprotozoal

INDICATIONS: Prevention and treatment of mild to moderate *Pneumocystis carinii* pneumonia (PCP) in those intolerant to trimethoprim-sulfamethoxazole.

DOSAGE: *Adults:* Take with food. Prevention: 1500mg qd. Treatment: 750mg bid for 21 days.

Pediatrics: 13-16 yrs: Take with food. Prevention: 1500mg qd. Treatment: 750mg bid for 21 days.

HOW SUPPLIED: Sus: 750mg/5mL (5mL, 42^s; 210mL)

WARNINGS/PRECAUTIONS: Monitor with severe hepatic impairment. Absorption significantly increased with food.

ADVERSE REACTIONS: Rash, nausea, GI effects, cough increased, rhinitis, asthenia, infection, dyspnea, insomnia, asthenia, pruritus.

INTERACTIONS: Significantly decreased plasma levels with rifampin. Caution with other highly protein-bound drugs.

PREGNANCY: Category C, caution in nursing.

Meridia
sibutramine HCl monohydrate (Abbott) — CIV

THERAPEUTIC CLASS: Dopamine/norepinephrine/serotonin reuptake inhibitor

INDICATIONS: To induce and maintain weight loss in obese patients with an initial BMI ≥30kg/m^2 or ≥27kg/m^2 with risk factors (eg, HTN, diabetes, dyslipidemias)

DOSAGE: *Adults:* Initial: 10mg qd. Titrate: May increase after 4 weeks to 15mg qd. Max: 15mg/day. Use 5mg/day in patients unable to tolerate 10mg/day. May continue for up to 2 yrs.

Pediatrics: ≥16 yrs: Initial: 10mg qd. Titrate: May increase after 4 weeks to 15mg qd. Use 5mg/day in patients unable to tolerate 10mg/day. Max: 15mg/day. May continue for up to 2 yrs.

HOW SUPPLIED: Cap: 5mg, 10mg, 15mg

CONTRAINDICATIONS: Concomitant MAOIs or centrally acting appetite suppressants, anorexia nervosa.

WARNINGS/PRECAUTIONS: May increase BP and/or pulse. Avoid with uncontrolled or poorly controlled HTN, CAD, CHF, arrhythmias, stroke, severe hepatic or renal dysfunction. Monitor BP and pulse before therapy and regularly thereafter. Caution with narrow angle glaucoma, mild-moderate renal impairment, seizures and if predisposed to bleeding. Exclude organic causes of obesity. Gallstones precipitated with weight loss.

ADVERSE REACTIONS: Anorexia, constipation, increased appetite, nausea, dyspepsia, dry mouth, insomnia, dizziness, nervousness, HTN, tachycardia, dysmenorrhea, headache.

INTERACTIONS: Avoid excess alcohol, CNS-active drugs, other serotonergic agents (eg, SSRIs, migraine therapy agents, certain opioids), within 14 days of MAOI use. Caution with drugs affecting hemostasis or platelet function, ephedrine, pseudoephedrine, and other agents that increase BP, heart rate. Possible decreased metabolism with ketoconazole and erythromycin.

PREGNANCY: Category C, not for use in nursing

MERREM RX
meropenem (AstraZeneca LP)

THERAPEUTIC CLASS: Carbapenem

INDICATIONS: Treatment of intra-abdominal infections, bacterial meningitis, and complicated skin and skin structure infections (cSSSI).

DOSAGE: *Adults:* IV: Intra-abdominal: 1g q8h. CrCl 26-50mL/min: 1g q12h. CrCl 10-25mL/min: 500mg q12h. CrCl <10mL/min: 500mg q24h. SSSI: 500mg q8h. CrCl 26-50mL/min: 500mg q12h. CrCl 10-25mL/min: 250mg q12h. CrCl <10mL/min: 250mg q24h.

Pediatrics: IV: ≥3 months: >50kg: Intra-abdominal: 1g q8h. Meningitis: 2g q8h. SSSI: 500mg q8h. ≤50kg: Intra-abdominal: 20mg/kg q8h. Max: 1g q8h. Meningitis: 40mg/kg q8h. Max: 2g q8h. SSSI: 10mg/kg q8h. Max: 500mg q8h.

HOW SUPPLIED: Inj: 500mg, 1g

CONTRAINDICATIONS: Hypersensitivity to beta-lactams.

WARNINGS/PRECAUTIONS: Severe and fatal hypersensitivity reactions reported; increased risk with allergens and/or penicillin sensitivity. Pseudomembranous colitis reported. Seizures and other CNS effects reported particularly with pre-existing CNS disorders, bacterial meningitis, and renal dysfunction. Thrombocytopenia reported with severe renal impairment. Prolonged use may result in superinfection. Use as monotherapy for meningitis caused by penicillin nonsusceptible strains of *Streptococcus pneumoniae* has not been established.

ADVERSE REACTIONS: Headache, rash, local reactions, diarrhea, nausea, vomiting, constipation.

INTERACTIONS: Probenecid inhibits renal excretion; avoid concomitant use. May reduce valproic acid levels.

PREGNANCY: Category B, caution in nursing.

MERUVAX II RX
rubella vaccine live (Merck)

THERAPEUTIC CLASS: Vaccine

INDICATIONS: Vaccination against rubella.

DOSAGE: *Adults:* 0.5mL SQ in outer aspect of upper arm.

Pediatrics: Primary Vaccination at 12-15 months: 0.5mL SQ in outer aspect of upper arm. Revaccinate with MMR II prior to elementary school entry.

HOW SUPPLIED: Inj: 1000 TCID$_{50}$

CONTRAINDICATIONS: Avoid pregnancy for 3 months after vaccine, anaphylactic reaction to neomycin, febrile/active respiratory illness, immunosuppressive therapy (except corticosteroids as replacement therapy), blood dyscrasias, leukemia, lymphoma, malignant neoplasms affecting bone marrow or lymphatic system, immunodeficiency states.

WARNINGS/PRECAUTIONS: May worsen thrombocytopenia. Defer vaccination for at least 3 months after blood or plasma transfusions, immune globulin (except susceptible postpartum patients with follow-up HI titer after 6-8 weeks). Do not vaccinate with active untreated TB. Temperature elevation may occur after vaccination. Contains albumin, remote risk of viral infection transmission. Have epinephrine (1:1000) available.

ADVERSE REACTIONS: Fever, syncope, headache, dizziness, malaise, irritability, thrombocytopenia, arthritis, vasculitis, diarrhea, local reactions.

INTERACTIONS: Do not give with immune globulin. May depress TB skin sensitivity, administer test either simultaneously or before. Do not give <1 month before or after other live viral vaccines. Do not give simultaneously with DTP or oral poliovirus vaccine.

PREGNANCY: Category C, contraindicated in pregnancy and caution in nursing.

METADATE CD
methylphenidate HCl (Celltech)

CII

THERAPEUTIC CLASS: Sympathomimetic amine

INDICATIONS: Treatment of attention deficit hyperactivity disorder (ADHD).

DOSAGE: *Pediatrics:* ≥6 yrs: Usual: 20mg qam before breakfast. Titrate: Increase weekly by 20mg depending on tolerability/efficacy. Max: 60mg/day. Reduce dose or discontinue if paradoxical aggravation of symptoms occur. Discontinue if no improvement after appropriate dose adjustments over 1 month. Swallow whole with liquids or open and sprinkle on 1 tbs applesauce followed by water. Do not crush, chew, or divide.

HOW SUPPLIED: Cap, Extended-Release: 10mg, 20mg, 30mg

CONTRAINDICATIONS: Marked anxiety, tension, and agitation; glaucoma; motor tics, family history or diagnosis of Tourette's syndrome, severe hypertension, angina pectoris, cardiac arrhythmias, heart failure, recent MI, hyperthyroidism or thyrotoxicosis; during or within 14 days of MAOI use.

WARNINGS/PRECAUTIONS: Monitor growth in children. Not for severe depression or fatigue. May exacerbate symptoms of behavior disturbance and thought disorder in psychotic patients. Caution when using stimulants to treat patients with comorbid bipolar disorder because of concern for possible induction of mixed/manic episode in such patients. Stimulants at usual doses can cause treatment emergent psychotic or manic symptoms (eg, hallucinations, delusional thinking, mania) in children and adolescents without prior history of psychotic illness. Aggressive behavior or hostility reported in clinical trials and postmarketing experience of some medications indicated for the treatment of ADHD. May lower seizure threshold, especially in known EEG abnormalities. Caution with HTN, conditions affected by BP or HR elevation, history of drug abuse or alcoholism. Monitor during withdrawal from abusive use. Visual disturbances may occur (rare). Monitor CBC, differential, and platelets with prolonged use. Avoid with serious structural cardiac abnormalities, cardiomyopathy, serious heart rhythm abnormalities, CAD, or other serious cardiac problems.

ADVERSE REACTIONS: Headache, abdominal pain, anorexia, insomnia.

INTERACTIONS: See Contraindications. Potentiates anticoagulants, anticonvulsants (eg, phenobarbital, phenytoin, primidone), TCAs, and SSRIs. Caution with α_2-agonist (eg, clonidine) and pressor agents.

PREGNANCY: Category C, caution in nursing.

METADATE ER
methylphenidate HCl (Celltech)

CII

THERAPEUTIC CLASS: Sympathomimetic amine

INDICATIONS: Treatment of attention deficit disorder and narcolepsy.

DOSAGE: *Adults:* (Immediate-Release Methylphenidate) 10-60mg/day given bid-tid 30-45 minutes ac. Take last dose before 6 pm if insomnia occurs. (Tab, Extended Release) May use in place of immediate release tabs when the 8 hr dose corresponds to the titrated 8 hr immediate release dose. Swallow whole; do not chew or crush.

Pediatrics: ≥6 yrs: (Immediate-Release Methylphenidate) Initial: 5mg bid before breakfast and lunch. Titrate: Increase gradually by 5-10mg weekly. Max: 60mg/day. (Tab, Extended Release) May use in place of immediate release tabs when the 8 hr dose corresponds to the titrated 8 hr immediate release dose. Swallow whole; do not chew or crush. Reduce dose or discontinue if paradoxical aggravation of symptoms occur. Discontinue if no improvement after appropriate dose adjustment over 1 month.

HOW SUPPLIED: Tab, Extended Release: 10mg, 20mg

CONTRAINDICATIONS: Marked anxiety, tension, and agitation; glaucoma; motor tics or family history or diagnosis of Tourette's syndrome; during or within 14 days of MAOI use.

WARNINGS/PRECAUTIONS: Monitor growth in children. Not for severe depression or fatigue. May exacerbate symptoms of behavior disturbance and thought disorder in psychotic children. May lower seizure threshold, especially in known EEG abnormalities.

METAPROTERENOL

Caution with HTN, emotionally-unstable patients. Monitor during withdrawal. Visual disturbances may occur (rare). Monitor CBC, differential, and platelets with prolonged use. Periodically d/c to assess condition.

ADVERSE REACTIONS: Nervousness, insomnia, hypersensitivity reactions, anorexia, nausea, dizziness, palpitations, headache, dyskinesia, drowsiness, BP and pulse changes, tachycardia, angina, arrhythmia, abdominal pain.

INTERACTIONS: See Contraindications. May decrease hypotensive effect of guanethidine. Caution with pressor agents. Potentiates anticoagulants, anticonvulsants (eg, phenobarbital, phenytoin, primidone), phenylbutazone, TCAs (eg, imipramine, clomipramine, desipramine).

PREGNANCY: Safety in pregnancy and nursing not known.

Metaproterenol RX
metaproterenol sulfate (Various)

OTHER BRAND NAME: Alupent (Boehringer Ingelheim)

THERAPEUTIC CLASS: Beta$_2$ agonist

INDICATIONS: For bronchial asthma and reversible bronchospasm. (Sol, Inhalation 5%) Treatment of acute asthmatic attacks in children ≥6 years.

DOSAGE: *Adults:* (MDI) 2-3 inh q3-4h. Max: 12 inh/day. (Sol 5%) Nebulizer or IPPB: 0.2-0.3mL (dilute in 2.5mL saline) tid-qid. Hand-bulb Nebulizer: 5-15 inh (undiluted) tid-qid. (Sol 0.4%, 0.6%) 2.5mL by IPPB tid-qid, up to q4h. (Syr, Tab) 20mg tid-qid.
Pediatrics: (MDI) ≥12 yrs: 2-3 inh q3-4h. Max: 12 inh/day. (Sol 5%) ≥12 yrs: Nebulizer or IPPB: 0.2-0.3mL (dilute in 2.5mL saline) tid-qid. Hand-bulb Nebulizer: 5-15 inh (undiluted) tid-qid. 6-12 yrs: Nebulizer: 0.1-0.2mL (dilute in 3mL saline) tid-qid. (Sol 0.4%, 0.6%) ≥12 yrs: 2.5mL by IPPB tid-qid, up to q4h. (Syr, Tab) >9 yrs or >60 lbs: 20mg tid-qid. 6-9 yrs or <60 lbs: 10mg tid-qid.

HOW SUPPLIED: MDI: 0.65mg/inh (14g); Sol, Inhalation: 0.4% (2.5mL), 0.6% (2.5mL); Syrup: 10mg/5mL (480mL); Tab: 10mg, 20mg

CONTRAINDICATIONS: Cardiac arrhythmias associated with tachycardia.

WARNINGS/PRECAUTIONS: Caution with cardiovascular disorders, (eg, ischemic heart disease, HTN, arrhythmias), hyperthyroidism, diabetes, convulsive disorders. Fatalities reported with excessive use. Can produce paradoxical bronchospasm. Monitor BP. Nebulized solution single dose may not abort an asthma attack.

ADVERSE REACTIONS: Headache, dizziness, HTN, GI distress, throat irritation, cough, asthma exacerbation, nervousness, tremor, nausea, vomiting.

INTERACTIONS: Avoid other aerosol β$_2$ agonists. Vascular effects may be potentiated by MAOIs, TCAs, and sympathomimetics.

PREGNANCY: Category C, caution in nursing.

Methotrexate Sodium RX
methotrexate sodium (Various)

> Only for life-threatening neoplastic disease, or in severe RA, and psoriasis unresponsive to other therapies. Death, fetal death/congenital anomalies, lung disease, tumor lysis syndrome, fatal skin reactions, PCP reported. Monitor for bone marrow, liver, lung, and kidney toxicities. Bone marrow suppression, aplastic anemia and GI toxicity reported with NSAIDs. Hepatotoxicity, fibrosis, and cirrhosis with prolonged use. Interrupt therapy with diarrhea, ulcerative stomatitis. Reduced elimination with renal dysfunction, ascites, or pleural effusion. Increased risk of soft tissue necrosis and osteonecrosis with radiotherapy. Malignant lymphoma may occur. Extreme caution with high dose regimen for osteosarcoma. Do not use formulations/diluents with preservatives for intrathecal or high dose therapy.

OTHER BRAND NAME: Rheumatrex (Stada)

THERAPEUTIC CLASS: Dihydrofolic acid reductase inhibitor

INDICATIONS: Treatment of neoplastic diseases (eg, acute lymphocytic leukemia, gestational choriocarcinoma, chorioadenoma destruens, hydatidiform mole, breast cancer, epidermoid cancer of the head and neck, advanced mycosis fungoides, lung cancer, advanced stage non-Hodgkin's lymphomas). Prophylaxis and treatment of meningeal leukemia, and maintenance with other chemotherapeutics. For prolonging relapse-free survival in non-metastatic osteosarcoma followed by leucovorin. Symptomatic control of severe, recalcitrant, disabling psoriasis, and management of rheumatoid arthritis (RA) or polyarticular-course juvenile rheumatoid arthritis (JRA) unresponsive to other therapies.

DOSAGE: *Adults:* Choriocarcinoma/Trophoblastic disease: 15-30mg qd PO/IM for 5 days. May repeat 3-5 times as required with rest period of ≥1 week. Leukemia: Induction: 3.3mg/m^2 with prednisone 60mg/m^2 qd. Remission Maintenance: 15mg/m^2 PO/IM twice weekly or 2.5mg/kg IV every 14 days. Burkitt's Tumor: Stages I-II: 10-25mg/day PO for 4-8 days. Administer several courses with rest periods of 7-10 days in between. Lymphosarcoma: Stage III: 0.625-2.5mg/kg/day with other antitumor agents. Mycosis Fungoides: 5-50mg once weekly. If poor response, give 15-37.5mg twice weekly. Adjust dose based on response and hematologic monitoring. Osteosarcoma: Initial: 12g/m^2 IV, increase to 15g/m^2 if peak serum levels of 1000 micromolar not reached at end of infusion. Meningeal Leukemia: Dilute preservative free MTX to 1mg/mL. Give 12mg intrathecally at 2-5 day intervals. Psoriasis: Initial: 10-25mg weekly until response or use divided oral dose schedule, 2.5mg at 12 hr intervals for 3 doses. Titrate: Increase gradually until optimal response. Maint: Reduce to lowest effective dose. Max: 30mg/week. Rheumatoid Arthritis: Initial: 7.5mg PO once weekly, or 2.5mg q12h for 3 doses given as a course once weekly. Titrate: Gradual increase. Max: 20mg weekly. After response, reduce dose to lowest effective amount of drug.
Pediatrics: Meningeal Leukemia: Dilute preservative free MTX to 1mg/mL. <1 yr: 6mg. 1 yr: 8mg. 2 yrs: 10mg. ≥ 3yrs: 12mg. Give intrathecally at 2-5 day intervals. JRA: 2-16 yrs: Initial: 10mg/m^2 once weekly. Adjust dose gradually to achieve optimal response.

HOW SUPPLIED: Inj: (Generic) 20mg, 25mg/mL, 1g; Tab: (Rheumatrex) 2.5mg* (Dose Pack 15mg, 4 x 6 tabs; 12.5mg, 4 x 5 tabs; 10mg, 4 x 4 tabs; 7.5mg, 4 x 3 tabs; 5mg, 4 x 2 tabs) *scored

CONTRAINDICATIONS: Pregnancy, nursing. Psoriasis or RA patients with alcoholism, alcoholic liver disease, chronic liver disease, immunodeficiency syndrome, and pre-existing blood dyscrasias.

WARNINGS/PRECAUTIONS: Monitor closely; toxicity may be related to dose and frequency of administration. When reactions do occur, doses should be reduced or discontinued and corrective measures should be taken. Avoid pregnancy if either partner is receiving therapy. Avoid intrathecal administration or high-dose therapy. Injection contains benzyl alcohol; avoid use in neonates (<1 month), may cause gasping syndrome.

ADVERSE REACTIONS: Ulcerative stomatitis, leukopenia, nausea, abdominal distress, malaise, fatigue, chills, fever, dizziness, decreased resistance to infection.

INTERACTIONS: Avoid NSAIDs with high doses. Caution with nephrotoxic agents (eg, cisplatin), NSAIDs, probenecid, and highly protein bound drugs (eg, sulfonamides, phenytoin, phenylbutazone, salicylates). Oral antibiotics (eg, tetracycline, chloramphenicol) may decrease absorption or interfere with enterohepatic circulation. Penicillins may decrease clearance. Closely monitor with hepatotoxins (eg, azathioprine, retinoids, sulfasalazine). Folic acid may decrease response to MTX. TMP/SMZ may increase bone marrow suppression. Decreased theophylline clearance.

PREGNANCY: Category X, contraindicated in nursing.

METHYLDOPA
methyldopa (Various)

RX

THERAPEUTIC CLASS: Central alpha-adrenergic agonist

INDICATIONS: Treatment of hypertension.

DOSAGE: *Adults:* Initial: 250mg bid-tid for 48 hrs. Adjust dose at intervals of not less than 2 days. Maint: 500mg-2g/day given bid-qid. Max: 3g/day. Concomitant Antihypertensives (other than thiazides): Initial: Limit to 500mg/day. Renal Impairment: May respond to lower doses.
Pediatrics: Initial: 10mg/kg/day given bid-qid. Max: 65mg/kg/day or 3g/day, whichever is less.

HOW SUPPLIED: Tab: 125mg, 250mg, 500mg

CONTRAINDICATIONS: Active hepatic disease, history of methyldopa associated liver disorder, concomitant MAOIs.

Methyldopate HCl

WARNINGS/PRECAUTIONS: Positive Coombs test, hemolytic anemia, and liver disorders may occur. Fever reported within the 1st 3 weeks of therapy. HTN has recurred after dialysis. Caution with liver disease or dysfunction. D/C if signs of heart failure, or involuntary choreoathetotic movements develop. Edema and weight gain reported. Blood count, Coombs test and LFTs prior to therapy and periodically thereafter.

ADVERSE REACTIONS: Sedation, headache, asthenia, edema/weight gain, hepatic disorders, vomiting, diarrhea, nausea, sore or "black" tongue, blood dyscrasias, BUN increase, gynecomastia, impotence.

INTERACTIONS: See Contraindications. May potentiate other antihypertensives. Anesthetics may need dose reduction. Monitor for lithium toxicity. Ferrous sulfate and ferrous gluconate may decrease bioavailability; avoid coadministration.

PREGNANCY: Category B, caution in nursing.

Methyldopate HCl   RX
methyldopate HCl (American Regent)

THERAPEUTIC CLASS: Central alpha-adrenergic agonist

INDICATIONS: Treatment of hypertension and hypertensive crises.

DOSAGE: *Adults:* 250-500mg IV q6h as needed. Max: 1gm q6h. Elderly/Renal Dysfunction: May reduce dose. Switch to oral therapy once BP is controlled.
Pediatrics: 20-40mg/kg/day IV given q6h. Max: 65mg/kg/day or 3 g/day, whichever is less. Switch to oral therapy once BP is controlled.

HOW SUPPLIED: Inj: 50mg/mL

CONTRAINDICATIONS: Hypersensitivity to sulfites, active hepatic disease, liver disorders previously associated with methyldopa therapy, concomitant MAOIs.

WARNINGS/PRECAUTIONS: Positive Coombs test, hemolytic anemia, and liver disorders may occur. Fever reported within the first 3 weeks of therapy. HTN has recurred after dialysis. Caution with liver disease or dysfunction. D/C if signs of heart failure develop. Edema and weight gain reported. Blood count, Coombs test and LFTs prior to therapy and periodically thereafter. Caution with cerebrovascular disease.

ADVERSE REACTIONS: Sedation, headache, asthenia, weakness, edema, weight gain, liver disorders, vomiting, diarrhea, nausea, sore or "black" tongue, blood dyscrasias, BUN increase, gynecomastia, impotence.

INTERACTIONS: See Contraindications. May potentiate other antihypertensives. Anesthetics may need dose reduction. May increase lithium levels. Ferrous sulfate and ferrous gluconate may decrease bioavailability; avoid coadministration.

PREGNANCY: Category C, caution in nursing.

Methylin   CII
methylphenidate HCl (Mallinckrodt)

OTHER BRAND NAME: Methylin ER (Mallinckrodt)

THERAPEUTIC CLASS: Sympathomimetic amine

INDICATIONS: Treatment of attention deficit disorder and narcolepsy.

DOSAGE: *Adults:* (Sol/Tab/Tab, Chewable) 10-60mg/day given bid-tid 30-45 min ac. Take last dose before 6 pm if insomnia occurs. (Tab, Extended-Release) May use in place of immediate release tabs when the 8 hr dose corresponds to the titrated 8 hr immediate release dose. Swallow whole; do not chew or crush.
Pediatrics: ≥6 yrs: (Sol/Tab/Tab, Chewable) Initial: 5mg bid before breakfast and lunch. Titrate: Increase gradually by 5-10mg weekly. Max: 60mg/day. (Tab, Extended-Release) May be used in place of immediate release tabs when the 8 hr dose corresponds to the titrated 8 hr immediate release dose. Swallow whole; do not chew or crush. Reduce dose or discontinue if paradoxical aggravation of symptoms occur. Discontinue if no improvement after appropriate dose adjustment over 1 month.

HOW SUPPLIED: Sol: 5mg/5mL (500mL), 10mg/5mL (500mL); Tab: 5mg, 10mg, 20mg; Tab, Chewable: 2.5mg, 5mg, 10mg; Tab, Extended-Release: 10mg, 20mg

CONTRAINDICATIONS: Marked anxiety, tension, and agitation; glaucoma; motor tics or family history or diagnosis of Tourette's syndrome, during or within 14 days of MAOI use.

WARNINGS/PRECAUTIONS: Monitor growth in children. Not for severe depression or fatigue. May exacerbate symptoms of behavior disturbance or thought disorder in psychotic children. Caution when using stimulants to treat patients with comorbid bipolar disorder because of concern for possible induction of mixed/manic episode in such patients. Stimulants at usual doses can cause treatment emergent psychotic or manic symptoms (hallucinations, delusional thinking, mania) in children and adolescents without prior history of psychotic illness. Aggressive behavior or hostility has been reported in clinical trials and the postmarketing experience of some medications indicated for the treatment of ADHD. May lower seizure threshold, especially in known EEG abnormalities. Caution with HTN, heart failure, recent MI, ventricular arrhythmia, or emotionally-unstable patients. Monitor during withdrawal. Visual disturbances may occur (rare). Monitor CBC, differential, and platelets with prolonged use. Periodically d/c to assess condition. Avoid with serious structural cardiac abnormalities, cardiomyopathy, serious heart rhythm abnormalities, CAD, or other serious cardiac problems. Caution in emotionally unstable patients with history of drug dependence or alcoholism.

ADVERSE REACTIONS: Nervousness, insomnia, hypersensitivity reactions, anorexia, nausea, dizziness, palpitations, headache, dyskinesia, drowsiness, BP and pulse changes, tachycardia, angina, arrhythmia, abdominal pain.

INTERACTIONS: May decrease hypotensive effect of guanethidine. Caution with pressor agents. Avoid during or within 14 days of MAOI use. Potentiates anticoagulants, anticonvulsants (phenobarbital, diphenylhydantoin, primidone), phenylbutazone, TCAs (imipramine, clomipramine, desipramine).

PREGNANCY: Safety in pregnancy and nursing not known.

METOCLOPRAMIDE RX
metoclopramide HCl (Various)

OTHER BRAND NAMES: Reglan (Schwarz) - Reglan Injection (Baxter)

THERAPEUTIC CLASS: Dopamine antagonist/prokinetic

INDICATIONS: (PO) Symptomatic treatment of gastroesophageal reflux in patients who fail to respond to conventional therapy. (Inj, PO) Symptomatic relief of diabetic gastroparesis. (Inj) Prevention of post-op and chemo-induced nausea/vomiting. Diagnostic aid during radiological examination and facilitates intubation of small intestine.

DOSAGE: *Adults:* GERD: PO: 10-15mg qid 30 minutes ac and hs. Elderly: 5 mg qid. Max: 12 weeks of therapy. Intermittent Symptoms: Up to 20mg single dose prior to provoking situation. Gastroparesis: 10mg PO 30 minutes ac and hs for 2-8 weeks. Severe Gastroparesis: May give same doses IV/IM for up to 10 days if needed. Antiemetic: (Postoperative) 10-20mg IM near end of surgery. (Chemotherapy-Induced) 1-2mg/kg 30 minutes before chemotherapy then q2h for two doses, then q3h for three doses. Give 2mg/kg for highly emetogenic drugs for initial 2 doses. Small Bowel Intubation/Radiological Exam: 10mg IV single dose. CrCl <40mL/min: 50% of normal dose.

Pediatrics: Small Bowel Intubation: 6-14 yrs: 2.5-5mg IV single dose. <6 yrs: 0.1mg/kg IV single dose. CrCl <40mL/min: 50% of normal dose.

HOW SUPPLIED: Inj: 5mg/mL; Syr: 5mg/5mL; Tab: 5mg, 10mg* *scored

CONTRAINDICATIONS: Where GI mobility stimulation is dangerous (eg, perforation, obstruction, hemorrhage), pheochromocytoma, seizure disorder, concomitant drugs that cause EPS effects.

WARNINGS/PRECAUTIONS: Caution with HTN, Parkinson's disease, depression. EPS, tardive dyskinesia, Parkinsonian-like symptoms, neuroleptic malignant syndrome reported. Administer IV injection slowly. Risk of developing fluid retention and volume overload especially with cirrhosis or CHF; d/c if these occur. May increase pressure of suture lines.

ADVERSE REACTIONS: Restlessness, drowsiness, fatigue, EPS effects (acute dystonic reactions), galactorrhea, hyperprolactinemia, hypotension, arrhythmia, diarrhea, dizziness, urinary frequency.

INTERACTIONS: See Contraindications. May decrease gastric absorption of drugs (eg, digoxin) and increase intestinal absorption of drugs (eg, APAP, tetracycline, levodopa,

MEVACOR

ethanol, and cyclosporine). Additive sedation with alcohol, hypnotics, narcotics, or tranquilizers. Caution with MAOIs. Antagonized by anticholinergics, narcotics. Insulin dose or timing of dose may need adjustment to prevent hypoglycemia.

PREGNANCY: Category B, caution with nursing.

MEVACOR
lovastatin (Merck)

RX

THERAPEUTIC CLASS: HMG-CoA reductase inhibitor

INDICATIONS: To reduce risk of MI, unstable angina, and coronary revascularization procedures in patients without symptomatic coronary disease, average to moderately elevated total-C and LDL-C, and below average HDL-C. To slow coronary atherosclerosis progression in patients with coronary heart disease to reduce total-C and LDL-C. Adjunct to diet to lower total-C and LDL-C in primary hypercholesterolemia (Types IIa and IIb). Adjunct to diet to lower total-C, LDL-C and apolipoprotein B in adolescents at least 1-yr postmenarchal with heterozygous familial hypercholesterolemia.

DOSAGE: *Adults:* Initial: 20mg qd at dinner (10mg/day if need LDL-C reduction <20%). Usual: 10-80mg/day given qd or bid. May adjust every 4 weeks. Max: 80mg/day. Concomitant Cyclosporine: Initial: 10mg/day. Max: 20mg/day. Fibrates/Niacin (≥1g/day): Max: 20mg/day. Concomitant Amiodarone/Verapamil: Max: 40mg/day. CrCl <30mL/min: Consider dose increase of >20mg/day carefully and implement cautiously.

Pediatrics: Heterozygous Familial Hypercholesterolemia: 10-17 yrs (at least 1-yr postmenarchal): Initial: If <20% LDL-C Reduction Needed: 10mg qd. If ≥20% LDL-C Reduction Needed: 20mg qd. May adjust every 4 weeks. Max: 40mg/day. Concomitant Cyclosporine: Initial: 10mg/day. Max: 20mg/day. Fibrates/Niacin (≥1g/day): Max: 20mg/day. Concomitant Amiodarone/Verapamil: Max: 40mg/day. CrCl <30mL/min: Consider dose increase of >20mg/day carefully and implement cautiously.

HOW SUPPLIED: Tab: 20mg, 40mg

CONTRAINDICATIONS: Active liver disease, unexplained persistent elevations of serum transaminases, pregnancy, nursing mothers.

WARNINGS/PRECAUTIONS: May increase serum transaminases and CPK levels; consider in differential diagnosis of chest pain. D/C if AST or ALT ≥3X ULN persist, or if myopathy diagnosed or suspected. Monitor LFTs prior to therapy, at 6 weeks, 12 weeks, then periodically or with dose elevation. Caution with heavy alcohol use and/or history of hepatic disease. Caution with dose escalation in renal insufficiency. Less effective with homozygous familial hypercholesterolemia. Rhabdomyolysis (rare), myopathy reported. D/C a few days before elective major surgery and when any major acute medical or surgical condition supervenes.

ADVERSE REACTIONS: Headache, constipation, flatulence, dizziness, rash, elevated transaminases or CK levels, GI upset, blurred vision.

INTERACTIONS: Increased risk of myopathy with CYP3A4 inhibitors (eg, cyclosporine, itraconazole, ketoconazole, erythromycin, clarithromycin, telithromycin, protease inhibitors, nefazodone, >1 quart/day of grapefruit juice), verapamil, amiodarone, fibrates (eg, gemfibrozil), danazol, and ≥1g/day of niacin. Monitor anticoagulants. Caution with drugs that diminish levels or activity of steroid hormones (eg, ketoconazole, spironolactone, cimetidine).

PREGNANCY: Category X, not for use in nursing.

MILTOWN
meprobamate (MedPointe)

CIV

THERAPEUTIC CLASS: Carbamate derivative

INDICATIONS: Management of anxiety disorders or short-term relief of symptoms of anxiety.

DOSAGE: *Adults:* Usual: 1200-1600mg/day given tid-qid. Max: 2400mg/day. Elderly: >65 yrs: Start at low end of dosing range.

Pediatrics: 6-12 yrs: 200-600mg/day given bid-tid.

HOW SUPPLIED: Tab: 200mg, 400mg

CONTRAINDICATIONS: Porphyria, allergic or idiosyncratic reactions to carisoprodol, mebutamate, tybamate, carbromal.

WARNINGS/PRECAUTIONS: Physical and psychological dependence reported. Avoid abrupt withdrawal after prolonged or excessive use. Increased risk of congenital malformations with use during 1st trimester of pregnancy. Caution with liver or renal dysfunction, and in elderly. May precipitate seizures in epileptic patients. Prescribe small quantities in suicidal patients.

ADVERSE REACTIONS: Drowsiness, ataxia, slurred speech, vertigo, weakness, nausea, vomiting, diarrhea, tachycardia, transient ECG changes, rash, leukopenia, petechiae.

INTERACTIONS: Administration with other CNS depressants, alcohol, psychotropics have additive effects.

PREGNANCY: Safety in pregnancy and nursing not known.

Minocin
minocycline HCl (Triax)

RX

THERAPEUTIC CLASS: Tetracycline derivative

INDICATIONS: Treatment of inclusion conjunctivitis, nongonococcal urethritis, and other infections (eg, respiratory tract, endocervical, rectal, urinary tract, skin and skin structure) caused by susceptible strains of microorganisms. Alternative treatment, when penicillin is contraindicated, in certain other infections (eg, urethritis, gonococcal, syphilis, anthrax). Adjunctive therapy in acute intestinal amebiasis and severe acne. Treatment of *Mycobacterium marinum* and asymptomatic carriers of *Neisseria meningitidis*.

DOSAGE: *Adults:* Usual: 200mg initially, then 100mg q12h; alternative is 100-200mg initially, then 50mg qid. Uncomplicated Gonococcal Infection (Men, other than urethritis and anorectal infections): 200mg initially, then 100mg q12h for minimum 4 days. Uncomplicated Gonococcal Urethritis (Men): 100mg q12h for 5 days. Syphilis: Administer usual dose for 10-15 days. Meningococcal Carrier State: 100mg q12h for 5 days. *Mycobacterium marinum:* 100mg q12h for 6-8 weeks. Uncomplicated Urethral, Endocervical, or Rectal Infection Caused by *Chlamydia trachomatis* or *Ureaplasma urealyticum:* 100mg q12h for at least 7 days. Gonorrhea in Patients Sensitive to PCN: 200mg initially, then 100mg q12h for at least 4 days, with post-therapy cultures within 2-3 days. Take with plenty of fluids. Renal Dysfunction: Max: 200mg/24hrs.

Pediatrics: >8 yrs: 4mg/kg initially followed by 2mg/kg q12h, not to exceed adult dose. Take with plenty of fluids. Renal Dysfunction: Max: 200mg/24hrs.

HOW SUPPLIED: Cap: 50mg, 100mg; Inj: 100mg; Sus: 50mg/5mL (60mL)

WARNINGS/PRECAUTIONS: May cause fetal harm during pregnancy. Use during tooth development (last half of pregnancy, infancy, <8yrs) may cause permanent discoloration of the teeth or enamel hypoplasia; avoid use during this period. Renal toxicity, hepatotoxicity, photosensitivity, increased BUN, superinfection, pseudotumor cerebri may occur; perform hematopoietic, renal, and hepatic monitoring. Caution with hepatic dysfunction. Caution in renal impairment; may lead to azotemia, hyperphosphatemia, and acidosis. Use alternate form of contraception other than oral contraceptives. May decrease bone growth in premature infants. If *clostridium difficile* associated diarrhea (CDAD) develops, appropriate therapy should be initiated.

ADVERSE REACTIONS: Anorexia, nausea, vomiting, diarrhea, dysphagia, enterocolitis, pancreatitis, increased LFTs, renal toxicity, rash, exfoliative dermatitis, Stevens-Johnson syndrome, skin and mucous membrane pigmentation, blood dyscrasias, headache, tooth discoloration.

INTERACTIONS: May require downward adjustments of anticoagulant dosage. May interfere with bactericidal action of penicillin; avoid concurrent use when possible. May decrease efficacy of oral contraceptives. Impaired absorption with antacids containing aluminum, calcium, or magnesium and iron-containing products. Fatal renal toxicity

MINOXIDIL
minoxidil (Par) — RX

> May cause pericardial effusion, occasionally progressing to tamponade, and angina pectoris may be exacerbated. Only for nonresponders to maximum therapeutic doses of two other antihypertensives and a diuretic. Administer under supervision with a β-blocker and diuretic. Monitor in hospital for a decrease in BP in those receiving guanethidine with malignant hypertension.

THERAPEUTIC CLASS: Peripheral vasodilator

INDICATIONS: Treatment of hypertension that is symptomatic or associated with target organ damage and is not manageable with maximum therapeutic doses of diuretic plus two other antihypertensive drugs.

DOSAGE: *Adults:* Initial: 5mg qd. Titrate: Increase by no less than 3 days; may increase every 6 hrs if closely monitored. Usual: 10-40mg/day. Max: 100mg/day. Frequency: Give qd if diastolic BP is reduced to <30 mmHg and if reduced to >30 mmHg give bid. Give with a diuretic (eg, HCTZ 50mg bid, furosemide 40mg bid) and a β-blocker (equivalent to propranolol 80-160mg/day) or methyldopa (250-750mg bid starting 24 hrs before therapy). Renal Failure/Dialysis: Reduce dose.

Pediatrics: >12 yrs: Initial: 5mg qd. Titrate: Increase by no less than 3 days; may increase every 6 hrs if closely monitored. Usual: 10-40mg/day. Max: 100mg/day. Frequency: Give qd if diastolic BP is reduced to <30 mmHg and if reduced to >30 mmHg give bid. Give with a diuretic (eg, HCTZ 50mg bid, furosemide 40mg bid) and a β-blocker (equivalent to propranolol 80-160mg/day) or methyldopa (250-750mg bid starting 24 hrs before therapy). <12 yrs: 0.2mg/kg qd. Titrate: May increase by 50-100% increments. Usual: 0.25-1mg/kg/day. Max: 50mg/day. Renal Failure/Dialysis: Reduce dose.

HOW SUPPLIED: Tab: 2.5mg*, 10mg* *scored

CONTRAINDICATIONS: Pheochromocytoma.

WARNINGS/PRECAUTIONS: Administer with a diuretic and β-blocker. Pericarditis, pericardial effusion and tamponade reported. With renal failure or dialysis, reduce dose to prevent renal failure exacerbation and precipitation of cardiac failure. Avoid rapid control with severe HTN. Monitor body weight, fluid and electrolyte balance. Extreme caution with post-MI. Hypersensitivity reactions reported.

ADVERSE REACTIONS: Salt and water retention, pericarditis, pericardial effusion, tamponade, hypertrichosis, nausea, vomiting, rash, ECG changes, hemodilution effects.

INTERACTIONS: Severe orthostatic hypotension with guanethidine.

PREGNANCY: Category C, not for use in nursing.

MINTEZOL
thiabendazole (Merck) — RX

THERAPEUTIC CLASS: Vermicidal and/or vermifugal agent

INDICATIONS: Treatment of strongyloidiasis (threadworm), cutaneous larva migrans (creeping eruption), visceral larva migrans, and trichinosis. Second line or adjunct treatment for uncinariasis, trichuriasis, ascariasis (intestinal roundworms).

DOSAGE: *Adults:* 100 lbs: 1g or 10mL bid. 125 lbs: 1.25g or 12.5mL bid. ≥150 lbs: 1.5g or 15mL bid. Max: 3g/day. Take with meals. Treatment Duration: Strongyloidiasis/Cutaneous Larva Migrans/Intestinal Roundworms: 2 days. Trichinosis: 2-4 days. Visceral Larva Migrans: 7 days.

Pediatrics: 30 lbs: 250mg or 2.5mL bid. 50 lbs: 500mg or 5mL bid. 75 lbs: 750mg or 7.5mL bid. Max: 3g/day. Take with meals. Treatment Duration: Strongyloidiasis/Cutaneous Larva Migrans/Intestinal Roundworms: 2 days. Trichinosis: 2-4 days. Visceral Larva Migrans: 7 days.

HOW SUPPLIED: Sus: 500mg/5mL (120mL); Tab, Chewable: 500mg* *scored

CONTRAINDICATIONS: Prophylactic treatment for pinworm infestation.

WARNINGS/PRECAUTIONS: D/C if hypersensitivity reactions occurs. Erythema multiforme and Stevens-Johnson syndrome, jaundice, cholestasis, and parenchymal hepatic damage reported. Prolonged use may cause abnormal sensation in eyes, xanthopsia, and blurred vision. Not for mixed infections with ascaris, prophylaxis, or first line treatment of enterobiasis. Monitor with hepatic or renal dysfunction.

ADVERSE REACTIONS: Anorexia, nausea, vomiting, diarrhea, weariness, drowsiness, dizziness, abnormal sensation in eyes, xanthopsia, hypotension, hyperglycemia, leukopenia, hematuria, pruritus, fever.

INTERACTIONS: Decreases metabolism of xanthine derivatives; monitor blood levels and/or reduce dose.

PREGNANCY: Category C, not for use in nursing.

MiraLax   OTC
polyethylene glycol 3350 (Schering-Plough)

THERAPEUTIC CLASS: Osmotic laxative

INDICATIONS: Treatment of occasional constipation.

DOSAGE: *Adults:* Stir and dissolve 17g in 4-8 oz of beverage and drink qd. Use no more than 7 days.
Pediatrics: ≥17 yrs: Stir and dissolve 17g in 4-8 oz of beverage and drink qd. Use no more than 7 days.

HOW SUPPLIED: Powder: 17g/dose (119g, 238g)

WARNINGS/PRECAUTIONS: Avoid in kidney disease; talk to your doctor before use if you have nausea, vomiting, abdominal pain, sudden change in bowel habits for ≥2 weeks, or IBS.

Moban   RX
molindone HCl (Endo)

THERAPEUTIC CLASS: Dihydroindolone

INDICATIONS: Management of psychotic disorders.

DOSAGE: *Adults:* Initial: 50-75mg/day. Titrate: Increase to 100mg/day in 3-4 days; adjust to patient response. Maint: Mild: 5-15mg tid-qid. Moderate: 10-25mg tid-qid. Severe: 225mg/day.
Pediatrics: ≥12 yrs: Initial: 50-75mg/day. Titrate: Increase to 100mg/day in 3-4 days; adjust to patient response. Maint: Mild: 5-15mg tid-qid. Moderate: 10-25mg tid-qid. Severe: 225mg/day.

HOW SUPPLIED: Tab: 5mg, 10mg, 25mg*, 50mg* *scored

CONTRAINDICATIONS: Severe CNS depression (alcohol, barbiturates, narcotics), comatose states.

WARNINGS/PRECAUTIONS: Tardive dyskinesia, NMS may occur. Concentrate contains sulfites. Caution with activities requiring alertness. Convulsions, increased activity reported. May obscure signs of intestinal obstruction or brain tumor. May elevate prolactin levels.

ADVERSE REACTIONS: Drowsiness, depression, hyperactivity, euphoria, extrapyramidal reactions, akathisia, Parkinson's syndrome, blurred vision, nausea, dry mouth.

INTERACTIONS: Tabs contain calcium sulfate; may interfere with phenytoin sodium and tetracycline absorption.

PREGNANCY: Safety in pregnancy and nursing not known.

Mobic   RX
meloxicam (Boehringer Ingelheim)

> NSAIDs may cause an increased risk of serious cardiovascular thrombotic events, MI, stroke and serious GI adverse events including bleeding, ulceration, and perforation of the stomach or intestines. Contraindicated for the treatment of peri-operative pain in the setting of coronary artery bypass graft (CABG) surgery.

THERAPEUTIC CLASS: NSAID

Monistat

INDICATIONS: Relief of signs and symptoms of osteoarthritis (OA) and rheumatoid arthritis (RA). Relief of the signs and symptoms of pauciarticular or polyarticular course juvenile rheumatoid arthritis (JRA) in patients >2 yrs.

DOSAGE: *Adults:* ≥18 yrs: OA/RA: Initial/Maint: 7.5mg qd. Max: 15mg/day.
Pediatrics: >2 yrs: JRA: 0.125mg/kg qd. Max: 7.5mg/day.

HOW SUPPLIED: Sus: 7.5mg/5mL; Tab: 7.5mg, 15mg

CONTRAINDICATIONS: ASA or other NSAID allergy that precipitates asthma, urticaria, or allergic-type. Treatment of peri-operative pain in the setting of CABG surgery.

WARNINGS/PRECAUTIONS: May lead to onset of new HTN or worsening of pre-existing HTN; monitor BP closely. Fluid retention and edema reported; caution with fluid retention, HTN, or heart failure. Renal papillary necrosis, renal insufficiency, acute renal failure, and other renal injury reported after long-term use. Not recommended for use with advanced renal disease; if therapy must be initiated, monitor renal function. Anaphylactoid reactions may occur. May cause serious skin adverse events (eg, exfoliative dermatitis, Stevens-Johnson syndrome, and toxic epidermal necrolysis). Avoid in late pregnancy; may cause premature closure of ductus arteriosis. May cause elevations of LFTs; d/c if liver disease develops or systemic manifestations occur. Caution with considerable dehydration and in elderly. Anemia may occur; with long-term use, monitor Hgb/Hct if signs or symptoms of anemia develop. May inhibit platelet aggregation and prolong bleeding time; monitor with coagulation disorders. Caution with asthma and avoid with aspirin-sensitive asthma.

ADVERSE REACTIONS: Abdominal pain, constipation, diarrhea, dyspepsia, nausea, vomiting, headache, anemia, arthralgia, insomnia, upper respiratory tract infection, UTI.

INTERACTIONS: May decrease antihypertensive effects of ACE inhibitors. Potentiates GI bleeds with ASA; avoid concomitant use. Increased clearance with cholestyramine. May decrease natriuretic effects of furosemide, thiazides. Decreased lithium clearance/ increased serum levels. Monitor PT/INR with warfarin. Caution with methotrexate.

PREGNANCY: Category C, not for use in nursing.

Monistat   OTC
miconazole nitrate (Personal Products Company)

OTHER BRAND NAMES: Monistat 3 (Personal Products Company) - Monistat 7 (Personal Products Company)

THERAPEUTIC CLASS: Azole antifungal

INDICATIONS: Treatment of vaginal yeast infections.

DOSAGE: *Adults:* 100mg sup or 2% cream intravaginally qhs for 7 days or 200mg sup or 4% cream intravaginally qhs for 3 days.
Pediatrics: ≥12 yrs: 100mg sup or 2% cream intravaginally qhs for 7 days or 200mg sup or 4% cream intravaginally qhs for 3 days.

HOW SUPPLIED: (Monistat 3) Cre: 4% (15g, 25g); Sup: 200mg (3s); (Monistat 7) Cre: 2% (35g, 45g); Sup: 100mg (7s)

WARNINGS/PRECAUTIONS: Avoid or d/c if abdominal pain, fever (>100°F), shoulder pain, back pain, or foul smelling discharge occurs. Do not use with tampons. Do not rely on condoms or diaphragm to prevent STDs or pregnancy.

ADVERSE REACTIONS: Vulvovaginal burning.

PREGNANCY: Safety in pregnancy and nursing not known.

Monistat 1 Combination Pack   OTC
miconazole nitrate (Personal Products Company)

THERAPEUTIC CLASS: Azole antifungal

INDICATIONS: (Cre) Relief of external vulvular itching and irritation associated with a yeast infection. (Sup) Topical treatment of vulvovaginal candidiasis.

DOSAGE: *Adults:* 1200mg intravaginally qhs for 1 day. Apply 2% cream bid for up to 7 days for external itching.

Pediatrics: ≥12 yrs: 1200mg intravaginally qhs for 1 day. Apply 2% cream bid for up to 7 days for external itching.

HOW SUPPLIED: Cre: 2% (9g); Sup: 1200mg

WARNINGS/PRECAUTIONS: Do not rely on condoms or diaphragm to prevent STDs or pregnancy until 3 days after last use. Do not use tampons, douches, or spermicides until 7 days after last use. Confirm diagnosis by KOH smears and/or cultures; reconfirm if no response.

ADVERSE REACTIONS: Female genitalia burning and irritation, external female genitalia pruritus, female genitalia discharge.

PREGNANCY: Category C, caution in nursing.

Monodox   RX
doxycycline monohydrate (Watson)

THERAPEUTIC CLASS: Tetracycline derivative

INDICATIONS: Treatment of respiratory tract, urinary tract, skin and skin structure, uncomplicated urethral/endocervical/rectal infection caused by *C.trachomatis*, nongonococcal urethritis caused by *C.trachomatis* and *U.urealyticum*, lymphogranuloma, psittacosis, trachoma, chancroid, plague, cholera, brucellosis. Treatment of uncomplicated gonorrhea, syphilis, listeriosis, anthrax, *Clostridium* species when PCN is contraindicated. Adjunct therapy for amebicides and severe acne.

DOSAGE: *Adults:* Usual: 100mg q12h or 50mg q6h for 1 day, then 100mg/day. Severe Infection: 100mg q12h. Uncomplicated Gonococcal Infections (except anorectal infections in men): 100mg bid for 7 days or 300mg stat, then repeat in 1 hr. Acute Epididymo-Orchitis caused by *N.gonorrhea* or *C.trachomatis:* 100mg bid for at least 10 days. Primary/Secondary Syphilis: 300mg/day in divided dose for at least 10 days. Uncomplicated Urethral/Endocervical/Rectal Infection caused by *C.trachomatis:* 100mg bid for at least 7 days. Nongonococcal Urethritis caused by *C.trachomatis* and *U.urealyticum:* 100mg bid for at least 7 days. Take with full glass of water. Take with food if GI upset occurs.

Pediatrics: >8 yrs:≤100 lbs: 2mg/lb divided in 2 doses for 1 day, then 1mg/lb daily in single or 2 divided doses. Severe Infection: May use up to 2mg/lb/day. >100 lbs: 100mg q12h or 50mg q6h for 1 day, then 100mg/day. Severe Infection: 100mg q12h. Take with a full glass of water. Take with food if GI upset occurs.

HOW SUPPLIED: Cap: 50mg, 100mg

WARNINGS/PRECAUTIONS: Avoid direct sunlight or UV light. May cause permanent tooth discoloration during tooth development (last half of pregnancy and children <8 years). Monitor renal/hepatic function, and blood with long-term therapy. May increase BUN. Photosensitivity, pseudotumor cerebri reported. D/C if superinfection occurs. Bulging fontanels in infants and intracranial HTN in adults reported.

ADVERSE REACTIONS: GI effects, photosensitivity, rash, blood dyscrasias, hypersensitivity reactions.

INTERACTIONS: Carbamazepine, barbiturates, phenytoin decrease half-life of doxycycline. May decrease PT; adjust anticoagulants. May decrease bactericidal agents (eg, penicillin). May decrease effects of oral contraceptives. Take 1 hr before or 2 hrs after dairy products. Aluminum-, calcium-, iron- and magnesium-containing products impair absorption. Fatal renal toxicity may occur with methoxyflurane.

PREGNANCY: Category D, not for use in nursing.

Motrin   RX
ibuprofen (Pharmacia & Upjohn)

> NSAIDs may cause an increased risk of serious cardiovascular thrombotic events, MI, stroke and serious GI adverse events including bleeding, ulceration, and perforation of the stomach or intestines. Contraindicated for the treatment of peri-operative pain in the setting of coronary artery bypass graft (CABG) surgery.

THERAPEUTIC CLASS: NSAID

Motrin IB

INDICATIONS: Adults: Relief of mild-to-moderate pain. Dysmenorrhea. Rheumatoid arthritis (RA) Osteoarthritis (OA). Pediatrics: Fever. Relief of mild-to-moderate pain. Juvenile arthritis (JA).

DOSAGE: *Adults:* Pain: 400mg q4-6h prn. Dysmenorrhea: 400mg q4h prn. RA/OA: 300mg qid or 400mg, 600mg or 800mg tid-qid. Max: 3200mg/day. Take with meals/milk. Renal Impairment: Reduce dose.
Pediatrics: Fever: 6 months-12 yrs: 5mg/kg for temp <102.5°F; 10mg/kg if temp ≥102.5°F q6-8h. Max: 40mg/kg/day. Pain: 6 months-12 yrs: 10mg/kg q6-8h. Max: 40mg/kg/day. JA: 30-40mg/kg/day divided into 3 or 4 doses. Milder disease may use 20mg/kg/day.

HOW SUPPLIED: Sus: 100mg/5mL (120mL, 480mL); Tab: 400mg, 600mg, 800mg

CONTRAINDICATIONS: Syndrome of nasal polyps, angioedema, and bronchospastic reactions to ASA or other NSAIDs. Treatment of peri-operative pain in the setting of CABG surgery.

WARNINGS/PRECAUTIONS: May lead to onset of new HTN or worsening of pre-existing HTN; monitor BP closely. Fluid retention and edema reported; caution with fluid retention or heart failure. Renal papillary necrosis and other renal injury reported after long-term use. Not recommended for use with advanced renal disease; if therapy must be initiated, monitor renal function. Anaphylactoid reactions may occur. May cause serious skin adverse events (eg, exfoliative dermatitis, Stevens-Johnson syndrome, and toxic epidermal necrolysis). Avoid in late pregnancy; may cause premature closure of ductus arteriosus. May cause elevations of LFTs; d/c if liver disease develops or systemic manifestations occur. Caution in elderly. Anemia may occur; with long-term use, monitor Hgb/Hct if signs or symptoms of anemia develop. May inhibit platelet aggregation and prolong bleeding time; monitor with coagulation disorders. Caution with asthma and avoid with aspirin-sensitive asthma. D/C if visual disturbances occur. Aseptic meningitis with fever and coma reported.

ADVERSE REACTIONS: Nausea, epigastric pain, heartburn, dizziness, rash.

INTERACTIONS: Use caution with anticoagulants. May enhance methotrexate toxicity. May decrease the natriuretic effects of furosemide or thiazides. Avoid use with aspirin. Decrease lithium clearance; monitor for toxicity.

PREGNANCY: Category C, not for use in nursing.

Motrin IB OTC
ibuprofen (McNeil Consumer)

THERAPEUTIC CLASS: NSAID

INDICATIONS: Temporary relief of headache, muscular aches, minor pain of arthritis, toothache, backache, minor aches and pains. Fever.

DOSAGE: *Adults:* 200mg q4-6h. 400mg if symptoms do not respond. Max: 1200mg/24hrs.
Pediatrics: ≥12 yrs: 200mg q4-6h. 400mg if symptoms do not respond. Max: 1200mg/24hrs.

HOW SUPPLIED: Tab: 200mg

WARNINGS/PRECAUTIONS: Do not take for >10 days for pain or >3 days for fever. May cause severe allergic reaction. Do not use if history of allergic reaction to other pain relievers/fever reducers.

INTERACTIONS: Avoid other ibuprofen-containing products.

PREGNANCY: Safety in pregnancy and nursing not known.

Motrin, Children's OTC
ibuprofen (McNeil Consumer)

OTHER BRAND NAMES: Motrin, Junior (McNeil Consumer) - Motrin, Infants (McNeil Consumer)

THERAPEUTIC CLASS: NSAID

INDICATIONS: To temporarily reduce fever, relief of minor aches and pains associated with the common cold, flu, sore throat, headaches and toothaches.

MUCINEX DM

DOSAGE: *Pediatrics:* Infant Drops: 6-11 months (12-17lbs): 1.25mL q6-8h. 12-23 months (18-23lbs): 1.875mL q6-8h. Use only with enclosed dropper. Sus: 2-3 yrs (24-35lbs): 5mL q6-8h. 4-5 yrs (36-47lbs): 7.5mL q6-8h. 6-8 yrs (48-59lbs): 10mL q6-8h. 9-10 yrs (60-71lbs): 12.5mL q6-8h. 11 yrs (72-95lbs): 15mL q6-8h. Use only with enclosed measuring cup. Children's Chewable Tab: 4-5 yrs (36-47lbs): 150mg q6-8h. 6-8 yrs (48-59lbs): 200mg q6-8h. 9-10 yrs (60-71lbs): 250mg q6-8h. 11 yrs (72-95lbs): 300mg q6-8h. Junior Tab/Chewable Tab: 6-8 yrs (48-59lbs): 200mg q6-8h. 9-10 yrs (60-71lbs): 250mg q6-8h. 11 yrs (72-95lbs): 300mg q6-8h. Max: 4 doses/24hrs. Take with food/milk to avoid upset stomach. Take chewable tabs with food/water to avoid mouth/throat burning.

HOW SUPPLIED: Infant Drops: 50mg/1.25mL (15mL); Children's Sus: 100mg/5mL (60mL, 120mL); Children's Tab, Chewable: 50mg; Junior Tab/Tab, Chewable: 100mg

WARNINGS/PRECAUTIONS: May cause severe allergic reaction (eg, hives, facial swelling, wheezing, shock). Avoid with history of allergic reaction to any other pain reliever/fever reducer. Not for use >2-3 days.

INTERACTIONS: Caution with other products that contain ibuprofen or any other pain reliever/fever reducer.

PREGNANCY: Safety in pregnancy and nursing not known.

MUCINEX
guaifenesin (Adams)

OTC

THERAPEUTIC CLASS: Expectorant

INDICATIONS: To help loosen phlegm, thin bronchial secretions and make coughs more productive.

DOSAGE: *Adults:* 1-2 tabs every 12hrs. Max: 4 tabs/24hrs. Take with a full glass of water. Do not crush, chew, or break tab.

Pediatrics: ≥12 yrs: 1-2 tabs every 12hrs. Max: 4 tabs/24hrs. Take with a full glass of water. Do not crush, chew, or break tab.

HOW SUPPLIED: Tab, Extended Release: 600mg

WARNINGS/PRECAUTIONS: Discontinue if cough lasts >7 days, recurs, or occurs with fever, rash, or persistent headache.

PREGNANCY: Safety in pregnancy or nursing not known.

MUCINEX D
guaifenesin - pseudoephedrine HCl (Adams)

OTC

THERAPEUTIC CLASS: Expectorant/nasal decongestant

INDICATIONS: Help loosen phlegm and thin bronchial secretions. Temporarily relieve nasal congestion due to common cold, hay fever, or upper respiratory allergies. Promote nasal and sinus drainage. Temporarily relieve sinus congestion and pressure.

DOSAGE: *Adults:* 2 tabs every 12hrs. Max: 4 tabs/24hrs. Do not crush, chew, or break.

Pediatrics: ≥12 yrs: 2 tabs every 12hrs. Max: 4 tabs/24hrs. Do not crush, chew, or break.

HOW SUPPLIED: Tab, Extended Release: (Guaifenesin-Pseudoephedrine HCl) 600mg-60mg

WARNINGS/PRECAUTIONS: Avoid use during or for 2 weeks after stopping MAOI therapy. Caution with heart disease, high BP, thyroid disease, diabetes, difficulty urinating due to enlarged prostate, persistent or chronic cough. D/C if cough lasts >7 days, or occurs with fever, rash or persistent headache.

INTERACTIONS: See Warnings and Precautions.

PREGNANCY: Safety in pregnancy and nursing not known.

MUCINEX DM
guaifenesin - dextromethorphan hydrobromide (Adams)

OTC

THERAPEUTIC CLASS: Cough suppressant/expectorant

INDICATIONS: To help loosen phlegm, thin bronchial secretions and makes coughs more productive. Temporarily relieves cough.

Mucomyst

DOSAGE: *Adults:* 1-2 tabs q12hrs. Max: 4 tabs/24hrs. Take with a full glass of water. Do not crush, chew, or break tab.

Pediatrics: ≥12 yrs: 1-2 tabs q12hrs. Max: 4 tabs/24hrs. Take with a full glass of water. Do not crush, chew, or break tab.

HOW SUPPLIED: Tab: (Dextromethorphan-Guaifenesin) 30mg-600mg

WARNINGS/PRECAUTIONS: Discontinue if cough lasts >7 days, recurs, or occurs with fever, rash, or persistent headache. Avoid during or within 14 days of MAOIs.

INTERACTIONS: See Warnings and Precautions.

PREGNANCY: Safety in pregnancy or nursing not known.

Mucomyst   RX
acetylcysteine (Sandoz)

THERAPEUTIC CLASS: Acetaminophen antidote/Mucolytic

INDICATIONS: Adjunctive mucolytic therapy in acute and chronic bronchopulmonary disease; pulmonary complications of cystic fibrosis and surgery; tracheostomy care; during anesthesia; post-traumatic chest conditions; atelectasis; diagnostic bronchial studies. Antidote for acute acetaminophen (APAP) toxicity.

DOSAGE: *Adults:* Antidote: Empty stomach by lavage or emesis before administration. Administer immediately, regardless of quantity, if APAP ingestion ≤24hrs. LD: 140mg/kg PO then 70mg/kg PO q4h for 17 doses starting 4 hours after LD. Discontinue if predetoxification APAP level is in the nontoxic range and overdose occurred at least 4 hrs before assay. Obtain 2nd plasma level if range is nontoxic and time of ingestion is unknown or <4 hrs. Mucolytic: Nebulization (face mask, mouth piece, tracheostomy): 1-10mL of 20% or 2-10mL of 10% q2-6h. Usual: 3-5mL of 20% or 6-10mL of 10% 3-4 times/day. Closed Tent or Croupette: Up to 300mL of 10% or 20%. Direct Instillation: 1-2 mL of 10% or 20% q1-4h. Percutaneous Intratracheal Catheter: 1-2mL of 20% or 2-4mL of 10% q1-4h. Diagnostic Bronchograms: Give before procedure. 2-3 doses of 1-2mL of 20% or 2-4mL of 10%.

Pediatrics: Antidote: Empty stomach by lavage or emesis before administration. Administer immediately, regardless of quantity, if APAP ingestion ≤24hrs. LD: 140mg/kg PO then 70mg/kg PO q4h for 17 doses starting 4 hours after LD. Discontinue if predetoxification APAP level is in the nontoxic range and overdose occurred at least 4 hrs before assay. Obtain 2nd plasma level if range is nontoxic and time of ingestion is unknown or <4 hrs. Mucolytic: Nebulization (face mask, mouth piece, tracheostomy): 1-10mL of 20% or 2-10mL of 10% q2-6h. Usual: 3-5mL of 20% or 6-10mL of 10% 3-4 times/day. Closed Tent or Croupette: Up to 300mL of 10% or 20%. Direct Instillation: 1-2 mL of 10% or 20% q1-4h. Percutaneous Intratracheal Catheter: 1-2mL of 20% or 2-4mL of 10% q1-4h. Diagnostic Procedures: Give before procedure. 2-3 doses of 1-2mL of 20% or 2-4mL of 10%.

HOW SUPPLIED: Sol: 10%, 20%

WARNINGS/PRECAUTIONS: (Oral) Discontinue if generalized urticaria or encephalopathy due to hepatic failure develops. May aggravate vomiting; evaluate with risk of gastric hemorrhage. (Inhalation) Monitor asthmatics. Discontinue if bronchospasm progresses.

ADVERSE REACTIONS: (Oral) Nausea, vomiting, other GI symptoms. (Inhalation) Stomatitis, nausea, vomiting, fever, rhinorrhea, drowsiness, clamminess, chest tightness, bronchoconstriction.

PREGNANCY: Category B, caution in nursing.

Mumpsvax   RX
mumps virus vaccine live (Merck)

THERAPEUTIC CLASS: Vaccine

INDICATIONS: Vaccination against mumps.

DOSAGE: *Adults:* 0.5mL SQ into outer aspect of upper arm.

Pediatrics: ≥12 mos: 0.5mL SQ in outer aspect of upper arm. Give primary vaccine at 12-15 months. Revaccinate prior to elementary school.

HOW SUPPLIED: Inj: 20,000 TCID$_{50}$

CONTRAINDICATIONS: Avoid pregnancy for 3 months after vaccine, anaphylactic reaction to neomycin, febrile/active respiratory illness, immunosuppressive therapy (except corticosteroids as replacement therapy), blood dyscrasias, leukemia, lymphoma, malignant neoplasms affecting the bone marrow or lymphatic system, immunodeficiency states.

WARNINGS/PRECAUTIONS: Caution with hypersensitivity to eggs and neomycin. May worsen thrombocytopenia. Defer vaccine for at least 3 months after blood or plasma transfusion and immune globulin. Do not revaccinate with active untreated TB. Monitor for temperature elevation after administration. Contains albumin, remote risk of viral infection transmission. Have epinephrine (1:1000) available.

ADVERSE REACTIONS: Fever, syncope, irritability, diarrhea, diabetes, purpura, cough, febrile seizures, local site reactions.

INTERACTIONS: Do not give with immune globulin. May depress TB skin sensitivity, administer test either simultaneously or before. Do not give <1 month before or after other live viral vaccines. Do not give simultaneously with DTP or oral poliovirus vaccine.

PREGNANCY: Category C, caution in nursing.

MYAMBUTOL
ethambutol HCl (Elan)
RX

THERAPEUTIC CLASS: Cell metabolism inhibitor

INDICATIONS: Adjunct treatment of pulmonary tuberculosis (TB) with at least one other anti-TB drug.

DOSAGE: *Adults:* Initial: 15mg/kg q24h. Retreatment: 25mg/kg q24h. After 60 days, decrease to 15mg/kg q24h. Renal Dysfunction: Reduce dose.
Pediatric: ≥13 yrs: Initial: 15mg/kg q24h. Retreatment: 25mg/kg q24h. After 60 days, decrease to 15mg/kg q24h. Renal Dysfunction: Reduce dose.

HOW SUPPLIED: Tab: 100mg, 400mg* *scored

CONTRAINDICATIONS: Optic neuritis. Patients unable to appreciate and report visual side effects or changes in vision.

WARNINGS/PRECAUTIONS: Test visual acuity before and periodically during therapy; monthly with dose >15mg/kg/day. Liver toxicity reported; monitor hepatic function at baseline and periodically. Evaluate renal and hematopoietic functions periodically.

ADVERSE REACTIONS: Decreased visual acuity, optic neuropathy, anaphylactic reactions, dermatitis, pruritus, joint pain, GI effects, malaise, dizziness, elevated uric acid levels, pulmonary infiltrates, abnormal LFTs, eosinophilia.

PREGNANCY: Category C, safety in nursing not known.

MYCELEX TROCHE
clotrimazole (Ortho-McNeil)
RX

THERAPEUTIC CLASS: Triazole antifungal

INDICATIONS: Treatment of oropharyngeal candidiasis. To prevent oropharyngeal candidiasis in immunocompromised conditions (eg, chemotherapy, radiotherapy or steroid therapy).

DOSAGE: *Adults:* Treatment: Slowly dissolve 1 troche in mouth 5 times/day for 14 days. Prophylaxis: Slowly dissolve 1 troche in mouth tid for duration of chemotherapy or until steroids are reduced.
Pediatrics: ≥3 yrs: Treatment: Slowly dissolve 1 troche in mouth 5 times/day for 14 days.

HOW SUPPLIED: Loz/Troche: 10mg (70 loz, 140 loz)

WARNINGS/PRECAUTIONS: Not for systemic mycoses. May cause abnormal LFTs; monitor hepatic function. Only use in patients mentally and physically able to dissolve the troche. Confirm diagnosis by KOH smear and/or culture.

ADVERSE REACTIONS: Abnormal LFTs, nausea, vomiting, unpleasant mouth sensations, pruritus.

PREGNANCY: Category C, safety in nursing is not known.

MYCELEX-3
butoconazole nitrate (Bayer Healthcare)
OTC

THERAPEUTIC CLASS: Azole antifungal

INDICATIONS: Treatment of vaginal yeast infection.

Mycelex-7

DOSAGE: *Adults:* Insert 1 applicatorful vaginally qhs for 3 days.
Pediatrics: ≥12 yrs: Insert 1 applicatorful vaginally qhs for 3 days.
HOW SUPPLIED: Cre: 2% (5g, 20g)
WARNINGS/PRECAUTIONS: Do not use if abdominal pain, fever, foul smelling discharge, pregnancy, diabetes, HIV positive and AIDS patients. Avoid tampons. Do not rely on condoms or diaphragms to prevent STDs or pregnancy while on therapy; use alternate birth control method.
PREGNANCY: Safety in pregnancy or nursing not known.

Mycelex-7
clotrimazole (Bayer Healthcare)
OTC

THERAPEUTIC CLASS: Azole antifungal
INDICATIONS: (Cre, Combination Pack) Treatment of vaginal yeast infection. (Combination Pack) For relief of external vulvar itching and irritation associated with vaginal yeast infections.
DOSAGE: *Adults:* (Cre) Insert 1 applicatorful vaginally qhs for 7 days. (Combination Pack) 1 insert vaginally qhs for 7 days. Apply small amount of cream onto irritated area of vulva qd-bid for up to 7 days.
Pediatrics: ≥12 yrs: (Cre) Insert 1 applicatorful vaginally qhs for 7 days. (Combination Pack) 1 insert vaginally qhs for 7 days. Apply small amount of cream onto irritated area of vulva qd-bid for up to 7 days.
HOW SUPPLIED: Cre: 1% (45g); (Combination Pack) Cre: 1% (7g), Vaginal Insert: 100 mg (7s)
WARNINGS/PRECAUTIONS: Do not use if abdominal pain, fever, foul smelling discharge, during pregnancy. Avoid tampons. May reduce effectiveness of condoms, diaphragm or vaginal spermicides.
PREGNANCY: Safety in pregnancy or nursing not known.

Mycolog-II
nystatin - triamcinolone acetonide (Apothecon)
RX

THERAPEUTIC CLASS: Polyene antifungal/corticosteroid
INDICATIONS: Topical treatment of cutaneous candidiasis.
DOSAGE: *Adults:* Apply bid (am and pm). Max: 25 days of treatment.
Pediatrics: Apply bid (am and pm). Max: 25 days of treatment.
HOW SUPPLIED: Cre, Oint: (Nystatin-Triamcinolone) 100,000 U/g-0.1% (15g, 30g, 60g)
WARNINGS/PRECAUTIONS: Avoid occlusive dressing. Monitor periodically for HPA axis suppression with prolonged use or when applied over a large area. Discontinue if develop hypersensitivity or irritation. Systemic absorption with topical corticosteroids reported; children are more prone to systemic toxicity. May cause Cushing's syndrome, hyperglycemia, and glucosuria.
ADVERSE REACTIONS: Acneform eruption, burning, itching, irritation, secondary infection.
PREGNANCY: Category C, caution in nursing.

Mycostatin Topical
nystatin (Westwood-Squibb)
RX

THERAPEUTIC CLASS: Polyene antifungal
INDICATIONS: Treatment of cutaneous or mucocutaneous mycotic infections caused by susceptible *Candida* species.
DOSAGE: Adults: (Cre) Apply to affected area bid until healing is complete. (Powder) Apply to lesions bid-tid until healing is complete. For fungal infections of the feet, dust powder on feet and in shoes also.

Pediatrics: Neonates and Older: (Cre) Apply to affected area bid until healing is complete. (Powder) Apply to lesions bid-tid until healing is complete. For fungal infections of the feet, dust powder on feet and in shoes also.

HOW SUPPLIED: Cre: 100,000 U/g (30g); Powder, Topical: 100,000 U/g (15g)

WARNINGS/PRECAUTIONS: Discontinue if irritation or sensitization occurs. Confirm diagnosis. Not for systemic, oral, intravaginal, or ophthalmic use. For fungal infections of the feet, dust powder on feet as well as in all footwear. Moist lesions are best treated with topical dusting powder.

ADVERSE REACTIONS: Allergic reactions, burning, itching, rash, eczema, pain at application site.

PREGNANCY: Category C, caution in nursing.

Myfortic RX
mycophenolic acid (Novartis)

> Increased susceptibility to infection. Possible development of lymphoma and other neoplasms.

THERAPEUTIC CLASS: Inosine monophosphate dehydrogenase inhibitor

INDICATIONS: Prophylaxis of organ rejection in patients receiving allogeneic renal transplants, administered in combination with cyclosporine and corticosteroids.

DOSAGE: *Adults:* 720mg bid on empty stomach, 1 hr before or 2 hrs after food intake. *Pediatrics:* 400mg/m^2 bid. Max: 720mg bid. BSA 1.19-1.58m^2: 540mg bid. BSA >1.58m^2: 720mg bid. BSA <1.19m^2 cannot be accurately adminsitered with current formulations.

HOW SUPPLIED: Tab, Delayed Release: 180mg, 360mg

WARNINGS/PRECAUTIONS: Risk of lymphomas and other malignancies, especially of the skin. Avoid sunlight to decrease risk of skin cancer. May cause fetal harm during pregnancy. Must have negative serum/urine pregnancy test within 1 week before therapy. Two reliable forms of contraception required before and during therapy, and 6 weeks following discontinuation. Monitor for bone marrow suppression. Risk of GI ulceration, hemorrhage, and perforation; caution with active digestive system disease. Caution with delayed renal graft function post-transplant. Oral suspension contains phenylalanine; caution with phenylketonurics. Monitor CBC weekly during the 1st month, twice monthly for the 2nd and 3rd months, and then monthly through 1st year. Avoid with rare hereditary deficiency of hypoxanthine-guanine phosphoribosyl-transferase (eg, Lesch-Nyhan and Kelley-Seegmiller syndrome).

ADVERSE REACTIONS: Infections, diarrhea, leukopenia, sepsis, vomiting, GI bleeding, pain, abdominal pain, fever, headache, asthenia, chest pain, back pain, anemia, leukopenia, thrombocytopenia.

INTERACTIONS: Additive bone marrow suppression with azathioprine; avoid use. Reduced efficacy with drugs that interfere with enterohepatic recirculation (eg, cholestyramine). Efficacy/safety with other immunosuppressive agents not determined. Avoid live attenuated vaccines. Increased levels of both drugs with acyclovir, ganciclovir. Decreased levels with magnesium- and aluminum-containing antacids; space dosing. Decreased effects of oral contraceptives. Increased levels with probenecid. Other drugs that compete for renal tubular secretion may raise levels of both drugs.

PREGNANCY: Category C, not for use in nursing.

Mylanta Maximum Strength Liquid OTC
simethicone - aluminum hydroxide - magnesium hydroxide (J&J -- Merck)

OTHER BRAND NAME: Mylanta Regular Strength Liquid (J&J -- Merck)

THERAPEUTIC CLASS: Antacid/antigas

MYLERAN

INDICATIONS: For the relief of heartburn, acid indigestion, sour stomach, upset stomach, pressure and bloating.

DOSAGE: *Adults:* ≥12 yrs: 2-4 tsp between meals or at bedtime. Max: 24 tsp/day for 2 weeks. Shake well.

Pediatrics: ≥12 yrs: 2-4 tsp between meals or at bedtime. Max: 24 tsp/day for 2 weeks. Shake well.

HOW SUPPLIED: Liq: (Aluminum Hydroxide-Magnesium Hydroxide-Simethicone) Maximum Strength: 400mg/5mL-400mg/5mL-40mg/5mL. Regular Strength: 200mg/5mL-200mg/5mL-20mg/5mL

MYLERAN RX
busulfan (GlaxoSmithKline)

> Do not use unless CML diagnosis is established. May induce severe bone marrow hypoplasia. Reduce dose or discontinue if unusual depression occurs.

THERAPEUTIC CLASS: Alkylating agent

INDICATIONS: Palliative treatment of chronic myelogenous leukemia (CML).

DOSAGE: *Adults:* 60mcg/kg/day or 1.8mg/m^2/day. Range: 4-8mg/day. Reserve dose >4mg/day for the most compelling symptoms.

Pediatrics: 60mcg/kg/day or 1.8mg/m^2/day. Range: 4-8mg/day. Reserve dose >4mg/day for the most compelling symptoms.

HOW SUPPLIED: Tab: 2mg* *scored

CONTRAINDICATIONS: Lack of definitive diagnosis of CML.

WARNINGS/PRECAUTIONS: Induction of bone marrow failure resulting in severe pancytopenia reported. Bronchopulmonary dysplasia with pulmonary fibrosis, cellular dysplasia, malignant tumors, acute leukemias, hepatic veno-occlusive disease reported. Ovarian suppression and amenorrhea with menopausal symptoms have occurred. Cardiac tamponade in patients with thalassemia and seizures reported. Caution with compromised bone marrow reserve from prior irradiation/chemotherapy.

ADVERSE REACTIONS: Myelosuppression, pulmonary fibrosis, cardiac tamponade, hyperpigmentation, weakness, fatigue, weight loss, nausea, vomiting, melanoderma, hyperuricemia, myasthenia gravis, hepatic veno-occlusive disease.

INTERACTIONS: Additive myelosuppression with myelosuppressive drugs. Additive pulmonary toxicity with myelotoxic drugs. Reduced clearance with cyclophosphamide. Reduced clearance with itraconazole; monitor for signs of toxicity.

PREGNANCY: Category D, not for use in nursing.

MYOZYME RX
alglucosidase alfa (Genzyme)

> Risk of hypersensitivity reactions. Life threatening anaphylactic reactions, including anaphylactic shock observed during infusion. Appropriate medical support should be readily available when administered.

THERAPEUTIC CLASS: Enzyme

INDICATIONS: Treatment of Pompe Disease.

DOSAGE: *Adults:* 20 mg/kg IV every 2 weeks. Administer over 4 hrs.

Pediatrics: 20 mg/kg IV every 2 weeks. Administer over 4 hrs.

HOW SUPPLIED: Inj: 50 mg

WARNINGS/PRECAUTIONS: See Black Box Warning. Risk of cardiac arrhythmia, sudden cardiac death during general anesthesia for central venous catheter placement, and acute cardiorespiratory failure. Infusion reactions observed. Caution with acutely ill patients.

ADVERSE REACTIONS: Pyrexia, cough, respiratory distress/failure, pneumonia, otitis media, upper respiratory tract infection, gastroenteritis, pharyngitis, diarrhea, vomiting, rash, decreased oxygen saturation, anemia, oral candidiasis.

PREGNANCY: Category B, caution in nursing.

Mysoline
primidone (Valeant) — RX

THERAPEUTIC CLASS: Pyrimidinedione derivative

INDICATIONS: For control of grand mal, psychomotor, and focal epileptic seizures.

DOSAGE: *Adults:* Initial: Day 1-3: 100-125mg qhs. Day 4-6: 100-125mg bid. Day 7-9: 100-125mg tid. Day 10-Maint: 250mg tid. Max: 500mg qid. Effective serum level is 5-12mcg/mL. Prior Anticonvulsant Therapy: Initial: 100-125mg qhs. Titrate: Increase gradually to maintenance dose as other drug is discontinued over 2 weeks.

Pediatrics: ≥8 yrs: Initial: Day 1-3: 100-125mg qhs. Day 4-6: 100-125mg bid. Day 7-9: 100-125mg tid. Day 10-Maint: 250mg tid. Max: 500mg qid. <8 yrs: Day 1-3: 50mg qhs. Day 4-6: 50mg bid. Day 7-9: 100mg bid. Day 10-Maint: 125-250mg tid or 10-25mg/kg/day in divided doses. Effective serum level is 5-12mcg/mL. Prior Anticonvulsant Therapy: Initial: 100-125mg qhs. Titrate: Increase gradually to maintenance dose as other drug is discontinued over 2 weeks.

HOW SUPPLIED: Tab: 50mg*, 250mg* *scored

CONTRAINDICATIONS: Porphyria, phenobarbital hypersensitivity.

WARNINGS/PRECAUTIONS: Avoid abrupt withdrawal. May take several weeks to assess therapeutic efficacy. Pregnant women should receive prophylactic vitamin K_1 therapy for one month prior to, and during delivery. Perform CBC and a SMA-12 test every 6 months. Phenobarbital is a metabolite of primidone.

ADVERSE REACTIONS: Ataxia, vertigo, nausea, anorexia, vomiting, fatigue, hyperirritability, emotional disturbances, sexual impotency, diplopia, nystagmus, drowsiness, morbilliform skin eruptions.

PREGNANCY: Safety in pregnancy not known, caution in nursing.

Naloxone
naloxone HCl (Various) — RX

OTHER BRAND NAME: Narcan (Endo)

THERAPEUTIC CLASS: Opioid antagonist

INDICATIONS: For complete or partial opioid depression reversal induced by natural and synthetic opioids. Diagnosis of suspected opioid tolerance or acute opioid overdose. Adjunct in management of septic shock to increase blood pressure.

DOSAGE: *Adults:* Opioid Overdose: Initial: 0.4-2mg IV every 2-3 minutes up to 10mg. IM/SQ if IV route not available. Post-op Opioid Depression: 0.1-0.2mg IV every 2-3 minutes to desired response. May repeat in 1-2 hr intervals. Supplemental IM doses last longer. Narcan Challenge Test: IV: 0.1-0.2mg, observe 30 secs for signs of withdrawal, then 0.6mg, observe for 20 minutes. SQ: 0.8mg, observe for 20 minutes.

Pediatrics: Opioid Overdose: Initial: 0.01mg/kg IV. Inadequate Response: repeat 0.01mg/kg once. IM/SQ in divided doses if IV route not available. Post-op Opioid Depression: 0.005-0.01mg IV every 2-3 minutes to desired response. May repeat in 1-2 hr intervals. Supplemental IM doses last longer. Neonates: Opioid-induced Depression: 0.01mg/kg IV/IM/SQ, may repeat every 2-3 minutes until desired response.

HOW SUPPLIED: Inj: 0.4mg/mL, 1mg/mL

WARNINGS/PRECAUTIONS: Caution in patients including newborns of mothers known or suspected of opioid physical dependence. May precipitate acute withdrawal syndrome. Have other resuscitative measures available. Caution with cardiac, renal, or hepatic disease. Monitor patients satisfactorily responding due to extended opioid duration of action. Abrupt postoperative opioid depression reversal may result in serious adverse effects leading to death.

ADVERSE REACTIONS: HTN, hypotension, ventricular tachycardia and fibrillation, dyspnea, pulmonary edema, cardiac arrest, nausea, vomiting, sweating, seizures, body aches, fever, nervousness.

INTERACTIONS: Caution using drugs with potential adverse cardiac effects. Reversal of buprenorphine-induced respiratory depression may be incomplete.

PREGNANCY: Category B, caution in nursing.

NAPHCON-A OTC
naphazoline HCl - pheniramine maleate (Alcon)

THERAPEUTIC CLASS: H_1 antagonist/alpha-agonist (imidazoline)

INDICATIONS: Temporary relief of ocular itching and redness caused by ragweed, pollen, grass, animal hair and dander.

DOSAGE: *Adults:* 1-2 drops up to 4 times daily.

Pediatrics: ≥6 yrs: 1-2 drops up to 4 times daily.

HOW SUPPLIED: Sol: (Pheniramine-Naphazoline) 0.3%-0.025% (15mL)

CONTRAINDICATIONS: Heart disease, high BP, enlargement of the prostate, narrow-angle glaucoma.

WARNINGS/PRECAUTIONS: Do not use if solution changes color or becomes cloudy. D/C with eye pain, changes in vision, continued redness or irritation, and if the condition worsens or persists for more than 72 hrs. Remove contact lenses before use. Supervision required with heart disease, high BP, difficulty in urination due to prostate enlargement or narrow angle glaucoma.

PREGNANCY: Safety in pregnancy and nursing not known.

NAPROSYN RX
naproxen (Roche Labs)

> NSAIDs may cause an increased risk of serious cardiovascular thrombotic events, MI, stroke and serious GI adverse events including bleeding, ulceration, and perforation of the stomach or intestines. Contraindicated for the treatment of peri-operative pain in the setting of coronary artery bypass graft (CABG) surgery.

OTHER BRAND NAME: EC-Naprosyn (Roche Labs)

THERAPEUTIC CLASS: NSAID

INDICATIONS: (Naprosyn, EC-Naprosyn) Relief of signs and symptoms of rheumatoid arthritis (RA), osteoarthritis (OA), ankylosing spondylitis and juvenile arthritis (JA). (Naprosyn) Relief of signs and symtoms of tendinitis, bursitis, and acute gout. Management of pain and primary dysmenorrhea. EC-Naprosyn is not recommended for initial treatment of acute pain.

DOSAGE: *Adults:* RA/OA/Ankylosing Spondylitis: Naprosyn: 250, 375, or 500mg bid; EC-Naprosyn: 375 or 500mg bid. Max: 1500mg/day. Acute Gout: Naprosyn: 750mg followed by 250mg q8h until attack subsides. Pain/Dysmenorrhea/Tendinitis/Bursitis: Naprosyn: 500mg followed by 500mg q12h or 250mg q6-8h prn. Max: 1250mg day 1, then 1000mg/day. EC-Naprosyn should not be chewed, crushed, or broken.

Pediatrics: ≥2 yrs: JA: (Sus) 5mg/kg bid. Max: 15mg/kg/day.

HOW SUPPLIED: (Naproxen) Sus: 25mg/mL; Tab: 250mg*, 375mg, 500mg*; Tab, Delayed Release: (EC-Naprosyn) 375mg, 500mg *scored

CONTRAINDICATIONS: History of ASA or NSAID allergy that cause symptoms of asthma, rhinitis, nasal polyps, and hypotension. Treatment of peri-operative pain in the setting of CABG surgery.

WARNINGS/PRECAUTIONS: May lead to onset of new HTN or worsening of pre-existing HTN; monitor BP closely. Fluid retention, edema, and peripheral edema reported; caution with fluid retention, HTN, or heart failure. Renal papillary necrosis and other renal injury reported after long-term use. Not recommended for use with advanced renal disease; if therapy must be initiated, monitor renal function. Anaphylactoid reactions may occur. May cause serious skin adverse events (eg, exfoliative dermatitis, Stevens-Johnson syndrome, and toxic epidermal necrolysis). Avoid in late pregnancy; may cause premature closure of ductus arteriosis. Monitor Hgb levels with long-term therapy if initial Hgb ≤10g. Monitor for visual changes or disturbances. May cause elevations of LFTs; d/c if liver disease develops or systemic manifestations occur. Caution with high doses in chronic alcoholic liver disease and elderly. Anemia may occur; with long-term use, monitor Hgb/Hct if signs or symptoms of anemia develop. May inhibit platelet aggregation and prolong bleeding time; monitor with coagulation disorders. Caution with asthma and avoid with aspirin-sensitive asthma.

ADVERSE REACTIONS: Edema, drowsiness, dizziness, constipation, heartburn, abdominal pain, nausea, headache, tinnitus, dyspnea, pruritus, skin eruptions, ecchymoses.

INTERACTIONS: (Naprosyn, EC-Naprosyn) Avoid with other products containing naproxen. Decreased plasma levels with ASA. May reduce tubular secretion of methotrexate; monitor for toxicity. May increase nephrotoxicity of cyclosporine; caution when co-administering. May diminish antihypertensive effect and potentiate renal disease with ACE inhibitors. May reduce natriuretic effect of furosemide and thiazides; monitor for renal failure. May increase lithium levels; monitor for toxicity. Synergistic effects on GI bleeding with warfarin. Observe for dose adjustment with hydantoins, sulfonamides, or sulfonylureas. May reduce antihypertensive effects of propranolol and other β-blockers. Probenecid may increase half-life. (EC-Naprosyn) Avoid with H_2-blockers, sucralfate, or intensive antacid therapy.

PREGNANCY: Category C, not for use in nursing.

Nasacort AQ   RX
triamcinolone acetonide (Sanofi-Aventis)

OTHER BRAND NAME: Nasacort HFA (Sanofi-Aventis)

THERAPEUTIC CLASS: Corticosteroid

INDICATIONS: Nasal treatment of seasonal and perennial allergic rhinitis symptoms.

DOSAGE: *Adults:* (AQ Spray) Initial/Max: 2 sprays per nostril qd. With improvement, may reduce dose to 1 spray per nostril qd. (HFA Aerosol) Initial: 2 sprays per nostril qd. Max: 4 sprays per nostril qd.

Pediatrics: ≥12 yrs: (AQ Spray) Initial/Max: 2 sprays per nostril qd. With improvement, may reduce dose to 1 spray per nostril qd. (HFA Aerosol) Initial: 2 sprays per nostril qd. Max: 4 sprays per nostril qd. 6-12 yrs: (AQ Spray) Initial: 1 spray per nostril qd. Max: 2 sprays per nostril qd. 6-11 yrs: (HFA Aerosol) 2 sprays per nostril qd.

HOW SUPPLIED: AQ Spray: 55mcg/spray (16.5g); HFA Aerosol: 55mcg/spray (9.3g)

WARNINGS/PRECAUTIONS: Risk of adrenal insufficiency and withdrawal symptoms when replacing systemic corticosteroid with a topical corticosteroids. Caution with active or quiescent TB, ocular herpes simplex, or untreated bacterial, fungal and systemic viral infections. Avoid with recent nasal trauma, surgery or septum ulcers. Risk for more severe/fatal course of infections (eg, chickenpox, measles) and for *Candida* infections of the nose and pharynx. Potential for growth velocity reduction in pediatrics.

ADVERSE REACTIONS: Pharyngitis, epistaxis, infection, otitis media, headache, sneezing, rhinitis, nasal irritation, cough, sinusitis, vomiting.

PREGNANCY: Category C, caution in nursing.

Nasarel   RX
flunisolide (Ivax)

THERAPEUTIC CLASS: Corticosteroid

INDICATIONS: Relief of seasonal or perennial rhinitis.

DOSAGE: *Adults:* Initial: 2 sprays per nostril bid. Titrate: May increase to 2 sprays per nostril tid. Max: 8 sprays per nostril/day.

Pediatrics: 6-14 yrs: Initial: 1 spray per nostril tid or 2 sprays per nostril bid. Max: 4 sprays per nostril/day.

HOW SUPPLIED: Spray: 29mcg/spray (25mL)

CONTRAINDICATIONS: Untreated localized infection of the nasal mucosa.

WARNINGS/PRECAUTIONS: Risk of adrenal insufficiency and withdrawal symptoms when replacing systemic corticosteroids with a topical corticosteroids. Caution with active or quiescent TB, ocular herpes simplex, or untreated bacterial, fungal and systemic viral infections. Avoid with recent nasal trauma, surgery or septum ulcers. Risk for more severe/fatal course of infections (eg, chickenpox, measles) and for *Candida* infections of the nose and pharynx. Potential for growth velocity reduction in pediatrics.

ADVERSE REACTIONS: Aftertaste, nasal burning/stinging, cough, epistaxis, nasal dryness.

NASONEX

INTERACTIONS: Concomitant systemic corticosteroids increases risk of hypercorticism and/or HPA axis suppression.

PREGNANCY: Category C, caution in nursing.

NASONEX RX
mometasone furoate monohydrate (Schering)

THERAPEUTIC CLASS: Corticosteroid

INDICATIONS: Treatment of the nasal symptoms of seasonal and perennial allergic rhinitis. Prophylaxis of the nasal symptoms of seasonal allergic rhinitis. Treatment of nasal polyps in patients 18 years of age and older.

DOSAGE: *Adults:* Allergic Rhinitis: Treatment/Prophylaxis: 2 sprays per nostril qd. For prophylaxis, start 2-4 weeks before allergy season. Nasal Polyps: 2 sprays per nostril bid.

Pediatrics: ≥12 yrs: Treatment/Prophylaxis: 2 sprays per nostril qd. For prophylaxis, start 2-4 weeks before allergy season. 2-11 yrs: Treatment: 1 spray per nostril qd.

HOW SUPPLIED: Spray: 50mcg/spray (17g)

WARNINGS/PRECAUTIONS: Risk of adrenal insufficiency and withdrawal symptoms when replacing systemic corticosteroids with a topical corticosteroids. Caution with active or quiescent TB, ocular herpes simplex, or untreated bacterial, fungal and systemic viral infections. Avoid with recent nasal trauma, surgery or septum ulcers. Risk for more severe/fatal course of infections (eg, chickenpox, measles) and for *Candida* infections of the nose and pharynx. Potential for growth velocity reduction in pediatrics.

ADVERSE REACTIONS: Headache, viral infection, pharyngitis, epistaxis, cough, upper respiratory tract infection, dysmenorrhea, myalgia, sinusitis.

PREGNANCY: Category C, caution with nursing.

NAVANE RX
thiothixene (Pfizer)

THERAPEUTIC CLASS: Thioxanthene

INDICATIONS: Management of schizophrenia.

DOSAGE: *Adults:* Mild Condition: Initial: 2mg tid. Titrate: May increase to 15mg/day. Severe Condition: Initial: 5mg bid. Usual: 20-30mg/day. Max: 60mg/day.

Pediatrics: ≥12yrs: Mild Condition: Initial: 2mg tid. Titrate: May increase to 15mg/day. Severe Condition: Initial: 5mg bid. Usual: 20-30mg/day. Max: 60mg/day.

HOW SUPPLIED: Cap: 2mg, 5mg, 10mg, 20mg

CONTRAINDICATIONS: Circulatory collapse, comatose states, CNS depression, blood dyscrasias.

WARNINGS/PRECAUTIONS: May develop tardive dyskinesia, NMS. May mask symptoms of overdose of toxic drugs. May obscure conditions such as intestinal obstruction and brain tumor. May lower seizure threshold. Monitor for pigmentary retinopathy and lenticular pigmentation. Caution with cardiovascular disease, extreme heat exposure, activities requiring alertness. May elevate prolactin levels.

ADVERSE REACTIONS: Tachycardia, hypotension, lightheadedness, syncope, drowsiness, agitation, insomnia, hyperreflexia, cerebral edema, pseudoparkinsonism, LFT elevation, blood dyscrasias, rash, photosensitivity, dry mouth, blurred vision.

INTERACTIONS: Possible additive effects including hypotension with CNS depressants, alcohol. Caution with atropine or related drugs. Paradoxical effects with pressor agents.

PREGNANCY: Safety in pregnancy and nursing not known.

NEGGRAM RX
nalidixic acid (Sanofi-Aventis)

THERAPEUTIC CLASS: Fluoroquinolone

INDICATIONS: Treatment of urinary tract infection.

DOSAGE: *Adults:* Initial: 1g qid with fluids for 1-2 weeks. Prolonged Therapy: Reduce to 2g/day after initial therapy.
Pediatrics: >12 yrs: Initial: 1g qid with fluids for 1-2 weeks. Prolonged Therapy: Reduce to 2g/day after initial therapy. 3 months-12 yrs: Initial: 25mg/lb/day given qid. Prolonged Therapy: Reduce dose to 15mg/lb/day after initial therapy. Use only in patients <18 yrs if potential benefit justifies the potential risk of cartilage erosion in weight-bearing joints and other signs of arthropathy.
HOW SUPPLIED: Sus: 250mg/5mL; Tab: 250mg*, 500mg*, 1g* *scored
CONTRAINDICATIONS: History of convulsive disorder.
WARNINGS/PRECAUTIONS: Convulsions, increased intracranial pressure, and toxic psychosis reported; caution with CNS disorders (eg, epilepsy, severe cerebral arteriosclerosis). May cause CNS stimulation (eg, tremor, lightheadedness, confusion, hallucinations). Pseudomembranous colitis and serious, fatal hypersensitivity reactions reported. If therapy ≥2 weeks, monitor blood counts and hepatic and liver function. Photosensitivity reaction reported; avoid excessive sunlight. D/C if phototoxicity occurs.
ADVERSE REACTIONS: Drowsiness, weakness, headache, dizziness, vertigo, abdominal pain, nausea, vomiting, diarrhea, rash, pruritus, angioedema.
INTERACTIONS: May potentiate theophylline, caffeine, oral anticoagulants, and cyclosporine. Diminished effects with nitrofurantoin, antacid containing magnesium, aluminum or calcium, sucralfate, iron, multivitamins containing zinc, didanosine; separate dose by 2 hrs.
PREGNANCY: Category C, not for use in nursing.

Nembutal Sodium
pentobarbital sodium (Ovation)

CII

THERAPEUTIC CLASS: Barbiturate
INDICATIONS: Short-term treatment of insomnia; sedation; preoperative anesthesia; anticonvulsant in the emergency control of certain acute convulsive episodes.
DOSAGE: *Adults:* Usual: 150-200mg as a single IM injection. IV: 100mg (commonly used initial dose for 70kg adult); if needed additional small increments may be given up to 200-500mg total dose. Rate of IV injection should not exceed 50mg/min. Elderly/Debilitated/Renal or Hepatic Impairment: Reduce dose.
Pediatrics: 2-6mg/kg as a single IM injection. Max: 100mg. IV: Proportional reduction in dosage. Slow IV injection is essential.
HOW SUPPLIED: Inj: 50mg/mL
CONTRAINDICATIONS: History of manifest or latent porphyria.
WARNINGS/PRECAUTIONS: May be habit forming; avoid abrupt cessation after prolonged use. Avoid rapid administration. Tolerance to hypnotic effect can occur. Prehepatic coma use not recommended. Use with caution in patients with chronic or acute pain, mental depression, suicidal tendencies, history of drug abuse or hepatic impairment. Monitor blood, liver and renal function. May impair mental/physical abilities. Avoid alcohol.
ADVERSE REACTIONS: Agitation, confusion, hyperkinesia, ataxia, CNS depression, somnolence, bradycardia, hypotension, nausea, vomiting, constipation, headache, hypersensitivity reactions, liver damage.
INTERACTIONS: May produce additive CNS depression with other CNS depressants (eg, other sedatives/hypnotics, antihistamines, tranquilizers, alcohol). May decrease levels of oral anticoagulants, corticosteroids, griseofulvin, and doxycycline. Dosage adjustments may be required for anticoagulants and corticosteroids. Variable effects on phenytoin and increased levels with valproic acid, sodium valproate; monitor blood levels and adjust dose appropriately. May decrease effects of estradiol; alternative contraceptive method should be suggested. Prolonged effect with MAOIs.
PREGNANCY: Category D, caution with nursing.

Neosar
cyclophosphamide (Teva)

RX

THERAPEUTIC CLASS: Nitrogen mustard alkylating agent
INDICATIONS: Treatment of malignant lymphomas, Hodgkin's disease, lymphocytic lymphoma, mixed-cell type or histiocytic lymphoma, Burkitt's lymphoma, multiple

myeloma, chronic lymphocytic leukemia, chronic granulocytic leukemia, acute myelogenous and monocytic leukemia, acute lymphoblastic leukemia in children, mycosis fungoides, neuroblastoma, ovary adenocarcinoma, retinoblastoma, breast carcinoma. Treatment of biopsy proven "minimal change" nephrotic syndrome in children, but not as primary therapy.

DOSAGE: *Adults:* Malignant Diseases (Without Hematologic Deficiency): Monotherapy: Initial: 40-50mg/kg IV in divided doses over 2-5 days, or 10-15mg/kg IV given every 7-10 days, or 3-5mg/kg twice weekly. Oral Cyclophosphamide: Initial/Maint: 1-5mg/kg/day PO. Adjust dose according to antitumor activity and/or leukopenia. May need to reduce dose when combined with other cytotoxic drugs.

Pediatrics: Malignant Diseases (Without Hematologic Deficiency): Monotherapy: Initial: 40-50mg/kg IV in divided doses over 2-5 days, or 10-15mg/kg IV given every 7-10 days, or 3-5mg/kg twice weekly. Oral Cyclophosphamide: Initial/Maint: 1-5mg/kg/day PO. Adjust dose according to antitumor activity and/or leukopenia. May need to reduce dose when combined with other cytotoxic drugs. Nephrotic Syndrome: 2.5-3mg/kg/day PO for 60-90 days.

HOW SUPPLIED: Inj: 100mg, 200mg, 500mg, 1g, 2g

CONTRAINDICATIONS: Severely depressed bone marrow function.

WARNINGS/PRECAUTIONS: Second malignancies, cardiac dysfunction, testicular atrophy, urinary bladder and ovarian fibrosis reported. Force fluid intake to prevent hemorrhagic cystitis. May cause fetal harm in pregnancy. Serious, fatal infections may develop if severely immunosuppressed. Discontinue or reduce dose with infection. Monitor for toxicity with leukopenia, thrombocytopenia, tumor cell infiltration of bone marrow, previous X-ray therapy or cytotoxic therapy, and impaired hepatic and/or renal function. Monitor hematologic profile and examine urine for red blood cells. Possible cross-sensitivity with other alkylating agents. May cause sterility. May interfere with normal wound healing. Consider dose adjustment with adrenalectomy.

ADVERSE REACTIONS: Impairment of fertility, amenorrhea, nausea, vomiting, anorexia, abdominal discomfort, diarrhea, alopecia, leukopenia, thrombocytopenia, hemorrhagic ureteritis, interstitial pneumonitis, malaise, asthenia, renal tubular necrosis, skin rash, fever, SIADH, anaphylactic reactions.

INTERACTIONS: Increased metabolism and leukopenic activity with chronic, high doses of phenobarbital. Potentiates succinylcholine chloride effects and doxorubicin-induced cardiotoxicity. Alert anesthesiologist if treated within 10 days of general anesthesia.

PREGNANCY: Category D, not for use in nursing.

Neosporin + Pain Relief Maximum Strength   OTC
neomycin - bacitracin - polymyxin B - pramoxine HCl (McNeil)

THERAPEUTIC CLASS: Antibacterial/analgesic

INDICATIONS: To help prevent infection and provide temporary relief of pain or discomfort in minor cuts, scrapes, and burns.

DOSAGE: *Adults:* Clean area and apply a small amount qd-tid. May cover with sterile bandage.

Pediatrics: ≥2 yrs: Clean area and apply a small amount qd-tid. May cover with sterile bandage.

HOW SUPPLIED: Cre: (Neomycin-Polymyxin-Pramoxine) 3.5mg-10,000 U-10mg/g (15g); Oint: (Bacitracin-Neomycin-Polymyxin-Pramoxine) 500 U-3.5mg-10,000 U-10mg/g (15g, 30g)

WARNINGS/PRECAUTIONS: Avoid eyes. Do not use over large areas. Discontinue if condition worsens, if develop rash or other allergic reaction, if symptoms persist >1 week, or if symptoms clear up and re-occur within a few days.

Neosporin Ointment   OTC
neomycin - bacitracin zinc - polymyxin B sulfate (McNeil)

THERAPEUTIC CLASS: Antibacterial combination

INDICATIONS: To help prevent infection in minor cuts, scrapes, and burns.

DOSAGE: *Adults:* Clean area and apply a small amount qd-tid. May cover with sterile bandage.

Pediatrics: Clean area and apply a small amount qd-tid. May cover with sterile bandage.

HOW SUPPLIED: Oint: (Neomycin-Polymyxin-Bacitracin) 3.5mg-5000 U-400 U/g (15g, 30g), (Neo To Go, 10 x 0.9g packets)

WARNINGS/PRECAUTIONS: Avoid eyes. Do not use over large areas. Discontinue if condition persists, worsens, or if a rash or other allergic reaction develops.

PREGNANCY: Safety in pregnancy and nursing not known.

Neo-Synephrine Ophthalmic   RX
phenylephrine HCl (Sanofi-Aventis)

THERAPEUTIC CLASS: Sympathomimetic

INDICATIONS: Use as a decongestant, vasoconstrictor, and pupil dilator in uveitis (posterior synechiae), wide angle glaucoma, before surgery, refraction, ophthalmoscopic exam, and diagnostic procedures.

DOSAGE: *Adults:* Vasoconstriction/Pupil Dilation: 1 drop 10% on upper limbus. May repeat after 1 hr. May precede by topical anesthetic. Uveitis: 1 drop 10% to upper surface of cornea. May repeat next day. Apply hot compresses tid for 5-10 minutes, with 1 drop atropine sulfate before and after compresses. Glaucoma: 1 drop 10% on upper surface of cornea, repeat prn. Surgery: Apply 2.5% or 10% drops 30-60 minutes before surgery. Refraction: 1 drop of cycloplegic, then 1 drop 2.5% after 5 minutes, then repeat cycloplegic 10 minutes later. Eyes ready for refraction in 50-60 minutes. "One Application Method": Combine 2.5% solution with cycloplegic for synergistic action. Consider increasing cycloplegic concentration. Ophthalmoscopic Exam: 1 drop 2.5% per eye. Diagnostic Procedures: Test for Angle Block with Glaucoma: Measure IOP before and after 2.5% solution. Shadow Test: Use 2.5% solution. Blanching Test: 1-2 drops 2.5% to injected eye.

Pediatrics: Refraction: 1 drop of atropine 1%, then 1 drop 2.5% after 10-15 minutes, then repeat 1 drop of atropine in 5-10 minutes. Eyes ready for refraction in 1-2 hrs.

HOW SUPPLIED: Sol: 2.5% (15mL), 10% (5mL)

CONTRAINDICATIONS: Narrow angle glaucoma, (10%) infants, (10%) aneurysm.

WARNINGS/PRECAUTIONS: (10%) Associated with cardiovascular reactions (eg, ventricular arrhythmias, MI) in elderly with pre-existing cardiovascular disease. May cause BP elevation; caution in low body weight children, elderly, insulin-dependent diabetes, HTN, hyperthyroidism, generalized arteriosclerosis, cardiovascular disease. (2.5%, 10%) Systemic vasopressor response may occur when exceed recommended doses or apply to instrumented, traumatized, diseased or postsurgical eye, adnexa, or in suppressed lacrimation.

ADVERSE REACTIONS: Rebound miosis (elderly), eye pain.

INTERACTIONS: TCAs, propranolol, reserpine, guanethidine, methyldopa, atropine-like drugs may potentiate pressor response. MAOIs during or up to 21 days after, may exaggerate adrenergic effects. Acute HTN and congenital cerebral aneurysm rupture reported with 10% solution and systemic β-blockers. May potentiate cardiovascular depressant effects of potent inhalation anesthetics.

PREGNANCY: Category C, caution in nursing.

Nesacaine   RX
chloroprocaine HCl (Abraxis)

OTHER BRAND NAME: Nesacaine-MPF (Abraxis)

THERAPEUTIC CLASS: Local anesthetic

INDICATIONS: (Nesacaine) Production of local anesthesia by infiltration and peripheral nerve block. (Nesacaine-MPF) Production of local anesthesia by infiltration, peripheral and central nerve block, including lumbar and caudal epidural blocks.

DOSAGE: *Adults:* Dosage varies depending on procedure, vascularity of tissues, depth and duration of anesthesia, degree of muscle relaxation required, and patient physical

NEURONTIN

condition. Max: 11mg/kg (800mg total dose) without epinephrine or 14mg/kg (1000mg total dose) with epinephrine. MPF: Caudal/Lumbar Epidural Block: Test dose: 3mL of 3% or 5mL of 2% prior to complete block. Caudal Epidural: 15-25mL of 2% or 3% solution. Repeat dose may be given at 40-60 minute intervals. Lumbar Epidural: 2-2.5mL/ segment of 2% or 3% solution. Usual: 15-25mL. Repeat doses of 2-6mL less than original dose at 40-50 minute intervals. Elderly/Debilitated/Acutely Ill/Cardiac or Liver Disease: Reduce dose.

Pediatrics: >3 yrs: Max: 11mg/kg. Use 0.5-1% for infiltration and 1-1.5% for nerve block.

HOW SUPPLIED: Inj: 1%, 2%; (MPF) 2%, 3%

CONTRAINDICATIONS: Extreme caution with lumbar and caudal epidural anesthesia in existing neurological disease, spinal deformities, septicemia, severe HTN.

WARNINGS/PRECAUTIONS: Acidosis, cardiac arrest, death reported from delay in toxicity management. Nesacaine contains methylparaben and should not be used for lumbar or caudal epidural anesthesia. MPF formulation contains no preservative; discard any unused injection after initial use. Use lowest effective dose. Perform syringe aspiration to avoid intravascular injection. Caution with hepatic disease or impaired cardiovascular function. Monitor cardiovascular and respiratory vital signs and state of consciousness after each injection. Caution when local anesthetic injections containing a vasoconstrictor are used in areas of the body supplied by end arteries or having otherwise compromised blood supply; ischemic injury or necrosis may result with peripheral or hypertensive vascular disease due to exaggerated vasoconstrictor response. Do not rely on lack of corneal sensation after retrobulbar block to determine if patient is ready for surgery.

ADVERSE REACTIONS: Restlessness, anxiety, dizziness, tinnitus, blurred vision, tremors, convulsions, drowsiness, hypotension, bradycardia, ventricular arrhythmias, urticaria, pruritus, nausea, vomiting, loss of bladder/bowel control, loss of sexual function.

INTERACTIONS: Caution regarding toxic equivalence when using local anesthetic mixtures. Vasopressors, ergot-type oxytocic drugs may cause severe, persistent HTN or CVA. Anesthetic solutions containing epinephrine or norepinephrine with MAOIs, TCAs, or phenothiazines may produce severe, prolonged hypotension or HTN. Avoid sulfonamides.

PREGNANCY: Category C, caution in nursing.

NEURONTIN RX
gabapentin (Parke-Davis)

THERAPEUTIC CLASS: GABA analog

INDICATIONS: Adjunct therapy for partial seizures with or without secondary generalization in patients ≥12 yrs. Adjunct therapy for partial seizures in pediatrics 3-12 yrs. Management of postherpetic neuralgia (PHN).

DOSAGE: *Adults:* Epilepsy: Initial: 300mg tid. Titrate: Increase up to 1800mg/day. Max: 3600mg/day. PHN: 300mg single dose on Day 1, then 300mg bid on Day 2, and 300mg tid on Day 3. Increase further prn pain. Max: 600mg tid. Renal Impairment: CrCl 30-59mL/min: 400-1400 mg/day. CrCl 15-29mL/min: 200-700 mg/day. CrCl 15mL/min: 100-300mg/day. CrCl <15 mL/min: Reduce dose in proportion to CrCl. Hemodialysis: Maint: Base on CrCl. Give supplemental dose (125-350mg) after 4 hrs of hemodialysis. Refer to prescribing information for dose-adjustment.

Pediatrics: Epilepsy: >12 yrs: Initial: 300mg tid. Titrate: Increase up to 1800mg/day. Max: 3600mg/day. 3-12 yrs: Initial: 10-15mg/kg/day given tid. Titrate: Increase over 3 days. Usual: 3-4 yrs: 40mg/kg/day given tid. ≥5 yrs: 25-35mg/kg/day given tid. Max: 50mg/kg/day. Renal Impairment: ≥12 yrs: CrCl 30-59mL/min: 400-1400 mg/day. CrCl 15-29mL/min: 200-700 mg/day. CrCl 15mL/min: 100-300mg/day. CrCl <15 mL/min: Reduce dose in proportion to CrCl. Hemodialysis: Maint: Base on CrCl. Give supplemental dose (125-350 mg) after 4 hrs of hemodialysis. Refer to prescribing information for dose-adjustment.

HOW SUPPLIED: Cap: 100mg, 300mg, 400mg; Sol: 250mg/5mL; Tab: 600mg*, 800mg*
*scored

WARNINGS/PRECAUTIONS: Avoid abrupt withdrawal. Possible tumorigenic potential. Sudden and unexplained deaths reported. Neuropsychiatric adverse events in pediatrics (3-12 yrs).

ADVERSE REACTIONS: Somnolence, dizziness, ataxia, nystagmus, fatigue, tremor, rhinitis, weight gain, nausea, vomiting, viral infection, fever, dysarthria, diplopia.

INTERACTIONS: Take 2 hrs after antacids. Increased levels with controlled-release morphine.

PREGNANCY: Category C, caution in nursing.

Nexium RX
esomeprazole magnesium (AstraZeneca LP)

THERAPEUTIC CLASS: Proton pump inhibitor

INDICATIONS: Symptomatic treatment of GERD; healing and maintenance treatment of erosive esophagitis. Reduction in the occurrence of gastric ulcers associated with continuous NSAID therapy in patients at risk for developing gastric ulcers. Adjunct therapy (with amoxicillin and clarithromycin) for *H. pylori* eradication to reduce the risk of duodenal ulcer recurrence. Long-term treatment of pathological hypersecretory conditions including Zollinger-Ellison Syndrome.

DOSAGE: *Adults:* Erosive Esophagitis: Healing: 20-40mg qd for 4-8 weeks; may extend treatment for 4-8 weeks if not healed. Maint: 20mg qd for up to 6 months. Risk Reduction of NSAID-Associated Gastric Ulcer: 20-40mg qd for up to 6 months. Symptomatic GERD: 20mg qd for 4 weeks; may extend treatment for 4 weeks if symptoms do not resolve. *H. pylori:* Triple Therapy: 40mg qd + amoxicillin 1000mg bid + clarithromycin 500mg bid, all for 10 days. Zollinger-Ellison Syndrome: 40mg bid. Severe Hepatic Dysfunction: Max: 20mg/day. Take 1 hr before meals. Swallow capsule whole. Contents may be mixed with soft food (eg, applesauce, yogurt) that does not require chewing.
Pediatrics: 12-17 yrs: GERD: 20-40mg qd for up to 8 weeks. Severe Hepatic Dysfunction: Max: 20mg/day. Take 1 hr before meals. Swallow capsule whole. Contents may be mixed with soft food (eg, applesauce, yogurt) that does not require chewing.

HOW SUPPLIED: Cap, Delayed Release: 20mg, 40mg; Sus, Delayed Release: 20mg, 40mg (granules/packet).

CONTRAINDICATIONS: Hypersensitivity to substituted benzimidazoles. Clarithromycin is contraindicated with pimozide.

WARNINGS/PRECAUTIONS: Atrophic gastritis may occur. Symptomatic response does not preclude gastric malignancy.

ADVERSE REACTIONS: Headache, diarrhea, abdominal pain, constipation, nausea, flatulence, dry mouth.

INTERACTIONS: Potentiates diazepam. May alter absorption of pH-dependent drugs (eg, ketoconazole, digoxin, and iron salts). May reduce levels of atazanavir when used concomitantly. Increased levels with amoxicillin and clarithromycin. Clarithromycin is contraindicated with pimozide.

PREGNANCY: Category B, not for use in nursing.

Niferex OTC
iron (Ther-Rx)

THERAPEUTIC CLASS: Iron supplement

INDICATIONS: Treatment of uncomplicated iron deficiency anemias.

DOSAGE: *Adults:* 1-2 tabs bid or 5-10mL qd.
Pediatrics: ≥6 yrs: 1-2 tabs qd or 5mL qd. <6 yrs: (Sol): Individualize dose.

HOW SUPPLIED: Cap: 60mg; Sol: 100mg/5mL

WARNINGS/PRECAUTIONS: Fatal poisoning reported in children <6 yrs with accidental overdose of iron-containing products.

PREGNANCY: Safety in pregnancy and nursing not known.

Nimbex RX
cisatracurium besylate (Abbott)

THERAPEUTIC CLASS: Skeletal muscle relaxant (nondepolarizing)

INDICATIONS: Adjunct to general anesthesia, to facilitate tracheal intubation, and to provide skeletal muscle relaxation during surgery/mechanical ventilation.

Nix

DOSAGE: *Adults:* Initial: 0.15mg/kg (3 x ED_{95}) or 0.20mg/kg (4 x ED_{95}) IV. Serious Cardiovascular Disease: Up to 8 x ED_{95}. Maint/Prolonged Surgical Procedures: 0.03mg/kg IV (for 20 minute blockade) 40-50 minutes after initial 0.15mg/kg, and 50-60 minutes after initial 0.20mg/kg. Operating Room Infusion: After initial bolus dose, give 3mcg/kg/min to counteract recovery from bolus, then 1-2mcg/kg/min. ICU: 3mcg/kg/min IV; dose requirements may increase/decrease with time.

Pediatrics: >12 yrs: Initial: 0.15mg/kg (3 x ED_{95}) or 0.20mg/kg (4 x ED_{95}) IV. Serious Cardiovascular Disease: Up to 8 x ED_{95}. Maint/Prolonged Surgical Procedures: 0.03mg/kg IV (for 20 minute blockade) 40-50 minutes after initial 0.15mg/kg, and 50-60 minutes after initial 0.20mg/kg. 2-12 yrs: Initial: 0.10mg/kg over 5-10 seconds during halothane or opioid anesthesia. ≥2 yrs: Operating Room Infusion: After initial bolus dose, give 3mcg/kg/min to counteract recovery from bolus, then 1-2mcg/kg/min.

HOW SUPPLIED: Inj: 2mg/mL, 10mg/mL

CONTRAINDICATIONS: Hypersensitivity to bis-benzylisoquinolinium agents and benzyl alcohol.

WARNINGS/PRECAUTIONS: Avoid administration before unconsciousness has been induced. Use in facility with resuscitation and life support, and have antagonist available. Monitor neuromuscular function with peripheral nerve stimulator during administration. Multi-dose vials contain benzyl alcohol. Not for rapid sequence endotracheal intubation. May have profound effect with neuromuscular diseases (eg, myasthenia gravis, carcinomatosis); monitor neuromuscular function with peripheral nerve stimulator. Resistance may develop in burn victims; consider increasing dose. Resistance with hemiparesis or paraparesis. Acid-base and/or serum electrolyte abnormalities may potentiate or antagonize effect. Monitor for malignant hyperthermia.

ADVERSE REACTIONS: Bradycardia, hypotension, flushing, bronchospasm, rash, muscle weakness, myopathy, prolonged/inadequate neuromuscular blockade.

INTERACTIONS: Prolonged duration of action and required infusion rate decreased with isoflurane or enflurane with nitrous oxide/oxygen. Enhanced neuromuscular blocking action with certain antibiotics (eg, aminoglycosides, tetracyclines, bacitracin, polymyxins, lincomycin, clindamycin, colistin, sodium colistimethate), magnesium salts, lithium, local anesthetics, procainamide, and quinidine. Antagonized effect with phenytoin and carbamazepine. May not be compatible with pH >8.5 alkaline solutions (eg, barbiturate solutions).

PREGNANCY: Category B, caution in nursing.

Nix OTC
permethrin (Insight Pharmaceuticals)

THERAPEUTIC CLASS: Pyrethroid pediculicide

INDICATIONS: (Liquid) Treatment of head lice and prophylactic use during epidemics (at least 20% of population are infested). (Spray) To kill lice on bedding and furniture. Not for use in humans.

DOSAGE: *Adults:* (Liquid) Treatment: Wash then towel dry hair. Apply liquid and saturate hair and scalp. Rinse with water after 10 minutes. Remove nits with comb provided. Repeat after 7 days if live lice is observed. Prophylaxis: Same as treatment. Repeat therapy after 2 weeks in epidemic setting. (Spray) Use from an 8-10 inch distance. Treat only garments, bedding, and furniture that cannot be washed or dry cleaned. Allow area to dry completely.

Pediatrics: ≥2 months: (Liquid) Treatment: Wash and dry hair, then saturate hair and scalp. Rinse with water after 10 minutes. Remove nits with comb provided. Repeat after 7 days if observe lice. Prophylaxis: Same as treatment. Do not use nit comb.

HOW SUPPLIED: Liq: (Creme Rinse) 1% (60mL); Spray: 0.25% (148mL)

WARNINGS/PRECAUTIONS: (Liquid) Protect from getting into eyes, inside nose, mouth, or vagina. May cause breathing difficulty or asthmatic episodes in susceptible persons. Discontinue if skin irritation persists or infection develops. (Spray) Do not use in food serving areas or while food is exposed. Do not apply in classrooms while in use.

ADVERSE REACTIONS: Itching, redness, swelling of the scalp.

PREGNANCY: Safety in pregnancy and nursing not known.

NIZORAL

ketoconazole (Janssen)

RX

> Risk of fatal hepatotoxicity. Concomitant terfenadine, astemizole and cisapride are contraindicated due to serious cardiovascular adverse events.

THERAPEUTIC CLASS: Azole antifungal

INDICATIONS: Treatment of systemic fungal infections including candidiasis, chronic mucocutaneous candidiasis, oral thrush, candiduria, blastomycosis, coccidioidomycosis, histoplasmosis, chromomycosis, and paracoccidioidomycosis. Treatment of severe recalcitrant cutaneous dermatophyte infections not responsive to topical therapy or oral griseofulvin. Not for treatment of fungal meningitis.

DOSAGE: *Adults:* Initial: 200mg qd. Max: 400mg qd.
Pediatrics: >2 yrs: 3.3-6.6mg/kg/day.

HOW SUPPLIED: Tab: 200mg* *scored

CONTRAINDICATIONS: Concomitant terfenadine, astemizole, cisapride or triazolam.

WARNINGS/PRECAUTIONS: Hepatotoxicity reported. Monitor LFTs prior to therapy and periodically thereafter. Serum testosterone levels may be lowered. Hypersensitivity reactions reported. Tablets require acidity for dissolution. Not for use in children unless benefit outweighs risk.

ADVERSE REACTIONS: Nausea, vomiting, abdominal pain, pruritus.

INTERACTIONS: Give antacids, anticholinergics, and H_2 blockers 2 hrs after ketoconazole. Contraindicated with terfenadine, astemizole, and cisapride due to cardiac adverse effects. May potentiate midazolam, triazolam, oral hypoglycemics. May enhance anticoagulant effect of coumarin-like drugs. Avoid rifampin, isoniazid. Monitor digoxin, phenytoin. May alter metabolism of cyclosporine, tacrolimus, methylprednisolone and drugs metabolized by CYP3A4.

PREGNANCY: Category C, not for use in nursing.

NIZORAL A-D

ketoconazole (McNeil Consumer)

OTC

THERAPEUTIC CLASS: Azole antifungal

INDICATIONS: Controls flaking, scaling and itching associated with dandruff.

DOSAGE: *Adults:* Wet hair. Apply and lather. Rinse thoroughly and repeat. Apply every 3-4 days up to 8 weeks if needed.
Pediatrics: >12 yrs: Wet hair. Apply and lather. Rinse thoroughly and repeat. Apply every 3-4 days up to 8 weeks if needed.

HOW SUPPLIED: Shampoo: 1% (4 oz, 7 oz)

CONTRAINDICATIONS: Scalp that is broken or inflamed.

WARNINGS/PRECAUTIONS: Avoid eyes. D/C if rash appears, or if condition worsens or does not improve in 2-4 weeks.

PREGNANCY: Use in pregnancy and nursing not known.

NORDITROPIN

somatropin (Novo Nordisk)

RX

OTHER BRAND NAME: Norditropin Nordiflex (Novo Nordisk)

THERAPEUTIC CLASS: Human growth hormone

INDICATIONS: (Adults) Replacement of endogenous growth hormone deficiency who meet either of the following criteria: (1) adult onset-patients with growth hormone deficiency, either alone or associated with multiple hormone deficiencies (hypopituitarism), as a result of pituitary disease, hypothalamic disease, surgery, radiation therapy, or trauma; or (2) childhood onset-patients who were growth hormone deficient during childhood should have growth hormone deficiency confirmed as an adult before

NORPACE

replacement therapy is started. (Pediatrics) Long-term treatment of children with growth failure due to inadequate growth hormone secretion. Treatment of children with short stature associated with Noonan syndrome.

DOSAGE: *Adults:* Initial: No more than 0.004mg/kg/day. Increase to no more than 0.016mg/kg/day after 6 weeks.

Pediatrics: Growth Hormone Deficiency: 0.024-0.034mg/kg SQ 6-7x/week. Noonan Syndrome: Dose up to 0.066mg/kg/day.

HOW SUPPLIED: Inj: (Norditropin (cartridge) and Norditropin Nordiflex (prefilled pen)) 5mg/1.5mL, 10mg/1.5ml, 15mg/1.5mL

CONTRAINDICATIONS: Presence of active neoplasia; acute critical illness due to complications following open heart or abdominal surgery, multiple accidental trauma or acute respiratory failure; proliferative or preproliferative diabetic retinopathy; closed epiphyses; and Prader-Willi syndrome with severe obesity or severe respiratory impairment.

WARNINGS/PRECAUTIONS: Monitor for recurrence or progression of underlying disease in growth hormone deficiency secondary to intracranial lesions. Hypothyroidism reported. May develop slipped capital epiphyses. Intracranial HTN with papilledema, visual changes, headache, nausea, and vomiting reported. Progression of scholiosis may occur in rapid growth. Monitor for any form of malignant skin lesion prior to and during therapy. May decrease insulin sensitivity; monitor blood sugar.

ADVERSE REACTIONS: *Pediatric:* Headache, injection site reaction, localized muscle pain, rash, weakness, mild hyperglycemia, glucosuria, arthralgia, leukemia. *Adults:* Edema, arthralgia, myalgia, infection, parasthesia, skeletal pain, headache, bronchitis.

INTERACTIONS: Diminished effects with glucocorticoid therapy. Insulin resistance reported. May reduce plasma levels of oral estrogens.

PREGNANCY: Category C, caution in nursing.

NORPACE RX
disopyramide phosphate (Pharmacia & Upjohn)

OTHER BRAND NAME: Norpace CR (Pharmacia & Upjohn)

THERAPEUTIC CLASS: Class I antiarrhythmic

INDICATIONS: Treatment of documented life-threatening ventricular arrhythmias.

DOSAGE: *Adults:* Usual: 400-800mg/day in divided dose. Recommended: 150mg q6h immediate-release (IR) or 300mg q12h extended-release (CR). Adjust dose with anticholinergic effects. Weight <110lbs/Moderate Hepatic or Renal Insufficiency (CrCl >40mL/min): 100mg q6h IR or 200mg q12h CR. Severe Renal Insufficiency (with or without initial 150mg LD): CrCl 30-40mL/min: 100mg q8h IR. CrCl 30-15mL/min: 100mg q12h IR. CrCl <15mL/min: 100mg q24h IR. Rapid Control of Ventricular Arrhythmia: LD: 300mg IR (200mg if <110lbs). Follow with maint dose. Cardiomyopathy/Cardiac Decompensation: Initial: 100mg q6-8h IR. Adjust gradually. See labeling if no response or toxicity occurs. Elderly: Start at low end of dosing range.

Pediatrics: <1 yr: 10-30mg/kg/day. 1-4 yrs: 10-20mg/kg/day. 4-12 yrs: 10-15mg/kg/day. 12-18 yrs: 6-15mg/kg/day. Give in equally divided doses q6h. Hospitalize patient during initial therapy. Start dose titration at lower end of range.

HOW SUPPLIED: Cap: (Norpace) 100mg, 150mg; Cap, Extended Release: (Norpace CR) 100mg, 150mg

CONTRAINDICATIONS: Cardiogenic shock, 2nd- or 3rd-degree AV block (if no pacemaker present), congenital QT prolongation.

WARNINGS/PRECAUTIONS: Proarrhythmic; reserve for life-threatening ventricular arrhythmias. May cause or worsen CHF and produce hypotension due to negative inotropic properties. Reduce dose if 1st-degree heart block occurs. Avoid with urinary retention, glaucoma, and myasthenia gravis unless adequate overriding measures taken. Atrial flutter/fibrillation; digitalize first. Monitor closely or withdraw if QT prolongation >25% occurs and ectopy continues. Discontinue if QRS widening >25% occurs. Avoid LD with cardiomyopathy or cardiac decompensation. Correct K^+ abnormalities before therapy. Reduce dose with renal/hepatic dysfunction; monitor ECG. Avoid CR formulation with CrCl ≤40mL/min. Caution with sick sinus syndrome, Wolff-Parkinson-White syndrome, bundle branch block, in elderly. May significantly lower blood glucose.

ADVERSE REACTIONS: Dry mouth, urinary retention/frequency/urgency, constipation, blurred vision, GI effects, dizziness, fatigue, headache.

INTERACTIONS: Avoid type IA and IC antiarrhythmics, and propranolol except in unresponsive, life-threatening arrhythmias. Hepatic enzyme inducers may lower levels. Avoid within 48 hrs before or 24 hrs after verapamil. Possible fatal interactions with CYP3A4 inhibitors. Monitor blood glucose with β-blockers, alcohol.

PREGNANCY: Category C, not for use in nursing.

Norvasc   RX
amlodipine besylate (Pfizer)

THERAPEUTIC CLASS: Calcium channel blocker (dihydropyridine)

INDICATIONS: Treatment of hypertension and Coronary Artery Disease (CAD) including chronic stable or vasospastic angina (Prinzmetal's or Variant Angina).

DOSAGE: *Adults:* HTN: Initial: 5mg qd. Titrate over 7-14 days. Max: 10mg qd. Small, Fragile, or Elderly/Hepatic Dysfunction/Concomitant Antihypertensive: Initial: 2.5mg qd. Angina: 10mg qd. Elderly/Hepatic Dysfunction: 5mg qd. CAD: 5-10mg qd.
Pediatrics: 6-17 yrs: HTN: 2.5-5mg qd.

HOW SUPPLIED: Tab: 2.5mg, 5mg, 10mg

WARNINGS/PRECAUTIONS: May increase angina or MI with severe obstructive CAD. Caution with severe aortic stenosis, CHF, severe hepatic impairment, and in elderly.

ADVERSE REACTIONS: Edema, flushing, palpitation, dizziness, headache, fatigue.

PREGNANCY: Category C, not for use in nursing.

Norvir   RX
ritonavir (Abbott)

> Use with certain non-sedating antihistamines, sedative hypnotics, antiarrhythmics, or ergot alkaloids may result in life-threatening adverse events.

THERAPEUTIC CLASS: Protease inhibitor

INDICATIONS: Treatment of HIV infection in combination with other antiretrovirals.

DOSAGE: *Adults:* Initial: 300mg bid. Titrate: Increase every 2-3 days by 100mg bid. Maint: 600mg bid. If combined with saquinavir, adjust dose to 400mg bid. Elderly: Start at low end of dosing range. Take with meals if possible.
Pediatrics: >1 month: Initial: 250mg/m^2 po bid. Titrate: Increase by 50mg/m^2 every 2-3 days. Maint: 350-400mg/m^2 po bid or highest tolerated dose. Max: 600mg bid.

HOW SUPPLIED: Cap: 100mg; Sol: 80mg/mL (240mL)

CONTRAINDICATIONS: Alfuzosin, amiodarone, bepridil, flecainide, propafenone, quinidine, voriconazole, astemizole, terfenadine, ergot derivatives, midazolam, triazolam, cisapride, pimozide.

WARNINGS/PRECAUTIONS: Allergic reactions (eg, urticaria, mild skin eruptions, bronchospasm, and angioedema), pancreatitis, new onset/exacerbation of pre-existing diabetes mellitus, hyperglycemia, immune reconstitution syndrome, hepatic transaminase elevations and hepatic dysfunction reported. Caution with moderate to severe hepatic impairment and in elderly. Monitor LFTs, especially first 3 months. Increased bleeding may occur with hemophilia A and B. Possible redistribution or accumulation of body fat. May increase total triglyceride and cholesterol levels.

ADVERSE REACTIONS: Diarrhea, anorexia, vomiting, nausea, abdominal pain, taste perversion, circumoral, peripheral paresthesia.

INTERACTIONS: See Contraindications. Avoid use with rifampin, St. John's wort; may cause loss of virologic response and resistance. Avoid use with lovastatin and simvastatin; risk of myopathy and rhabdomyolysis. Neurologic and cardiac events reported with disopyramide, mexiletine, nefazodone, fluoxetine, and β-blockers. May increase levels of saquinavir, desipramine, indinavir, rifabutin. May increase levels of

Novacort

clarithromycin with renal impairment; reduce clarithromycin dose by 50% if CrCl 30-60mL/min and by 75% if CrCl<30mL/min. May increase ketoconazole levels; avoid ketoconazole doses >200mg/day. May increase sildenafil levels; do not exceed sildenafil 25mg/48hrs. May increase levels of tramadol, propoxyphene, disopyramide, lidocaine, mexilitene, carbamazepine, clonazepam, ethosuximide, bupropion, nefazodone, SSRIs, TCAs, dronabinol, itraconazole, quinine, metoprolol, timolol, diltiazem, nifedipine, verapamil, atorvastatin, cyclosporine, tacrolimus, sirolimus, perphenazine, risperidone, thioridazine, clorazepate, diazepam, estazolam, flurazepam, zolpidem, dexamethasone, fluticasone, prednisone, methamphetamine. May increase levels of trazodone; use with caution and consider lower trazodone dose. Decreases levels of theophylline, meperidine, methadone. May decrease levels of phenytoin, divalproex, lamotrigine, and atovaquone. Separate dosing with didanosine by 2.5 hrs. May increase plasma levels of drugs metabolized by CYP3A or CYP2D6. May decrease ethinyl estradiol levels; use alternative contraceptive measures. Monitor PT/INR with warfarin. Contains alcohol; may produce disulfiram-like reactions with disulfiram, metronidazole.

PREGNANCY: Category B, not for use in nursing.

Novacort RX
pramoxine HCl - hydrocortisone acetate (Primus)

THERAPEUTIC CLASS: Corticosteroid/anesthetic

INDICATIONS: Relief of the inflammatory and pruritic manifestations of corticosteroid-responsive dermatoses.

DOSAGE: *Adults:* Apply to affected area(s) tid-qid. May use occlusive dressings for psoriasis or recalcitrant conditions. Discontinue dressings if infection develops.

Pediatrics: Apply to affected area(s) tid-qid. May use occlusive dressings for psoriasis or recalcitrant conditions. Discontinue dressings if infection develops.

HOW SUPPLIED: Gel: (Hydrocortisone-Pramoxine) 2%-1% (29g)

WARNINGS/PRECAUTIONS: May produce reversible HPA axis suppression, manifestations of Cushing's syndrome, hyperglycemia, and glucosuria. Caution when applied to large surface areas, under occlusive dressings, or with prolonged use. Use appropriate antifungal or antibacterial agent with dermatological infections; discontinue if infection does not clear. Pediatrics may be more susceptible to systemic toxicity. Discontinue if irritation develops. Avoid eyes.

ADVERSE REACTIONS: Burning, itching, irritation, dryness, folliculitis, hypertrichosis, acneiform eruptions, hypopigmentation, perioral dermatitis, allergic dermatitis, skin maceration, secondary infection, skin atrophy, striae, miliaria.

PREGNANCY: Category C, caution in nursing.

Novarel RX
chorionic gonadotropin (Ferring)

THERAPEUTIC CLASS: Human chorionic gonadotropin

INDICATIONS: For prepubertal cryptorchidism not due to anatomic obstruction. For hypogonadotropic hypogonadism (secondary to a pituitary deficiency) in males. To induce ovulation (OI) and pregnancy in anovulatory, infertile women in whom anovulation is not due to primary ovarian failure and pretreated with human menotropins.

DOSAGE: *Adults:* Hypogonadism: 500-1000 U IM 3x/week (TIW) for 3 weeks, then twice weekly for 3 weeks; or 4000 U IM TIW for 6-9 months, then reduce to 2000 U TIW for 3 months. OI: 5000-10,000 U IM 1 day after last dose of menotropins.

Pediatrics: ≥4 yrs: Cryptorchidism: 4000 U IM TIW for 3 weeks; or 5000 U IM every 2nd day for 4 doses; or 15 doses of 500-1000 U over 6 weeks; or 500 U TIW for 4-6 weeks (if treatment fails, give 1000 U/injection starting 1 month later). Initiate therapy between 4-9 yrs. Hypogonadism: 500-1000 U IM TIW for 3 weeks, then twice weekly for 3 weeks; or 4000 U IM TIW for 6-9 months, then reduce to 2000 U TIW for 3 months.

HOW SUPPLIED: Inj: 10,000 U

Novolin 70/30

CONTRAINDICATIONS: Precocious puberty, prostatic carcinoma or other androgen-dependent neoplasms, pregnancy.

WARNINGS/PRECAUTIONS: Potential ovarian hyperstimulation, enlargement or rupture of ovarian cysts, multiple births, and arterial thromboembolism with infertility treatment. D/C if precocious puberty occurs in cryptorchidism patients. Caution with cardiac or renal disease, epilepsy, migraine, asthma. Not effective treatment for obesity.

ADVERSE REACTIONS: Headache, irritability, restlessness, depression, fatigue, edema, precocious puberty, gynecomastia, injection site pain.

PREGNANCY: Category C, caution in nursing.

Novolin OTC
insulin, human regular - insulin, human isophane - insulin human, rDNA origin (Novo Nordisk)

OTHER BRAND NAMES: Novolin N (Novo Nordisk) - Novolin R (Novo Nordisk)

THERAPEUTIC CLASS: Insulin

INDICATIONS: To control hyperglycemia in diabetes.

DOSAGE: *Adults:* Individualize dose.
Pediatrics: Individualize dose.

HOW SUPPLIED: Inj: 100U/mL (Novolin N, Novolin R); PenFill: 100U/mL (Novolin N, Novolin R); Prefilled: 100U/mL (Novolin N, Novolin R)

WARNINGS/PRECAUTIONS: Human insulin differs from animal source insulin. Any change of insulin should be made cautiously. Changes in strength, manufacturer, type or method of manufacture may result in the need for a change in dosage. Hypoglycemia may occur with taking too much insulin, missing or delaying meals, exercising or working more than usual. An infection or illness (especially with diarrhea or vomiting) may change insulin requirements. Administration of insulin SQ can result in lipoatrophy. Novolin R is not recommended for use in insulin pumps.

ADVERSE REACTIONS: Hypoglycemia, sweating, dizziness, palpitation, tremor, hunger, restlessness, lightheadedness, inability to concentrate, headache, injection site reaction, allergic reaction.

INTERACTIONS: Increased insulin requirements with oral contraceptives, corticosteroids, or thyroid replacement therapy. Reduced insulin requirements with oral hypoglycemics, salicylates, sulfa antibiotics, and certain antidepressants. Alcoholic beverages may change insulin requirements. β-blockers may mask symptoms of hypoglycemia.

PREGNANCY: Pregnancy category is not known.

Novolin 70/30 OTC
insulin human, rDNA origin - insulin, human (isophane/regular) (Novo Nordisk)

THERAPEUTIC CLASS: Insulin

INDICATIONS: To control hyperglycemia in diabetes.

DOSAGE: *Adults:* Individualize dose. Administer SQ.
Pediatrics: Individualize dose. Administer SQ.

HOW SUPPLIED: (Isophane/Regular) Inj: 70U-30U/mL; PenFill: 70U-30U/mL; Prefilled: 70U-30U/mL

WARNINGS/PRECAUTIONS: Human insulin differs from animal source insulin. Any change of insulin should be made cautiously. Changes in strength, manufacturer, type or method of manufacture may result in the need for a change in dosage. Hypoglycemia may occur with taking too much insulin, missing or delaying meals, exercising or working more than usual. An infection or illness (especially with diarrhea or vomiting) may change insulin requirements. Caution with diseases of adrenal, pituitary, or thyroid glands, or progression of kidney or liver disease. Administration of insulin SQ can result in lipoatrophy.

ADVERSE REACTIONS: Hypoglycemia, sweating, dizziness, palpitation, tremor, hunger, restlessness, lightheadedness, inability to concentrate, headache, injection site reaction, allergic reaction.

Novolog

INTERACTIONS: Increased insulin requirements with oral contraceptives, corticosteroids, or thyroid replacement therapy. Reduced insulin requirements with oral hypoglycemics, salicylates, sulfa antibiotics, and certain antidepressants. Alcoholic beverages may change insulin requirements. β-blockers may mask symptoms of hypoglycemia.

PREGNANCY: Pregnancy category is not known.

Novolog RX
insulin aspart (Novo Nordisk)

THERAPEUTIC CLASS: Insulin

INDICATIONS: To control hyperglycemia in diabetes.

DOSAGE: *Adults:* Individualize dose. Inject SQ within 5-10 minutes before a meal. Draw first when mixing with NPH human insulin; inject immediately. Do not mix with crystalline zinc insulins, animal source insulins, or other manufacturer insulins. External Insulin Pump: Do not dilute or mix with other insulins.

Pediatrics: Individualize dose. Inject SQ within 5-10 minutes before a meal. Draw first when mixing with NPH human insulin; inject immediately. Do not mix with crystalline zinc insulins, animal source insulins, or other manufacturer insulins. External Insulin Pump: Do not dilute or mix with other insulins.

HOW SUPPLIED: Inj: 100 U/mL; PenFill: 100 U/mL; Prefilled: 100 U/mL

CONTRAINDICATIONS: Hypoglycemia.

WARNINGS/PRECAUTIONS: Any change of insulin should be made cautiously. Changes in strength, manufacturer, type or method of manufacture may result in the need for a change in dosage. Hypoglycemia may occur with taking too much insulin, missing or delaying meals, exercising or working more than usual, diseases of adrenal, pituitary, or thyroid glands, or progression of kidney or liver disease. Dosage adjustments may be needed with hepatic or renal dysfunction, during any infection, illness (especially with diarrhea or vomiting) or pregnancy. A longer-acting insulin is usually required to maintain adequate glucose control. Infusion sets and the insulin in the infusion sets should be changed q48h or sooner. Do not use in quick-release infusion sets or cartridge adapters.

ADVERSE REACTIONS: Hypoglycemia, hypokalemia, lipodystrophy, hypersensitivity reaction, injection site reactions, pruritus, rash.

INTERACTIONS: Increased glucose lowering effects with ACE inhibitors, disopyramide, fibrates, fluoxetine, MAOIs, propoxyphene, salicylates, somatostatin analog, sulfonamide antibiotics and other antidiabetic agents. Decreased blood glucose lowering effects with corticosteroids, niacin, danazol, diuretics, sympathomimetic agents, isoniazid, phenothiazine derivatives, somatropin, thyroid hormones, estrogens, progesterones. Pentamidine may cause hypoglycemia followed by hyperglycemia. β-blockers, clonidine, lithium salts, and alcohol may potentiate or weaken glucose lowering effect. Masked or reduced hypoglycemic symptoms with β-blockers, clonidine, guanethidine, and reserpine.

PREGNANCY: Category B, caution in nursing.

Noxafil RX
posaconazole (Schering)

THERAPEUTIC CLASS: Triazole antifungal

INDICATIONS: Prophylaxis of invasive *Aspergillus* and *Candida* infections in patients, ≥13 yrs, who are at high risk of developing these infections due to being severely immunocompromised. Treatment of oropharyngeal candidiasis, including oropharyngeal candidiasis refractory to itraconazole and/or fluconazole.

DOSAGE: *Adults:* Prophylaxis of Invasive Fungal Infections: 200mg (5mL) tid. Base duration of therapy on recovery from neutropenia or immunosuppression. Oropharyngeal

Candidiasis: LD: 100mg (2.5mL) bid on 1st day, then 100mg qd for 13 days. Oropharyngeal Candidiasis Refractory to Itraconazole and/or Fluconazole: 400mg (10mL) bid. Base duration of therapy on severity of underlying disease and clinical response. Give each dose with full meal or nutritional supplement.

Pediatrics: ≥13 yrs: Prophylaxis of Invasive Fungal Infections: 200mg (5mL) tid. Base duration of therapy on recovery from neutropenia or immunosuppression. Oropharyngeal Candidiasis: LD: 100mg (2.5mL) bid on 1st day, then 100mg qd for 13 days. Oropharyngeal Candidiasis Refractory to Itraconazole and/or Fluconazole: 400mg (10mL) bid. Base duration of therapy on severity of underlying disease and clinical response. Give each dose with full meal or nutritional supplement.

HOW SUPPLIED: Susp: 40mg/mL

CONTRAINDICATIONS: Concomitant ergot alkaloids, terfenadine, astemizole, cisapride, pimozide, halofantrine, or quinidine.

WARNINGS/PRECAUTIONS: Hepatic reactions (eg, mild-to-moderate elevations in ALT, AST, alkaline phosphatase, total bilirubin, and/or clinical hepatitis) reported; monitor LFTs at start of and during therapy. Caution with hepatic impairment. Monitor closely with severe renal impairment. Prolongation of QT interval reported; caution with potentially proarrhythmic conditions.

ADVERSE REACTIONS: Fever, headache, rigors, hypertension, anemia, neutropenia, diarrhea, nausea, vomiting, abdominal pain, constipation, hypokalemia, thrombocytopenia, coughing, dyspnea.

INTERACTIONS: See Contraindications. May elevate cyclosporine and tacrolimus levels; consider dose reduction and more frequent clinical monitoring of cyclosporine, tacrolimus, and sirolimus when therapy is initiated. Avoid use with drugs that are known to prolong the QTc interval and are metabolized through CYP3A4. Avoid concurrent use of cimetidine, rifabutin, and phenytoin unless benefits outweigh risks. If concomitant phenytoin is required, monitor closely and consider phenytoin dose reduction. If concomitant rifabutin is required, monitor CBC and adverse events. Monitor adverse events with concomitant benzodiazepines metabolized by CYP3A4; consider dose reduction of these benzodiazepines during co-administration. May increase levels of vinca alkaloids; consider dose adjustment of vinca alkaloid. Consider dose reduction of concomitant HMG-CoA reductase inhibitors (statins). Monitor for adverse events and toxicity with concomitant calcium channel blockers; dose reduction of calcium channel blockers may be needed.

PREGNANCY: Category C, not for use in nursing.

NUCOFED
codeine phosphate - pseudoephedrine HCl (King)

`CIII`

THERAPEUTIC CLASS: Antitussive/decongestant

INDICATIONS: Relief of cough and congestion associated with respiratory infections, bronchitis, influenza, and sinusitis.

DOSAGE: *Adults:* 1 cap q6h. Max: 4 caps/24 hrs.

Pediatrics: ≥12 yrs: 1 cap q6h. Max: 4 caps/24 hrs.

HOW SUPPLIED: (Codeine-Pseudoephedrine) Cap: 20mg-60mg; Syrup: 20mg-60mg/5mL

WARNINGS/PRECAUTIONS: Not for cough associated with smoking, emphysema, asthma, or excessive secretions. May cause constipation. Caution with pulmonary disease, shortness of breath, HTN, heart disease, DM, thyroid disease, prostatic hypertrophy, Addison's disease, children, ulcerative colitis, drug dependence, liver or kidney dysfunction. May impair alertness.

ADVERSE REACTIONS: Nervousness, restlessness, insomnia, drowsiness, dysuria, dizziness, headache, nausea, vomiting, constipation, trembling, dyspnea, sweating, paleness, weakness, heart rate changes.

INTERACTIONS: β-blockers, MAOIs, sympathomimetics may increase the effects of pseudoephedrine. Avoid within 14 days of MAOI use. TCAs may antagonize effects of pseudoephedrine. Caution with CNS depressants, general anesthetics, alcohol. Anticholinergics may cause paralytic ileus. Digitalis glycosides may cause cardiac arrhythmias. Decreases effects of antihypertensive agents.

PREGNANCY: Category C, caution in nursing.

Nucofed Pediatric Expectorant
guaifenesin - codeine phosphate - pseudoephedrine HCl (King)

OTHER BRAND NAME: Mytussin DAC (Morton Grove)

THERAPEUTIC CLASS: Antitussive/expectorant/decongestant

INDICATIONS: Relief of cough and congestion associated with respiratory infections, bronchitis, influenza, and sinusitis.

DOSAGE: *Adults:* 10mL q6h. Max: 40mL/24 hrs.
Pediatrics: ≥12 yrs: 10mL q6h. Max: 40mL/24hrs. 6 to <12 yrs: 5mL q6h. Max: 20mL/24hrs. 2 to <6 yrs: 2.5mL q6h. Max: 10mL/24hrs.

HOW SUPPLIED: (Codeine-Guaifenesin-Pseudoephedrine) Syrup: 10mg-100mg-30mg/5mL

WARNINGS/PRECAUTIONS: Not for cough associated with smoking, emphysema, asthma, or excessive secretions. May cause constipation. Caution with pulmonary disease, shortness of breath, HTN, heart disease, DM, thyroid disease, prostatic hypertrophy, Addison's disease, children, ulcerative colitis, drug dependence, liver or kidney dysfunction. May impair alertness.

ADVERSE REACTIONS: Nervousness, restlessness, insomnia, drowsiness, dysuria, dizziness, headache, nausea, vomiting, constipation, trembling, dyspnea, sweating, paleness, weakness, heart rate changes.

INTERACTIONS: β-blockers, MAOIs, sympathomimetics may increase the effects of pseudoephedrine. Avoid within 14 days of MAOI use. TCAs may antagonize effects of pseudoephedrine. Caution with CNS depressants, general anesthetics, alcohol. Anticholinergics may cause paralytic ileus. Digitalis glycosides may cause cardiac arrhythmias. Decreases effects of antihypertensive agents.

PREGNANCY: Category C, caution in nursing.

NuLev
hyoscyamine sulfate (Schwarz)

RX

THERAPEUTIC CLASS: Anticholinergic

INDICATIONS: Adjunct treatment of peptic ulcer, irritable bowel syndrome, neurogenic bladder, and neurogenic bowel disturbances. Management of functional intestinal disorders (eg, mild dysenteries, diverticulitis). To control gastric secretion, visceral spasm, and hypermotility in spastic colitis, spastic bladder, cystitis, pylorospasm, and associated abdominal cramps. Symptomatic relief of biliary and renal colic with concomitant morphine or other narcotics. "Drying agent" for symptomatic relief of acute rhinitis. To reduce rigidity and tremors of Parkinson's disease and control associated sialorrhea and hyperhidrosis. For anticholinesterase poisoning.

DOSAGE: *Adults:* 0.125-0.25mg q4h or prn. Max: 1.5mg/24hrs. Take with or without water.
Pediatrics: ≥12 yrs: 0.125-0.25mg q4h or prn. Max: 1.5mg/24hrs. 2 to <12 yrs: 0.0625-0.125mg q4h or prn. Max: 0.75mg/24hrs. Take with or without water.

HOW SUPPLIED: Tab, Disintegrating: 0.125mg

CONTRAINDICATIONS: Glaucoma, obstructive uropathy, GI tract obstruction, paralytic ileus; intestinal atony of elderly/debilitated, unstable cardiovascular status in acute hemorrhage, toxic megacolon complicating ulcerative colitis, myasthenia gravis.

WARNINGS/PRECAUTIONS: Risk of heat prostration with high environmental temperature. Avoid activities requiring mental alertness. Psychosis has been reported in sensitive patients. Caution with diarrhea, autonomic neuropathy, hyperthyroidism, coronary heart disease, CHF, arrhythmias/tachycardia, HTN, renal disease, and hiatal hernia associated with reflux esophagitis. Contains phenylalanine.

ADVERSE REACTIONS: Anticholinergic effects, drowsiness, headache, nervousness.

INTERACTIONS: Additive effects with other antimuscarinics, amantadine, haloperidol, phenothiazines, MAOIs, TCAs, and some antihistamines. Antacids interfere with absorption; take ac and antacids pc.

PREGNANCY: Category C, caution in nursing.

NuLYTELY   RX
sodium chloride - potassium chloride - sodium bicarbonate - polyethylene glycol 3350 (Braintree)

OTHER BRAND NAME: Trilyte (Schwarz Pharma)

THERAPEUTIC CLASS: Bowel cleanser

INDICATIONS: Bowel cleansing prior to colonoscopy.

DOSAGE: *Adults:* Oral: 240mL every 10 minutes until fecal discharge is clear or 4L is consumed. Nasogastric Tube: 20-30mL/minute (1.2-1.8L/hr). Patient should fast at least 3-4 hours before administration.

Pediatrics: ≥6 months: Oral/Nasogastric Tube: 25mL/kg/hr until fecal discharge is clear. Patient should fast at least 3-4 hours before administration.

HOW SUPPLIED: Sol: (Polyethylene Glycol-Potassium Chloride-Sodium Bicarbonate-Sodium Chloride) 420g-1.48g-5.72g-11.2g (4000mL)

CONTRAINDICATIONS: GI obstruction, gastric retention, bowel perforation, toxic colitis, toxic megacolon, ileus.

WARNINGS/PRECAUTIONS: Do not add additional ingredients (eg, flavorings). Caution with severe ulcerative colitis. Monitor therapy with impaired gag reflex, unconsciousness/semiconsciousness and patients prone to regurgitation and aspiration. Temporarily d/c if develop severe bloating, distention, or abdominal pain. Monitor for hypoglycemia in pediatrics <2 yrs of age.

ADVERSE REACTIONS: Nausea, abdominal fullness/cramps, bloating, vomiting, anal irritation.

INTERACTIONS: Oral medications taken within 1 hr of start of administration may not be absorbed from GI tract.

PREGNANCY: Category C, caution in nursing.

Nutropin   RX
somatropin (Genentech)

OTHER BRAND NAME: Nutropin AQ (Genentech)

THERAPEUTIC CLASS: Human growth hormone

INDICATIONS: (Adults) Replacement of endogenous growth hormone (GH) in GH deficiency (GHD). (Pediatrics) Long-term treatment of growth failure due to lack of adequate endogenous GH secretion, in short-stature associated with Turner Syndrome, and in idiopathic short stature (ISS). Treatment of growth failure associated with chronic renal insufficiency (CRI) up to the time of renal transplantation.

DOSAGE: *Adults:* GHD: Initial: Up to 0.006mg/kg/day SQ. Max: <35 yrs: 0.025mg/kg/day. ≥35 yrs: 0.0125mg/kg/day.

Pediatrics: GHD: Usual: 0.30mg/kg/week divided into daily SQ doses. Pubertal Patients: Up to 0.7mg/kg/week divided into daily SQ doses. CRI: 0.35mg/kg/week divided into daily SQ doses. Continue until renal transplantation. Hemodialysis: Give qhs or 3-4 hrs post dialysis. Chronic Cycling Peritoneal Dialysis: Give in am after dialysis. Chronic Ambulatory Peritoneal Dialysis: Give qhs during overnight exchange. Turner Syndrome: Up to 0.375mg/kg/week SQ in divided doses 3-7x/week. ISS: 0.3mg/kg/week divided into daily SQ doses.

HOW SUPPLIED: Inj: 5mg, 10mg, (AQ) 5mg/mL

CONTRAINDICATIONS: Acute critical illness after serious surgeries (eg, open heart or abdominal surgery, accidental trauma, acute respiratory failure), closed epiphyses in pediatrics, active neoplasia, evidence of recurrence or progression of an intracranial tumor, benzyl alcohol sensitivity. Prader-Willi syndrome (unless also diagnosed with GH deficiency) with severe obesity or respiratory impairment.

Nystop

WARNINGS/PRECAUTIONS: Caution with epiphyseal closure in adults treated with GH-replacement therapy in childhood. Recurrence/progression reported with intracranial lesions. Renal osteodystrophy may occur with growth failure secondary to renal impairment. Scoliosis and slipped capital femoral epiphysis may develop in rapid growth. Caution with Turner syndrome and ISS.Intracranial hypertension with papilledema, visual changes, headache, nausea, and/or vomiting has beed reported. Funduscopic exam should be done before and during treatment. Slipped capital femoral epiphysis may occur. Monitor for malignant transformation of skin lesions.Injecting SQ in the same site over a long period of time may cause tissue atrophy. May decrease insulin sensitivity, monitor blood sugar.

ADVERSE REACTIONS: Antibodies to the protein, leukemia, transient peripheral edema, arthralgia, carpal tunnel syndrome, malignant transformations, gynecomastia, pancreatitis.

INTERACTIONS: Decreased effects with glucocorticoids. May reduce insulin sensitivity; may need insulin adjustment.

PREGNANCY: Category C, caution in nursing.

Nystop RX
nystatin (Paddock)

THERAPEUTIC CLASS: Polyene antifungal

INDICATIONS: Treatment of cutaneous and mucocutaneous mycotic infections caused by susceptible *Candida* species.

DOSAGE: *Adults:* Apply to lesions bid-tid until healing is complete. For fungal infections of the feet, dust powder on feet and also in shoes.

Pediatrics: Neonates and Older: Apply to lesions bid-tid until healing is complete. For fungal infections of the feet, dust powder on feet and in shoes also.

HOW SUPPLIED: Powder, Topical: 100,000 U/g (15g, 30g, 60g)

WARNINGS/PRECAUTIONS: D/C if irritation or sensitization occurs. Confirm diagnosis. Not for systemic, oral, intravaginal, or ophthalmic use.

ADVERSE REACTIONS: Allergic reactions, burning, itching, rash, eczema, pain at application site.

PREGNANCY: Safety in pregnancy and nursing not known.

Ocuflox RX
ofloxacin (Allergan)

THERAPEUTIC CLASS: Fluoroquinolone

INDICATIONS: Management of bacterial infections in conjunctivitis and corneal ulcers.

DOSAGE: *Adults:* Conjunctivitis: 1-2 drops q2-4h for 2 days, then 1-2 drops qid for 5 days. Corneal Ulcer: 1-2 drops every 30 minutes while awake and 1-2 drops 4-6 hrs after retiring for 2 days, then 1-2 drops q1h while awake for 5-7 days, then 1-2 drops qid for 2 days or until treatment completion.

Pediatrics: ≥1 yr: Conjunctivitis: 1-2 drops q2-4h for 2 days, then 1-2 drops qid for 5 days. Corneal Ulcer: 1-2 drops every 30 minutes while awake and 1-2 drops 4-6 hrs after retiring for 2 days, then 1-2 drops q1h while awake for 5-7 days, then 1-2 drops qid for 2 days or until treatment completion.

HOW SUPPLIED: Sol: 0.3% (5mL, 10mL)

WARNINGS/PRECAUTIONS: Not for injection into eye. Do not inject subconjunctivally nor into the eye's anterior chamber. Superinfection may result with prolonged use. Fatal hypersensitivity reactions reported after 1st dose of systemic quinolone therapy. Avoid allowing tip of container to contact fingers, eye or surrounding structures.

ADVERSE REACTIONS: Transient ocular burning or discomfort, stinging, redness, itching, keratitis, ocular periocular/facial edema, photophobia, blurred vision, tearing, dryness, eye pain.

INTERACTIONS: Systemic quinolone therapy may increase theophylline levels, interfere with caffeine metabolism, enhance warfarin effects, and elevate serum creatinine with cyclosporine.

PREGNANCY: Category C, not for use in nursing.

OLUX
clobetasol propionate (Stiefel)
RX

THERAPEUTIC CLASS: Corticosteroid

INDICATIONS: Short-term treatment of inflammatory and pruritic manifestations of moderate to severe corticosteroid responsive dermatoses of the scalp. Short-term treatment of mild to moderate plaque-type psoriasis of non-scalp regions excluding the face and intertriginous areas.

DOSAGE: *Adults:* Apply to affected area bid (am and pm). No more than 1.5 capfuls/application. Limit to 2 consecutive weeks. Do not use with occlusive dressings. Max 50g/week.

Pediatrics: ≥12 yrs: Apply to affected area bid (am and pm). No more than 1.5 capfuls/application. Limit to 2 consecutive weeks. Do not use with occlusive dressings. Max 50g/week.

HOW SUPPLIED: Foam: 0.05% (50g, 100g)

WARNINGS/PRECAUTIONS: May produce reversible HPA axis suppression, manifestations of Cushing's syndrome, hyperglycemia, and glucosuria. Caution when applied to large surface areas or under occlusive dressings. Use appropriate antifungal or antibacterial agent with dermatological infections; discontinue if infection does not clear. Pediatrics may be more susceptible to systemic toxicity. Avoid eyes. Discontinue if irritation occurs.

ADVERSE REACTIONS: Burning/stinging, pruritus, irritation, erythema, folliculitis, cracking/fissuring of skin, numbness of fingers, telangiectasia, skin atrophy.

PREGNANCY: Category C, caution in nursing.

OLUX-E
clobetasol propionate (Stiefel)
RX

THERAPEUTIC CLASS: Corticosteroid

INDICATIONS: Treatment of inflammatory and pruritic manifestations of corticosteroid-responsive dermatoses.

DOSAGE: *Adults:* Apply thin layer to affected area bid (am and pm). Limit to 2 consecutive weeks. Avoid with occlusive dressings. Max: 50g/week.

Pediatrics: ≥12 yrs: Apply thin layer to affected area bid (am and pm). Limit to 2 consecutive weeks. Avoid with occlusive dressings. Max: 50g/week.

HOW SUPPLIED: Foam: 0.05% (100g)

WARNINGS/PRECAUTIONS: May produce reversible HPA axis suppression, Cushing's syndrome, hyperglycemia, and glucosuria. Caution when applied to large surface area or under occlusive dressings. Use appropriate antifungal or antibacterial agent with dermatological infections; discontinue if infection does not clear. Pediatrics may be more susceptible to systemic toxicity. Discontinue if irritation occurs. Should not be used to treat rosacea or perioral dermatitis. Avoid use on face, groin, axillae, or other intertriginous areas.

ADVERSE REACTIONS: Folliculitits, acneiform eruptions, hypopigmentation, perioral dermatitis, allergic contact dermatitis, secondary infection, irritation, striae, miliaria.

PREGNANCY: Category C, caution in nursing.

OMNARIS
ciclesonide (Altana)
RX

THERAPEUTIC CLASS: Corticosteroid

INDICATIONS: Treatment of nasal symptoms associated with seasonal and perennial allergic rhinitis.

DOSAGE: *Adults:* 2 sprays (50mcg/spray) in each nostril qd. Max: 2 sprays/nostril/day (200mcg/day).

Pediatrics: ≥12 yrs: 2 sprays (50mcg/spray) in each nostril qd. Max: 2 sprays/nostril/day (200mcg/day).

HOW SUPPLIED: Spray: 50mcg/spray (12.5g)

WARNINGS/PRECAUTIONS: Risk of adrenal insufficiency and withdrawal symptoms when replacing systemic corticosteroids with a topical corticosteroids; monitor closely. Risk for more severe/fatal course of infections (eg, chickenpox, measles); avoid exposure in patients who have not had disease or been properly immunized. Potential for growth velocity reduction in pediatrics. Avoid with recent nasal septal ulcers, nasal surgery, or nasal trauma until healed. Symptoms of hypercorticism may occur with excessive use or in highly sensitive patients.

ADVERSE REACTIONS: Headache, epistaxis, nasopharyngitis, ear pain.

INTERACTIONS: Ketoconazole may increase levels of the pharmacologically active metabolite des-ciclesonide; co-administer with caution.

PREGNANCY: Category C, caution in nursing.

OMNICEF — RX
cefdinir (Abbott)

THERAPEUTIC CLASS: Cephalosporin (3rd generation)

INDICATIONS: Community acquired pneumonia (CAP), acute exacerbations of chronic bronchitis (AECB), acute maxillary sinusitis, pharyngitis/tonsillitis, uncomplicated skin and structure infections (SSSI), and acute bacterial otitis media.

DOSAGE: *Adults:* (Cap) SSSI/CAP: 300mg q12h for 10 days. AECB/Pharyngitis/Tonsillitis: 300mg q12h for 5-10 days or 600mg q24h for 10 days. Sinusitis: 300mg q12h or 600mg q24h for 10 days. CrCl <30mL/min: 300mg qd.
Pediatrics: (Sus) 6 months-12 yrs: Otitis Media/Pharyngitis/Tonsillitis: 7mg/kg q12h for 5-10 days or 14mg/kg q24h for 10 days. Sinusitis: 7mg/kg q12h or 14mg/kg q24h for 10 days. SSSI: 7mg/kg q12h for 10 days. (Cap) ≥13 yrs: CAP/SSSI: 300mg q12h for 10 days. AECB/Pharyngitis/Tonsillitis: 300mg q12h for 5-10 days or 600mg q24h for 10 days. Sinusitis: 300mg q12h or 600mg q24h for 10 days. CrCl <30mL/min/1.73m^2: 7mg/kg qd. Max: 300mg qd.

HOW SUPPLIED: Cap: 300mg; Sus: 125mg/5mL, 250mg/5mL (60mL, 100mL)

WARNINGS/PRECAUTIONS: Cross sensitivity to penicillins and other cephalosporins may occur. Pseudomembranous colitis reported. Positive direct Coombs' tests may occur. Caution with renal dysfunction, history of colitis. Suspension contains 2.86g/5mL of sucrose; caution in diabetes. False (+) for urine glucose with Clinitest® and Benedict's or Fehling's solution.

ADVERSE REACTIONS: Diarrhea, vaginal moniliasis, nausea, headache, abdominal pain, superinfection (prolonged use).

INTERACTIONS: Iron-fortified foods, iron supplements, and aluminum- or magnesium-containing antacids reduce absorption; separate doses by 2 hrs. Probenecid inhibits the renal excretion. Reddish stools reported with iron-containing products.

PREGNANCY: Category B, caution in nursing.

OMNITROPE — RX
somatropin (Sandoz)

THERAPEUTIC CLASS: Human growth hormone

INDICATIONS: Long-term treatment of pediatric patients who have growth failure due to an inadequate secretion of endogenous growth hormone. Long-term replacement therapy in adults with growth hormone deficiency (GHD) of either childhood- or adult-onset etiology.

DOSAGE: *Adults:* Individualize dose. GHD: ≤0.04mg/kg/week. May increase at 4-8 week intervals. Max: 0.08mg/kg/week. Divide dose into daily SQ injections (give preferably in the evening).
Pediatrics: Individualize dose. GHD: 0.16-0.24mg/kg/week. Divide dose into daily SQ injections (give preferably in the evening).

HOW SUPPLIED: Inj: 1.5mg, 5.8mg

CONTRAINDICATIONS: Evidence of neoplastic activity. Pediatrics with fused epiphyses. Acute critical illness due to complications after open heart or abdominal surgery, multiple accidental trauma, or with acute respiratory failure. Patients with Prader-Willi syndrome who are severely obese or have severe respiratory impairment.

WARNINGS/PRECAUTIONS: Contains benzyl alcohol; avoid use in newborns. Patients with GHD secondary to an intracranial lesion should be monitored closely for progression or recurrence of underlying disease process. Monitor closely for any malignant transformation of skin lesions, scoliosis progression, or gait abnormalities. Monitor closely with DM, glucose intolerance, hypopituitarism. Intracranial HTN reported. Funduscopic exam recomended at initiation, and periodically during course of therapy.

ADVERSE REACTIONS: Hypothyroidism, elevated HbA1c, eosinophilia, hematoma, headache, hypertriglyceridemia, leg pain.

INTERACTIONS: Growth promoting effects may be inhibited by glucocorticoids. May alter clearance of CYP450 substrates (eg, corticosteroids, sex steroids, anticonvulsants, cyclosporine); monitor closely. May need insulin dose adjustment.

PREGNANCY: Category B, caution in nursing.

ONCASPAR
pegaspargase (Enzon)

RX

THERAPEUTIC CLASS: Protein synthesis inhibitor

INDICATIONS: Acute lymphoblastic leukemia in patients who have developed hypersensitivity to the native forms of L-asparaginase. May be given as monotherapy if multiagent therapy is inappropriate.

DOSAGE: *Adults:* Usual: 2500 IU/m^2 IM every 14 days.
Pediatrics: BSA ≥0.6m^2: 2500 IU/m^2 every 14 days. BSA <0.6m^2: 82.5 IU/kg every 14 days.

HOW SUPPLIED: Inj: 750 IU/mL (5mL)

CONTRAINDICATIONS: Pancreatitis. History of pancreatitis, significant hemorrhagic events, or serious thrombosis with prior L-asparaginase therapy.

WARNINGS/PRECAUTIONS: May be a contact irritant. Avoid inhalation or contact with skin or mucous membranes. Serious allergic reaction, pancreatitis, or glucose intolerance can occur. Increased prothrombin time, partial thromboplastin time, and hypofibrinogenemia can occur; monitor coagulation parameters. May predispose to infections, bleeding, thrombosis. D/C in patients with serious thrombotic event including sagittal sinus thrombosis.

ADVERSE REACTIONS: Allergic reactions, SGPT increase, nausea, vomiting, fever, malaise.

INTERACTIONS: May increase toxicity of protein bound drugs. May interfere with the action of drugs that require cell replication for their lethal effects (eg, methotrexate), and the enzymatic detoxification of other drugs, particularly in the liver. Caution with concomitant anticoagulants (eg, coumadin, heparin, dipyridamole, aspirin or NSAIDs), hepatotoxic agents.

PREGNANCY: Category C, not for use in nursing.

OPCON-A
naphazoline HCl - pheniramine maleate (Bausch & Lomb)

OTC

THERAPEUTIC CLASS: H$_1$ antagonist/alpha-agonist (imidazoline)

INDICATIONS: Temporary relief of redness and itching of the eye due to various allergens.

DOSAGE: *Adults:* 1-2 drops up to qid.
Pediatrics: ≥6 yrs: 1-2 drops up to qid.

HOW SUPPLIED: Sol: (Pheniramine-Naphazoline) 0.3%-0.027% (15mL)

CONTRAINDICATIONS: Cardiovascular disease, HTN, narrow angle glaucoma, BPH.

OPTICROM

WARNINGS/PRECAUTIONS: D/C if pain, vision changes, no improvement, condition worsens or persists >72 hrs. Remove contact lens before use. Overuse may produce increased redness of eye. Supervision required with heart disease, high BP, difficulty in urination due to prostate enlargement, or narrow angle glaucoma.

ADVERSE REACTIONS: Brief tingling sensation.

PREGNANCY: Safety in pregnancy and nursing not known.

OPTICROM
cromolyn sodium (Allergan)

RX

THERAPEUTIC CLASS: Mast cell stabilizer

INDICATIONS: Treatment of vernal keratoconjunctivitis, vernal conjunctivitis, and vernal keratitis.

DOSAGE: *Adults:* 1-2 drops 4-6x/day at regular intervals.

Pediatrics: ≥4 yrs: 1-2 drops 4-6x/day at regular intervals.

HOW SUPPLIED: Sol: 4% (10mL)

WARNINGS/PRECAUTIONS: Do not wear contacts during therapy. Do not exceed recommended frequency.

ADVERSE REACTIONS: Transient burning or stinging.

PREGNANCY: Category B, caution in nursing.

OPTIVAR
azelastine HCl (MedPointe)

RX

THERAPEUTIC CLASS: H_1 antagonist

INDICATIONS: Treatment of itching of the eye associated with allergic conjunctivitis.

DOSAGE: *Adults:* 1 drop bid.

Pediatrics: ≥3 yrs: 1 drop bid.

HOW SUPPLIED: Sol: 0.05% (6mL)

WARNINGS/PRECAUTIONS: Not for injection or oral use. Do not wear contact lens if the eye is red. Not for treatment of contact lens irritation. Wait 10 minutes after instilling drops to insert contact lens.

ADVERSE REACTIONS: Transient eye burning/stinging, headaches, asthma, conjunctivitis, dyspnea, eye pain, fatigue, influenza like symptoms, pharyngitis, pruritus, rhinitis, temporary blurring.

PREGNANCY: Category C, caution in nursing.

ORAP
pimozide (Gate)

RX

THERAPEUTIC CLASS: Diphenylbutylperidine

INDICATIONS: Suppression of motor and phonic tics in Tourette's Syndrome in patients that failed standard therapy.

DOSAGE: *Adults:* Initial: 1-2mg/day in divided doses. May increase every other day. Maint: <0.2mg/kg/day or 10mg/day, whichever is less. Max: 0.2mg/kg/day or 10mg/day.

Pediatrics: >12 yrs: Initial: 0.05mg/kg qhs. Titrate: May increase every 3 days. Max: 0.2mg/kg/day or 10mg/day.

HOW SUPPLIED: Tab: 1mg*, 2mg* *scored

CONTRAINDICATIONS: Severe CNS depression, comatose states, congenital long QT syndrome, history of cardiac arrhythmias, hypokalemia, hypomagnesemia, simple tics or tics not associated with Tourette's Syndrome. CYP3A4 inhibitors (eg, nefazadone, macrolide antibiotics, azole antifungals, protease inhibitors), sertraline, and drugs that cause motor and phonic tics (eg, pemoline, methylphenidate, amphetamines) or prolong the QT interval.

WARNINGS/PRECAUTIONS: May cause tardive dyskinesia, NMS, hyperpyrexia. Caution with history of seizures, EEG abnormalities, severe hepatic/renal impairment. Perform ECG before therapy, periodically thereafter, with dose adjustment. Produces anticholinergic effects. Sudden death reported. May impair mental/physical abilities.

ADVERSE REACTIONS: Akinesia, QT prolongation, tardive dyskinesia, sedation, impotence, constipation, dry mouth, visual disturbances, headache, asthenia, increased salivation.

INTERACTIONS: May potentiate CNS depressants (eg, analgesics, sedatives, anxiolytics, alcohol). Bradycardia reported with fluoxetine. Avoid grapefruit juice, CYP3A4 inhibitors (eg, azole antifungal drugs, macrolides, protease inhibitors, zileuton, fluvoxamine), sertraline. May interact with CYP1A2 inhibitors. Avoid other drugs that may potentiate QT prolongation such as phenothiazines, TCAs, antiarrhythmics, sparfloxacin, gatifloxacin, moxifloxacin, halofantrine, mefloquine, pentamidine, arsenic trioxide, levomethadyl acetate, dolasetron mesylate, probucol, tacrolimus, ziprasidone.

PREGNANCY: Category C, not for use in nursing.

ORAPRED RX
prednisolone sodium phosphate (Biomarin)

THERAPEUTIC CLASS: Glucocorticoid

INDICATIONS: Steroid responsive dermatoses.

DOSAGE: *Adults:* Initial: 5-60mg/day depending on disease and response. Maint: Decrease dose by small amounts to lowest effective dose. MS Exacerbations: 200mg qd for 1 week, then 80mg every other day for 1 month.
Pediatrics: Initial: 0.14-2mg/kg/day, depending on disease and response, given tid-qid. Nephrotic Syndrome: 20mg/m^2 tid for 4 weeks, then 40mg/m^2 every other day for 4 weeks. Uncontrolled Asthma: 1-2mg/kg/day in single or divided doses until peak expiratory flow rate of 80% is achieved (usually 3-10 days).

HOW SUPPLIED: Sol: 15mg/5mL (237mL)

CONTRAINDICATIONS: Systemic fungal infections.

WARNINGS/PRECAUTIONS: May produce reversible HPA axis suppression. Adjust dose during stress or change in thyroid status. May mask signs of infection or cause new infections. May activate latent amebiasis. Avoid with cerebral malaria. Avoid exposure to chickenpox or measles. Not for treatment of optic neuritis or active ocular herpes simplex. May cause elevation of BP or IOP, cataracts, glaucoma, optic nerve damage, Kaposi's sarcoma, psychic derangements, salt/water retention, increased excretion of potassium and/or calcium, osteoporosis, growth suppression in children, secondary ocular infections. Caution with Strongyloides, CHF, diverticulitis, HTN, renal insufficiency, fresh intestinal anastomoses, active or latent peptic ulcer, ulcerative colitis. Enhanced effect in hypothyroidism or cirrhosis. Avoid abrupt withdrawal.

ADVERSE REACTIONS: Edema, fluid/electrolyte disturbances, osteoporosis, muscle weakness, pancreatitis, peptic ulcer, impaired wound healing, increased intracranial pressure, cushingoid state, hirsutism, menstrual irregularities, growth suppression in children, glaucoma, nausea, weight gain.

INTERACTIONS: Enhanced metabolism with barbiturates, phenytoin, ephedrine, and rifampin. Use with cyclosporine may increase activity of both drugs; convulsions reported with concomitant use. Decreased metabolism with estrogens or ketoconazole. May inhibit response to warfarin. Increased risk of GI side effects with ASA or other NSAIDs. May increase clearance of salicylates. High doses or concurrent neuromuscular drugs may cause acute myopathy. Enhanced possibility of hypokalemia when given with potassium-depleting agents. May produce severe weakness in myasthenia gravis patients on anticholinesterase agents. Avoid live vaccines with immunosuppressive doses. Possible diminished response with killed or inactivated vaccines. May increase blood glucose; adjust antidiabetic agents. May suppress reactions to skin tests.

PREGNANCY: Category C, caution in nursing.

ORFADIN

nitisinone (Rare Disease Therapeutics) — RX

THERAPEUTIC CLASS: 4-hydroxyphenylpyruvate dioxygenase inhibitor

INDICATIONS: Adjunct to dietary restriction of tyrosine and phenylalanine in the treatment of hereditary tyrosinemia type I.

DOSAGE: *Adults:* Initial: 1mg/kg/day in divided doses, qam and qpm. Titrate: Increase to 1.5mg/kg/day if biochemical parameters (except plasma succinylacetone) are not normalized within 1 month. Max: 2mg/kg/day. Take at least 1 hr before a meal. May sprinkle contents of capsule in small amount of water, formula or apple sauce immediately before use.

Pediatrics: Initial: 1mg/kg/day in divided doses, qam and qpm. Titrate: Increase to 1.5mg/kg/day if biochemical parameters (except plasma succinylacetone) are not normalized within 1 month. Max: 2mg/kg/day. Take at least 1 hr before a meal. May sprinkle contents of capsule in small amount of water, formula or apple sauce immediately before use.

HOW SUPPLIED: Cap: 2mg, 5mg, 10mg

WARNINGS/PRECAUTIONS: Inadequate restriction of tyrosine and phenylalanine can result in elevated tyrosine levels. Maintain tyrosine levels <500µmol/L to avoid toxicity. Transient thrombocytopenia and leucopenia reported; monitor platelet and WBC count. Perform slit-lamp eye examination before initiation and if patient develops photophobia, eye pain or inflammation. Do not adjust dose further to lower tyrosine levels; may deteriorate patients condition; use diet restriction instead. Increased risk of porphyric crises, liver failure, or hepatic neoplasms; monitor liver by imaging and lab tests including serum alpha-fetoprotein. Monitor urine succinylacetone levels to guide dose-adjustment. Monitor serum phosphate to screen for renal involvement.

ADVERSE REACTIONS: Hepatic neoplasm, liver failure, conjunctivitis, corneal opacity, keratitis, photophobia, thrombocytopenia, leucopenia.

PREGNANCY: Category C, caution in nursing.

ORTHO TRI-CYCLEN

norgestimate - ethinyl estradiol (Ortho-McNeil) — RX

OTHER BRAND NAMES: Tri-Previfem (Teva) - Tri-Sprintec (Barr)

THERAPEUTIC CLASS: Estrogen/progestogen combination

INDICATIONS: Prevention of pregnancy. Treatment of acne vulgaris in females ≥15 yrs who want contraception, have achieved menarche and are unresponsive to topical acne agents.

DOSAGE: *Adults:* Contraception/Acne: 28-day: 1 tab qd for 28 days, then repeat. Start 1st Sunday after menses begin or 1st day of menses.

Pediatrics: Contraception (postpubertal adolescents)/Acne: 28-day: 1 tab qd for 28 days, then repeat. Start 1st Sunday after menses begin or 1st day of menses.

HOW SUPPLIED: Tab: (Ethinyl Estradiol-Norgestimate) 0.035mg-0.18mg, 0.035mg-0.215mg, and 0.035mg-0.25mg

CONTRAINDICATIONS: Thrombophlebitis, deep vein thrombophlebitis, thromboembolic disorders, pregnancy, cerebrovascular or coronary artery disease, migraine with focal aura, acute or chronic hepatocellular disease with abnormal liver function, undiagnosed abnormal genital bleeding, cholestatic jaundice of pregnancy or jaundice with prior pill use, hepatic adenomas or carcinomas, breast cancer, endometrium carcinoma, or other estrogen-dependent neoplasia.

WARNINGS/PRECAUTIONS: Cigarette smoking increases risk of serious cardiovascular side effects. This risk increases with age (especially >35 yrs) and heavy smoking. Increased risk of MI, vascular disease, thromboembolism, stroke, and gallbladder disease. Retinal thrombosis, hepatic neoplasia, carcinoma of breast and reproductive organs reported. May cause glucose intolerance, fluid retention, breakthrough bleeding, and spotting. May increase BP, elevate LDL levels, or cause other lipid changes. May cause or exacerbate migraine. May develop visual changes with contact lens. Increased risk of morbidity and mortality with HTN, hyperlipidemia, obesity, and diabetes. D/C if jaundice, significant depression, or ophthalmic irregularities develop. Perform annual physical exam. Use before menarche is not indicated. May affect certain endocrine, LFTs, and blood components.

ADVERSE REACTIONS: Nausea, vomiting, breakthrough bleeding, spotting, amenorrhea, migraine, depression, vaginal candidiasis, edema, weight changes.

INTERACTIONS: Reduced effects, increased breakthrough bleeding, and menstrual irregularities with rifampin, barbiturates, phenylbutazone, phenytoin, carbamazepine, griseofulvin, topiramate, St. John's wort, and possibly with ampicillin and tetracyclines.

PREGNANCY: Category X, not for use in nursing.

OVIDE RX
malathion (Taro)

THERAPEUTIC CLASS: Organophosphate/cholinesterase inhibitor

INDICATIONS: For infections of *Pediculus humanus capitis* (head lice and their ova) of scalp hair.

DOSAGE: *Adults:* Apply sufficient amount on dry hair to thoroughly wet hair and scalp. Allow hair to dry naturally. Shampoo after 8-12 hrs. Rinse and use a fine-toothed comb to remove dead lice and eggs. Repeat with 2nd application if lice present after 7-9 days.

Pediatrics: ≥6 yrs: Apply sufficient amount on dry hair to thoroughly wet hair and scalp. Allow hair to dry naturally. Shampoo after 8-12 hrs. Rinse and use a fine-toothed comb to remove dead lice and eggs. Repeat with 2nd application if lice present after 7-9 days.

HOW SUPPLIED: Lot: 0.5% (59mL)

CONTRAINDICATIONS: Neonates, infants.

WARNINGS/PRECAUTIONS: Lotion is flammable; do not expose lotion or wet hair to open flames or electric heat sources (eg, hair dryers, electric curlers). If contact with eyes, flush immediately with water. If skin irritation develops, d/c until irritation clears. Slight stinging sensations reported. Adult supervision is required with use in children.

ADVERSE REACTIONS: Skin and scalp irritation, mild conjunctivitis (with eye contact).

PREGNANCY: Category B, caution in nursing.

OXANDRIN CIII
oxandrolone (Savient)

THERAPEUTIC CLASS: Anabolic steroid

INDICATIONS: Adjunctive therapy to promote weight gain after weight loss following extensive surgery, chronic infections, severe trauma, and for those who fail to gain or maintain normal weight without pathophysiologic reasons, to offset protein catabolism associated with prolonged administration of corticosteroids, for the relief of osteoporotic bone pain.

DOSAGE: *Adults:* Usual: 2.5-20mg/day given bid-qid for 2-4 weeks. May repeat course intermittently as indicated. Elderly: 5mg bid.

Pediatrics: ≤0.1mg/kg/day. May repeat intermittently as indicated.

HOW SUPPLIED: Tab: 2.5mg*, 10mg *scored

CONTRAINDICATIONS: Carcinoma of the prostate or breast, carcinoma of the breast in females with hypercalcemia, pregnancy, nephrosis, hypercalcemia.

WARNINGS/PRECAUTIONS: D/C if peliosis hepatis, liver cell tumors, cholestatic hepatitis, jaundice, LFT abnormalities, hypercalcemia or signs of virilization (females) occur. Edema, with or without CHF, may occur with pre-existing cardiac, renal, or hepatic disease. Monitor bone growth in children every 6 months. Increased risk of prostatic hypertrophy/carcinoma in the elderly. May decrease levels of thyroxine-binding globulin, suppress clotting factors II, V, VII, and X and increase PT. Caution with CAD and history of MI. Lower dose recommended in elderly.

ADVERSE REACTIONS: Cholestatic jaundice, gynecomastia, edema, CNS effects, acne, phallic enlargement, increased frequency/persistence of erections, inhibition of testicular function, chronic priapism, epididymitis, impotence, testicular atrophy, oligospermia, bladder irritability, menstrual irregularities, virilization.

INTERACTIONS: Increased sensitivity to oral anticoagulants (eg, warfarin). May increase edema with adrenal cortical steroids or ACTH. May inhibit metabolism of oral hypoglycemics.

PREGNANCY: Category X, not for use in nursing.

Oxistat RX
oxiconazole nitrate (GlaxoSmithKline)

THERAPEUTIC CLASS: Azole antifungal

INDICATIONS: (Cre/Lot) Topical treatment of tinea pedis, tinea cruris and tinea corporis due to *Trichophyton rubrum*, *Trichophyton mentagrophytes*, or *Epidermophyton floccosum*. (Cre) Topical treatment of tinea versicolor due to *Malassezia furfur*.

DOSAGE: *Adults:* (Cre/Lot) T.pedis/T.corporis/T.cruris: Apply qd-bid. (Cre) T.versicolor: Apply qd. Treat t.pedis for 1 month and other infections for 2 weeks.

Pediatrics: ≥12 yrs: (Cream) T.pedis/T.corporis/T.cruris: Apply qd-bid. T.versicolor: Apply qd. Treat t.pedis for 1 month and other infections for 2 weeks.

HOW SUPPLIED: Cre: 1% (15g, 30g, 60g); Lot: 1% (30mL)

WARNINGS/PRECAUTIONS: Not for ophthalmic or intravaginal use. D/C if irritation or sensitivity occurs.

ADVERSE REACTIONS: Pruritus, burning/stinging.

PREGNANCY: Category B, caution in nursing.

Oxsoralen RX
methoxsalen (Valeant)

THERAPEUTIC CLASS: Psoralen

INDICATIONS: As a topical repigmenting agent in vitiligo with controlled doses of UVA (320-400nm) or sunlight.

DOSAGE: *Adults:* Apply to small well defined lesions before UVA exposure. Determine treatment intervals by erythema response; generally 1 week or less often.

Pediatrics: ≥12 yrs: Apply to small well defined lesions before UVA exposure. Determine treatment intervals by erythema response; generally 1 week or less often.

HOW SUPPLIED: Lot: 1% (30mL)

CONTRAINDICATIONS: Current or history of melanoma, invasive skin carcinoma, photosensitive diseases (eg, acute lupus erythematosus, porphyria, xeroderma pigmentosum), patients <12 yrs.

WARNINGS/PRECAUTIONS: May develop serious burns if exceed recommended dose or exposure. Protect treated areas from sunlight. Increased risk of skin cancer in fair-skinned patients or prior coal tar UVA treatment, ionizing radiation, or taken arsenical compounds. Protect treated areas from light by using protective clothing or sunscreen.

ADVERSE REACTIONS: Minor blistering, severe burns (from overexposure to UVA).

INTERACTIONS: Caution with photosensitizers such as anthralin, coal tar and its derivatives, griseofulvin, phenothiazines, nalidixic acid, halogenated salicylanilides, sulfonamides, tetracyclines, thiazides, and certain organic staining dyes (eg, methylene blue, toluidine blue, rose bengal, methyl orange).

PREGNANCY: Category C, caution in nursing.

Palgic RX
carbinoxamine maleate (PamLab)

THERAPEUTIC CLASS: H_1 antagonist

INDICATIONS: Seasonal and perennial allergic rhinitis, vasomotor rhinitis, allergic conjunctivitis, urticaria, angioedema, dermatographism, allergic reactions to blood or plasma. Adjunct in anaphylaxis.

DOSAGE: *Adults:* Usual: 4mg prn. Max: 24mg/day given q6-8h.
Pediatrics: ≥6 yrs: Usual: 4mg prn. Max: 24mg/day given q6-8h. 1-6 yrs: Usual: 2mg prn. May increase to 0.2-0.4mg/kg/day given q6-8h.

HOW SUPPLIED: Sol: 4mg/5mL; Tab: 4mg* *scored

CONTRAINDICATIONS: Concomitant MAOIs, newborns, premature infants, lower respiratory tract disorders (eg, asthma), nursing mothers.

WARNINGS/PRECAUTIONS: Caution in narrow angle glaucoma, stenosing peptic ulcer, symptomatic prostatic hypertrophy, bladder neck or pyloroduodenal obstruction, history of bronchial asthma, increased IOP, hyperthyroidism, CVD, HTN, and elderly. May impair mental/physical abilities.

ADVERSE REACTIONS: Sedation, sleepiness, dizziness, disturbed coordination, epigastric distress, thickening of bronchial secretions, excitation, diminished mental alertness.

INTERACTIONS: See Contraindications. Intensified anticholinergic effects with MAOIs; avoid concurrent use. Additive effects with alcohol, other CNS depressants (eg, hypnotics, sedatives, tranquilizers).

PREGNANCY: Category C, not for use in nursing.

PANCREASE   RX
lipase - amylase - protease (McNeil Consumer)

OTHER BRAND NAME: Pancrease MT (McNeil Consumer)

THERAPEUTIC CLASS: Pancreatic enzyme supplement

INDICATIONS: Treatment of steatorrhea secondary to pancreatic insufficiency such as cystic fibrosis (CF) and chronic alcoholic pancreatitis.

DOSAGE: *Adults:* Initial: 400 U lipase/kg/meal. Max: 2500 U lipase/kg/meal. Adjust dose based on 3-day fecal fat studies. Take with plenty of water. Do not chew/crush caps. May add capsule contents to soft food (pH <7.3) and swallow immediately without chewing.
Pediatrics: ≤12 months: 2000-4000 U lipase/120mL formula or per breast feeding. 13 months-3 yrs: Initial: 1000 U lipase/kg/meal. Max: 2500 U lipase/kg/meal. ≥4 yrs: Initial: 400U lipase/kg/meal. Max: 2500 U lipase/kg/meal. Adjust dose based on 3-day fecal fat studies. Take with plenty of water. Do not chew/crush caps. May add capsule contents to soft food (pH <7.3) and swallow immediately without chewing.

HOW SUPPLIED: Cap, Extended Release: (Amylase-Lipase-Protease) 20,000 U-4500 U-25,000 U, (MT 4) 12,000 U-4000 U-12,000 U, (MT 10) 30,000 U-10,000 U-30,000 U, (MT 16) 48,000 U-16,000 U-48,000 U, (MT 20) 56,000 U-20,000 U-44,000 U

CONTRAINDICATIONS: Pork protein hypersensitivity.

WARNINGS/PRECAUTIONS: May cause fibrotic strictures in colon of primarily CF patients. Caution when changing dose or brand of medication.

ADVERSE REACTIONS: Diarrhea, abdominal pain, intestinal obstruction, vomiting, flatulence, nausea, constipation, melena, perianal irritation, weight loss, pain.

PREGNANCY: Category B, safety in nursing not known.

PANCURONIUM   RX
pancuronium bromide (Various)

> Administer by adequately trained individuals familiar with actions, characteristics, and hazards.

THERAPEUTIC CLASS: Skeletal muscle relaxant (nondepolarizing)

INDICATIONS: Adjunct to general anesthesia, to facilitate endotracheal intubation, and to provide skeletal muscle relaxation during surgery or mechanical ventilation.

DOSAGE: *Adults:* Individualize dose. Initial: 0.04-0.1mg/kg IV. Late incremental doses of 0.01mg/kg may be used. Skeletal Muscle Relaxation For Endotracheal Intubation: 0.06-0.1mg/kg bolus.
Pediatrics: Individualize dose. Initial: 0.04-0.1mg/kg IV. Late incremental doses of 0.01mg/kg may be used. Skeletal Muscle Relaxation For Endotracheal Intubation: 0.06-0.1mg/kg bolus. Neonates: Use test dose of 0.02mg/kg.

PANIXINE

HOW SUPPLIED: Inj: 1mg/mL, 2mg/mL

WARNINGS/PRECAUTIONS: May have profound effect in myasthenia gravis or myasthenic (Eaton Lambert) syndrome; use small test dose and monitor closely. Contains benzyl alcohol; caution in neonates. Use peripheral nerve stimulator to monitor neuromuscular blocking effect. Caution with pre-existing pulmonary, hepatic, or renal disease. Conditions associated with slower circulation time in cardiovascular disease, old age, and edematous states may delay onset time; dosage should not be increased. Possible slower onset, higher total dosage, and prolongation of neuromuscular blockade with hepatic and/or biliary tract disease. In ICU, long-term use may be associated with prolonged paralysis and/or skeletal muscle weakness; monitor closely. Severe obesity and neuromuscular disease may pose airway or ventilatory problems. Electrolyte imbalances may alter neuromuscular blockade.

ADVERSE REACTIONS: Skeletal muscle weakness and paralysis, salivation, rash.

INTERACTIONS: Prior administration of succinylcholine may enhance neuromuscular blocking effect. Avoid use with vercuronium, atracurium, d-tubocurarine, metocurine, gallamine. Enhanced neuromuscular blockade with enflurane, isoflurane, halothane, aminoglycosides, tetracyclines, bacitracin, polymyxin B, colistin, sodium colistimethate, and magnesium salts. Quinidine injection during recovery from use of other muscle relaxants suggests that recurrent paralysis may occur.

PREGNANCY: Category C, safety in nursing not known.

PANIXINE RX
cephalexin (Ranbaxy)

THERAPEUTIC CLASS: Cephalosporin (1st generation)

INDICATIONS: Skin and skin structure (SSSI), bone, genitourinary and respiratory tract infections, otitis media, acute prostatitis.

DOSAGE: *Adults*: ≥15 yrs: Usual: 250mg q6h. Streptococcal pharyngitis/SSSI: 500mg q12h. Cystitis: 500mg q12h for minimum of 7-14 days. Max: 4g/day. Do not crush, cut, or chew tab. Treat β-hemolytic streptococcal infections for ≥10 days.
Pediatrics: Usual: 25-50mg/kg/day in divided doses. Streptococcal Pharyngitis (>1 yr)/SSS: May divide into 2 doses, give q12h. Otitis Media: 75-100mg/kg/day given qid. Treat β-hemolytic streptococcal infections for ≥10 days.

HOW SUPPLIED: Tab, Dispersible: 125mg, 250mg

WARNINGS/PRECAUTIONS: Caution with markedly impaired renal function, history of GI disease. Cross-sensitivity with cephalosporins and penicillins. Pseudomembranous colitis reported. False (+) direct Coombs' tests reported. False (+) for urine glucose with Benedict's, Fehling's solution, and Clinitest® tablets.

ADVERSE REACTIONS: Diarrhea, dyspepsia, gastritis, abdominal pain, allergic reactions, genital and anal pruritus, moniliasis, vaginitis, dizziness, fatigue, headache, superinfection (prolonged use).

INTERACTIONS: Probenecid inhibits excretion. Concomitant usage with metformin may require monitoring and dose adjustment.

PREGNANCY: Category B, caution in nursing.

PARLODEL RX
bromocriptine mesylate (Novartis)

THERAPEUTIC CLASS: Dopamine receptor agonist

INDICATIONS: Management of hyperprolactinemia including amenorrhea with or without galactorrhea, infertility, or hypogonadism. Treatment of prolactin-secreting adenomas, acromegaly, and symptoms of Parkinson's disease.

DOSAGE: *Adults:* Take with food. Parkinson's Disease: Initial: 1.25mg bid. Titrate: if needed, increase by 2.5mg/day every 2-4 weeks. Max: 100mg/day.
Hyperprolactinemia: Initial: 1.25mg-2.5mg qd. Titrate: If needed, increase by 2.5mg every 2-7 days. Usual: 2.5-15mg/day. Acromegaly: Initial: 1.25-2.5mg qhs for 3 days.

Titrate: Increase by 1.25-2.5mg every 3-7 days until optimal response. Usual: 20-30mg/day. Max: 100mg/day. Withdraw for 4-8 weeks every year in patients treated with pituitary irradiation.

Pediatrics: Take with food. 11-15 yrs: Prolactin-Secreting Pituitary Adenomas: Initial: 1.25-2.5mg/day. Titrate: Increase as tolerated. Usual: 2.5-10mg/day.

HOW SUPPLIED: Cap: 5mg; Tab: 2.5mg* *scored

CONTRAINDICATIONS: Uncontrolled HTN, ergot alkaloid sensitivity, postpartum with CVD unless withdrawal is medically contraindicated, pregnancy if treating hyperprolactinemia, HTN in pregnancy.

WARNINGS/PRECAUTIONS: Caution with renal or hepatic dysfunction, psychosis, CVD, peptic ulcer, dementia. Discontinue with macroadenomas associated with rapid regrowth of tumor and increased prolactin levels and if severe headache or HTN develops. Risk of pulmonary infiltrates, pleural effusion, thickening of pleura, and retroperitoneal fibrosis with long-term use. Not for prevention of physiological lactation. Monitor BP for symptomatic hypotension and HTN.

ADVERSE REACTIONS: Headache, dizziness, GI effects, orthostatic hypotension, fatigue, arrhythmia, insomnia, hallucinations, abnormal involuntary movements, depression, syncope.

INTERACTIONS: Decreased effects with dopamine antagonists (eg, butyrophenones, haloperidol, phenothiazines, pimozide, metoclopramide). Levodopa may cause hallucinations. Caution with antihypertensives. Alcohol may potentiate side effects. Not for use with other ergot alkaloids.

PREGNANCY: Category B, not for use in nursing.

PASER
aminosalicylic acid (Jacobus)

RX

THERAPEUTIC CLASS: Hydroxybenzoic acid derivative

INDICATIONS: Treatment of tuberculosis in combination with other agents.

DOSAGE: *Adults:* 4g tid. Sprinkle on apple sauce, yogurt, or mix with tomato or orange juice.

Pediatrics: Use correspondingly smaller doses to the adult dose.

HOW SUPPLIED: Packet: 4g

CONTRAINDICATIONS: Severe renal disease.

WARNINGS/PRECAUTIONS: Monitor for rash, or signs of intolerance during 1st 3 months. D/C if hypersensitivity occurs. Can desensitize by administering small, gradually increasing doses.

ADVERSE REACTIONS: Diarrhea, nausea, vomiting, abdominal pain, fever, dermatitis, lymphoma-like syndrome, agranulocytosis, thrombocytopenia, anemia, jaundice, hepatitis, hypoglycemia.

INTERACTIONS: Reduces acetylation of isoniazid, especially in rapid acetylators. Decreases vitamin B_{12} absorption; consider vitamin B_{12} maintenance treatment. Decreases digoxin levels.

PREGNANCY: Category C, safety in nursing not known.

PATANOL
olopatadine HCl (Alcon)

RX

THERAPEUTIC CLASS: H_1 antagonist and mast cell stabilizer

INDICATIONS: Allergic conjunctivitis.

DOSAGE: *Adults:* 1 drop bid, q6-8h.

Pediatrics: ≥3 yrs: 1 drop bid, q6-8h.

HOW SUPPLIED: Sol: 0.1% (5mL)

WARNINGS/PRECAUTIONS: May reinsert contact lens 10 minutes after dosing if eye is not red.

PCE

ADVERSE REACTIONS: Headache, asthenia, blurred vision, burning, stinging, cold syndrome, dry eye, foreign body sensation, hyperemia, hypersensitivity, keratitis, lid edema, nausea, pharyngitis, pruritus, rhinitis, sinusitis, taste perversion.

PREGNANCY: Category C, caution in nursing.

PCE
erythromycin (Abbott)

RX

THERAPEUTIC CLASS: Macrolide antibiotic

INDICATIONS: Mild to moderate upper and lower respiratory tract and skin and skin structure infections, listeriosis, pertussis, diphtheria, erythrasma, intestinal amebiasis, acute pelvic inflammatory disease (PID) (*N.gonorrhea*), primary syphilis in PCN allergy, Legionnaires' disease, chlamydial infections (eg, newborn conjunctivitis urethral, endocervical, or rectal, etc), and nongonococcal urethritis. Prophylaxis of rheumatic fever.

DOSAGE: *Adults:* Usual: 333mg q8h or 500mg q12h without food. Max: 4g/day. Do not take bid when dose is ≥1g/day. Treat strep infections for 10 days. Chlamydial Urogenital Infection During Pregnancy: 500mg qid or 666mg q8h for 7 days, or 500mg q12h, 333mg q8h or 250mg q6h for 14 days. Urethral/Endocervical/Rectal Chlamydial Infections and Nongonococcal Urethritis: 500mg qid or 666mg q8h for at least 7 days. Primary Syphilis: 30-40g in divided doses for 10-15 days. Acute PID: 500mg (erythromycin lactobionate) IV q6h for 3 days, then 500mg PO q12h or 333mg q8h for 7 days. Streptococcal Infection Long-Term Prophylaxis of Rheumatic Fever: 250mg bid. Intestinal Amebiasis: 500mg q12h, or 333mg q8h or 250mg q6h for 10-14 days. Pertussis: 40-50mg/kg/day in divided doses for 5-14 days. Legionnaires' Disease: 1-4g/day in divided doses.
Pediatrics: Usual: 30-50mg/kg/day in divided doses without food. Max: 4g/day. Severe Infections: Double dose up to 4g/day. Treat strep infections for 10 days. Chlamydial Conjunctivitis of Newborns and Chlamydial Pneumonia in Infancy: 12.5mg/kg qid for 2 weeks and 3 weeks, respectively. Intestinal Amebiasis: 30-50mg/kg/day in divided doses for 10-14 days. Long-Term Prophylaxis of Rheumatic Fever: 250mg bid. Pertussis: 40-50mg/kg/day in divided doses for 5-14 days. Legionnaires' Disease: 1-4g/day in divided doses.

HOW SUPPLIED: Tab, Extended Release: 333mg, 500mg

CONTRAINDICATIONS: Concomitant terfenadine, astemizole, cisapride, pimozide.

WARNINGS/PRECAUTIONS: Pseudomembranous colitis, hepatic dysfunction reported. May aggravate myasthenia gravis. Erythromycin does not reach adequate concentrations in fetus to prevent congenital syphilis.

ADVERSE REACTIONS: Nausea, vomiting, abdominal pain, diarrhea, anorexia, hepatic dysfunction, abnormal LFTs, allergic reactions, superinfection (prolonged use).

INTERACTIONS: Rhabdomyolysis reported with lovastatin. May increase levels of theophylline, digoxin, drugs metabolized by CYP450 (eg, carbamazepine, cyclosporine, phenytoin, alfentanil, disopyramide, lovastatin, bromocriptine, valproate, etc). Increases effects of oral anticoagulants, triazolam, midazolam. Risk of acute ergot toxicity with ergotamine or dihydroergotamine. May potentiate sildenafil. Avoid terfenadine, astemizole, cisapride, pimozide.

PREGNANCY: Category B, caution in nursing.

Pediapred
prednisolone sodium phosphate (Celltech)

RX

THERAPEUTIC CLASS: Glucocorticoid

INDICATIONS: Steroid responsive dermatoses.

DOSAGE: *Adults:* Initial: 5-60mg/day depending on disease and response. Maint: Decrease dose by small amounts to lowest effective dose. MS Exacerbations: 200mg qd for 1 week, then 80mg every other day for 1 month.
Pediatrics: Initial: 0.14-2mg/kg/day given tid-qid. Nephrotic Syndrome: 20mg/m^2 tid for 4 weeks, then 40mg/m^2 every other day for 4 weeks. Uncontrolled Asthma: 1-2mg/kg/day in single or divided doses peak expiratory rate of 80% is achieved (usually 3-10 days).

HOW SUPPLIED: Sol: 5mg/5mL (120mL)

CONTRAINDICATIONS: Systemic fungal infections.

WARNINGS/PRECAUTIONS: May produce reversible HPA axis suppression. Adjust dose during stress or change in thyroid status. May mask signs of infection or cause new infections. May activate latent amebiasis. Avoid with cerebral malaria. Avoid exposure to chickenpox or measles. Not for treatment of optic neuritis or active ocular herpes simplex. May cause elevation of BP or IOP, cataracts, glaucoma, optic nerve damage, Kaposi's sarcoma, psychic derangements, salt/water retention, increased excretion of potassium and/or calcium, osteoporosis, growth suppression in children, secondary ocular infections. Caution with Strongyloides, CHF, diverticulitis, HTN, renal insufficiency, fresh intestinal anastomoses, active or latent peptic ulcer, ulcerative colitis. Enhanced effect in hypothyroidism or cirrhosis. Avoid abrupt withdrawal. Use with caution in elderly, increased risk of corticosteroid-induced side effects; start at low end of dosing range; monitor bone mineral density.

ADVERSE REACTIONS: Edema, fluid/electrolyte disturbances, osteoporosis, muscle weakness, pancreatitis, peptic ulcer, impaired wound healing, increased intracranial pressure, cushingoid state, hirsutism, menstrual irregularities, growth suppression in children, glaucoma, nausea, weight gain.

INTERACTIONS: Enhanced metabolism with barbiturates, phenytoin, ephedrine, and rifampin. Use with cyclosporine may increase activity of both drugs; convulsions reported with concomitant use. Decreased metabolism with estrogens or ketoconazole. May inhibit response to warfarin. Increased risk of GI side effects with ASA or other NSAIDs. May increase clearance of salicylates. High doses or concurrent neuromuscular drugs may cause acute myopathy. Enhanced possibility of hypokalemia when given with potassium-depleting agents. May produce severe weakness in myasthenia gravis patients on anticholinesterase agents. Avoid live vaccines with immunosuppressive doses. Possible diminished response with killed or inactivated vaccines. May increase blood glucose; adjust antidiabetic agents. May suppress reactions to skin tests.

PREGNANCY: Category C, caution in nursing.

Pediarix   RX
tetanus toxoid - diphtheria toxoid - hepatitis B (recombinant) - pertussis vaccine, acellular - poliovirus vaccine, inactivated (GlaxoSmithKline)

THERAPEUTIC CLASS: Vaccine/toxoid combination

INDICATIONS: Active immunization against diphtheria, tetanus, pertussis, hepatitis B, and poliomyelitis (polioviruses Types 1, 2, and 3).

DOSAGE: *Pediatrics:* ≥6 weeks-up to 7 yrs: 3 doses of 0.5mL IM at 6-8 week intervals. Start at 2 months old or as early as 6 weeks old if necessary. May use to complete primary series in infants who have received 1 or 2 doses of Infanrix® or IPV or to complete a hepatitis B vaccine (Recombinant) series. Not recommended for completion of the first 3 doses of the DTaP vaccination series initiated with a DTaP vaccine from a different manufacturer.

HOW SUPPLIED: Inj: 0.5mL

CONTRAINDICATIONS: Hypersensitivity to yeast, neomycin, and polymyxin B. Anaphylaxis associated with previous dose or encephalopathy within 7 days of previous vaccine, progressive neurologic disorder (including infantile spasms, uncontrolled epilepsy, progressive encephalopathy).

WARNINGS/PRECAUTIONS: Higher rates of fever reported. Tip cap and plunger contains latex. Caution if within 48 hrs of previous whole-cell DTP or vaccine containing an acellular pertussis component, fever ≥105°F not due to another identifiable cause, collapse or shock-like state, or inconsolable crying lasting ≥3 hrs occurs, or if seizures occur within 3 days. Re-evaluate need if Guillain-Barre syndrome occurs within 6 weeks of receipt of tetanus toxoid-containing vaccine. Defer vaccination with moderate or severe illness, with or without fever. Administer antipyretic for initial 24 hours for those with higher risk for seizures. Caution with bleeding disorders (eg, hemophilia, thrombocytopenia). Have epinephrine available. Suboptimal response may occur in immunocompromised patients.

ADVERSE REACTIONS: Local injection-site reactions, fever, fussiness.

INTERACTIONS: Avoid with anticoagulants unless benefit outweighs risk. Immunosuppressive therapy (eg, irradiation, antimetabolites, alkylating agents, cytotoxic drugs, large doses of corticosteroids) may decrease response. Do not mix with other vaccines in same syringe/vial. Tetanus immune globulin or diphtheria antitoxin should be given at separate site with separate needle/syringe.

PREGNANCY: Category C, safety in nursing not known.

PEDIAZOLE RX
sulfisoxazole acetyl - erythromycin ethylsuccinate (Ross)

THERAPEUTIC CLASS: Macrolide antibiotic/sulfonamide

INDICATIONS: Acute otitis media caused by *H.influenzae*.

DOSAGE: *Pediatrics:* ≥2 months: Dose based on 50mg/kg/day erythromycin or 150mg/kg/day sulfisoxazole given tid-qid for 10 days. Max: 6g/day sulfisoxazole.

HOW SUPPLIED: Sus: (Erythromycin Ethylsuccinate-Sulfisoxazole Acetyl) 200mg-600mg/5mL (100mL, 150mL, 200mL)

CONTRAINDICATIONS: Pediatrics <2 months old, pregnant women at term, mothers nursing infants <2 months old, concomitant terfenadine.

WARNINGS/PRECAUTIONS: Pseudomembranous colitis, hepatic dysfunction reported. Severe, fatal allergic reactions reported with sulfonamides. Caution with hepatic or renal dysfunction, bronchial asthma, and severe allergies. May aggravate myasthenia gravis. Erythromycin does not reach adequate concentrations in fetus' to prevent congenital syphilis. Hemolysis may occur in G6P-deficiency patients. Sulfonamides not for treatment of group A beta-hemolytic infections.

ADVERSE REACTIONS: Nausea, vomiting, abdominal pain, diarrhea, anorexia, hepatic dysfunction, abnormal LFTs, allergic reactions, tachycardia, syncope, blood dyscrasias, BUN elevation, edema, superinfection.

INTERACTIONS: Rhabdomyolysis reported with lovastatin. May increase levels of theophylline, digoxin, methotrexate, drugs metabolized by CYP450 (eg, carbamazepine, cyclosporine, tacrolimus, phenytoin, alfentanil, disopyramide, lovastatin, bromocriptine, valproate, etc). Increases effects of oral anticoagulants, triazolam, midazolam, sulfonylureas. Risk of acute ergot toxicity with ergotamine or dihydroergotamine. Avoid terfenadine. May require less thiopental for anesthesia. May have cross-sensitivity with thiazides, acetazolamide, and oral hypoglycemics.

PREGNANCY: Category C, not for use in nursing.

PEDIOTIC RX
hydrocortisone - neomycin sulfate - polymyxin B sulfate (King)

THERAPEUTIC CLASS: Antibacterial/corticosteroid combination

INDICATIONS: Superficial bacterial infections of the external auditory canal. Infections of mastoidectomy and fenestration cavities.

DOSAGE: *Adults:* Clean and dry ear canal. Instill 4 drops tid-qid. Max: 10 days.
Pediatrics: Clean and dry ear canal. Instill 4 drops tid-qid. Max: 10 days.

HOW SUPPLIED: Sus: (Neomycin-Hydrocortisone-Polymyxin B) 0.35%-1%-10,000 U/mL (7.5mL)

CONTRAINDICATIONS: Herpes simplex, vaccinia, and varicella infections.

WARNINGS/PRECAUTIONS: Caution with perforated eardrum or chronic otitis media; ototoxicity may develop. Re-evaluate if no improvement after 10 days.

ADVERSE REACTIONS: Allergic sensitization, superinfection.

INTERACTIONS: Cross-reactivity with kanamycin, paromomycin, streptomycin, and gentamycin.

PREGNANCY: Category C, caution in nursing.

PENICILLIN VK
penicillin V potassium (Various)

RX

OTHER BRAND NAME: Veetids (Sandoz)

THERAPEUTIC CLASS: Acid-stable penicillin

INDICATIONS: Mild to moderately severe bacterial infections including conditions of the respiratory tract, oropharynx, skin and soft tissue. Prevention of recurrence following rheumatic fever and/or chorea.

DOSAGE: *Adults:* Usual: Streptococcal Infections (Scarlet Fever, Erysipelas, Upper Respiratory Tract): 125-250mg q6-8h for 10 days. Pneumococcal Infections (Otitis media, Respiratory Tract): 250-500mg q6h until afebrile for at least 2 days. Staphylococcus Infections (Skin/Soft Tissue): 250-500mg q6-8h. Fusospirochetosis Infections (Oropharnyx): 250-500mg q6-8h. Rheumatic Fever/Chorea Prevention: 125-250mg bid.

Pediatrics: ≥12 yrs: Usual: Streptococcal Infections (Scarlet fever, Erysipelas, Upper Respiratory Tract): 125-250mg q6-8h for 10 days. Pneumococcal Infections (Otitis media, Respiratory Tract): 250-500mg q6h until afebrile for at least 2 days. Staphylococcus Infections (Skin/Soft Tissue): 250-500mg q6-8h. Fusospirochetosis Infections (Oropharnyx): 250-500mg q6-8h. Rheumatic Fever/Chorea Prevention: 125-250mg bid.

HOW SUPPLIED: Sus: 125mg/5mL, 250mg/5mL (100mL, 200mL); Tab: 250mg, 500mg

WARNINGS/PRECAUTIONS: Not for severe pneumonia, empyema, bacteremia, pericarditis, meningitis and arthritis during the acute stage. Serious, fatal anaphylactic reactions reported. Pseudomembranous colitis reported. Oral administration may not be effective with severe illnesses, nausea, vomiting, gastric dilation, cardiospasm, intestinal hypermobility. Cross-sensitivity with cephalosporins. Caution with asthma and allergies.

ADVERSE REACTIONS: Nausea, vomiting, epigastric distress, diarrhea, hypersensitivity reactions, black hairy tongue, anaphylaxis, superinfection (prolonged use).

PREGNANCY: Category B, caution in nursing.

PEPCID
famotidine (Merck)

RX

OTHER BRAND NAME: Pepcid RPD (Merck)

THERAPEUTIC CLASS: H_2 blocker

INDICATIONS: (PO/Inj) Short term treatment of active duodenal ulcer (DU), active benign gastric ulcer (GU), gastroesophageal reflux disease (GERD) and esophagitis due to GERD. Maintenance therapy for DU. Treatment of hypersecretory conditions (eg, Zollinger-Ellison syndrome). (Inj) For hospitalized patients with hypersecretory conditions or intractable ulcers. As an alternative in patients unable to take oral forms.

DOSAGE: *Adults:* (PO) Acute DU: 40mg qhs or 20mg bid for 4-8 weeks. Maint DU: 20mg qhs. GU: 40mg qhs. GERD: 20mg bid up to 6 weeks. GERD with Esophagitis: 20-40mg bid up to 12 weeks. Hypersecretory Conditions: Initial: 20mg q6h. Max: 160mg q6h. (Inj) 20mg IV q12h, hypersecretory conditions may require higher doses. CrCl <50mL/min: Reduce to 1/2 dose, or increase interval to q36-48h.

Pediatrics: 1-16 yrs: (PO) DU/GU: Usual: 0.5mg/kg/day qhs or divided bid. Max: 40mg/day. GERD With or Without Esophagitis: 0.5mg/kg PO bid. Max: 40mg bid. (Inj) 0.25mg/kg IV q12h up to 40mg/day. Base duration of therapy on clinical response, and/or pH, and endoscopy. (PO) GERD: 3 months-1yr: 0.5mg/kg bid for up to 8 weeks. <3 months: 0.5mg/kg qd for up to 8 weeks. CrCl <50mL/min: Reduce to 1/2 dose, or increase interval to q36-48h.

HOW SUPPLIED: Inj: 0.4mg/mL, 10mg/mL; Sus: 40mg/5mL (50mL); Tab: 20mg, 40mg; Tab, Disintegrating: (RPD) 20mg, 40mg

CONTRAINDICATIONS: Hypersensitivity to other H_2 antagonists.

WARNINGS/PRECAUTIONS: CNS adverse effects reported with moderate to severe renal insufficiency; adjust dose. Disintegrating tabs contain phenylalanine; caution in phenylketonurics. Symptomatic response does not preclude the presence of gastric malignancy.

ADVERSE REACTIONS: Headache, dizziness, constipation, diarrhea.

Pepcid AC

INTERACTIONS: May give with antacids.
PREGNANCY: Category B, not for use in nursing.

Pepcid AC OTC
famotidine (J&J - Merck)

THERAPEUTIC CLASS: H_2 blocker
INDICATIONS: Relief and prevention of heartburn, acid indigestion, and sour stomach.
DOSAGE: *Adults:* Relief: 1 tab/cap prn. Max: 2 doses/24 hrs. Prevention: 1 tab/cap 15-60 minutes before food or beverages that cause heartburn. Max: 2 doses/24 hrs.
Pediatrics: ≥12yrs: 1 tab/cap prn. Max: 2 doses/24 hrs. Prevention: 1 tab/cap 15-60 minutes before food or beverages that cause heartburn. Max: 2 doses/24 hrs.
HOW SUPPLIED: Cap: 10mg; Tab: 10mg, 20mg; Tab, Chewable: 10mg
INTERACTIONS: Avoid with other acid reducers.

Pepcid Complete OTC
famotidine - calcium carbonate - magnesium hydroxide (J&J - Merck)

THERAPEUTIC CLASS: H_2 blocker/antacid
INDICATIONS: To relieve heartburn associated with acid indigestion and sour stomach.
DOSAGE: *Adults:* Chew 1 tab to relieve symptoms. Max: 2 tabs/24hrs.
Pediatrics: ≥12 yrs: Chew 1 tab to relieve symptoms. Max: 2 tabs/24hrs.
HOW SUPPLIED: Tab, Chewable: (Famotidine-Calcium Carbonate-Magnesium Hydroxide) 10mg-800mg-165mg
WARNINGS/PRECAUTIONS: Not for use in those with trouble swallowing. Avoid use if allergic to other acid reducers.
PREGNANCY: Safety in pregnancy and nursing not known.

Pepto-Bismol OTC
bismuth subsalicylate (Procter & Gamble)

OTHER BRAND NAME: Pepto-Bismol Maximum Strength (Procter & Gamble)
THERAPEUTIC CLASS: Antimicrobial
INDICATIONS: To control diarrhea within 24 hours, relieving associated abdominal cramps; soothes heartburn, and indigestion without constipation; and relieves nausea and upset stomach.
DOSAGE: *Adults:* (Sus) 30mL every 0.5-1 hr prn. Max: 8 doses/24hrs. (Sus, Max Strength) 30mL hourly prn. Max: 4 doses/24 hrs. (Tab; Tab, Chewable) 2 tabs every 0.5-1 hr prn. Max: 8 doses/24hrs. Drink plenty of clear fluids.
Pediatrics: (Sus) 9-12 yrs: 15mL every 0.5-1 hr prn. 6-9 yrs: 10mL every 0.5-1 hr prn. 3-6 yrs: 5mL every 0.5-1 hr. Max: 8 doses/24hrs. (Sus, Max Strength) 9-12 yrs: 15mL hourly prn. 6-9 yrs: 10mL hourly prn. 3-6 yrs: 5mL hourly prn. Max: 4 doses/24hrs. (Tab; Tab, Chewable) 9-12 yrs: 1 tab every 0.5-1 hr prn. 6-9 yrs: 2/3 tab every 0.5-1 hr prn. 3-6 yrs: 1/3 tab every 0.5-1 hr prn. Max: 8 doses/24 hrs. Drink plenty of clear fluids.
HOW SUPPLIED: Sus: 262mg/15mL; Sus, Maximum Strength: 525mg/15mL; Tab: 262mg; Tab, Chewable: 262mg
WARNINGS/PRECAUTIONS: Avoid in children and teenagers with or recovering from chickenpox or flu. Do not give with aspirin or non-aspirin salicylate allergy. May cause temporary darkening of tongue or stool. Product may contain small amounts of naturally occurring lead.
INTERACTIONS: May cause ringing in the ears with aspirin; discontinue if this occurs. Caution with anticoagulants, antidiabetic, and antigout agents.
PREGNANCY: Safety in pregnancy and nursing not known.

Peri-Colace OTC
senna - docusate sodium (Purdue Products)

THERAPEUTIC CLASS: Stool softener/laxative combination
INDICATIONS: Management of constipation.

DOSAGE: *Adults:* 2-4 tabs daily

Pediatrics: ≥12yrs: 2-4 tabs daily. 6-<12yrs: 1-2 tabs daily. 2-<6yrs: Max of 1 tab daily.

HOW SUPPLIED: (Docusate Sodium-Sennosides) Tab: 50mg-8.6mg

WARNINGS/PRECAUTIONS: Caution with use >1 week.

INTERACTIONS: Caution with mineral oil.

PREGNANCY: Safety in pregnancy and nursing not known.

PERMAPEN
penicillin G benzathine (Pfizer)

RX

THERAPEUTIC CLASS: Penicillin

INDICATIONS: Treatment of microorganisms susceptible to low and very prolonged serum levels in upper respiratory tract infections (streptococci group A - without bacteremia), syphilis, yaws, bejel, and pinta. Prophylaxis for rheumatic fever and/or chorea. Follow-up prophylactic therapy for rheumatic heart disease and acute glomerulonephritis.

DOSAGE: *Adults:* Streptococcal Infection: 1.2MU IM single dose. Primary/Secondary/Latent Syphilis: 1MU IM single dose. Late (Tertiary/Neurosyphilis) Syphilis: 3MU IM every 7 days for total of 6-9MU. Yaws/Bejel/Pinta: 1.2MU IM single dose. Rheumatic Fever/Glomerulonephritis Prophylaxis: 1.2MU IM once monthly or 600,000U IM twice monthly. Use upper outer quadrant of buttock. Rotate injection site.

Pediatrics: ≤12 yrs: Adjust dose according to age and weight and severity of infection. Streptococcal Infection: 900,000U IM single dose in older children. Congenital Syphilis: <2 yrs: 50,000U/kg IM single dose. 2-12 yrs: Adjust dose based on adult schedule. Use midlateral aspect of thigh in infants and small children. May divide dose between 2 buttocks in peds <2 yrs. Rotate injection site.

HOW SUPPLIED: Inj: 600,000U/mL

WARNINGS/PRECAUTIONS: Caution in newborns; evaluate organ system function frequently. Evaluate renal, hepatic and hematopoietic systems with prolonged therapy. Serious, fatal anaphylactic reactions reported; increased risk with hypersensitivity to penicillins, cephalosporins, and other allergens. Avoid IV, intra-arterial administration, or injection into/near major peripheral nerves or blood vessels may cause severe neurovascular damage. May result in overgrowth of nonsusceptible organisms. Avoid subcutaneous and fat-layer injections. Take culture after therapy completion to determine streptococci eradication.

ADVERSE REACTIONS: Skin eruptions, urticaria, laryngeal edema, anaphylaxis, fever, eosinophilia.

INTERACTIONS: Bacteriostatic agents (eg, tetracycline, erythromycin) may diminish effects. Prolonged levels with probenecid.

PREGNANCY: Category B, caution in nursing.

PERPHENAZINE
perphenazine (Various)

RX

THERAPEUTIC CLASS: Phenothiazine

INDICATIONS: Treatment of schizophrenia. To control severe nausea and vomiting.

DOSAGE: *Adults:* Moderately Disturbed Non-Hospitalized With Schizophrenia: Initial: 4-8mg tid. Maint: Reduce to minimum effective dose. Hospitalized Psychotic Patients With Schizophrenia: 8-16mg bid-qid. Max: 64mg/day. Severe Nausea/Vomiting: 8-16mg/day in divided doses. Max: 24mg/day. Elderly: Lower dosages recommended.

Pediatrics: ≥12 yrs: Use lowest limits of adult dose.

HOW SUPPLIED: Tab: 2mg, 4mg, 8mg, 16mg

CONTRAINDICATIONS: Comatose or greatly obtunded patients, large doses of CNS depressants (eg, barbiturates, alcohol, narcotics, analgesics, or antihistamines), blood dyscrasias, bone marrow depression, liver damage, subcortical brain damage with or without hypothalamic involvement.

PFIZERPEN

WARNINGS/PRECAUTIONS: Tardive dyskinesia may develop. NMS, photosensitivity reported. May lower convulsive threshold; caution with alcohol withdrawal. Caution with psychic depression, renal impairment, respiratory impairment. May impair mental/physical abilities. May mask signs of overdosage to other drugs. May obsure diagnosis of intestinal obstruction, brain tumor. Severe hypotension may occur in surgery. May elevate prolactin levels. Monitor hepatic/renal functions, blood counts. Increased risk of liver damage, jaundice, corneal and lenticular deposits, and irreversible dyskinesias with long-term use.

ADVERSE REACTIONS: Aching/numbness of the limbs, motor restlessness, cerebral edema, seizures, drowsiness, dry mouth, salivation, nausea, vomiting, diarrhea, lactation, postural hypotension, tachycardia.

INTERACTIONS: See Contraindications. Additive effects with CNS depressants and phenothiazine; use reduced amount of added drug. Additive anticholinergic effects with atropine/atropine-like drugs, exposure to phosphorous insecticide. Additive effects and hypotension may occur with alcohol. Cytochrome P450 2D6 inhibitors (TCAs, SSRIs) may increase levels; lower doses may be required.

PREGNANCY: Safety in pregnancy and nursing not known.

PFIZERPEN RX
penicillin G potassium (Pfizer)

THERAPEUTIC CLASS: Penicillin

INDICATIONS: For therapy of severe infections when rapid and high blood levels of penicillin required. Management of streptococcal, pneumococcal, staphylococcal, clostridial, fusospirochetal, listeria, and gram negative bacillary, and pasteurella infections. For anthrax, actinomycosis, diphtheria, erysipeloid, meningitis, endocarditis, bacteremia, rat-bite fever, syphilis, and gonorrheal endocarditis and arthritis. With combined oral therapy, prophylaxis against endocarditis in patients with congenital heart disease, rheumatic, or other acquired valvular heart disease undergoing dental procedures or surgical procedures of upper respiratory tract.

DOSAGE: *Adults:* Anthrax/Gonorrheal Endocarditis/Severe Infections (Streptococci, Pneumococci, Staphylococci): Minimum of 5MU/day. Syphilis: Administer in hospital. Determine dose and duration based on age and weight. Meningococcic Meningitis: 1-2MU IM q2h or 20-30MU/day continuous IV. Actinomycosis: 1-6MU/day for cervicofacial cases; 10-20MU/day for thoracic and abdominal disease. Clostridial Infections: 20MU/day (adjunct to antitoxin). Fusospirochetal Severe Infections: 5-10MU/day for oropharynx, lower respiratory tract, and genital area infection. Rat-bite Fever: 12-15MU/day for 3-4 weeks. Listeria Endocarditis: 15-20MU/day for 4 weeks. Pasteurella Bacteremia/Meningitis: 4-6MU/day for 2 weeks. Erysipeloid Endocarditis: 2-20MU/day for 4-6 weeks. Gram Negative Bacillary Bacteremia: 20-80MU/day. Diphtheria (carrier state): 0.3-0.4MU/day in divided doses for 10-12 days. Endocarditis Prophylaxis: 1MU IM mixed with 0.6MU procaine penicillin G 0.5-1 hr before procedure. Renal/Cardiac/Vascular Dysfunction: Consider dose reduction. For streptococcal infection, treat for minimum 10 days.

Pediatrics: Listeria Infections: Neonates: 0.5-1MU/day. Congenital Syphilis: Administer in hospital. Determine dose and duration based on age and weight. Endocarditis Prophylaxis: 30,000U/kg IM mixed with 0.6MU procaine penicillin G 0.5-1 hr before procedure. For streptococcal infection, treat for minimum 10 days.

HOW SUPPLIED: Inj: 1MU, 5MU, 20MU

WARNINGS/PRECAUTIONS: Serious, fatal anaphylactic reactions reported; increased risk with hypersensitivity to penicillins, cephalosporins, and other allergens. Avoid IV, intra-arterial administration, or injection into/near major peripheral nerves or blood vessels; may cause severe neurovascular damage. Take culture after therapy completion to determine streptococci eradication. Caution with history of significant allergies or asthma. May result in overgrowth of nonsusceptible organisms. Evaluate renal, hepatic and hematopoietic systems with prolonged therapy. Administer slowly to avoid electrolyte imbalance from potassium or sodium content; monitor electrolytes and consider dose reductions with renal, cardiac, or vascular dysfunction. Caution in newborns; evaluate organ system function frequently.

ADVERSE REACTIONS: Skin rash (eg, maculopapular eruption, exfoliative dermatitis) urticaria, chills, fever, edema, arthralgia, prostration, anaphylaxis, arrhythmias, cardiac arrest, Jarisch-Herxheimer reaction.

INTERACTIONS: Bacteriostatic agents (eg, tetracycline, erythromycin) may diminish effects. Prolonged levels with probenecid.

PREGNANCY: Category B, caution in nursing.

Phenergan Injection   RX
promethazine HCl (Baxter)

THERAPEUTIC CLASS: Phenothiazine derivative

INDICATIONS: For blood or plasma allergic reactions, allergic reactions where oral therapy is not possible, sedation, and special surgical situations (eg, repeated bronchoscopy). Adjunct for anaphylactic reactions and postoperative pain. Treatment of motion sickness. Prevention and control of nausea and vomiting in surgery.

DOSAGE: *Adults:* (IM/IV) IM is preferred. Allergy: Initial: 25mg, may repeat within 2 hrs. Sedation: 25-50mg qhs. Nausea/Vomiting: 12.5-25mg q4h. Preoperative/Postoperative: 25-50mg. Obstetrics: 50mg in early labor, 25-75mg in established labor, may repeat once or twice q4h. Max: 100mg/24 hrs of labor. Do not give IV administration >25mg/mL and at a rate >25mg/minute.

Pediatrics: ≥2 yrs: Dose should not exceed half of adult dose. Premedication: Usual: 0.5mg/lb. Do not give IV administration >25mg/mL and at a rate >25mg/minute.

HOW SUPPLIED: Inj: 25mg/mL, 50mg/mL

CONTRAINDICATIONS: Comatose states, intra-arterial or subcutaneous injection. Hypersensitivity to other phenothiazines.

WARNINGS/PRECAUTIONS: Caution in patients ≥2 yrs. Not recommended for uncomplicated vomiting in pediatrics. May cause marked drowsiness; caution with operating machinery. Fatal respiratory depression reported; avoid with respiratory dysfunction (eg, COPD, sleep apnea). Avoid prolonged sun exposure. May lower seizure threshold. Caution with bone marrow depression. NMS reported. Caution in acutely ill pediatric patients. Avoid in pediatrics with Reye's syndrome or hepatic disease. Avoid perivascular extravasation or inadvertent intra-arterial injection. Caution with narrow-angle glaucoma, prostatic hypertrophy, stenosing peptic ulcer, bladder-neck or pyloroduodenal obstruction, cardiovascular disease, hepatic dysfunction. Cholestatic jaundice reported. Alters HCG pregnancy test reading. May increase blood glucose.

ADVERSE REACTIONS: Drowsiness, dizziness, tinnitus, blurred vision, dry mouth, increased or decreased blood pressure, urticaria, nausea, vomiting, blood dyscrasia.

INTERACTIONS: Added sedative effects with CNS depressants (eg, alcohol, narcotics, narcotic analgesics, sedatives, hypnotics, general anesthetics, tranquilizers, TCAs); reduce dose or eliminate these agents. Reduce barbiturate dose by one-half and analgesic depressant dose by one-quarter to one-half. Caution with drugs that alter seizure threshold (eg, narcotics, local anesthetics). Do not use epinephrine for promethazine injection overdose. Caution with anticholinergics. Possible adverse reactions with MAOIs.

PREGNANCY: Category C, caution in nursing.

Phenobarbital   CIV
phenobarbital (Various)

THERAPEUTIC CLASS: Barbiturate

INDICATIONS: Treatment of generalized, tonic-clonic and cortical focal seizures. For relief of anxiety, tension and apprehension. Short-term treatment of insomnia.

DOSAGE: *Adults:* Sedation: 30-120mg/day given bid-tid. Max: 400mg/24h. Hypnotic: 100-200mg. Seizures: 60-200mg/day. Elderly/Debilitated/Renal or Hepatic Dysfunction: Reduce dosage.

Pediatrics: Seizures: 3-6mg/kg/day.

HOW SUPPLIED: Elixir: 20mg/5mL; Tab: 15mg, 30mg, 32.4mg, 60mg, 64.8mg, 100mg

PHENYTEK

CONTRAINDICATIONS: Respiratory disease with dyspnea or obstruction, porphyria, severe liver dysfunction. Large doses with nephritic patients.

WARNINGS/PRECAUTIONS: May be habit forming. Avoid abrupt withdrawal. Caution with acute or chronic pain; may mask symptoms or paradoxical excitement may occur. Cognitive deficits reported in children with febrile seizures. May cause excitement in children and excitement, depression or confusion in elderly, debilitated. Caution with hepatic dysfunction, borderline hypoadrenal function, depression.

ADVERSE REACTIONS: Drowsiness, residual sedation, lethargy, vertigo, somnolence, respiratory depression, hypersensitivity reactions, nausea, vomiting, headache.

INTERACTIONS: May be potentiated by MAOIs, antihistamines, alcohol, tranquilizers, sedative/hypnotics, other CNS depressants. Decreases effects of oral anticoagulants. Increases corticosteroid metabolism. Decreases effects of oral contraceptives. Decreases absorption of griseofulvin. Decreases half-life of doxycycline. May alter phenytoin metabolism. Increased levels with sodium valproate and valproic acid.

PREGNANCY: Category D, caution in nursing.

PHENYTEK
phenytoin sodium (Mylan Bertek)

RX

THERAPEUTIC CLASS: Hydantoin

INDICATIONS: Control of generalized tonic-clonic (grand mal) and complex partial (psychomotor, temporal lobe) seizures. Prevention and treatment of neurosurgically induced seizures.

DOSAGE: *Adults:* No Previous Treatment: Initial: 100mg extended phenytoin sodium capsule tid. Titrate: May increase at 7-10 day intervals. Usual: 100mg tid-qid. May increase up to 200mg Phenytek tid. Once Daily Dosing: 300mg Phenytek qd may replace 100mg extended phenytoin sodium capsule tid if seizures are controlled. LD (clinic/hospital): 1g in 3 divided doses (400mg, 300mg, 300mg) given 2 hrs apart. Start maintenance 24 hrs later. Avoid LD with renal and hepatic disease.

Pediatrics: Initial: 5mg/kg/day given bid-tid. Titrate: May increase at 7-10 day intervals. Maint: 4-8mg/kg/day. Max: 300mg/day. >6 yrs: May require the minimum adult dose (300mg/day).

HOW SUPPLIED: Cap, Extended Release: 200mg, 300mg

WARNINGS/PRECAUTIONS: Avoid abrupt discontinuation. Caution with porphyria, hepatic dysfunction, elderly, diabetes, debilitated. Discontinue if rash occurs. Lymphadenopathy reported. Serum sickness may occur with lymph node involvement. Gingival hyperplasia reported; maintain proper dental hygiene. Hyperglycemia, birth defects and osteomalacia reported. Monitor levels. Confusional states reported with toxic levels. Increased seizure frequency during pregnancy. Neonatal coagulation defects reported within first 24 hrs of birth; give Vitamin K to mother before delivery and to neonate after birth. Avoid use with seizures due to hypoglycemia or other metabolic causes.

ADVERSE REACTIONS: Nystagmus, ataxia, slurred speech, decreased coordination, confusion, dizziness, insomnia, transient nervousness, motor twitchings, headaches, nausea, vomiting, constipation, rash, hypersensitivity reactions.

INTERACTIONS: Increased levels with acute alcohol intake, amiodarone, chloramphenicol, chlordiazepoxide, diazepam, dicumarol, disulfiram, estrogens, H_2-antagonists, halothane, isoniazid, methylphenidate, phenothiazines, phenylbutazone, salicylates, succinamides, sulfonamides, tolbutamide, trazodone. Decreased levels with chronic alcohol abuse, carbamazepine, reserpine, sucralfate. Decreases effects of corticosteroids, coumarin anticoagulants, digitoxin, doxycycline, estrogens, furosemide, oral contraceptives, quinidine, rifampin, theophylline, vitamin D. Phenobarbital, sodium valproate, valproic acid may increase or decrease levels. May increase or decrease levels of phenobarbital, sodium valproate, valproic acid. Calcium antacids decrease absorption; space dosing. Moban® contains calcium ions which interfere with absorption. TCAs may precipitate seizures. Increased risk of phenytoin hypersensitivity with barbiturates, succinamides, oxazolidinediones.

PREGNANCY: Possibly teratogenic, weigh benefits versus risk; not for use in nursing.

pHisoHex
hexachlorophene (Sanofi-Aventis)

RX

THERAPEUTIC CLASS: Detergent cleanser

INDICATIONS: As a surgical scrub and a bacteriostatic skin cleanser. Also to control outbreak of gram-positive infection, when other infection control methods failed.

DOSAGE: *Adults:* Surgical Scrub: Apply 5mL with water and lather over hands and forearms. Scrub well with a wet brush for 3 minutes, including nails and interdigital spaces. Rinse thoroughly then repeat. Bacteriostatic Cleansing: Apply 5mL with water and lather, apply to areas that need cleansing. Rinse thoroughly.
Pediatrics: Bacteriostatic Cleansing: Apply 5mL with water and lather, apply to areas that need cleansing. Rinse thoroughly. Do not use routinely for bathing infants.

HOW SUPPLIED: Liq: 3% (150mL, 480mL, 3840mL)

CONTRAINDICATIONS: Burned/denuded skin. Should not use as wet pack, vaginal pack, tampon, occlusive dressing, lotion, on mucous membranes, or as a routine prophylactic bath. Light sensitivity to halogenated phenol derivatives.

WARNINGS/PRECAUTIONS: D/C promptly if cerebral irritability occurs. Infants are more susceptible to CNS toxicity. Avoid skin lesions; may cause toxic blood levels. Do not apply to burns; may cause neurotoxicity and death. Avoid eye contact.

ADVERSE REACTIONS: Dermatitis, photosensitivity, redness, mild scaling, dryness.

INTERACTIONS: Skin products containing alcohol may decrease efficacy.

PREGNANCY: Category C, not for use in nursing.

Phospholine Iodide
echothiophate iodide (Wyeth)

RX

THERAPEUTIC CLASS: Cholinesterase inhibitor

INDICATIONS: Treatment of glaucoma and accommodative esotropias.

DOSAGE: *Adults:* Early Chronic Simple Glaucoma: (0.3%) 1 drop bid, am and hs. Advanced Chronic Simple Glaucoma/Glaucoma Secondary to Cataract Surgery: Initial: (0.3%) 1 drop bid, am and hs. Titrate: Increase to higher strengths as needed.
Pediatrics: Accommodative Esotropia: Diagnosis: (0.125%) 1 drop qhs for 2-3 weeks. Treatment: Decrease dose to 1 drop (0.125%) every other day or (0.6%) 1 drop qd. Titrate: Decrease strength gradually. Max: (0.125%) 1 drop qd.

HOW SUPPLIED: Sol: 0.125% (5mL)

CONTRAINDICATIONS: Active uveal inflammation, angle-closure glaucoma.

WARNINGS/PRECAUTIONS: Avoid with quiescent uveitis. Should hold nose for 1-2 minutes to prevent absorption. Discontinue with cardiac irregularities, salivation, urinary incontinence, diarrhea, profuse sweating, muscle weakness, or respiratory difficulties. Caution with vagotonia, bronchial asthma, spastic GI disturbance, peptic ulcer, bradycardia, hypotension, recent MI, epilepsy, parkinsonism, retinal detachment. Tolerance may develop.

ADVERSE REACTIONS: Stinging, burning, lacrimation, lid muscle twitching, conjunctival and ciliary redness, browache, induced myopia, visual blurring.

INTERACTIONS: Risk of respiratory or cardiovascular collapse with succinylcholine during general anesthesia. Potentiates effects of other cholinesterase inhibitors (eg, succinylcholine, organophosphate, carbamate insecticides, myasthenia gravis drugs).

PREGNANCY: Category C, not for use in nursing.

Phrenilin Forte
butalbital - acetaminophen (Amarin)

RX

OTHER BRAND NAME: Phrenilin (Amarin)
THERAPEUTIC CLASS: Barbiturate/analgesic
INDICATIONS: Tension or muscle contraction headaches.

PHYTONADIONE

DOSAGE: *Adults:* (Phrenilin Forte) 1 cap q4h. (Phrenilin) 1-2 tabs q4h. Max: 6 caps/tabs/day.

Pediatrics: ≥12 yrs: (Phrenilin Forte) 1 cap q4h. (Phrenilin) 1-2 tabs q4h. Max: 6 caps/tabs/day.

HOW SUPPLIED: (Butalbital-APAP) Cap: (Phrenilin Forte) 50mg-650mg; Tab: (Phrenilin)50mg-325mg.

CONTRAINDICATIONS: Porphyria.

WARNINGS/PRECAUTIONS: Abuse potential. Caution in elderly/debilitated, severe renal/hepatic impairment, and acute abdominal conditions.

ADVERSE REACTIONS: Drowsiness, lightheadedness, dizziness, sedation, shortness of breath, nausea, vomiting, abdominal pain, intoxicated feeling.

INTERACTIONS: Enhanced CNS effects with MAOIs. May enhance CNS depression effects of narcotic analgesics, alcohol, general anesthetics, tranquilizers (eg, chlordiazepoxide, sedative hypnotics, CNS depressants).

PREGNANCY: Category C, not for use in nursing.

PHYTONADIONE RX
phytonadione (Various)

> Severe, fatal reactions reported during or immediately after IV or IM use. Only use IV or IM route when SC route is not feasible.

THERAPEUTIC CLASS: Vitamin K derivative

INDICATIONS: For coagulation disorders caused by vitamin K deficiency or interference with vitamin K activity, including prophylaxis and therapy of hemorrhagic disease of the newborn; anticoagulant-induced prothrombin deficiency caused by coumarin or indanedione derivatives; and hypoprothrombinemia caused by antibacterials, secondary factors that limit absorption or synthesis of vitamin K (obstructive jaundice, biliary fistula), or by drugs that interfere with vitamin K metabolism (eg, salicylates).

DOSAGE: *Adults:* Administer SQ when possible. Anticoagulant-Induced PT Deficiency: Initial: 2.5-10mg up to 25mg (rarely 50mg). May repeat if PT is still elevated 6-8 hrs after initial dose. Hypoprothrombinemia Due to Other Causes: 2.5-25mg or more (rarely up to 50mg); route depends on severity of condition and response.

Pediatrics: Prophylaxis of Hemorrhagic Disease in Newborn: 0.5-1mg IM within 1 hr of birth. Treatment of Hemorrhagic Disease in Newborn: 1mg SQ/IM (may need higher dose if mother has received oral anticoagulants).

HOW SUPPLIED: Inj: 1mg/0.5 mL, 10mg/mL

WARNINGS/PRECAUTIONS: Contains benzyl alcohol; toxicity in newborns may occur. Takes 1-2 hrs to observe improvement in PT. Maintain lowest possible dose to prevent original thromboembolic events. Avoid repeated large doses with hepatic disease. Failure to respond may indicate a congenital coagulation defect or a condition unresponsive to vitamin K. Monitor PT regularly.

ADVERSE REACTIONS: Anaphylactoid reactions, flushing, peculiar taste sensations, dizziness, rapid and weak pulse, profuse sweating, hypotension, dyspnea, cyanosis, injection site tenderness or swelling, hyperbilirubinemia (in newborns).

INTERACTIONS: Does not counteract anticoagulant effects of heparin. Temporary resistance to prothrombin-depressing anticoagulants, especially with large doses.

PREGNANCY: Category C, caution in nursing.

PIPERACILLIN RX
piperacillin sodium (Various)

THERAPEUTIC CLASS: Broad-spectrum penicillin

INDICATIONS: Treatment of serious intra-abdominal, urinary tract, gynecologic, lower respiratory tract, skin and skin structure, bone and joint, and gonococcal infections, septicemia, and perioperative surgical prophylaxis.

DOSAGE: *Adults:* Usual: 3-4g IM/IV q4-6h. Max: 24g/day; IM: 2g/site. Serious Infections: 200-300mg/kg/day IV divided q4-6h. Complicated UTI: 125-200mg/kg/day IV divided q6-8h. Uncomplicated UTI/Community Acquired Pneumonia: 100-125mg/kg/day IM/IV divided q6-12h. Uncomplicated Gonorrhea: 2g IM single dose with 1g PO probenecid 1/2 hr before injection. Surgical Prophylaxis: 2g IV 20-30 minute just prior to anesthesia (See labeling for follow-up dosing). C-section: 2g IV after cord is clamped, then 2g 4 hrs and 8 hrs after 1st dose. Renal Impairment: Uncomplicated/Complicated UTI: CrCl <20mL/min: 3g q12h. Complicated UTI: CrCl 20-40mL/min: 3g q8h. Serious Infection: CrCl 20-40mL/min: 4g q8h. CrCl <20mL/min: 4g q12h. Hemodialysis: Give 1g additional dose after each dialysis. Max: 2g q8h. Usual treatment is for 7-10 days; treat gynecologic infections for 3-10 days; treat *S.pyogenes* infections for at least 10 days.

Pediatrics: ≥12 yrs: Usual: 3-4g IM/IV q4-6h. Max: 24g/day; IM: 2g/site. Serious Infections: 200-300mg/kg/day IV divided q4-6h. Complicated UTI: 125-200mg/kg/day IV divided q6-8h. Uncomplicated UTI/Community Acquired Pneumonia: 100-125mg/kg/day IM/IV divided q6-12h. Uncomplicated Gonorrhea: 2g IM single dose with 1g PO probenecid 1/2 hr before injection. Surgical Prophylaxis: 2g IV 20-30 minute just prior to anesthesia (See labeling for follow-up dosing). C-section: 2g IV after cord is clamped, then 2g 4 hrs and 8 hrs after 1st dose. Renal Impairment: Uncomplicated/Complicated UTI: CrCl <20mL/min: 3g q12h. Complicated UTI: CrCl 20-40mL/min: 3g q8h. Serious Infection: CrCl 20-40mL/min: 4g q8h. CrCl <20mL/min: 4g q12h. Hemodialysis: Give 1g additional dose after each dialysis. Max: 2g q8h. Usual treatment is for 7-10 days; treat gynecologic infections for 3-10 days; treat *S.pyogenes* infections for at least 10 days.

HOW SUPPLIED: Inj: 2g, 3g, 4g

CONTRAINDICATIONS: Hypersensitivity to cephalosporins.

WARNINGS/PRECAUTIONS: Serious hypersensitivity reactions reported; increased risk with sensitivity to multiple allergens. Cross sensitivity to cephalosporins. Monitor renal, hepatic and hematopoietic functions with prolonged use. D/C if bleeding manifestations occur; increased risk with renal failure. Prolonged use may cause superinfections. May experience neuromuscular excitability or convulsions with higher than recommended doses. Contains 1.85mEq/g sodium; caution with salt restriction. Monitor electrolytes periodically with low potassium levels. May mask symptoms of syphilis. Increased incidence of rash and fever in cystic fibrosis. Continue treatment for at least 48-72 hrs after patient becomes asymptomatic.

ADVERSE REACTIONS: Thrombophlebitis, erythema and pain at injection site, diarrhea, headache, dizziness, anaphylaxis, rash, superinfections.

INTERACTIONS: Do not mix with aminoglycoside in a syringe or infusion bottle; may cause inactivation of aminoglycoside. May prolong neuromuscular blockade of nondepolarizing muscle relaxants (eg, vecuronium). Increased risk of hypokalemia with cytotoxic therapy or diuretics. May reduce methotrexate clearance. Probenecid may increase levels. Monitor coagulation parameters closely with concomitant anticoagulants.

PREGNANCY: Category B, caution in nursing.

PLAQUENIL
hydroxychloroquine sulfate (Sanofi-Aventis)

RX

Be familiar with complete prescribing information before prescribing hydroxychloroquine.

THERAPEUTIC CLASS: Quinine derivative

INDICATIONS: Suppression and treatment of acute attacks of malaria in adults and children. Treatment of discoid and systemic lupus erythematosus and rheumatoid arthritis (RA) in adults.

DOSAGE: *Adults:* Malaria Suppression: 400mg weekly. Begin 2 weeks before exposure and continue for 8 weeks after leaving endemic area. Give 400mg q6h for 2 doses if therapy is not begun before exposure. Acute Attack: 800mg, then 400mg 6-8 hrs later, then 400mg for 2 more days. RA: Initial: 400-600mg qd with food or milk; increase until optimum response. Maint: After 4-12 weeks, 200-400mg qd with food or milk. Lupus Erythematosus: Initial: 400mg qd-bid for several weeks depending on response. Maint: 200-400mg/day.

PLEXION

Pediatrics: Malaria Suppression: 5mg/kg (base) weekly, max 400mg/dose. Begin 2 weeks before exposure and continue for 8 weeks after leaving endemic area. q6h for 2 doses if therapy is not begun before exposure. Acute Attack: 10mg base/kg, max 800mg/dose; then 5mg base/kg, max 400mg/dose at 6, 24 and 48 hrs after 1st dose.

HOW SUPPLIED: Tab: 200mg (200mg tab=155mg base)

CONTRAINDICATIONS: Long term therapy in children or if retinal/visual field changes due to 4-aminoquinoline compounds.

WARNINGS/PRECAUTIONS: Caution with hepatic disease, G6PD deficiency, alcoholism, psoriasis, and porphyria. Perform baseline and periodic (3 months) ophthalmologic exams and blood cell counts with prolonged therapy. Test periodically for muscle weakness. Discontinue if blood disorders occur. Avoid if possible in pregnancy. Discontinue after 6 months if no improvement in rheumatoid arthritis.

ADVERSE REACTIONS: Headache, dizziness, diarrhea, loss of appetite, muscle weakness, nausea, abdominal cramps, bleaching of hair, dermatitis, ocular toxicity, visual field defects.

INTERACTIONS: Caution with hepatotoxic drugs.

PREGNANCY: Safety in pregnancy and nursing not known.

PLEXION RX
sulfur - sulfacetamide sodium (Medicis)

OTHER BRAND NAMES: Plexion TS (Medicis) - Plexion SCT (Medicis)

THERAPEUTIC CLASS: Sulfonamide/sulfur combination

INDICATIONS: Topical treatment of acne vulgaris, acne rosacea, and seborrheic dermatitis.

DOSAGE: *Adults:* (Cleanser) Wash qd-bid. Massage into skin for 10-20 seconds, then rinse and dry. (TS) Apply qd-tid. (Cre) Apply to wet skin. Rinse off with water after 10 minutes or if dry.

Pediatrics: ≥12 yrs: (Cleanser) Wash qd-bid. Massage into skin for 10-20 seconds, then rinse and dry. (TS) Apply qd-tid. (Cre) Apply to wet skin. Rinse off with water after 10 minutes or if dry.

HOW SUPPLIED: Cleanser: (Sulfacetamide-Sulfur) 10%-5% (170.3g, 340.2g); Cre: (SCT) 10%-5% (120g); Lot: (TS) 10%-5% (30g); Pads: 10%-5% (30's)

CONTRAINDICATIONS: Kidney disease.

WARNINGS/PRECAUTIONS: D/C if irritation occurs. Avoid eye contact or mucous membranes. Caution with denuded or abraded skin, patients prone to topical sulfonamide hypersensitivity. Can cause reddening and scaling of epidermis.

ADVERSE REACTIONS: Local irritation.

PREGNANCY: Category C, caution in nursing.

PNEUMOVAX 23 RX
pneumococcal vaccine (Merck)

THERAPEUTIC CLASS: Vaccine

INDICATIONS: Immunization against pneumococcal disease caused by those pneumococcal types included in the vaccine.

DOSAGE: *Adults:* Usual: 0.5mL SQ/IM in deltoid muscle or lateral mid-thigh.

Pediatrics: ≥2 yrs: 0.5mL SQ/IM in deltoid muscle or lateral mid-thigh.

HOW SUPPLIED: Inj: 575mcg/0.5mL

WARNINGS/PRECAUTIONS: Vaccination timing is critical for chemotherapy or immunosuppressive therapy. Suboptimal response may occur in immunocompromised patients. Caution with severely compromised cardiovascular or pulmonary function where systemic reaction would be a significant risk. Delay vaccine with febrile respiratory illness or other active infection. Do not revaccinate immunocompetent patients. Continue prophylaxis pneumococcal antibiotics. May not prevent pneumococcal meningitis with chronic CSF leakage.

ADVERSE REACTIONS: Local injection site reactions (eg, soreness, warmth, erythema, swelling, induration), fever (≤102°F).

PREGNANCY: Category C, caution use in nursing.

POLYTRIM
polymyxin B sulfate - trimethoprim sulfate (Allergan)

RX

THERAPEUTIC CLASS: Dihydrofolate reductase inhibitor/antibiotic

INDICATIONS: Surface ocular bacterial infections, including blepharoconjunctivitis, acute bacterial conjunctivitis.

DOSAGE: *Adults:* Mild-Moderate Infections: 1 drop q3h for 7-10 days. Max: 6 doses/day.
Pediatrics: ≥2 months: Mild-Moderate Infections: 1 drop q3h for 7-10 days. Max: 6 doses/day.

HOW SUPPLIED: Sol: (Trimethoprim-Polymyxin B) 1mg-10,000U/mL (10mL)

WARNINGS/PRECAUTIONS: Not indicated for the prophylaxis or treatment of ophthalmia neonatorum.

ADVERSE REACTIONS: Local irritation, lid edema, itching, increased redness, tearing, burning, stinging, circumocular rash, superinfection (prolonged use).

PREGNANCY: Category C, caution in nursing.

POLY-VI-FLOR
sodium fluoride - multiple vitamin (Mead Johnson)

RX

THERAPEUTIC CLASS: Multiple vitamin/fluoride supplement

INDICATIONS: Vitamin supplement. Fluoride supplement for caries prophylaxis in areas where water contains less than optimal fluoride levels.

DOSAGE: *Pediatrics:* (Sol) 6 months-3 yrs and <0.3 ppm Fluoride or 3-6 yrs and 0.3-0.6 ppm Fluoride: 1mL (0.25mg) qd. 3-6 yrs and <0.3 ppm Fluoride or >6 yrs and 0.3-0.6 ppm Fluoride: 1mL (0.5mg) qd. (Tab) 4-6 yrs and 0.3-0.6 ppm Fluoride: 0.25mg qd. 4-6 yrs and <0.3 ppm Fluoride or ≥6 yrs and 0.3-0.6 ppm Fluoride: 0.5mg qd. 6-16 yrs and <0.3 ppm Fluoride: 1mg qd.

HOW SUPPLIED: Sol: Vitamin A 1500 IU-Vitamin C 35mg-Vitamin D 400 IU-Vitamin E 5 IU-Thiamin 0.5mg-Riboflavin 0.6mg-Niacin 8mg-Vitamin B_6 0.4mg-Vitamin B_{12} 2mcg. 0.25mg drops contains 0.25mg Fluoride (50mL), 0.5mg drops contain 0.5mg Fluoride (50mL); Tab, Chewable: Vitamin A 2500 IU-Vitamin C 60mg-Vitamin D 400 IU-Vitamin E 15 IU-Thiamin 1.05mg-Riboflavin 1.2mg-Niacin 13.5mg-Vitamin B_6 1.05mg-Folate 0.3mg-Vitamin B_{12} 4.5mcg. 0.25mg tabs contain 0.25mg Fluoride; 0.5mg tabs contain 0.5mg Fluoride; 1mg tabs contain 1mg Fluoride

WARNINGS/PRECAUTIONS: Must chew tab; not for pediatrics <4yrs. Risk of dental fluorosis from ingestion of large amounts of fluoride. Children up to 16 yrs, in areas where water contains less than optimal fluoride levels, should receive daily fluoride supplementation.

ADVERSE REACTIONS: Allergic rash.

PREGNANCY: Safety in pregnancy and nursing not known.

PONSTEL
mefenamic acid (Sciele)

RX

> NSAIDs may cause an increased risk of serious cardiovascular thrombotic events, MI, stroke and serious GI adverse events including bleeding, ulceration, and perforation of the stomach or intestines. Contraindicated for the treatment of peri-operative pain in the setting of coronary artery bypass graft (CABG) surgery.

THERAPEUTIC CLASS: NSAID (fenamate derivative)

INDICATIONS: Relief of mild to moderate pain in patients ≥14 yrs, when therapy will not exceed 7 days. Treatment of primary dysmenorrhea.

POTABA

DOSAGE: *Adults:* Acute Pain: Usual: 500mg, then 250mg q6h prn up to 1 week. Primary Dysmenorrhea: Usual: 500mg, then 250mg q6h up to 3 days. Take with food.

Pediatrics: ≥14 yrs: Acute Pain: Usual: 500mg, then 250mg q6h prn, up to 1 week. Primary Dysmenorrhea: Usual: 500mg, then 250mg q6h up to 3 days. Take with food.

HOW SUPPLIED: Cap: 250mg

CONTRAINDICATIONS: Pre-existing renal disease, active ulceration or chronic inflammation of the GI tract. Allergic-type reactions, including asthma and urticaria, after taking ASA or other NSAIDs. Treatment of peri-operative pain in the setting of CABG surgery.

WARNINGS/PRECAUTIONS: May lead to onset of new HTN or worsening of pre-existing HTN; monitor BP closely. Fluid retention and edema reported; caution with fluid retention or heart failure. Renal papillary necrosis and other renal injury reported after long-term use. Not recommended for use with advanced renal disease. Anaphylactoid reactions may occur. May cause serious skin adverse events (eg, exfoliative dermatitis, Stevens-Johnson syndrome, and toxic epidermal necrolysis). Avoid in late pregnancy; may cause premature closure of ductus arteriosis. May cause elevations of LFTs; d/c if liver disease develops or systemic manifestations occur. Caution in elderly. Anemia may occur; with long-term use, monitor Hgb/Hct if signs or symptoms of anemia develop. May inhibit platelet aggregation and prolong bleeding time; monitor with coagulation disorders. Caution with asthma and avoid with aspirin-sensitive asthma.

ADVERSE REACTIONS: Abdominal pain, constipation, diarrhea, dyspepsia, flatulence, gross bleeding/perforation, heartburn, nausea, GI ulcers, vomiting, abnormal renal function, anemia, dizziness, edema, elevated liver enzymes, headache, increased bleeding time, pruritus, rash, tinnitus.

INTERACTIONS: ASA may increase adverse effects; avoid use. Warfarin may increase GI bleeding. May prolong PT with oral anticoagulants. May enhance methotrexate toxicity. Decrease effects of ACE inhibitors, furosemide and thiazides; monitor for renal toxicity. Increase in lithium levels. Magnesium hydroxide may increase mefenamic acid levels. Caution with CYP2C9 inhibitors including fluconazole, lovastatin and trimethoprim.

PREGNANCY: Category C, not for use in nursing.

POTABA RX
potassium p-aminobenzoate (Glenwood)

THERAPEUTIC CLASS: Vitamin B complex

INDICATIONS: Possibly effective for the treatment of Peyronie's disease, dermatomyositis, linear scleroderma, pemphigus.

DOSAGE: *Adults:* Usual: 12g/day, in 4 to 6 divided doses. Take with meals or snacks. Tabs should be taken with plenty of liquid. Dissolve powder in water or juice.

Pediatrics: 1g/day for each 10 lbs of body weight given in divided doses. Dissolve powder in water or juice. Take with food and plenty of liquid.

HOW SUPPLIED: Cap: 0.5g; Pow: 2g/envule (50^s); Tab: 0.5g

CONTRAINDICATIONS: Concomitant sulfonamides.

WARNINGS/PRECAUTIONS: Suspend therapy if anorexia, nausea, occurs. D/C if hypersensitivity reaction develops. Caution with renal disease.

ADVERSE REACTIONS: Anorexia, nausea, fever, rash.

PREGNANCY: Safety in pregnancy or nursing not known.

PRAMOSONE RX
pramoxine HCl - hydrocortisone acetate (Ferndale)

THERAPEUTIC CLASS: Corticosteroid/anesthetic

INDICATIONS: Relief of the inflammatory and pruritic manifestations of corticosteroid-responsive dermatoses.

DOSAGE: *Adults:* Apply tid-qid. May use occlusive dressings for psoriasis or recalcitrant conditions. D/C dressings if infection develops.

Pediatrics: Apply tid-qid. May use occlusive dressings for psoriasis or recalcitrant conditions. D/C dressings if infection develops.

HOW SUPPLIED: (Pramoxine-Hydrocortisone) Cre: 1%-1%, 1%-2.5% (30g, 60g); Lot: 1%-1% (60mL, 120mL, 240mL), 1%-2.5% (60mL, 120mL); Oint: 1%-1%, 1%-2.5% (30g)

WARNINGS/PRECAUTIONS: May produce reversible HPA axis suppression, manifestations of Cushing's syndrome, hyperglycemia, and glucosuria. Caution when applied to large surface areas or under occlusive dressings. Use appropriate antifungal or antibacterial agent with dermatological infections; d/c if infection does not clear. Peds may be more susceptible to systemic toxicity. Avoid eyes. D/C if irritation occurs.

ADVERSE REACTIONS: Burning, itching, irritation, dryness, folliculitis, hypertrichosis, acneiform eruptions, hypopigmentation, perioral dermatitis, allergic dermatitis, skin maceration, secondary infection, skin atrophy, striae, miliaria.

PREGNANCY: Category C, caution in nursing.

PRAVACHOL
pravastatin sodium (Bristol-Myers Squibb)

RX

THERAPEUTIC CLASS: HMG-CoA reductase inhibitor

INDICATIONS: As adjunct to diet, to reduce elevated total-C, LDL-C, Apo B, TG levels, and to increase HDL-C in primary hypercholesterolemia and mixed dyslipidemia (Type IIa and IIb). Treatment of primary dysbetalipoproteinemia (Type III) and heterozygous familial hypercholesterolemia. To reduce elevated serum TG levels (Type IV). In hypercholesterolemic patients without coronary heart disease, to reduce risk of: MI, undergoing myocardial revascularization procedures, and cardiovascular mortality with no increase in death from non-cardiovascular causes. In patients with coronary heart disease, to reduce risk of: mortality by reducing coronary death, undergoing myocardial revascularization procedures, MI, stroke, and TIA; and to slow progression of coronary atherosclerosis.

DOSAGE: *Adults:* ≥18 yrs: Initial: 40mg qd. Perform lipid tests within 4 weeks and adjust according to response and guidelines. Titrate: May increase to 80mg qd if needed. Significant Renal/Hepatic Dysfunction: Initial: 10mg qd. Concomitant Immunosuppressives (eg, Cyclosporine): Initial: 10mg qhs. Max: 20mg/day.
Pediatrics: Heterozygous Familial Hypercholesterolemia: 14-18 yrs: Initial: 40mg qd. 8-13 yrs: Initial: 20mg qd. Concomitant Immunosuppressives (eg, Cyclosporine): Initial: 10mg qhs. Max: 20mg/day.

HOW SUPPLIED: Tab: 10mg, 20mg, 40mg, 80mg

CONTRAINDICATIONS: Active liver disease, unexplained persistent elevations of LFTs, pregnancy, nursing mothers.

WARNINGS/PRECAUTIONS: Perform LFTs before therapy, before dose increases, and if clinically indicated. Risk of myopathy, myalgia, and rhabdomyolysis. D/C if AST or ALT ≥3X ULN persists, if elevated CPK levels occur, or if myopathy diagnosed or suspected. Less effective with homozygous familial hypercholesterolemia. Monitor for endocrine dysfunction. Closely monitor with heavy alcohol use, recent history or signs of hepatic disease, or renal dysfunction.

ADVERSE REACTIONS: Rash, nausea, vomiting, diarrhea, headache, chest pain, influenza, abdominal pain, dizziness, increases ALT, AST, CPK.

INTERACTIONS: Risk of myopathy with fibrates, niacin, cyclosporine, erythromycin. Increased levels with gemfibrozil, itraconazole. Avoid fibrates unless benefit outweighs drug combination risk. Decreased levels with concomitant cholestyramine/colestipol; take 1 hr before or 4 hrs after resins. Caution with drugs that diminish levels or activity of steroid hormones (eg, ketoconazole, spironolactone, cimetidine).

PREGNANCY: Category X, not for use in nursing.

PREDNISONE
prednisone (Roxane)

RX

OTHER BRAND NAME: Deltasone (Pharmacia & Upjohn)
THERAPEUTIC CLASS: Glucocorticoid

PREGNYL

INDICATIONS: Steroid responsive disorders.

DOSAGE: *Adults:* Initial: 5-60mg/day depending on disease and response. Maint: Decrease dose by small amounts to lowest effective dose.
Pediatrics: Initial: 5-60mg/day depending on disease and response. Maint: Decrease dose by small amounts to lowest effective dose.

HOW SUPPLIED: Sol: 5mg/mL, 5mg/5mL; Tab: 1mg, 2.5mg*, 5mg*, 10mg*, 20mg*, 50mg* *scored

CONTRAINDICATIONS: Systemic fungal infections.

WARNINGS/PRECAUTIONS: May need to increase dose before, during, and after stressful situations. May mask signs of infection or cause new infections. Prolonged use may produce glaucoma, optic nerve damage, secondary ocular infections. Increases BP, salt/water retention, potassium excretion. More severe/fatal course of infections reported with chickenpox, measles. Caution with latent TB, hypothyroidism, cirrhosis, ocular herpes simplex, HTN, diverticulitis, fresh intestinal anastomosis, ulcerative colitis, osteoporosis, myasthenia gravis, renal insufficiency, peptic ulcer disease. Growth and development of children on prolonged therapy should be monitored. Monitor for psychic disturbances. Avoid abrupt withdrawal.

ADVERSE REACTIONS: Fluid and electrolyte disturbances, HTN, osteoporosis, muscle weakness, cushingoid state, menstrual irregularities, nervousness, insomnia, impaired wound healing, DM, ulcerative esophagitis, excessive sweating, increases intracranial pressure, carbohydrate intolerance, glaucoma, cataracts, weight gain, nausea, malaise.

INTERACTIONS: Increases clearance of high dose ASA; caution in hypoprothrombinemia. Increased insulin and oral hypoglycemic requirements in DM. Avoid small pox vaccine, and live vaccines with immunosuppressive doses. Possible decreased vaccine response with killed or inactivated vaccines with immunosuppressive doses. Increased clearance with hepatic enzyme inducers. Decreased metabolism with troleandomycin, ketoconazole. Variable effect on oral anticoagulants.

PREGNANCY: Safety in pregnancy and nursing not known.

PREGNYL   RX
chorionic gonadotropin (Organon)

THERAPEUTIC CLASS: Human chorionic gonadotropin

INDICATIONS: For prepubertal cryptorchidism not due to anatomic obstruction. For hypogonadotropic hypogonadism (secondary to a pituitary deficiency) in males. To induce ovulation (OI) and pregnancy in anovulatory, infertile women in whom anovulation is not due to primary ovarian failure and pretreated with human menotropins.

DOSAGE: *Adults:* Hypogonadism: 500-1000 U IM 3x/week (TIW) for 3 weeks, then twice weekly for 3 weeks; or 4000 U IM TIW for 6-9 months, then reduce to 2000 U TIW for 3 months. OI: 5000-10,000 U IM 1 day after last dose of menotropins.
Pediatrics: Cryptorchidism: 4000 U IM TIW for 3 weeks; or 5000 U IM every 2nd day for 4 doses; or 15 doses of 500-1000 U over 6 weeks; or 500 U TIW for 4-6 weeks (if treatment fails, give 1000 U/injection starting 1 month later). Initiate therapy between 4-9 yrs. Hypogonadism: 500-1000 U IM TIW for 3 weeks, then twice weekly for 3 weeks; or 4000 U IM TIW for 6-9 months, then reduce to 2000 U TIW for 3 months.

HOW SUPPLIED: Inj: 10,000 U

CONTRAINDICATIONS: Precocious puberty, prostatic carcinoma or other androgen-dependent neoplasms, pregnancy.

WARNINGS/PRECAUTIONS: Potential ovarian hyperstimulation, enlargement or rupture of ovarian cysts, multiple births, and arterial thromboembolism with infertility treatment. D/C if precocious puberty occurs in cryptorchidism patients. Caution with cardiac or renal disease, epilepsy, migraine, asthma. Not effective treatment for obesity.

ADVERSE REACTIONS: Headache, irritability, restlessness, depression, fatigue, edema, precocious puberty, gynecomastia, injection site pain.

PREGNANCY: Safety in pregnancy and nursing not known.

PRELONE   RX
prednisolone (Muro)

THERAPEUTIC CLASS: Glucocorticoid
INDICATIONS: Treatment of steroid responsive disorders.

DOSAGE: *Adults:* Initial: 5-60mg/day depending on disease and response. Maint: Decrease dose by small amounts to lowest effective dose.

Pediatrics: Initial: 5-60mg/day depending on disease and response. Maint: Decrease dose by small amounts to lowest effective dose.

HOW SUPPLIED: Syrup: 5mg/5mL (120mL), 15mg/5mL (240mL, 480mL)

CONTRAINDICATIONS: Systemic fungal infections.

WARNINGS/PRECAUTIONS: Adjust dose during stress or change in thyroid status. May mask signs of infection or or cause new infections. Prolonged use may produce glaucoma, optic nerve damage, secondary ocular infections. Increases BP, salt/water retention, potassium excretion. Avoid exposure to chickenpox, measles. Caution with latent TB, hypothyroidism, cirrhosis, ocular herpes simplex, HTN, diverticulitis, fresh intestinal anastomosis, ulcerative colitis, osteoporosis, myasthenia gravis, renal insufficiency, peptic ulcer disease. Growth and development of children on prolonged therapy should be monitored. Monitor for psychic disturbances. Avoid abrupt withdrawal.

ADVERSE REACTIONS: Fluid and electrolyte disturbances, osteoporosis, muscle weakness, cushingoid state, menstrual irregularities, nervousness, insomnia, impaired wound healing, excessive sweating, carbohydrate intolerance, glaucoma, cataracts, weight gain, nausea, malaise.

INTERACTIONS: Avoid ASA with hypoprothrombinemia. May increase blood glucose; adjust antidiabetic agents. Avoid smallpox vaccination, and live vaccines with immunosuppressive doses. Possible decreased vaccine response with killed or inactivated vaccines with immunosuppressive doses.

PREGNANCY: Safety in pregnancy and nursing not known.

PREVACID
lansoprazole (TAP)

RX

OTHER BRAND NAMES: Prevacid IV (TAP) - Prevacid Solutab (TAP)

THERAPEUTIC CLASS: Proton pump inhibitor

INDICATIONS: (PO) Treatment of active duodenal ulcer (DU), active benign gastric ulcer (GU), erosive esophagitis, symptomatic GERD. Maintain healing of erosive esophagitis and duodenal ulcers. Treatment of pathological hypersecretory conditions (eg, Zollinger-Ellison syndrome). Combination therapy with amoxicillin +/- clarithromycin for *H.pylori* eradication in duodenal ulcer disease, to reduce risk of ulcer recurrence. Treatment and risk reduction in NSAID induced gastric ulcer. (Inj) Short-term treatment of erosive esophagitis.

DOSAGE: *Adults:* >17 yrs: (PO) DU: 15mg qd for 4 weeks. Maint: 15mg qd. GU: 30mg qd up to 8 weeks. GERD: 15mg qd up to 8 weeks. Erosive Esophagitis: 30mg qd up to 8 weeks. May repeat for 8 weeks if needed. Maint: 15mg qd. NSAID Induced GU: 30mg qd for 8 weeks. Reduce Risk of NSAID Induced GU: 15mg qd for 12 weeks. Hypersecretory Conditions: Initial: 60mg qd, then adjust. Max: 90mg bid. Divide dose if >120mg/day. *H.pylori:* Triple Therapy: 30mg + clarithromycin 500mg + amoxicillin 1000mg, all bid (q12h) for 10-14 days. Dual Therapy: 30mg + amoxicillin 1000mg both tid (q8h) for 14 days. Take before eating. Caps: Swallow whole or sprinkle cap contents on 1 tbsp of applesauce, ENSURE® pudding, cottage cheese, yogurt, strained pears, or in 60mL orange juice or tomato juice; swallow immediately. Sus: Do not chew or crush. Mix packet with 30mL of water; stir well and drink immediately; not for use with NG tube. Solutab: Place on tongue with or without water. Oral Syringe: (SoluTab) Place 15mg tab in oral syringe and draw up 4mL of water, or 30mg tab in oral syringe and draw up 10mL of water. Shake contents and administer after tablet has dispersed within 15 mins. Refill syringe with 2mL (5mL for 30mg tab) of water, shake, and give any remaining contents. NG Tube: (Cap) Mix cap contents with 40mL apple juice and inject into NG tube; flush with additional juice to clear tube. (SoluTab) Place 15mg tab and draw up 4mL of water, or 30mg tab and draw up 10mL of water. Shake contents and after tablet has dispersed, inject through NG tube into stomach within 15 mins. Refill syringe with 5mL of water, shake, and flush NG tube. (Inj) Erosive Esophagitis: 30mg IV qd over 30 mins for 7 days. May switch to PO formulation for total of 6 to 8 weeks of therapy once patient is able to take oral medications. Severe Hepatic Impairment: Adjust dose.

PreviDent

Pediatrics: 12-17 yrs: Short-Term Symptomatic GERD: 15mg qd for up to 8 weeks. Erosive Esophagitis: 30mg qd for up to 8 weeks. 1-11 yrs: Short-Term Symptomatic GERD/Erosive Esophagitis: ≤30kg: 15mg qd for up to 12 weeks. >30kg: 30mg qd for up to 12 weeks. Titrate: May increase up to 30mg bid after 2 weeks if symptomatic. Severe Hepatic Impairment: Adjust dose. Take before eating. Caps: Swallow whole or sprinkle contents on 1 tbsp of applesauce, ENSURE® pudding, cottage cheese, yogurt, strained pears, or in 60mL orange juice or tomato juice; swallow immediately. Sus: Do not chew or crush. Mix packet with 30mL water; stir well and drink immediately; not for use with NG tube. Solutab: Place on tongue with or without water. Oral Syringe: (SoluTab) Place 15mg tab in oral syringe and draw up 4mL of water, or 30mg tab in oral syringe and draw up 10mL of water. Shake contents and administer after tablet has dispersed within 15 mins. Refill syringe with 2mL (5mL for 30mg tab) of water, shake, and give any remaining contents. NG Tube: (Cap) Mix cap contents with 40mL apple juice and inject into NG tube; flush with additional juice to clear tube. (SoluTab) Place 15mg tab and draw up 4mL of water, or 30mg tab and draw up 10mL of water. Shake contents and after tablet has dispersed, inject through NG tube into stomach within 15 mins. Refill syringe with 5mL of water, shake, and flush NG tube.

HOW SUPPLIED: Cap, Delayed Release: 15mg, 30mg; Inj: 30mg; Sus, Delayed Release: 15mg, 30mg (granules/packet); Tab, Disintegrating (SoluTab): 15mg, 30mg.

WARNINGS/PRECAUTIONS: Symptomatic response does not preclude the presence of gastric malignancy. Adjust dose with hepatic impairment.

ADVERSE REACTIONS: Abdominal pain, constipation, diarrhea, nausea.

INTERACTIONS: May alter absorption of pH-dependent drugs (eg, ketoconazole, ampicillin esters, digoxin, and iron salts). Give at least 30 minutes prior to sucralfate. Theophylline may need dose adjustment. Concomitant use with warfarin may increase INR and prothrombin time.

PREGNANCY: Category B, not for use in nursing.

PreviDent
sodium fluoride (Colgate Oral)

RX

OTHER BRAND NAME: PreviDent 5000 Plus (Colgate Oral)

THERAPEUTIC CLASS: Fluoride preparation

INDICATIONS: Prevention of dental caries.

DOSAGE: *Adults:* Apply thin ribbon to teeth with toothbrush or mouth tray qhs for at least 1 minute with the gel and 2 minutes with the cream after regular brushing. Expectorate after use. Do not eat, drink or rinse for 30 minutes.
Pediatrics: 6-16 yrs: Apply thin ribbon to teeth with toothbrush or mouth tray qhs for at least 1 minute with the gel and 2 minutes with the cream after regular brushing. Expectorate and rinse mouth thoroughly after use.

HOW SUPPLIED: Gel: (PreviDent) 1.1%; Cre: (PreviDent 5000 Plus) 1.1%

CONTRAINDICATIONS: Not for children <6 years of age, unless recommended by dentist or physician.

WARNINGS/PRECAUTIONS: Prolonged ingestion may lead to dental fluorosis in children <6 years of age. Not for systemic treatment. Do not swallow.

ADVERSE REACTIONS: Allergic reactions.

PREGNANCY: Category B, caution in nursing.

Priftin
rifapentine (Sanofi-Aventis)

RX

THERAPEUTIC CLASS: Rifamycin derivative

INDICATIONS: Treatment of pulmonary tuberculosis. Do not use alone, as initial or retreatment.

DOSAGE: *Adults:* Intensive Phase: Initial: 600mg twice weekly with an interval of not <3 days (72 hrs) between doses. Continue for 2 months. Maint: 600mg once weekly for 4 months. Elderly: Start at low end of dosing range.

Pediatrics: ≥12 yrs: Intensive Phase: Initial: 600mg twice weekly with an interval of not <3 days (72 hrs) between doses. Continue for 2 months. Maint: 600mg once weekly for 4 months.

HOW SUPPLIED: Tab: 150mg

WARNINGS/PRECAUTIONS: Give with pyridoxine in the malnourished, if predisposed to neuropathy (eg, alcoholics, diabetics), and adolescents. Caution with hepatic impairment; monitor LFTs before and every 2-4 weeks during therapy. May cause postnatal hemorrhages in mother and infant during last weeks of pregnancy; monitor clotting parameters; may need vitamin K. May produce a red-orange discoloration of body tissues, fluids. May stain/discolor contact lenses, breast milk or dentures. Pseudomembranous colitis reported. Avoid with porphyria. Caution in elderly.

ADVERSE REACTIONS: Hyperuricemia, increased ALT/AST, neutropenia, pyuria, proteinuria, lymphopenia, urinary casts, rash, pruritus, acne, anorexia, anemia.

INTERACTIONS: Antagonizes drugs metabolized by CYP3A4, CYP2C8, and CYP2C9 due to enzyme induction (eg, anticonvulsants, antiarrhythmics, oral anticoagulants, antibiotics, antifungals, barbiturates, benzodiazepines, β-blockers, calcium channel blockers, corticosteroids, cardiac glycosides, clofibrate, hormonal contraceptives, oral hypoglycemics, haloperidol, immunosuppressants, levothyroxine, narcotic analgesics, progestins, quinine, reverse transcriptase inhibitors, sildenafil, theophylline, TCAs). Increases indinavir metabolism; extreme caution with protease inhibitors. Avoid hormonal contraceptives. Consider hepatotoxic effects of other antituberculosis drug therapy (eg, isoniazid, pyrazinamide).

PREGNANCY: Category C, not for use in nursing.

PRILOSEC

RX

omeprazole (AstraZeneca LP)

THERAPEUTIC CLASS: Proton pump inhibitor

INDICATIONS: Active duodenal ulcer, active benign gastric ulcer, erosive esophagitis, symptomatic GERD. Maintain healing of erosive esophagitis. Long-term treatment of pathological hypersecretory conditions (eg, Zollinger-Ellison syndrome). Combination therapy with clarithromycin +/- amoxicillin for H.pylori eradication in duodenal ulcer disease, and to reduce risk of ulcer recurrence.

DOSAGE: *Adults:* Duodenal Ulcer: 20mg qd for 4-8 weeks. Gastric Ulcer: 40mg qd for 4-8 weeks. GERD: 20mg qd up to 4 weeks without esophageal lesions and 4-8 weeks with erosive esophagitis. Treatment Erosive Esophagitis with GERD: 20mg qd for 4-8 weeks. Maint: 20mg qd. Hypersecretory Conditions: Initial: 60mg qd, then adjust if needed. Divide dose if >80mg/day. Doses up to 120mg tid have been given. H.pylori Triple Therapy: 20mg + clarithromycin 500mg + amoxicillin 1g, all bid for 10 days. Give additional 18 days of omeprazole 20mg every morning if ulcer present initially. Dual Therapy: 40mg qd + clarithromycin 500mg tid for 14 days. Give additional 14 days of omeprazole 20mg every morning if ulcer present initially. Do not crush or chew. Take before eating. Can add contents of caps to applesauce if difficulty swallowing; swallow immediately without chewing.

Pediatrics: ≥2 yrs: GERD/Erosive Esophagitis: >20kg: 20mg qd. <20kg: 10mg qd. Do not crush or chew. Take before eating. Can add contents of caps to applesauce if difficulty swallowing; swallow immediately without chewing.

HOW SUPPLIED: Cap, Delayed Release: 10mg, 20mg, 40mg;

WARNINGS/PRECAUTIONS: Atrophic gastritis reported with long-term use. Symptomatic response does not preclude the presence of gastric malignancy.

ADVERSE REACTIONS: Headache, diarrhea, abdominal pain, asthenia, nausea, vomiting.

INTERACTIONS: May potentiate diazepam, warfarin, phenytoin and drugs metabolized by oxidation. May alter absorption of pH-dependent drugs (eg, ketoconazole, ampicillin esters, and iron salts). Monitor drugs metabolized by CYP450 (eg, cyclosporine, disulfiram, benzodiazepines). Increased levels with clarithromycin. Increases levels of clarithromycin.

PREGNANCY: Category C, not for use in nursing.

PRIMAXIN I.M.
imipenem - cilastatin (Merck)

RX

THERAPEUTIC CLASS: Thienamycin/dehydropeptidase I inhibitor

INDICATIONS: Treatment of lower respiratory tract (LRTI), skin and skin structure (SSSI), intra-abdominal, and gynecologic infections caused by susceptible strains of microorganisms. Not for severe or life-threatening infections.

DOSAGE: *Adults:* Dose according to imipenem. Mild to Moderate LRTI/SSSI/Gynecologic Infection: 500mg or 750mg IM q12h depending on severity. Intra-Abdominal Infection: 750mg IM q12h. Continue for at least 2 days after symptoms resolve. Elderly: Start at low end of dosing range. Continue for at least 2 days after symptoms resolve; do not treat >14 days. Max: 1500mg/day. Avoid if CrCl <20mL/min.

Pediatrics: ≥12 yrs: Dose according to imipenem. Mild to Moderate LRTI/SSSI/Gynecologic Infection: 500mg or 750mg IM q12h depending on severity. Intra-abdominal Infection: 750mg IM q12h. Continue for at least 2 days after symptoms resolve; do not treat >14 days. Max: 1500mg/day. Avoid if CrCl <20mL/min.

HOW SUPPLIED: Inj: (Imipenem-Cilastatin) 500mg-500mg, 750-750

CONTRAINDICATIONS: Severe shock, heart block, hypersensitivity to local anesthetics of amide type (due to lidocaine diluent).

WARNINGS/PRECAUTIONS: Serious, fatal hypersensitivity reactions reported. Increased incidence of reactions with previous hypersensitivity to cephalosporins, penicillins, other β-lactams, and other allergens. Pseudomembranous colitis reported. Prolonged use may result in overgrowth of non-susceptible organisms. Avoid injection into blood vessel. Caution in elderly. CNS adverse events (eg, myoclonic activity, confusion, seizures) reported most commonly with CNS disorders and renal dysfunction; d/c if these occur.

ADVERSE REACTIONS: Injection site pain, nausea, diarrhea, fever, vomiting, rash, hypotension, seizures, dizziness, pruritus, urticaria, somnolence.

INTERACTIONS: Avoid probenecid. Do not mix or physically add with other antibiotics. May give concomitantly with other antibiotics.

PREGNANCY: Category C, caution in nursing.

PRIMAXIN I.V.
imipenem - cilastatin (Merck)

RX

THERAPEUTIC CLASS: Thienamycin/dehydropeptidase I inhibitor

INDICATIONS: Treatment of serious lower respiratory tract, urinary tract (UTI), intra-abdominal, gynecologic, skin and skin structure, bone and joint, septicemia, endocarditis, and polymicrobic infections caused by susceptible strains of microorganisms..

DOSAGE: *Adults:* ≥70kg and CrCl >70mL/min: Dose based on imipenem component. Uncomplicated UTI: 250mg q6h. Complicated UTI: 500mg q6h. Mild Infection: 250-500mg q6h. Moderate Infection: 500mg q6-8h or 1g q8h. Severe, Life Threatening Infection: 500mg-1g q6h or 1g q8h. Max dose: 50mg/kg/day or 4g/day, whichever is lower. Renal Impairment and/or <70kg: Refer to prescribing information. CrCl 6-20mL/min: 125-250mg q12h. CrCl ≤5mL/min: Administer hemodialysis within 48 hrs of dose.

Pediatrics: ≥3 months: Dose based on imipenem component. Non-CNS Infections: 15-25mg/kg q6h. Max: 2g/day if susceptible or 4g/day if moderately susceptible. May use up to 90mg/kg/day in older cystic fibrosis children. 4 weeks-3 months and ≥1500g: 25mg/kg q6h. 1-4 weeks and ≥1500g: 25mg/kg q8h. <1 week and ≥1500g: 25mg/kg q12h. Not recommended with CNS infection, and <30kg with impaired renal function.

HOW SUPPLIED: Inj: (Imipenem-Cilastatin) 250mg-250mg, 500mg-500mg

WARNINGS/PRECAUTIONS: Serious, fatal hypersensitivity reactions reported. Increased incidence of reactions with previous hypersensitivity to cephalosporins, penicillins, other β-lactams, and other allergens. Pseudomembranous colitis reported. Prolonged use may result in overgrowth of non-susceptible organisms. CNS adverse events (eg, myoclonic activity, confusion, seizures) reported most commonly with CNS disorders and renal dysfunction.

ADVERSE REACTIONS: Phlebitis/thrombophlebitis, nausea, diarrhea, vomiting, rash, fever, hypotension, seizures, dizziness, pruritus, urticaria, somnolence, hepatitis (including fulminant hepatitis), hepatic Failure.

INTERACTIONS: Seizures reported with ganciclovir; avoid concomitant use. Avoid probenecid. Do not mix or physically add to other antibiotics. May give concomitantly with other antibiotics.

PREGNANCY: Category C, caution in nursing.

Primsol
trimethoprim HCl (FSC Laboratories)

RX

THERAPEUTIC CLASS: Tetrahydrofolic acid inhibitor

INDICATIONS: Treatment of acute otitis media in pediatrics and urinary tract infection (UTI) in adults.

DOSAGE: *Adults:* UTI: Usual: 100mg q12h or 200mg q24h for 10 days. CrCl: 15-30mL/min: Give 50% of usual dose.
Pediatrics: Otitis Media: ≥6 months: 5mg/kg q12h for 10 days. CrCl: 15-30mL/min: Give 50% of usual dose.

HOW SUPPLIED: Sol: 50mg/5mL

CONTRAINDICATIONS: Megaloblastic anemia due to folate deficiency.

WARNINGS/PRECAUTIONS: May interfere with hematopoiesis. Serious blood disorders; monitor for sore throat, fever, pallor, and purpura. Caution with folate deficiency and renal/hepatic impairment, diarrhea, rash.

ADVERSE REACTIONS: Epigastric distress, nausea, vomiting, anemia, methemoglobinemia, hyperkalemia, hyponatremia, fever, elevation of serum transaminases and bilirubin, increases BUN and serum creatinine.

INTERACTIONS: May inhibit phenytoin metabolism.

PREGNANCY: Category C, caution in nursing.

ProAir HFA
albuterol sulfate (Ivax)

RX

THERAPEUTIC CLASS: Beta$_2$ agonist

INDICATIONS: Prevention and treatment of bronchospasm with reversible obstructive airway disease; prevention of exercise-induced bronchospasm (EIB) in patients ≥12 yrs.

DOSAGE: *Adults:* Bronchospasm or Asthmatic Symptoms: 2 inh q4-6h or 1 inh q4h. EIB: 2 inh 15-30 min before activity.
Pediatrics: ≥12 yrs: Bronchospasm or Asthmatic Symptoms: 2 inh q4-6h or 1 inh q4h. EIB: 2 inh 15-30 min before activity.

HOW SUPPLIED: MDI: 90mcg/inh (8.5g)

WARNINGS/PRECAUTIONS: Hypersensitivity reactions reported. Monitor for worsening asthma. Fatalities reported with excessive use. Caution with cardiovascular disorders, especially coronary insufficiency, arrhythmias and HTN. May need concomitant corticosteroids. Can produce paradoxical bronschospasm. Caution with DM, hyperthyroidism, and seizures. May cause transient hypokalemia.

ADVERSE REACTIONS: Pharyngitis, headache, rhinitis, dizziness, pain, tachycardia, tremor, nervousness.

INTERACTIONS: Avoid other sympathomimetic agents. Extreme caution with MAOIs and TCAs, and β-blockers. Monitor digoxin. May worsen ECG changes and/or hypokalemia with nonpotassium-sparing diuretics.

PREGNANCY: Category C, not for use in nursing.

Probenecid
probenecid (Various)

RX

THERAPEUTIC CLASS: Uricosuric

INDICATIONS: Treatment of hyperuricemia associated with gout and gouty arthritis. Adjunct to penicillin, ampicillin, methicillin, oxacillin, cloxacillin, or nafcillin for elevation and prolongation of plasma levels.

PROCRIT

DOSAGE: *Adults:* Gout: Initial: 250mg bid for 1 week. Titrate: May increase by 500mg every 4 weeks. Maint: 500mg bid. Max: 2g/day. May reduce by 500mg every 6 months if acute attack has been absent ≥6 months and serum urate levels are normal. Renal Impairment: Usual: 1g/day. Adjunct Antibiotic Therapy: 500mg qid. Elderly/Renal Impairment: Reduce dose. Decrease dose with gastric intolerance. May not be effective if CrCl ≤30mL/min.
Pediatrics: 2-14 yrs: Adjunct Antibiotic Therapy: Initial: 25mg/kg. Maint: 10mg/kg qid. ≥50kg: 500mg qid.

HOW SUPPLIED: Tab: 500mg

CONTRAINDICATIONS: Blood dyscrasias, uric acid kidney stones and children <2 yrs. Do not use in acute gout attack.

WARNINGS/PRECAUTIONS: Initiate therapy when acute gout attack subsides. Exacerbation of gout may occur; treat with colchicine. Use APAP if analgesic needed. Severe allergic reactions and anaphylaxis reported. D/C if hypersensitivity occurs. Caution with peptic ulcer. Monitor for glycosuria. Maintain liberal fluid intake and alkalization of urine.

ADVERSE REACTIONS: Headache, acute gouty arthritis, dizziness, hepatic necrosis, vomiting, nausea, anorexia, sore gums, nephrotic syndrome, uric acid stones, renal colic, costovertebral pain, urinary frequency, anaphylaxis, fever, urticaria, pruritus, blood dyscrasias, dermatitis, alopecia, flushing.

INTERACTIONS: Probenecid increases plasma levels of penicillin and other β-lactams; psychic disturbances reported. Avoid use with penicillin in the presence of renal impairment. Salicylates and pyrazinamide antagonize uricosuric effects. Increased plasma levels of methotrexate, sulfonamides, sulfonylureas, thiopental or ketamine-induced anesthesia, some NSAIDs (eg, indomethacin, naproxen), lorazepam, APAP, and rifampin. Possible false high plasma levels of theophylline.

PREGNANCY: Safety in pregnancy and nursing is not known.

PROCRIT   RX
epoetin alfa (Ortho Biotech)

> Erythropoiesis-stimulating agents (ESAs) may increase risk for death and/or serious cardiovascular events when administered to a target Hgb >12g/dL. Use lowest dose that will gradually increase Hgb concentration to lowest level sufficient to avoid need for RBC transfusion. When ESAs are used preoperatively for reduction of allogenic RBC transfusions, a higher incidence of DVT was reported in patients not receiving prophylactic anticoagulation. Antithrombotic prophylaxis should be strongly considered when ESAs are used to reduce allogenic RBC transfusions.

THERAPEUTIC CLASS: Erythropoiesis stimulator

INDICATIONS: Treatment of anemia of chronic renal failure (CRF), anemia related to zidovudine-treatment of HIV, chemotherapy-induced anemia in non-myeloid malignancies, and reduction of allogeneic blood transfusions in anemic patients (>10 to ≤13g/dL) scheduled for elective, noncardiac, nonvascular surgery.

DOSAGE: *Adults:* CRF: Initial: 50-100U/kg IV/SQ 3x/week. IV is preferred route in dialysis patients. Titrate: Reduce if Hgb approaches 12g/dL or if Hgb increases >1g/dL in any 2-week period. Increase when Hgb does not increase by 2g/dL after 8 weeks of therapy and Hgb is below target range (10-12g/dL). Maint: Individually titrate. Zidovudine-Treated HIV Patients: If serum erythropoietin levels ≤500mU/mL and zidovudine ≤4200mg/week give 100U/kg IV/SQ 3x/week for 8 weeks. Titrate: Increase by 50-100U/kg 3x/week after 8 weeks if necessary. Maint: If Hgb >13g/dL, discontinue until Hgb <12g/dL, then reduce dose by 25% when resume therapy. Max: 300U/kg 3x/week. Chemotherapy Induced Anemia: Initial: 150U/kg SQ 3x/week. Titrate: Reduce by 25% when Hgb approaches 12g/dL or Hgb increases >1g/dL in any 2-week period. If Hgb >13g/dL, withhold until Hgb <12g/dL then restart at 25% below previous dose. May increase to 300U/kg 3x/week if no response after 8 weeks of therapy. Max: 300U/kg 3x/week. Weekly Dosing: 40,000U SQ weekly. Titrate: If Hgb not increased by ≥1g/dL after 4 weeks, increase to 60,000U weekly. If Hgb >13g/dL, withhold until Hgb <12g/dL then restart with 25% dose reduction. Reduce dose by 25% if very rapid Hgb response (eg, increase >1g/dL in any 2-week period. Max: 60,000U weekly. Surgery: 300U/kg/day

SQ for 10 days before surgery, on surgery day, and 4 days post-op or 600U/kg SQ once weekly on 21, 14, and 7 days before surgery and a 4th dose on surgery day, with adequate iron supplement.

Pediatrics: CRF: Initial: 50U/kg 3x/week IV/SQ. Titrate: Reduce if Hgb approaches 12g/dL or if Hgb increases by >1g/dL in any 2-week period. Increase if Hgb does not increase by 2g/dL after 8 weeks of therapy and Hgb is below target range (10-12g/dL). Maint: Individually titrate.

HOW SUPPLIED: Inj: 2000U/mL, 3000U/mL, 4000U/mL, 10,000U/mL, 20,000U/mL, 40,000U/mL

CONTRAINDICATIONS: Uncontrolled HTN. Hypersensitivity to mammalian cell-derived products and albumin (human).

WARNINGS/PRECAUTIONS: Pure red cell aplasia and severe anemia (with or without other cytopenias) may occur. Caution with porphyria, HTN, or history of seizures. Evaluate iron stores before and during therapy; most patients need iron supplementation. Monitor Hgb, BP, iron levels, serum chemistry, and CBC. Menses may resume. Multidose formulation contains benzyl alcohol that has been associated with an increased incidence of neurological and other complications in premature infants which are sometimes fatal.

ADVERSE REACTIONS: HTN, headache, fatigue, arthralgias, nausea, vomiting, diarrhea, edema, rash, pyrexia, constipation, respiratory congestion, dyspnea, asthenia, skin reaction.

INTERACTIONS: Adjust anticoagulant dose in dialysis patients.

PREGNANCY: Category C, caution in nursing

Proctocort Cream
hydrocortisone (Salix)

RX

THERAPEUTIC CLASS: Corticosteroid

INDICATIONS: Corticosteroid responsive dermatoses.

DOSAGE: *Adults:* Apply bid-qid. May use occlusive dressings for psoriasis or recalcitrant conditions; discontinue dressings if infection develops.

Pediatrics: Apply bid-qid. May use occlusive dressings for psoriasis or recalcitrant conditions; discontinue dressings if infection develops.

HOW SUPPLIED: Cre: 1% (30g)

WARNINGS/PRECAUTIONS: May produce reversible HPA axis suppression, manifestations of Cushing's syndrome, hyperglycemia, and glucosuria. Caution when applied to large surface areas or under occlusive dressings. Use appropriate therapy with infections. Pediatrics may be more susceptible to systemic toxicity. Discontinue if irritation occurs. Avoid eyes.

ADVERSE REACTIONS: Burning, itching, irritation, dryness, folliculitis, hypertrichosis, acneiform eruptions, hypopigmentation, perioral dermatitis, allergic contact dermatitis, maceration skin, secondary infection, skin atrophy, striae, miliaria.

PREGNANCY: Category C, caution in nursing.

ProctoFoam-HC
pramoxine HCl - hydrocortisone acetate (Schwarz Pharma)

RX

THERAPEUTIC CLASS: Corticosteroid/anesthetic

INDICATIONS: Corticosteroid responsive dermatoses of the anal region.

DOSAGE: *Adults:* Apply to anal/perianal area tid-qid.

Pediatrics: Apply to anal/perianal area tid-qid.

HOW SUPPLIED: Foam: (Hydrocortisone-Pramoxine) 1%-1% (10g)

WARNINGS/PRECAUTIONS: Discontinue if no improvement in 2-3 weeks. May produce reversible HPA axis suppression, manifestations of Cushing's syndrome, hyperglycemia, and glucosuria. Caution when applied to large surface areas or under occlusive dressings. Use appropriate therapy if infections develop; discontinue steroid if favorable response does not occur promptly. Discontinue if irritation develops. Pediatrics may be more susceptible to systemic toxicity. Avoid eyes.

ADVERSE REACTIONS: Burning, itching, irritation, dryness, folliculitis, hypertrichosis, acneiform eruptions, hypopigmentation, perioral dermatitis, allergic contact dermatitis, skin maceration, secondary infection, skin atrophy, striae, miliaria.

PREGNANCY: Category C, caution in nursing.

PROFASI
chorionic gonadotropin (Serono)

RX

THERAPEUTIC CLASS: Human chorionic gonadotropin

INDICATIONS: For prepubertal cryptorchidism not due to anatomic obstruction. For hypogonadotropic hypogonadism (secondary to a pituitary deficiency) in males. To induce ovulation (OI) and pregnancy in anovulatory, infertile women in whom anovulation is not due to primary ovarian failure and pretreated with human menotropins.

DOSAGE: *Adults:* Hypogonadism: 500-1000 U IM 3x/week (TIW) for 3 weeks, then twice weekly for 3 weeks; or 4000 U IM TIW for 6-9 months, then reduce to 2000 U TIW for 3 months. OI: 5000-10,000 U IM 1 day after last dose of menotropins.
Pediatrics: ≥4 yrs: Cryptorchidism: 4000 U IM TIW for 3 weeks; or 5000 U IM every 2nd day for 4 doses; or 15 doses of 500-1000 U over 6 weeks; or 500 U TIW for 4-6 weeks (if treatment fails, give 1000 U/injection starting 1 month later). Initiate therapy between 4-9 yrs. Hypogonadism: 500-1000 U IM TIW for 3 weeks, then twice weekly for 3 weeks; or 4000 U IM TIW for 6-9 months, then reduce to 2000 U TIW for 3 months.

HOW SUPPLIED: Inj: 10,000 U

CONTRAINDICATIONS: Precocious puberty, prostatic carcinoma or other androgen-dependent neoplasms, pregnancy.

WARNINGS/PRECAUTIONS: Potential ovarian hyperstimulation, enlargement or rupture of ovarian cysts, multiple births, and arterial thromboembolism with infertility treatment. D/C if precocious puberty occurs in cryptorchidism patients. Caution with cardiac or renal disease, epilepsy, migraine, asthma. Diluent contains benzyl alcohol. Not effective treatment for obesity.

ADVERSE REACTIONS: Headache, irritability, restlessness, depression, fatigue, edema, precocious puberty, gynecomastia, injection site pain, hypersensitivity reactions.

PREGNANCY: Category X, caution in nursing.

PROGRAF
tacrolimus (Astellas)

RX

> Increased susceptibility to infection and development of lymphoma.

THERAPEUTIC CLASS: Macrolide immunosuppressant

INDICATIONS: Prophylaxis of organ rejection in allogenic liver, kidney, or heart transplants with concomitant adrenal corticosteroids. In heart transplant patients, azathioprine or mycophenolate mofetil co-administration is recommended.

DOSAGE: *Adults:* Initial (6h after transplantation): 0.03-0.05mg/kg/day (liver, kidney) or 0.01mg/kg/day (heart) IV infusion if cannot tolerate PO. Hepatic Transplant: 0.05-0.075mg/kg PO q12h with grapefruit juice; start 8-12 hrs after last IV dose. Kidney Transplant: 0.1mg/kg PO q12h, 24 hrs after transplant or until renal function recovered. Heart Transplant: 0.0375mg/kg PO q12h; start 8-12 hrs after last IV dose. Renal/Hepatic Impairment: Give lowest recommended dose. Severe Hepatic Impairment (Pugh ≥10): May require lower doses. Wait at least 48 hrs with post-op oliguria.

Pediatrics: Liver Transplant: Initial: 0.03-0.05mg/kg/day IV or 0.15-0.2mg/kg/day PO. Severe Hepatic Impairment (Pugh ≥10): May require lower doses.

HOW SUPPLIED: Cap: 0.5mg, 1mg, 5mg; Inj: 5mg/mL

CONTRAINDICATIONS: Hypersensitivity to HCO-60.

WARNINGS/PRECAUTIONS: Insulin-dependent post-transplant DM, HTN, myocardial hypertrophy, neurotoxicity, hyperkalemia, nephrotoxicity reported. Monitor drug levels frequently to prevent organ rejection and/or reduce potential toxicity. Monitor for anaphylaxis with infusion. Monitor levels closely with hepatic impairment.

ADVERSE REACTIONS: HTN, headache, insomnia, fever, pruritus, hyperglycemia, hyperkalemia, hypomagnesemia, diarrhea, nausea, vomiting, increased BUN, anorexia, constipation, tremor, rash, pleural effusion, gastroenteritis.

INTERACTIONS: CYP450 3A inducers (eg, carbamazepine, phenobarbital, phenytoin, rifabutin, rifampin, St. John's wort, etc.) may decrease plasma levels. Caution with other nephrotoxic drugs (eg. aminoglycosides, amphotericin B, cisplatin). May affect drugs metabolized by CYP450 3A. Avoid grapefruit juice. CYP450 3A inhibitors (eg, diltiazem, nicardipine, nifedipine, verapamil, azole antifungal, macrolides, cisapride, metoclopramide, etc) may increase plasma levels. Vaccination may be less effective. Avoid live vaccines, cyclosporine (when switching to tacrolimus, wait at least 24 hrs. after last cyclosporine dose), and K^+ sparing diuretics.

PREGNANCY: Category C, not for use in nursing.

PROMETHAZINE
promethazine HCl (Various)

RX

OTHER BRAND NAMES: Phenergan (Wyeth) - Promethegan (G & W Labs)

THERAPEUTIC CLASS: Phenothiazine derivative

INDICATIONS: Allergic and vasomotor rhinitis, allergic conjunctivitis, blood or plasma allergic reactions, dermographism, urticaria, angioedema. Pre- and postoperative sedation. Adjunct in anaphylaxis, postoperative pain. Prevention and control of nausea, vomiting, and motion sickness.

DOSAGE: *Adults:* Allergy: 25mg qhs or 12.5mg ac and hs. Motion Sickness: Initial: 25mg 30-60 minutes before travel, then 25mg 8-12 hrs later if needed. Maint: 25mg bid. Prevention/Control of Nausea/Vomiting: 25mg initially, then 12.5-25mg q4-6h prn. Sedation: 25-50mg qhs. Preoperative: 50mg night before surgery, then 50mg preoperatively. Postoperative: 25-50mg.

Pediatrics: ≥2 yrs: Allergy: 25mg or 0.5mg/lb qhs or 6.25-12.5 tid. Motion Sickness: 12.5-25mg bid. Prevention/Control of Nausea/Vomiting: 25mg or 0.5mg/lb initially then 12.5-25mg or 0.5mg/lb q4-6h prn. Sedation: 12.5-25mg hs. Preoperative: 12.5-25mg night before surgery, then 0.5mg/lb preoperatively. Postoperative: 12.5-25mg.

HOW SUPPLIED: Sup: (Promethegan, Phenergan, Promethazine)12.5mg, 25mg, 50mg; Tab: (Phenergan, Promethazine)12.5mg*, 25mg*, 50mg *scored

CONTRAINDICATIONS: Treatment of lower respiratory tract symptoms (eg, asthma). Pediatric patients <2 yrs.

WARNINGS/PRECAUTIONS: Potential for fatal respiratory depression in pediatric patients <2 yrs. Caution in patients ≥2 yrs. Avoid with compromised respiratory function (eg, COPD, sleep apnea). Caution with bone marrow depression, narrow-angle glaucoma, stenosing peptic ulcer, bladder or pyloroduodenal obstruction, prostatic hypertrophy, CVD, hepatic dysfunction. Cholestatic jaundice reported. Alters HCG pregnancy tests. May lower seizure threshold, increase blood glucose, cause sun sensitivity. May impair mental/physical abilities.

ADVERSE REACTIONS: Drowsiness, sedation, blurred vision, dizziness, increased or decreased blood pressure, urticaria, dry mouth, nausea, vomiting.

INTERACTIONS: Additive sedative effects with CNS depressants (eg, alcohol, narcotic analgesics, sedatives, hypnotics, tranquilizers); reduce dose or eliminate these agents. Reduce barbiturate dose by one-half and analgesic depressant dose by one-quarter to one-half. Caution with drugs that alter seizure threshold (eg, narcotics, local anesthetics). Avoid sedatives and CNS depressants with sleep apnea.

PREGNANCY: Category C, not for use in nursing.

Promethazine DM
promethazine HCl - dextromethorphan HBr (Various)
RX

THERAPEUTIC CLASS: Phenothiazine derivative/antitussive

INDICATIONS: For relief of coughs and upper respiratory symptoms associated with allergy or colds.

DOSAGE: *Adults:* 5mL q4-6h. Max: 30mL/24 hr.
Pediatrics: ≥12 yrs: 5mL q4-6h. Max: 30mL/24hr. 6-11 yrs: 2.5-5mL q4-6h. Max: 20mL/24hr. 2-5 yrs: 1.25-2.5mL q4-6h. Max: 10mL/24hr.

HOW SUPPLIED: Syrup: (Promethazine-Dextromethorphan) 6.25mg-15mg/5mL

CONTRAINDICATIONS: Treatment of lower respiratory tract symptoms (eg, asthma), concomitant MAOIs.

WARNINGS/PRECAUTIONS: May lower seizure threshold. Avoid with sleep apnea. Caution with narrow-angle glaucoma, stenosing peptic ulcer, atopic children, bladder or pyloroduodenal obstruction, cardiovascular disease, hepatic dysfunction. Cholestatic jaundice reported. Alters HCG pregnancy test reading. May increase blood glucose.

ADVERSE REACTIONS: Drowsiness, dizziness, sedation, GI disturbance, blurred vision, dry mouth, increased or decreased blood pressure, rash, nausea, vomiting.

INTERACTIONS: Hyperpyrexia, hypotension and death associated with MAOIs. Added sedative effects with alcohol, narcotic analgesics, sedatives, hypnotics, TCAs, and tranquilizers. Reduce barbiturate dose by one-half and narcotic analgesics by one-quarter to one-half.

PREGNANCY: Category C, caution in nursing.

Promethazine VC
promethazine HCl - phenylephrine HCl (Various)
RX

THERAPEUTIC CLASS: Phenothiazine derivative/ sympathomimetic

INDICATIONS: For relief of upper respiratory symptoms (eg, nasal congestion) associated with allergy or colds.

DOSAGE: *Adults:* 5mL q4-6h. Max: 30mL/24 hr.
Pediatrics: ≥12 yrs: 5mL q4-6h. Max: 30mL/24 hr. 6-11 yrs: 2.5-5mL q4-6h. Max: 30mL/24 hr. 2-5 yrs: 1.25-2.5mL q4-6h.

HOW SUPPLIED: Syrup: (Promethazine-Phenylephrine) 6.25mg-5mg/5mL

CONTRAINDICATIONS: Treatment of lower respiratory tract symptoms (eg, asthma), HTN, peripheral vascular insufficiency, concomitant MAOIs.

WARNINGS/PRECAUTIONS: May lower seizure threshold. Avoid with sleep apnea. Caution with thyroid disease, diabetes, elderly, poor cerebral or coronary circulation, narrow-angle glaucoma, stenosing peptic ulcer, bladder or pyloroduodenal obstruction, cardiovascular disease, hepatic dysfunction. Cholestatic jaundice reported. Alters HCG pregnancy test reading. May increase blood glucose. Avoid prolonged exposure to sunlight.

ADVERSE REACTIONS: Drowsiness, dizziness, anxiety, tremor, sedation, blurred vision, dry mouth, increased or decreased blood pressure, rash, nausea, vomiting.

INTERACTIONS: Added sedative effects with alcohol, narcotic analgesics, sedatives, hypnotics, TCAs, tranquilizers. Reduce barbiturate dose by one-half and narcotic analgesics by one-quarter to one-half. Possible hypertensive crisis with MAOIs. Pressor response increased with TCAs. Excessive rise in BP with ergot alkaloids. Arrhythmias with other sympathomimetics. β-blockers block cardiostimulating effects. Reflex bradycardia blocked and pressor response enhanced with atropine. Pressor response decreased with β-blockers. Synergistic adrenergic response with amphetamines.

PREGNANCY: Category C, caution in nursing.

Promethazine VC/Codeine
promethazine HCl - codeine phosphate - phenylephrine HCl (Various)
CV

THERAPEUTIC CLASS: Phenothiazine derivative/antitussive/sympathomimetic

INDICATIONS: For relief of cough and upper respiratory symptoms (eg, nasal congestion) associated with allergy or colds.

DOSAGE: *Adults:* 5mL q4-6h. Max: 30mL/24hr.

Pediatrics: ≥12 yrs: 5mL q4-6h. Max: 30mL/24hr. 6-11 yrs: 2.5-5mL q4-6h. Max: 30mL/24hr. 2-5 yrs: 1.25-2.5mL q4-6h. Max: 18kg: 9mL/24hr. 16kg: 8mL/24hr. 14kg: 7mL/24hr. 12kg: 6mL/24hr.

HOW SUPPLIED: Syrup: (Promethazine-Codeine-Phenylephrine) 6.25mg-10mg-5mg/5mL

CONTRAINDICATIONS: Treatment of lower respiratory tract symptoms (eg, asthma), HTN, peripheral vascular insufficiency, concomitant MAOIs.

WARNINGS/PRECAUTIONS: May lower seizure threshold. Avoid with sleep apnea, asthma, acute febrile illness with productive cough, atopic children. Caution with acute abdominal conditions, convulsive disorders, significant renal dysfunction, fever, thyroid disease, diabetes, Addison's disease, ulcerative colitis, prostatic hypertrophy, recent GI or urinary tract surgery, elderly, debilitated, narrow-angle glaucoma, stenosing peptic ulcer, bladder or pyloroduodenal obstruction, cardiovascular disease, hepatic dysfunction. Cholestatic jaundice reported. Alters HCG pregnancy test reading. May increase blood glucose. Respiratory depressant effects may be exacerbated with head injury or increased intracranial pressure.

ADVERSE REACTIONS: Drowsiness, dizziness, sedation, tremor, anxiety, blurred vision, dry mouth, increased or decreased blood pressure, rash, nausea, vomiting, constipation, urinary retention.

INTERACTIONS: Added sedative effects with alcohol, narcotic analgesics, sedatives, hypnotics, TCAs, tranquilizers. Reduce barbiturate dose by one-half and narcotic analgesics by one-quarter to one-half. Possible hypertensive crisis with MAOIs. Pressor response increased with TCAs. Excessive rise in BP with ergot alkaloids. Arrhythmias with other sympathomimetics. β-blockers block cardiostimulating effects. Reflex bradycardia blocked and pressor response enhanced with atropine. Pressor response decreased with β-blockers. Synergistic adrenergic response with amphetamines.

PREGNANCY: Category C, caution in nursing.

PROMETHAZINE W/CODEINE CV
promethazine HCl - codeine phosphate (Various)

THERAPEUTIC CLASS: Phenothiazine derivative/antitussive

INDICATIONS: For relief of coughs and upper respiratory symptoms associated with allergy or colds.

DOSAGE: *Adults:* 5mL q4-6h. Max: 30mL/24 hr.

Pediatrics: ≥12 yrs: 5mL q4-6h. Max: 30mL/24 hr. 6 to <12 yrs: 2.5-5mL q4-6h. Max: 30mL/24 hr. 2 to <6 yrs: 1.25-2.5mL q4-6h. Max: 2 to <6 yrs: 18kg: 9mL/24 hr. 16kg: 8mL/24 hr. 14kg: 7mL/24 hr. 12kg: 6mL/24 hr.

HOW SUPPLIED: Syrup: (Promethazine-Codeine) 6.25mg-10mg/5mL

CONTRAINDICATIONS: Treatment of lower respiratory tract symptoms (eg, asthma).

WARNINGS/PRECAUTIONS: Avoid prolonged sun exposure. May lower seizure threshold. Avoid with sleep apnea, asthma, acute febrile illness with productive cough, atopic children. Caution with acute abdominal conditions, convulsive disorders, significant renal dysfunction, fever, hypothyroidism, Addison's disease, ulcerative colitis, prostatic hypertrophy, recent GI or urinary tract surgery, elderly, debilitated, narrow-angle glaucoma, stenosing peptic ulcer, bladder or pyloroduodenal obstruction, cardiovascular disease, hepatic dysfunction. Cholestatic jaundice reported. Alters HCG pregnancy test reading. May increase blood glucose. Respiratory depressant effects may be exacerbated with head injury or increased intracranial pressure.

ADVERSE REACTIONS: Drowsiness, dizziness, sedation, blurred vision, dry mouth, increased or decreased blood pressure, rash, nausea, vomiting, constipation, urinary retention.

INTERACTIONS: Added sedative effects with alcohol, narcotic analgesics, sedatives, hypnotics, TCAs, and tranquilizers. Reduce barbiturate dose by one-half and narcotic analgesics by one-quarter to one-half. Possible adverse reactions with MAOIs.

PREGNANCY: Category C, caution in nursing.

PROPYLTHIOURACIL RX
propylthiouracil (Various)

THERAPEUTIC CLASS: Thiourea-derivative antithyroid agent

INDICATIONS: Treatment of hyperthyroidism.

ProQuad

DOSAGE: *Adults:* Initial: 300mg/day in 3 divided doses, q8h. Severe Hyperthyroidism/Very Large Goiters: Initial: 400mg/day in 3 divided doses; may give up to 600-900mg/day if needed. Maint: 100-150mg/day.

Pediatrics: 6-10 yrs: Initial: 50-150mg/day. ≥10 yrs: Initial: 150-300mg/day. Maint: Determine by patient response.

HOW SUPPLIED: Tab: 50mg

CONTRAINDICATIONS: Nursing mothers.

WARNINGS/PRECAUTIONS: Discontinue with agranulocytosis, aplastic anemia, hepatitis, fever, or exfoliative dermatitis. Rare reports of severe hepatic reactions exist. Discontinue with significant hepatic abnormality, including transaminases >3X ULN. Caution with pregnancy, may cause fetal harm. Monitor PT and TFTs.

ADVERSE REACTIONS: Agranulocytosis, skin rash, urticaria, nausea, vomiting, epigastric distress, arthralgia, paresthesias, loss of taste, myalgia, headache, pruritus, drowsiness, neuritis, edema, vertigo, jaundice.

INTERACTIONS: May potentiate anticoagulant effects. Hyperthyroidism increases clearance of β-blockers; reduce β-blocker dose when patient becomes euthyroid. Increased digitalis glycoside levels when patient becomes euthyroid; reduce digitalis dose. Decreased theophylline clearance when patient becomes euthyroid; reduce theophylline dose. Caution with other drugs that cause agranulocytosis.

PREGNANCY: Category D, contraindicated in nursing.

ProQuad RX
mumps vaccine live - measles vaccine live - rubella vaccine live - varicella virus vaccine live (Merck)

THERAPEUTIC CLASS: Vaccine

INDICATIONS: Vaccination against measles, mumps, rubella, and varicella in children 12 months to 12 yrs of age.

DOSAGE: *Pediatrics:* 12 months-12 yrs: 0.5mL SQ. At least 1 month should elapse between dose of measles-containing vaccine and a dose of ProQuad. If for any reason a second dose of varicella-containing vaccine is required, at least 3 months should elapse between doses.

HOW SUPPLIED: Inj: 0.5mL

CONTRAINDICATIONS: Anaphylactic reactions to neomycin; hypsensitivity to gelatin; blood dyscrasias, leukemia, lymphomas, or other malignant neoplasms affecting the bone marrow or lymphatic system; immunosuppressive therapy; primary and acquired immunodeficiency states (e.g., AIDS/HIV); congenital or hereditary immunodeficiency; active untreated tuberculosis; active afebrile illness with fever >101.3°F; pregnant.

WARNINGS/PRECAUTIONS: Caution with egg allergy. May cause thrombocytopenia. Contains albumin, remote risk of viral infection transmission. Have epinephrine (1:1000) available.

ADVERSE REACTIONS: Injection Site: Pain/tenderness/soreness, erythema, swelling. Systemic: Fever, irritability, measles-like rash

INTERACTIONS: Do not give with immune globulin. Avoid use of salicylates for 6 weeks after vaccination. Avoid use of immunosuppressive doses of corticosteriods or other immunosuppressive drugs.

PREGNANCY: Category C, not for use in nursing.

Prosed EC RX
methenamine - benzoic acid - methylene blue - phenyl salicylate - atropine sulfate - hyoscyamine sulfate (Esprit)

OTHER BRAND NAME: Prosed DS (Star)

THERAPEUTIC CLASS: Urinary tract analgesic

INDICATIONS: Relief of lower urinary tract discomfort due to hypermotility. Treatment of formaldehyde-susceptible cystitis, urethritis, trigonitis.

DOSAGE: *Adults:* 1 tab qid with plenty of fluid.

Pediatrics: >12 yrs: Individualize dose. Take with plenty of fluid.

HOW SUPPLIED: Tab, Enteric Coated: Atropine 0.06mg-Benzoic Acid 9mg-Hyoscyamine 0.06mg-Methenamine 81.6mg-Methylene Blue 10.8mg-Phenyl Salicylate 36.2mg

CONTRAINDICATIONS: Risk-benefit assessment in glaucoma, urinary bladder neck obstruction, pyloric or duodenal obstruction, cardiospasm.

WARNINGS/PRECAUTIONS: Discontinue if tachycardia, dizziness, or blurred vision occurs. Delay in gastric emptying time may obscure gastric ulcer therapy.

ADVERSE REACTIONS: Rapid pulse, flushing, blurred vision, dizziness, shortness of breath, difficult micturition, acute urinary retention, dry mouth, nausea, vomiting.

INTERACTIONS: May decrease absorption of other oral agents (dose 2 hrs after ketoconazole). Reduced effectiveness with urinary alkaliners, thiazide diuretics, antacids/antidiarrheals (space dosing by 1 hr). Antimuscarinic effects potentiated with other antimuscarinics, MAOIs. Caution with antimyasthenics. Increased risk of constipation with opioids. Increased risk of crystalluria with sulfonamides.

PREGNANCY: Category C, caution in nursing.

PROSTIN VR PEDIATRIC   RX
alprostadil (Pharmacia & Upjohn)

> Apnea occurs in about 10-12% of neonates, usually appearing during the 1st hr of drug infusion. Monitor respiratory status throughout treatment.

THERAPEUTIC CLASS: Prostaglandin E_1

INDICATIONS: Palliative therapy to maintain patency of the ductus arteriosus until corrective surgery in neonates with congenital heart defects.

DOSAGE: *Pediatrics:* Initial: 0.05-0.1mcg/kg/min IV. Maint: 0.025-0.01mcg/kg/min IV. Max: 0.4mcg/kg/min.

HOW SUPPLIED: Inj: 0.5mg/mL

WARNINGS/PRECAUTIONS: May cause gastric outlet obstruction secondary to antral hyperplasia, monitor closely after 120 hrs of therapy. Limit infusion to minimum effective dose and time. May inhibit platelet aggregation; caution with bleeding tendencies. Cortical proliferation of long bones, localized and aneurysmal dilatations, vessel wall edema, intimal lacerations, decrease in medial muscularity and disruption of medial and internal lamina reported. Avoid in respiratory distress syndrome. Monitor arterial pressure intermittently; decrease rate of infusion with significant fall in pressure.

ADVERSE REACTIONS: Apnea, fever, seizures, bradycardia, flushing, diarrhea, hypotension, tachycardia.

PREGNANCY: Safety in pregnancy and nursing not known.

PROTOPIC   RX
tacrolimus (Astellas)

THERAPEUTIC CLASS: Macrolide immunosuppressant

INDICATIONS: Short-term and intermittent long-term therapy of moderate to severe atopic dermatitis intolerant or unresponsive to conventional therapy.

DOSAGE: *Adults:* (0.03% or 0.1%) Apply thin layer bid. Rub in gently. Continue for 1 week after symptoms clear.

Pediatrics: ≥16 yrs: (0.03% or 0.1%) Apply thin layer bid. Rub in gently. Continue for 1 week after symptoms clear. 2-15 yrs: (0.03%) Apply thin layer bid. Rub in gently. Continue for 1 week after symptoms clear.

HOW SUPPLIED: Oint: 0.03%, 0.1% (30g, 60g, 100g)

WARNINGS/PRECAUTIONS: Do not use with occlusive dressings. Increased risk of varicella zoster, herpes simplex, or eczema herpeticum. Lymphadenopathy reported; monitor closely. Discontinue if unknown etiology of lymphadenopathy or presence of acute infectious mononucleosis. Avoid in Netherton's syndrome. Minimize or avoid exposure to natural or artificial sunlight. Long-term safety has not been established. Rare cases of malignancy (eg, skin and lymphoma) have been reported with topical calcineurin

PROVENTIL HFA

inhibitors; therefore, continuous long-term use should be avoided and application limited to areas of involvement. Not indicated for use in children <2 yrs. Only 0.03% ointment is indicated for use in children 2-15 yrs.

ADVERSE REACTIONS: Skin burning, pruritus, flu-like symptoms, allergic reaction, skin erythema, headache, skin infection, fever, herpes simplex, rhinitis.

INTERACTIONS: Caution with CYP3A4 inhibitors (eg, erythromycin, itraconazole, ketoconazole, fluconazole, calcium channel blockers, cimetidine) in widespread and/or erythrodermic disease. Increased risk for lymphomas in transplant patients receiving other immunosuppressive therapy.

PREGNANCY: Category C, not for use in nursing.

PROVENTIL HFA   RX
albuterol sulfate (Schering)

THERAPEUTIC CLASS: Beta$_2$ agonist

INDICATIONS: Prevention and treatment of bronchospasm with reversible obstructive airway disease; prevention of exercise-induced bronchospasm (EIB) in patients ≥4 yrs old.

DOSAGE: *Adults:* Bronchospasm: 2 inh q4-6h or 1 inh q4h. EIB: 2 inh 15-30 min before activity.
Pediatrics: ≥4 yrs: Bronchospasm: 2 inh q4-6h or 1 inh q4h. EIB: 2 inh 15-30 min before activity.

HOW SUPPLIED: HFA: 90mcg/inh (6.7g)

WARNINGS/PRECAUTIONS: Hypersensitivity reactions reported. Monitor for worsening asthma. fatalities reported with excessive use. Caution with cardiovascular disorders, especially coronary insufficiency, arrhythmias and HTN. May need concomitant corticosteroids. Can produce paradoxical bronschospasm. Caution with DM, hyperthyroidism, and seizures. May cause transient hypokalemia.

ADVERSE REACTIONS: Tachycardia, tremor, dizziness, nausea/vomiting, palpitations, rihinitis, upper respiratory tract infection, fever, inhalation site and taste sensation, back pain, and nervousness.

INTERACTIONS: Avoid other sympathomimetic agents. Extreme caution wtih MAOIs and TCAs. Monitor digoxin. May worsen ECG changes and/or hypokalemia with nonpotassium-sparing diuretics. Antagonized by β-blockers.

PREGNANCY: Category C, not for use in nursing.

PROVIGIL   CIV
modafinil (Cephalon)

THERAPEUTIC CLASS: Wakefulness-promoting agent

INDICATIONS: To improve wakefulness in patients with excessive daytime sleepiness associated with narcolepsy, obstructive sleep apnea/hypopnea syndrome (OSAHS), shiftwork sleep disorder (SWSD). As adjunct treatment for underlying obstruction in OSAHS.

DOSAGE: *Adults:* 200mg qd. Narcolepsy/OSAHS: Take in AM. SWSD: Take 1 hr prior to start of work shift. Hepatic Dysfunction: 100mg qd. Elderly: Consider dose reduction.
Pediatrics: ≥16 yrs: 200mg qd. Narcolepsy/OSAHS: Take in AM. SWSD: Take 1 hr prior to start of work shift. Hepatic Dysfunction: 100mg qd.

HOW SUPPLIED: Tab: 100mg, 200mg* *scored

WARNINGS/PRECAUTIONS: Avoid in history of left ventricular hypertrophy, ischemic ECG changes, chest pain, arrhythmia or other manifestations of mitral valve prolapse with CNS stimulants. Caution if recent MI, unstable angina, history of psychosis. Monitor hypertensive patients.

ADVERSE REACTIONS: Headache, infection, nausea, nervousness, anxiety, insomnia.

INTERACTIONS: Methylphenidate may delay absorption. May reduce efficacy of steroidal contraceptives up to 1 month after discontinuation. Caution with MAOIs. CYP3A4 inducers (eg, carbamazepine, phenobarbital, rifampin) may decrease levels. CYP3A4 inhibitors (eg, ketoconazole, itraconazole) may increase levels. May increase levels of drugs metabolized by CYP2C19 (eg, diazepam, propranolol, phenytoin) or CYP2C9 (eg, warfarin). Monitor for toxicity with phenytoin and PT with warfarin. May increase levels of clomipramine, desipramine. May decrease levels of drugs metabolized by CYP3A4 (eg, cyclosporine, steroidal contraceptives, theophylline). Avoid alcohol.

PREGNANCY: Category C, caution in nursing.

Prozac
fluoxetine HCl (Lilly)

RX

> Antidepressants increased the risk of suicidal thinking and behavior (suicidality) in short-term studies in children and adolescents with Major Depressive Disorder (MDD) and other psychiatric disorders. Fluoxetine is approved for use in pediatric patients with MDD and Obsessive Compulsive Disorder (OCD).

THERAPEUTIC CLASS: Selective serotonin reuptake inhibitor

INDICATIONS: Treatment of MDD, OCD, bulimia nervosa, panic disorder with or without agoraphobia.

DOSAGE: *Adults:* MDD: Daily Dosing: Initial: 20mg qam; increase dose if no improvement after several weeks. Doses >20mg/day, give qam or bid (am and noon). Max: 80mg/day. OCD: Initial: 20mg/day. Maint: 20-60mg/day given qd-bid, am and noon. Max: 80mg/day. Bulimia Nervosa: 60mg qam. Max: 60mg/day. Panic Disorder: Initial: 10mg/day. May increase to 20mg/day after 1 week. May increase further after several weeks if no clinical improvement. Max: 60mg/day. Hepatic Impairment/Elderly: Use lower or less frequent dosage.

Pediatrics: MDD: ≥8 yrs: Higher Weight Peds: Initial: 10 or 20mg/day. After 1 week at 10mg/day, may increase to 20mg/day. Lower Weight Peds: Initial: 10mg/day. Titrate: May increase to 20mg/day after several weeks if clinical improvement not observed. OCD: ≥7 yrs: Adolescents and Higher Weight Peds: Initial: 10mg/day. Titrate: Increase to 20mg/day after 2 weeks. Consider additional dose increases after several more weeks if clinical improvement not observed. Usual: 20-60mg/day. Lower Weight Peds: Initial: 10mg/day. Titrate: Consider additional dose increases after several weeks if clinical improvement not observed. Usual: 20-30mg/day. Max: 60mg/day.

HOW SUPPLIED: Cap: 10mg, 20mg, 40mg; Sol: 20mg/5mL (120mL); Tab: 10mg* *scored

CONTRAINDICATIONS: During or within 14 days of MAOI therapy. Thioridazine within 5 weeks of discontinuation. Concomitant use of pimozide.

WARNINGS/PRECAUTIONS: D/C if unexplained allergic reaction occurs. Monitor for symptoms of mania/hypomania. Caution with diseases or conditions that could affect metabolism or hemodynamic responses, diabetes, history of seizures, suicidal tendencies. Altered platelet function, hyponatremia reported. Periodically monitor height and weight in pediatrics. Monitor for clinical worsening and/or suicidality, especially at initiation of therapy or dose changes. Avoid abrupt withdrawal. Monitor for discontinuation symptoms. Caution in third trimester of pregnancy due to risk of serious neonatal complications.

ADVERSE REACTIONS: Nausea, diarrhea, insomnia, anxiety, nervousness, dizziness, somnolence, tremor, decreased libido, sweating, anorexia, asthenia, dry mouth, dyspepsia, headache.

INTERACTIONS: See Contraindications. Antidiabetic drugs may need adjustment. May shift concentrations with plasma-bound drugs (eg, coumadin, digitoxin). May alter warfarin effects. May increase benzodiazepine, phenytoin, carbamazepine levels. Increased adverse effects with tryptophan. Caution with CNS drugs. Lithium levels may increase/decrease; monitor lithium levels. May potentiate drugs metabolized by CYP2D6, antipsychotics (eg, haloperidol, clozapine), other antidepressants. Avoid alcohol. Caution with drugs that interfere with hemostasis (eg, non-selective NSAIDs, aspirin, warfarin) due to increased risk of bleeding. Serotonin syndrome reported with use of an SSRI and a triptan; monitor closely.

PREGNANCY: Category C, not for use in nursing.

PULMICORT
budesonide (AstraZeneca LP)
RX

OTHER BRAND NAMES: Pulmicort Respules (AstraZeneca LP) - Pulmicort Flexhaler (AstraZeneca LP)

THERAPEUTIC CLASS: Corticosteroid

INDICATIONS: (Respules) Treatment of asthma and as prophylactic therapy in children 12 months to 8 years of age. (Flexhaler) Maintenance treatment of asthma as prophylactic therapy in patients ≥6 years and to reduce or eliminate the need for oral systemic corticosteroidal therapy.

DOSAGE: *Adults:* (Flexhaler) Initial: 180-360mcg bid. Max: 720mcg bid. Individualize dose.

Pediatrics: (Flexhaler) ≥6 yrs: Initial: 180-360mcg bid. Max: 360mcg bid. Individualize dose. (Respules) 1-8 yrs: Previous Bronchodilator Only: Initial: 0.5mg qd or 0.25mg bid. Administer via jet nebulizer. Max: 0.5mg/day. Previous Inhaled Corticosteroid: 0.5mg qd or 0.25mg bid. Max: 1mg/day. Previous Oral Corticosteroid: 1mg qd or 0.5mg bid. Max: 1mg/day. Gradually reduce PO corticosteroid after 1 week of budesonide.

HOW SUPPLIED: Powder, Inhalation: (Flexhaler) 90mcg/dose, 180mcg/dose; Sus, Inhalation: (Respules) 0.25mg/2mL; 0.5mg/2mL (2mL, 30^s)

CONTRAINDICATIONS: Primary treatment of status asthmaticus or other acute episodes of asthma where intensive measures are required.

WARNINGS/PRECAUTIONS: Deaths due to adrenal insufficiency have occurred with transfer from systemic corticosteroids to inhaled corticosteroids. Resume oral corticosteroids during stress or severe asthma attack. Transferring from oral to inhalation therapy may unmask allergic conditions (eg, rhinitis, conjunctivitis, arthritis, eosinophilic conditions, eczema). Observe for adrenal insufficiency, systemic corticosteroid withdrawal effects, and growth suppression (children). More susceptible to infections. Not for acute bronchospasm. D/C if bronchospasm occurs after dosing. Caution with TB of respiratory tract; untreated systemic fungal, bacterial, viral or parasitic infections; or ocular herpes simplex. *Candida* infection of mouth and pharynx reported.

ADVERSE REACTIONS: Nasopharyngitis, pharyngitis, headache, fever, sinusitis, pain, bronchospasm, bronchitis, respiratory infection, moniliasis.

INTERACTIONS: Oral ketoconazole increases plasma levels. CYP3A4 inhibitors (eg, itraconazole, clarithromycin, erythromycin) may inhibit metabolism and increase systemic exposure. (Respules) Slight decrease in clearance and increase in oral bioavailabilty with cimetidine.

PREGNANCY: (Respules) Category B, caution in nursing; (Flexhaler) Category B, not for use in nursing.

PURINETHOL
mercaptopurine (Gate)
RX

THERAPEUTIC CLASS: Purine analog

INDICATIONS: Remission induction and maintenance therapy of acute lymphatic leukemia (ALL).

DOSAGE: *Adults:* Induction: Initial: 2.5mg/kg/day. Calculate to nearest multiple of 25mg. Titrate: If no improvement after 4 weeks, increase to 5mg/kg/day. Discontinue with large rise or rapid fall in leukocytes or platelets. Resume when counts remain constant for 2-3 days or rises. Maint: 1.5-2.5mg/kg/day. Renal/Hepatic Impairment: Reduce dose.

Pediatrics: Induction: Initial: 2.5mg/kg qpm. Calculate to nearest multiple of 25mg. Titrate: If no improvement after 4 weeks, increase to 5mg/kg/day. Discontinue with large rise or rapid fall in leukocytes or platelets. Resume when counts remain constant for 2-3 days or rises. Maint: 1.5-2.5mg/kg/day. Renal/Hepatic Impairment: Reduce dose.

HOW SUPPLIED: Tab: 50mg* *scored

CONTRAINDICATIONS: Lack of definitive diagnosis of ALL. Prior resistance to mercaptopurine or thioguanine.

WARNINGS/PRECAUTIONS: Risk of dose-related bone marrow suppression. Monitor weekly platelet counts, Hgb, Hct, total WBC with differential; increase frequency during induction phase. Monitor closely for life-threatening infection or bleeding. Risk of hepatotoxicity, anorexia, diarrhea, jaundice, and ascites (especially with >2.5mg/kg dose). Perform LFTs weekly initially, then monthly; monitor more frequently with hepatotoxic drugs or pre-existing liver disease.

ADVERSE REACTIONS: Bone marrow toxicity, hepatotoxicity, hyperuricemia (reduce incidence by prehydration, urine alkalinization, prophylactic allopurinol), intestinal ulceration, rash, hyperpigmentation, alopecia, transient oligospermia.

INTERACTIONS: Reduce to 1/3-1/4 of usual dose with allopurinol to avoid toxicity. Reduce dose with myelosuppressants. Bone marrow suppression reported with trimethoprim-sulfamethoxazole. Cross-resistance with thioguanine.

PREGNANCY: Category D, not for use in nursing.

PYRAZINAMIDE RX
pyrazinamide (Wyeth)

THERAPEUTIC CLASS: Nicotinamide analogue

INDICATIONS: Adjunctive initial treatment of active tuberculosis (TB). For use after treatment failure with other primary drugs in active TB.

DOSAGE: *Adults:* Usual: 15-30mg/kg qd. Max: 3g/day. (CDC recommends Max: 2g/day). Alternate Regimen: 50-70mg/kg twice weekly. Dose based on lean body weight. Take initial 2 months of 6 month or longer regimen.

Pediatrics: Usual: 15-30mg/kg qd. Max: 3g/day. (CDC recommends Max: 2g/day). Alternate Regimen: 50-70mg/kg twice weekly. Dose based on lean body weight. Take initial 2 months of 6 month or longer regimen.

HOW SUPPLIED: Tab: 500mg* *scored

CONTRAINDICATIONS: Severe hepatic damage and active gout.

WARNINGS/PRECAUTIONS: Obtain baseline serum uric acid and LFTs before therapy. Caution with hepatic dysfunction or those at risk for drug-related hepatitis (eg, alcoholics) and DM. D/C if hyperuricemia with gouty arthritis or hepatocellular damage occurs. Inhibits renal excretion of urates.

ADVERSE REACTIONS: Gout, hepatotoxicity, nausea, vomiting, anorexia, arthralgia, myalgia, rash, urticaria, pruritus.

PREGNANCY: Category C, caution in nursing.

QUESTRAN RX
cholestyramine (Par)

OTHER BRAND NAME: Questran Light (Par)

THERAPEUTIC CLASS: Bile acid sequestrant

INDICATIONS: Adjunct to reduce elevated cholesterol in primary hypercholesterolemia not responding to diet or to reduce LDL in hypertriglyceridemia. Relief of pruritus associated with partial biliary obstruction.

DOSAGE: *Adults:* Initial: 1 packet or scoopful qd or bid. Maint: 2-4 packets or scoopfuls/day, given bid. Titrate: Adjust at no less than 4 week intervals. Max: 6 packets/day or 6 scoopfuls/day. May also give as 1-6 doses/day. Mix with fluid or highly fluid food.

Pediatrics: Usual: 240mg/kg/day of anhydrous cholestyramine resin in 2-3 divided doses. Max: 8g/day.

HOW SUPPLIED: Powder: 4g/packet (60^s, 378g), (Light) 4g/scoopful (60^s, 268g)

CONTRAINDICATIONS: Complete biliary obstruction.

Quinidine Gluconate Injection

WARNINGS/PRECAUTIONS: May produce hyperchloremic acidosis with prolonged use. Caution in renal insufficiency, volume depletion. Chronic use may produce or worsen constipation. Avoid constipation with symptomatic CAD. May increase bleeding tendency due to vitamin K deficiency. Serum or red cell folate reduced with chronic use. Constipation may aggravate hemorrhoids. Light formulation contains phenylalanine. Measure cholesterol during 1st few months; periodically thereafter. Measure TG periodically.

ADVERSE REACTIONS: Constipation, heartburn, nausea, vomiting, abdominal pain, flatulence, diarrhea, anorexia, osteoporosis, rash, hyperchloremic acidosis (children), vitamin A and D deficiency, steatorrhea, hypoprothrombinemia (vitamin K deficiency).

INTERACTIONS: May interfere with absorption of fat-soluble vitamins (A, D, E, K), drugs that undergo enterohepatic circulation, and oral phosphate supplements. Take concomitant drugs 1hr before or 4-6 hrs after. Additive effects with HMG-CoA reductase inhibitors and nicotinic acid. Caution with spironolactone. May reduce or delay absorption of phenylbutazone, warfarin, thiazide diuretics, propranolol, tetracycline, penicillin G, phenobarbital, thyroid and thyroxine agents, estrogens, progestins, digitalis.

PREGNANCY: Category C, caution in nursing.

Quinidine Gluconate Injection RX
quinidine gluconate (Various)

THERAPEUTIC CLASS: Class IA antiarrhythmic/schizonticide antimalarial

INDICATIONS: Treatment of life-threatening Plasmodium flacipurum malaria. Conversion of atrial fibrillation/flutter (A-Fib/Flutter) to normal sinus rhythm. Treatment of ventricular arrhythmias.

DOSAGE: *Adults:* Malaria: LD: 15mg/kg base (24mg/kg gluconate) over 4 hrs. Maint: After 8 hrs, 7.5mg/kg (12mg/kg gluconate) IV q8h for 7 days. Alternate: Initial: 6.25mg/kg base (10mg/kg/min gluconate) IV over 1-2 hrs. Maint: 12.5mcg/kg/min base (20mcg/kg/min gluconate) for 72h. Switch to PO therapy when possible. A-Fib/Flutter and Ventricular Arrhythmia: 0.25mg/kg/minute. Max: 5-10mg/kg. Consider alternate therapy if conversion to sinus rhythm not achieved. Renal/Hepatic Impairment or CHF: Reduce dose. Elderly: Start at low end of dosing range.

Pediatrics: Malaria: LD: 15mg/kg base (24mg/kg gluconate) over 4 hrs. Maint: After 8 hrs, 7.5mg/kg (12mg/kg gluconate) IV q8h for 7 days. Alternate: Initial: 6.25mg/kg base (10mg/kg/min gluconate) IV over 1-2 hrs. Maint: 12.5mcg/kg/min base (20mcg/kg/min gluconate) for 72h. Switch to PO therapy when possible.

HOW SUPPLIED: Inj: 80mg/mL

CONTRAINDICATIONS: Cardiac rhythm dependent upon a junctional or idioventricular pacemaker (absent of functioning pacemaker), thrombocytopenic purpura with previous treatment, patients adversely affected by anticholinergics (eg, myasthenia gravis).

WARNINGS/PRECAUTIONS: Rapid infusion can cause peripheral vascular collapse and hypotension. May prolong QTc interval. Paradoxical increase in ventricular rate in A-Fib/Flutter. Caution in those at risk of complete AV block without implanted pacemakers, renal/hepatic dysfunction, elderly, and CHF. Physical/pharmacologic maneuvers to terminate paroxysmal supraventricular tachycardia may be ineffective. Exacerbated bradycardia in sick sinus syndrome.

ADVERSE REACTIONS: GI distress, lightheadedness, fatigue, palpitations, weakness, visual problems, nausea, vomiting, diarrhea, sleep disturbances, rash, headache, cinchonism, hepatotoxicity, autoimmune/inflammatory syndromes.

INTERACTIONS: Urine alkalinizers (eg, carbonic anhydrase inhibitors, sodium bicarbonate, thiazide diuretics) reduce renal elimination. CYP3A4 inducers (eg, phenobarbital, phenytoin, rifampin) may accelerate elimination. Verapamil, diltiazem decrease clearance. Caution with drugs metabolized by CYP2D6 (eg, mexiletine, phenothiazines, polycyclic antidepressants, codeine, hydrocodone) or by CYP3A4 (eg, nifedipine, felodipine, nicardipine, nimodipine). β-blockers may decrease clearance. May slow metabolism of nifedipine. Increases levels of digoxin, digitoxin, procainamide and haloperidol. Increased levels with ketoconazole, amiodarone, cimetidine. Potentiates warfarin, depolarizing and nondepolarizing neuromuscular blockers. Additive effects with anticholinergics, vasodilators, and negative inotropes. Antagonistic effects with cholinergics, vasoconstrictors, and positive inotropes.

PREGNANCY: Category C, not for use in nursing.

QUIXIN
levofloxacin (Vistakon)

RX

THERAPEUTIC CLASS: Fluoroquinolone

INDICATIONS: Treatment of bacterial conjunctivitis.

DOSAGE: *Adults:* Days 1-2: 1-2 drops q2h while awake, up to 8x/day. Days 3-7: 1-2 drops q4h while awake, up to qid.
Pediatrics: ≥1 yr: Days 1-2: 1-2 drops q2h while awake, up to 8x/day. Days 3-7: 1-2 drops q4h while awake, up to qid.

HOW SUPPLIED: Sol: 0.5% (5mL)

WARNINGS/PRECAUTIONS: Discontinue if hypersensitivity or superinfection occurs. Avoid contact lenses with conjunctivitis.

ADVERSE REACTIONS: Transient ocular burning, decreased vision, fever, foreign body sensation, headache, ocular pain, pharyngitis, photophobia.

INTERACTIONS: Systemic quinolone therapy may increase theophylline levels, interfere with caffeine metabolism, enhance warfarin effects, and elevate serum creatinine with cyclosporine.

PREGNANCY: Category C, caution in nursing.

QVAR
beclomethasone dipropionate (Ivax)

RX

THERAPEUTIC CLASS: Corticosteroid

INDICATIONS: Maintenance treatment of asthma as prophylactic therapy in patients ≥5 tears; to reduce or eliminate the need for oral corticosteroidal therapy.

DOSAGE: *Adults:* Previous Bronchodilator Only: 40-80mcg bid. Max: 320mcg bid. Previous Inhaled Corticosteroid Therapy: 40-160mcg bid. Max: 320mcg bid. Maint With Oral Corticosteroids: May attempt gradual reduction of oral dose after 1 week on inhaled therapy.
Pediatrics: Adolescents: Previous Bronchodilator Only: 40-80mcg bid. Max: 320mcg bid. Previous Inhaled Corticosteroid Therapy: 40-160mcg bid. Max: 320mcg bid. 5-11 yrs: Previous Bronchodilator Only or Inhaled Corticosteroid Therapy: 40mcg bid. Max: 80mcg bid. ≥5 yrs: Maint With Oral Corticosteroids: May attempt gradual reduction of oral dose after 1 week on inhaled therapy.

HOW SUPPLIED: MDI: 40mcg/inh, 80mcg/inh (7.3g)

CONTRAINDICATIONS: Status asthmaticus, acute asthmatic attacks.

WARNINGS/PRECAUTIONS: Deaths due to adrenal insufficiency have occurred with transfer from systemic corticosteroids to inhaled corticosteroids. Resume oral corticosteroids during stress or severe asthma attack. Risk of adrenal insufficiency and withdrawal symptoms when replacing systemic corticosteroids. May unmask allergic conditions previously suppressed by systemic steroid therapy. Caution with TB, ocular herpes simplex, or untreated systemic bacterial, fungal, parasitic or viral infections. May suppress growth in children. Exposure to chickenpox or measles requires prophylaxis treatment. Not for rapid relief of bronchospasm.

ADVERSE REACTIONS: Headache, pharyngitis, upper respiratory tract infection, rhinitis, increased asthma symptoms, sinusitis.

PREGNANCY: Category C, not for use in nursing.

RAPAMUNE
sirolimus (Wyeth)

RX

> Increased susceptibility to infection and development of lymphoma.

THERAPEUTIC CLASS: Macrocyclic lactone immunosuppressant

Rebetol

INDICATIONS: Prophylaxis of organ rejection in renal transplant patients. Recommended to be used initially with cyclosporine and corticosteroids. In low-moderate risk patients, withdraw cyclosporine 2-4 months after transplantation and increase sirolimus dose to reach recommended blood levels.

DOSAGE: *Adults:* LD: 6mg. Maint: 2mg qd. Hepatic Impairment: Reduce maintenance dose by one-third.

Pediatrics: ≥13 yrs and <40kg: LD: 3mg/m^2 Maint: 1mg/m^2/day. Hepatic Impairment: Reduce maintenance dose by one-third. Take 4 hrs after cyclosporine.

HOW SUPPLIED: Sol: 1mg/mL (60mL); Tab: 1mg, 2mg

WARNINGS/PRECAUTIONS: Increased cholesterol and triglycerides that may require treatment. Reduction in renal function due to long-term concomitant cyclosporine. Increased risk of lymphocele. Provide 1 year prophylaxis for *pneumocystis carinii* pneumonia and 3 months for cytomegalovirus after transplant. Limit exposure to sunlight and UV light. Not for use in liver or lung transplants. Interstitial lung disease reported. Increased susceptability to infection and the possible development of lymphoma and malignancy, especially of the skin, may result from immnosupression. Avoid in liver or lung transplant patients. Increased risk of angioedema, caution with concomitant use of angioedema-causing drugs, such as ACEI.

ADVERSE REACTIONS: Hypercholesterolemia, hyperlipemia, HTN, rash, acne, anemia, leukopenia, arthralgia, diarrhea, hypokalemia, thrombocytopenia, fever, abdominal pain, headache, constipation, creatinine increase, arthralgia, insomnia, dyspnea, upper respiratory infection, anaphylactic/anaphylactoid reactions, angioedema, hypersensitivity vasculitis.

INTERACTIONS: Increased levels with diltiazem. CYP3A4 inhibitors (eg, calcium channel blockers, antifungals, macrolide antibiotics) may increase levels of sirolimus, while CYP3A4 inducers (eg, anticonvulsants, rifabutin, St. John's wort) may decrease levels. Avoid live vaccines, grapefruit juice, rifampin, ketoconazole. Caution with other nephrotoxic drugs (eg, aminoglycosides, amphotericin B). Hepatic artery thrombosis reported with cyclosporine or tacrolimus, and increased death rate and graft loss with tacrolimus in liver transplant patients. Bronchial anastomotic dehiscence reported with immunosupressives in lung transplant patients. Cyclosporine is a substrate and inhibitor of CYP3A4 and P-gp. Caution with dosing. Monitor for rhabdomyolysis with cyclosporine and HMG Co-A reductase inhibitors/fibrates. Monitor renal function with cyclosporine. Grapefruit juice reduces CYP3A4 medicated drug metabolism, should not be administered with rapamune or used for dilution. Increased risk of deterioration of renal function, serum lipid abnormalities, and urinary tract infections with calcineurin inhibitors and corticosteriods.

PREGNANCY: Category C, not for use in nursing.

Rebetol
ribavirin (Schering)

RX

> Not for monotherapy treatment of chronic hepatitis C. Primary toxicity is hemolytic anemia. Avoid with significant or unstable cardiac disease. Contraindicated in pregnancy and male partners of pregnant women. Use 2 forms of contraception during therapy and for 6 months after discontinuation.

THERAPEUTIC CLASS: Nucleoside analogue

INDICATIONS: In combination with Intron A® for treatment of chronic hepatitis C in patients ≥3 yrs with compensated liver disease previously untreated with alpha interferon or in patients ≥18 yrs who relapsed after alpha interferon therapy. In combination with Peg-Intron® for treatment of chronic hepatitis C in patients ≥18 yrs with compensated liver disease previously untreated with interferon alpha.

DOSAGE: *Adults:* ≥18 yrs: With Intron A: ≤75kg: 400mg qam and 600mg qpm. >75kg: 600mg qam and 600mg qpm. Treat for 24-48 weeks interferon-naive; 24 weeks in relapse. With PEG-INTRON: 400mg bid, qam and qpm with food. Reduce to 600mg qd if Hgb <10g/dL with no cardiac history, or if Hgb decreases by ≥2g/dL during a 4 week-period with a cardiac history. D/C if Hgb <8.5g/L with no cardiac history or if Hgb <12g/dL after 4 weeks of dose reduction with a cardiac history. CrCl <50mL/min: Avoid use.

Pediatrics: ≥3 yrs: 15mg/kg/day in divided doses qam and qpm. Use sol if ≤25kg or cannot swallow caps. With Intron A: 25-36kg: 200mg bid, qam and qpm. 37-49kg: 200mg qam and 400mg qpm. 50-61kg: 400mg bid, qam and qpm. >61kg: Dose as adult. Genotype 1: Treat for 48 weeks. Genotype 2/3: Treat for 24 weeks.

HOW SUPPLIED: Cap: 200mg; Sol: 40mg/mL (120mL)

CONTRAINDICATIONS: Pregnancy, male partners of pregnant women, hemoglobinopathies (eg, thalassemia major, sickle cell anemia). When used with Intron A or PEG-Intron, refer to the individual monograph.

WARNINGS/PRECAUTIONS: Severe depression, suicidal ideation, bone marrow suppression, autoimmune and infectious disorders, pulmonary dysfunction, pancreatitis, and DM reported. Assess for underlying cardiac disease (obtain EKG); fatal and nonfatal MI reported with anemia. Hemolytic anemia reported; monitor Hgb or Hct initially then at Week 2 and 4 (or more if needed) of therapy. Suspend therapy if symptoms of pancreatitis arise. Avoid if CrCl <50mL/min. Obtain negative pregnancy test prior to initiation then monthly, and for 6 months post-therapy.

ADVERSE REACTIONS: Hemolytic anemia, headache, fatigue, rigors, fever, nausea, anorexia, myalgia, arthralgia, insomnia, irritability, depression, dyspnea, alopecia.

INTERACTIONS: Dental and periodontal disorders reported with interferon or peginterferon combination therapy.

PREGNANCY: Category X, not for use in nursing.

Recombivax HB
hepatitis B (recombinant) (Merck)

RX

OTHER BRAND NAMES: Recombivax HB Adult (Merck) - Recombivax HB Dialysis (Merck) - Recombivax HB Pediatric/Adolescent (Merck)

THERAPEUTIC CLASS: Vaccine

INDICATIONS: Vaccination against hepatitis B virus.

DOSAGE: *Adults:* Give IM into deltoid muscle. Give SQ if risk of hemorrhage. ≥20 yrs: 3-Dose Regimen: 10mcg at 0,1,6 months. Predialysis/Dialysis (Dialysis Formulation): 40mcg at 0,1,6, months; consider booster if anti-HBs level <10MIU/mL.

Pediatrics: Give IM into anterolateral thigh in infants/young children. Give SQ if risk of hemorrhage. 0-19 yrs: 3-Dose Regimen (Pediatric/Adolescent Formulation) 5mcg at 0,1,6 months. 11-15 yrs: 2-Dose Regimen (Adult Formulation): 10mcg 1st dose, 10mcg 4-6 months later. Infants Born to HBsAg Positive/Unknown Status Mothers: Give 3-dose regimen vaccine and 0.5mL HBIG in opposite anterolateral thigh.

HOW SUPPLIED: Inj: (Pediatric/Adolescent-Preservative Free) 5mcg/0.5mL, (Adult) 10mcg/mL, (Dialysis) 40mcg/mL

CONTRAINDICATIONS: Yeast hypersensitivity.

WARNINGS/PRECAUTIONS: Do not continue therapy if hypersensitivity occurs after injection. May not prevent hepatitis B with unrecognized infection. Caution with severely compromised cardiopulmonary status and those where febrile or systemic reaction is a significant risk. May delay use with serious active infection (eg, febrile illness). Have epinephrine available. Do not give intradermally or IV.

ADVERSE REACTIONS: Irritability, fever, diarrhea, fatigue/weakness, diminished appetite, rhinitis, injection site reactions.

PREGNANCY: Category C, caution in nursing.

Regranex
becaplermin (Ortho-McNeil)

RX

THERAPEUTIC CLASS: Platelet-derived growth factor (recombinant human)

INDICATIONS: Treatment of lower extremity diabetic neuropathic ulcers that extend into the subcutaneous tissue or beyond and have an adequate blood supply.

DOSAGE: *Adults:* Amount applied will vary depending on ulcer size. Measure the greatest length by the greatest width of the ulcer to determine amount of gel to apply. To calculate in inches: (For 15g or 7.5g tube) length x width x 0.6; (For 2g tube) length x width x 1.3. To calculate in centimeters: (For 15g or 7.5g tube) length x width/4; (For 2g

RELENZA

tube) length x width/2. Adjust amount weekly or biweekly depending on the change in ulcer area. Squeeze gel onto clean measuring surface (eg, wax paper), then apply to ulcer with an application aid. Apply 1/16 of an inch thickness over entire ulcer area qd, then cover with moist saline dressing for 12 hrs. Remove dressing, rinse off residual gel with saline or water and cover again with moist saline dressing for 12 hrs and repeat. Reassess if ulcer does not decrease by 30% after 10 weeks or is not completely healed in 20 weeks.

Pediatrics: ≥16 yrs: Amount applied will vary depending on ulcer size. Measure the greatest length by the greatest width of the ulcer to determine amount of gel to apply. To calculate in inches: (For 15g or 7.5g tube) length x width x 0.6; (For 2g tube) length x width x 1.3. To calculate in centimeters: (For 15g or 7.5g tube) length x width/4; (For 2g tube) length x width/2. Adjust amount weekly or biweekly depending on the change in ulcer area. Squeeze gel onto clean measuring surface (eg, wax paper), then apply to ulcer with an application aid. Apply 1/16 of an inch thickness over entire ulcer area qd, then cover with moist saline dressing for 12 hrs. Remove dressing, rinse off residual gel with saline or water and cover again with moist saline dressing for 12 hrs and repeat. Reassess if ulcer does not decrease by 30% after 10 weeks or is not completely healed in 20 weeks.

HOW SUPPLIED: Gel: 0.01% (15g)

CONTRAINDICATIONS: Known neoplasm at application site.

WARNINGS/PRECAUTIONS: Do not use in wounds that close by primary intention.

ADVERSE REACTIONS: Erythematous rash.

PREGNANCY: Category C, caution in nursing.

RELENZA RX
zanamivir (GlaxoSmithKline)

THERAPEUTIC CLASS: Neuraminidase inhibitor

INDICATIONS: Treatment of uncomplicated acute illness due to influenza A and B virus in patients symptomatic for ≤2 days. Prophylaxis of influenza.

DOSAGE: *Adults:* Treatment: Usual: 2 inh (10mg) q12h for 5 days. Take 2 doses at least 2 hrs apart on 1st day. Prophylaxis: Household Setting: 2 inh (10mg) qd for 10 days. Community Setting: 2 inh (10mg) qd for 28 days. Administer at same time every day.

Pediatrics: Treatment: ≥7 yrs: Usual: 2 inh (10mg) q12h for 5 days. Take 2 doses at least 2 hrs apart on 1st day. Prophylaxis: ≥5 yrs: Household Setting: 2 inh (10mg) qd for 10 days. Community Setting: 2 inh (10mg) qd for 28 days. Administer at same time every day.

HOW SUPPLIED: Inh: 5mg/inh (20 blisters)

WARNINGS/PRECAUTIONS: Not recommended for use with underlying airways disease (eg, asthma, COPD). Serious cases of bronchospasm have been reported during treatment; d/c in any patient if bronchospasm or decline in respiratory function develops. D/C if allergic reaction occurs.

ADVERSE REACTIONS: Dizziness, headaches, diarrhea, nausea, sinusitis, bronchitis, cough, ear/nose/throat infections, nasal symptoms.

INTERACTIONS: Use inhaled bronchodilator before zanamivir.

PREGNANCY: Category C, caution in nursing

REMICADE RX
infliximab (Centocor)

> Reports of TB, invasive fungal infections, and other opportunistic infections. Evaluate for latent TB and treat if necessary prior to initiation of therapy.

THERAPEUTIC CLASS: Monoclonal antibody/TNF-alpha receptor blocker

INDICATIONS: In combination with methotrexate (MTX), for reducing signs/symptoms, inhibiting structural damage progression and improving physical function in moderately to severely active rheumatoid arthritis (RA). For reducing signs/symptoms and inducing and maintaining clinical remission of moderately to severely active Crohn's disease, when response to conventional therapy is inadequate. For reducing the number of draining enterocutaneous and rectovaginal fistulas and maintaining fistula closure in fistulizing Crohn's disease. For reducing signs/symptoms in patients with active ankylosing spondylitis (AS). For reducing signs/symptoms of active arthritis, inhibiting structural damage progression, and improving physical function in patients with psoriatic arthritis. For reducing signs/symptoms, inducing and maintaining clinical remission and mucosal healing, and eliminating corticosteroid use in patients with moderately to severely active ulcerative colitis (UC) who have inadequate response to conventional therapy. Treatment of patients with chronic, severe plaque psoriasis who are candidates for systemic therapy and when other systemic therapies are medically less appropriate.

DOSAGE: *Adults:* RA (Combo with MTX): 3mg/kg as IV infusion; repeat at 2 and 6 weeks. Maint: 3mg/kg every 8 weeks. Incomplete Response: May increase to 10mg/kg or give every 4 weeks. Crohn's Disease/Fistulizing Crohn's Disease: Induction Regimen: 5mg/kg IV at 0, 2, and 6 weeks. Maint: 5mg/kg every 8 weeks. For patients who respond then lose their response, may increase to 10mg/kg. Consider discontinuing therapy if no response to by Week 14. Ankylosing Spondylitis: 5mg/kg as IV infusion; repeat at 2 and 6 weeks. Maint: 5mg/kg every 6 weeks. Psoriatic Arthritis: 5mg/kg as IV infusion; repeat at 2 and 6 weeks. Maint: 5mg/kg every 8 weeks. May be used with or without MTX. Ulcerative Colitis: 5mg/kg at 0, 2, and 6 weeks. Maint: 5mg/kg every 8 weeks. Plaque Psoriasis: 5mg/kg IV infusion; repeat at 2 and 6 weeks. Maint: 5mg/kg every 8 weeks.

Pediatrics: ≥6 yrs: Crohn's Disease: Induction Regimen: 5mg/kg IV at 0, 2, and 6 weeks. Maint: 5mg/kg every 8 weeks.

HOW SUPPLIED: Inj: 100mg

CONTRAINDICATIONS: Hypersensitivity to murine proteins. Moderate or severe CHF (NYHA Class III/IV) with doses >5mg/kg.

WARNINGS/PRECAUTIONS: Leukopenia, neutropenia, thrombocytopenia, and pancytopenia reported. Serious infections, including sepsis and pneumonia, reported. Avoid with active infection. Monitor for signs of infection during and after therapy; d/c if serious infection develops. Caution in patients who have resided in areas where histoplasmosis or coccidioidomycosis are endemic. Hypersensitivity reactions reported. Caution with optic neuritis, chronic and recurrent infections, CNS demyelinating disease (eg, MS) and seizure disorder. May result in autoantibody formation; d/c if lupus-like syndrome develops. Monitor closely and discontinue if new or worsening symptoms of heart failure appear. Lymphoma reported; caution with malignancies. Severe hepatic reactions, including acute liver failure, jaundice, hepatitis and cholestasis have been reported rarely. Caution in elderly.

ADVERSE REACTIONS: Nausea, infections, infusion reactions, headache, sinusitis, pharyngitis, coughing, abdominal pain, diarrhea, bronchitis, dyspepsia, fatigue, rhinitis, pain, arthralgia, hepatotoxicity.

INTERACTIONS: Do not give concurrently with live vaccines. May increase risk of serious infections and neutropenia with anakinra.

PREGNANCY: Category B, not for use in nursing.

RESCRIPTOR
delavirdine mesylate (Pfizer)

RX

THERAPEUTIC CLASS: Non-nucleoside reverse transcriptase inhibitor

INDICATIONS: Treatment of HIV-1 infection in combination with other antiretrovirals.

DOSAGE: *Adults:* Usual: 400mg tid. May disperse 100mg tab in ≥3 oz of water (200mg tab is not dispersible). Take with acidic beverage (eg, orange juice) if achlorhydria.

Pediatrics: ≥16yrs: Usual: 400mg tid. May disperse 100mg tab in at least 3 oz of water (200mg tab is not dispersible). Take with acidic beverage (eg, orange juice) if achlorhydria.

HOW SUPPLIED: Tab: 100mg, 200mg

CONTRAINDICATIONS: Contraindicated with drugs that are highly dependent on CYP3A for clearance (eg, astemizole, terfenadine, dihdroergotamine, egonovine, ergotamine, methylergonovine, cisapride, pimozide, alprazolam, midazolam, triazolam).

RESTASIS

WARNINGS/PRECAUTIONS: Caution with hepatic dysfunction. D/C if severe rash develops. May cause immune reconstitution syndrome. May confer cross-resistance to other NNRTIs. May cause body fat redistribution/accumulation.

ADVERSE REACTIONS: Headache, fatigue, nausea, diarrhea, vomiting, increased ALT and AST, rash, maculopapular rash, pruritus, erythema, insomnia, upper respiratory infection.

INTERACTIONS: See Contraindications. Antacids decrease absorption; separate doses by 1 hr. H_2 antagonists reduce absorption; avoid chronic use. CYP3A inducers (eg, carbamazepine, phenobarbital, phenytoin, rifabutin, rifampin) may decrease plasma levels; avoid concomitant use. Increased plasma levels of drugs metabolized by CYP3A and 2C9 and amprenavir. Certain nonsedating antihistamines, sedative hypnotics, antiarrhythmics, calcium channel blockers, ergot agents, amphetamines, cisapride, and sildenafil (max of 25mg/48hrs of sildenafil) may result in potentially serious and/or life-threatening adverse events. Reduced effects of both delavirdine and didanosine; separate doses by 1 hr. Monitor LFTs with saquinavir. Increases indinavir plasma levels; reduce indinavir dose to 600mg tid.

PREGNANCY: Category C, not for use in nursing.

RESTASIS RX
cyclosporine (Allergan)

THERAPEUTIC CLASS: Topical immunomodulator

INDICATIONS: To increase tear production in patients with suppressed tear production due to ocular inflammation associated with keratoconjunctivitis sicca.

DOSAGE: *Adults:* 1 drop bid, q12h. Concomitant Artificial Tears: Space by 15 minutes. *Pediatrics:* ≥16 yrs: 1 drop bid, q12h. Concomitant Artificial Tears: Space by 15 minutes.

HOW SUPPLIED: Emul: 0.05% (0.4mL 32^s)

CONTRAINDICATIONS: Active ocular infections.

WARNINGS/PRECAUTIONS: Not studied in patients with a history of herpes keratitis. Not to be given while wearing contact lenses; lenses may be reinserted 15 minutes following administration.

ADVERSE REACTIONS: Ocular burning, conjunctival hyperemia, discharge, epiphora, eye pain, foreign body sensation, pruritus, stinging, visual disturbance (eg, blurring).

PREGNANCY: Category C, caution in nursing

RETIN-A RX
tretinoin (Ortho Neutrogena)

OTHER BRAND NAME: Retin-A Micro (Ortho Neutrogena)

THERAPEUTIC CLASS: Retinoic acid derivative

INDICATIONS: Topical treatment of acne vulgaris.

DOSAGE: *Adults:* Cleanse area thoroughly, then apply qhs. May temporarily d/c or reduce dosing frequency if irritation occurs.
Pediatrics: ≥12 yrs: (Gel 0.04%, 0.1%) Cleanse area thoroughly, then apply qhs. May temporarily d/c or reduce dosing frequency if irritation occurs.

HOW SUPPLIED: (Retin-A) Cre: 0.025%, 0.05%, 0.1% (20g, 45g); Gel: 0.01%, 0.025% (15g, 45g); Sol: 0.05% (28mL); (Retin-A Micro) Gel: 0.04%, 0.1% (20g, 45g)

WARNINGS/PRECAUTIONS: Avoid eyes, lips, paranasal creases, mucous membranes, and sunburned skin. Acne exacerbation during 1st weeks of therapy may occur. D/C if sensitivity or irritation occurs. Severe irritation with eczematous skin. Causes photosensitivity. Extreme weather (eg, cold, wind) may irritate skin.

ADVERSE REACTIONS: Local skin reactions (red, edematous, blistered, crusted), photosensitivity, temporary skin pigmentation changes.

INTERACTIONS: Caution with topical agents with strong drying effects, high concentration of alcohol, astringents, spices, or lime. Caution with sulfur, resorcinol, or salicylic acid, allow effects of these agents to subside before application of tretinoin.

PREGNANCY: Category C, caution in nursing.

Retrovir
zidovudine (GlaxoSmithKline)

RX

> Associated with hematologic toxicity (eg, neutropenia, severe anemia), especially with advanced HIV disease. Prolonged use associated with symptomatic myopathy. Lactic acidosis and severe, possibly fatal hepatomegaly with steatosis reported.

THERAPEUTIC CLASS: Nucleoside analogue

INDICATIONS: Treatment of HIV infection in combination with other antiretrovirals. Prevention of maternal-fetal HIV transmission.

DOSAGE: *Adults:* (Tab) 600mg/day in divided doses. (Inj) 1mg/kg IV over 1 hr 5-6 times/day. Prevention of Maternal-Fetal HIV Transmission: >14 weeks pregnancy: 100mg PO five times/day until start of labor. During labor and delivery: 2mg/kg IV over 1 hr followed by 1mg/kg/hr IV infusion until clamping of umbilical cord. End-Stage Renal Disease/Dialysis: 100mg PO q6-8h or 1mg/kg IV q6-8h. Significant Anemia/Neutropenia: May require dose interruption and adjunctive epoetin therapy. Less Severe Anemia/Neutropenia: Reduce daily dose.

Pediatrics: 6 weeks-12 yrs: 160mg/m^2 PO q8h. Max: 200mg PO q8h. Prevention of Maternal-Fetal HIV Transmission: Neonates: 2mg/kg PO q6h (or 1.5mg/kg IV over 30 min q6h) starting within 12 hrs after birth and continue through 6 weeks of age. End-Stage Renal Disease/Dialysis: 100mg PO q6-8h or 1mg/kg IV q6-8h. Significant Anemia/Neutropenia: May require dose interruption and adjunctive epoetin therapy. Pronounced Anemia: Reduce daily dose. Mild to Moderate Hepatic Impairment: Monitor for hematologic toxicity and reduce dose if needed.

HOW SUPPLIED: Cap: 100mg; Inj: 10mg/mL; Syrup: 50mg/5mL (240mL); Tab: 300mg

WARNINGS/PRECAUTIONS: Adverse reactions increase with disease progression. Caution with compromised bone marrow or in elderly. Monitor for hematologic toxicity; reduce dose or stop therapy. Myopathy and myositis with pathological changes associated with prolonged use. Caution with obesity and liver disease; increased risk of lactic acidosis and hepatomegaly with steatosis. Increased risk of toxicity with prolonged exposure to nucleosides, in women, obesity, advanced HIV disease, severe hepatic impairment. Possible redistribution or accumulation of body fat. Hepatic decompensation has occurred in HIV/HCV co-infected patients receiving combination antiretroviral therapy for HIV and interferon alfa with or without ribavirin; monitor for treatment associated toxicities. Immune reconstitution syndrome has been reported with combination antiretroviral therapy.

ADVERSE REACTIONS: Headache, nausea, malaise, anorexia, vomiting, asthenia, constipation, anemia, neutropenia.

INTERACTIONS: Increased risk of hematologic toxicities with ganciclovir, interferon-alpha, bone marrow suppressives and cytotoxic drugs. Possible increased levels with phenytoin, atovaquone, fluconazole, methadone, probenecid, valproic acid. Possible decreased levels with nelfinavir, ritonavir, rifampin. Avoid with stavudine, ribavirin, doxorubicin, other combination products containing zidovudine. Prolonged exposure to antiretroviral nucleoside analogues increases risk of lactic acidosis and hepatomegaly with steatosis. May decrease phenytoin levels.

PREGNANCY: Category C, not for use in nursing.

Rhinocort Aqua
budesonide (AstraZeneca LP)

RX

THERAPEUTIC CLASS: Corticosteroid

INDICATIONS: Management of seasonal or perennial allergic rhinitis.

DOSAGE: *Adults:* 1 spray per nostril qd. Max: 4 sprays/nostril/day.

Pediatrics: ≥6 yrs: 1 spray per nostril qd. Max: 6-12 yrs: 2 sprays/nostril/day. >12 yrs: 4 sprays/nostril/day.

HOW SUPPLIED: Spray: 32mcg/spray (8.6g)

WARNINGS/PRECAUTIONS: Risk of adrenal insufficiency and withdrawal symptoms when replacing systemic corticosteroids with a topical corticosteroids. Caution with active or quiescent TB, ocular herpes simplex, or untreated bacterial, fungal and systemic viral infections. Avoid with recent nasal trauma, surgery or septum ulcers. Risk for more severe/fatal course of infections (eg, chickenpox, measles) and for *Candida* infections of the nose and pharynx. Potential for growth velocity reduction in pediatrics.

ADVERSE REACTIONS: Nasal irritation, pharyngitis, cough, epistaxis.

INTERACTIONS: Oral ketoconazole and cimetidine increase plasma levels. CYP3A inhibitors (eg, itraconazole, clarithromycin, erythromycin) may decrease metabolism and increase systemic exposure. Concomitant systemic corticosteroids increases risk of hypercorticism and/or HPA axis suppression.

PREGNANCY: Category B, caution in nursing.

RIFADIN RX
rifampin (Sanofi-Aventis)

THERAPEUTIC CLASS: Rifamycin derivative

INDICATIONS: Treatment of all forms of tuberculosis (TB). Treatment of asymptomatic carriers of *Neisseria meningitidis* to eliminate meningococci from the nasopharynx.

DOSAGE: *Adults:* TB: 10mg/kg PO/IV qd. Max: 600mg/day. Meningococcal Carriers: 600mg bid for 2 days. Take 1 hr before or 2 hrs after a meal with a full glass of water.

Pediatrics: TB: 10-20mg/kg PO/IV qd. Max: 600mg/day. Meningococcal Carriers: ≥1 month: 10mg/kg q12h for 2 days. Max: 600mg/dose. <1 month: 5mg/kg q12h for 2 days. Take 1 hr before or 2 hrs after a meal with a full glass of water.

HOW SUPPLIED: Cap: 150mg, 300mg; Inj: 600mg

WARNINGS/PRECAUTIONS: May produce liver dysfunction. May cause hyperbilirubinemia. Not for treatment of meningococcal disease. May produce reddish coloration of the urine, sweat, sputum, and tears. May permanently stain soft contact lenses.

ADVERSE REACTIONS: GI distress, thrombocytopenia, visual disturbances, menstrual disturbances, edema of face and extremities, elevated BUN and serum uric acid levels.

INTERACTIONS: May accelerate elimination of drugs metabolized by CYP450 (eg, anticonvulsants, antiarrhythmics, anticoagulants, azole antifungals, barbiturates, β-blockers, calcium channel blockers, chloramphenicol, clarithromycin, corticosteroids, cyclosporine, cardiac glycosides, clofibrate, oral or systemic contraceptives, dapsone, diazepam, doxycycline, fluoroquinolones, haloperidol, oral hypoglycemics, levothyroxine, methadone, narcotics, nortriptyline, progestins, quinine, tacrolimus, theophylline, TCAs, and zidovudine). Give antacids at least 1 hr before rifampin. Increased hepatotoxicity with halothane or isoniazid. Increased serum levels with probenecid and cotrimoxazole. Caution with other hepatotoxic agents. Concomitant ketoconazole decreases both drug serum levels. Decreased levels of enalapril, atovaquone. Increased levels with atovaquone.

PREGNANCY: Category C, not for use in nursing.

RIFATER RX
rifampin - isoniazid - pyrazinamide (Sanofi-Aventis)

> Isoniazid associated with severe and sometimes fatal hepatitis. Monitor LFTs on a monthly basis.

THERAPEUTIC CLASS: Isonicotinic acid hydrazide/rifamycin derivative/nicotinamide analogue

INDICATIONS: For initial phase of pulmonary tuberculosis treatment.

DOSAGE: *Adults:* ≤44kg: 4 tabs single dose qd. 45-54kg: 5 tabs single dose. ≥55kg: 6 tabs single dose. Give pyridoxine in malnourished, if predisposed to neuropathy (eg, alcoholics, diabetics), and adolescents. Take 1 hr before or 2 hrs after meals with full glass of water. Treatment usually lasts 2 months.

Pediatrics: ≥15 yrs: ≤44kg: 4 tabs single dose qd. 45-54kg: 5 tabs qd single dose. ≥55kg: 6 tabs qd single dose. Give pyridoxine in malnourished, if predisposed to neuropathy (eg, alcoholics, diabetics), and adolescents. Take 1 hr before or 2 hrs after meals with full glass of water. Treatment usually lasts 2 months.

HOW SUPPLIED: Tab: (Isoniazid-Pyrazinamide-Rifampin) 50mg-300mg-120mg

CONTRAINDICATIONS: Severe hepatic damage, adverse reactions to isoniazid (eg, drug fever, chills, arthritis), acute liver disease, acute gout.

WARNINGS/PRECAUTIONS: Liver dysfunction, hyperbilirubinemia, and hyperuricemia with acute gouty arthritis reported. Monitor LFTs (every 2-4 weeks), serum uric acid. Perform regular ophthalmologic exams. Caution with DM, severe renal dysfunction. May produce reddish coloration of urine, sweat, sputum, and tears. May permanently stain soft contact lenses.

ADVERSE REACTIONS: GI effects, cutaneous reactions, musculoskeletal pain, hepatitis, CNS and cardiorespiratory effects.

INTERACTIONS: Rifampin may accelerate metabolism of anticonvulsants (eg, phenytoin), antiarrhythmics (eg, disopyramide, mexiletine, quinidine, tocainide), anticoagulants, antifungals (eg, fluconazole, itraconazole, ketoconazole), barbiturates, β-blockers, calcium channel blockers (eg, diltiazem, nifedipine, verapamil), chloramphenicol, ciprofloxacin, corticosteroids, cyclosporine, cardiac glycosides, clofibrate, oral contraceptives, dapsone, diazepam, haloperidol, oral hypoglycemics (eg, sulfonylureas), methadone, narcotic analgesics, nortriptyline, progestins, theophylline. Antacids may reduce rifampin absorption. Avoid foods containing tyramine and histamine (eg, cheese, red wine, tuna). Anticoagulants may need dose increase. Higher incidence of isoniazid hepatitis with daily alcohol ingestion. Avoid halothane. INH inhibits certain CYP450 enzymes; monitor with anticonvulsants, benzodiazepines, haloperidol, ketoconazole, warfarin. Decreased levels with corticosteroids. Exaggerates CNS effects of meperidine, cycloserine, disulfiram. Excess catecholamine stimulation with L-dopa.

PREGNANCY: Category C, not for use in nursing.

RISPERDAL RX
risperidone (Janssen)

> Elderly patients with dementia-related psychosis treated with atypical antipsychotic drugs are at an increased risk of death; most appeared to be cardiovascular (eg, heart failure, sudden death) or infectious (eg, pneumonia) in nature. Risperidone is not approved for the treatment of patients with dementia-related psychosis.

OTHER BRAND NAME: Risperdal M-Tab (Janssen)

THERAPEUTIC CLASS: Benzisoxazole derivative

INDICATIONS: Treatment of schizophrenia. Short-term treatment of acute manic or mixed episodes associated with bipolar I disorder as monotherapy or with lithium or valproate. Treatment of irritability associated with autistic disorder in children and adolescents, including symptoms of aggression towards others, deliberate self-injuriousness, temper tantrums, and quickly changing moods.

DOSAGE: *Adults:* Schizophrenia: Initial: 1mg bid. Titrate: Increase by 1mg bid on the 2nd and 3rd day until target dose of 3mg bid by third day. Adjust further at intervals of at least 1 week. Usual: 4-8mg/day. Max: 16mg/day. Doses up to 8mg can be taken once daily. Bipolar Mania: Initial: 2-3mg qd. Titrate: Increase/Decrease by 1mg qd. Usual: 1-6mg/day. Max: 6mg/day. Elderly/Debilitated/Hypotension/Severe Renal or Hepatic Impairment: Initial: 0.5mg bid. Titrate: Increase by no more than 0.5mg bid. Increase at intervals of at least 1 week for dosages >1.5mg bid. Reassess periodically to determine maintenance treatment.

Pediatrics: 5-16 yrs: Irritability with Autistic Disorder: Initial: <20kg: 0.25mg/day; ≥20kg: 0.5mg/day. Titrate after at least 4 days: <20kg: Increase by 0.5mg/day; ≥20kg: 1mg/day. Maint: For minimum of 14 days. Inadequate Response: Increase at ≥2-wk intervals: <20kg: Increase by 0.25mg/day; ≥20kg: Increase by 0.5mg/day. Caution in patients <15kg. Max: <20kg: 1mg/day; ≥20kg: 2.5mg/day; >45kg: 3mg/day.

HOW SUPPLIED: Sol: 1mg/mL (30mL); Tab: 0.25mg, 0.5mg, 1mg, 2mg, 3mg, 4mg; Tab, Disintegrating: (M-Tab) 0.5mg, 1mg, 2mg, 3mg, 4mg

WARNINGS/PRECAUTIONS: Neuroleptic malignant syndrome and/or tardive dyskinesia may occur. Monitor for hyperglycemia; perform fasting blood glucose testing if symptoms develop or with risk factors for DM. Cerebrovascular events (eg, stroke, TIA) reported in elderly with dementia-related psychosis. Not approved for the treatment of dementia-related psychosis. May induce orthostatic hypotension, elevate prolactin levels, have an antiemetic effect. Caution in elderly, renal/hepatic impairment, history of seizures, cardio- or cerebrovascular disease, suicidal tendencies, risk of aspiration pneu-

Ritalin

monia, conditions predisposing to hypotension (eg, hypovolemia, dehydration) or affecting metabolism or hemodynamic responses. May impair judgement, thinking, or motor skills; caution when operating hazardous machinery. May disrupt body temperature regulation; caution in patients exposed to temperature extremes. Re-evaluate periodically. Patients who receive antipsychotics are reported to have an increased sensitivity to antipsychotic medications.

ADVERSE REACTIONS: Insomnia, agitation, anxiety, somnolence, extrapyramidal symptoms, nausea, headache, dizziness, constipation, dyspepsia, rhinitis, diarrhea, akathisia, dystonia, parkinsonism.

INTERACTIONS: Caution with other CNS drugs or alcohol. May potentiate antihypertensives, antagonize levodopa and dopamine agonists, or increase valproate levels. Cimetidine and ranitidine may increase bioavailability. CYP3A4 inducers (eg, carbamazepine, phenytoin, rifampin, phenobarbital) may decrease levels. Clozapine, fluoxetine, and paroxetine may increase levels. Increased mortality with furosemide in elderly patients.

PREGNANCY: Category C, not for use in nursing.

Ritalin
methylphenidate HCl (Novartis) — CII

OTHER BRAND NAMES: Ritalin LA (Novartis) - Ritalin SR (Novartis)

THERAPEUTIC CLASS: Sympathomimetic amine

INDICATIONS: (Cap, Extended-Release, Tab, Tab Extended-Release) Treatment of attention deficit disorders. (Tab, Tab, Extended-Release) Treatment of narcolepsy.

DOSAGE: *Adults:* (Tab) 10-60mg/day given bid-tid 30-45 min ac. Take last dose before 6 pm if insomnia occurs. (Tab, Extended-Release) May use in place of immediate release (IR) when the 8 hr dose corresponds to the titrated 8 hr IR dose. Swallow whole; do not chew or crush.

Pediatrics: ≥6 yrs: (Tab) Initial: 5mg bid before breakfast and lunch. Titrate: Increase gradually by 5-10mg weekly. Max: 60mg/day. (Tab, Extended-Release) May use in place of immediate release (IR) when the 8 hr dose corresponds to the titrated 8 hr IR dose. Swallow whole; do not chew or crush. (Cap, ER) Initial: 10-20mg qam. Titrate: Adjust weekly by 10mg. Max: 60mg qam. Previous Methylphenidate Use: May use as qd in place of IR dosed bid or daily dose of methylphenidate-SR. Swallow whole or sprinkle over spoonful of applesauce. Do not crush, chew, or divide. Reduce dose or discontinue if paradoxical aggravation of symptoms occurs. Discontinue if no improvement after appropriate dose adjustment over 1 month.

HOW SUPPLIED: Cap, Extended-Release (Ritalin LA): 10mg, 20mg, 30mg, 40mg; Tab (Ritalin): 5mg, 10mg*, 20mg*; Tab, Extended-Release (Ritalin SR): 20mg *scored

CONTRAINDICATIONS: Marked anxiety, tension, and agitation; glaucoma; motor tics or family history or diagnosis of Tourette's syndrome; during or within 14 days of MAOI use.

WARNINGS/PRECAUTIONS: Monitor growth in children. Not for severe depression or fatigue. May exacerbate symptoms of behavior disturbance and thought disorder in psychotic children. Care should be taken in using stimulants to treat patients with comorbid bipolar disorder because of concern for possible induction of mixed/manic episode in such patients. Stimulants at usual doses can cause treatment emergent psychotic or manic symptoms (hallucinations, delusional thinking, mania) in children and adolescents without prior history of psychotic illness. Aggressive behavior or hostility reported in clinical trials and the postmarketing experience of some medications indicated for the treatment of ADHD. May lower seizure threshold, especially with prior history of seizures or with prior EEG abnormalities; d/c if seizures occur. Caution with HTN and other underlying conditions that may be compromised such as heart failure, recent MI, or hyperthyroidism. Visual disturbances may occur (rare). Monitor CBC, differential, and platelets with prolonged use. Caution with emotionally-unstable patients or prior history of drug dependence or alcoholism; chronic use may lead to tolerance and psychological dependence. Monitor during withdrawal. Periodically d/c to assess condition. Avoid with known structural cardiac abnormalities or other serious cardiac problems.

ADVERSE REACTIONS: Nervousness, insomnia, hypersensitivity reactions, anorexia, nausea, dizziness, palpitations, headache, dyskinesia, drowsiness, BP and pulse changes, tachycardia, angina, arrhythmia, abdominal pain.

INTERACTIONS: See Contraindications. May decrease hypotensive effect of guanethidine. Caution with α_2-agonist (eg, clonidine) and pressor agents. Potentiates anticoagulants, anticonvulsants (eg, phenobarbital, diphenylhydantoin, primidone), phenylbutazone, TCAs (eg, imipramine, clomipramine, desipramine); monitor plasma drug levels or PT/INR. (Cap, Extended-Release) Antacids or acid suppressants may alter release characteristics of cap.

PREGNANCY: (Tab, ER) Safety in pregnancy and nursing not known. (Cap, ER) Category C, caution in nursing.

ROBAXIN RX
methocarbamol (Schwarz)

OTHER BRAND NAMES: Robaxin-750 (Schwarz) - Robaxin Injection (Baxter)

THERAPEUTIC CLASS: Muscular analgesic (central-acting)

INDICATIONS: Adjunct for relief of acute, painful musculoskeletal conditions.

DOSAGE: *Adults:* (PO) Initial: (500mg tab) 1500mg qid for 2-3 days. Maint: 1000mg qid. Initial: (750mg tab) 1500mg qid for 2-3 days. Maint: 750mg q4h or 1500mg tid. Max: 6gm/d for 2-3 days; 8gm/d if severe. (Inj) Moderate Symptoms: 10mL IV/IM. IV Max Rate: 3mL undiluted drug/min. IM Max: 5mL into each gluteal region. Severe/Post-Op Condition: Max: 20-30mL/day up to 3 consecutive days. If feasible, continue with PO. Tetanus: 10-20mL up to 30mL. May repeat q6h until NG tube can be inserted. Continue with crushed tabs. Max: 24g/day PO.

Pediatrics: Tetanus: Initial: 15mg/kg. Repeat q6h prn. Administer through tubing or IV. Safety and effctiveness in pediatric patients have not been established except tetanus

HOW SUPPLIED: Inj: 100mg/mL; Tab: 500mg, 750mg

CONTRAINDICATIONS: (Inj) Renal pathology with injection due to propylene glycol content.

WARNINGS/PRECAUTIONS: May cause color interference in certain screening tests for 5-hydroxy-indoleacetic acid (5-HIAA) and vanillylmandelic acid (VMA). Caution in epilepsy with the injection. Injection rate should not exceed 3mL/min. Avoid extravasation with injection.

ADVERSE REACTIONS: Lightheadedness, dizziness, drowsiness, nausea, urticaria, pruritus, rash, conjunctivitis, nasal congestion, blurred vision, headache, fever, seizures, syncope, flushing.

INTERACTIONS: Additive adverse effects with alcohol and other CNS depressants. May inhibit effect of pyridostigmine; caution in patients with myasthemia gravis receiving anticholinergics.

PREGNANCY: Category C, caution in nursing.

ROBINUL RX
glycopyrrolate (Sciele)

OTHER BRAND NAME: Robinul Forte (Sciele)

THERAPEUTIC CLASS: Anticholinergic

INDICATIONS: Adjunct treatment of peptic ulcer.

DOSAGE: *Adults:* Usual: (Tab) 1mg tid (am, pm and hs); may increase to 2mg qhs if needed. Maint: 1mg bid. (Forte) 2mg bid-tid. Max: 8mg/day.

Pediatrics: ≥12 yrs: Usual: (Tab) 1mg tid (am, pm & hs); may increase to 2mg qhs if needed. Maint: 1mg bid. (Forte) 2mg bid-tid. Max: 8mg/day.

HOW SUPPLIED: Tab: 1mg*, (Forte) 2mg* *scored

Robinul Injection

CONTRAINDICATIONS: Glaucoma, obstructive uropathy, GI tract obstruction, paralytic ileus, intestinal atony of elderly or debilitated, unstable cardiovascular status in acute hemorrhage, severe ulcerative colitis, toxic megacolon complicating ulcerative colitis, myasthenia gravis.

WARNINGS/PRECAUTIONS: May produce drowsiness and blurred vision; avoid operating machinery. Risk of heat prostration with high environmental temperature. Diarrhea may be early symptom of incomplete intestinal obstruction especially with ileostomy or colostomy. Caution in elderly, autonomic neuropathy, hepatic/renal disease, ulcerative colitis, hyperthyroidism, coronary heart disease, CHF, tachyarrhythmias, tachycardia, HTN, prostatic hypertrophy, hiatal hernia associated with reflux esophagitis.

ADVERSE REACTIONS: Blurred vision, dry mouth, urinary retention and hesitancy, increased ocular tension, tachycardia, decreased sweating, xerostomia, loss of taste, headache.

PREGNANCY: Safety in pregnancy is not known; not for use in nursing.

Robinul Injection RX
glycopyrrolate (Baxter)

THERAPEUTIC CLASS: Anticholinergic

INDICATIONS: Preoperative antimuscarinic to reduce salivary tracheobronchial, and pharyngeal secretions; decrease gastric sections; and block cardiac vagal inhibitory reflexes during anesthesia induction and intubation. Intra-operatively to counteract drug-induced or vagal traction reflexes associated with arrhythmias. To protect against peripheral muscarinic effects of cholinergic agents. Adjunct therapy for treatment of peptic ulcer when rapid anticholinergic effect is desired or when oral medication is not tolerated.

DOSAGE: *Adults:* Preanesthesia: 0.002mg/lb IM 30-60 minutes before anesthesia induction or at the time of preanesthetic narcotic/sedative. Intraoperatively: 0.1mg IV, repeat prn every 2-3 minutes. Reverse Neuromuscular Blockade: 0.2mg IV for each 1mg neostigmine or 5mg pyridostigmine. Peptic Ulcer: 0.1mg IV/IM q4h, tid-qid. May use 0.2mg if needed.
Pediatrics: Preanesthesia: 1 month-12 yrs: 0.002mg/lb IM 30-60 minutes before anesthesia induction or at the time of preanesthetic narcotic/sedative. 1 month-2 yrs: May require up to 0.004mg/lb. Intraoperatively: 0.002mg/lb IV. Max: 0.1mg single dose. May repeat prn every 2-3 minutes. Reverse Neuromuscular Blockade: 0.2mg IV for each 1mg neostigmine or 5mg pyridostigmine. Peptic Ulcer: ≥12 yrs: 0.1mg IV/IM q4h, tid-qid. May use 0.2mg if needed.

HOW SUPPLIED: Inj: 0.2mg/mL

CONTRAINDICATIONS: Newborns (<1 month) due to benzyl alcohol content. For long treatment duration: Glaucoma, obstructive uropathy, obstructive disease of GI tract, paralytic ileus, intestinal atony of elderly or debilitated, unstable cardiovascular status in acute hemorrhage, severe ulcerative colitis, toxic megacolon complicating ulcerative colitis, myasthenia gravis.

WARNINGS/PRECAUTIONS: Caution with CAD, CHF, arrhythmias, HTN, hyperthyroidism, elderly, autonomic neuropathy, hepatic or renal disease, ulcerative colitis, or hiatal hernia. May produce drowsiness and blurred vision; caution when operating machinery. Risk of fever and heat stroke due to decreased sweating in high environmental temperature. Diarrhea may be early symptom of incomplete intestinal obstruction.

ADVERSE REACTIONS: Drowsiness, blurred vision, dry mouth, urinary retention and hesitancy, increased ocular tension, tachycardia, palpation, decreased sweating, loss of taste.

INTERACTIONS: Increased anticholinergic side effects with other anticholinergics, phenothiazines, antiparkinson drugs, TCAs. Increased severity of GI lesions with potassium chloride in a wax matrix.

PREGNANCY: Category B, caution in nursing.

Rocaltrol RX
calcitriol (Roche Labs)

THERAPEUTIC CLASS: Vitamin D analog

INDICATIONS: Predialysis: Management of secondary hyperparathyroidism and resultant metabolic bone disease with moderate to severe chronic renal failure (CrCl 15-55mL/

min). Dialysis: Management of hypocalcemia and resultant metabolic bone disease. Hypoparathyroidism: Management of hypocalcemia and manifestations of postsurgical hypoparathyroidism, idiopathic hypoparathyroidism, and pseudohypoparathyroidism.

DOSAGE: *Adults:* Predialysis: Initial: 0.25mcg/day. Max: 0.5mcg/day. Hypoparathyroidism: Initial: 0.25mcg/day every am. Titrate: May increase at 2-4 week intervals to 0.5-2mcg/day. Elderly: Start at low end of dosing range. Dialysis: Initial: 0.25mcg/day. Titrate: May increase by 0.25mcg/day every 4-8 weeks to 0.5-1mcg/day. Monitor serum calcium levels twice weekly during titration. Normal to slightly reduced serum calcium, give 0.25mcg every other day. Discontinue with hypercalcemia; when calcium levels return to normal continue therapy and decrease dose by 0.25 mcg.

Pediatrics: Predialysis: ≥3 yrs: Initial: 0.25mcg/day. Max: 0.5mcg/day. <3yrs: Initial: 10-15ng/kg/day. Hypoparathyroidism: ≥6 yrs: Initial: 0.25mcg/day every am. Titrate: May increase at 2-4 week intervals to 0.5-2mcg/day. 1-5yrs: Initial: 0.25mcg/day every am. Titrate: May increase at 2-4 week intervals up to 0.75mcg/day. Monitor serum calcium levels twice weekly during titration. Discontinue with hypercalcemia; when calcium levels return to normal continue therapy and decrease dose by 0.25 mcg.

HOW SUPPLIED: Cap: 0.25mcg, 0.5mcg; Sol: 1mcg/mL (15mL)

CONTRAINDICATIONS: Hypercalcemia or vitamin D toxicity.

WARNINGS/PRECAUTIONS: Use non-aluminum phosphate binders and low phosphate diet to control serum phosphate. Chronic hypercalcemia can cause calcification of soft tissues. Monitor calcium levels twice a week initially. Avoid dehydration. Monitor serum creatinine. Maintain adequate calcium intake of at least 600mg/day. Caution in elderly. If treatment switched from ergocalciferol, may take several months for ergocalciferol level to decrease to baseline. May increase inorganic phosphate levels; ectopic calcification reported with renal failure. Monitor phosphorus, magnesium, alkaline phosphatase, and 24-hour urine periodically.

ADVERSE REACTIONS: Weakness, nausea, vomiting, dry mouth, constipation, muscle and bone pain, metallic taste, polyuria, polydipsia, weight loss, pancreatitis, photophobia, pruritus, decreased libido.

INTERACTIONS: Avoid vitamin D products and derivatives during therapy. Hypermagnesemia may occur with magnesium-containing antacids, especially in chronic renal dialysis. Caution with digoxin; hypercalcemia may precipitate arrhythmias. Reduced intestinal absorption with cholestyramine. May need to increase dose if given with phenytoin or phenobarbital. Caution with thiazides; risk of hypercalcemia. Ketoconazole may effect metabolism. Corticosteroids antagonize activity. Changes in diet or uncontrolled intake of calcium preparations can cause hypercalcemia. Adjust dose phosphate-binding agents.

PREGNANCY: Category C, not for use in nursing.

Rocephin
ceftriaxone sodium (Roche Labs)

RX

THERAPEUTIC CLASS: Cephalosporin (3rd generation)

INDICATIONS: Treatment of lower respiratory tract infections, skin and skin structure infections, bone and joint infections, intra-abdominal infections, acute otitis media, uncomplicated gonorrhea, pelvic inflammatory disease, UTI, septicemia, and meningitis. For surgical prophylaxis.

DOSAGE: *Adults:* Usual: 1-2g/day IV/IM given qd-bid. Max: 4g/day. Gonorrhea: 250mg IM single dose. Surgical Prophylaxis: 1g IV 1/2-2 hrs before surgery.

Pediatrics: Skin Infections: 50-75mg/kg/day IV/IM given qd-bid. Max: 2g/day. Otitis Media: 50mg/kg (up to 1g) IM single dose. Serious Infections: 50-75mg/kg/day IM/IV given q12h. Max: 2g/day. Meningitis: Initial: 100mg/kg (up to 4g), then 100mg/kg/day given qd-bid for 7-14 days. Max: 4g/day.

HOW SUPPLIED: Inj: 250mg, 500mg, 1g, 2g, 10g

ROFERON-A

WARNINGS/PRECAUTIONS: Cross sensitivity to penicillins and other cephalosporins may occur. Pseudomembranous colitis reported. May result in overgrowth of nonsusceptible organisms. Altered PT, transient BUN, and serum creatinine elevations may occur. Do not exceed 2g/day and monitor blood levels with both hepatic and renal dysfunction. Caution with history of GI disease. D/C if develop gallbladder disease. May alter PT; monitor with impaired vitamin K synthesis or low vitamin K stores. Avoid in hyperbilirubinemic neonates, especially prematures.

ADVERSE REACTIONS: Injection site reactions, eosinophilia, thrombocytosis, diarrhea, SGOT and SGPT elevations.

PREGNANCY: Category B, caution in nursing.

ROFERON-A RX
interferon alfa-2a, recombinant (Roche Labs)

> May cause or aggravate fatal or life-threatening neuropsychiatric, autoimmune, ischemic, and infectious disorders. Monitor closely with periodic clinical and laboratory evaluations. D/C with persistently severe or worsening signs or symptoms of these conditions.

THERAPEUTIC CLASS: Biological response modifier

INDICATIONS: Treatment of chronic hepatitis C (HCV) and hairy cell leukemia. For chronic phase, Philadelphia chromosome positive chronic myelogenous leukemia (CML) in patients minimally pretreated.

DOSAGE: *Adults:* ≥18 yrs: HCV: 3MIU SQ 3x/week (TIW) for 48-52 weeks or 6MIU TIW for 12 weeks, then 3MIU TIW for 36 weeks. D/C if no response within 3 months. If intolerant to prescribed dose, temporarily reduce by 50%. May reinstate once adverse reactions resolve. Retreatment: 3MIU TIW or 6MIU TIW for 6-12 months. Hairy Cell Leukemia: Induction: 3MIU SQ qd for 16-24 weeks. Maint: 3MIU TIW. CML: 3MIU SQ qd for 3 days, 6MIU qd for 3 days, then to target dose of 9MIU qd. D/C or reduce dose or frequency of inj if severe adverse reactions occur.

Pediatrics: CML: 3MIU SQ qd for 3 days, 6MIU qd for 3 days, then to target dose of 9MIU qd. D/C or reduce dose or frequency of inj if severe adverse reactions occur.

HOW SUPPLIED: Inj: 3MIU/0.5mL, 6MIU/0.5mL, 9MIU/0.5mL

CONTRAINDICATIONS: Autoimmune hepatitis; hepatic decompensation (Child-Pugh class B & C) before or during treatment; neonates and infants (contains benzyl alcohol).

WARNINGS/PRECAUTIONS: Depression and suicidal behavior reported; extreme caution with history of depression. Cardiomyopathy reported; caution with cardiac disease or history of cardiac illness. Serious, acute hypersensitivity reactions reported. Transient liver abnormalities and/or GI hemorrhage reported. May suppress bone marrow function and result in severe cytopenias and anemia; caution with myelosuppression. May cause or aggravate hypothyroidism and hyperthyroidism. Hyperglycemia reported; monitor closely. May induce or aggravate dyspnea, pulmonary infiltrates, pneumonia, bronchiolitis obliterans, interstitial pneumonitis, and sarcoidosis; d/c with persistent or unexplained pulmonary infiltrates or pulmonary function impairment. Decrease/loss of vision and retinopathy reported; perform eye exam at baseline, if any ocular symptoms develop, and periodically with pre-existing disorder and d/c if new or worsening ophthalmologic disorders develop. Renal toxicities reported; monitor closely with impaired renal function and caution with CrCl <50mL/min. Development and exacerbation of autoimmune disease reported; monitor closely. Monitor CBC, platelets, and clinical chemistry tests before therapy and periodically thereafter. Severe infections reported; consider discontinuation. Pancreatitis reported; suspend if signs or symptoms observed; d/c if pancreatitis diagnosed.

ADVERSE REACTIONS: Depression, flu-like symptoms (fever, asthenia, fatigue, chills, myalgia), dizziness, headache, nausea, vomiting, diarrhea, rash, arthralgia, anorexia.

INTERACTIONS: May reduce theophylline clearance. Caution with agents that cause myelosuppression or are metabolized by CYP450. Synergistic myelosuppression with zidovudine. Anti-diabetic regimens may need adjustments. Use with interleukin-2 may increase risk of renal failure. May increase neurotoxic, hematotoxic or cardiotoxic effects of other drugs.

PREGNANCY: Category C, not for use in nursing.

ROMAZICON
flumazenil (Roche Labs)

RX

THERAPEUTIC CLASS: Benzodiazepine antagonist

INDICATIONS: Complete or partial reversal of sedative effects of benzodiazepines (BZDs) given with general anesthesia, or diagnostic and therapeutic procedures, and for the management of BZD overdose in adults. For reversal of BZD-induced conscious sedation in pediatrics (1-17 yrs old).

DOSAGE: *Adults:* Reversal of Conscious Sedation/General Anesthesia: Give IV over 15 seconds. Initial: 0.2mg. May repeat dose after 45 seconds and again at 60 second intervals up to a max of 4 additional times until reach desired level of consciousness. Max Total Dose: 1mg. In event of resedation, repeated doses may be given at 20-min intervals. Max: 1mg/dose (0.2mg/min) and 3mg/hr. BZD Overdose: Give IV over 30 seconds. Initial: 0.2mg. May repeat with 0.3mg after 30 seconds and then 0.5mg at 1-min intervals until reach desired level of consciousness. Max Total Dose: 3mg. In event of resedation, repeated doses may be given at 20-min intervals. Max: 1mg/dose (0.5mg/min); 3mg/hr.

Pediatrics: >1yr: Give IV over 15 seconds. Initial: 0.01mg/kg (up to 0.2mg). May repeat dose after 45 seconds and again at 60-second intervals up to a max of 4 additional times until reach desired level of consciousness. Max Total Dose: 0.05mg/kg or 1mg, whichever is lower.

HOW SUPPLIED: Inj: 0.1mg/mL

CONTRAINDICATIONS: Patients given BZDs for life-threatening conditions (eg, control of intracranial pressure or status epilepticus), signs of serious cyclic antidepressant overdose.

WARNINGS/PRECAUTIONS: Caution in overdoses involving multiple drug combinations. Risk of seizures, especially with long-term BZD-induced sedation, cyclic antidepressant overdose, concurrent major sedative-hypnotic drug withdrawal, recent therapy with repeated doses of parenteral BZDs, myoclonic jerking or seizure prior to flumazenil administration. Monitor for resedation, respiratory depression, or other residual BZD effects (up to 2 hrs). Avoid use in the ICU; increased risk of unrecognized BZD dependence. Caution with head injury, alcoholism, and other drug dependencies. Does not reverse respiratory depression/hypoventilation or cardiac depression. May provoke panic attacks with history of panic disorder. Adjust subsequent doses in hepatic dysfunction. Not for use as treatment for BZD dependence or for management of protracted abstinence syndromes. May trigger dose-dependent withdrawal syndromes.

ADVERSE REACTIONS: Nausea, vomiting, dizziness, injection site pain, increased sweating, headache, abnormal or blurred vision, agitation.

INTERACTIONS: Avoid use until neuromuscular blockade effects are reversed. Toxic effects (eg, convulsions, cardiac dysrhythmias) may occur with mixed drug overdose (eg, cyclic antidepressants).

PREGNANCY: Category C, caution in nursing.

RONDEC
pseudoephedrine HCl - carbinoxamine maleate (Biovail)

RX

OTHER BRAND NAMES: Rondec-TR (Biovail) - Rondec Oral Drops (Biovail)

THERAPEUTIC CLASS: Antihistamine/decongestant

INDICATIONS: (Drops) Seasonal/perennial allergic and vasomotor rhinitis. (Tab, Tab, Extended Release) Relief of upper respiratory symptoms associated with allergic rhinitis and the common cold.

DOSAGE: *Adults:* (Tab) 1 tab qid; (Tab, Extended Release) 1 tab bid.
Pediatrics: (Sol) Give qid. 12-24 months: 1mL. 6-12 months: 3/4mL. 3-6 months: 1/2mL. 1-3 months: 1/4mL. (Tab) ≥6 yrs:1 tab qid. (Tab, Extended Release) ≥12 yrs: 1 tab bid.

HOW SUPPLIED: (Carbinoxamine-Pseudoephedrine) Sol: 1mg-15mg/mL (30mL); Tab: 4mg-60mg; Tab, Extended Release: (Rondec TR) 8mg-120mg

CONTRAINDICATIONS: Severe HTN or CAD, MAOIs, narrow-angle glaucoma, urinary retention, peptic ulcer, during asthma attack.

Rondec Syrup

WARNINGS/PRECAUTIONS: Caution in asthma, DM, HTN, heart disease, hyperthyroidism, increased IOP, prostatic hypertrophy, elderly. May cause excitability, especially in children.

ADVERSE REACTIONS: Sedation, dizziness, diplopia, vomiting, diarrhea, dry mouth, headache, nervousness, nausea, convulsions, CNS stimulation, cardiac arrhythmias, respiratory difficulty, increased HR or BP.

INTERACTIONS: May enhance effects of TCAs, benzodiazepines, barbiturates, alcohol, other CNS depressants. Increased sympathomimetic effects with MAOIs, beta blockers. May reduce antihypertensive effects of reserpine, veratrum alkaloids, methyldopa, mecamylamine.

PREGNANCY: Category C, safety in nursing not known.

Rondec Syrup RX
pseudoephedrine HCl - brompheniramine maleate (Biovail)

THERAPEUTIC CLASS: Antihistamine/decongestant

INDICATIONS: Symptomatic relief of seasonal and perennial allergic rhinitis and vasomotor rhinitis.

DOSAGE: *Adults:* 5mL qid.
Pediatrics: ≥6 yrs: 5mL qid. 2-6 yrs: 2.5mL qid.

HOW SUPPLIED: (Brompheniramine-Pseudoephedrine) Syrup: 4mg-45mg/5mL

CONTRAINDICATIONS: Severe HTN or CAD, MAOIs, narrow-angle glaucoma, urinary retention, peptic ulcer, during asthma attack.

WARNINGS/PRECAUTIONS: Caution in asthma, DM, HTN, heart disease, hyperthyroidism, increased IOP, prostatic hypertrophy, elderly. May cause excitability, especially in children.

ADVERSE REACTIONS: Sedation, dizziness, diplopia, vomiting, diarrhea, dry mouth, headache, nervousness, nausea, convulsions, CNS stimulation, cardiac arrhythmias, respiratory difficulty, increased HR or BP.

INTERACTIONS: May enhance effects of TCAs, benzodiazepines, barbiturates, alcohol, other CNS depressants. Increased sympathomimetic effects with MAOIs, beta blockers. May reduce antihypertensive effects of reserpine, veratrum alkaloids, methyldopa, mecamylamine.

PREGNANCY: Category C, safety in nursing not known.

Rondec-DM Drops RX
pseudoephedrine HCl - dextromethorphan HBr - carbinoxamine maleate (Biovail)

THERAPEUTIC CLASS: Antihistamine/decongestant/antitussive

INDICATIONS: Relief of coughs and upper respiratory symptoms associated with allergy or the common cold.

DOSAGE: *Pediatrics:* Give qid. 12-24 months: 1mL. 6-12 months: 3/4mL. 3-6 months: 1/2mL. 1-3 months: 1/4mL.

HOW SUPPLIED: (Carbinoxamine-Dextromethorphan-Pseudoephedrine) Sol: 1mg-4mg-15mg/mL (30mL)

CONTRAINDICATIONS: Severe HTN or CAD, during or within 2 weeks of MAOIs, narrow-angle glaucoma, urinary retention, peptic ulcer, during asthma attack.

WARNINGS/PRECAUTIONS: Caution with HTN, DM, heart disease, asthma, hyperthyroidism, increased IOP, prostatic hypertrophy and in atopic children, elderly, sedated, debilitated, or confined to supine positions. May cause excitability especially in children.

ADVERSE REACTIONS: Sedation, drowsiness, dizziness, diplopia, nausea, vomiting, diarrhea, dry mouth, headache, nervousness, convulsions, CNS stimulation, arrhythmias, increased HR or BP, tremors.

INTERACTIONS: Avoid during or within 2 weeks of MAOIs. May enhance effects of TCAs, barbiturates, alcohol, other CNS depressants. May reduce antihypertensive effects of reserpine, veratrum alkaloids, methyldopa, mecamylamine. Increased sympathomimetic effect with MAOIs, beta-blockers. Additive cough-suppressant effect with narcotic antitussives.

PREGNANCY: Category C, safety in nursing not known.

Rondec-DM Syrup   RX
pseudoephedrine HCl - dextromethorphan HBr - brompheniramine maleate (Biovail)

OTHER BRAND NAMES: Cardec DM (Alpharma) - Carbofed DM (Hi-Tech)
THERAPEUTIC CLASS: Antihistamine/decongestant/antitussive
INDICATIONS: Relief of coughs and upper respiratory symptoms, including nasal congestion, associated with allergy or the common cold.
DOSAGE: *Adults:* 5mL qid.
Pediatrics: >6 yrs: 5mL qid. 2-6 yrs: 2.5mL qid.
HOW SUPPLIED: Syrup: (Brompheniramine-Dextromethorphan-Pseudoephedrine) 4mg-15mg-45mg/5mL (120mL, 480mL)
CONTRAINDICATIONS: Severe HTN or CAD, narrow-angle glaucoma, urinary retention, peptic ulcer, acute asthma attack, with MAOI therapy.
WARNINGS/PRECAUTIONS: Caution with HTN, DM, ischemic heart disease, hyperthyroidism, BPH, asthma, and increased IOP. May produce CNS stimulation with convulsion, cardiovascular collapse and hypotension. Excitability reported especially in children. Do not exceed recommended doses. Caution in atopic children, elderly, sedated/debilitated, and patients confined to supine positions.
ADVERSE REACTIONS: Sedation, drowsiness, dizziness, diplopia, nausea, vomiting, diarrhea, dry mouth, headache, arrhythmias, increased heart rate, tremors, nervousness, insomnia, heartburn, dysuria, polyuria, increased BP.
INTERACTIONS: May enhance effects of TCAs, barbiturates, alcohol, other CNS depressants. May diminish antihypertensive effects of reserpine, veratrum alkaloids, methyldopa, mecamylamine. Increased sympathomimetic effect with beta-blockers and MAOIs. Additive cough-suppressant effect with narcotic antitussives. Do not use within 14 days of MAOI therapy.
PREGNANCY: Category C, caution in nursing.

Rosac   RX
sulfur - sulfacetamide sodium (Stiefel)

THERAPEUTIC CLASS: Sulfonamide/sulfur combination
INDICATIONS: Topical control of acne vulgaris, acne rosacea and seborrheic dermatitis.
DOSAGE: *Adults:* Apply a thin film qd-tid.
Pediatrics: ≥12 yrs: Apply a thin film qd-tid.
HOW SUPPLIED: Cre: (Sulfacetamide-Sulfur) 10%-5% (45g)
CONTRAINDICATIONS: Kidney disease.
WARNINGS/PRECAUTIONS: Discontinue if irritation or hypersensitivity reaction occurs. Avoid contact with eyes. Caution if denuded or abraded skin. May cause reddening and scaling of epidermis.
ADVERSE REACTIONS: Local irritation.
PREGNANCY: Category C, caution in nursing.

Rosula   RX
sulfur - sulfacetamide sodium (Doak)

THERAPEUTIC CLASS: Sulfonamide/sulfur combination
INDICATIONS: Topical treatment of acne vulgaris, acne rosacea, and seborrheic dermatitis.

Rosula NS

DOSAGE: *Adults:* (Gel) Apply thin film qd-tid. (Cleanser) Wash for 10-20 seconds qd-bid. *Pediatrics:* ≥12 yrs: (Gel) Apply thin film qd-tid. (Cleanser) Wash for 10-20 seconds qd-bid.
HOW SUPPLIED: (Sulfacetamide-Sulfur) Gel: 10%-5% (45mL); Cleanser: 10%-5% (355mL)
CONTRAINDICATIONS: Kidney disease.
WARNINGS/PRECAUTIONS: Discontinue if irritation or hypersensitivity reaction occurs. Avoid contact with eyes, lips, and mucous membranes. Caution with denuded or abraded skin. Can cause reddening and scaling of epidermis.
ADVERSE REACTIONS: Local irritation.
PREGNANCY: Category C, caution in nursing.

Rosula NS RX
urea - sulfacetamide sodium (Doak)

THERAPEUTIC CLASS: Sulfonamide
INDICATIONS: Topical treatment of bacterial infections of the skin including *P.acne* and seborrheic dermatitis.
DOSAGE: *Adults:* Apply to affected area qd-bid.
Pediatrics: ≥12 yrs: Apply to affected area qd-bid.
HOW SUPPLIED: Swab: (Sulfacetamide-Urea) 10%-10% (30s)
CONTRAINDICATIONS: Kidney disease
WARNINGS/PRECAUTIONS: Discontinue if irritation or hypersensitivity reaction occurs. Avoid contact with eyes, lips, and mucous membranes. Caution with denuded or abraded skin. Cases of Stevens-Johnson syndrome and drug-induced systemic lupus erythematosus have been reported.
ADVERSE REACTIONS: Local hypersensitivity, instances of Stevens-Johnson syndrome.
INTERACTIONS: Incompatible with silver preparations.
PREGNANCY: Category C, caution in nursing.

RotaTeq RX
rotavirus vaccine, live (Merck)

THERAPEUTIC CLASS: Vaccine
INDICATIONS: Prevention of rotavirus gastroenteritis in infants and children caused by the serotypes G1, G2, G3, and G4 when administered as a 3-dose series to infants between the ages of 6-32 weeks. The first dose should be administered between 6-12 weeks of age.
DOSAGE: *Pediatrics:* Administer series of 3 doses orally starting at 6-12 weeks of age, with subsequent doses administered at 4-10 week intervals. Third dose should not be given after 32 weeks of age. Do not mix with any other vaccines or solutions. Do not reconstitute or dilute.
HOW SUPPLIED: Sus: 2mL
WARNINGS/PRECAUTIONS: Consider delaying use with febrile illness. Vaccination may not result in complete protection in all recipients. May increase risk of intussusception.
ADVERSE REACTIONS: Bronchiolitis, gastroenteritis, pneumonia, fever, UTI.
INTERACTIONS: Immunosuppressive therapies including irradiation, antimetabolites, alkylating agents, cytotoxic drugs, and corticosteroids (used in greater than physiologic doses) may reduce the immune response to vaccines.
PREGNANCY: Safety in pregnancy and nursing not known.

Rynatan Pediatric RX
phenylephrine tannate - Chlorpheniramine tannate (MedPointe)

THERAPEUTIC CLASS: Antihistamine/sympathomimetic
INDICATIONS: Symptomatic relief of coryza and nasal congestion with the common cold, sinusitis, allergic rhinitis, and other upper respiratory tract conditions.

DOSAGE: *Pediatrics:* >6 yrs: 5-10mL q12h. 2 to 6 yrs: 2.5-5mL q12h. <2 yrs: Titrate individually.

HOW SUPPLIED: Sus: (Chlorpheniramine-Phenylephrine) 4.5mg-5mg/5mL

CONTRAINDICATIONS: Newborns and nursing mothers.

WARNINGS/PRECAUTIONS: Caution with HTN, cardiovascular disease, hyperthyroidism, DM, narrow angle glaucoma, prostatic hypertrophy, and elderly. May impair mental alertness. Contains tartrazine.

ADVERSE REACTIONS: Drowsiness, sedation, dryness of mucous membranes, GI effects.

INTERACTIONS: Increased anticholinergic and sympathomimetic effects with MAOIs; avoid during or within 14 days of use. Additive CNS effects with alcohol or other CNS depressants (eg, sedative-hypnotics, tranquilizers).

PREGNANCY: Category C, not for use in nursing.

RYNATUSS   RX
ephedrine tannate - phenylephrine tannate - carbetapentane tannate - chlorpheniramine tannate (MedPointe)

OTHER BRAND NAME: Rynatuss Pediatric (MedPointe)

THERAPEUTIC CLASS: Antitussive/antihistamine/bronchodilator/ sympathomimetic combination

INDICATIONS: Symptomatic relief of cough associated with respiratory tract conditions such as the common cold, bronchial asthma, acute and chronic bronchitis.

DOSAGE: *Adults:* 1-2 tabs q12h.

Pediatrics: >6 yrs: 5-10mL q12h. 2-6 yrs: 2.5-5mL q12h.

HOW SUPPLIED: (Carbetapentane-Chlorpheniramine-Ephedrine-Phenylephrine) Sus: (Rynatuss Pediatric) 30mg-4mg-5mg-5mg/5mL (240mL 480mL); Tab: (Rynatuss) 60mg-5mg-10mg-10mg* *scored

CONTRAINDICATIONS: Newborns, nursing mothers.

WARNINGS/PRECAUTIONS: Caution with HTN, cardiovascular disease, hyperthyroidism, DM, narrow angle glaucoma, elderly or prostatic hypertrophy. Suspension contains FD&C Yellow No. 5 which may cause allergic-type reactions.

ADVERSE REACTIONS: Drowsiness, sedation, dryness of mucous membranes, GI effects.

INTERACTIONS: Avoid MAOI use within 14 days. Additive CNS effects with alcohol or other CNS depressants.

PREGNANCY: Category C, not for use in nursing.

SAIZEN   RX
somatropin (Serono)

THERAPEUTIC CLASS: Human growth hormone

INDICATIONS: Long-term treatment of children with growth failure due to inadequate secretion of endogenous growth hormone. For replacement of endogenous growth hormone in adults who have growth hormone deficiency either alone, or associated with multiple hormone deficiencies, as a result of pituitary disease, hypothalamic disease, surgery, radiation therapy or trauma; or in patients who were growth hormone deficient during childhood as a result of congenital, genetic, acquired or idiopathic causes.

DOSAGE: *Adults:* Initial: ≤0.005mg/kg/day SQ. Titrate: May increase after 4 weeks to ≤0.01mg/kg/day depending on patient tolerance. Without Consideration of Body Weight: Initial: 0.2mg/day (0.15-0.3mg/day) SQ. Titrate: May increase by increments of 0.1-0.2mg/day every 1-2 months. Consider dose reduction in elderly.

Pediatrics: Individualize dose. Usual: 0.06mg/kg IM/SQ 3x/week. If epiphyses are fused, d/c therapy.

HOW SUPPLIED: Inj: 4mg, 5mg, 8.8mg

CONTRAINDICATIONS: Acute critical illness due to complications following open heart or abdominal surgery, accidental trauma or acute respiratory failure. Active prolifera-

SANDIMMUNE

tive or severe non-proliferative diabetic retinopathy. Active malignancy, or evidence of progression or recurrence of intracranial tumor. Prader-Willi syndrome when severely obese or have severe respiratory impairment, and in pediatric patients with closed epiphyses. Avoid reconstitution with bacteriostatic water if sensitive to benzyl alcohol.

WARNINGS/PRECAUTIONS: See Contraindications. Benzyl alcohol associated with toxicity in newborns; if sensitivity occurs, may reconstitute with SWFI. Insulin resistance reported; use caution with DM or family history of DM. Hypothyroidism may occur; bone maturation should be carefully followed. Increased incidence of slipped capital femoral epiphysis may develop with endocrine disorders; monitor for limping or hip/knee pain. Intracranial hypertension (IH) reported; d/c treatment if papilledema observed. Patients with Turner syndrome, chronic renal insufficiency or Prader-Willi syndrome may have increased risk for IH. If idiopathic IH confirmed, may restart therapy at lower dose after signs/symptoms resolve. Alternate injection sites to reduce development of tissue atrophy. Monitor for any malignant transformation of skin lesions.

ADVERSE REACTIONS: Arthalgia, headache, influenza-like symptoms, peripheral edema, back pain, myalgia, rhinitis, dizziness, upper respiratory tract infection, paraesthesia, hypoaesthesia, insomnia, nausea, generalized edema, depression.

INTERACTIONS: Diminished effects with concomitant glucocorticoid; adjust dose of accordingly. May alter clearance of CYP450 substrates (eg, corticosteroids, sex steroids, anticonvulsants, cyclosporine). May increase dose if taking oral estrogen replacement concomitantly. Adjust dose of insulin/oral antidiabetics when initiating therapy.

PREGNANCY: Category B, caution in nursing.

SANDIMMUNE RX
cyclosporine (Novartis)

> Give with adrenal corticosteroids but not with other immunosuppressives. Increased susceptibility to infection and development of lymphoma. Sandimmune and Neoral are not bioequivalent. Monitor blood levels to avoid toxicity.

THERAPEUTIC CLASS: Cyclic polypeptide immunosuppressant

INDICATIONS: Prophylaxis of organ rejection in kidney, liver, and heart allogeneic transplants with concomitant adrenal corticosteroids. Treatment of chronic rejection in patients previously treated with other immunosuppressives.

DOSAGE: *Adults:* Initial: PO: 15mg/kg single dose 4-12 hrs before transplant; continue same dose qd for 1-2 weeks. Usual: Taper by 5% per week until 5-10mg/kg/day. May mix oral solution with milk, chocolate milk, or orange juice. IV: 1/3 PO dose. Initial: 5-6mg/kg/day single dose; begin 4 to 12 hrs prior to transplantation. Maint: Continue single daily dose until PO forms are tolerated. Due to risk of anaphylaxis, only use injection if unable to take oral agents.

Pediatrics: Initial: PO: 15mg/kg single dose 4-12 hrs before transplant; continue same dose qd for 1-2 weeks. Usual: Taper by 5% per week until 5-10mg/kg/day. May mix oral solution with milk, chocolate milk, or orange juice. IV: 1/3 PO dose. Initial: 5-6mg/kg/day single dose; begin 4 to 12 hrs prior to transplantation. Maint: Continue single daily dose until PO forms are tolerated. Due to risk of anaphylaxis, only use injection if unable to take oral agents.

HOW SUPPLIED: Cap: 25mg, 100mg; Inj: 50mg/mL; Sol: 100mg/mL (50mL)

CONTRAINDICATIONS: Hypersensitivity to Cremophor EL (polyoxyethylated castor oil).

WARNINGS/PRECAUTIONS: May cause hepatotoxicity and nephrotoxicity. Convulsions, elevated serum creatinine, and BUN levels reported. Thrombocytopenia and microangiopathic hemolytic anemia may develop. Monitor for hyperkalemia. Increases risk for development of lymphomas and other malignancies. Observe for 30 minutes after the start of infusion and frequently thereafter. Caution with malabsorption.

ADVERSE REACTIONS: Renal dysfunction, tremor, hirsutism, HTN, gum hyperplasia, HTN, glomerular capillary thrombosis, cramps, acne, convulsions, headache, diarrhea, hepatotoxicity, abdominal discomfort, paresthesia, flushing.

INTERACTIONS: Ciprofloxacin, gentamicin, tobramycin, vancomycin, SMZ/TMP, amphotericin B, ketoconazole, melphalan, diclofenac, azapropazon, sulindac, naproxen, colchicine, cimetidine, ranitidine, tacrolimus, bezafirate, fenofibrate may potentiate renal dysfunction. Diltiazem, nicardipine, colchicine, fluconazole, itraconazole, ketoconazole, verapamil, azithromycin, clarithromycin, erythromycin, quinupristin/dalfopristin, allopurinol, amiodarone, bromocriptine, danazol, imatinib, metoclopramide, oral contraceptives, HIV protease inhibitors may increase levels. St. John's wort, grapefruit juice, carbamazepine, phenobarbital, phenytoin, rifampin, sulfinpyrazone, octreotide, orlistat, terbinafine, ticlopidine, and nafcillin may decrease levels. Avoid with potassium-sparing diuretics. Caution with ACEIs, angiotensin II blockers, NSAIDs. Digitalis toxicity reported. Myotoxicity with statins, frequent gingival hyperplasia with nifedipine, and convulsions with high dose methylprednisolone reported. Increased levels of sirolimus; give 4 hrs after cyclosporine. Avoid live vaccines during therapy.

PREGNANCY: Category C, not for use in nursing.

SECONAL SODIUM
secobarbital sodium (Ranbaxy)

CII

THERAPEUTIC CLASS: Barbiturate

INDICATIONS: Hypnotic, for the short-term treatment of insomnia (may lose effectiveness after 2 weeks); Preanesthetic.

DOSAGE: *Adults:* Hypnotic: 100mg hs; Preoperatively: 200-300mg, 1-2 hrs before surgery; Elderly/Debilitated/Renal or Hepatic Dysfunction: Reduce dose.
Pediatrics: Preoperatively: 2-6mg/kg. Max: 100mg.

HOW SUPPLIED: Cap: 100mg

CONTRAINDICATIONS: History of manifest or latent porphyria, marked impairment of liver function, or respiratory disease in which dyspnea or obstruction is evident.

WARNINGS/PRECAUTIONS: May be habit-forming; avoid abrupt cessation after prolonged use. Tolerance, psychological and physical dependence may occur with continued use. Use with caution, if at all, in patients who are mentally depressed, have suicidal tendencies, or have a history of drug abuse. In patients with hepatic damage, use with caution and initially reduce dose. Caution when administering to patients with acute or chronic pain. May impair mental and/or physical abilities. Avoid alcohol.

ADVERSE REACTIONS: Agitation, confusion, hyperkinesia, ataxia, CNS depression, somnolence, bradycardia, hypotension, nausea, vomiting, constipation, headache, hypersensitivity reactions, liver damage.

INTERACTIONS: May increase metabolism and decrease response to oral anticoagulants and enhance metabolism of exogenous corticosteroids. May interfere with absorption of griseofulvin, decreasing its blood level. May shorten half-life of doxycycline for up to 2 weeks after being discontinued. Variable effect on phenytoin and increased levels with sodium valproate and valproic acid; monitor blood levels and adjust dose appropriately. May cause additive depressant effects with other CNS depressants (eg, sedatives/hypnotics, antihistamines, tranquilizers, alcohol). Prolonged effects with MAOIs. May decrease effect of estradiol; alternative contraceptive methods should be suggested.

PREGNANCY: Category D, caution in nursing.

SEMPREX-D
acrivastine - pseudoephedrine HCl (Celltech)

RX

THERAPEUTIC CLASS: Antihistamine/decongestant

INDICATIONS: Relief of symptoms associated with seasonal allergic rhinitis.

DOSAGE: *Adults:* 1 cap q4-6h, qid.
Pediatrics: ≥12 yrs: 1 cap q4-6h, qid.

HOW SUPPLIED: Cap: (Acrivastine-Pseudoephedrine) 8mg-60mg

CONTRAINDICATIONS: Severe HTN, CAD, MAOIs during or within 14 days of use. Hypersensitivity to alkylamine antihistamines.

WARNINGS/PRECAUTIONS: Not for use >14 days. Caution with HTN, DM, increased IOP, ischemic heart disease, hyperthyroidism, BPH, renal impairment, peptic ulcer, pyloroduodenal obstruction, and elderly. Sedation reported. Avoid with CrCl ≤48mL/min.

Senokot

ADVERSE REACTIONS: Somnolence, headache, dry mouth, insomnia, dizziness, nervousness.

INTERACTIONS: MAOIs and β-agonists increase effects of sympathomimetics; avoid use during or within 14 days of MAOIs. Increased sedation with CNS depressants, alcohol.

PREGNANCY: Category B, caution in nursing.

Senokot   OTC
senna (Purdue Products)

THERAPEUTIC CLASS: Stimulant laxative

INDICATIONS: To relieve functional constipation. Senokot-S also contains a stool softener.

DOSAGE: *Adults:* Take at bedtime. (Senokot/Senokot-S) 2 tabs qd. Max: 4 tabs bid. (SenokotXTRA) 1 tab qd. Max: 2 tabs bid. (Granules) 5mL qd. Max: 15mL bid. Granules may be eaten plain, mixed with liquids, or sprinkled on food.

Pediatrics: Take at bedtime. (Senokot/Senokot-S) ≥12 yrs: 2 tabs qd. Max: 4 tabs bid. 6-12 yrs: 1 tab qd. Max: 2 tabs bid. 2-6 yrs: 1/2 tab qd. Max: 1 tab bid. (SenokotXTRA) ≥12 yrs: 1 tab qd. Max: 2 tabs bid. 6-12 yrs: 1/2 tab qd. Max: 1 tab bid. (Granules) ≥12 yrs: 1 tsp qd. Max: 2 tsp bid. 6-12 yrs: 1/2 tsp qd. Max: 1 tsp bid. 2-6 yrs: 1/4 tsp qd. Max: 1/2 tsp bid. Granules may be eaten plain, mixed with liquids, or sprinkled on food.

HOW SUPPLIED: Granules: 15mg/dose; Tab (Sennoside A and B): (Senokot) 8.6mg, (SenokotXTRA) 17mg; (Docusate Sodium-Sennoside A and B) (Senokot-S) 50mg-8.6mg

WARNINGS/PRECAUTIONS: Do not use with abdominal pain, nausea, or vomiting. Should not be used for longer than 1 week. Rectal bleeding or failure to have a bowel movement after use may indicate serious condition.

INTERACTIONS: Avoid mineral oil with Senokot-S.

PREGNANCY: Safety in pregnancy and nursing not known.

Sensorcaine   RX
bupivacaine HCl (Abraxis)

OTHER BRAND NAME: Sensorcaine-MPF (Abraxis)

THERAPEUTIC CLASS: Local anesthetic

INDICATIONS: Production of local or regional anesthesia for surgery, oral surgery procedures, diagnostic and therapeutic procedures, and for obstetrical procedures. Only 0.25% and 0.5% are indicated for obstetrical anesthesia.

DOSAGE: *Adults:* Individualize dose. Dosage varies depending on procedure, area to be anesthetized, vascularity of tissues, number of neural segments to be blocked, depth and duration of anesthesia, degree of muscle relaxation required, and patient tolerance and physical condition. Single Dose Max: 175mg. May repeat once every 3 hrs. Total Daily Dose Max: 400mg. Epidural Anesthesia: 0.5% or 0.75% in 3-5mL increments. In obstetrics, use only 0.25% or 0.5%. Use 3-5mL increments of 0.5% solution not to exceed 50-100mg at any dosing interval. Repeat doses should be preceded by test dose containing epinephrine if not contraindicated. Young/Elderly/Debilitated/Cardiac or Liver Disease: Reduce dose.

Pediatrics: ≥12 yrs: Individualize dose. Dosage varies depending on procedure, area to be anesthetized, vascularity of tissues, number of neural segments to be blocked, depth and duration of anesthesia, degree of muscle relaxation required, and patient tolerance and physical condition. Single Dose Max: 175mg. May repeat once every 3 hrs. Total Daily Dose Max: 400mg. Epidural Anesthesia: 0.5% in 3-5mL increments. In obstetrics, use only 0.25% or 0.5%. Use 3-5mL increments of 0.5% solution not to exceed 50-100mg at any dosing interval. Repeat doses should be preceded by test dose containing epinephrine if not contraindicated.

HOW SUPPLIED: Inj: 0.25%, 0.5%; (MPF) 0.25%, 0.5%, 0.75%

CONTRAINDICATIONS: Obstetrical paracervical block anesthesia.

WARNINGS/PRECAUTIONS: The 0.75% strength is not recommended for obstetrical anesthesia. Acidosis, cardiac arrest, death reported from delay in toxicity management. Local anesthetic solutions containing antimicrobial preservatives should not be used for epidural or caudal anesthesia. Not recommended for IV regional anesthesia. Monitor cardiovascular and respiratory vital signs and state of consciousness after each injection. Caution with hepatic disease and impaired cardiovascular function. Monitor circulation and respiration with injections into head and neck area. Respiratory arrest following local anesthetic injection during retrobulbar blocks has been reported.

ADVERSE REACTIONS: Restlessness, anxiety, dizziness, tinnitus, blurred vision, tremors, convulsions, nausea, vomiting, chills, hypotension, bradycardia, ventricular arrhythmias, urticaria, pruritus, erythema, edema.

INTERACTIONS: Avoid use with any other local anesthetics.

PREGNANCY: Category C, not for use in nursing.

SENSORCAINE WITH EPINEPHRINE RX
epinephrine - bupivacaine HCl (Abraxis)

OTHER BRAND NAME: Sensorcaine-MPF w/Epinephrine (Abraxis)

THERAPEUTIC CLASS: Local anesthetic

INDICATIONS: Production of local or regional anesthesia for surgery, oral surgery procedures, diagnostic and therapeutic procedures, and for obstetrical procedures. Only 0.25% and 0.5% are indicated for obstetrical anesthesia.

DOSAGE: *Adults:* Individualize dose. Dosage varies depending on procedure, area to be anesthetized, vascularity of tissues, number of neural segments to be blocked, depth and duration of anesthesia, degree of muscle relaxation required, and patient tolerance and physical condition. Single Dose Max: 225mg. May repeat once every 3 hrs. Total Daily Dose Max: 400mg. Epidural Anesthesia: 0.5% or 0.75% in 3-5mL increments. In obstetrics, use only 0.25% or 0.5%. Use 3-5mL increments of 0.5% solution not to exceed 50-100mg at any dosing interval. Repeat doses should be preceded by test dose containing epinephrine if not contraindicated. Young/Elderly/Debilitated/Cardiac or Liver Disease: Reduce dose.

Pediatrics: ≥12 yrs: Individualize dose. Dosage varies depending on procedure, area to be anesthetized, vascularity of tissues, number of neural segments to be blocked, depth and duration of anesthesia, degree of muscle relaxation required, and patient tolerance and physical condition. Single Dose Max: 225mg. May repeat once every 3 hrs. Total Daily Dose Max: 400mg. Epidural Anesthesia: 0.5% or 0.75% in 3-5mL increments. In obstetrics, use only 0.25% or 0.5%. Use 3-5mL increments of 0.5% solution not to exceed 50-100mg at any dosing interval. Repeat doses should be preceded by test dose containing epinephrine if not contraindicated.

HOW SUPPLIED: Inj: (Bupivacaine-Epinephrine) 0.25%/1:200,000, 0.5%/1:200,000; (MPF) 0.25%/1:200,000, 0.5%/1:200,000, 0.75%/1:200,000

CONTRAINDICATIONS: Obstetrical paracervical block anesthesia.

WARNINGS/PRECAUTIONS: The 0.75% strength is not recommended for obstetrical anesthesia. Acidosis, cardiac arrest, death reported from delay in toxicity management. Local anesthetic solutions containing antimicrobial preservatives should not be used for epidural or caudal anesthesia. Not recommended for IV regional anesthesia. Bupivacaine with epinephrine solutions contain sodium metabisulfite which may cause allergic-type reactions in susceptible people. Monitor cardiovascular and respiratory vital signs and state of consciousness after each injection. Caution when local anesthetic solutions containing a vasoconstrictor are used in areas of the body supplied by end arteries or having otherwise compromised blood supply; ischemic injury or necrosis may result with hypertensive vascular disease. Caution with hepatic disease and impaired cardiovascular function. Monitor circulation and respiration with injections into head and neck area. Respiratory arrest following local anesthetic injection during retrobulbar blocks has been reported.

ADVERSE REACTIONS: Restlessness, anxiety, dizziness, tinnitus, blurred vision, tremors, convulsions, nausea, vomiting, chills, hypotension, bradycardia, ventricular arrhythmias, urticaria, pruritus, erythema, edema.

INTERACTIONS: Avoid use with any other local anesthetics. Anesthetic solutions containing epinephrine or norepinephrine with MAOIs or TCAs may produce severe, prolonged HTN; avoid concurrent use or monitor closely if concurrent use is necessary. Concurrent administration of vasopressors and ergot-type oxytocic drugs may cause severe, persistent HTN or CVA. Phenothiazines and butyrophenones may reduce or reverse the pressor effect of epinephrine. Serious dose-related cardiac arrhythmias may occur with use during or following administration of potent inhalation anesthetics.

PREGNANCY: Category C, not for use in nursing.

SEPTOCAINE RX
epinephrine - articaine HCl (Septodont)

THERAPEUTIC CLASS: Anesthetic

INDICATIONS: For local, infiltrative, or conductive anesthesia in both simple and complex dental and periodontal procedures.

DOSAGE: *Adults:* Submucosal Infiltration: 0.5-2.5mL. Nerve Block: 0.5-3.4mL. Oral Surgery: 1-5.1mL. Max: 7mg/kg (0.175mL/kg) or 3.2mg/lb (0.0795mL/lb).
Pediatrics: ≥4 yrs: Submucosal Infiltration/Nerve Block/Oral Surgery: up to 7mg/kg (0.175mL/kg) or 3.2mg/lb (0.0795mL/lb).

HOW SUPPLIED: Inj: (Articaine-Epinephrine) 4%-1:100,000/1.7mL, 4%-1:200,000/1.7ml.

CONTRAINDICATIONS: Hypersensitivity to sodium metabisulfite.

WARNINGS/PRECAUTIONS: Avoid intravascular injection; aspirate needle before use. Intravascular injection is associated with convulsions, followed by CNS or cardiorespiratory depression and coma progressing to respiratory arrest. Epinephrine can cause local tissue necrosis or systemic toxicity. Contains sodium metabisulfite which can cause allergic reactions. Exaggerated vasoconstrictive response may occur with peripheral vascular disease and hypertensive vascular disease. CNS or cardiovascular effects may occur with systemic absorption. Local anesthetics are capable of producing methemoglobinemia, with signs of cyanosis, fatigue, and weakness.

ADVERSE REACTIONS: Face edema, headache, infection, pain, gingivitis, swelling, paresthesia, trismus.

INTERACTIONS: MAOIs or TCAs may produce severe, prolonged HTN. Phenothiazines and butyrphenones may reduce or reverse pressor effect of epinephrine.

PREGNANCY: Category C, caution in nursing.

SEPTRA RX
trimethoprim - sulfamethoxazole (King)

OTHER BRAND NAMES: Septra DS (King) - Sulfatrim Pediatric (Alpharma)

THERAPEUTIC CLASS: Sulfonamide/tetrahydrofolic acid inhibitor

INDICATIONS: (Inj, Susp, Tab) Treatment of urinary tract infection (UTI), pneumocystitis carinii pneumonia (PCP) and enteritis caused by *Shigella*. (Susp, Tab). Treatment of acute exacerbation of chronic bronchitis (AECB), travelers' diarrhea, and acute otitis media.

DOSAGE: *Adults:* (Sus, Tab) UTI: 800mg-160mg PO q12h for 10-14 days. Shigellosis/Traveler's Diarrhea: 800mg-160mg PO q12h for 5 days. AECB: 800mg-160mg PO q12h for 14 days. PCP Treatment: 15-20mg/kg TMP and 75-100mg/kg SMX per 24 hrs given PO q6h for 14-21 days PCP Prophylaxis: 800mg-160mg PO qd. (Inj) Severe UTI: 8-10mg/kg TMP IV given in divided doses q6, 8 or 12h for up to 14 days. PCP Treatment: 15-20mg/kg TMP IV given in divided doses q6-8h for up to 14 days. Shigellosis: 8-10mg/kg TMP IV given in divided doses q6, 8 or 12h for 5 days. (Inj, Sus, Tab) Renal Impairment: CrCl 15-30mL/min: 50% usual dose. CrCl <15mL/min: Not recommended.
Pediatrics: (Sus, Tab) ≥2 months: UTI/Otitis Media: 4mg/kg TMP and 20mg/kg SMX q12h for 10 days. Shigellosis/Traveler's Diarrhea: 4mg/kg TMP and 20mg/kg SMX q12h for 5 days. PCP Treatment: 15-20mg/kg TMP and 75-100mg/kg SMX/24 hrs given q6h for 14-21 days. PCP Prophylaxis: 150mg/m^2/day TMP and 750mg/m^2/day SMX PO given bid, on 3 consecutive days per week. Max: 320mg TMP and 1600mg SMX per day. (Inj) Severe UTI: 8-10mg/kg TMP IV given in divided doses q6, 8 or 12h for up to 14 days. PCP Treatment: 15-20mg/kg TMP IV given in divided doses q6-8h for up to 14 days. Shigellosis: 8-10mg/kg TMP IV given in divided doses q6, 8 or 12h for 5 days. (Inj, Sus, Tab) Renal Impairment: CrCl 15-30mL/min: 50% usual dose. CrCl <15mL/min: Not recommended.

HOW SUPPLIED: (Sulfamethoxazole (SMX)-Trimethoprim (TMP)) Inj: (Septra) 80mg-16mg/mL; Sus: (Sulfatrim Pediatric, Septra) 200mg-40mg/5mL (100mL, 473mL); Tab: (Septra) 400mg-80mg*; Tab, DS: (Septra) 800mg-160mg* *scored

CONTRAINDICATIONS: Megaloblastic anemia due to folate deficiency, pregnancy at term, nursing, infants <2 months old.

WARNINGS/PRECAUTIONS: Fatal hypersensitivity reactions (eg, Stevens-Johnson syndrome, toxic epidermal necrolysis, fulminant hepatic necrosis, agranulocytosis, aplastic anemia) may occur. Pseudomembranous colitis, cough, SOB, and pulmonary infiltrates reported. Avoid with group A β-hemolytic streptococcal infections. Caution with hepatic/renal impairment, elderly, folate deficiency (eg, chronic alcoholics, anticonvulsants, malabsorption, malnutrition), bronchial asthma, and other allergies. In G6PD deficiency, hemolysis may occur. Increased incidence of adverse events in AIDS patients. Maintain adequate fluid intake.

ADVERSE REACTIONS: Anorexia, nausea, vomiting, rash, urticaria, cholestatic jaundice, agranulocytosis, anemia, hyperkalemia, renal failure, interstitial nephritis, hyponatremia, convulsions, arthralgia, myalgia, weakness.

INTERACTIONS: Increase risk of thrombocytopenia with purpura with diuretics (especially thiazides) in the elderly. Caution with warfarin; may prolong PT. Increased effects of phenytoin, methotrexate.

PREGNANCY: Category C, contraindicated in nursing.

SEREVENT
salmeterol xinafoate (GlaxoSmithKline)

RX

> Long-acting $β_2$-adrenergic agonists, such as salmeterol, may increase the risk of asthma-related deaths.

THERAPEUTIC CLASS: Beta$_2$ agonist

INDICATIONS: Long-term maintenance treatment of asthma and COPD. Prevention of bronchospasm with reversible obstructive airway disease (including nocturnal asthma) when regular treatment with inhaled short-acting $β_2$-agonists is required. Prevention of exercise-induced bronchospasm (EIB).

DOSAGE: *Adults:* Asthma/COPD: 1 inh bid, am and pm (12 hrs apart). EIB Prevention: 1 inh 30 minutes before exercise (do not give preventive doses if already on bid dose). *Pediatrics:* ≥4 yrs: Asthma: 1 inh bid, am and pm (12 hrs apart). EIB Prevention: 1 inh 30 minutes before exercise (do not give preventive doses if already on bid dose).

HOW SUPPLIED: Disk: 50mcg (28, 60 blisters)

WARNINGS/PRECAUTIONS: Avoid with significantly worsening or acutely deteriorating asthma. Not for acute treatment or substitute for oral/inhaled corticosteroids. Monitor for increasing use of inhaled $β_2$ agonists. QTc interval prolongation reported when exceeded recommended dose. D/C if paradoxical bronchospasm occurs. Immediate hypersensitivity and upper airway symptom reactions reported. Caution with cardiovascular disorder (eg, coronary insufficiency, arrhythmia, HTN), convulsive disorders, thyrotoxicosis, if usually unresponsive to sympathomimetic amines. May cause hypokalemia.

ADVERSE REACTIONS: Nasal/sinus congestion, pallor, rhinitis, headache, tracheitis/bronchitis, influenza, throat irritation.

INTERACTIONS: Caution with non-potassium-sparing diuretics. Extreme caution within 14 days of using MAOIs or TCAs. Avoid with β-blockers. Caution with >8 inhalations of short-acting $β_2$-agonists.

PREGNANCY: Category C, not for use in nursing.

SIMULECT
basiliximab (Novartis)

RX

> Manage patient in facility with adequate lab and supportive resources. Prescribing physician should be experienced with immunosuppressives and transplantation. Physician should have complete information requisite for patient follow-up.

THERAPEUTIC CLASS: Monoclonal antibody/IL-2R alpha (CD25) blocker

SINGULAIR

INDICATIONS: Prophylaxis of acute organ rejection in renal transplantation.

DOSAGE: *Adults:* 20mg within 2 hrs prior to transplant, repeat 4 days after transplant. Withhold 2nd dose if graft loss or complications occur.

Pediatrics: ≥35kg: 20mg within 2 hrs prior to transplant, repeat 4 days after transplant. <35kg: 10mg within 2 hrs prior to transplant, repeat 4 days after transplant. Withhold 2nd dose if graft loss or complications occur.

HOW SUPPLIED: Inj: 10mg, 20mg

WARNINGS/PRECAUTIONS: Only administer under qualified medical supervision. Increased risk of developing lymphoproliferative disorder and opportunistic infections. Anaphylaxis and other severe hypersensitivity reactions (eg, hypotension, cardiac failure, bronchospasm, respiratory failure, etc) reported and may necessitate discontinuation. Anti-idiotype antibodies may develop.

ADVERSE REACTIONS: GI effects, peripheral edema, fever, viral infection, hyperkalemia, hypokalemia, hyperglycemia, hypercholesterolemia, hypophosphatemia, hyperuricemia, UTI, dyspnea, upper respiratory infection, acne, HTN, headache, tremor, insomnia, anemia.

PREGNANCY: Category B, not for use in nursing.

SINGULAIR
montelukast sodium (Merck)

RX

THERAPEUTIC CLASS: Leukotriene receptor antagonist

INDICATIONS: Prophylaxis and chronic treatment of asthma (≥12 months). Relief of symptoms of seasonal allergic rhinitis (≥2 yrs) and perennial allergic rhinitis (≥6 months). Prevention of exercise-induced bronchoconstriction (EIB) (≥15 yrs).

DOSAGE: *Adults:* Asthma: 10mg qpm. Allergic Rhinitis: 10mg qd. EIB: 10mg 2 hrs before exercise. Do not take additional dose within 24 hrs of previous dose.

Pediatrics: Asthma: ≥15 yrs: 10mg qpm. 6-14 yrs: 5mg qpm. 2-5 yrs: 4mg qpm. 12-23 months: 4mg qpm. Seasonal/Perennial Allergic Rhinitis: ≥15 yrs: 10mg qd. 6-14 yrs: 5mg qd. 2-5 yrs: 4mg qd. Perennial Allergic Rhinitis: 6-23 months: 4mg qd. EIB: ≥15 yrs: 10mg 2 hrs before exercise. Do not take additional dose within 24 hrs of previous dose. Granules may be mixed with applesauce, carrots, rice or ice cream; give within 15 minutes of opening packet.

HOW SUPPLIED: Granules: 4mg/packet; Tab, Chewable: 4mg, 5mg; Tab: 10mg

WARNINGS/PRECAUTIONS: Not for treatment of acute asthma attacks. Do not abruptly substitute for inhaled or oral corticosteroids. Eosinophilic conditions reported (rare).

ADVERSE REACTIONS: (Adults, Pediatrics) Headache, cough. (Pediatrics) Pharyngitis, fever, flu, nausea, diarrhea, dyspepsia, rhinorrhea, upper respiratory infection.

INTERACTIONS: Monitor with potent CYP450 inducers (eg, phenobarbital, rifampin).

PREGNANCY: Category B, caution in nursing.

SKELAXIN
metaxalone (King)

RX

THERAPEUTIC CLASS: Muscular analgesic (central-acting)

INDICATIONS: Adjunct for acute, painful musculoskeletal conditions.

DOSAGE: *Adults:* 800mg tid-qid.
Pediatrics: >12 yrs: 800mg tid-qid.

HOW SUPPLIED: Tab: 800mg* *scored

CONTRAINDICATIONS: Tendency for drug-induced, hemolytic, and other anemias. Significant renal or hepatic impairment.

WARNINGS/PRECAUTIONS: Caution with pre-existing liver damage. Monitor hepatic function. False-positive Benedict's test reported.

ADVERSE REACTIONS: Nausea, vomiting, GI upset, drowsiness, dizziness, headache, nervousness, leukopenia, hemolytic anemia, jaundice.

INTERACTIONS: May enhance the effects of alcohol, barbiturates and other CNS depressants.

PREGNANCY: Not for use in pregnancy or nursing.

Solaquin Forte RX
hydroquinone (Valeant)

THERAPEUTIC CLASS: Depigmenting agent

INDICATIONS: For the gradual bleaching of hyperpigmented skin conditions (eg, chloasma, melasma, freckles, senile lentigines).

DOSAGE: *Adults:* Apply bid.

Pediatrics: ≥12 yrs: Apply bid.

HOW SUPPLIED: Cre: 4% (28.4g); Gel: 4% (28.4g)

WARNINGS/PRECAUTIONS: Avoid sun exposure on bleached skin. Solaquin Forte contains sunscreen. May produce unwanted cosmetic effects if not used as directed. Test for skin sensitivity. Discontinue if no lightening effect after 2 months. Contains sodium metabisulfite, may cause serious allergic type reactions. Limit treatment to small areas of body at one time. Avoid contact with eyes.

ADVERSE REACTIONS: Cutaneous hypersensitivity (contact dermatitis).

PREGNANCY: Category C, caution in nursing.

Solodyn RX
minocycline HCl (Medicis)

THERAPEUTIC CLASS: Tetracycline derivative

INDICATIONS: Treatment of inflammatory lesions of non-nodular moderate to severe acne vulgaris in patients ≥12 yrs.

DOSAGE: *Adults:* 1mg/kg qd for 12 weeks. Reduce dose with renal impairment.

Pediatrics: ≥12 yrs: 1mg/kg qd for 12 weeks. Reduce dose with renal impairment.

HOW SUPPLIED: Tab, Extended Release: 45mg, 90mg, 135mg.

WARNINGS/PRECAUTIONS: May cause fetal harm during pregnancy. Use during tooth development (last half of pregnancy, infancy, <8yrs) may cause permanent discoloration of the teeth or enamel hypoplasia; avoid use during this period. May decrease bone growth in premature infants. May cause pseudomembarnous colitis. Renal toxicity, hepatotoxicity, photosensitivity, increased BUN, superinfection, pseudotumor cerebri may occur. Caution in renal impairment; may lead to azotemia, hyperphosphatemia, and acidosis. Long-term use has been associated with lupus-like syndrome, autoimmune hepatitis and vasculitis. May cause serum sickness. May induce hyperpigmentation.

ADVERSE REACTIONS: Headache, fatigue, dizziness, pruritus, malaise, mood alteration.

INTERACTIONS: May require downward regulation of anticoagulant therapy. May interfere with bactericidal action of penicillin; avoid concurrent. May decrease efficacy of oral contraceptives. Impaired absorption with antacids containing aluminum, calcium or magnesium, and iron-containing preparations. Fatal renal toxicity with methoxyflurane reported.

PREGNANCY: Category D, not for use in nursing.

Solu-Cortef RX
hydrocortisone sodium succinate (Pharmacia & Upjohn)

THERAPEUTIC CLASS: Corticosteroid

INDICATIONS: Steroid responsive disorders.

DOSAGE: *Adults:* Initial: 100-500mg IV/IM, depending on condition severity. May repeat dose at 2, 4, or 6 hrs based on clinical response. High dose therapy usually not >48-72 hrs; may use antacids prophylactically.

Solu-Medrol

Pediatrics: Use lower adult doses. Determine dose by severity of condition and response. Dose should not be <25mg/day.

HOW SUPPLIED: Inj: 100mg, 250mg, 500mg, 1g

CONTRAINDICATIONS: Premature infants, systemic fungal infections.

WARNINGS/PRECAUTIONS: May need to increase dose before, during, and after stressful situations. May mask signs of infection or cause new infections. Prolonged use may produce glaucoma, optic nerve damage, secondary ocular infections. Increases BP, salt/water retention, potassium and calcium excretion. More severe/fatal course of infections reported with chickenpox, measles. Enhanced effect with hypothyroidism or cirrhosis. Caution with Strongyloides, latent TB, ocular herpes simplex, HTN, diverticulitis, fresh intestinal anastomoses, ulcerative colitis, osteoporosis, myasthenia gravis, renal insufficiency, peptic ulcer disease. Kaposi's sarcoma reported. Monitor for psychic disturbances. Acute myopathy with high doses. Avoid abrupt withdrawal. Monitor growth and development of children on prolonged therapy. Hypernatremia may occur with high dose therapy >48-72 hrs.

ADVERSE REACTIONS: Fluid and electrolyte disturbances, HTN, osteoporosis, muscle weakness, cushingoid state, menstrual irregularities, vertigo, headache, impaired wound healing, DM, ulcerative esophagitis, peptic ulcer, pancreatitis, increased sweating, increases intracranial pressure, carbohydrate intolerance, glaucoma, cataracts.

INTERACTIONS: Reduced efficacy and increased clearance with hepatic enzyme inducers (eg, phenobarbital, phenytoin, and rifampin). Increases clearance of chronic high dose ASA. Caution with ASA in hypoprothrombinemia. Effects on oral anticoagulants are variable; monitor PT/INR. Increased insulin and oral hypoglycemic requirements in DM. Avoid live vaccines with immunosuppressive doses. Possible decreased vaccine response with killed or inactivated vaccines with immunosuppressive doses. Decreased clearance with ketoconazole and troleandomycin.

PREGNANCY: Safety in pregnancy and nursing not known.

Solu-Medrol RX
methylprednisolone sodium succinate (Pharmacia & Upjohn)

THERAPEUTIC CLASS: Glucocorticoid

INDICATIONS: Steroid responsive disorders.

DOSAGE: *Adults:* Usual: Initial: 10-40mg IV over several minutes. May repeat IV/IM dose at intervals based on clinical response. High Dose Therapy: 30mg/kg IV over at least 30 minutes, may repeat q4-6h for 48 hrs. High dose therapy usually not >48-72 hrs. Give antacids prophylactically. Multiple Sclerosis: (4mg methylprednisolone=5mg prednisolone): 200mg/day prednisolone for 1 week, then 80mg every other day for 1 month.
Pediatrics: Use lower adult doses. Determine dose by severity of condition and response. Dose should not be <0.5mg/kg q24h.

HOW SUPPLIED: Inj: 40mg, 125mg, 500mg, 1g, 2g

CONTRAINDICATIONS: Premature infants (due to benzyl alcohol diluent) and systemic fungal infections.

WARNINGS/PRECAUTIONS: May need to increase dose before, during, and after stressful situations. May mask signs of infection or cause new infections. Prolonged use may produce cataracts, glaucoma, secondary ocular infections. Increases BP, salt/water retention, calcium/potassium excretion. More severe/fatal course of infections reported with chickenpox, measles. Caution with latent TB, hypothyroidism, cirrhosis, ocular herpes simplex, HTN, diverticulitis, fresh intestinal anastomoses, ulcerative colitis, osteoporosis, myasthenia gravis, renal insufficiency, peptic ulcer disease. Kaposi's sarcoma reported. Growth and development of children on prolonged therapy should be monitored. Monitor for psychic disturbances. Avoid abrupt withdrawal. Reports of cardiac arrhythmias, circulatory collapse, cardiac arrest following rapid administration of large IV doses. Effectiveness not established for the treatment of sepsis syndrome and septic shock. Bradycardia reportedwith high doses.

ADVERSE REACTIONS: Fluid and electrolyte disturbances, HTN, osteoporosis, muscle weakness, cushingoid state, menstrual irregularities, insomnia, impaired wound healing, DM, ulcerative esophagitis, excessive sweating, increases intracranial pressure, carbohydrate intolerance, glaucoma, cataracts, nausea.

INTERACTIONS: Reduced efficacy with hepatic enzyme inducers (eg, phenobarbital, phenytoin, and rifampin). Increases clearance of chronic high dose ASA. Caution with ASA in hypoprothrombinemia. Effects on oral anticoagulants are variable; monitor PT/INR. Increased insulin and oral hypoglycemic requirements in DM. Avoid live vaccines with immunosuppressive doses. Possible decreased vaccine response with killed or inactivated vaccines with immunosuppressive doses. Mutual inhibition of metabolism with cyclosporine; convulsions reported. Decreased clearance with ketoconazole and troleandomycin.

PREGNANCY: Safety in pregnancy and nursing not known.

SOMA
carisoprodol (MedPointe)

RX

THERAPEUTIC CLASS: Skeletal muscle relaxant (central-acting)

INDICATIONS: Adjunct for relief of discomfort associated with acute, painful musculoskeletal conditions.

DOSAGE: *Adults:* 350mg tid and hs.
Pediatrics: ≥12 yrs: 350mg tid and hs.

HOW SUPPLIED: Tab: 350mg

CONTRAINDICATIONS: Acute intermittent porphyria. Allergic or idiosyncratic reactions to meprobamate.

WARNINGS/PRECAUTIONS: May have sedative properties. Cases of drug abuse, dependence and withdrawal have been reported. Caution in addiction-prone patients. First-dose idiosyncratic reactions reported (rare). Occasionally within the period of teh fisrt to fourth dose, allergic reactions have occured. Rare reports of seizures in post-marketing surveillance. Caution with liver or renal dysfunction.

ADVERSE REACTIONS: Drowsiness, dizziness, nausea, vomiting, tachycardia, postural hypotension, idiosyncratic reactions.

INTERACTIONS: Additive effects with alcohol, other CNS depressants, and psychotropic drugs.

PREGNANCY: Safety in pregnancy and nursing not known.

SOMA CMPD/CODEINE
aspirin - carisoprodol - codeine phosphate (MedPointe)

CIII

THERAPEUTIC CLASS: Central muscle relaxant/analgesic

INDICATIONS: Adjunct for pain, muscle spasm, and limited mobility associated with acute, painful musculoskeletal conditions.

DOSAGE: *Adults:* 1-2 tabs qid.
Pediatrics: ≥12 yrs: 1-2 tabs qid.

HOW SUPPLIED: Tab: (Carisoprodol-Codeine-Aspirin) 200mg-16mg-325mg

CONTRAINDICATIONS: Acute intermittent porphyria, bleeding disorders.

WARNINGS/PRECAUTIONS: First-dose idiosyncratic reactions reported (rare). Caution with liver or renal dysfunction, elderly, peptic ulcer, gastritis, addiction-prone patients and anticoagulant therapy. Contains sulfites.

ADVERSE REACTIONS: Drowsiness, dizziness, vertigo, ataxia, nausea, vomiting, gastritis, occult bleeding, constipation, diarrhea, miosis.

INTERACTIONS: Enhances methotrexate toxicity and hypoglycemia with oral antidiabetics. Corticosteroids and antacids decrease plasma levels. Increases GI bleeding risk with alcohol. Potentiated by urine acidifiers (eg, ammonium chloride). Antagonizes uricosuric effects of probenecid, sulfinpyrazone. Additive effects with alcohol, other CNS depressants, psychotropic drugs. Increases bleeding risk with anticoagulants.

PREGNANCY: Category C, not for use in nursing.

SOMA COMPOUND
aspirin - carisoprodol (MedPointe)
RX

THERAPEUTIC CLASS: Central muscle relaxant/analgesic

INDICATIONS: Adjunct for pain, muscle spasm and limited mobility associated with acute, painful musculoskeletal conditions.

DOSAGE: *Adults:* 1-2 tabs qid.
Pediatrics: ≥12 yrs: 1-2 tabs qid.

HOW SUPPLIED: Tab: (Carisoprodol-ASA) 200mg-325mg

CONTRAINDICATIONS: Acute intermittent porphyria, bleeding disorders.

WARNINGS/PRECAUTIONS: First-dose idiosyncratic reactions reported (rare). Caution with liver or renal dysfunction, elderly, peptic ulcer, gastritis, addiction-prone patients and anticoagulant therapy.

ADVERSE REACTIONS: Drowsiness, dizziness, vertigo, ataxia, nausea, vomiting, gastritis, occult bleeding, constipation, diarrhea.

INTERACTIONS: Enhances methotrexate toxicity and hypoglycemia with oral antidiabetics. Corticosteroids and antacids decrease plasma levels. Increases GI bleeding risk with alcohol. Potentiated by urine acidifiers (eg, ammonium chloride). Antagonizes uricosuric effects of probenecid, sulfinpyrazone. Additive effects with alcohol, other CNS depressants, psychotropic drugs. Increases bleeding risk with anticoagulants.

PREGNANCY: Category C, not for use in nursing.

SPECTRACEF
cefditoren pivoxil (Purdue Pharmaceutical)
RX

THERAPEUTIC CLASS: Cephalosporin (3rd generation)

INDICATIONS: Treatment of acute bacterial exacerbations of chronic bronchitis (ABECB), pharyngitis/tonsillitis, community acquired pneumonia (CAP), and uncomplicated skin and skin-structure infections (SSSI).

DOSAGE: *Adults:* ABECB: 400mg bid for 10 days. Pharyngitis/Tonsillitis/SSSI: 200mg bid for 10 days. CAP: 400mg bid for 14 days. CrCl 30-49mL/min: 200mg bid. CrCl <30mL/min: 200mg qd. Take with meals.
Pediatrics: ≥12 yrs: ABECB: 400mg bid for 10 days. Pharyngitis/Tonsillitis/SSSI: 200mg bid for 10 days. CAP: 400mg bid for 14 days. CrCl 30-49mL/min: 200mg bid. CrCl <30mL/min: 200mg qd. Take with meals.

HOW SUPPLIED: Tab: 200mg

CONTRAINDICATIONS: Milk protein hypersensitivity, carnitine deficiency.

WARNINGS/PRECAUTIONS: Cross sensitivity to penicillins and other cephalosporins may occur. Pseudomembranous colitis reported. Not recommended for prolonged antibiotic therapy. Prolonged therapy may cause superinfection. May decrease PT.

ADVERSE REACTIONS: Diarrhea, nausea, vaginal moniliasis.

INTERACTIONS: Avoid antacids. H2 receptor antagonists may reduce absorption. Increased plasma levels with probenecid.

PREGNANCY: Category B, caution in nursing.

STRATTERA
atomoxetine HCl (Lilly)
RX

> Increased risk of suicidal ideation in short-term studies in children or adolescents with ADHD. Closely monitor for suicidality, clinical worsening, or unusual changes in behavior. Close observation/communication with prescriber by families and caregivers is advised.

THERAPEUTIC CLASS: Selective norepinephrine reuptake inhibitor

INDICATIONS: Treatment of attention-deficit hyperactivity disorder (ADHD).

DOSAGE: *Adults:* Initial: 40mg/day given qam or evenly divided doses in the am and late afternoon/early evening. Titrate: Increase after minimum of 3 days to target dose of about 80mg/day. After 2-4 weeks, may increase to max of 100mg/day. Max: 100mg/day. Hepatic Insufficiency: Moderate (Child-Pugh Class B): Reduce initial and target doses to 50% of normal dose. Severe (Child-Pugh Class C): Reduce initial and target doses to 25% of normal dose. Concomitant CYP450 2D6 inhibitor (eg, paroxetine, fluoxetine, quinidine): Initial: 40mg/day. Titrate: Only increase to 80mg/day if symptoms fail to improve after 4 weeks.

Pediatrics: ≥6 yrs: ≤70kg: Initial: 0.5mg/kg/day given qam or evenly divided doses in the am and late afternoon or early evening. Titrate: Increase after minimum of 3 days to target dose of about 1.2mg/kg/day. Max: 1.4mg/kg/day or 100mg, whichever is less. >70kg: Initial: 40mg/day given qam or evenly divided doses in the am and late afternoon/early evening. Titrate: Increase after minimum of 3 days to target dose of about 80mg/day. After 2-4 weeks, may increase to max of 100mg/day. Max: 100mg/day. Hepatic Insufficiency: Moderate (Child-Pugh Class B): Reduce initial and target doses to 50% of the normal dose. Severe (Child-Pugh Class C): Reduce initial and target doses to 25% of normal dose. Concomitant CYP450 2D6 inhibitor (eg, paroxetine, fluoxetine, quinidine): ≥6 yrs: ≤70kg: Initial: 0.5mg/kg/day. Titrate: Only increase to 1.2mg/kg/day if symptoms fail to improve after 4 weeks. >70kg: Initial: 40mg/day. Titrate: Only increase to 80mg/day if symptoms fail to improve after 4 weeks.

HOW SUPPLIED: Cap: 10mg, 18mg, 25mg, 40mg, 60mg

CONTRAINDICATIONS: During or within 14 days of MAOI use; narrow angle glaucoma.

WARNINGS/PRECAUTIONS: Allergic reactions and orthostatic hypotension reported. Monitor growth. May increase BP and HR; caution with HTN, tachycardia, cardiovascular or cerebrovascular disease. May increase urinary retention and urinary hesitation. May cause severe liver injury in rare cases; monitor liver enzymes and d/c with jaundice or liver injury. Reports of MI, stroke and sudden death in adults. Avoid with known structural cardiac abnormalities or other serious cardiac problems. Physical exam and evaluation of patient history is necessary. Stimulants at usual doses can cause treatment emergent psychotic or manic symptoms (eg, hallucinations, delusional thinking, mania) in children and adolescents without prior history of psychotic illness.

ADVERSE REACTIONS: (Adults) Dry mouth, headache, insomnia, nausea, decreased appetite, constipation, dysmenorrhea, ejaculation failure/disorder, urinary retention. (Pediatrics) Upper abdominal pain, headache, vomiting, decreased appetite, cough, irritability, dizziness, somnolence.

INTERACTIONS: See Contraindications. May potentiate the cardiovascular effects of albuterol or other β^2 agonists. Caution with pressor agents. Increased levels in extensive metabolizers with CYP2D6 inhibitors (eg, paroxetine, fluoxetine, quinidine); atomoxetine may need dose adjustment.

PREGNANCY: Category C, caution in nursing.

STREPTOMYCIN RX
streptomycin sulfate (Various)

> Risk of severe neurotoxic reactions (eg, vestibular and cochlear disturbances) increased significantly with renal dysfunction or pre-renal azotemia. Optic nerve dysfunction, peripheral neuritis, arachnoiditis, and encephalopathy may occur. Monitor renal function; reduce dose with renal impairment and/or nitrogen retention. Do not exceed peak serum level of 20-25mcg/mL with kidney damage. Avoid other neurotoxic and/or nephrotoxic drugs (eg, neomycin, kanamycin, gentamicin, cephaloridine, paromomycin, viomycin, polymyxin B, colistin, tobramycin, cyclosporine). Respiratory paralysis can occur, especially if given soon after anesthesia or muscle relaxants. Reserve parenteral form when adequate lab and audiometric testing is available.

THERAPEUTIC CLASS: Aminoglycoside

INDICATIONS: Treatment of moderate to severe infections such as mycobacterium tuberculosis (TB) and non-TB infections (eg, plague, tularemia, chancroid, granuloma inguinale, *H.influenzae* and *K.pneumoniae* infections, UTI, gram-negative bacillary bacteremia, endocardial infections).

STROMECTOL

DOSAGE: *Adults:* IM only. TB: 15mg/kg/day (Max: 1g), or 25-30mg/kg twice weekly (Max: 1.5g), or 25-30mg/kg three times weekly (Max: 1.5g). Do not exceed a total dose of 120g over the course of therapy unless no other therapeutic options exist. Elderly (>60 yrs): Reduce dose. Treat for minimum of 1 year if possible. Tularemia: 1-2g/day in divided doses for 7-14 days until afebrile for 5-7 days. Plague: 1g bid for minimum of 10 days. Streptococcal Endocarditis: With PCN, 1g bid for week 1, then 500mg bid for week 2. Elderly (>60 yrs): 500mg bid for 2 weeks. Enterococcal Endocarditis: With PCN, 1g bid for 2 weeks, then 500mg bid for 4 weeks. Renal Impairment: Reduce dose. Moderate/Severe Infections: 1-2g/day in divided doses q6-12h. Max: 2g/day.

Pediatrics: IM only. TB: 20-40mg/kg/day (Max: 1g), or 25-30mg/kg twice weekly (Max: 1.5g), or 25-30mg/kg three times weekly (Max: 1.5g). Do not exceed a total dose of 120g over the course of therapy unless no other therapeutic options exist. Treat for minimum of 1 year if possible. Moderate/Severe Infections: 20-40mg/kg/day (8-20mg/lb/day) in divided doses q6-12h.

HOW SUPPLIED: Inj: 1g

WARNINGS/PRECAUTIONS: Vestibular and auditory dysfunction may occur. Contains sodium metabisulfite. Can cause fetal harm in pregnancy. Caution with dose selection in renal impairment. Alkalinize urine to minimize or prevent renal irritation with prolonged therapy. CNS depression (eg, stupor, flaccidity) reported in infants with higher than recommended doses. If syphilis is suspected when treating venereal infections, perform dark field exam before initiate treatment, and monthly serologic tests for at least 4 months. Overgrowth of nonsusceptible organisms may occur. Terminate therapy when toxic symptoms appear, when impending toxicity is feared, when organisms become resistant, or when full treatment effect has been obtained.

ADVERSE REACTIONS: Vestibular ototoxicity (nausea, vomiting, vertigo), paresthesia of face, rash, fever, urticaria, angioneurotic edema, eosinophilia.

INTERACTIONS: See Black Box Warning. Increased ototoxicity with ethacrynic acid, furosemide, mannitol and possibly other diuretics.

PREGNANCY: Category D, not for use in nursing.

STROMECTOL RX
ivermectin (Merck)

THERAPEUTIC CLASS: Avermectins derivative

INDICATIONS: Treatment of strongyloidiasis of the intestinal tract due to *Strongyloides stercoralis*, and onchocerciasis due to *Onchocerca volvulus*. Has no activity against adult *Onchocerca volvulus* parasites.

DOSAGE: *Adults:* Strongyloidiasis: 200mcg/kg single dose. Onchocerciasis: 150mcg/kg single dose. For mass distribution in international treatment programs, the usual dosing interval is 12 months. Usual dosing interval for retreatment for individual patients can be as short as 3 months. Take on empty stomach with water. To verify eradication of infection perform follow-up stool exams.

Pediatrics: ≥15kg: Strongyloidiasis: 200mcg/kg single dose. Onchocerciasis: 150mcg/kg single dose. For mass distribution in international treatment programs, the usual dosing interval is 12 months. Usual dosing interval for retreatment for individual patients can be as short as 3 months. Take on empty stomach with water. To verify eradication of infection perform follow-up stool exams.

HOW SUPPLIED: Tab: 3mg, 6mg* *scored

WARNINGS/PRECAUTIONS: May cause cutaneous and/or systemic reactions of varying severity (the Mazzotti reaction) and ophthalmological reactions. Patients with hyperreactive onchodermatitis (sowda) may be more likely to experience severe advisers reactions, especially edema and aggravation of onchodermatitis. Risk of serious or even fatal encephalopathy with onchocerciasis and *Loa loa* infection. Pretreatment assessment for loiasis and careful posttreatment follow-up should be performed in patients who were exposed to *Loa loa*-endemic areas of West or Central Africa.

ADVERSE REACTIONS: Diarrhea, nausea, dizziness, pruritis, decrease in leukocyte count, arthralgia/synovitis, axillary/cervical/inguinal lymph node enlargement, rash, fever, peripheral edema, tachycardia

PREGNANCY: Category C, caution in nursing.

SUBLIMAZE
fentanyl citrate (Akorn) — CII

THERAPEUTIC CLASS: Opioid analgesic

INDICATIONS: For analgesic action of short duration during the anesthetic periods, premedication, induction and maintenance, and in the immediate postoperative period (recovery room) as the need arises. For use as a narcotic analgesic supplement in general or regional anesthesia. For administration with a neuroleptic as an anesthetic premedication, for the induction of anesthesia and as an adjunct in the maintenance of general and regional anesthesia. For use as an anesthetic agent with oxygen in selected high risk patients, such as those undergoing open heart surgery or certain complicated neurological or orthopedic procedures.

DOSAGE: *Adults:* ≥12 yrs: Individualize dose. Premedication: 50-100mcg IM 30-60 minutes prior to surgery. Adjunct to General Anesthesia: Low Dose: Total Dose: 2mcg/kg for minor surgery. Maint: 2mcg/kg. Moderate Dose: Total Dose: 2-20mcg/kg for major surgery. Maint: 2-20mcg/kg or 25-100mcg IM or IV if surgical stress or lightening of analgesia. High Dose: Total Dose: 20-50mcg/kg for open heart surgery, complicated neurosurgery, or orthopedic surgery. Maint: 20-50mcg/kg. Adjunct to Regional Anesthesia: 50-100mcg IM or slow IV over 1-2 minutes. Postoperative: 50-100mcg IM, repeat q 1-2 hrs as needed. General Anesthetic: 50-100mcg/kg with oxygen and a muscle relaxant, up to 150mcg/kg may be used.
Pediatrics: 2-12 yrs: Individualize dose. Induction/Maint: 2-3mcg/kg.

HOW SUPPLIED: Inj: 50mcg/mL

WARNINGS/PRECAUTIONS: Should only be administered by persons specifically trained in the use of IV anesthetics and management of the respiratory effects of potent opioids. An opioid antagonist, resuscitative and intubation equipment and oxygen should be readily available. Fluids and other countermeasures to manage hypotension should be available with tranquilizers. Initial dose reduction recommended with narcotic analgesia for recovery. May cause muscle rigidity particularly with muscles used for respiration. Adequate facilities should be available for postoperative monitoring and ventilation. Caution in respiratory depression susceptible patients (eg, comatose patients with head injury or brain tumor). Reduce dose for elderly and debilitated patients. Caution with obstructive pulmonary disease, decreased respiratory reserve, liver and kidney dysfunction, cardiac bradyarrhythmias. Monitor vital signs routinely.

ADVERSE REACTIONS: Respiratory depression, apnea, rigidity, bradycardia, HTN, hypotension, dizziness, blurred vision, nausea, emesis, diaphoresis, pruritus, urticaria, laryngospasms, anaphylaxis, euphoria, miosis, bradycardia, and bronchoconstriction.

INTERACTIONS: Severe and unpredictable potentiation by MAO inhibitors has been reported. Appropriate monitoring and availability of vasodilators and beta-blockers for the treatment of hypertension is indicated. Additive or potentiating effects with other CNS depressants (eg, barbiturates, tranquilizers, narcotics, general anesthetics). Reduce dose of other CNS depressants. Reports of cardiovascular depression with nitrous oxide. Alteration of respiration with certain forms of conduction anesthesia (eg, spinal anesthesia, some peridural anesthesia). Decreased pulmonary arterial pressure and hypotension with tranquilizers. Elevated blood pressure, with and without pre-existing hypertension, slower normalacy of EEG patterns with neuroleptics. Extreme caution with neuroleptics in the presense of risk factors for development of prolonged QT syndrome and torsade de pointes; ECG monitoring indicated.

PREGNANCY: Category C, caution with nursing.

SUBOXONE
naloxone - buprenorphine (Reckitt Benckiser) — CIII

OTHER BRAND NAME: Subutex (Reckitt Benckiser)
THERAPEUTIC CLASS: Partial opioid agonist/opioid antagonist
INDICATIONS: Opioid dependence.
DOSAGE: *Adults:* Give either agent SL as a single daily dose in the range of 12-16mg/day. Hold tabs under tongue until dissolved; swallowing tabs reduces bioavailability. Induction: Subutex: Give at least 4 hrs after last short-acting opioid (eg, heroin) use or

SUDAFED

preferably when early signs of opioid withdrawal appear. Maint: Suboxone: Range: 4mg-24mg/day. Target dose: 16mg/day. Titrate: Adjust by 2mg or 4mg to a level that maintains treatment and suppresses opioid withdrawal effects. Hepatic Impairment: Adjust dose and observe for precipitated opioid withdrawal. Concomitant CNS Depressants: Consider dose reduction.

Pediatrics: ≥16 yrs: Give either agent SL as a single daily dose in the range of 12-16mg/day. Hold tabs under tongue until dissolved; swallowing tabs reduces bioavailability. Induction: Subutex: Give at least 4 hrs after last short-acting opioid (eg, heroin) use or preferably when early signs of opioid withdrawal appear. Maint: Suboxone: Range: 4mg-24mg/day. Target dose: 16mg/day. Titrate: Adjust by 2mg or 4mg to a level that maintains treatment and suppresses opioid withdrawal effects. Hepatic Impairment: Adjust dose and observe for precipitated opioid withdrawal. Concomitant CNS Depressants: Consider dose reduction.

HOW SUPPLIED: Suboxone (Buprenorphine-Naloxone) Tab, SL: 2mg-0.5mg, 8mg-2mg. Subutex (Buprenorphine) Tab, SL: 2mg, 8mg

WARNINGS/PRECAUTIONS: Significant respiratory depression reported with buprenorphine; caution with compromised respiratory function. Naloxone may not be effective in reversing any respiratory depression produced by buprenorphine. Cytolytic hepatitis and hepatitis with jaundice reported. Obtain LFTs prior to initiation and periodically thereafter. Acute and chronic hypersensitivity reactions reported. May increase CSF pressure; caution with head injury, intracranial lesions. May cause miosis, changes in level of consciousness, and orthostatic hypotension. Caution with elderly, debilitated, myxedema, hypothyroidism, acute alcoholism, Addison's disease, CNS depression or coma, toxic psychoses, prostatic hypertrophy, urethral stricture, delirium tremens, kyphoscoliosis, biliary tract dysfunction or severe hepatic/renal/pulmonary impairment. Suboxone may cause opioid withdrawal symptoms. May obscure diagnosis of acute abdominal conditions. May produce dependence.

ADVERSE REACTIONS: Headache, infection, pain (general, abdomen, back), withdrawal syndrome, constipation, nausea, insomnia, sweating, asthenia, anxiety, depression, rhinitis.

INTERACTIONS: May need dose reduction with CYP3A4 inhibitors (eg, azole antifungals, macrolides and HIV protease inhibitors). General anesthetics, other narcotic analgesics, benzodiazepines, phenothiazines, other tranquilizers, sedative/hypnotics or other CNS depressants (including alcohol) may increase risk of CNS depression; consider dose reduction of one or both agents. Monitor closely with CYP3A4 inducers (eg, phenobarbital, carbamazepine, phenytoin, rifampicin).

PREGNANCY: Category C, not for use in nursing.

SUDAFED OTC
pseudoephedrine HCl (McNeil)

THERAPEUTIC CLASS: Decongestant

INDICATIONS: For the temporary relief of nasal congestion due to common cold, hay fever, or other upper respiratory allergies, and nasal congestion associated with sinusitus.

DOSAGE: *Adults:* Tab, ER: 120mg q12h or 240mg q24h. Max: 240mg/24h.

Pediatrics:>12 yrs: Liquid/Tab/Tab, Chew: 60mg q4-6h. Max 240mg/24hrs. Tab, ER: 120mg q12h or 240mg q24h. Max: 240mg/24hrs. 6 to <12 yo: (Liquid/Tab/Tab, Chew) 30mg q4-6h. Max: 4 doses/24hrs. 2 to <6 yo: (Liquid/Tab/Tab, Chew) 15mg q4-6h. Max: 4 doses/24hrs.

HOW SUPPLIED: Liq: 15mg/5mL; Tab: 30mg, 60mg; Tab, Chewable: 15mg; Tab, Extended Release: 120mg, 240mg

WARNINGS/PRECAUTIONS: Do not exceed recommended dosage. If nervousness, dizziness, or sleeplessness occurs, discontinue use. Do not take this product if you have heart disease, high BP, thyroid disease, diabetes, or difficulty in urination due to prostate enlargement.

INTERACTIONS: Do not take with a MAOI or 14d after discontinuation.

PREGNANCY: Not rated in pregnancy or nursing.

SUFENTA
sufentanil citrate (Akorn)

CII

THERAPEUTIC CLASS: Opioid analgesic

INDICATIONS: Analgesic adjunct in the maintenance of balanced general anesthesia in patients who are intubated and ventilated. Primary anesthetic agent of the induction and maintenance of anesthesia with 100% oxygen in patients undergoing major surgical procedures who are intubated or ventilated, such as cardiovascular surgery or neurosurgical procedures in the sitting position, to provide favorable myocardial and cerebral oxygen balance or when extended postoperative ventilation is anticipated. For epidural administrations an analgesic combined with low dose bupivacaine, usually 12.5mg per administration during labor and vaginal delivery.

DOSAGE: *Adults:* ≥12 yrs: Individualize dose. Premedication: Based on patients needs. Analgesic: Total Dose: 1-8mcg/kg. Maint: Incremental: 10-50mcg. Infusion: Based on induction dose not to exceed 1mcg/kg/hr. Anesthetic: Total Dose: 8-30mcg/kg. Maint: Incremental 0.5-10mcg/kg. Infusion: Based on induction dose not to exceed 30mcg/kg. Epidural: 10-15mcg with 10mL bupivacaine 0.125% with or without epinephrine. May repeat for a total of 3 doses in not less than 1 hour intervals.

Pediatrics: Individualize dose. 10-25mcg/kg with 100% oxygen. Maint: 25-50mcg supplemental doses.

HOW SUPPLIED: Inj: 50mcg/mL

WARNINGS/PRECAUTIONS: Should only be administered by persons specifically trained in the use of IV and epidural anesthetics and management of the respiratory effects of potent opioids. An opioid antagonist, resuscitation and intubation equipment and oxygen should be readily available. Prior to catheter insertion, the physician should be familiar with patient conditions (such as infection at the injection site, bleeding diathesis, anticoagulation therapy) which call for special evaluation of the benefit versus risk potential. May cause muscle rigidity of the neck and extremities. Adequate facilities should be available for postoperative monitoring and ventilation. Monitor vital signs routinely. Reduce dose for elderly and debilitated patients. Caution with pulmonary disease, decreased respiratory reserve, liver and kidney dysfunction, cardiac bradyarrhythmias. Reports of bradycardia responsive to atropine. May obscure clinical course of patients with head injuries.

ADVERSE REACTIONS: Respiratory depression, skeletal muscle rigidity, bradycardia, HTN, hypotension, chest wall rigidity, somnolence, pruritus, nausea, vomiting.

INTERACTIONS: Reports of cardiovascular depression with nitrous oxide. High doses of pancuronium may produce increase in heart rate. Reports of bradycardia and hypotension with other muscle relaxants. Greater incidence and degree of bradycardia and hypotension with chronic calcium channel blocker and beta-blocker therapy. Additive or potentiating effects with other CNS depressants (eg, barbiturates, tranquilizers, narcotics, general anesthetics). Reduce dose of either agent. Decrease in mean arterial pressure and systemic vascular resistance with benzodiazepines.

PREGNANCY: Category C, caution in nursing.

SULFACET-R
sulfur - sulfacetamide sodium (Dermik)

RX

THERAPEUTIC CLASS: Sulfonamide/sulfur combination

INDICATIONS: Topical treatment of acne vulgaris, acne rosacea, and seborrheic dermatitis.

DOSAGE: *Adults:* Shake well before use. Apply qd-tid. Expires after 4 months.

Pediatrics: ≥12 yrs: Shake well before use. Apply qd-tid. Expires after 4 months.

HOW SUPPLIED: Lot: (Sulfacetamide-Sulfur) 10%-5% (25g)

CONTRAINDICATIONS: Kidney disease.

SULFAMYLON

WARNINGS/PRECAUTIONS: D/C if irritation or hypersensitivity reaction occurs. Avoid eye contact. Contains sulfites. Caution with denuded or abraded skin. May cause reddening and scaling of epidermis.

ADVERSE REACTIONS: Local irritation.

PREGNANCY: Category C, caution in nursing.

SULFAMYLON
mafenide acetate (Mylan Bertek)

RX

THERAPEUTIC CLASS: Sulfonamide

INDICATIONS: (Cre) Adjunct therapy for 2nd- and 3rd-degree burns. (Sol) Adjunct therapy for excised burn wounds.

DOSAGE: *Adults:* (Cre) Clean and debride wound, then apply qd-bid. Cream should cover wound at all times. Continue application until healing is progressing well or until site is ready for grafting. (Sol) Cover grafted area with mesh gauze and wet with solution using irrigation syringe/tubing q4h or prn to keep wet. If irrigation tube is not used, moisten gauze q6-8h or prn to keep wet. May use solution up to 5 days with same dressing.

Pediatrics: (Cre) Clean and debride wound, then apply qd-bid. Cream should cover wound at all times. Continue application until healing is progressing well or until site is ready for grafting. (Sol) 3 months-16 yrs: Cover grafted area with mesh gauze and wet with solution using irrigation syringe/tubing q4h or prn to keep wet. If irrigation tube is not used, moisten gauze q6-8h or prn to keep wet. May use solution up to 5 days with same dressing.

HOW SUPPLIED: Cre: 85mg/g (60g, 120g, 453.6g); Sol: 50g/pkt (1^s, 5^s)

WARNINGS/PRECAUTIONS: Fatal hemolytic anemia with DIC related to G6PD deficiency reported. Cream contains sodium metabisulfite. Monitor acid-base balance with pulmonary or renal dysfunction; risk of metabolic acidosis due to carbonic anhydrase inhibition. Fungal colonization may occur. D/C if hypersensitivity occurs, and for 24-48 hrs if acidosis occurs. Caution with acute renal failure.

ADVERSE REACTIONS: Facial edema, rash, burning sensation, pruritus, erythema, swelling, hyperventilation, tachypnea, acidosis.

INTERACTIONS: Possible cross sensitivity to other sulfonamides.

PREGNANCY: Category C, not for use in nursing.

SUMYCIN
tetracycline HCl (Par)

RX

THERAPEUTIC CLASS: *Streptomyces* derived bacteriostatic agent

INDICATIONS: Treatment of respiratory tract, urinary tract, and skin and skin structure infections, lymphogranuloma, psittacosis, trachoma, uncomplicated urethral/endocervical/rectal infection caused by *Chlamydia*, nongonococcal urethritis, chancroid, plague, cholera, brucellosis, and others. When PCN is contraindicated, treatment of uncomplicated gonorrhea, syphilis, listeriosis, anthrax, *Clostridium* species, and others. Adjunct therapy for amebicides and severe acne.

DOSAGE: *Adults:* Mild-Moderate: 250mg qid or 500mg bid. Severe: 500mg qid. Continue for 24-48 hrs after symptoms subside (minimum 10 days with Group A β-hemolytic streptococci). Severe Acne: Initial: 1g/day in divided doses. Maint: After improvement, 125-500mg/day. Brucellosis: 500mg qid for 3 weeks plus streptomycin 1g IM bid for 1 week, then qd for 1 week. Syphilis: 30-40g equally divided over 10-15 days. Gonorrhea: 500mg q6h for 7 days. Chlamydia: 500mg qid for at least 7 days. Renal Dysfunction: Reduce dose or extend dose interval.

Pediatrics: >8 yrs: Usual: 25-50mg/kg divided bid-qid. Continue for 24-48 hrs after symptoms subside (minimum 10 days with Group A β-hemolytic streptococci). Severe Acne: Initial: 1g/day in divided doses. Maint: After improvement, 125-500mg/day. Renal Dysfunction: Reduce dose or extend dose interval.

HOW SUPPLIED: Sus: 125mg/5mL; Tab: 250mg, 500mg

WARNINGS/PRECAUTIONS: May cause fetal harm with pregnancy, permanent tooth discoloration during tooth development (last half of pregnancy and children <8 yrs). May increase BUN. Photosensitivity, enamel hypoplasia reported. Superinfection with prolonged use. Suspension contains sodium metabisulfite. Bulging fontanels in infants and benign intracranial HTN in adults reported. Monitor renal/hepatic and hematopoietic function with long-term use. Caution with history of asthma, hay fever, urticaria, and allergy.

ADVERSE REACTIONS: GI effects, photosensitivity, increased BUN, hypersensitivity reactions, blood dyscrasias, dizziness, headache.

INTERACTIONS: May decrease PT; adjust anticoagulants. May interfere with bactericidal agents (eg, penicillin). May decrease effects of oral contraceptives. Take 1 hr before or 2 hrs after dairy products. Aluminum-, calcium-, iron- and magnesium-containing products impair absorption. Fatal renal toxicity reported with concurrent methoxyflurane.

PREGNANCY: Category D, not for use in nursing.

SUPPRELIN LA   RX
histrelin acetate (Indevus)

THERAPEUTIC CLASS: Gonadotropin releasing hormone

INDICATIONS: Treatment of children with central precocious puberty.

DOSAGE: *Pediatrics:* ≥2 yrs: 50mg every 12 months. Inject SQ into inner aspect of upper arm. Remove after 12 months of therapy.

HOW SUPPLIED: Implant: 50mg

CONTRAINDICATIONS: Women who are or may become pregnant.

WARNINGS/PRECAUTIONS: Transient increase in estradiol in females and testosterone in both sexes with initial therapy. Proper surgical technique is critical during implant insertion and removal. Monitor LH, FSH, and estradiol or testosterone at 1 month post-implantation, then every 6 months. Assess height and bone age every 6-12 months.

ADVERSE REACTIONS: Implant site reactions, wound infection, dysmenorrhea, epistaxis, erythema, gynecomastia, headache, weight increase.

PREGNANCY: Category X, not for use in nursing.

SUPRANE   RX
desflurane (Baxter Anesthesia)

THERAPEUTIC CLASS: Inhalation anesthetic

INDICATIONS: Induction and/or maintenance of anesthesia for inpatient and outpatient surgery in adults. Maintenance of anesthesia in infants and children after induction of anesthesia with other agents and tracheal intubation.

DOSAGE: *Adults:* Individualize dose. MAC Values: 70 yrs: 5.2 with oxygen 100% or 1.7 with nitrous oxide 60%. 45 yrs: 6 with oxygen 100% or 2.8 with nitrous oxide 60%. 25 yrs: 7.3 with oxygen 100% or 4 with nitrous oxide 60%. With Fentanyl or Midazolam: 31-65 yrs: No Fentanyl: 6.3. With 3mcg/kg Fentanyl: 3.1. With 6mcg/kg Fentanyl: 2.3. No Midazolam: 5.9. With Midazolam 25mcg/kg: 4.9. With Midazolam 50mcg/kg: 4.9. 18-30 yrs: No Fentanyl: 6.4. With Fentanyl 3mcg/kg: 3.5. With Fentanyl 6mcg/kg: 3. No Midazolam: 6.9.

Pediatrics: Individualize dose. MAC Values: 7 yrs: 8.1 with oxygen 100%. 4 yrs: 8.6 with oxygen 100%. 3 yrs: 6.4 with nitrous oxide 60%. 2 yrs: 9.1 with oxygen 100%. 9 months: 10 with oxygen 100% or 7.5 with nitrous oxide 60%. 10 weeks: 9.4 with oxygen 100%. 2 weeks: 9.2 with oxygen 100%.

HOW SUPPLIED: Liq: (240mL)

CONTRAINDICATIONS: Known or suspected susceptibility to malignant hyperthermia.

WARNINGS/PRECAUTIONS: Not recommended for induction of general anesthesia via mask in infants or children. Produces dose-dependent decreases in BP. Concentrations >1 MAC may increase HR. Administer at 0.8 MAC or less, in conjunction with barbiturate induction and hyperventilation. Maintain normal hemodynamics with CAD. May cause sensitivity hepatitis in patients who have been sensitized by previous exposure to halogenated anesthetics. May trigger malignant hyperthermia. May produce a dose-

SUPRAX

dependent increase in CSF pressure when administered to patients with intracranial space occupying lesions. Not recommended for maintenence of anesthesia in non-intubated children.

ADVERSE REACTIONS: Coughing, breathholding, apnea, laryngospasm, oxyhemoglobin desaturation, increased secretions, bronchospasm, nausea, vomiting.

INTERACTIONS: Decreased MAC with benzodiazepines and opioids. May decrease the required dose of neuromuscular blocking agents.

PREGNANCY: Category B, caution in nursing.

SUPRAX
cefixime (Lupin)
RX

THERAPEUTIC CLASS: Cephalosporin (3rd generation)

INDICATIONS: Otitis media, pharyngitis, tonsillitis, acute bronchitis, acute exacerbation of chronic bronchitis, uncomplicated UTIs, and cervical/urethral gonorrhea caused by susceptible strains.

DOSAGE: *Adults:* Usual: 400mg qd. Gonorrhea: 400mg single dose. CrCl 21-60mL/min/Hemodialysis: Give 75% of standard dose. CrCl <20mL/min/CAPD: Give 50% of standard dose.
Pediatrics: >12 yrs or >50kg: (Tab/Sus) Usual: 400mg qd. ≥6 months: (Sus) 8mg/kg qd or 4mg/kg bid. Treat for at least 10 days with *S. pyogenes*. CrCl 21-60mL/min/Hemodialysis: Give 75% of standard dose. CrCl <20mL/min/CAPD: Give 50% of standard dose.

HOW SUPPLIED: Sus: 100mg/5mL (50mL, 75mL, 100mL)

WARNINGS/PRECAUTIONS: Caution with penicillin or other allergy, GI disease (eg, colitis). Anaphylactic/anaphylactoid reactions, pseudomembranous colitis reported. May cause false (+) direct Coombs, Benedict's, Fehling's solution, Clinitest.

ADVERSE REACTIONS: Diarrhea, abdominal pain, nausea, dyspepsia, flatulence, superinfection.

INTERACTIONS: May increase carbamazepine levels. Increased PT with anticoagulants (eg, warfarin).

PREGNANCY: Category B, not for use in nursing.

SURMONTIL
trimipramine maleate (Odyssey)
RX

> Antidepressants increased the risk of suicidal thinking and behavior (suicidality) in short-term studies in children and adolescents with Major Depressive Disorder (MDD) and other psychiatric disorders. Trimipramine is not approved for use in pediatric patients.

THERAPEUTIC CLASS: Tricyclic antidepressant

INDICATIONS: Relief of symptoms of depression.

DOSAGE: *Adults:* Outpatient: Initial: 75mg/day in divided doses. Titrate: Increase to 150mg/day. Maint: 50-150mg/day. Max: 200mg/day. Hospitalized Patients: Initial: 100mg/day in divided doses. Titrate: Increase gradually to 200mg/day. If no improvement after 2-3 weeks, may increase up to 250-300mg/day. Elderly: Initial: 50mg/day. Titrate: Increase gradually to 100mg/day. Take at bedtime for at least 3 months.
Pediatrics: Adolescents: Initial: 50mg/day. Titrate: Increase gradually to 100mg/day. Take at bedtime for at least 3 months.

HOW SUPPLIED: Cap: 25mg, 50mg, 100mg

CONTRAINDICATIONS: Acute recovery period post-MI, within 14 days of MAOI therapy.

WARNINGS/PRECAUTIONS: Caution with cardiovascular disease, increased IOP, urinary retention, narrow-angle glaucoma, hyperthyroidism, seizure disorder, liver dysfunction. May impair ability to operate machinery. May alter glucose levels. May activate psychosis in schizophrenia. Manic or hypomanic episodes may occur. May increase hazards with electroshock therapy.

ADVERSE REACTIONS: Hypotension, HTN, arrhythmia, confusion, insomnia, incoordination, GI complaints, allergic reactions, gynecomastia, blood dyscrasias, dry mouth, blurred vision, urinary retention.

INTERACTIONS: Cimetidine inhibits elimination. Alcohol may exaggerate effects. May potentiate catecholamine or anticholinergic effects. Potentiated by CYP2D6 inhibitors (eg, quinidine) and substrates (eg, other antidepressants, phenothiazines, propafenone, fleccainide). Caution with SSRIs; wait 5 weeks after fluoxetine withdrawal before initiating therapy. Avoid MAOIs.

PREGNANCY: Category C, safety in nursing not known.

SUSTIVA   RX
efavirenz (Bristol-Myers Squibb)

THERAPEUTIC CLASS: Non-nucleoside reverse transcriptase inhibitor

INDICATIONS: Treatment of HIV-1 infection in combination with other antiretrovirals.

DOSAGE: *Adults:* Initial: 600mg qd. Take on an empty stomach, preferably at bedtime. *Pediatrics:* ≥3 yrs: 10 to <15kg: 200mg qd. 15 to <20kg: 250mg qd. 20 to <25kg: 300mg qd. 25 to <32.5kg: 350mg qd. 32.5 to <40kg: 400mg qd. ≥40kg: 600mg qd. Take on an empty stomach, preferably at bedtime.

HOW SUPPLIED: Cap: 50mg, 100mg, 200mg; Tab: 600mg

CONTRAINDICATIONS: Concomitant astemizole, bepridil, cisapride, midazolam, pimozide, triazolam, ergot derivatives, or standard doses of voriconazole.

WARNINGS/PRECAUTIONS: Not for monotherapy. Severe skin rash reported. Avoid pregnancy; use barrier contraception with other contraception methods and obtain (-) pregnancy test before therapy. Monitor LFTs with known or suspected hepatitis B or C. Monitor cholesterol and triglycerides. High fat meals may increase absorption. Possible redistribution or accumulation of body fat. Serious psychiatric adverse experiences and central nervous symptoms (dizziness, insomnia, impaired concentration, somnolence, abnormal dreams, hallucinations) have been reported.

ADVERSE REACTIONS: CNS symptoms (eg, dizziness, insomnia, impaired concentration, somnolence, abnormal dreams), psychiatric symptoms (eg, severe depression), rash, GI effects.

INTERACTIONS: Avoid astemizole, cisapride, midazolam, triazolam, voriconazole, St. John's wort, or ergot derivatives. St. John's wort decreases efavirenz to suboptimal levels; increases risk of resistance. Significantly decreased levels of voriconazole. CYP3A4 inducers (eg, phenobarbital, rifampin, rifabutin) may decrease plasma levels. Increased levels of ethinyl estradiol. Decreased levels of clarithromycin; consider alternative. Decreased levels of indinavir and rifabutin; adjust doses. Increased levels of ritonavir and efavirenz with concomitant use; monitor LFTs. Decreased levels of saquinavir, sertraline. May decrease methadone levels; monitor for signs of withdrawal. May affect warfarin levels. May decrease itraconazole, ketoconazole, amprenavir levels. Decreased levels of anticonvulsants (eg, phenytoin, phenobarbital, carbamazepine) and efavirenz; monitor anticonvulsant levels.

PREGNANCY: Category D, not for use in nursing.

SYMBICORT   RX
formoterol - budesonide fumarate dihydrate (AstraZeneca)

> Long-acting beta2-adrenergic agonists (formoterol) may increase the risk of asthma-related death.

THERAPEUTIC CLASS: Corticosteroid/beta$_2$ agonist

INDICATIONS: Long-term maintenance treatment of asthma in patients ≥12 yrs.

DOSAGE: *Adults:* Current Medium to High Doses Inhaled CS: 2 inh bid of 160/4.5. Current Low to Medium Doses Inhaled CS: 2 inh bid of 80/4.5. No Current Inhaled CS: 2 inh bid of 80/4.5 or 160/4.5 depending on asthma severity. Max: 640mcg/18mcg (2 inh bid of 160/4.5). Patients not responding to the starting dose after 1-2 weeks of therapy with 80/4.5, replace with 160/4.5 for better asthma control. Rinse mouth after use.

SYMMETREL

Pediatrics: ≥12 yrs: Current Medium to High Doses Inhaled CS: 2 inh bid of 160/4.5. Current Low to Medium Doses Inhaled CS: 2 inh bid of 80/4.5. No Current Inhaled CS: 2 inh bid of 80/4.5 or 160/4.5 depending on asthma severity. Max: 640mcg/18mcg (2 inh bid of 160/4.5). Patients not responding to the starting dose after 1-2 weeks of therapy with 80/4.5, replace with 160/4.5 for better asthma control. Rinse mouth after use.

HOW SUPPLIED: MDI: (Budesonide-Formoterol) 80mcg-4.5mcg/inh, 160mcg-4.5mcg/inh (10.2g)

CONTRAINDICATIONS: Primary treatment of status asthmaticus or other acute asthma attacks.

WARNINGS/PRECAUTIONS: Do not use in patients with significantly worsening or acutely deteriorating asthma. Not for acute treatment of symptoms. Monitor for increasing use of inhaled, short-acting beta$_2$-agonists. Deaths due to adrenal insufficiency have occured with transfer from systemic corticosteroids to inhaled corticosteroids. Resume oral corticosteroids during stress or severe asthma attack. Transferring from oral to inhalation therapy may unmask allergic conditions (eg, rhinitis, conjunctivitis, eczema). Observe for adrenal insufficiency, systemic corticosteroid withdrawal effects, and growth suppression (children). More susceptible to infections. Not for acute bronchospasm. Do not use any additional inhaled long-acting beta$_2$-agonist for prevention of exercise induced bronchospasm or the maintenance treatment of asthma. D/C if paradoxical bronchospasm occurs. Immediate hypersensitivity and upper airway symptom reactions reported. Caution with cardiovascular disorder (eg, coronary insufficiency, arrythmia, HTN). QTc interval prolongation reported.

ADVERSE REACTIONS: Nasopharyngitis, headache, upper respiratory tract infections, sinusitis, back pain, nasal/sinus congestion, oral candidiasis, influenza, rhinitis, pharyngolaryngeal pain, vomiting.

INTERACTIONS: Oral ketoconazole increases plasma levels. CYP3A4 inhibitors (eg, itraconazole, clarithromycin, erythromycin) may inhibit metabolism and increase systemic exposure. Caution with non-potassium-sparing diuretics. Extreme caution within 14 days of using MAOIs or TCAs. Avoid with β-blockers.

PREGNANCY: Category C, caution in nursing.

SYMMETREL
amantadine HCl (Endo)

RX

THERAPEUTIC CLASS: Dopamine agonist

INDICATIONS: Prophylaxis and treatment of uncomplicated influenza A infections. Treatment of parkinsonism and drug-induced extrapyramidal reactions.

DOSAGE: *Adults:* Influenza A Virus Prophylaxis/Treatment: 200mg qd or 100mg bid. Elderly: ≥65 yrs: 100mg qd. Parkinsonism: Initial: 100mg qd. Serious Associated Illness/Concomitant High Dose Antiparkinson Agent: Initial: 100mg qd. Titrate: May increase to 100mg bid after 1 to several weeks. Max: 400mg/day. Drug-Induced Extrapyramidal Reactions: 100mg bid. Titrate: May increase to 300mg/day in divided doses. CrCl 30-50mL/min: 200mg on Day 1, then 100mg qd. CrCl 15-29mL/min: 200mg on Day 1, then 100mg every other day. CrCl <15mL/min/Hemodialysis: 200mg every 7 days.
Pediatrics: Influenza A Virus Prophylaxis/Treatment: 9-12 yrs: 100mg bid. 1-9 yrs: 4.4-8.8mg/kg/day. Max: 150mg/day.

HOW SUPPLIED: Syrup: 50mg/5mL; Tab: 100mg

WARNINGS/PRECAUTIONS: Deaths reported from overdose. Suicide attempts, NMS reported. Caution with CHF, peripheral edema, orthostatic hypotension, renal or hepatic dysfunction, recurrent eczematoid rash, uncontrolled psychosis or severe psychoneurosis. Avoid in untreated angle closure glaucoma. Do not d/c abruptly in Parkinson's disease. May increase seizure activity.

ADVERSE REACTIONS: Nausea, dizziness, insomnia, depression, anxiety, hallucinations, confusion, anorexia, dry mouth, constipation, ataxia, livedo reticularis, peripheral edema, orthostatic hypotension, agranulocytosis.

INTERACTIONS: Caution with CNS stimulants. Anticholinergic agents may potentiate the anticholinergic side effects. Increased tremor in elderly Parkinson's patients with thioridazine. Increased plasma levels with trimethoprim-sulfamethoxazole, quinine, or quinidine. Avoid use of Attenuated Influenza Vaccine within 2 weeks before or 48 hours after.

PREGNANCY: Category C, not for use in nursing.

SYNAGIS
palivizumab (MedImmune)

RX

THERAPEUTIC CLASS: Monoclonal antibody/RSV F-protein blocker

INDICATIONS: Prevention of serious lower respiratory tract disease caused by respiratory syncytial virus (RSV) in pediatrics at high risk of RSV.

DOSAGE: *Pediatrics:* 15mg/kg IM; give 1st dose before start of RSV season (November-April), then monthly throughout season. Give monthly also if develop RSV infection. Safety and efficacy established in infants with bronchopulmonary dysplasia (BPD) and infants with history of prematurity (≤35 weeks gestational age).

HOW SUPPLIED: Inj: 50mg, 100mg

WARNINGS/PRECAUTIONS: Anaphylactoid reactions reported. Caution with thrombocytopenia or any coagulation disorder due to IM injection. Safety and efficacy not demonstrated for treatment of established RSV disease.

ADVERSE REACTIONS: Upper respiratory infection, otitis media, rash, pharyngitis, cough, bronchiolitis, pneumonia, bronchitis, asthma, croup, dyspnea, apnea, diarrhea, vomiting, nervousness, liver function abnormality, anemia.

PREGNANCY: Category C, safety in nursing not known.

SYNALAR
fluocinolone acetonide (Medicis)

RX

THERAPEUTIC CLASS: Corticosteroid

INDICATIONS: Corticosteroid responsive dermatoses.

DOSAGE: *Adults:* Apply bid-qid. May use occlusive dressings for psoriasis or recalcitrant conditions; d/c dressings if infection develops.
Pediatrics: Apply bid-qid. May use occlusive dressings for psoriasis or recalcitrant conditions; d/c dressings if infection develops.

HOW SUPPLIED: Cre, Oint: 0.025% (15g, 60g); Sol: 0.01% (20mL, 60mL)

WARNINGS/PRECAUTIONS: May produce reversible HPA axis suppression, manifestations of Cushing's syndrome, hyperglycemia, and glucosuria. Caution when applied to large surface areas or under occlusive dressings. Use appropriate antifungal or antibacterial agent with dermatological infections; d/c if infection does not clear. Peds may be more susceptible to systemic toxicity. Avoid eyes. D/C if irritation occurs.

ADVERSE REACTIONS: Burning, itching, irritation, dryness, folliculitis, hypertrichosis, acneiform eruptions, premolar dermatitis, hypopigmentation, allergic dermatitis, skin maceration, secondary infection, skin atrophy.

PREGNANCY: Category C, caution with nursing.

SYNALGOS-DC
aspirin - caffeine - dihydrocodeine bitartrate (Women First)

CIII

THERAPEUTIC CLASS: Opioid analgesic

INDICATIONS: Relief of moderate to moderately severe pain.

DOSAGE: *Adults:* 2 caps q4h prn pain. Elderly: Start at low end of dosing range.
Pediatrics: >12 yrs: 2 caps q4h prn pain.

HOW SUPPLIED: Cap: (Dihydrocodeine-ASA-Caffeine) 16mg-356.4mg-30mg (Painpak, 12 caps)

WARNINGS/PRECAUTIONS: Caution in elderly, debilitated, and with peptic ulcer or coagulation abnormalities. May impair mental or physical abilities. Abuse potential.

ADVERSE REACTIONS: Lightheadedness, dizziness, drowsiness, sedation, nausea, vomiting, constipation, pruritus, skin reactions.

INTERACTIONS: Additive CNS depression with narcotic analgesics, general anesthetics, tranquilizers, sedative hypnotics, alcohol, and other CNS depressants. Enhanced effects of anticoagulants. Inhibits effects of uricosuric agents.

PREGNANCY: Safety in pregnancy and nursing is not known.

SYNAREL — RX
nafarelin acetate (Searle)

THERAPEUTIC CLASS: Gonadotropin-releasing hormone analog

INDICATIONS: Management of endometriosis, including pain relief and reduction of lesions. Treatment of central precocious puberty (CPP) (gonadotropin-dependent precocious puberty) in children of both sexes.

DOSAGE: (Endometriosis) *Adults:* ≥18 yrs: 1 spray (200mcg) into one nostril qam and 1 spray into other nostril qpm. Initiate therapy between days 2-4 of menstrual cycle. Increase to 1 spray per nostril qam and qpm after 2 months (800mcg/day) if amenorrhea has not occurred. Treat for 6 months.

(CPP) *Pediatrics:* Usual: 2 sprays (400mcg) per nostril qam and qpm. Total Daily Dose: 1600mcg. Increase to 3 sprays into alternating nostrils tid (1800mcg daily) if needed 30 seconds should elapse between sprays. Continue until resumption of puberty is desired.

HOW SUPPLIED: Spray: 200mcg/inh (8mL)

CONTRAINDICATIONS: Pregnancy, women who may become pregnant, nursing, undiagnosed abnormal vaginal bleeding.

WARNINGS/PRECAUTIONS: (Endometriosis) Ovarian cysts reported in adult women. Caution if risk factors for decreased bone mineral content present. Avoid sneezing during or after administration. Use nonhormonal methods of contraception. (CPP) Determine diagnosis before initiating therapy. Monitor regularly. Assess growth and bone age velocity within 3 to 6 months of initiation. Avoid sneezing during or after administration.

ADVERSE REACTIONS: (Endometriosis) Hot flashes, decreased libido, vaginal dryness, headache, emotional lability, myalgia, acne, nasal irritation, reduced breast size, insomnia, edema, seborrhea, weight gain, depression, hirsutism. (CPP) Acne, breast enlargement, vaginal bleeding, emotional lability, transient increase in pubic hair, rhinitis, body odor, seborrhea, white or brownish vaginal discharge.

INTERACTIONS: Avoid topical decongestants within 2 hrs after dosing.

PREGNANCY: Category X, not for use in nursing.

SYNERA — RX
lidocaine - tetracaine (Tapemark)

THERAPEUTIC CLASS: Acetamide local anesthetic

INDICATIONS: For use on intact skin to provide local dermal analgesia for superficial venous access and superficial dermatological procedures such as excision, electrodessication, and shave biopsy of skin lesions.

DOSAGE: *Adults:* Venipuncture or IV Cannulation: Apply to intact skin for 20-30 minutes prior to procedure. Superficial Dermatological Procedures: Apply to intact skin for 30 minutes prior to the procedure.

Pediatrics: ≥3 yrs: Venipuncture or IV Cannulation: Apply to intact skin for 20-30 minutes prior to procedure. Superficial Dermatological Procedure: Apply to intact skin for 30 minutes prior to the procedure.

HOW SUPPLIED: Patch: (Lidocaine-Tetracaine) 70mg-70mg

CONTRAINDICATIONS: PABA hypersensitivity.

WARNINGS/PRECAUTIONS: Serious adverse events may occur in children or pets if ingested. Caution in acutely ill or debilitated. Risk of allergic/anaphylactoid reactions (urticaria, angioedema, bronchospasm, shock). Increased risk of toxicity in severe hepatic disease. Avoid broken or inflamed skin, eye contact, larger area or longer duration than recommended.

ADVERSE REACTIONS: Erythema, blanching, edema, urticaria, angioedema, bronchospasm, shock.

INTERACTIONS: Additive toxic effect with concomitant Class I antiarrhythmics (eg, tocainide, mexiletine). Consider total amount absorbed from all formulations with other local anesthetics.

PREGNANCY: Category B, caution in nursing.

SYNERCID
dalfopristin - quinupristin (King)

RX

THERAPEUTIC CLASS: Streptogramin

INDICATIONS: Treatment of serious or life-threatening infections associated with vancomycin-resistant *Enterococcus faecium* (VREF) bacteremia and complicated skin and skin structure infections (SSSI) caused by *Staphylococcus aureus* (methicillin susceptible) or *Streptococcus pyogenes*.

DOSAGE: *Adults:* VREF: 7.5mg/kg IV q8h. Duration depends on site and severity of infection. Complicated SSSI: 7.5mg/kg IV q12h for at least 7 days. Hepatic Cirrhosis (Child Pugh A or B): May need dose reduction.

Pediatrics: ≥16 yrs: VREF: 7.5mg/kg IV q8h. Duration depends on site and severity of infection. Complicated SSSI: 7.5mg/kg IV q12h for at least 7 days. Hepatic Cirrhosis (Child Pugh A or B): May need dose reduction.

HOW SUPPLIED: Inj: (Dalfopristin-Quinupristin) 350mg-150mg per 500mg vial

WARNINGS/PRECAUTIONS: Pseudomembranous colitis reported. Flush vein with 5% dextrose after infusion to minimize venous irritation. Arthralgia, myalgia, and bilirubin elevation reported.

ADVERSE REACTIONS: Infusion site reactions (inflammation, pain, edema), nausea, diarrhea, rash.

INTERACTIONS: Significant inhibition of CYP3A4; caution with drugs metabolized by this system (eg, cyclosporin A, tacrolimus, midazolam, nifedipine, verapamil, diltiazem astemizole, terfenadine, delavirdine, nevirapine, indinavir, ritonavir, vinca alkaloids, docetaxel, paclitaxel, diazepam, HMG-CoA reductase inhibitors, methylprednisolone, carbamazepine, quinidine, lidocaine, disopyramide). Monitor cyclosporine levels. Avoid drugs metabolized by CYP3A4 that prolong QTc interval. May inhibit digoxin's gut metabolism.

PREGNANCY: Category B, caution in nursing.

SYNTHROID
levothyroxine sodium (Abbott)

RX

THERAPEUTIC CLASS: Thyroid replacement hormone

INDICATIONS: Hypothyroidism. As a pituitary TSH suppressant in the treatment and prevention of euthyroid goiters, including thyroid nodules, lymphocytic thyroiditis, and multinodular goiter. Adjunct to surgery and radioiodine therapy for thyrotropin-dependent well-differentiated thyroid cancer.

DOSAGE: *Adults:* Hypothyroidism: Usual: 1.7mcg/kg/day PO. Titrate: May increase by 12.5-25mcg every 6-8 weeks until euthyroid. >200mcg/day (seldom). Elderly/Cardiovascular Disease: Initial: 12.5-50mcg qd PO. Titrate: Increase by 12.5-25mcg every 3-6 weeks until euthyroid. Give 1/2 of oral dose for IV/IM. Pregnancy: May require increased doses. Subclinical Hypothyroidism: Lower doses required.

Pediatrics: Hypothyroidism: 0-3 months: 10-15mcg/kg/day. 3-6 months: 8-10mcg/kg/day. 6-12 months: 6-8mcg/kg/day. 1-5 yrs: 5-6mcg/kg/day. 6-12 yrs: 4-5mcg/kg/day. >12 yrs (growth/puberty complete): 2-3mcg/kg/day. Cardiac Risk: Lower starting dose. Infants with Serum T_4 <5mcg/dL: Initial: 50mcg/day. Chronic/Severe Hypothyroidism: Children: Initial: 25mcg/day. Titrate: Increase by 25mcg for 2 weeks then every 2-4 weeks until euthyroid. May crush tab and sprinkle over food (applesauce) or mix with 5-10mL water, formula (non-soy), or breast milk.

Talwin NX

HOW SUPPLIED: Tab: 25mcg*, 50mcg*, 75mcg*, 88mcg*, 100mcg*, 112mcg*, 125mcg*, 137mcg*, 150mcg*, 175mcg*, 200mcg*, 300mcg* *scored

CONTRAINDICATIONS: Untreated thyrotoxicosis, uncorrected adrenal insufficiency.

WARNINGS/PRECAUTIONS: Do not use in the treatment of obesity; larger doses in euthyroid patients can cause serious or even life threatening toxicity. Caution with cardiovascular disorders, angina, CAD, HTN and the elderly. May aggravate DM, diabetes insipidus, or adrenal cortical insufficiency. Treatment of myxedema coma may require glucocorticoids. May lower seizure threshold.

ADVERSE REACTIONS: Craniosynostosis in infants, transient hair loss, pseudotumor cerebri in pediatrics (rare), hypersensitivity reactions, seizures (rare).

INTERACTIONS: Increased risk of coronary insufficiency with sympathomimetics and CAD. May potentiate oral anticoagulant effects; adjust dose and monitor PT/INR. Lithium blocks release of T_4 and T_3. Antidiabetic agents may need adjustment. Decreased absorption with cholestyramine resin, colestipol, ferrous sulfate, aluminum hydroxide, sodium polystyrene sulfonate, soybean flour (infant formula), sucralfate. Altered protein binding with clofibrate, estrogens, androgens/anabolic hormones, asparaginase, 5-FU, furosemide, glucocorticoids, meclofenamic acid, mefenamic acid, methadone, perphenazine, phenytoin, phenylbutazone, tamoxifen, salicylates. Altered thyroid hormone or TSH levels with aminoglutethimide, p-aminosalicyclic acid, amiodarone, androgens/anabolic hormones, complex anions (eg, thiocyanate, perchlorate, pertechnetate), antithyroid drugs, β-adrenergic blockers, carbamazepine, chloral hydrate, diazepam, dopamine/dopamine agonists, ethionamide, glucocorticoids, heparin, hepatic enzyme inducers, insulin, iodinated cholestographic agents, iodine-containing compounds, levodopa, lovastatin, lithium, 6-mercaptopurine, metoclopramide, mitotane, nitroprusside, phenobarbital, phenytoin, resorcinol, rifampin, somatostatin analogs, sulfonamides, sulfonylureas, thiazide diuretics. Adrenocorticoid clearance is decreased with hypothyroidism and increased with hyperthyroidism. May potentiate anticoagulants. Cytokines, amiodarone may induce hypo- or hyperthyroidism. Increased risk of arrhythmias with maprotiline. HTN and tachycardia reported with ketamine. Sympathomimetics may increase risk of coronary insufficiency with CAD. Adverse effects of both drugs with TCAs. Decreased clearance of theophylline with hypothyroidism. Impaired β-blocker effects. Decreased digitalis effects. Decreased uptake of iodine-containing radiolabeled ions. Altered levels of theophylline may occur. Use with somatrem/somatropin may accelerate epiphyseal closure. Additive effects of both agents with TCAs. Avoid mixing crushed tabs with foods/formula with large amounts of iron, soybean or fiber.

PREGNANCY: Category A, caution in nursing.

Talwin NX   CIV
naloxone HCl - pentazocine HCl (Sanofi-Aventis)

> For oral use only. Severe, potentially lethal reactions may result from misuse by injection alone, or in combination with other agents.

THERAPEUTIC CLASS: Opioid agonist-antagonist analgesic

INDICATIONS: Relief of moderate to severe pain.

DOSAGE: *Adults:* Usual: 1 tab q3-4h. May increase to 2 tabs q3-4h. Max: 12 tabs/day. *Pediatrics:* ≥12 yrs: Usual: 1 tab q3-4h. May increase to 2 tabs q3-4h. Max: 12 tabs/day.

HOW SUPPLIED: Tab: (Pentazocine-Naloxone) 50mg-0.5mg* *scored

WARNINGS/PRECAUTIONS: Caution with elderly, drug dependence, head injury, increased intracranial pressure, certain respiratory conditions, acute CNS manifestations, renal or hepatic dysfunction, biliary surgery, and MI.

ADVERSE REACTIONS: Hypotension, tachycardia, hallucinations, dizziness, sedation, euphoria, sweating, nausea, vomiting, constipation, diarrhea, anorexia, facial edema, dermatitis, visual problems, chills, insomnia, urinary retention, paresthesia.

INTERACTIONS: Increased CNS depressant effects with alcohol. Withdrawal symptoms with narcotics.

PREGNANCY: Category C, caution in nursing.

TAMBOCOR
flecainide acetate (Graceway)
RX

THERAPEUTIC CLASS: Class IC antiarrhythmic

INDICATIONS: Prevention of paroxysmal supraventricular tachycardias (PSVT), paroxysmal atrial fibrillation/flutter (PAF) associated with disabling symptoms in patients without structural heart disease. Prevention of life-threatening ventricular arrhythmias (VT).

DOSAGE: *Adults:* PSVT/PAF: Initial: 50mg q12h. Titrate: May increase by 50mg bid every 4 days. Max: 300mg/day. Sustained VT: Initial: 100mg q12h. Titrate: May increase by 50mg bid every 4 days. Max: 400mg/day. CrCl ≤35mL/min: Initial: 100mg qd or 50mg bid. Reduce dose by 50% with amiodarone.

Pediatrics: <6 months: Initial: 50mg/m^2/day given bid-tid. ≥6 months: Initial: 100mg/m^2/day given bid-tid. Max: 200mg/m^2/day. Reduce dose by 50% with amiodarone.

HOW SUPPLIED: Tab: 50mg, 100mg*, 150mg* *scored

CONTRAINDICATIONS: Right bundle branch block associated with left hemiblock (without a pacemaker), pre-existing 2nd- or 3rd-degree AV block, cardiogenic shock.

WARNINGS/PRECAUTIONS: Avoid with non-life-threatening ventricular arrhythmias. Increased mortality and non-cardiac arrests reported. Ventricular proarrhythmic effects may occur with atrial fibrillation/flutter. May cause or worsen CHF, arrhythmias. Slows cardiac conduction; dose related increases in PR, QRS, and QT intervals reported. Conduction changes may cause sinus pause, sinus arrest, bradycardia, 2nd- or 3rd-degree AV block. Extreme caution with sick sinus syndrome. May increase endocardial pacing thresholds and suppress ventricular escape with pacemakers. Correct hypokalemia or hyperkalemia before therapy. Monitor with significant hepatic impairment. Initiate treatment of sustained VT in the hospital.

ADVERSE REACTIONS: Arrhythmias, hepatic dysfunction, cardiac arrest, CHF, flushing, anxiety, vomiting, diarrhea, tinnitus.

INTERACTIONS: Additive negative inotropic effects with β-blockers (eg, propranolol). Potentiated by cimetidine, amiodarone, CYP2D6 inhibitors (eg, quinidine). Increases digoxin levels. Increased elimination with phenytoin, phenobarbital, carbamazepine. Diltiazem, nifedipine, verapamil, disopyramide not recommended.

PREGNANCY: Category C, safety in nursing unknown.

TAMIFLU
oseltamivir phosphate (Roche Labs)
RX

THERAPEUTIC CLASS: Neuraminidase inhibitor

INDICATIONS: Treatment of uncomplicated acute illness due to influenza in adults and children ≥1 yr who have been symptomatic for no more than 2 days. Prophylaxis of influenza in adults and children ≥1 yr.

DOSAGE: *Adults:* Prophylaxis: Begin within 2 days of exposure to infection. 75mg qd for at least 10 days, up to 6 weeks with community outbreak. CrCl 10-30mL/min: 75mg every other day. Treatment: Begin therapy within 2 days of symptom onset. 75mg bid for 5 days. CrCl 10-30mL/min: 75mg qd for 5 days.

Pediatrics: Prophylaxis: ≥13 yr: Begin within 2 days of exposure to infection. 75mg qd for at least 10 days, up to 6 weeks with community outbreak. ≥1 yr: (Sus) ≤15kg: 30mg qd. >15-23kg: 45mg qd. >23-40kg: 60mg qd. >40kg: 75mg qd. Duration: 10 days. Treatment: ≥13 yrs: Begin therapy within 2 days of symptom onset. 75mg bid for 5 days. ≥1 yr: (Sus) ≤15kg: 30mg bid. >15-23kg: 45mg bid. >23-40kg: 60mg bid. >40kg: 75mg bid. Duration: 5 days.

HOW SUPPLIED: Cap: 75mg; Sus: 12mg/mL (25mL)

WARNINGS/PRECAUTIONS: Efficacy not known with chronic cardiac disease, respiratory disease, and immunocompromised. Not a substitute for influenza vaccine. Adjust dose with renal dysfunction. Postmarketing neuropsychiatric events (self-injury & delirium) reported.

ADVERSE REACTIONS: Nausea, vomiting, diarrhea, cough, headache, fatigue, toxic epidermal necrolysis, hepatitis, abnormal LFTs.

INTERACTIONS: Avoid admininstration of attenuated influenza vaccine within 2 weeks before or 48 hours after; may inhibit repliaction of live vaccine virus.

PREGNANCY: Category C, caution in nursing.

Tapazole
methimazole (King)
RX

THERAPEUTIC CLASS: Thyroid hormone synthesis inhibitor

INDICATIONS: Treatment of hyperthyroidism. To ameliorate hyperthyroidism prior to subtotal thyroidectomy or radioactive iodine therapy. Also indicated when thyroidectomy is contraindicated or not advisable.

DOSAGE: *Adults:* Initial: Mild Hyperthyroidism: 5mg q8h. Moderately Severe Hyperthyroidism: 30-40mg/day, in divided doses q8h. Severe Hyperthyroidism: 20mg q8h. Maint: 5-15mg/day.

Pediatrics: Initial: 0.4mg/kg/day, in divided doses q8h. Maint: 1/2 of initial dose.

HOW SUPPLIED: Tab: 5mg*, 10mg* *scored

CONTRAINDICATIONS: Nursing mothers.

WARNINGS/PRECAUTIONS: Can cause fetal harm. Agranulocytosis, leukopenia, thrombocytopenia, aplastic anemia may occur; monitor bone marrow function. Discontinue with agranulocytosis, aplastic anemia, or exfoliative dermatitis. Discontinue with liver abnormality (eg, hepatitis) including transaminases >3X ULN. Monitor thyroid function periodically. May cause hypoprothrombinemia and bleeding; monitor PT.

ADVERSE REACTIONS: Rash, urticaria, nausea, vomiting, arthralgia, paresthesia, myalgia, neuritis, vertigo, edema, altered taste, hair loss, lymphadenopathy, lupuslike syndrome, insulin autoimmune syndrome.

INTERACTIONS: May potentiate anticoagulants. β-blockers, digitalis, theophylline may need dose reduction when patient becomes euthyroid. Caution with other drugs that cause agranulocytosis.

PREGNANCY: Category D, contraindicated in nursing.

Tavist Allergy
clemastine fumarate (Novartis Consumer)
OTC

THERAPEUTIC CLASS: Antihistamine

INDICATIONS: Temporarily reduces symptoms of common cold, hay fever or other respiratory allergies.

DOSAGE: *Adults:* 1 tab q12h. Max: 2 tabs/24 hrs.

Pediatrics: ≥12 yrs: 1 tab q12h. Max: 2 tabs/24 hrs.

HOW SUPPLIED: Tab: 1.34mg* *scored

WARNINGS/PRECAUTIONS: May cause excitability in children. Caution with respiratory problems (eg, emphysema, chronic bronchitis), glaucoma, and enlarged prostate gland. May impair mental/physical abilities.

ADVERSE REACTIONS: Drowsiness, dizziness.

INTERACTIONS: Alcohol, sedatives, and tranquilizers may increase drowsiness.

PREGNANCY: Safety in pregnancy and nursing not known.

Taxotere
docetaxel (Sanofi-Aventis)
RX

> Increased treatment-related mortality reported with hepatic dysfunction, high-dose therapy, and in non-small cell lung carcinoma previously treated with platinum-based chemotherapy with docetaxel 100mg/m^2. Avoid if neutrophils <1500cells/mm^3, bilirubin >ULN, or SGOT/SGPT >1.5X ULN with alkaline phosphatase >2.5X ULN. Severe hypersensitivity reactions reported.

THERAPEUTIC CLASS: Antimicrotubule agent

INDICATIONS: Treatment of locally advanced or metastatic breast cancer and non-small cell lung cancer (NSCLC) after failure of prior chemotherapy. In combination with doxorubicin and cyclophosphamide for the adjuvant treatment of operable, node-positive breast cancer. In combination with cisplatin for treatment of unresectable, locally advanced or metastatic NSCLC in those previously untreated with chemotherapy. Treatment of androgen independent (hormone refractory) metastatic prostate cancer in combination with prednisone. In combination with cisplatin and fluorouracil for the treatment of advanced gastric adenocarcinoma, including adenocarcinoma of the gastroesophageal junction, in patients who have not received prior chemotherapy for advanced disease. In combination with cisplatin and fluorouracil for the induction treatment of patients with inoperable locally advanced squamous cell carcinoma of the head and neck (SCCHN).

DOSAGE: *Adults:* Premedicate with oral corticosteroids. Adjust dose based on febrile neutropenia, neutrophil count, cutaneous reactions, peripheral neuropathy, neurosensory signs/symptoms, or GI toxicities (see package insert). Breast Cancer: 60-100mg/m^2 IV over 1 hr every 3 weeks. Adjuvant Treatment Operable Node-Positive Breast CA: 75mg/m^2 1 hr after doxorubicin 50mg/m^2 and cyclophosphamide 500mg/m^2 every 3 weeks for 6 courses. NSCLC: 75mg/m^2 IV over 1 hr every 3 weeks. Prostate Cancer: 75mg/m^2 every 3 weeks over 1 hr with prednisone 5mg bid. Gastric Adenocarcinoma: Premedicate with antiemetics and appropriate hydration. 75mg/m^2 IV over 1 hr, followed by cisplatin 75mg/m^2 IV over 1-3 hrs (both on Day 1 only), followed by fluorouracil 750mg/m^2/day IV over 24 hrs for 5 days, starting at end of cisplatin infusion. Repeat treatment every 3 weeks. SCCHN: 75mg/m^2 IV over 1 hr, followed by cisplatin 75mg/m^2 IV over 1 hr, on Day 1, followed by fluorouracil as a continuous IV infusion at 750mg/m^2/day for five days administered every 3 weeks for 4 cycles.

Pediatrics: ≥16 yrs: Premedicate with oral corticosteroids. Adjust dose based on febrile neutropenia, neutrophil count, cutaneous reactions, peripheral neuropathy, neurosensory signs/symptoms, or GI toxicities (see package insert). Breast Cancer: 60-100mg/m^2 IV over 1 hr every 3 weeks. Adjuvant Treatment Operable Node-Positive Breast CA: 75mg/m^2 1 hr after doxorubicin 50mg/m^2 and cyclophosphamide 500mg/m^2 every 3 weeks for 6 courses. NSCLC: 75mg/m^2 IV over 1 hr every 3 weeks. Prostate Cancer: 75mg/m^2 every 3 weeks over 1 hr with prednisone 5mg bid. Gastric Adenocarcinoma: Premedicate with antiemetics and appropriate hydration. 75mg/m^2 IV over 1 hr, followed by cisplatin 75mg/m^2 IV over 1-3 hrs (both on Day 1 only), followed by fluorouracil 750mg/m^2/day IV over 24 hrs for 5 days, starting at end of cisplatin infusion. Repeat treatment every 3 weeks. SCCHN: 75mg/m^2 IV over 1 hr, followed by cisplatin 75mg/m^2 IV over 1 hr, on Day 1, followed by fluorouracil as a continuous IV infusion at 750mg/m^2 per day for five days administered every 3 weeks for 4 cycles.

HOW SUPPLIED: Inj: 20mg/0.5mL

CONTRAINDICATIONS: Neutrophils <1500cells/mm^3, hypersensitivity to polysorbate 80.

WARNINGS/PRECAUTIONS: Toxic deaths, febrile neutropenia, neutropenia, localized erythema of extremities with edema and desquamation, severe neurosensory symptoms, severe asthenia reported. Monitor for hypersensitivity reactions. Can cause fetal harm. Caution in elderly. Monitor CBC frequently; avoid subsequent cycles until neutrophils recover to >1500 cells/mm^3 and platelets recover to >100,000cells/mm^3.

ADVERSE REACTIONS: Arthralgia, myalgia, alopecia, stomatitis, nausea, vomiting, diarrhea, nail changes, cutaneous and neurosensory reactions, fluid retention, hypersensitivity reaction, leukopenia, thrombocytopenia, anemia, neutropenia, fever.

INTERACTIONS: Caution with agents that induce, inhibit, or are metabolized by CYP450 3A4 (eg, ketoconazole, erythromycin, terfenadine, astemizole, cyclosporine).

PREGNANCY: Category D, not for use in nursing.

TAZICEF
ceftazidime (Hospira) — RX

THERAPEUTIC CLASS: Cephalosporin (3rd generation)

INDICATIONS: Treatment of lower respiratory tract (eg, pneumonia), skin and skin structure (SSSI), bone and joint, gynecologic, CNS (eg, meningitis), intra-abdominal, and urinary tract infections (UTI), and septicemia. For use in sepsis.

DOSAGE: *Adults:* Usual: 1g IM/IV q8-12h. Uncomplicated UTI: 250mg IM/IV q12h. Complicated UTI: 500mg IM/IV q8-12h. Bone and Joint Infection: 2g IV q12h. Uncomplicated Pneumonia/SSSI: 500mg-1g IM/IV q8h. Gynecological/Intra-Abdominal/Meningitis/

TAZIDIME

Severe Life-Threatening Infection: 2g IV q8h. Lung Infection caused by Pseudomonas in Cystic Fibrosis (normal renal function): 30-50mg/kg IV q8h. Max: 6g/day. Renal Impairment: CrCl 31-50mL/min: 1g q12h. CrCl 16-30mL/min: 1g q24h. CrCl 6-15mL/min: 500mg q24h. CrCl <5mL/min: 500mg q48h. For severe infections (6g/day), increase renal impairment dose by 50% or increase dosing interval. Apply reduced dosage recommendations after initial 1g LD is given. Hemodialysis: Give 1g before and 1g after each hemodialysis. Intra-Peritoneal Dialysis/Continuous Ambulatory Peritoneal Dialysis: Give 1g followed by 500mg q24h, or add to fluid at 250mg/2L.

Pediatrics: Neonates (0-4 weeks): 30mg/kg IV q12h. 1 month-12 yrs: 30-50mg/kg IV q8h. Max: 6g/day. Higher doses for patients with cystic fibrosis or when treating meningitis. Renal impairment: CrCl 31-50mL/min: 1g q12h. CrCl 16-30mL/min: 1g q24h. CrCl 6-15mL/min: 500mg q24h. CrCl <5mL/min: 500mg q48h. For severe infections (6g/day), increase renal impairment dose by 50% or increase dosing interval. Apply reduced dosage recommendations after initial 1g LD is given. Hemodialysis: Give 1g before and 1g after each hemodialysis. Intra-Peritoneal Dialysis/Continuous Ambulatory Peritoneal Dialysis: Give 1g followed by 500mg q24h, or add to fluid at 250mg/2L.

HOW SUPPLIED: Inj: 1g, 2g, 6g

WARNINGS/PRECAUTIONS: Monitor renal function; potential for nephrotoxicity. May result in overgrowth of nonsusceptible organisms. Possible cross-sensitivity between penicillins, cephalosporins, and other beta-lactams. Pseudomembranous colitis reported. Elevated levels with renal insufficiency can lead to seizures, encephalopathy, asterixis, and neuromuscular excitability. Possible decrease in PT; caution with renal or hepatic impairment, poor nutritional state; monitor PT and give vitamin K if needed. Caution with colitis and other GI diseases. Distal necrosis can occur after inadvertent intra-arterial administration. Continue for 2 days after signs and symptoms of infection resolve, but may require longer therapy with complicated infections. Caution in elderly.

ADVERSE REACTIONS: Phlebitis and inflammation at injection site, pruritus, rash, fever, diarrhea, anaphylaxis.

INTERACTIONS: Nephrotoxicity reported with aminoglycosides or potent diuretics (eg, furosemide). Avoid with chloramphenicol; may decrease effect of beta-lactam antibiotics.

PREGNANCY: Category B, caution in nursing.

TAZIDIME   RX
ceftazidime (Lilly)

THERAPEUTIC CLASS: Cephalosporin (3rd generation)

INDICATIONS: Treatment of lower respiratory tract (eg, pneumonia), skin and skin structure (SSSI), bone and joint, gynecologic, CNS (eg, meningitis), intra-abdominal, and urinary tract infections (UTI), and septicemia. For use in sepsis.

DOSAGE: *Adults:* Usual: 1g IM/IV q8-12h. Uncomplicated UTI: 250mg IM/IV q12h. Complicated UTI: 500mg IM/IV q8-12h. Bone and Joint Infection: 2g IV q12h. Uncomplicated Pneumonia/Skin and Skin Structure Infection: 500mg-1g IM/IV q8h. Gynecological/Intra-Abdominal/Meningitis/Severe Life-Threatening Infection: 2g IV q8h. Lung Infection caused by Pseudomonas spp. in Cystic Fibrosis (normal renal function): 30-50mg/kg IV q8h. Max: 6g/day. Renal impairment: CrCl 31-50mL/min: 1g q12h. CrCl 16-30mL/min: 1g q24h. CrCl 6-15mL/min: 500mg q24h. CrCl <5mL/min: 500mg q48h. For severe infections (6g/day), increase renal impairment dose by 50% or increase dosing interval. Apply reduced dosage recommendations after initial 1g LD is given. Hemodialysis: Give 1g before then 1g after each hemodialysis. Intra-Peritoneal Dialysis/Continuous Ambulatory Peritoneal Dialysis: Give 1g followed by 500mg q24h, or add to fluid at 250mg/2L.

Pediatrics: Neonates (0-4 weeks): 30mg/kg IV q12h. 1 month-12 yrs: 30-50mg/kg IV q8h. Max: 6g/day. Higher doses for cystic fibrosis and meningitis. Renal Impairment: CrCl 31-50mL/min: 1g q12h. CrCl 16-30mL/min: 1g q24h. CrCl 6-15mL/min: 500mg q24h. CrCl <5mL/min: 500mg q48h. For severe infections (6g/day), increase renal impairment dose by 50% or increase dosing interval. Apply reduced dosage recommendations after initial 1g LD is given. Hemodialysis: Give 1g before then 1g after each hemodialysis. Intra-Peritoneal Dialysis/Continuous Ambulatory Peritoneal Dialysis: Give 1g followed by 500mg q24h, or add to fluid at 250mg/2L.

HOW SUPPLIED: Inj: 1g, 2g, 6g

WARNINGS/PRECAUTIONS: Monitor renal function; potential for nephrotoxicity. Prolonged use may result in overgrowth of nonsusceptible organisms. Possible cross-sensitivity between penicillins, cephalosporins, and other beta-lactam antibiotics. Pseudomembranous colitis reported. Elevated levels with renal insufficiency can lead to seizures, encephalopathy, asterixis and neuromuscular excitability. Possible decrease in PT; caution with renal or hepatic impairment, poor nutritional state; monitor PT and give vitamin K if needed. Caution with colitis and other GI diseases. Distal necrosis can occur after inadvertent intra-arterial administration. Continue therapy for 2 days after the signs and symptoms of infection have disappeared, but in complicated infections longer therapy may be required.

ADVERSE REACTIONS: Phlebitis and inflammation at injection site, pruritus, rash, fever, diarrhea.

INTERACTIONS: Nephrotoxicity reported with aminoglycosides or potent diuretics (eg, furosemide). Avoid with chloramphenicol; may decrease effect of beta-lactam antibiotics.

PREGNANCY: Category B, caution in nursing.

TAZORAC
tazarotene (Allergan)

RX

THERAPEUTIC CLASS: Retinoic acid derivative

INDICATIONS: (Gel 0.05%, 0.1%) Stable plaque psoriasis of up to 20% body surface area involvement. (Cre 0.1%, Gel 0.1%) Acne vulgaris of mild to moderate severity. (Cre 0.05%, 0.1%) Treatment of plaque psoriasis.

DOSAGE: *Adults:* Cleanse and dry skin. Apply to skin qpm.
Pediatrics: ≥12 yrs: Cleanse and dry skin. Apply to acne or psoriatic lesions qpm.

HOW SUPPLIED: Cre: 0.05%, 0.1% (30g, 60g); Gel: 0.05%, 0.1% (30g, 100g)

CONTRAINDICATIONS: Women who are or may become pregnant.

WARNINGS/PRECAUTIONS: Use adequate birth control measures. Avoid mouth, eyes, eyelids, sunlight exposure (including sunlamps), or eczematous skin. Stop therapy with pruritus, burning, skin redness, or peeling. Weather extremes (eg, wind, cold) may be irritating.

ADVERSE REACTIONS: Pruritus, burning/stinging, erythema, worsening of psoriasis, irritation, skin pain, desquamation, dry skin, rash, fissuring, localized edema, skin discoloration.

INTERACTIONS: Avoid topical agents that have a strong drying effect. Caution with photosensitizers (eg, thiazides, tetracyclines, fluoroquinolones, phenothiazines, sulfonamides).

PREGNANCY: Category X, caution in nursing.

TEGRETOL
carbamazepine (Novartis)

RX

> Aplastic anemia and agranulocytosis reported. Obtain complete pretreatment hematological testing as a baseline. Discontinue if develop evidence of bone marrow depression.

OTHER BRAND NAME: Tegretol-XR (Novartis)

THERAPEUTIC CLASS: Carboxamide anticonvulsant

INDICATIONS: Treatment of partial seizures with complex symptomatology, general tonic-clonic seizures, and mixed seizure patterns of these or other partial or generalized seizures. Treatment of trigeminal or glossopharyngeal neuralgia pain.

DOSAGE: *Adults:* Epilepsy: Initial: (Immediate or Extended Release Tabs) 200mg bid or (Sus) 100mg qid. Titrate: (Immediate Release Tabs/Sus) Increase weekly by 200mg/day given tid-qid. (Extended Release Tabs) Increase weekly by 200mg/day given bid. Maint: 800-1200mg/day. Max: 1200mg/day. Trigeminal Neuralgia: Initial (Day 1): (Immediate or Extended Release Tabs) 100mg bid or (Sus) 50mg qid. Titrate: May increase by

TEMOVATE

100mg q12h (Tabs) or 50mg qid (Sus). Maint: 400-800mg/day. Max: 1200mg/day. Re-evaluate every 3 months. Swallow Extended Release Tabs whole; do not crush or chew.

Pediatrics: Epilepsy: >12 yrs: Initial: (Immediate or Extended Release Tabs) 200mg bid or (Sus) 100mg qid. Titrate: (Immediate Release Tabs/Sus) Increase weekly by 200mg/day given tid-qid. (Extended Release Tabs) Increase weekly by 200mg/day given bid. Max: 12-15 yrs: 1000mg/day. >15 yrs: 1200mg/day. 6-12 yrs: Initial: (Immediate or Extended Release Tabs) 100mg bid or (Sus) 50mg qid. Titrate: (Immediate Release Tabs/Sus) Increase weekly by 100mg/day given tid-qid. (Extended Release Tabs) Increase weekly by 100mg/day given bid. Maint: 400-800mg/day. Max: 1000mg/day. 6 months-6 yrs: Initial: (Immediate Release Tabs) 10-20mg/kg/day given bid-tid or (Sus) 10-20mg/kg/day given qid. Titrate: (Immediate Release Tabs/Sus) Increase weekly tid-qid. Max: 35mg/kg/day. Swallow Extended Release Tabs whole; do not crush or chew.

HOW SUPPLIED: Sus: 100mg/5mL; Tab: (Tegretol) 200mg*; Tab, Chewable: 100mg*; Tab, Extended Release: (Tegretol-XR) 100mg, 200mg, 400mg *scored

CONTRAINDICATIONS: History of bone marrow depression, MAOI use within 14 days, hypersensitivity to TCAs.

WARNINGS/PRECAUTIONS: Lyell's syndrome and Stevens-Johnson syndrome, multi-organ hypersensitivity reactions reported. Caution with history of adverse hematologic reaction to any drug, increased IOP, the elderly, mixed seizure disorder with atypical absence seizure. Fetal harm with pregnancy. May activate latent psychosis. Caution with cardiac, hepatic, or renal damage. Perform eye exam and monitor LFTs and renal function at baseline and periodically. Suspension produces higher peak levels than the tablet.

ADVERSE REACTIONS: Dizziness, drowsiness, unsteadiness, nausea, vomiting, bone marrow depression, rash, urticaria, hypersensitivity reactions, photosensitivity reactions, CHF, edema, HTN, hypotension.

INTERACTIONS: Do not give suspension with other medicinal liquids or diluents. Metabolism is inhibited by CYP3A4 inhibitors (eg, cimetidine, macrolides) and induced by CYP3A4 inducers (eg, rifampin, phenytoin). Decreases oral contraceptive effectiveness. Increases plasma levels of clomipramine, phenytoin and primidone. Decreases levels of APAP, alprazolam, clonazepam, clozapine, dicumarol, doxycycline, ethosuximide, haloperidol, lamotrigine, methsuximide, oral contraceptives, phensuximide, phenytoin, theophylline, tiagabine, topiramate, valproate, and warfarin. Increased risk of neurotoxic side effects with lithium. Avoid MAOIs.

PREGNANCY: Category D, not for use in nursing.

TEMOVATE   RX
clobetasol propionate (GlaxoSmithKline)

OTHER BRAND NAMES: Temovate-E (GlaxoSmithKline) - Temovate Scalp (GlaxoSmithKline)

THERAPEUTIC CLASS: Corticosteroid

INDICATIONS: Corticosteroid responsive dermatoses. Temovate-E is also used to treat moderate to severe plaque-type psoriasis.

DOSAGE: *Adults:* Apply bid. Max: 50g/week or 50mL/week. Moderate-Severe Psoriasis: (Temovate-E) Apply bid for up to 4 weeks. May use on 5-10% of BSA. Max: 50g/week. Limit treatment to 2 consecutive weeks. Avoid with occlusive dressings.

Pediatrics: ≥12 yrs: Apply bid. Max: 50g/week or 50mL/week. Moderate-Severe Psoriasis: ≥16 yrs: (Temovate-E) Apply bid for up to 4 weeks. May use on 5-10% of BSA. Max: 50g/week. Limit treatment to 2 consecutive weeks. Avoid with occlusive dressings.

HOW SUPPLIED: (Temovate) Cre, Oint: 0.05% (15g, 30g, 45g, 60g); Gel: 0.05% (15g, 30g, 60g); Sol: 0.05% (25mL); (Temovate-E) Cre: 0.05% (15g, 30g, 60g); (Temovate Scalp) Sol: 0.05% (25mL, 50mL).

CONTRAINDICATIONS: (Scalp Sol) Primary scalp infections.

WARNINGS/PRECAUTIONS: Not for use on face, groin, or axillae, or for treatment of rosacea or perioral dermatitis. May produce reversible HPA axis suppression, manifestations of Cushing's syndrome, hyperglycemia, and glucosuria. Use appropriate antifungal or antibacterial agent with dermatological infections; d/c if infection does not clear. Peds may be more susceptible to systemic toxicity. Avoid eyes. D/C if irritation occurs.

ADVERSE REACTIONS: Burning, stinging, pruritus, skin atrophy, cracking/fissuring of the skin, erythema, folliculitis, numbness of fingers, telangiectasia, tingling (Sol), folliculitis (Sol).

PREGNANCY: Category C, caution in nursing.

Tenuate
diethylpropion HCl (Watson) — CIV

OTHER BRAND NAME: Tenuate Dospan (Watson)

THERAPEUTIC CLASS: Sympathomimetic amine

INDICATIONS: Short term adjunct for exogenous obesity in patients with an initial BMI$\geq$30kg/m^2.

DOSAGE: *Adults:* (Tab) 25mg tid 1 hour before meals, and mid-evening if needed for night hunger. (Tab, ER): 75mg at qd in mid-morning, swallowed whole.

Pediatrics: $\geq$16 yrs: (Tab) 25mg tid 1 hour before meals, and mid-evening if needed for night hunger. (Tab, ER): 75mg at qd in mid-morning, swallowed whole.

HOW SUPPLIED: Tab: (Tenuate) 25mg; Tab, Extended Release: (Tenuate Dospan) 75mg

CONTRAINDICATIONS: Advanced arteriosclerosis, hyperthyroidism, glaucoma, pulmonary HTN, severe HTN, within 14 days of MAOI use, agitated states, history of drug abuse, other concomitant anorectics.

WARNINGS/PRECAUTIONS: Possible risk of pulmonary hypertension and valvular heart disease. Caution in HTN, symptomatic cardiovascular disease. Avoid with heart murmur, valvular heart disease, severe HTN. May increase convulsions with epilepsy. Prolonged use may induce dependence with withdrawal symptoms. Discontinue if tolerance develops or if insignificant weight loss after 4 weeks of therapy.

ADVERSE REACTIONS: Palpitations, tachycardia, arrhythmias, blurred vision, dizziness, anxiety, insomnia, depression, urticaria, gynecomastia, nausea, vomiting, GI disturbances, bone marrow depression, impotence.

INTERACTIONS: MAOIs may cause hypertensive crisis. Avoid with other anorectic agents (prescription, OTC, herbal products) or if used within prior year. Phenothiazines may antagonize anorectic effects. Potential for arrhythmias with general anesthetics. May interfere with antihypertensives (eg, guanethidine, methyldopa). Adverse reactions with alcohol. Antidiabetic drug requirements may be altered. Valvular heart disease reported with fenfluramine or dexfenfluramine.

PREGNANCY: Category B, caution in nursing.

Terbutaline
terbutaline sulfate (Various) — RX

THERAPEUTIC CLASS: Beta$_2$ agonist

INDICATIONS: Prevention and reversal of bronchospasm in asthma, and reversible bronchospasm in bronchitis and emphysema.

DOSAGE: *Adults:* (PO) Usual: 5mg tid. May reduce to 2.5mg tid. Max: 15mg/24hrs. (Inj) Usual: 0.25mg SQ into lateral deltoid area. May repeat within 15-30 minutes if no improvement. Max: 0.5mg/4hrs.

Pediatrics: (PO) 12-15 yrs: Usual: 2.5mg tid. Max: 7.5mg/24hrs. (Inj) $\geq$12 yrs: Usual: 0.25mg SQ into lateral deltoid area. May repeat within 15-30 minutes if no improvement. Max: 0.5mg/4hrs.

HOW SUPPLIED: Inj: 1mg/mL (1mL); Tab: 2.5mg*, 5mg* *scored

CONTRAINDICATIONS: Hypersensitivity to sympathomimetic amines.

TESSALON

WARNINGS/PRECAUTIONS: Caution with ischemic heart disease, HTN, arrhythmias, hyperthyroidism, DM, seizures. Not approved for tocolysis. Hypersensitivity and exacerbation of bronchospasm reported. Monitor for transient hypokalemia.

ADVERSE REACTIONS: Nervousness, tremor, headache, somnolence, palpitations, dizziness, tachycardia, nausea.

INTERACTIONS: Avoid other sympathomimetic agents (except aerosol bronchodilators). Extreme caution with MAOIs and TCAs during or within 14 days of treatment. Decreased effects with β-blockers. Possible ECG changes and hypokalemia with loop or thiazide diuretics.

PREGNANCY: Category B, caution in nursing.

TESSALON — RX
benzonatate (Forest)

THERAPEUTIC CLASS: Non-narcotic antitussive

INDICATIONS: Symptomatic relief of cough.

DOSAGE: *Adults:* Usual: 100-200mg tid as needed. Max: 600mg/day.
Pediatrics: >10 yrs: Usual: 100-200mg tid as needed. Max: 600mg/day.

HOW SUPPLIED: Cap: 100mg, 200mg

WARNINGS/PRECAUTIONS: Severe hypersensitivity reactions; confusion and hallucinations reported in combination with other prescribed drugs. Swallow capsules without sucking/chewing to avoid local anesthesia adverse effects.

ADVERSE REACTIONS: Sedation, headache, dizziness, confusion, hallucinations, constipation, nausea, GI upset, pruritus.

PREGNANCY: Category C, caution in nursing.

TESTRED — CIII
methyltestosterone (Valeant)

THERAPEUTIC CLASS: Androgen

INDICATIONS: Testosterone replacement therapy in males with primary hypogonadism or hypogonadotrophic hypogonadism. To stimulate puberty in males with delayed puberty. Secondary treatment of advancing inoperable metastatic (skeletal) breast cancer in females 1-5 yrs postmenopausal.

DOSAGE: *Adults:* Dose based on age, sex and diagnosis. Adjust dose according to clinical response and adverse events. Male Replacement Therapy: 10-50mg/day. Breast Carcinoma: 50-200mg/day.
Pediatrics: Dose based on age, sex and diagnosis. Adjust dose according to clinical response and adverse events. Delayed Puberty: Use lower range of 10-50mg/day for 4-6 months. Caution in children.

HOW SUPPLIED: Cap: 10mg

CONTRAINDICATIONS: Pregnancy. Males with breast or prostate carcinoma.

WARNINGS/PRECAUTIONS: D/C if hypercalcemia occurs in breast cancer; monitor calcium levels. Monitor for virilization in females. Risk of compromised stature in children; monitor bone growth every 6 months. Risk of hepatic damage with long-term use. D/C if jaundice, cholestatic hepatitis occurs. Risk of edema; caution with pre-existing cardiac, renal or hepatic disease. Caution in the elderly; increased risk of prostatic hypertrophy and prostatic carcinoma. Should not be used for enhancement of athletic performance. Monitor LFTs, Hct, and Hgb periodically.

ADVERSE REACTIONS: Amenorrhea, virilization, menstrual irregularities, gynecomastia, excessive frequency/duration of penile erections, male pattern baldness, increased/decreased libido, oligospermia, hirsutism, acne, fluid and electrolyte disturbances, nausea, hypercholesterolemia, clotting factor suppression, polycythemia, altered LFTs, priapism, anxiety, depression.

INTERACTIONS: Potentiates oral anticoagulants and oxyphenbutazone. May decrease blood glucose and insulin requirements in diabetics.

PREGNANCY: Category X, not for use in nursing.

Tetanus & Diphtheria Toxoids Adsorbed RX
tetanus toxoid - diphtheria toxoid (Sanofi Pasteur)

THERAPEUTIC CLASS: Toxoid combination

INDICATIONS: Active immunization against tetanus and diphtheria (Td).

DOSAGE: *Adults:* 0.5mL IM in the vastus lateralis or deltoid. Repeat 4-8 weeks later. Give 3rd dose 6-12 months after 2nd dose. Booster: 0.5mL IM every 10 yrs.
Pediatrics: >7 yrs: 0.5mL IM in the vastus lateralis or deltoid. Repeat 4-8 weeks later. Give 3rd dose 6-12 months after 2nd dose. Booster: 0.5mL IM every 10 yrs.

HOW SUPPLIED: Inj: 5LFU-2LFU/0.5mL

CONTRAINDICATIONS: Neurological or systemic allergic reaction to previous dose. Defer during febrile illness, acute infection, or an outbreak of poliomyelitis. Thimerosal hypersensitivity.

WARNINGS/PRECAUTIONS: Suboptimal response may occur in immunocompromised patients. Avoid booster more frequently than every 10 yrs especially with Arthus-type hypersensitivity reactions or temperature >39.4°C after a previous dose of tetanus toxoid. Caution with IM injection in thrombocytopenia or any coagulation disorder. Increased risk of local/systemic reactions to boosters doses. Have epinephrine available.

ADVERSE REACTIONS: Injection site reaction, fever, malaise, hypotension, nausea, arthralgia.

INTERACTIONS: Immunosuppressive therapy may reduce response to active immunization. Caution with anticoagulants.

PREGNANCY: Category C, safety in nursing not known.

Tetanus Toxoid Adsorbed RX
tetanus toxoid (Sanofi Pasteur)

THERAPEUTIC CLASS: Toxoid

INDICATIONS: Active immunization against tetanus.

DOSAGE: *Adults:* Primary Immunization: 0.5mL IM. Repeat 4-8 weeks later. Give 3rd dose 6-12 months after 2nd dose. Booster: 0.5mL IM every 10 yrs.
Pediatrics: <1 yr: 3 doses of 0.5mL IM 4 to 8 weeks apart, then 4th dose (0.5mL) 6 to 12 months after the 3rd dose. Last dose before 4 yrs. Give booster of 0.5mL at 4-6 yrs. No booster needed if last primary dose was given after 4 yrs. ≥1 yrs: Primary Immunization: 0.5mL IM. Repeat 4-8 weeks later. Give 3rd dose 6-12 months after 2nd dose. Booster: 0.5mL IM every 10 yrs.

HOW SUPPLIED: Inj: 5 LFU/0.5mL

CONTRAINDICATIONS: Neurological or systemic allergic reaction to previous dose. Defer during febrile illness, acute infection, or an outbreak of poliomyelitis. Thimerosal hypersensitivity.

WARNINGS/PRECAUTIONS: Suboptimal response may occur in immunocompromised patients. Avoid booster more frequently than every 10 yrs especially with Arthus-type hypersensitivity reactions or temperature >103°F after a previous dose of tetanus toxoid. Caution with IM injections in thrombocytopenia or any coagulation disorders. Have epinephrine injection available. Increased incidence of local/systemic reaction to booster doses.

ADVERSE REACTIONS: Local erythema, malaise, transient fever, pain, hypotension, nausea, arthralgia.

INTERACTIONS: Caution with anticoagulants. Immunosuppresive therapy (eg, radiation, corticosteroids, chemotherapy) may reduce antibody response to vaccine; defer routine vaccination. Separate syringes and sites should be used when Tetanus Immune Globulin (human) and vaccine are given concurrently.

PREGNANCY: Category C, safety in nursing not known.

Tev-Tropin RX
somatropin (Gate)

THERAPEUTIC CLASS: Human growth hormone

INDICATIONS: Long-term treatment of children who have growth failure due to an inadequate secretion of normal endogenous growth hormone.

THALOMID

DOSAGE: *Pediatrics:* 0.1mg/kg (0.3 IU/kg) SQ 3x week.

HOW SUPPLIED: Inj: 5mg

CONTRAINDICATIONS: Prader-Willi syndrome (PWS) with severe obesity or severe respiratory impairment. Growth failure due to PWS. Acute critical illness due to complications following open heart or abdominal surgery, multiple accidental traumas, acute respiratory failure; closed epiphyses; progression of an underlying intracranial lesion; active neoplasia, benzyl alcohol sensitivity.

WARNINGS/PRECAUTIONS: Reports of fatalities in pediatric patients with PWS. In PWS, evaluate for upper airway obstruction prior to initiation; monitor weight, for sleep apnea, signs of upper airway obstruction (eg, suspend therapy with onset of or increased snoring), respiratory infections (treat early and aggressively if occur). Monitor GHD secondary to intracranial lesion for progression/recurrence; glucose intolerance; hypothyroidism; intracranial hypertension (perform fundoscopic exam at start and periodically). Slipped capital femoral epiphysis may occur. Monitor for malignant transformation of any skin lesion. When injected SQ in the same site over a long period of time, may cause tissue atrophy; rotate injection site.

ADVERSE REACTIONS: Headaches, injection site reactions (pain, bruise), leukemia.

INTERACTIONS: Decreased effects with glucocorticoids.

PREGNANCY: Category C, caution with nursing.

THALOMID
thalidomide (Celgene)

RX

> Severe, life-threatening human birth defects if taken during pregnancy. Women of childbearing potential should have a pregnancy test before starting therapy, then weekly for 1st month, and monthly thereafter. Males must use latex condoms in sexual intercourse with females of childbearing potential. Only prescribers and pharmacists registered with the S.T.E.P.S.® distribution program can prescribe and dispense. The use of thalidomide in multiple myeloma results in an increased risk of venous thromboembolic events, such as deep vein thrombosis and pulmonary embolus.

THERAPEUTIC CLASS: Immunomodulatory agent

INDICATIONS: Acute treatment of the cutaneous manifestations of moderate to severe erythema nodosum leprosum (ENL). Maintenance therapy for prevention and suppression of the cutaneous manifestations of ENL recurrence. In combination with dexamethasone for the treatment of newly diagnosed multiple myeloma.

DOSAGE: *Adults:* Acute ENL: Initial: 100-300mg qhs with water at least 1 hr after evening meal. <50kg: Start therapy at lower end of dosing range. Severe Cutaneous ENL: Initial: 400mg qhs with water at least 1 hr after evening meal. Use with corticosteroids in moderate to severe neuritis with severe ENL. Taper steroid where neuritis is ameliorated. Duration of therapy is usually 2 weeks. Taper Dose: Decrease by 50mg every 2-4 weeks. Maintenance Therapy for Prevention/Suppression of ENL Recurrence: Use minimum dose to control reaction. Taper Dose: Every 3-6 months, attempt to decrease dose by 50mg every 2-4 weeks. Multiple Myeloma: 200mg qhs at least 1 hr after evening meal. Give with dexamethasone in 28 day treatment cycles.

Pediatrics: ≥12 yrs: Acute ENL: Initial: 100-300mg qhs with water at least 1 hr after evening meal. <50kg: Start therapy at lower end of dosing range. Severe Cutaneous ENL: Initial: 400mg qhs with water at least 1 hour after evening meal. Use with corticosteroids in moderate to severe neuritis with severe ENL. Taper steroid where neuritis is ameliorated. Duration of therapy is usually 2 weeks. Taper Dose: Decrease by 50mg every 2-4 weeks. Maintenance Therapy for Prevention/Suppression of ENL Recurrence: Use minimum dose to control reaction. Taper Dose: Every 3-6 months, attempt to decrease dose by 50mg every 2-4 weeks. Multiple Myeloma: 200mg qhs at least 1 hr after evening meal. Give with dexamethasone in 28 day treatment cycles.

HOW SUPPLIED: Cap: 50mg, 100mg, 200mg

CONTRAINDICATIONS: Women of childbearing potential unless alternative therapies are considered inappropriate and if precautions are taken to avoid pregnancy. Sexually mature males unless they comply with the S.T.E.P.S.® program and mandatory contraceptive measures.

WARNINGS/PRECAUTIONS: See Black Box Warning. If hypersensitivity reaction occurs such as rash, fever, or tachycardia, d/c drug. Stevens-Johnson syndrome and toxic epidermal necrolysis reported. May cause severe birth defects. Drowsiness and somnolence reported, caution when operating machinery. May cause neuropathy, monitor for symptoms. If symptoms of neuropathy arise, d/c immediately. Do not initiate if ANC <750/mm^3. Measure viral load of HIV patients after 1st and 3rd month of therapy and every 3 months thereafter.

ADVERSE REACTIONS: Drowsiness, somnolence, peripheral neuropathy, dizziness, orthostatic hypotension, neutropenia, increased HIV viral load, rash, constipation, hypocalcemia, thrombosis/embolism, dyspnea.

INTERACTIONS: Enhanced sedation with barbiturates, alcohol, chlorpromazine, and reserpine. Caution with drugs associated with peripheral neuropathy.

PREGNANCY: Category X, not for use in nursing.

THEO-24
theophylline (UCB Pharma)
RX

THERAPEUTIC CLASS: Xanthine bronchodilator

INDICATIONS: Treatment of symptoms and reversible airflow obstruction associated with chronic asthma and other chronic lung diseases.

DOSAGE: *Adults:* Initial: 300-400mg/day. Titrate: After 3 days increase to 400-600mg/day if tolerated. May increase to >600mg/day if needed and tolerated after 3 more days. Renal/Liver Dysfunction/Elderly/CHF: Max: 400mg/day. May give in divided doses q12h in fast metabolizers. Swallow tab whole with full glass of water, do not crush. Dose should be titrated based on serum levels.
Pediatrics: 12-15 yrs: <45kg: Initial: 12-14mg/kg/day. Max: 300mg/day. Titrate: After 3 days increase to 16mg/kg/day. Max: 400mg/day. May increase to 20mg/kg/day if tolerated and needed after 3 more days. Max: 600mg/day. 12-15 yrs (>45kg): Follow adult dose schedule. Renal/Liver Dysfunction/CHF: Max: 16mg/kg/day or 400mg/day. May give in divided doses q12h in fast metabolizers. Swallow tab whole with full glass of water, do not crush. Dose should be titrated based on serum levels.

HOW SUPPLIED: Cap, Extended Release: 100mg, 200mg, 300mg, 400mg

WARNINGS/PRECAUTIONS: Extreme caution in peptic ulcer disease, seizure disorders and/or cardiac arrhythmias (except bradycardia). Caution in neonates, children <1 yr, and the elderly. Caution in pulmonary edema, CHF, fever ≥102°F for 24 hrs, corpulmonale, hypothyroidism, liver disease, reduced renal function, sepsis, shock, and HTN. If toxicity develops (eg, repetitive vomiting) monitor serum levels and adjust dosage.

ADVERSE REACTIONS: Diarrhea, nausea, vomiting, abdominal pain, nervousness, headache, insomnia, seizures, dizziness, tremor, tachycardia, arrhythmias, restlessness, tremor, transient diuresis.

INTERACTIONS: Potentiated by propranolol, allopurinol, erythromycin, cimetidine, interferon, ciprofloxacin, clarithromycin, disulfiram, enoxacin, methotrexate, beta adrenergic blockers, oral contraceptives, fluvoxamine, calcium channel blockers, corticosteroid, thyroid hormones, thiabendazole, ticlopidine, troleadomycin, carbamazepine, pentoxifylline, diuretics, tacrine, and isoniazid. Diminishes the effects of adenosine, diazepam, lithium, lorazepam, midazolam, and pancuronium. Synergistic CNS effects with ephedrine. Diminished effects with aminoglutethimide, phenytoin, phenobarbital, carbamazepine, rifampin, barbiturates, hydantoins, ketoconazole, diuretics sympathomimetics, and isoproterenol.

PREGNANCY: Category C, caution in nursing.

THEOLAIR
theophylline (Graceway)
RX

THERAPEUTIC CLASS: Xanthine bronchodilator

INDICATIONS: Treatment of symptoms and reversible airflow obstruction associated with chronic asthma and other chronic lung diseases (eg, emphysema, chronic bronchitis).

THIOGUANINE

DOSAGE: *Adults:* Initial: 300mg/day divided q6-8h. Titrate: if tolerated, after 3 days, increase to 400mg/day divided q6-8h. May increase to 600mg/day divided q6-8h if needed and tolerated after 3 more days.
Pediatrics: ≥1 yr and <45kg: Initial: 12-14mg/kg/day divided q4-6h. Max: 300mg/day. Titrate: If tolerated after 3 days, increase to 16mg/kg/day divided q6-8h. Max: 400mg/day. May increase to 20mg/kg/day divided q6-8h if tolerated and needed after 3 more days. Max: 600mg/day. ≥1 yr and >45kg: Follow adult dosage schedule.

HOW SUPPLIED: Tab: 125mg*, 250mg* *scored

WARNINGS/PRECAUTIONS: Extreme caution in peptic ulcer disease, seizure disorders and/or cardiac arrhythmias (except bradycardia). Caution in neonates, children <1 yr, and the elderly. Caution in pulmonary edema, CHF, fever ≥102°F for 24 hrs, cor-pulmonale, hypothyroidism, liver disease, reduced renal function, sepsis, shock, and HTN. If toxicity develops (eg repetitive vomiting) monitor serum levels and adjust dosage.

ADVERSE REACTIONS: Nausea, vomiting, headache, insomnia, cardiac arrhythmias, intractable seizures, diarrhea, irritability, restlessness, fine skeletal muscle tremors, transient diuresis.

INTERACTIONS: Alcohol, propranolol, allopurinol, erythromycin, cimetidine, interferon, ciprofloxacin, clarithromycin, disulfiram, enoxacin, methotrexate, mexiletine, estrogen-containing oral contraceptives, propafenone, propranolol, verapamil, fluvoxamine, thiabendazole, ticlopidine, troleadomycin, pentoxifylline, and tacrine may increase levels. Diminishes the effects of adenosine, diazepam, flurazepam, lithium, lorazepam, midazolam, and pancuronium. Synergistic CNS effects with ephedrine. Aminoglutethemide, phenytoin, phenobarbital, carbamazepine, rifampin, barbiturates, hydantoins, moricizine, sulfinpyrazone and isoproterenol may decrease levels. Increased risk of ventricular arrhythmias with halothane. Ketamine may lower theophylline seizure threshold.

PREGNANCY: Category C, caution in nursing.

THIOGUANINE RX
thioguanine (GlaxoSmithKline)

THERAPEUTIC CLASS: Purine analog

INDICATIONS: For remission induction, remission consolidation, and maintenance therapy of acute nonlymphocytic leukemias.

DOSAGE: *Adults:* Monotherapy: 2mg/kg/day. After 4 weeks, may increase to 3mg/kg/day if no improvement and leukocyte or platelet depression. Usual therapy is with other agents in combination.
Pediatrics: Monotherapy: 2mg/kg/day. After 4 weeks, may increase to 3mg/kg/day if no improvement and leukocyte or platelet depression. Usual therapy is with other agents in combination.

HOW SUPPLIED: Tab: 40mg* *scored

CONTRAINDICATIONS: Prior resistance to this drug.

WARNINGS/PRECAUTIONS: Dose-related bone marrow suppression. Increased sensitivity to myelosuppression with thiopurine methyltransferase (TPMT) deficiency. D/C temporarily at 1st sign of abnormally large fall in any formed elements of the blood. Withhold therapy with toxic hepatitis or biliary stasis. Monitor Hgb, Hct, platelets, WBCs, and differential frequently. Monitor LFTs weekly at start of therapy, monthly thereafter.

ADVERSE REACTIONS: Myelosuppression, hyperuricemia, hepatotoxicity, nausea, vomiting, anorexia, stomatitis.

INTERACTIONS: May be cross-resistant with mercaptopurine. Caution with TPMT inhibitors such as aminosalicylate derivatives (eg, olsalazine, mesalazine, sulfasalazine); increased sensitivity to myelosuppression. May need dose reduction with other drugs whose primary toxicity is myelosuppression. Esophageal varices reported with busulfan. Veno-occlusive liver disease reported with combination chemotherapy.

PREGNANCY: Category D, not for use in nursing.

THIORIDAZINE RX
thioridazine HCl (Various)

> Prolongation of QTc interval reported in a dose related manner. Associated with torsade de pointes and sudden death; reserve for patients who fail to respond to or cannot tolerate other antipsychotics.

THERAPEUTIC CLASS: Piperidine phenothiazine

INDICATIONS: Management of schizophrenia in patients not responsive to or intolerant to other antipsychotics.

DOSAGE: *Adults:* Initial: 50-100mg tid. Titrate: Increase gradually. Usual: 200-800mg/day given bid-qid. Max: 800mg/day.
Pediatrics: Initial: 0.6mg/kg/day given in divided doses. Titrate: Increase gradually. Max: 3mg/kg/day.

HOW SUPPLIED: Tab: 10mg, 15mg, 25mg, 50mg, 100mg, 150mg, 200mg

CONTRAINDICATIONS: Severe CNS depression, comatose states, severe hypo- or hypertensive heart disease. Drugs that prolong QTc interval, congenital long QT syndrome, cardiac arrhythmias, drugs that inhibit CYP450 2D6 (eg, fluoxetine, paroxetine), patients with reduced activity of CYP450 2D6.

WARNINGS/PRECAUTIONS: Perform baseline ECG and measure baseline potassium level; monitor periodically thereafter. May develop tardive dyskinesia. NMS, seizures, leukopenia, agranulocytosis reported. Caution with activities requiring alertness. May elevate prolactin levels.

ADVERSE REACTIONS: Tardive dyskinesia, ECG changes, drowsiness, dry mouth, blurred vision, peripheral edema, galactorrhea, nausea, vomiting, gynecomastia, impotence, constipation, diarrhea.

INTERACTIONS: See Contraindications. May potentiate CNS depressants, alcohol, atropine, and phosphorus insecticides. Propranolol, fluvoxamine, pindolol increases thioridazine plasma levels; avoid concomitant use. Avoid CYP2D6 inhibitors (eg, fluoxetine, paroxetine); increased risk of arrhythmias.

PREGNANCY: Safety in pregnancy and nursing not known.

THYROLAR RX
liotrix (Forest)

THERAPEUTIC CLASS: Thyroid replacement hormone

INDICATIONS: Hypothyroidism. As a pituitary TSH suppressant in the treatment or prevention of euthyroid goiters. Diagnostic agent in suppression tests to differentiate suspected hyperthyroidism or thyroid gland autonomy. Management of thyroid cancer.

DOSAGE: *Adults:* Hypothyroidism: Usual: 12.5mcg-50mcg to 25mcg-100mcg qd. Elderly/Coronary Artery Disease: Initial: 6.25mcg-25mcg qd. Chronic Myxedema: 3.1mcg-12.5mcg qd. Titrate: Increase by 3.1mcg-12.5mcg/d q 2-3 weeks. Reduce dose if angina occurs. Myxedema Coma: 400mcg IV levothyroxine sodium (100mcg/mL rapidly) followed by 100-200mcg/day IV. Switch to PO when stable. Thyroid Suppression: 1.56mg/kg/d levothyroxine (T_4) for 7-10 days.
Pediatrics: Hypothyroidism: >12 yrs: 18.75mcg-75mcg qd. 6-12 yrs: 12.5mcg-50mcg to 18.75mcg-75mcg qd. 1-5 yrs: 9.35mcg-37.5mcg to 12.5mcg-50mcg qd. 6-12 months: 6.25mcg-25mcg to 9.35mcg-37.5mcg qd. 0-6 months: 3.1mcg-12.5mcg to 6.25mcg-25mcg qd.

HOW SUPPLIED: (T3-T4) Tab: (1/4) 3.1mcg-12.5mcg, (1/2) 6.25mcg-25mcg, (1) 12.5mcg-50mcg, (2) 25mcg-100mcg, (3) 37.5mcg-150mcg

CONTRAINDICATIONS: Untreated thyrotoxicosis, uncorrected adrenal cortical insufficiency.

WARNINGS/PRECAUTIONS: Do not use in the treatment of obesity; larger doses in euthyroid patients can cause serious or even life threatening toxicity. Caution with angina pectoris and elderly; use lower doses. May aggravate diabetes mellitus or insipidus and adrenal cortical insufficiency. Excessive doses may cause craniosynostosis. Extreme caution with long standing myxedema especially with cardiovascular impairment.

INTERACTIONS: May increase insulin or oral hypoglycemic requirements. Decreased absorption with cholestyramine and colestipol; space dosing by 4-5 hrs. Altered effect of oral anticoagulants; monitor PT/INR. Estrogens increase thyroxine-binding globulin; increase in thyroid dose may be needed. Serious or life-threatening side effects can occur with sympathomimetic amines. Androgens, corticosteroids, estrogens, iodine-containing preparations, and salicylates may interfere with thyroid lab tests.

PREGNANCY: Category A, caution in nursing.

TILADE RX
nedocromil sodium (King)

THERAPEUTIC CLASS: Pyranoquinoline anti-inflammatory agent
INDICATIONS: Maintenance therapy for mild to moderate asthma.

TIMENTIN

DOSAGE: *Adults:* 2 inh qid. May reduce to bid-tid once desired response is observed. *Pediatrics:* ≥6 yrs: 2 inh qid. May reduce to bid-tid once desired response is observed.

HOW SUPPLIED: MDI: 1.75mg/inh (16.2g)

WARNINGS/PRECAUTIONS: Not for treatment of acute bronchospasm or status asthmaticus. Monitor when reducing systemic or inhaled steroid therapy. Stop therapy if bronchospasm occurs.

ADVERSE REACTIONS: Unpleasant taste, nausea, vomiting, dyspepsia, abdominal pain, pharyngitis, headache, cough, rhinitis.

PREGNANCY: Category B, caution with nursing

TIMENTIN RX
ticarcillin disodium - clavulanate potassium (GlaxoSmithKline)

THERAPEUTIC CLASS: Broad-spectrum penicillin/beta-lactamase inhibitor

INDICATIONS: Treatment of lower respiratory tract, bone and joint, skin and skin structure, urinary tract (UTI), gynecologic, and intra-abdominal infections, and septicemia.

DOSAGE: *Adults:* ≥60kg: UTI/Systemic Infection: 3g-100mg (3.1g vial) IV q4-6h. Gynecologic Infections: Moderate: 200mg/kg/day ticarcillin IV given q6h. Severe: 300mg/kg/day ticarcillin IV given q4h. <60kg: Usual: 200-300mg/kg/day ticarcillin IV given q4-6h. UTI: 3g-200mg (3.2g vial) q8h. Renal Impairment (based on ticarcillin): CrCl 60-30mL/min: 2g IV q4h. CrCl 30-10mL/min: 2g IV q8h. CrCl <10mL/min: 2g IV q12h (2g IV q24h with hepatic dysfunction). Peritoneal Dialysis: 3.1g IV q12h. Hemodialysis: 2g IV q12h, and 3.1g after each dialysis. Apply reduced dosage after initial 3.1g LD is given.

Pediatrics: ≥3 months: ≥60kg: Mild to Moderate: 3g-100mg (3.1g vial) IV q6h. Severe: 3g-100mg (3.1g vial) IV q4h. <60 kg: Mild to Moderate: 50mg/kg ticarcillin IV q6h. Severe: 50mg/kg ticarcillin IV q4h. Renal Impairment (based on ticarcillin): CrCl 60-30mL/min: 2g IV q4h. CrCl 30-10mL/min: 2g IV q8h. CrCl <10mL/min: 2g IV q12h (2g IV q24h with hepatic dysfunction). Peritoneal Dialysis: 3.1g IV q12h. Hemodialysis: 2g IV q12h, and 3.1g after each dialysis. Apply reduced dosage after initial 3.1g LD is given.

HOW SUPPLIED: Inj: (Ticarcillin-Clavulanate) 3g-100mg, 3g-100mg/100mL, 30g-1g

WARNINGS/PRECAUTIONS: Prolonged use may result in overgrowth of nonsusceptible organisms. Caution with penicillin, cephalosporin, and other allergen sensitivities. Pseudomembranous colitis reported. Risk of convulsions with high doses especially with renal impairment. Monitor renal, hepatic, hematopoietic functions, and serum K+ with prolonged therapy. Caution with fluid and electrolyte imbalance; hypokalemia reported. Clotting time, platelet aggregation, and PT abnormalities may occur especially with renal impairment; discontinue therapy. Continue therapy for at least 2 days after signs/symptoms disappear. Caution in elderly patient with impaired renal function.

ADVERSE REACTIONS: Hypersensitivity reactions, headache, giddiness, taste/smell disturbances, stomatitis, flatulence, nausea, vomiting, diarrhea, hematologic disturbances, hepatic/renal function tests abnormalities, local reactions.

INTERACTIONS: May inactivate aminoglycoside if mixed together in parenteral solution. Increased serum levels and prolonged half-life with probenecid.

PREGNANCY: Category B, caution in nursing.

TINDAMAX RX
tinidazole (Presutti)

> Avoid unnecessary use. Reserve only for indicated conditions.

THERAPEUTIC CLASS: Antiprotozoal agent

INDICATIONS: Treatment of trichomoniasis caused by *Trichomonas vaginalis*, giardiasis caused by *Giardia duodenalis*, intestinal amebiasis and amebic liver abscess caused by *Entamoeba histolytica*, and bacterial vaginosis in non-pregnant women.

DOSAGE: *Adults:* Take with food. Trichomoniasis/Giardiasis: 2g single dose. Amebiasis: Intestinal: 2g qd for 3 days. Amebic Liver Abscess: 2g qd for 3-5 days. Hemodialysis: Give additional dose equivalent to one-half of recommended dose at the end of dialysis. For trichomoniasis, treat sexual partner with the same dose. Bacterial Vaginosis: 2g qd for 2 days or 1g qd for 5 days.

Pediatrics: >3 yrs: Take with food. Giardiasis: 50mg/kg single dose. Amebiasis: Intestinal: 50mg/kg qd for 3 days. Amebic Liver Abscess: 50mg/kg qd for 3-5 days. Max (for all): 2g/day. May crush tabs in cherry syrup.

HOW SUPPLIED: Tab: 250mg*, 500mg* *scored

CONTRAINDICATIONS: Treatment during 1st trimester of pregnancy.

WARNINGS/PRECAUTIONS: Seizures, peripheral neuropathy reported. Discontinue if abnormal neurological signs occur. Caution with hepatic impairment, blood dyscrasias, or CNS diseases.

ADVERSE REACTIONS: Metallic/bitter taste, nausea, anorexia.

INTERACTIONS: Avoid alcohol during and for 3 days after use and within 2 weeks of disulfiram. May potentiate oral anticoagulants. May reduce clearance of phenytoin (IV), fluorouracil. May increase levels of lithium, cyclosporine, tacrolimus, fluorouracil. Separate dosing with cholestyramine. Phenobarbital, rifampin, phenytoin, other hepatic enzyme inducers may decrease levels. Cimetidine, ketoconazole, other hepatic enzyme inhibitors may increase levels. Antagonized by oxytetracycline.

PREGNANCY: Category C, not for use in nursing.

TIROSINT
levothyroxine sodium (IBSA)

RX

THERAPEUTIC CLASS: Thyroid replacement hormone

INDICATIONS: Replacement or supplemental therapy in congenital or acquired hypothyroidism of any etiology, except transient hypothyroidism during the recovery phase of subacute thyroiditis, including primary, secondary, tertiary and subclinical hypothyroidism. Treatment or prevention of various euthyroid goiters including thyroid nodules, subacute or chronic lymphocytic throiditis (Hashimoto's thyroiditis) and multinodular goiter. Adjunct to surgery and radioiodine therapy in the management of thyrotropin-dependent well-differentiated thyroid cancer.

DOSAGE: *Adults:* Take in AM 1/2-1 hr before breakfast. Hypothyroidism: Usual: 1.7mcg/kg/day PO. Titrate: Adjust in 12.5-25mcg increments until patient is euthyroid. Elderly with Cardiac Disease: Initial: 12.5-25mcg qd PO. Titrate: May increase by 12.5-25mcg every 4-6 weeks until euthyroid. >50 yrs or <50 yrs with Underlying Cardiac Disease: Initial: 25-50mcg/day. Titrate: Gradual increments at 6-8 week intervals prn. Severe Hypothyroidism: Initial: 12.5-25mcg/day. Titrate: May increase by 25mcg/day every 2-4 weeks until TSH normalized. Pregnancy: May require increased doses. Subclinical Hypothyroidism: May require lower doses. Do not crush, cut or dissolve content in water.

Pediatrics: Take in AM 1/2-1hr before breakfast. Hypothyroidism: 0-3 months: 10-15mcg/kg/day. 3-6 months: 8-10mcg/kg/day. 6-12 months: 6-8mcg/kg/day. 6-12 yrs: 4-5mcg/kg/day. >12 yrs (growth/puberty incomplete): 2-3mcg/kg/day. >12 yrs (growth/puberty complete): 1.7mcg/kg/day. To minimize hyperactivity in older children give 1/4 of full replacement dose initially, then increase dose by same amount weekly until full replacement dose is achieved. Chronic/Severe Hypothyroidism: Initial: 25mcg/day. Titrate: Increase by 25mcg every 2-4 weeks until euthyroid. Do not crush, cut or dissolve content in water.

HOW SUPPLIED: Cap: 25mcg, 50mcg, 75mcg, 100mcg, 125mcg, 150mcg

CONTRAINDICATIONS: Untreated subclinical (suppressed serum TSH level with normal T_3 and T_4 levels) or overt thyrotoxicosis of any etiology, acute MI, uncorrected adrenal insufficiency or inability to swallow capsules.

WARNINGS/PRECAUTIONS: Do not use in treatment of obesity. Should not be used in treatment of male or female infertility unless condition is associated with hypothyroidism. Carefully titrate dose to avoid over/under treatment. Decreased bone mineral

TOBI

density with long term use. Caution with cardiovascular disease especially in elderly, adrenal insufficiency, non-toxic diffuse goiter or nodular thyroid disease and hypothalamic pituitary hormone deficiencies. Chronic autoimmune thyroiditis may occur in association with other autoimmune disorders; treat patients with concomitant adrenal insufficiency with replacement glucocorticoids before therapy. Infants with congenital hypothyroidism may be at increased risk for other congenital abnormalities.

ADVERSE REACTIONS: Hyperthyroidism (increased appetite, weight loss, heat intolerance, hyperactivity, tremors, palpitations, tachycardia, diarrhea, vomiting, hair loss), pseudotumor cerebri, craniosynostosis and premature closure of the epiphyses in children.

INTERACTIONS: Dopamine/dopamine agonists, glucocorticoids and octreotide may result in transient reduction in TSH secretion. Aminogluthetimide, amiodarone, iodide (including iodine-containing radiographic contrast agents), lithium, methimazole, propylthiouracil, sulfonamides and tolbutamide may decrease thyroid hormone secretion. Amiodarone and iodide (including iodine-containing radiographic contrast agents) may increase thyroid hormone secretion. Antacids (eg, aluminum/magnesium), hydroxides (simethicone), bile acid sequestrants (cholestyramine, colestipol), calcium carbonate, cation exchange resins (kayexalate), ferrous sulfate and sucralfate may decrease T4 absorption. Clofibrate, estrogen-containing oral contraceptives, oral estrogens, heroin/methadone, 5-fluorouracil, mitotane and tamoxifen may increase serum TBG levels. Androgens/anabolic steroids, asparaginase, glucocorticoids and slow release nicotinic acid may decrease serum TBG levels. Furosemide (>80mg IV), heparin, hydantoins, NSAIDs (eg, fenamates, phenylbutazone) and salicylates (>2g/day) may cause protein-binding site displacement. Carbamazepine, hydantoins, phenobarbital and rifampin may increase hepatic metabolism. Amiodarone, β-adrenergic antagonists (eg, propranolol >160mg/day), glucocorticoids (eg, dexamethasone ≥4mg/day) and PTU may decrease T4 5'-deiodinase activity. Sympathomimetics may increase risk of coronary insufficiency with CAD. May potentate anticoagulants. Concurrent use of tri/tetracyclic antidepressants may increase effects of both agents; SSRIs (eg, sertraline) may result in increased levothyroxine requirements. May require higher doses of antidiabetic therapy. May decrease effect of digitalis glycosides. Cytokines (interferon-α, interleukin-2) may induce hypo/hyperthyroidism. Excessive use with somatrem or somatropin may accelerate epiphyseal closure. Concurrent use with ketamine may produce HTN and tachycardia. May decrease theophylline clearance. Chloral hydrate, diazepam, ethionamide, lovastatin, metoclopramide, 6-mercaptopurine, nitroprusside, para-aminosalicylate sodium, perphenazine, resorcinol (excessive topical use) and thiazide diuretics associated with thyroid hormone and/or TSH level alterations. May reduce the uptake of radiographic agents. Soybean flour (infant formula), cotton seed meal, walnuts, and dietary fiber may bind and decrease absorption of levothyroxine from GI tract.

PREGNANCY: Category A, caution in nursing.

TOBI
tobramycin (Chiron)

RX

THERAPEUTIC CLASS: Aminoglycoside

INDICATIONS: Management of cystic fibrosis patients with *P.aeruginosa*.

DOSAGE: *Adults:* Inhale via nebulizer 300mg q12h for 28 days, then stop for 28 days. Resume therapy for next 28 day on/28 day off cycle.

Pediatrics: ≥6 yrs: Inhale via nebulizer 300mg q12h for 28 days, then stop for 28 days. Resume therapy for next 28 day on/28 day off cycle.

HOW SUPPLIED: Sol: 60mg/mL (300mg/amp)

WARNINGS/PRECAUTIONS: Caution with muscular disorders (eg, myasthenia gravis, Parkinson's disease), and renal, auditory, vestibular, or neuromuscular dysfunction. May cause hearing loss, bronchospasm. Can cause fetal harm in pregnancy. D/C if nephrotoxicity occurs until serum level <2mcg/mL.

ADVERSE REACTIONS: Voice alteration, taste perversion, tinnitus.

INTERACTIONS: Avoid neurotoxic or ototoxic drugs. Hearing loss reported with previous or concomitant systemic aminoglycosides. Avoid ethacrynic acid, furosemide, urea, and mannitol.

PREGNANCY: Category D, not for use in nursing.

TobraDex
tobramycin - dexamethasone (Alcon)

RX

THERAPEUTIC CLASS: Aminoglycoside/corticosteroid

INDICATIONS: Ocular inflammation associated with infection or risk of infection.

DOSAGE: *Adults:* (Sus) 1-2 drops q4-6h. May increase to 1-2 drops q2h for first 24-48 hrs. (Oint) Apply 1/2 inch in conjunctival sac up to tid-qid. Max: 20mL or 8g for initial RX.
Pediatrics: ≥2 yrs: (Sus) 1-2 drops q4-6h. May increase to 1-2 drops q2h for first 24-48 hrs. (Oint) Apply 1/2 inch in conjunctival sac up to tid-qid. Max: 20mL or 8g for initial RX.

HOW SUPPLIED: Oint: (Tobramycin-Dexamethasone) 0.3-0.1% (3.5g); Sus: 0.3-0.1% (2.5mL, 5mL, 10mL)

CONTRAINDICATIONS: Viral diseases of the cornea and conjunctiva including epithelial herpes simplex keratitis, vaccinia, and varicella. Mycobacterial infection and fungal diseases of the eye.

WARNINGS/PRECAUTIONS: Not for injection into the eye. Prolonged use may result in glaucoma, optic nerve damage, visual acuity and fields of vision defects, cataracts, secondary ocular infections (eg, fungal infections).

ADVERSE REACTIONS: Conjunctival erythema, hypersensitivity, lid itching and swelling, secondary infection.

PREGNANCY: Category C, caution in nursing.

Tobramycin Sulfate
tobramycin sulfate (Various)

RX

> Potential ototoxicity, nephrotoxicity, and neurotoxicity. Monitor peak and trough serum levels to avoid toxicity. Avoid prolonged serum levels >12mcg/mL. Rising trough levels (>2mcg/mL) may indicate tissue accumulation. Tissue accumulation, excessive peak levels, advanced age, and cumulative dose may contribute to ototoxicity and nephrotoxicity. Monitor urine, BUN, serum creatinine, and CrCl periodically. Obtain serial audiograms. D/C or adjust dose with renal, vestibular, or auditory dysfunction. Caution in premature and neonatal infants, advanced age, and dehydration. Avoid other neurotoxic or nephrotoxic agents, particularly other aminoglycosides, cephaloridine, viomycin, polymyxin B, colistin, cisplatin, and vancomycin. Avoid potent diuretics (eg, ethacrynic acid, furosemide). Risk of fetal harm during pregnancy.

THERAPEUTIC CLASS: Aminoglycoside

INDICATIONS: Treatment of serious lower respiratory tract, CNS (eg, meningitis), intra-abdominal, bone, skin and skin structure, and complicated/recurrent urinary tract infections, and septicemia.

DOSAGE: *Adults:* IM/IV: Serious Infections: 3mg/kg/day given q8h. Life-Threatening Infections: Up to 5mg/kg/day given tid-qid. Reduce to 3mg/kg/day as soon as clinically indicated. Max: 5mg/kg/day unless serum levels monitored. Treat for 7-10 days; may need longer course in difficult and complicated infections. Severe Cystic Fibrosis: Initial: 10mg/kg/day given qid. Measure levels to determine subsequent doses. Renal Impairment: LD: 1mg/kg, followed by reduced doses given q8h or normal doses given at prolonged intervals based on either CrCl or serum creatinine. Do not use either method during dialysis. Obese Patients: Calculate dose based on estimated lean body weight plus 40% of the excess as the basic weight on which to figure mg/kg. ADD-Vantage vials are not for IM use.
Pediatrics: >1 week: IM/IV: 6-7.5mg/kg/day given tid-qid (eg, 2-2.5mg/kg q8h or 1.5-1.89mg/kg q6h). ≤1 week: Up to 2mg/kg q12h. Treat for 7-10 days; may need longer course in difficult and complicated infections. Severe Cystic Fibrosis: Initial: 10mg/kg/day given qid. Measure levels to determine subsequent doses. Renal Impairment: LD: 1mg/kg, followed by reduced doses given q8h or normal doses given at prolonged intervals based on either CrCl or serum creatinine. Do not use either method during

TOFRANIL

dialysis. Obese Patients: Calculate dose based on estimated lean body weight plus 40% of the excess as the basic weight on which to figure mg/kg. ADD-Vantage vials are not for IM use.

HOW SUPPLIED: Inj: 10mg/mL, 40mg/mL, 1.2g

CONTRAINDICATIONS: History of serious toxic reactions to aminoglycosides.

WARNINGS/PRECAUTIONS: Increased risk of ototoxicity, nephrotoxicity, and neurotoxicity if treatment >10 days. Contains sodium bisulfite. D/C if allergic reaction occurs. Monitor serum calcium, magnesium, and sodium. For peak levels, measure about 30 minutes after IV infusion or 1 hr after IM injection. For trough levels, measure at 8 hrs or just before next dose. Prolonged or secondary apnea may occur with massive transfusions of citrated blood. Caution with muscular disorders (eg, myasthenia gravis, parkinsonism). Increased risk of neurotoxicity and nephrotoxicity after absorption from body surfaces with local irrigation or application. Not for intraocular and/or subconjunctival use. Overgrowth of nonsusceptible organisms may occur.

ADVERSE REACTIONS: Neurotoxicity (eg, dizziness, tinnitus, hearing loss, numbness, skin tingling, muscle twitching, convulsions), nephrotoxicity (eg, rising BUN/nonprotein nitrogen/serum creatinine, oliguria, cylindruria, increased proteinuria), blood dyscrasias, fever, rash, exfoliative dermatitis, urticaria, nausea, vomiting, diarrhea, headache, lethargy, injection site pain, confusion, disorientation, increased serum transaminases.

INTERACTIONS: Increased nephrotoxicity with cephalosporins. Do not premix with other drugs; administer separately. Possibility of prolonged or secondary apnea in anesthetized patients receiving neuromuscular blockers (eg, succinylcholine, tubocurarine, decamethonium). See Black Box Warning.

PREGNANCY: Category D, safety not known in nursing.

TOFRANIL RX
imipramine HCl (Mallinckrodt)

> Antidepressants increased the risk of suicidal thinking and behavior (suicidality) in short-term studies in children and adolescents with Major Depressive Disorder (MDD) and other psychiatric disorders. Imipramine HCl is not approved for use in pediatric patients except for patients with nocturnal enuresis.

THERAPEUTIC CLASS: Tricyclic antidepressant

INDICATIONS: Treatment of depression. Temporary adjunct in childhood enuresis in ≥6 years of age.

DOSAGE: *Adults:* Depression: Initial: (Inpatient) 100mg/day in divided doses. Titrate: Increase to 200mg/day; up to 250-300mg/day after 2 weeks if needed. (Outpatient) 75mg/day. Titrate: Increase to 150mg/day. Maint: 50-150mg/day. Max: 200mg/day. Elderly/Adolescents: Initial: 30-40mg/day. Max: 100mg/day.

Pediatrics: Depression: Adolescents: Initial: 30-40mg/day. Max: 100mg/day. Enuresis: ≥6 years old: Initial: 25mg/day 1 hour before bedtime. Titrate: 6-12 yrs: If inadequate response in 1 week, increase to 50mg before bedtime. ≥12 yrs: Increase to 75mg before bedtime after 1 week if needed. Max: 2.5mg/kg/day.

HOW SUPPLIED: Tab: 10mg, 25mg, 50mg

CONTRAINDICATIONS: Within 14 days of MAOI therapy, or during acute recovery period following MI.

WARNINGS/PRECAUTIONS: Caution with elderly, serious depression, cardiovascular disease, hyperthyroidism, urinary retention, narrow-angle glaucoma, increased IOP, seizure disorders, renal and hepatic impairment. May activate psychosis in schizophrenia; reduce dose. Limit electroshock therapy. May alter blood glucose levels. Photosensitivity reported. Discontinue prior to elective surgery, or with hypomanic or manic episodes. Discontinue with pathological neutrophil depression.

ADVERSE REACTIONS: Orthostatic hypotension, HTN, confusion, hallucinations, numbness, tremors, dry mouth, urticaria, nausea, vomiting, diarrhea, gynecomastia (male), breast enlargement (female), galactorrhea.

INTERACTIONS: See Contraindications. Increased levels with methylphenidate, CYP2D6 inhibitors (eg, quinidine, cimetidine, SSRIs) and enzyme substrates (eg, phenothiazines, other antidepressants, propafenone, flecainide). Wait 5 weeks after discontinuing SSRIs before initiating TCAs. Decreased levels with enzyme inducers (eg, barbiturates, phenytoin). Blocks effects of clonidine, guanethidine. Additive effects with anticholinergics,

CNS depressants, alcohol. Caution with drugs that lower BP and thyroid drugs. Paralytic ileus with anticholinergics. Avoid preparations that contain a sympathomimetic amine (eg, epinephrine, norepinephrine); may potentiate catecholamine effect.

PREGNANCY: Safety in pregnancy not known; not for use in nursing.

TOFRANIL-PM
imipramine pamoate (Mallinckrodt)

RX

> Antidepressants increased the risk of suicidal thinking and behavior (suicidality) in short-term studies in children and adolescents with Major Depressive Disorder (MDD) and other psychiatric disorders. Imipramine is not approved for use in pediatric patients.

THERAPEUTIC CLASS: Tricyclic antidepressant

INDICATIONS: Treatment of depression.

DOSAGE: *Adults:* (Inpatient) Initial: 100-150mg/day. Titrate: May increase to 200mg/day. After 2 weeks may increase up to 250-300mg/day if needed. (Outpatient) Initial: 75mg/day. Titrate: May increase to 150mg/day. Max: 200mg/day. (Inpatient/Outpatient) Maint: Following remission, maintain at lowest possible dose. Usual: 75-150mg/day. Elderly/Adolescents: Initiate with Tofranil 25-50mg/day. Switch to Tofranil-PM with doses ≥75mg. Max: 100mg/day.
Pediatrics: Adolescents: Initiate with Tofranil 25-50mg/day. Switch to Tofranil-PM with doses ≥75mg. Max: 100mg/day.

HOW SUPPLIED: Cap: 75mg, 100mg, 125mg, 150mg

CONTRAINDICATIONS: Within 14 days of MAOI therapy or during acute recovery period following MI.

WARNINGS/PRECAUTIONS: Caution with elderly, serious depression, cardiovascular disease, hyperthyroidism, urinary retention, narrow-angle glaucoma, increased IOP, seizure disorders, renal and hepatic impairment. May activate psychosis in schizophrenia; reduce dose. Limit electroshock therapy. May alter blood glucose levels. Photosensitivity reported. Discontinue prior to elective surgery, or with hypomanic or manic episodes. Discontinue with pathological neutrophil depression.

ADVERSE REACTIONS: Orthostatic hypotension, HTN, confusion, hallucinations, numbness, tremors, dry mouth, urticaria, nausea, vomiting, diarrhea, gynecomastia (male), breast enlargement (female), galactorrhea.

INTERACTIONS: See Contraindications. Increased levels with methylphenidate, CYP2D6 inhibitors (eg, quinidine, cimetidine, SSRIs) and enzyme substrates (eg, phenothiazines, other antidepressants, propafenone, flecainide). Wait 5 weeks after discontinuing SSRIs before initiating TCAs. Decreased levels with enzyme inducers (eg, barbiturates, phenytoin). Blocks effects of clonidine, guanethidine. Additive effects with anticholinergics, CNS depressants, alcohol. Caution with drugs that lower BP and thyroid drugs. Paralytic ileus with anticholinergics. Avoid preparations that contain a sympathomimetic amine (eg, epinephrine, norepinephrine); may potentiate catecholamine effect.

PREGNANCY: Safety in pregnancy not known; not for use in nursing.

TOLMETIN
tolmetin sodium (Various)

RX

> NSAIDs may cause an increased risk of serious cardiovascular thrombotic events, MI, stroke, and serious GI adverse events including bleeding, ulceration and perforation of the stomach or intestines. Contraindicated for the treatment of peri-operative pain in the setting of coronary artery bypass graft (CABG) surgery.

OTHER BRAND NAME: Tolectin (Ortho-McNeil)

THERAPEUTIC CLASS: NSAID

INDICATIONS: Rheumatoid arthritis (RA). Osteoarthritis (OA). Juvenile rheumatoid arthritis (JRA). Fever. Relief of mild-to-moderate pain.

DOSAGE: *Adults:* OA/RA: Initial: 400mg tid. Usual: 200-600mg tid. Max: 1800mg/day. Take with antacids other than sodium bicarbonate if GI upset occurs.

TOPAMAX

Pediatrics: JRA: ≥2 yrs: Initial: 20mg/kg/day given tid-qid. Usual: 15-30mg/kg/day. Max: 30mg/kg/day. Take with antacids other than sodium bicarbonate if GI upset occurs.

HOW SUPPLIED: Cap: (DS) 400mg; Tab: 200mg*, 600mg *scored

CONTRAINDICATIONS: ASA or other NSAID allergy that precipitates asthma, rhinitis, urticaria, or allergic-type reactions. Treatment of peri-operative pain in the setting of CABG surgery.

WARNINGS/PRECAUTIONS: May cause adverse ocular events. Prolongs bleeding time. Risk of renal toxicity with heart failure, liver dysfunction, and elderly. Caution with compromised cardiac function, HTN, or other conditions predisposing to fluid retention. Borderline LFT elevations may occur. Decreased bioavailability with milk or food. Can cause serious skin adverse reactions such as exfoliative dermatitis, SJS, and TEN, which can be fatal. Avoid with aspirin-sensitive asthma and caution with preexisting asthma. Cannot be expected to substitute for corticosteroids or to treat corticosteroid insufficiency. Notable elevations of ALT or AST have been reported. Rare cases of severe hepatic reactions, including jaundice and fatal fulminant hepatitis, liver necrosis, and hepatic failure. Patients on long term treatment should have Hgb or Hct checked if exhibit signs or symptoms of anemia.

ADVERSE REACTIONS: Dyspepsia, GI distress, diarrhea, flatulence, vomiting, headache, asthenia, elevated blood pressure, dizziness, edema.

INTERACTIONS: Increased PT and bleeding with warfarin. May enhance methotrexate toxicity. May diminish the antihypertensive effect of ACEIs. Concomitant administration with aspirin is not recommended; potential for increased adverse effects. Can reduce the natriuretic effect of furosemide and thiazides. Can produce an elevation of plasma lithium levels and a reduction in renal lithium clearance.

PREGNANCY: Category C, not for use in nursing.

TOPAMAX   RX
topiramate (Ortho-McNeil)

THERAPEUTIC CLASS: Sulfamate-substituted monosaccharide antiepileptic

INDICATIONS: Monotherapy therapy in patients 10 yrs of age and older with partial onset or primary generalized tonic-clonic seizures. Adjunct therapy in patients 2-16 yrs of age and older with partial onset seizures, primary generalized tonic-clonic seizures, and seizures associated with Lennox-Gastaut syndrome. Migraine prophylaxis in adults.

DOSAGE: *Adults:* Seizures: Monotherapy: Initial: 25mg qam and qpm for one week. Titrate: Increase am and pm dose by 25mg every week until 200mg/day, then increase by 50mg every week until 400mg/day. Adjunct Therapy: ≥17 yrs: Initial: 25-50mg/day. Titrate: Increase by 25-50mg/week. Usual: Partial: 100-200mg bid. Tonic-Clonic: 200mg bid. Max: 1600mg/day. Migraine Prophylaxis: Titrate: Week 1: 25mg qpm. Week 2: 25mg bid. Week 3: 25mg qam and 50mg qpm. Week 4: 50mg bid. Usual: 50mg bid. Renal Dysfunction: 50% of usual dose. Swallow caps whole or sprinkle over food.

Pediatrics: Seizures: Monotherapy: ≥10 yrs: Initial: 25mg qam and qpm for one week. Titrate: Increase am and pm dose by 25mg every week until 200mg/day, then increase by 50mg every week until 400mg/day. Adjunct Therapy: 2-16 yrs: Initial: 1-3mg/kg nightly for 1 week. Titrate: Increase by 1-3mg/kg/day every 1-2 weeks. Usual: 2.5-4.5mg/kg bid. Swallow caps whole or sprinkle over food.

HOW SUPPLIED: Cap: 15mg, 25mg; Tab: 25mg, 50mg, 100mg, 200mg

WARNINGS/PRECAUTIONS: Hyperchloremic, non-anion gap, metabolic acidosis reported; obtain baseline and periodic serum bicarbonate levels. Withdraw gradually. Psychomotor slowing, difficulty with concentration, speech/language problems, paresthesia, acute myopia with secondary angle closure glaucoma, oligohidrosis, hyperthermia, and dose related depression or mood problems reported. May cause hyperammonemia and encephalopathy if used concomitantly with valproic acid. Risk of kidney stones; maintain adequate fluid intake. Caution with renal or hepatic dysfunction.

ADVERSE REACTIONS: Somnolence, fatigue, dizziness, ataxia, speech disorders, psychomotor slowing, abnormal vision, memory difficulty, paresthesia, diplopia, depression, anorexia, anxiety, mood problems, pancreatitis, hepatic failure.

INTERACTIONS: Phenytoin, carbamazepine, valproic acid decrease levels. Increases phenytoin, decreases valproic acid levels. May decrease AUC of digoxin. May potentiate CNS depression with alcohol, other CNS depressants. Increased risk of kidney stones with carbonic anhydrase inhibitors. May increase metformin levels; monitor diabetics regularly.

PREGNANCY: Category C, caution in nursing.

TOPICORT
desoximetasone (Taro)

RX

OTHER BRAND NAME: Topicort LP (Taro)

THERAPEUTIC CLASS: Corticosteroid

INDICATIONS: Corticosteroid responsive dermatoses.

DOSAGE: *Adults:* Apply bid.

Pediatrics: (Cre, Gel) Apply bid. ≥10 yrs: (Oint) Apply bid.

HOW SUPPLIED: Cre: (LP) 0.05% (15g, 60g), 0.25% (15g, 60g); Gel: 0.05% (15g, 60g); Oint: 0.25% (15g, 60g)

WARNINGS/PRECAUTIONS: May produce reversible HPA axis suppression, manifestations of Cushing's syndrome, hyperglycemia, and glucosuria. Caution when applied to large surface areas or under occlusive dressings. Use appropriate antifungal or antibacterial agent with dermatological infections; d/c if infection does not clear. Peds may be more susceptible to systemic toxicity. Avoid eyes. D/C if irritation occurs.

ADVERSE REACTIONS: Burning, itching, irritation, dryness, folliculitis, hypertrichosis, acneiform eruptions, hypopigmentation, perioral dermatitis, allergic contact dermatitis, skin maceration, secondary infection, skin atrophy, striae, miliaria.

PREGNANCY: Category C, caution in nursing.

TRACLEER
bosentan (Actelion)

RX

> Potential liver injury; monitor LFTs before therapy, then monthly. Contraindicated in pregnancy; obtain monthly pregnancy tests. Prescribe through Tracleer Access Program.

THERAPEUTIC CLASS: Endothelin receptor antagonist

INDICATIONS: Treatment of pulmonary arterial hypertension in patients with WHO Class III or IV symptoms, to improve exercise ability and decrease rate of clinical worsening.

DOSAGE: *Adults:* Initial: 62.5mg bid. Titrate/Maint: Increase to 125mg bid after 4 weeks. Low Weight (<40kg): Initial/Maint: 62.5mg bid. Adjust if Develop LFT Abnormality: >3 to ≤5X ULN: Reconfirm LFTs. Reduce dose or interrupt therapy. Monitor LFTs every 2 weeks. If LFTs return to pre-treatment levels, reintroduce or continue therapy. >5 to ≤8X ULN: Reconfirm LFTs. Stop treatment and monitor LFTs every 2 weeks. If LFTs return to pre-treatment values, may reintroduce therapy. >8X ULN: Stop treatment, do not reintroduce.

Pediatrics: >12 yrs; <40kg: Initial/Maint: 62.5mg bid.

HOW SUPPLIED: Tab: 62.5mg, 125mg

CONTRAINDICATIONS: Pregnancy, cyclosporine A, glyburide.

WARNINGS/PRECAUTIONS: May decrease Hgb and Hct; monitor 1 and 3 months after initiation, then every 3 months. Caution in elderly or mild hepatic impairment. Avoid with moderate to severe hepatic impairment, or LFTs >3X ULN. Discontinue gradually. Patients with severe chronic heart failure had an increased incidence of hospitalization for CHF associated with weight gain and increased leg edema during the first 4-8 weeks of treatment with tracleer. Should considered intervention with a diuretic, fluid management, or hospitalization for decompensating heart failure. If the signs of pulmonary edema occur when tracleer is administered the possibility of associated Pulmonary Veno-Occlusive Disease should be considered. Discontinue tracleer.

ADVERSE REACTIONS: Headache, nasopharyngitis, flushing, hepatic dysfunction, lower limb edema, hypotension, palpitations, dyspepsia, edema, fatigue, pruritus, thrombocytopenia.

TRACRIUM

INTERACTIONS: Do not rely on hormonal contraception alone. Cyclosporine A increases levels. Glyburide increases risk of elevated LFTs. May reduce statin efficacy; monitor cholesterol levels. May decrease levels of drugs metabolized by CYP450 3A4 (eg, statins) and 2C9. CYP450 3A4 inhibitors (eg, ketoconazole) increase levels.
PREGNANCY: Category X, not for use in nursing.

TRACRIUM RX
atracurium besylate (Hospira)

THERAPEUTIC CLASS: Skeletal muscle relaxant (nondepolarizing)

INDICATIONS: Adjunct to general anesthesia to facilitate endotracheal intubation and to provide skeletal muscle relaxation during surgery or mechanical ventilation.

DOSAGE: *Adults:* Initial: 0.4-0.5mg/kg IV bolus. Prolonged Procedure: Maint: 0.08-0.1mg/kg at regular intervals to meet needs; give after 1st dose. Operating Room Infusion: Initial: 0.3-0.5mg/kg IV bolus. Maint: 9-10mcg/kg/min initial infusion to counteract recovery from bolus followed by 5-9mcg/kg/min. ICU: 11-13mcg/kg/min IV. Isoflurane/Enflurane at Steady State: Reduce dose by 1/3. Significant Cardiovascular Disease/Histamine Release Sensitive Patients: Initial: 0.3-0.4mg/kg IV slowly or in divided doses. Following Succinylcholine: Initial: 0.3-0.4mg/kg IV.
Pediatrics: >2 yrs: Initial: 0.4-0.5mg/kg IV bolus. Prolonged Procedure: Maint: 0.08-0.1mg/kg at regular intervals to meet needs; give after 1st dose. Operating Room Infusion: Initial: 0.3-0.5mg/kg IV bolus. Maint: 9-10mcg/kg/min initial infusion to counteract recovery from bolus followed by 5-9mcg/kg/min. Isoflurane/Enflurane at Steady State: Reduce dose by 1/3. 1 month-2 yrs (under halothane): Initial: 0.3-0.4mg/kg IV bolus. Maint: Slightly greater frequency than adults. ≥1 month: Significant Cardiovascular Disease/Histamine Release Sensitive Patients: Initial: 0.3-0.4mg/kg IV slowly or in divided doses.

HOW SUPPLIED: Inj: 10mg/mL

WARNINGS/PRECAUTIONS: Avoid IM administration or administration before unconsciousness has been induced. Use with adequate anesthesia. The 10mL vial contains benzyl alcohol. May release histamines; caution in those where substantial histamine release would be hazardous (eg, severe cardiovascular disease) or if at a greater risk of histamine release (eg, anaphylactoid reactions, asthma). Use peripheral nerve stimulators to assess neuromuscular block in myasthenia gravis, Eaton-Lambert syndrome, other neuromuscular diseases, severe electrolyte disorders, elderly, carcinomatosis. Malignant hyperthermia (rare) reported. Resistance may develop in burn patients; increase dose. Monitor neuromuscular transmission of ICU patients continuously with a nerve stimulator.

ADVERSE REACTIONS: Allergic reactions, inadequate/prolonged block, hypotension, vasodilation (flushing), tachycardia, bradycardia, dyspnea, bronchospasm, laryngospasm, rash, urticaria, injection site pain.

INTERACTIONS: Enhanced neuromuscular blocking action with enflurane, isoflurane, halothane, certain antibiotics (eg, aminoglycosides, polymyxins), lithium, magnesium salts, procainamide, quinidine. Possible synergistic or antagonistic effects with other muscle relaxants. Prior succinylcholine may quicken onset and increase depth of neuromuscular block. Do not mix with alkaline solutions.

PREGNANCY: Category C, caution in nursing.

TRANXENE-SD CIV
clorazepate dipotassium (Ovation)

OTHER BRAND NAMES: Tranxene T-Tab (Ovation) - Tranxene-SD Half Strength (Ovation)

THERAPEUTIC CLASS: Benzodiazepine

INDICATIONS: Management of anxiety disorders. Adjunct therapy for partial seizures. Symptomatic relief of acute alcohol withdrawal.

DOSAGE: *Adults:* Anxiety: Initial: (Tab) 15mg qhs. Usual: 30mg/day in divided doses. Max: 60mg/day. Elderly/Debilitated: Initial: 7.5-15mg/day. (Tab, Extended-Release) 22.5mg q24h, (may substitute for 7.5mg tid) or 11.25mg q24h (may substitute for 3.75mg tid). Do not use Extended-Release for initial therapy. Alcohol Withdrawal: Day 1: (Tab)

30mg, then 30-60mg/day. Day 2: 45-90mg/day. Day 3: 22.5-45mg/day. Day 4: 15-30mg. Give in divided doses. Reduce dose and continue with 7.5-15mg/day; discontinue when stable. Max: 90mg/day. Antiepileptic Adjunct: Initial: (Tab) 7.5mg tid. Titrate: Increase by no more than 7.5mg/week. Max: 90mg/day.

Pediatrics: >9 yrs: Anxiety: Initial: (Tab) 15mg qhs. Usual: 30mg/day in divided doses. Max: 60mg/day. (Tab, Extended-Release) 22.5mg q24h, (may substitute for 7.5mg tid) or 11.25mg q24h (may substitute for 3.75mg tid). Do not use Extended-Release for initial therapy. >12 yrs: Antiepileptic Adjunct: Initial: (Tab) 7.5mg tid. Titrate: Increase by no more than 7.5mg/week. Max: 90mg/day. 9-12 yrs: Initial: 7.5mg bid. Titrate: Increase by no more than 7.5mg/week. Max: 60mg/day.

HOW SUPPLIED: Tab: (Tranxene T-Tab) 3.75mg*, 7.5mg*, 15mg*; Tab, Extended Release: (Tranxene-SD) 22.5mg, (Tranxene-SD Half Strength) 11.25mg *scored

CONTRAINDICATIONS: Acute narrow-angle glaucoma.

WARNINGS/PRECAUTIONS: Avoid with depressive neuroses or psychotic reactions. Withdrawal symptoms with abrupt withdrawal; taper gradually. Caution with known drug dependency, renal/hepatic impairment. Suicidal tendencies reported; give lowest effective dose. Monitor LFTs and blood counts periodically with long-term therapy. Use lowest effective dose in elderly.

ADVERSE REACTIONS: Drowsiness, dizziness, GI complaints, nervousness, blurred vision, dry mouth, headache, mental confusion.

INTERACTIONS: Additive CNS depression with CNS depressants, alcohol. Potentiated by barbiturates, narcotics, phenothiazines, MAOIs, other antidepressants. Increased sedation with hypnotics.

PREGNANCY: Safety in pregnancy not known, not for use in nursing.

TRAUMEEL
botanical/mineral substances (Heel)   RX

THERAPEUTIC CLASS: Homeopathic Complex

INDICATIONS: Treatment of symptoms associated with inflammatory, exudative, and degenerative processes due to acute trauma (eg, contusions, lacerations, fractures, sprains, post-op wounds), repetitive or overuse injuries (eg, tendonitis, bursitis, epicondylitis), and for minor aches and pains associated with such conditions. Treatment of minor aches and pains associated with backache, muscular aches, and minor pain from rheumatoid arthritis, osteoarthritis, gouty arthritis, and anklyosing spondylitis.

DOSAGE: *Adults:* 1 amp qd for acute disorders or 1-2 amps 1-3 times weekly. May administer IV, IM, SQ, or intradermally.

Pediatrics: >6 yrs: 1 amp qd for acute disorder or 1-2 amps 1-3 times weekly. 2-6 yrs: Half the adult dosage. May administer IV, IM, SQ, or intradermally.

HOW SUPPLIED: Inj: 2mL amps (10^5)

WARNINGS/PRECAUTIONS: Carefully re-evaluate if pain persists or worsens, if new symptoms occur, or if redness or swelling is present.

ADVERSE REACTIONS: Allergic reactions, anaphylactic reactions.

PREGNANCY: Category C, caution in nursing.

TRAUMEEL TOPICAL
botanical/mineral substances (Heel)   OTC

THERAPEUTIC CLASS: Homeopathic Complex

INDICATIONS: Treatment of symptoms associated with inflammatory, exudative, and degenerative processes due to acute trauma (eg, contusions, lacerations, fractures, sprains, post-op wounds), repetitive or overuse injuries (eg, tendonitis, bursitis, epicondylitis), and for minor aches and pains associated with such conditions. Treatment of minor aches and pains associated with backache, muscular aches, and minor pain from rheumatoid arthritis, osteoarthritis, gouty arthritis, and anklyosing spondylitis.

TRECATOR

DOSAGE: *Adults:* Individualize dose. Oint: Apply to affected area(s) morning and evening or more often if needed. Max: 5x/day. May also apply oint dressing. Gel: Apply to affected area(s) 1-2x/day or more often if needed. Max: 5x/day. May apply using mild compression and/or occlusive bandaging.

Pediatrics: Individualize dose. Oint: Apply to affected area(s) morning and evening or more often if needed. Max: 5x/day. May also apply oint dressing. Gel: Apply to affected area(s) 1-2x/day or more often if needed. Max: 5x/day. May apply using mild compression and/or occlusive bandaging.

HOW SUPPLIED: Gel (50g, 250g); Oint (50g, 100g)

WARNINGS/PRECAUTIONS: Avoid administration for pain for >10 days for adults or 5 days for children. Persistent or worsening pain, occurrence of new symptoms, or presence of redness or swelling may signify a serious condition. Avoid applying over larger areas. Only apply to unbroken skin. Ointment contains cetylstearyl alcohol which may cause local skin reactions (eg, contact dermatitis).

ADVERSE REACTIONS: Hypersensitivity reactions, local allergic reactions (cutaneous inflammation, redness, swelling, pruritus).

PREGNANCY: Safety in pregnancy not known, caution in nursing.

TRECATOR
ethionamide (Wyeth)
RX

THERAPEUTIC CLASS: Peptide synthesis inhibitor

INDICATIONS: Treatment of active tuberculosis in patients with *M.tuberculosis* resistant to isoniazid or rifampin, or where there is intolerance to other drugs.

DOSAGE: *Adults:* 15-20mg/kg qd with food. May give in divided doses with poor GI tolerance. Max: 1g/day. Alternate Regimen: Initial: 250mg qd then titrate gradually to optimal doses as tolerated, or 250mg qd for 1-2 days, then 250mg bid for 1-2 days, then 1g/day in 3-4 divided doses. Continue therapy until bacteriological conversion has become permanent and maximal clinical improvement occurred.

Pediatrics: ≥12 yrs: 10-20 mg/kg/day in divided doses given bid or tid with food, or 15mg/kg/day as single dose. Continue therapy until bacteriological conversion has become permanent and maximal clinical improvement occurred.

HOW SUPPLIED: Tab: 250mg

CONTRAINDICATIONS: Severe hepatic impairment.

WARNINGS/PRECAUTIONS: Rapid development of resistance if used alone; should be used with at least 1 or 2 other drugs. Perform ophthalmologic exams before and periodically during therapy. Measure serum transaminases prior to initiation and monthly thereafter. Risk of hypoglycemia in diabetics; monitor blood glucose prior to initiation then periodically. Hypothroidism reported; monitor TFTs.

ADVERSE REACTIONS: Nausea, vomiting, diarrhea, abdominal pain, excessive salivation, metallic taste, stomatitis, anorexia, psychotic disturbances, drowsiness, dizziness, hypersensitivity reactions, increase in serum bilirubin, SGOT or SGPT.

INTERACTIONS: Discontinue all antituberculous medication with elevated serum transaminases until resolved; reintroduce sequentially to determine which drug is responsible. May raise isoniazid levels. May potentiate adverse effects of other antituberculous drugs. Convulsions reported with cycloserine. Risk of psychotic reactions with excessive ethanol ingestion. Give with pyridoxine.

PREGNANCY: Category C, not for use in nursing.

TRIFLUOPERAZINE HCL
trifluoperazine HCl (Various)
RX

THERAPEUTIC CLASS: Piperazine phenothiazine

INDICATIONS: Management of psychotic disorders (eg, schizophrenia) and for short-treatment of generalized non-psychotic anxiety (not as initial therapy).

DOSAGE: *Adults:* Psychotic Disorders: Initial: 2-5mg PO bid. Usual: 15-20mg/day. Max: 40mg/day or more if needed. Non-Psychotic Anxiety: 1-2mg bid. Max: 6mg/day or >12 weeks. Elderly: Lower dose and increase more gradually.

Pediatrics: Psychotic Disorders: 6-12 yrs: Initial: 1mg PO qd-bid. Titrate: Increase gradually until symptoms controlled. Usual: 15mg/day.

HOW SUPPLIED: Tab: 1mg, 2mg, 5mg, 10mg

CONTRAINDICATIONS: Comatose or greatly depressed states due to CNS depressants, bone marrow depression, blood dyscrasias, hepatic damage.

WARNINGS/PRECAUTIONS: May develop tardive dyskinesia, neuroleptic malignant syndrome. May elevate prolactin levels; caution with prolactin-dependent tumors. May mask drug toxicity and drug overdose due to antiemetic effects. May obscure diagnosis and treatment of intestinal obstruction, brain tumor, and Reye's syndrome. Risk of hypotension; avoid large doses and IV use with cardiovascular disease. Caution with glaucoma, angina, and elderly. May cause retinopathy; discontinue if retinal changes occur. Evaluate therapy periodically with prolonged use. May interfere with thermoregulatory mechanism; caution in extreme heat. Solution contains sodium bisulfite. Jaundice, hepatic damage reported. May cause false-positive PKU test.

ADVERSE REACTIONS: EPS, motor restlessness, dystonias, pseudo-parkinsonism, tardive dyskinesia, convulsions, dryness of mouth, headache, nausea, blood dyscrasias.

INTERACTIONS: Additive CNS depression with other CNS depressants (eg, sedatives, narcotics, anesthetics, tranquilizers, alcohol). May decrease effects of guanethidine, oral anticoagulants. Propranolol may increase levels of both drugs. Thiazide diuretics may potentiate orthostatic hypotension. May lower seizure threshold; adjust anticonvulsants. May cause phenytoin toxicity. May potentiate α-adrenergic blockade. Risk of encephalopathic syndrome with lithium. Avoid with Amipaque®; discontinue 48 hrs before myelography, resume 24 hrs post procedure.

PREGNANCY: Safety in pregnancy not known. Not for use in nursing.

TRILEPTAL
oxcarbazepine (Novartis)

RX

THERAPEUTIC CLASS: Dibenzazepine

INDICATIONS: Monotherapy or adjunct therapy in adults and children 4-16 yrs with partial seizures.

DOSAGE: *Adults:* Monotherapy: Initial: 300mg bid. Titrate: Increase by 300mg/day every 3rd day. Maint: 1200mg/day. Adjunct Therapy: Initial: 300mg bid. Titrate: Increase weekly by a maximum of 600mg/day. Maint: 600mg bid. Conversion to Monotherapy: Initial: 300mg bid while reducing other AEDs. Titrate: Increase weekly by 600mg/day. Withdraw other AEDs over 3-6 weeks. Maint: 2400mg/day. Renal Impairment: CrCl <30mL/min: Initial: 300mg qd. Titrate: Increase gradually.

Pediatrics: 4-16yrs: Monotherapy: Initial: 4-5mg/kg bid. Titrate: Increase by 5mg/kg/day every 3rd day. Maint (mg/day): 20kg: Initial: 600mg. Max: 900mg. 25-30kg: Initial: 900mg. Max: 1200mg. 35-40kg: Initial: 900mg. Max: 1500mg. 45kg: Initial: 1200mg. Max: 1500mg. 50-55kg: Initial: 1200mg. Max: 1800mg. 60-65kg: Initial: 1200mg. Max: 2100mg. 70kg: Initial: 1500mg. Max: 2100mg. Adjunct Therapy: Initial: 4-5mg/kg bid. Max: 600mg/day. Titrate: Increase over 2 weeks. Maint (mg/day): 20-29kg: 900mg. 29.1-39kg: 1200mg. >39kg: 1800mg. Conversion to Monotherapy: Initial: 4-5mg/kg bid while reducing other AEDs. Titrate: Increase weekly by max of 10mg/kg/day to target dose. Withdraw other AEDs over 3-6 weeks. Renal Impairment: CrCl <30mL/min: Initial: 300mg qd. Titrate: Increase gradually.

HOW SUPPLIED: Sus: 300mg/5mL (250mL); Tab: 150mg*, 300mg*, 600mg* *scored

WARNINGS/PRECAUTIONS: Risk of hyponatremia. Cross sensitivity with carbamazepine. Avoid abrupt withdrawal. Adjust dose in renal impairment. Reports of serious dermatologic reactions (eg, Stevens-Johnson syndrome, toxic epidermal necrolysis). CNS effects reported (eg, psychomotor slowing, concentration difficulty, speech or language problems, somnolence or fatigue, coordination abnormalities). Reports of multi-organ hypersensitivity reactions in close temporal association to initiation of therapy.

ADVERSE REACTIONS: Dizziness, somnolence, diplopia, nausea, vomiting, asthenia, nystagmus, ataxia, abnormal vision, tremor, abnormal gait, headache.

TRILISATE

INTERACTIONS: Additive sedative effect with alcohol. Verapamil, carbamazepine, phenytoin, phenobarbital, valproic acid may decrease levels. Decreased plasma levels of felodipine and oral contraceptives. Increased plasma levels of phenytoin, phenobarbital.

PREGNANCY: Category C, not for use in nursing.

TRILISATE   RX
choline magnesium trisalicylate (Purdue Frederick)

THERAPEUTIC CLASS: Salicylate (non-acetylated)

INDICATIONS: Osteoarthritis, rheumatoid arthritis, acute painful shoulder, fever and mild-to-moderate pain.

DOSAGE: *Adults:* Initial: 1500mg bid. Max: 3g/d. Renal Dysfunction: Monitor salicylate level, adjust dose. Elderly: 750mg tid.
Pediatrics: >37kg: 2250mg/day given bid. 12-37kg: 50mg/kg/d given bid.

HOW SUPPLIED: Liq: 500mg/5mL (240mL); Tab: 500mg*, 750mg*, 1000mg* *scored

WARNINGS/PRECAUTIONS: Caution with renal or hepatic dysfunction, gastritis and peptic ulcer disease. Avoid with chickenpox, influenza or flu symptoms due to development of Reye syndrome in children and teenagers. Heavy alcohol use increases risk for adverse GI events.

ADVERSE REACTIONS: Tinnitus, nausea, vomiting, indigestion, heartburn, constipation, diarrhea, epigastric pain.

INTERACTIONS: Rise in urine pH (with chronic antacid use) increases salicylate clearance. Urine acidification decreases salicylate clearance. May potentiate anticoagulants, sulfonylureas, insulin, methotrexate, phenytoin, valproic acid and carbonic anhydrase inhibitors. Corticosteroids decrease salicylate levels. Salicylates may decrease effects of uricosuric agents.

PREGNANCY: Category C, caution with nursing.

TRIPEDIA   RX
tetanus toxoid - diphtheria toxoid - pertussis vaccine, acellular (Sanofi Pasteur)

THERAPEUTIC CLASS: Vaccine/toxoid combination

INDICATIONS: Active immunization against diphtheria, tetanus, and pertussis in pediatrics 6 weeks to 7 yrs of age (prior to 7th birthday). Combined with ActHIB for active immunization in pediatrics 15-18 months previously immunized against diphtheria, tetanus, and pertussis with 3 doses of whole-cell pertussis DTP or acellular pertussis vaccine and 3 or fewer doses of ActHIB® within 1st year of life for prevention of H. influenzae type b, diphtheria, tetanus, and pertussis.

DOSAGE: *Pediatrics:* <7 yrs: Primary Series: 3 doses of 0.5mL IM at 4-8 week intervals. 1st dose usually at 2 months, but can give at 6 weeks up to 7th birthday. Booster: 4th dose (0.5mL IM) at 15-20 months, at least 6 months after 3rd dose, 5th dose at 4-6 yrs; prior to school entry. May give to complete the 4th or 5th dose of primary series of 3 doses of whole-cell pertussis DTP (4th dose at 15-20 months and 5th dose before school if 4th dose not given on or before 4th birthday). May combine with ActHIB® for 4th dose at 15-18 months.

HOW SUPPLIED: Inj: (Diphtheria-Pertussis-Tetanus) 6.7LFU-46.8mcg-5LFU/0.5mL

CONTRAINDICATIONS: Hypersensitivity to thimersal and gelatin, immediate anaphylactic reaction associated with previous dose, encephalopathy not due to an identifiable cause within 7 days of prior pertussis immunization. Defer during poliomyelitis outbreak or acute febrile illness.

WARNINGS/PRECAUTIONS: Caution if within 48 hrs of previous whole-cell DTP or acellular DTP vaccine, fever ≥105°F not due to another identifiable cause, collapse or shock-like state, or inconsolable crying lasting ≥3 hrs occurs, or if convulsions occur within 3 days. For high seizure risk, give APAP at time of vaccination and q4-6h for 24 hrs. Caution with neurologic or CNS disorders. Avoid with coagulation disorders. Have epinephrine available. Suboptimal response may occur in immunocompromised patients.

ADVERSE REACTIONS: Local erythema and swelling, irritability, drowsiness, anorexia, fever.

INTERACTIONS: Avoid with anticoagulants. Immunosuppressive therapy (eg, irradiation, antimetabolites, alkylating agents, cytotoxic drugs, corticosteroids) may decrease response. Do not combine through reconstitution with any vaccine for infants <15 months.

PREGNANCY: Category C, safety in nursing not known.

TRISENOX RX
arsenic trioxide (Cell Therapeutics)

> Acute promyelocytic leukemia (APL) differentiation syndrome reported. Can cause QT interval prolongation and complete AV block. Perform ECG and assess serum electrolytes and creatinine before therapy.

THERAPEUTIC CLASS: DNA fragmentation agent

INDICATIONS: For induction of remission and consolidation of APL refractory to or relapsed from retinoid and anthracycline chemotherapy, and has t(15;17) translocation or PML/RAR-alpha gene expression.

DOSAGE: *Adults:* Induction: 0.15mg/kg IV qd until bone marrow remission. Max: 60 doses. Consolidation: 0.15mg/kg IV qd for 25 doses over 5 weeks. Begin 3-6 weeks after complete induction therapy.
Pediatrics: ≥5 yrs: Induction: 0.15mg/kg IV qd until bone marrow remission. Max: 60 doses. Consolidation: 0.15mg/kg IV qd for 25 doses over 5 weeks. Begin 3-6 weeks after complete induction therapy.

HOW SUPPLIED: Inj: 1mg/mL

WARNINGS/PRECAUTIONS: Hyperleukocytosis, QT interval prolongation, torsade de pointes, and complete AV block reported. Caution with renal failure. Monitor electrolyte, hematologic, and coagulation profiles at least twice weekly, and more frequently in unstable patients during induction. Obtain ECG weekly, and more frequently for unstable patients.

ADVERSE REACTIONS: Fatigue, pyrexia, edema, chest pain, injection site pain, nausea, vomiting, abdominal pain, constipation, hypokalemia, hypomagnesemia, hyperglycemia, increased ALT, headache, insomnia, dyspnea.

INTERACTIONS: Caution with agents that prolong the QT interval (eg, certain antiarrhythmics, thioridazine) or lead to electrolyte abnormalities (eg, diuretics, amphotericin B).

PREGNANCY: Category D, not for use in nursing.

TRIZIVIR RX
lamivudine - zidovudine - abacavir sulfate (GlaxoSmithKline)

> Fatal hypersensitivity reactions reported; discontinue if hypersensitivy reaction suspected and do not restart. Hematologic toxicities, lactic acidosis, and severe hepatomegaly with steatosis (including fatal cases) reported. Severe exacerbations of hepatitis B in patients co-infected with HIV upon discontinuation; monitor hepatic function.

THERAPEUTIC CLASS: Nucleoside analog combination

INDICATIONS: Treatment of HIV-1 infection alone or in combination with other antiretrovirals.

DOSAGE: *Adults:* >40kg and CrCl >50mL/min: 1 tab bid.
Pediatrics: Adolescents: >40kg and CrCl >50mL/min: 1 tab bid.

HOW SUPPLIED: Tab: (Abacavir-Lamivudine-Zidovudine) 300mg-150mg-300mg

WARNINGS/PRECAUTIONS: Hypersensitivity; discontinue if suspected and register patients by calling 1-800-270-0425. Caution with bone marrow compromise. Prolonged use associated with myopathy and myositis with pathological changes. Avoid with mild to moderate hepatic impairment or liver cirrhosis. Recurrent hepatitis upon discontinuation of lamivudine reported in hepatitis B patients. Lamivudine-resistant hepatitis B virus reported.

TRUSOPT

ADVERSE REACTIONS: Nausea, vomiting, diarrhea, loss of appetite, insomnia, fever, chills, fatigue.

INTERACTIONS: Ethanol decreases elimination. Ganciclovir, interferon alpha, and other bone marrow suppressants or cytotoxic agents may increase hematologic toxicity. Antagonistic effects with stavudine. Increased lamivudine exposure with trimethoprim 160mg/sulfamethoxazole 800mg. Avoid zalcitabine. Hepatic decompensation reported in patients on combination antiretroviral therapy for HIV and interferon alfa with or without ribavarin; monitor closely for treatment-associated toxicities.

PREGNANCY: Category C, not for use in nursing.

Trusopt   RX
dorzolamide HCl (Merck)

THERAPEUTIC CLASS: Carbonic anhydrase inhibitor

INDICATIONS: Treatment of open-angle glaucoma and ocular hypertension.

DOSAGE: *Adults:* 1 drop tid. Space dosing other ophthalmic drugs by 10 minutes.

Pediatrics: 1 drop tid. Space dosing other ophthalmic drugs by 10 minutes.

HOW SUPPLIED: Sol: 2% (5mL, 10mL)

WARNINGS/PRECAUTIONS: Systemically absorbed. Avoid with sulfonamide allergy or severe renal impairment. Caution with hepatic impairment. Not studied in acute angle-closure glaucoma. Local ocular adverse effects (conjunctivitis, lid reactions) reported with chronic use. Bacterial keratitis reported with contaminated containers.

ADVERSE REACTIONS: Ocular burning, stinging, discomfort, superficial punctate keratitis, bitter taste, blurred vision, eye redness, tearing, dryness, photophobia, ocular allergic reactions, lid reactions, conjunctivitis.

INTERACTIONS: Caution with high-dose salicylates. Acid-base disturbances with oral carbonic anhydrase inhibitors. Avoid oral carbonic anhydrase inhibitors due to additive effects. Wait 10 minutes before using another ophthalmic drug.

PREGNANCY: Category C, not for use in nursing.

Tucks Ointment   OTC
mineral oil - zinc oxide - pramoxine HCl (McNeil)

THERAPEUTIC CLASS: Anesthetic agent

INDICATIONS: Temporary relief of pain, soreness, burning, and itching associated with hemorrhoids and anorectal disorders.

DOSAGE: *Adults:* Cleanse area with soap and water, then rinse and dry. Apply externally to affected area. Max: 5 times/day for 7 days. To use dispensing cap, attach it to tube, lubricate well, then gently insert part way into anal canal. Squeeze tube to deliver medication.

Pediatrics: ≥12 yrs: Cleanse area with soap and water, then rinse and dry. Apply externally to affected area. Max: 5 times/day for 7 days. To use dispensing cap, attach it to tube, lubricate well, then gently insert part way into anal canal. Squeeze tube to deliver medication.

HOW SUPPLIED: Oint: (Mineral Oil-Pramoxine-Zinc Oxide) 46.6%-1%-12.5%

WARNINGS/PRECAUTIONS: Allergic reactions may develop. D/C if redness, irritation, swelling, pain, or other symptoms develop or increase. Do not administer into rectum by using fingers or any mechanical device or applicator.

PREGNANCY: Safety in pregnancy and nursing not known.

Tucks Suppositories   OTC
starch (McNeil)

THERAPEUTIC CLASS: Anesthetic agent

INDICATIONS: To give temporary relief from itching, burning, and discomfort associated with hemorrhoids and other anorectal disorders.

DOSAGE: *Adults:* Cleanse area with soap and water, then rinse and dry. Insert 1 sup rectally. Max: 6 times/day for 7 days.

Pediatrics: ≥12 yrs: Cleanse area with soap and water, then rinse and dry. Insert 1 sup rectally. Max: 6 times/day for 7 days.

HOW SUPPLIED: Sup: 51%

PREGNANCY: Safety in pregnancy and nursing not known.

Tussend CIII
pseudoephedrine HCl - hydrocodone bitartrate - chlorpheniramine maleate (King)

THERAPEUTIC CLASS: Cough suppressant

INDICATIONS: Relief of cough and congestion of the respiratory tract. Relief of hay fever symptoms.

DOSAGE: *Adults:* 1 tab or 10mL q4-6h. Max: 4 doses/24 hrs.

Pediatrics: >12 yrs: 1 tab or 10mL q4-6h. Max: 4 doses/24 hrs. 6-12 yrs: 1/2 tab or 5mL q4-6h. Max: 4 doses/24 hrs.

HOW SUPPLIED: (Hydrocodone-Chlorpheniramine-Pseudophedrine) Syrup: 2.5mg-2mg-30mg/5mL; Tab: 5mg-4mg-60mg

CONTRAINDICATIONS: Severe CAD, MAOI therapy, narrow-angle glaucoma, urinary retention, peptic ulcer, during an asthma attack, nursing mothers and infants. Hypersensitivity to other sympathomimetic amines.

WARNINGS/PRECAUTIONS: Caution with HTN, ischemic heart disease, DM, asthma, increased IOP, elderly/debilitated, severe impairment of hepatic or renal function, hyperthyroidism, or prostatic hypertrophy. Caution with head injury, intracranial lesions or pre-existing increase in intracranial pressure. May obscure the diagnosis/clinical course with acute abdominal conditions. May impair the mental and physical abilities.

ADVERSE REACTIONS: Lightheadedness, dizziness, sedation, nausea, vomiting, constipation, urethral spasm, urinary retention.

INTERACTIONS: Narcotics, antipsychotics, antianxiety agents, alcohol, and other CNS depressants may potentiate CNS depression. Increased effect of antidepressant or hydrocodone with MAOIs or TCAs. Anticholinergics may produce paralytic ileus. Digitalis glycosides may increase risk of cardiac arrhythmias. Decreased hypotensive effects of guanethidine, mecamylamine, methyldopa, reserpine, and veratrum alkaloids. TCAs may antagonize the effects of pseudoephedrine. Risk of hypertensive crises with pseudoephedrine and MAOIs, indomethacin, or with β-adrenergic blockers and methyldopa.

PREGNANCY: Category C, not for use in nursing.

Tussend Expectorant CIII
guaifenesin - pseudoephedrine HCl - hydrocodone bitartrate (King)

THERAPEUTIC CLASS: Cough suppressant/expectorant/decongestant

INDICATIONS: For exhausting, nonproductive cough accompanying respiratory tract congestion associated with the common cold, influenza, sinusitis and bronchitis.

DOSAGE: *Adults:* 10mL q4-6h. Max: 10mL qid prn. May take with meals.

Pediatrics: 6-12 yrs: 5mL q4-6h. Max: 5mL qid prn. May take with meals.

HOW SUPPLIED: Sol: (Hydrocodone-Guaifenesin-Pseudophedrine) 2.5mg-100mg-30mg/5mL

CONTRAINDICATIONS: Severe HTN, severe CAD, MAOI therapy and nursing women. Hypersensitivity to sympathomimetics and phenanthrene derivatives.

WARNINGS/PRECAUTIONS: Caution with severe respiratory impairment, HTN, DM, ischemic heart disease, hyperthyroidism, increased IOP, prostatic hypertrophy, and in elderly or debilitated patients. May impair mental and physical abilities. May produce drug dependence of the morphine type.

ADVERSE REACTIONS: GI upset, nausea, drowsiness, constipation, tachycardia, palpitations, headache, dizziness.

Tussi-12 (continued)

INTERACTIONS: Hydrocodone may potentiate effects of narcotics, general anesthetics, tranquilizers, sedatives and hypnotics, alcohol, and other CNS depressants. Increased effect of antidepressant or hydrocodone with MAOIs or TCAs. Decreased hypotensive effects of mecamylamine, methyldopa, reserpine, and veratrum alkaloids. MAOIs and β-adrenergic blockers potentiate the sympathomimetic effect of pseudoephedrine.

PREGNANCY: Category C, not for use in nursing.

Tussi-12   RX
carbetapentane tannate - chlorpheniramine tannate (Wallace)

THERAPEUTIC CLASS: Antitussive/antihistamine

INDICATIONS: Symptomatic relief of cough.

DOSAGE: *Adults:* 1-2 tabs q12h.
Pediatrics: >6 yrs: 5-10mL q12h. 2-6 yrs: 2.5-5mL q12h.

HOW SUPPLIED: (Carbetapentane-Chlorpheniramine) Sus: 30mg-4mg/5mL (118mL); Tab: 60mg-5mg* *scored

CONTRAINDICATIONS: Newborns, nursing mothers.

WARNINGS/PRECAUTIONS: Caution with HTN, cardiovascular disease, hyperthyroidism, DM, elderly, narrow angle glaucoma, or prostatic hypertrophy. Excitation in children may occur. Suspension contains tartrazine.

ADVERSE REACTIONS: Drowsiness, sedation, dryness of mucous membranes, GI effects.

INTERACTIONS: Avoid with or within 14 days of discontinuation of MAOIs. Additive CNS effects with alcohol, CNS depressants.

PREGNANCY: Category C, not for use in nursing.

Tussionex Pennkinetic
hydrocodone polistirex - chlorpheniramine polistirex (UCB)

THERAPEUTIC CLASS: Opioid antitussive/antihistamine

INDICATIONS: Relief of cough and upper respiratory symptoms associated with allergy and cold.

DOSAGE: *Adults:* 5mL q12h. Max: 10mL/24 hrs.
Pediatrics: >12 yrs: 5mL q12h. Max: 10mL/24 hrs. 6-12 yrs: 2.5mL q12h. Max: 5mL/24 hrs.

HOW SUPPLIED: Sus: (Hydrocodone-Chlorpheniramine) 10mg-8mg/5mL

WARNINGS/PRECAUTIONS: May produce dose-related respiratory depression. Caution with pulmonary disease, post-surgery, head injury, intracranial lesions or pre-existing increase in intracranial pressure, narrow angle glaucoma, asthma, BPH, elderly, debilitated, impaired hepatic/renal functions, hypothyroidosis, Addison's disease or urethral stricture. May mask acute abdominal conditions and the clinical course of head injuries. May cause obstructive bowel disease. Consider risk/benefit ratio in pediatrics especially in croup. Impairment of mental and physical performance.

ADVERSE REACTIONS: Sedation, drowsiness, lethargy, anxiety, dysphoria, euphoria, dizziness, psychotic dependence, rash, pruritus, nausea, vomiting, ureteral spasm, urinary retention, respiratory depression, dryness of the pharynx, tightness of the chest.

INTERACTIONS: Additive CNS depression with narcotics, antipsychotics, antianxiety agents, and alcohol. Increased effect of antidepressant or hydrocodone with MAOIs or TCAs. Concurrent anticholinergics may cause paralytic ileus.

PREGNANCY: Category C, not for use in nursing.

Tussi-Organidin DM NR   RX
guaifenesin - dextromethorphan hydrobromide (MedPointe)

OTHER BRAND NAMES: Gani-Tuss-DM NR (Cypress) - Tussi-Organidin DM S NR (MedPointe)

THERAPEUTIC CLASS: Antitussive/expectorant

INDICATIONS: Temporary relief of cough due to minor throat and bronchial irritation.

DOSAGE: *Adults:* 10mL q4h. Max: 60mL/24hrs.

Pediatrics: ≥12 yrs: 10mL q4h. Max: 60mL/24hrs. 6 to <12 yrs: 5mL q4h. Max: 30mL/24hrs. 2 to <6 yrs: 2.5mL q4h. Max: 15mL/24hrs. 6 months to <2 yrs: 0.6-1.25mL q4h or 2.5mL q6-8h. Max: 7.5mL/24hrs.

HOW SUPPLIED: Liq: (Dextromethorphan-Guaifenesin) 10mg/5mL-100mg/5mL

CONTRAINDICATIONS: MAOIs.

ADVERSE REACTIONS: Drowsiness, GI disturbance.

INTERACTIONS: Avoid MAOIs use during or within 2 weeks of discontinuation. Additive CNS depression with alcohol, antihistamines, psychotropics, or other CNS depressants.

PREGNANCY: Category C, not for use in nursing.

TWINJECT   RX
epinephrine (Verus)

THERAPEUTIC CLASS: Sympathomimetic catecholamine

INDICATIONS: Emergency treatment of severe allergic reactions (type 1) including anaphylaxis to insect stings or bites, allergens, foods, drugs, diagnostic testing substances, as well as idiopathic or exercise-induced anaphylaxis.

DOSAGE: *Adults:* Administer SQ or IM into thigh. 15-30kg: (Twinject 0.15mg) 0.15mg. May repeat if needed. ≥30kg: (Twinject 0.3mg) 0.3mg. May repeat if needed.

Pediatrics: Administer SQ or IM into thigh. 15-30kg: (Twinject 0.15mg) 0.15mg. May repeat if needed. ≥30kg: (Twinject 0.3mg) 0.3mg. May repeat if needed.

HOW SUPPLIED: Inj: (Twinject 0.15mg, Twinject 0.3mg) 1mg/mL

WARNINGS/PRECAUTIONS: Inject into anterolateral aspect of thigh; avoid injecting into hands, feet, or buttock. Avoid IV use. Contains sodium bisulfite. Caution with cardiac arrhythmias, coronary artery or organic heart disease, or hypertension. May precipitate/aggravate angina pectoris or produce ventricular arrhythmias with coronary insufficiency or ischemic heart disease. Light sensitive; store in tube provided.

ADVERSE REACTIONS: Anxiety, apprehensiveness, restlessness, tremor, weakness, dizziness, sweating, palpitations, pallor, nausea, vomiting, headache, respiratory difficulties, hypertension.

INTERACTIONS: Monitor for cardiac arrhythmias with cardiac glycosides or diuretics. Effects may be potentiated by TCAs, MAOIs, levothyroxine, and certain antihistamines (notably chlorpheniramine, tripelennamine, diphenhydramine). Cardiostimulating and bronchodilating ffects antagonized by beta-adrenergic blockers (eg, propranolol). Vasoconstricting and hypertensive effects antagonized by alpha-adrenergic blockers (eg, phentolamine). Ergot alkaloids and phenothiazines may reverse pressor effects.

PREGNANCY: Category C, safety in nursing not known.

TYLENOL   OTC
acetaminophen (McNeil Consumer)

OTHER BRAND NAMES: Tylenol 8 Hour (McNeil Consumer) - Tylenol Junior (McNeil Consumer) - Tylenol Infant's (McNeil Consumer) - Tylenol Children's (McNeil Consumer) - Tylenol Arthritis Pain (McNeil Consumer) - Tylenol Extra Strength (McNeil Consumer) - Tylenol Regular Strength (McNeil Consumer)

THERAPEUTIC CLASS: Analgesic

INDICATIONS: Temporary relief of minor aches and pains. Temporary reduction of fever.

DOSAGE: *Adults:* ≥12 yrs: (Regular Strength) 650mg q4-6h prn. Max: 3900mg/day. (Extra Strength Tabs, Caplets, or Geltabs) 1000mg q4-6h prn. Max: 4000mg/day. (Arthritis Pain, 8 Hour) 2 caplets or geltabs q8h with water. Max: 6 caplets or geltabs/day.

Pediatrics: Max: 5 doses/day. 0-3 mths (6-11 lbs): 40mg q4h prn. 4-11 mths (12-17 lbs): 80mg q4h prn. 12-23 mths (18-23 lbs): 120mg q4h prn. 2-3 yrs (24-35 lbs): 160mg q4h

Tylenol with Codeine

prn. 4-5 yrs (36-47 lbs): 240mg q4h prn. 6-8 yrs (48-59 lbs): 320mg q4h prn. 9-10 yrs (60-71 lbs): 400mg q4h prn. 11 yrs (72-95 lbs): 480mg q4h prn. 12 yrs (≥96 lbs): 640mg q4h prn. Older Children: Regular Strength: 6-11 yrs: 325mg q4-6h prn. Max: 1625mg/day.

HOW SUPPLIED: Caplets: (Arthritis Pain, 8 Hour) 650mg; Drops: (Infants') 80mg/0.8mL; Geltabs: (Arthritis Pain, 8 Hour) 650mg; Sol: (Extra Strength) 500mg/15mL; Sus: (Children's) 160mg/5mL; Tab: (Regular Strength) 325mg; (Extra Strength Tabs, EZ Tabs, GoTabs, Caplets, Cool Caplet, Geltabs, Rapid Release Gels) 500mg; Tab, Chewable: (Children's) 80mg, (Junior) 160mg

WARNINGS/PRECAUTIONS: May cause liver damage.

INTERACTIONS: Increased risk of hepatotoxicity with excessive alcohol use (≥3 drinks/day).

PREGNANCY: Safety in pregnancy or nursing not known.

Tylenol with Codeine   CIII
acetaminophen - codeine phosphate (Ortho-McNeil)

THERAPEUTIC CLASS: Opioid analgesic

INDICATIONS: Relief of mild to moderately severe pain.

DOSAGE: *Adults:* (Tab) Usual: 15-60mg codeine/dose and 300-1000mg APAP/dose up to q4h prn. Max: 60mg codeine/dose, 360mg codeine/day and 4g APAP/day. (Elixir): 15mL q4h prn.
Pediatrics: (Elixir): Usual: 7-12 yrs: 10mL tid-qid. 3-6 yrs: 5mL tid-qid.

HOW SUPPLIED: (Codeine-APAP) Elixir: (CV) 12-120mg/5mL; Tab: (#3, CIII) 30-300mg, (#4, CIII) 60-300mg

WARNINGS/PRECAUTIONS: Respiratory depressant effects may be exacerbated with head injury or increased intracranial pressure. May obscure head injuries, acute abdominal conditions. Caution in the elderly, debilitated, severe hepatic or renal dysfunction, hypothyroidism, Addison's disease, prostatic hypertrophy or urethral stricture. Potential for physical dependence, tolerance. Tabs contain sulfites.

ADVERSE REACTIONS: Lightheadedness, dizziness, sedation, shortness of breath, nausea, vomiting, allergic reactions, euphoria, dysphoria, constipation, abdominal pain, pruritus.

INTERACTIONS: Additive CNS depression with narcotic analgesics, antipsychotics, antianxiety agents, alcohol, other CNS depressants. Anticholinergics may produce paralytic ileus.

PREGNANCY: Category C, caution in nursing.

Tyzeka   RX
telbivudine (Novartis)

> Lactic acidosis and severe hepatomegaly with steatosis reported. Discontinuation may result in severe acute exacerbations of hepatitis; monitor hepatic function closely for at least several months following discontinuation of therapy.

THERAPEUTIC CLASS: Nucleoside analogue

INDICATIONS: Treatment of chronic hepatitis B.

DOSAGE: *Adults:* CrCl ≥50mL/min: 600mg qd. CrCl 30-49mL/min: 600mg every 48 hrs. CrCl <30mL/min (not requiring dialysis): 600mg every 72 hrs. ESRD: 600mg every 96 hrs.
Pediatrics: ≥16 yrs: CrCl ≥50mL/min: 600mg qd. CrCl 30-49mL/min: 600mg every 48 hrs. CrCl <30mL/min (not requiring dialysis): 600mg every 72 hrs. ESRD: 600mg every 96 hrs.

HOW SUPPLIED: Tab: 600mg

WARNINGS/PRECAUTIONS: Myopathy reported; interrupt therapy if myopathy suspected and d/c if myopathy diagnosed. Monitor renal function.

ADVERSE REACTIONS: Upper respiratory tract infection, fatigue, malaise, abdominal pain, nasopharyngitis, headache, elevated blood CPK, cough, nausea, vomiting, influenza, flu-like symptoms, diarrhea, loose stools, pharyngolaryngeal pain.

INTERACTIONS: Drugs that alter renal function may alter plasma concentrations of telbivudine.

PREGNANCY: Category B, not for use in nursing.

Ultane
sevoflurane (Abbott)
RX

THERAPEUTIC CLASS: Inhalation anesthetic

INDICATIONS: For induction and maintenance of general anesthesia in adult and pediatric patients for inpatient and outpatient surgery.

DOSAGE: *Adults:* Individualize dose. MAC Values: 80 yrs: 1.4% sevoflurane in oxygen or 0.7% sevoflurane in 65% nitrous oxide/35% oxygen. 60 yrs: 1.7% sevoflurane in oxygen or 0.9% sevoflurane in 65% nitrous oxide/35% oxygen. 40 yrs: 2.1% sevoflurane in oxygen or 1.1% sevoflurane in 65% nitrous oxide/35% oxygen. 25 yrs: 2.6% sevoflurane in oxygen or 1.4% sevoflurane in 65% nitrous oxide/35% oxygen.
Pediatrics: Individualize dose. MAC Values: 3-12 yrs: 2.5% sevoflurane in oxygen. 6 months-<3 yrs: 2.8% sevoflurane in oxygen or 2% sevoflurane in 65% nitrous oxide/35% oxygen. 1-<6 months: 3% sevoflurane in oxygen. 0-1 month: 3.3% sevoflurane in oxygen.

HOW SUPPLIED: Liq: (250mL)

CONTRAINDICATIONS: Susceptibility to malignant hyperthermia.

WARNINGS/PRECAUTIONS: Potential for renal injury. May be associated with glycosuria and proteinuria. May cause malignant hyperthermia. May cause perioperative hyperkalemia resulting in cardiac arrhythmias. May decrease BP. Rare cases of seizures have been reported. Transient changes in postoperative LFTs and very rare cases of postoperative hepatic dysfunction or hepatitis reported. Concomitant use of desiccated CO_2 absorbents (eg, potassium hydroxide) are not recommended, may result in rare cases of extreme heat, smoke, and/or spontaneous fire in anesthesia breathing circuit; replace CO_2 absorbent routinely.

ADVERSE REACTIONS: Bradycardia, hypotension, agitation, laryngospasm, airway obstruction, breathholding, cough, tachycardia, shivering, somnolence, dizziness, increased salivation, nausea, vomiting.

INTERACTIONS: Decreased anesthetic requirement with nitrous oxide. May increase both the intensity and duration of neuromuscular blockade induced by nondepolarizing muscle relaxants.

PREGNANCY: Category B, caution in nursing.

Ultiva
remifentanil HCl (Abbott)
CII

THERAPEUTIC CLASS: Opioid analgesic

INDICATIONS: As an analgesic agent for use during the induction and maintenance of general anesthesia. For continuation as an analgesic into the immediate postoperative period in adults under the direct supervision of an anesthesia practitioner in a postoperative anesthesia care unit or intensive care setting. As an analgesic component of monitored anesthesia care in adults.

DOSAGE: *Adults:* Continuous IV Infusion: Induction: 0.5-1mcg/kg/min. Maint: 0.4mcg/kg with nitrous oxide 66%; 0.25mcg/kg with isoflurane (0.4-1.25 MAC); 0.25 with propofol (100-200mcg/kg/min). Post-Op Continuation: 0.1mcg/kg/min. CABG: Induction/Maint/Continuation: 1mcg/kg/min. Elderly (>65 yrs): Use 50% of adult dose. Titrate carefully.
Pediatrics: Anesthesia Maint: Continuous IV Infusion: 1-12 yrs: 0.25mcg/kg/min with halothane (0.3-1.5 MAC), sevoflurane (0.3-1.5 MAC, or isoflurane (0.4-1.5 MAC). Range: 0.05-1.3mcg/kg/min. Birth-2 months: 0.4mcg/kg/min. Range: 0.4-1mcg/kg/min.

HOW SUPPLIED: Inj: 1mg, 2mg, 5mg

CONTRAINDICATIONS: Epidural or intrathecal administration, hypersensitivity to fentanyl analogs.

WARNINGS/PRECAUTIONS: Administer only with infusion device. IV bolus administration should be used only during the maintenance of general anesthesia. Interruption of infusion will result in rapid offset of effect. Use associated with apnea and respiratory

ULTRAVATE (continued)

depression. Not for use in diagnostic or therapeutic procedures outside the monitored anesthesia care setting. Resuscitative and intubation equipment, oxygen, and opioid antagonist must be readily available. May cause skeletal muscle rigidity and is related to the dose and speed of administration. Do not administer into the same IV tubing with blood due to potential inactivation by nonspecific esterases in blood products. Continuously monitor vital signs and oxygenation. Bradycardia, hypotension, intraoperative awareness reported. Not recommended as sole agent for induction of anesthesia.

ADVERSE REACTIONS: Nausea, vomiting, hypotension, muscle rigidity, bradycardia, shivering, fever, dizziness, visual disturbances, respiratory depression, apnea.

INTERACTIONS: Synergism with thiopental, propofol, isoflurane, midazolam; reduce doses of these drugs by up to 75%.

PREGNANCY: Category C, caution in nursing.

ULTRAVATE RX
halobetasol propionate (Westwood-Squibb)

THERAPEUTIC CLASS: Corticosteroid

INDICATIONS: Corticosteroid responsive dermatoses.

DOSAGE: *Adults:* Apply qd-bid. Rub in gently. Limit treatment to 2 weeks. Max: 50g/week.

Pediatrics: ≥12 yrs: Apply qd-bid. Rub in gently. Limit treatment to 2 weeks. Max: 50g/week.

HOW SUPPLIED: Cre, Oint: 0.05% (15g, 50g)

WARNINGS/PRECAUTIONS: Avoid face, groin, or axillae. Not for treatment of rosacea or perioral dermatitis. May produce reversible HPA axis suppression, manifestations of Cushing's syndrome, hyperglycemia, and glucosuria. Caution when applied to large surface areas or under occlusive dressings. Use appropriate antifungal or antibacterial agent with dermatological infections; discontinue if infection does not clear. Pediatrics may be more susceptible to systemic toxicity. Avoid eyes. Discontinue if irritation occurs. Reassess if no improvement after 2 weeks.

ADVERSE REACTIONS: Stinging, burning, itching, irritation, dryness, folliculitis, hypertrichosis, acneiform eruptions, hypopigmentation, perioral dermatitis, allergic contact dermatitis, skin maceration, secondary infection, skin atrophy, striae, miliaria.

PREGNANCY: Category C, caution in nursing.

UNASYN RX
sulbactam sodium - ampicillin sodium (Pfizer)

THERAPEUTIC CLASS: Semisynthetic penicillin/beta lactamase inhibitor

INDICATIONS: Treatment of skin and skin structure (SSSI), intra-abdominal, and gynecological infections caused by susceptible microorganisms.

DOSAGE: *Adults:* 1.5-3g (ampicillin+sulbactam) IM/IV q6h. Max: 4g/day sulbactam. Renal Impairment: CrCl ≥30mL/min: 1.5-3g q6-8h. CrCl 15-29mL/min: 1.5-3g q12h. CrCl 5-14mL/min: 1.5-3g q24h.

Pediatrics: ≥1 yr: SSSI: 1.5-3g (ampicillin+sulbactam) IM/IV q6h. Max: 4g/day sulbactam.

HOW SUPPLIED: Inj: (Ampicillin-Sulbactam) 1g-0.5g, 2g-1g, 10g-5g

WARNINGS/PRECAUTIONS: Serious, fatal hypersensitivity reactions reported. Pseudomembranous colitis reported. Increased risk of skin rash with mononucleosis, use alternate agent.

ADVERSE REACTIONS: Injection site pain, thrombophlebitis, diarrhea, rash, nausea, vomiting, malaise, headache, chest pain, flatulence, dysuria, edema, erythema, chills, epistaxis.

INTERACTIONS: Probenecid increases and prolongs blood levels. Increased incidence of rash with allopurinol. Do not reconstitute with aminoglycosides; may inactivate aminoglycosides.

PREGNANCY: Category B, caution in nursing.

UNIPHYL
theophylline (Purdue Pharmaceutical)

RX

THERAPEUTIC CLASS: Xanthine bronchodilator

INDICATIONS: Treatment of the symptoms and reversible airflow obstruction associated with chronic asthma and other chronic lung disease (eg, emphysema, chronic bronchitis).

DOSAGE: *Adults:* Initial: 300-400mg qd for 3 days with meals. Titrate: Increase to 400-600mg qd. After 3 days and if needed/tolerated, increase dose according to blood levels. Tab may be split in half; do not chew or crush. Renal Dysfunction/Elderly (>60 yrs): Max: 400mg/day. Conversion from Immediate-Release Theophylline: Give same daily dose as once daily.

Pediatrics: 12-15 yrs: (<45kg): Initial: 12-14mg/kg/day up to 300mg qd for 3 days with meals. Titrate: Increase to 16mg/kg/day up to 400mg qd. After 3 days if needed/tolerated increase to 20mg/kg/day up to 600mg qd. (>45kg): Follow adult dose schedule. Tab may be split in half; do not chew or crush. Conversion from Immediate-Release Theophylline: ≥12 yrs: Give same daily dose as once daily. Renal Dysfunction: Max: 400mg qd.

HOW SUPPLIED: Tab, Extended Release: 400mg*, 600mg* *scored

WARNINGS/PRECAUTIONS: Extreme caution in peptic ulcer disease, seizure disorders and/or cardiac arrhythmias (except bradycardia). Caution in neonates, children <1 yr, and the elderly. Caution in pulmonary edema, CHF, fever ≥102°F for 24 hrs, cor-pulmonale, hypothyroidism, liver disease, reduced renal function, sepsis, shock, and HTN. If toxicity develops (eg, repetitive vomiting) monitor serum levels and adjust dosage.

ADVERSE REACTIONS: Vomiting, headache, insomnia, diarrhea, restlessness, tremors, hematemesis, hypokalemia, hyperglycemia, tachycardia, hypotension/shock, nervousness, disorientation, arrhythmias, seizures.

INTERACTIONS: Diminished effects with charcoal broiled food, phenytoin, carbamazepine, phenobarbital, hydantoins, rifampin, ritonavir, aminoglutethimide, barbiturates, ketoconazole, sulfinpyrazone, INH, loop diuretics, sympathomimetics, high protein/low carbohydrate diet, St. John's wort. Potentiated by propranolol, allopurinol, erythromycin, troleandomycin, ciprofloxacin, quinolone antibiotics, oral contraceptives, calcium channel blockers, corticosteroids, disulfiram, ephedrine, influenza virus vaccine, interferon, macrolides, mexiletine, thiabendazole, thyroid hormones, carbamazepine, loop diuretics

PREGNANCY: Category C, caution in nursing.

UNISOM
doxylamine succinate (Chattem)

OTC

THERAPEUTIC CLASS: Antihistamine

INDICATIONS: As a sleep aid 30 minutes before retiring.

DOSAGE: *Adult:* 1 tab 30 minutes prior to going to bed. Max: 1 tab qhs.

Pediatrics: >12 yrs: 1 tab 30 minutes prior to going to bed. Max: 1 tab qhs.

HOW SUPPLIED: Tab: 25mg

CONTRAINDICATIONS: Pregnancy, nursing, asthma, glaucoma, prostate enlargement.

WARNINGS/PRECAUTIONS: Caution in emphysema, chronic bronchitis, glaucoma, and difficulty in urination due to BPH. Caution with alcohol. Re-evaluate therapy if sleeplessness persists >2 weeks.

ADVERSE REACTIONS: Anticholinergic effects.

PREGNANCY: Not for use in pregnancy or nursing.

UNITHROID RX
levothyroxine sodium (Lannett)

THERAPEUTIC CLASS: Thyroid replacement hormone

INDICATIONS: Hypothyroidism. As a pituitary TSH suppressant in the treatment and prevention of euthyroid goiters, including thyroid nodules, lymphocytic thyroiditis, and multinodular goiter. Adjunct to surgery and radioiodine therapy for thyrotropin-dependent well-differentiated thyroid cancer.

DOSAGE: *Adults:* Take in the AM at least 1/2-1 hr before food. Hypothyroid: Usual: 1.7mcg/kg/day. >200mcg/day (seldom). >50 yrs/<50 yrs with Cardiac Disease: Initial: 25-50mcg/day. Titrate: Increase by 12.5-25mcg/day every 6-8 weeks until euthyroid. Elderly with Cardiac Disease: Initial: 12.5-25mcg/day. Titrate: Increase by 12.5-25mcg/day every 4-6 weeks until euthyroid. Severe Hypothyroidism: Initial: 12.5-25mcg/day. Titrate: Increase by 25mcg/day every 2-4 weeks until euthyroid. Pregnancy: May increase dose requirements. Subclinical Hypothyroidism: Lower doses required.

Pediatrics: Take in the AM at least 1/2-1 hr before food. Hypothyroidism: 0-3 months: 10-15mcg/kg/day. 3-6 months: 8-10mcg/kg/day. 6-12 months: 6-8mcg/kg/day. 1-5 yrs: 5-6mcg/kg/day. 6-12 yrs: 4-5mcg/kg/day. >12 yrs: 2-3mcg/kg/day. Growth/Puberty Complete: 1.7mcg/kg/day. Cardiac Risk: Initial: Use lower dose. Titrate: Increase dose every 4-6 weeks until euthyroid. Infants with Serum T_4 <5mcg/dL: Initial: 50mcg/day. Chronic/Severe Hypothyroidism: Children: Initial: 25mcg/day. Titrate: Increase by 25mcg/day every 2-4 weeks until desired effect. Minimize Hyperactivity in Older Children: Initial: Give 1/4 of full replacement dose. Titrate: Increase by same amount weekly until full dose achieved. May crush tab and mix with 5-10mL water.

HOW SUPPLIED: Tab: 25mcg*, 50mcg*, 75mcg*, 88mcg*, 100mcg*, 112mcg*, 125mcg*, 150mcg*, 175mcg*, 200mcg*, 300mcg* *scored

CONTRAINDICATIONS: Untreated thyrotoxicosis, acute MI, uncorrected adrenal insufficiency.

WARNINGS/PRECAUTIONS: Do not use in the treatment of obesity; larger doses in euthyroid patients can cause serious or even life threatening toxicity. Caution with cardiovascular disease, CAD, adrenal insufficiency, autonomous thyroid tissue, hypothalamic/pituitary hormone deficiencies, and the elderly with risk of occult cardiac disease. Carefully titrate dose to avoid over or under treatment. Decreased bone mineral density with long term use. With adrenal insufficiency supplement with glucocorticoids before therapy.

INTERACTIONS: Sympathomimetics may increase risk of coronary insufficiency with CAD. Upward dose adjustments needed for insulin and oral hypoglycemic agents. Decreased absorption with soybean flour (infant formula), cotton seed meal, walnuts, and fiber. May potentiate oral anticoagulant effects; adjust dose and monitor PT/INR. May decrease levels and effects of digitalis glycosides. Cholestyramine, colestipol, ferrous sulfate, aluminum hydroxide, sodium polystyrene, soybean flour, sucralfate may decrease absorption. Reduced TSH secretion with dopamine/dopamine agonists, glucocorticoids, octreotide. Decreased thyroid hormone secretion with aminoglutethimide, amiodarone, iodine (including iodine-containing radiographic contrast agents), lithium, methimazole, PTU, sulfonamides, tolbutamide. Increased thyroid hormone secretion with amiodarone, iodide (including iodine-containing radiographic contrast agents). Decreased T_4 absorption with antacids (aluminum & magnesium hydroxides), simethicone, bile acid sequestrants (cholestyramine, colestipol), calcium carbonate, cation exchange resins (eg, Kayexalate), ferrous sulfate, sucralfate. Increased serum TBG concentration with clofibrate, estrogens, heroin/methadone, 5-FU, mitotane, tamoxifen. Decreased serum TBG concentration with androgens/anabolic steroids, asparaginase, glucocorticoids, nicotinic acid (slow-release). Protein-binding site displacement with furosemide, heparin, hydantoins, NSAIDs, salicylates. Increased hepatic metabolism with carbamazepine, hydantoins, phenobarbital, rifampin. Decreased conversion of T_4 to T_3 levels with amiodarone, β-adrenergic antagonists (propranolol >160mg/day), glucocorticoids (dexamethasone >4mg/day), PTU. Additive effects of both agents with antidepressants. Interferon-(alpha) may cause development of anti-thyroid microsomal antibodies causing transient hypothyroidism, hyperthyroidism, or both. Interleukin-2 has been associated with transient painless thyroiditis. Excessive use with growth hormones may accelerate epiphyseal closure. Ketamine use may produce marked HTN and tachycardia. May reduce uptake of iodine-containing radiographic contrast agents. Altered levels of thyroid hormone and/or TSH level with choral hydrate, diazepam, ethionamide, lovastatin, metoclopramide, 6-mercaptopurine, nitroprusside, para-aminosalicylate sodium, perphenazine, resorcinol (excessive topical use), thiazide diuretics.

PREGNANCY: Category A, caution in nursing.

URIMAX
RX
methenamine - methylene blue - phenyl salicylate - sodium biphosphate - hyoscyamine sulfate (Xanodyne)

THERAPEUTIC CLASS: anticholinergic/antibacterial/antiseptic/analgesic/Acidifier

INDICATIONS: Treatment of symptoms of irritative voiding. For relief of local symptoms that accompany lower urinary tract infections (eg, inflammation, hypermotility, pain). For relief of urinary tract symptoms caused by diagnostic procedures.

DOSAGE: *Adults:* 1 tab qid with plenty of fluid.
Pediatrics: >6 yrs: Individualize dose. Take with plenty of fluid.

HOW SUPPLIED: Tab, Extended Release: (Hyoscyamine-Methenamine-Methylene Blue-Phenyl Salicylate-Sodium Biphosphate) 0.12mg-81.6mg-10.8mg-36.2mg-40.8mg

CONTRAINDICATIONS: Consider risk-benefit with the following: cardiac disease, GI tract obstructive disease, glaucoma, myasthenia gravis, obstructive uropathy.

WARNINGS/PRECAUTIONS: Discontinue if rapid pulse, dizziness, or blurred vision occurs. Intolerance may occur if intolerant to belladonna alkaloids or salicylates. Delay in gastric emptying could complicate management of gastric ulcers. Infants and children are especially susceptible to toxic effect of belladonna alkaloids. Caution in elderly. Urine and feces may become blue to blue-green due to methylene blue.

ADVERSE REACTIONS: Rapid pulse, flushing, blurred vision, dizziness, shortness of breath, difficult micturition, acute urinary retention, dry mouth, nausea, vomiting.

INTERACTIONS: May decrease absorption of urinary alkalizers, thiazide diuretics, antimuscarinics, antacids/antidiarrheals. Space dosing by 1 hr with antimyasthenics, MAOIs, opioids, sulfonamides. Space dosing by 2 hrs with ketoconazole. Thiazide diuretics may decrease effectiveness of methenamine. Intensified antimuscarinic effects of hyoscyamine with antimuscarinics. Antacids/antidiarrheals may reduce absorption of hyoscyamine and may reduce effectiveness of methenamine.

PREGNANCY: Category C, caution in nursing.

URISED
RX
methenamine - benzoic acid - methylene blue - phenyl salicylate - atropine sulfate - hyoscyamine sulfate (PolyMedica)

THERAPEUTIC CLASS: anticholinergic/antiseptic/antibacterial/analgesic

INDICATIONS: Relief of lower urinary tract discomfort due to hypermotility. Treatment of formaldehyde-susceptible cystitis, urethritis, trigonitis.

DOSAGE: *Adults:* Usual: 2 tabs qid with plenty of fluid.
Pediatrics: ≥6 yrs: Individualize dose. Take with plenty of fluid.

HOW SUPPLIED: Tab: Atropine 0.03mg-Benzoic Acid 4.5mg-Hyoscyamine 0.03mg-Methenamine 40.8mg-Methylene Blue 5.4mg-Phenyl Salicylate 18.1mg

CONTRAINDICATIONS: Glaucoma, pyloric or duodenal obstruction, urinary bladder neck obstruction, or cardiospasm.

WARNINGS/PRECAUTIONS: Caution with cardiovascular disorders. May precipitate acute urinary retention in prostatic hypertrophy.

ADVERSE REACTIONS: Rash, dry mouth, flushing, difficult micturition, rapid pulse, dizziness, blurred vision, urine/feces discoloration.

INTERACTIONS: Avoid alkalinizing agents/foods. Sulfonamides may precipitate in the urine; avoid concomitant use.

PREGNANCY: Category C, caution in nursing.

URISPAS
flavoxate HCl (Ortho-McNeil)
RX

THERAPEUTIC CLASS: Smooth muscle antispasmodic

INDICATIONS: Relief of dysuria, urgency, nocturia, suprapubic pain, frequency and incontinence.

DOSAGE: *Adults:* 100-200mg tid-qid. Reduce dose with improvement.
Pediatrics: ≥12 yrs: 100-200mg tid-qid. Reduce dose with improvement.

HOW SUPPLIED: Tab: 100mg

CONTRAINDICATIONS: Pyloric or duodenal obstruction, obstructive intestinal lesions or ileus, achalasia, GI hemorrhage, and obstructive uropathies of the lower urinary tract.

WARNINGS/PRECAUTIONS: Caution with glaucoma and while operating machinery where alertness is required. Drowsiness, blurred vision may occur.

ADVERSE REACTIONS: Drowsiness, dry mouth, nausea, vomiting, tachycardia, leukopenia, vertigo, nervousness, confusion, fatigue, headache, hyperpyrexia, constipation, urticaria, blurred vision.

PREGNANCY: Category B, caution in nursing.

UROGESIC BLUE
methenamine - methylene blue - phenyl salicylate - sodium biphosphate - hyoscyamine sulfate (Edwards)
RX

THERAPEUTIC CLASS: anticholinergic/antibacterial/antiseptic/analgesic/Acidifier

INDICATIONS: Treatment of symptoms of irritative voiding. Relief of lower urinary tract discomfort.

DOSAGE: *Adults:* 1 tab qid with plenty of fluid.
Pediatrics: >6 yrs: Individualize dose. Take with plenty of fluid.

HOW SUPPLIED: Tab: Hyoscyamine 0.12mg-Methenamine 81.6mg-Methylene Blue 10.8mg-Phenyl Salicylate 36.2mg-Sodium Biphosphate 40.8mg

CONTRAINDICATIONS: Consider risk-benefit with: cardiac disease, GI tract obstructive disease, glaucoma, myasthenia gravis, obstructive uropathy.

WARNINGS/PRECAUTIONS: Discontinue if rapid pulse, dizziness, or blurred vision occurs. Delay in gastric emptying may obscure gastric ulcer therapy. Caution in elderly.

ADVERSE REACTIONS: Rapid pulse, flushing, blurred vision, dizziness, shortness of breath, difficult micturition, acute urinary retention, dry mouth, nausea, vomiting, urine/feces discoloration.

INTERACTIONS: May decrease absorption of other oral agents (dose 2 hrs after ketoconazole). Reduced effectiveness with urinary alkaliners, thiazide diuretics, antacids/antidiarrheals (space dosing by 1 hr). Antimuscarinic effects potentiated with other antimuscarinics, MAOIs. Caution with antimyasthenics. Increased risk of constipation with opioids. Sulfonamides may precipitate in the urine.

PREGNANCY: Category C, safety in nursing not known.

VAGISTAT-1
tioconazole (Novartis)
OTC

THERAPEUTIC CLASS: Azole antifungal

INDICATIONS: Treatment of recurrent vaginal yeast infections.

DOSAGE: *Adults:* Insert applicatorful intravaginally hs single dose.
Pediatrics: ≥12 yrs: Insert applicatorful intravaginally hs single dose.

HOW SUPPLIED: Oint: 6.5% (4.6g)

WARNINGS/PRECAUTIONS: Do not use if abdominal pain, fever (>100°F), chills, nausea, vomiting, diarrhea, or foul smelling discharge. Do not use with tampons. Do not rely on condoms or diaphragm to prevent STDs or pregnancy until 3 days after last use.

PREGNANCY: Not for use in pregnancy, safety in nursing not known.

VALIUM
diazepam (Roche Labs)

CIV

THERAPEUTIC CLASS: Benzodiazepine

INDICATIONS: Management of anxiety disorders and short-term relief of anxiety symptoms. Symptomatic relief of acute alcohol withdrawal. Adjunct therapy in skeletal muscle spasm and convulsive disorders.

DOSAGE: *Adults:* Anxiety: 2-10mg bid-qid. Alcohol Withdrawal: 10mg tid-qid for 24 hours. Maint: 5mg tid-qid prn. Skeletal Muscle Spasm: 2-10mg tid-qid: Seizure Disorders: 2-10mg bid-qid. Elderly/Debilitated: 2-2.5mg qd-bid initially; may increase gradually as needed and tolerated.

Pediatrics: ≥6 months: 1-2.5mg tid-qid initially; may increase gradually as needed and tolerated.

HOW SUPPLIED: Tab: 2mg*, 5mg*, 10mg* *scored

CONTRAINDICATIONS: Acute narrow angle glaucoma, untreated open angle glaucoma, patients <6 months.

WARNINGS/PRECAUTIONS: Monitor blood counts and LFTs in long-term use. Neutropenia and jaundice reported. Increase in grand mal seizures reported. Avoid abrupt withdrawal. Caution with kidney or hepatic dysfunction.

ADVERSE REACTIONS: Drowsiness, fatigue, ataxia, paradoxical reactions, minor EEG changes.

INTERACTIONS: Phenothiazines, narcotics, barbiturates, MAOIs, and other antidepressants may potentiate effects. Delayed clearance with cimetidine. Avoid alcohol and other CNS-depressants. Risk of seizure with flumazenil.

PREGNANCY: Not for use during pregnancy, safety in nursing not known.

VALTREX
valacyclovir HCl (GlaxoSmithKline)

RX

THERAPEUTIC CLASS: Nucleoside analogue

INDICATIONS: Treatment of herpes zoster (shingles) and herpes labialis (cold sores). Treatment or suppression of genital herpes in immunocompetent patients and for the suppression of recurrent genital herpes in HIV-infected patients.

DOSAGE: *Adults:* Herpes Zoster: 1g q8h for 7 days. Start within 48-72 hrs after onset of rash. CrCl 30-49mL/min: 1g q12h. CrCl 10-29mL/min: 1g q24h. CrCl <10mL/min: 500mg q24h. Genital Herpes: Initial: 1g q12h for 10 days. Start within 48-72 hrs after onset of symptoms. CrCl 10-29mL/min: 1g q24h. CrCl <10mL/min: 500mg q24h. Recurrent Episodes: Treatment: 500mg bid for 3 days. Start within 24 hrs after onset of symptoms. CrCl ≤29mL/min: 500mg q24h. Suppressive Therapy with Normal Immune Function:1g q24h. CrCl ≤29mL/min: 500mg q24h. Alternative: (≤9 episodes/yr) 500mg q24h. CrCl ≤29mL/min: 500mg q48h. Suppressive Therapy with HIV and CD4 ≥100cells/mm^3: 500mg q12h. CrCl ≤29mL/min: 500mg q24h. Herpes Labialis: 2g q12h for 1 day. Start at earliest symptom of cold sore. CrCl 30-49mL/min: 1g q12h. 10-29mL/min: 500mg q12h. <10mL/min: 500mg single dose. Administer therapy for 1 day. Initiate at earliest symptoms of a cold sore.

Pediatrics: Post-Pubertal: Herpes Zoster: 1g q8h for 7 days. Start within 48-72 hrs after onset of rash. CrCl 30-49mL/min: 1g q12h. CrCl 10-29mL/min: 1g q24h. CrCl <10mL/min: 500mg q24h. Genital Herpes: Initial: 1g q12h for 10 days. Start within 48-72 hrs after onset of symptoms. CrCl 10-29mL/min: 1g q24h. CrCl <10mL/min: 500mg q24h. Recur-

VANCOCIN

rent Episodes: Treatment: 500mg bid for 3 days. Start within 24 hrs after onset of symptoms. CrCl ≤29mL/min: 500mg q24h. Suppressive Therapy with Normal Immune Function:1g q24h. CrCl ≤29mL/min: 500mg q24h. Alternative: (≤9 episodes/yr) 500mg q24h. CrCl ≤29mL/min: 500mg q48h. Suppressive Therapy with HIV and CD4 ≥100cells/mm^3: 500mg q12h. CrCl ≤29mL/min: 500mg q24h. Herpes Labialis: 2g q12h for 1 day. Start at earliest symptom of cold sore. CrCl 30-49mL/min: 1g q12h. 10-29mL/min: 500mg q12h. <10mL/min: 500mg single dose. Administer therapy for 1 day. Initiate at earliest symptoms of a cold sore.

HOW SUPPLIED: Tab: 500mg, 1g
CONTRAINDICATIONS: Acyclovir hypersensitivity.
WARNINGS/PRECAUTIONS: Thrombotic thrombocytopenic purpura/hemolytic uremic syndrome reported with advanced HIV disease, allogenic bone marrow or renal transplants. Reduce dose with renal dysfunction. Possible renal and CNS toxicity in elderly.
ADVERSE REACTIONS: Nausea, headache, vomiting, dizziness, abdominal pain.
INTERACTIONS: Renal and CNS toxicity with nephrotoxic drugs.
PREGNANCY: Category B, caution in nursing.

VANCOCIN   RX
vancomycin HCl (Baxter)

THERAPEUTIC CLASS: Tricyclic glycopeptide antibiotic
INDICATIONS: Treatment of severe infections caused by susceptible strains of methicillin-resistant staphylococci. Indicated for penicillin-allergic patients, those who cannot receive or have failed to respond to other drugs, and for vancomycin-susceptible organisms that are resistant to other antimicrobials.
DOSAGE: *Adults:* Usual: 500mg IV q6h or 1g IV q12h. Mild to Moderate Renal Impairment: Initial: 15mg/kg/day. Maint: 1.9mg/kg/d. Administer 10mg/minute or over at least 60 minutes, whichever is longer. Renal Dysfunction: Initial: 15mg/kg. Dose is about 15x the GFR in mL/min (refer to table in labeling). Elderly: Require greater dose reduction. Functionally Anephric: Initial: 15mg/kg, then 1.9mg/kg/24hrs. Marked Renal Dysfunction: 250-1000mg every several days. Anuria: 1000mg every 7-10 days.
Pediatrics: Usual: 10mg/kg IV q6h. Infants/Neonates: Initial: 15mg/kg, then 10mg/kg q12h for neonates in the 1st week of life and q8h thereafter until 1 month of age. Administer over at least 60 minutes. Renal Dysfunction: Initial: 15mg/kg. Dose is about 15x the GFR in mL/min (refer to table in labeling). Premature Infants: Require greater dose reduction.
HOW SUPPLIED: Inj: 500mg/100mL, 1g/200mL
CONTRAINDICATIONS: Known allergy to corn or corn products because the solution contains dextrose.
WARNINGS/PRECAUTIONS: Only for colitis treatment; not systemically absorbed. Rapid bolus may cause hypotension, cardiac arrest (rare). Administer in a dilute solution over at least 60 minutes. Ototoxicity, pseudomembranous colitis reported. Adjust dose in renal dysfunction. Prolonged use may result in the overgrowth of nonsusceptible organisms. Monitor renal and auditory function. Reversible neutropenia reported; monitor leukocyte count periodically. Intrathecal safety has not been assessed.
ADVERSE REACTIONS: Infusion-related events, hypotension, wheezing, pruritus, pain, chest and head muscle spasm, dyspnea, urticaria, "Red Man Syndrome," nephrotoxicity, pseudomembranous colitis, ototoxicity, neutropenia, phlebitis.
INTERACTIONS: Infusion-related events (eg, erythema, flushing, anaphylactoid reactions) increases with anesthetic agents. Carefully monitor with other neurotoxic or nephrotoxic drugs (eg, amphotericin B, aminoglycosides, bacitracin, polymyxin B, colistin, or cisplatin).
PREGNANCY: Category C, not for use in nursing.

VANCOCIN ORAL   RX
vancomycin HCl (Viro Pharma)

THERAPEUTIC CLASS: Tricyclic glycopeptide antibiotic
INDICATIONS: Staphylococcal enterocolitis and antibiotic-associated pseudomembranous colitis caused by *C. difficile*.

DOSAGE: *Adults:* 500mg-2g/day given tid-qid for 7-10 days.

Pediatrics: 40mg/kg/day given tid-qid for 7-10 days. Max: 2g/day.

HOW SUPPLIED: Cap: 125mg, 250mg

WARNINGS/PRECAUTIONS: Not effective for other types of infection. Caution with inflammatory disorders of intestinal mucosa, renal impairment; increased risk of systemic absorption. Ototoxicity reported. Monitor auditory function.

ADVERSE REACTIONS: Nephrotoxicity, ototoxicity, reversible neutropenia, anaphylactoid reactions (hypotension, wheezing, "Red Man Syndrome," pruritus), superinfection.

INTERACTIONS: Monitor renal function with aminoglycosides.

PREGNANCY: Category B (Caps) or C (Susp), not for use in nursing.

VANIQA   RX
eflornithine HCl (SkinMedica)

THERAPEUTIC CLASS: Ornithine decarboxylase inhibitor

INDICATIONS: Reduction of unwanted facial hair in women. Usage is limited to the face and areas under the chin.

DOSAGE: *Adults:* Apply to affected areas bid, at least 8 hrs apart. Rub in thoroughly. May wash area after 4 hrs. May apply 5 minutes after other hair removal techniques. May apply sunscreen or cosmetics after cream dries.

Pediatrics: ≥12 yrs: Apply to affected areas bid, at least 8 hrs apart. Rub in thoroughly. May wash area after 4 hrs. May apply 5 minutes after other hair removal techniques. May apply sunscreen or cosmetics after cream dries.

HOW SUPPLIED: Cre: 13.9% (30g)

WARNINGS/PRECAUTIONS: Discontinue if hypersensitivity or continued irritation occurs. Transient stinging/burning with abraded/broken skin. Condition may return to pretreatment levels 8 weeks after discontinuation.

ADVERSE REACTIONS: Acne, stinging/tingling skin, burning/dry skin, pseudofolliculitis barbae, alopecia.

PREGNANCY: Category C, caution in nursing.

VANOS   RX
fluocinonide (Medicis)

THERAPEUTIC CLASS: Corticosteroid

INDICATIONS: Corticosteroid responsive dermatoses.

DOSAGE: *Adults:* Apply thin layer to affected area qd-bid. Max: 60g/week. Do not exceed 2 weeks.

Pediatrics: ≥12 yrs: Appy thin layer to affected area qd-bid. Max: 60g/week. Do not exceed 2 weeks.

HOW SUPPLIED: Cre: 0.1% (30g, 60g)

WARNINGS/PRECAUTIONS: May produce reversible HPA axis suppression, manifestations of Cushing's syndrome, hyperglycemia, and glucosuria. Caution when applied to large surface areas or under occlusal dressings. Use appropriate antifungal or antibacterial agent with dermatological infections. Discontinue if infection does not clear or if irritation develops. Do not use for more than 2 weeks at a time.

ADVERSE REACTIONS: Headache, application site burning, nasopharyngitis, nasal congestion, unspecified application site reaction.

PREGNANCY: Category C, not for use in nursing.

VANTIN   RX
cefpodoxime proxetil (Pharmacia & Upjohn)

THERAPEUTIC CLASS: Cephalosporin (3rd generation)

INDICATIONS: Acute otitis media, pharyngitis/tonsillitis, community acquired pneumonia (CAP), acute bacterial exacerbation of chronic bronchitis (ABECB), acute uncomplicated urethral and cervical gonorrhea, acute uncomplicated ano-rectal infections in women, uncomplicated skin and skin structure infections (SSSI), acute maxillary sinusitis, uncomplicated urinary tract infections (UTI).

DOSAGE: *Adults:* Take tabs with food. Pharyngitis/Tonsillitis: 100mg q12h for 5-10 days. CAP: 200mg q12h for 14 days. ABECB: 200mg q12h for 10 days. Uncomplicated Gonorrhea (men and women)/Rectal Gonococcal Infections (women): 200mg single dose. SSSI: 400mg q12h for 7-14 days. Sinusitis: 200mg q12h for 10 days. UTI: 100mg q12h for 7 days. CrCl <30mL/min: Increase interval to q24h. Hemodialysis: Dose 3 times weekly after dialysis.

Pediatrics: ≥12 yrs: Take tabs with food. Pharyngitis/Tonsillitis: 100mg q12h for 5-10 days. CAP: 200mg q12h for 14 days. ABECB: 200mg q12h for 10 days. Uncomplicated Gonorrhea (men and women)/Rectal Gonococcal Infections (women): 200mg single dose. SSSI: 400mg q12h for 7-14 days. Sinusitis: 200mg q12h for 10 days. UTI: 100mg q12h for 7 days. 2 months-11 yrs: Otitis Media: 5mg/kg q12h for 5 days. Max: 200mg/dose. Pharyngitis/Tonsillitis: 5mg/kg q12h for 5-10 days. Max: 100mg/dose. Sinusitis: 5mg/kg q12h for 10 days. Max: 200mg/dose. CrCl <30mL/min: Increase interval to q24h. Hemodialysis: Dose 3 times weekly after dialysis.

HOW SUPPLIED: Sus: 50mg/5mL (50mL, 100mL), 100mg/5mL (50mL, 75mL, 100mL); Tab: 100mg, 200mg

WARNINGS/PRECAUTIONS: Cross sensitivity to penicillins and other cephalosporins may occur. Pseudomembranous colitis reported. Positive direct Coombs' tests reported. Caution with renal dysfunction.

ADVERSE REACTIONS: Diarrhea, nausea, vaginal fungal infections, vulvovaginal infections, abdominal pain, headache, superinfection.

INTERACTIONS: Decreased plasma levels and absorption with antacids and H_2 blockers. Delayed peak plasma levels with anticholinergics. Probenecid inhibits renal excretion. Closely monitor renal function with nephrotoxic agents.

PREGNANCY: Category B, not for use in nursing.

VAQTA RX
hepatitis A vaccine (inactivated) (Merck)

THERAPEUTIC CLASS: Vaccine

INDICATIONS: Active immunization against hepatitis A virus in persons 12 months of age and older. Give primary immunization at least 2 weeks before expected exposure.

DOSAGE: *Adults:* ≥19 yrs: 1mL (50 U) IM followed by a booster of 1mL (50 U) 6-18 months later.

Pediatrics: 1-18 yrs: 0.5mL (25 U) IM followed by a booster of 0.5mL (25 U) 6-18 months later.

HOW SUPPLIED: Inj: 25 U/0.5mL, 50 U/mL

WARNINGS/PRECAUTIONS: Have epinephrine (1:1000) available. May not prevent hepatitis A with unrecognized infection. Caution with bleeding disorders. Defer use with acute infection or febrile illness. Suboptimal response may occur in immunocompromised patients.

ADVERSE REACTIONS: Injection-site pain, tenderness, erythema, swelling, warmth, fever.

INTERACTIONS: Immunosuppressive therapy may reduce response to active immunization.

PREGNANCY: Category C, caution in nursing.

VASOCON-A OTC
naphazoline HCl - antazoline phosphate (Novartis Ophthalmics)

THERAPEUTIC CLASS: Antihistamine/decongestant

INDICATIONS: Temporary relief of minor allergic symptoms of the eye, including itching and redness due to pollen and animal hair.

DOSAGE: *Adults:* 1-2 drops prn. Max: 4 doses/day.

Pediatrics: >6 yrs: 1-2 drops prn. Max: 4 doses/day.

HOW SUPPLIED: Sol: (Antazoline-Naphazoline) 0.5%-0.05% (15mL)

WARNINGS/PRECAUTIONS: Do not use if solution changes color or becomes cloudy. D/C if develop eye pain, vision changes, redness or irritaton continues, or if condition worsens or persists >72hrs. Supervision required with heart disease, HTN, or narrow angle glaucoma.

PREGNANCY: Safety in pregnancy and nursing not known.

VASOTEC RX
enalapril maleate (Merck)

> ACE inhibitors can cause death/injury to developing fetus during 2nd and 3rd trimesters. Stop therapy if pregnancy detected.

THERAPEUTIC CLASS: ACE inhibitor

INDICATIONS: Treatment of hypertension. Treatment of symptomatic CHF usually in combination with diuretics and digitalis. To decrease overt heart failure development and hospitalization in stable asymptomatic left ventricular dysfunction.

DOSAGE: *Adults:* HTN: If possible, discontinue diuretic 2-3 days prior to therapy. Initial: 5mg qd, 2.5mg qd with concomitant diuretic. Usual: 10-40mg/day given qd or bid. Resume diuretic if BP not controlled. CrCl ≤30mL/min: Initial: 2.5mg/day. Dialysis: 2.5mg/day on dialysis days. Heart Failure: Initial: 2.5mg/day. Usual: 2.5-20mg given bid. Max: 40mg/day. Left Ventricular Dysfunction: Initial: 2.5mg bid. Titrate: Increase to 20mg/day. Hyponatremia or SrCr 1.6mg/dL with Heart Failure: Initial: 2.5mg qd. Titrate: Increase to 2.5mg bid, then 5mg bid. Max: 40mg/day.

Pediatrics: HTN: 1 month-16 yrs: Initial: 0.08mg/kg (up to 5mg) qd. Titrate: Adjust according to response. Max: 0.58mg/kg/dose (or 40mg/dose). Avoid if GFR <30mL/min/1.73m^2. (To prepare 200mL of 1mg/mL sus: Add 50mL of Bicitra® to polyethylene terephthalate bottle with ten 20mg tabs and shake for at least 2 minutes. Let stand for 60 minutes, then shake again for 1 minute. Add 150mL of Ora-Sweet SF™ and shake, then refrigerate. Can store up to 30 days.)

HOW SUPPLIED: Tab: 2.5mg*, 5mg*, 10mg, 20mg *scored

CONTRAINDICATIONS: History of ACE inhibitor associated angioedema and hereditary or idiopathic angioedema.

WARNINGS/PRECAUTIONS: D/C if angioedema, jaundice, or if marked LFT elevation occurs. Risk of hyperkalemia with DM, renal dysfunction. Persistent nonproductive cough reported. Monitor WBCs in renal or collagen vascular disease. Anaphylactoid reactions reported. Fetal/neonatal morbidity and death reported. Monitor for hypotension in high risk patients (heart failure, surgery/anesthesia, hyponatremia, high dose diuretic therapy, severe volume and/or salt depletion, etc). Caution with CHF, obstruction to left ventricle outflow tract, renal dysfunction, and renal artery stenosis. Less effective on BP in blacks and more reports of angioedema than nonblacks.

ADVERSE REACTIONS: Fatigue, orthostatic effects, asthenia, diarrhea, nausea, headache, dizziness, cough, rash, hypotension, vomiting.

INTERACTIONS: May increase lithium levels. Hypotension risk with diuretics. May further decrease renal dysfunction with NSAIDs. Increase risk of hyperkalemia with K$^+$-sparing diuretics, K$^+$-containing salt substitutes or K$^+$ supplements. Augmented effect by antihypertensives that cause renin release (eg, thiazides). NSAIDs may diminish antihypertensive effect.

PREGNANCY: Category C (1st trimester) and D (2nd and 3rd trimesters), not for use in nursing.

VECURONIUM RX
vecuronium bromide (Various)

> Administer by adequately trained individuals familiar with actions, characteristics, and hazards.

THERAPEUTIC CLASS: Skeletal muscle relaxant (nondepolarizing)

INDICATIONS: Adjunct to general anesthesia, to facilitate endotracheal intubation, and to provide skeletal muscle relaxation during surgery or mechanical ventilation.

Ventolin HFA

DOSAGE: *Adults:* Individualize dose. Initial: 0.08-0.1mg/kg IV bolus. Maint: 0.01-0.015mg/kg IV within 25-40 minutes of initial dose. Administer subsequent doses at 12-15 minute intervals under balanced anesthesia and slightly longer with inhalation agents. Max: 0.15-0.28mg/kg. Prior Succinylcholine: Reduce dose to 0.04-0.06mg/kg with inhalation anesthesia and 0.05-0.06mg/kg with balanced anesthesia. Continuous Infusion: Initial: 1mcg/kg/min administered 20-40 minutes after intubating dose of 80-100mcg/kg. Administer infusion after evidence of recovery from bolus. Adjust infusion rate to maintain 90% suppression of twitch response. Maint: 0.8-1.2mcg/kg/min. Concurrent Steady-State Enflurane/Isoflurane: Reduce rate 25-60%, 45-60 minutes after intubating dose.

Pediatrics: 10-17 yrs: Individualize dose. Initial: 0.08-0.1mg/kg IV bolus. Maint: 0.01-0.015mg/kg IV within 25-40 minutes of initial dose. Administer subsequent dose at 12-15 minute intervals under balanced anesthesia and slightly longer with inhalation agents. Max: 0.15-0.28mg/kg. Prior Succinylcholine: Reduce dose to 0.04-0.06mg/kg with inhalation anesthesia and 0.05-0.06mg/kg with balanced anesthesia. Continuous Infusion: Initial: 1mcg/kg/min administered 20-40 minutes after intubating dose of 80-100mcg/kg. Administer infusion after evidence of recovery from bolus. Adjust infusion rate to maintain 90% suppression of twitch response. Maint: 0.8-1.2mcg/kg/min. Concurrent Steady-State Enflurane/Isoflurane: Reduce rate 25-60%, 45-60 minutes after intubating dose. 1-10 yrs: May require a slightly higher initial dose and may also require supplementation slightly more often than adults.

HOW SUPPLIED: Inj: 10mg, 20mg

WARNINGS/PRECAUTIONS: May have profound effect in myasthenia gravis or myasthenic (Eaton Lambert) syndrome; use small test dose and monitor closely. Prolongation of neuromuscular blockade may occur in anephric patients; consider lower initial dose. Conditions associated with slower circulation time in cardiovascular disease, old age, and edematous states may delay onset time; dosage should not be increased. Prolonged recovery time reported with cirrhosis or cholestasis. In ICU, long-term use may be associated with prolonged paralysis and/or skeletal muscle weakness. Monitor neuromuscular transmission of ICU patients continuously with a nerve stimulator. Severe obesity and neuromuscular disease may pose airway or ventilatory problems. Electrolyte imbalances may alter neuromuscular blockade.

ADVERSE REACTIONS: Skeletal muscle weakness and paralysis.

INTERACTIONS: Enhanced neuromuscular blocking action with pancuronium, d-tubocurarine, metocurine, gallamine, enflurane, isoflurane, halothane, aminoglycosides, tetracyclines, bacitracin, polymyxin B, colistin, sodium colistimethate, and magnesium salts. Possible synergistic or antagonistic effects with other muscle relaxants. Prior administration of succinylcholine may enhance neuromuscular blocking effect.

PREGNANCY: Category C, safety in nursing not known.

Ventolin HFA   RX
albuterol sulfate (GlaxoSmithKline)

THERAPEUTIC CLASS: Beta$_2$ agonist

INDICATIONS: Prevention and treatment of bronchospasm with reversible obstructive airway disease. Prevention of Exercise-Induced Bronchospasm (EIB).

DOSAGE: *Adults:* Bronchospasm: 2 inh q4-6h or 1 inh q4h. EIB: 2 inh 15-30 minutes before activity.

Pediatrics: ≥4 yrs: Bronchospasm: 2 inh q4-6h or 1 inh q4h. EIB: 2 inh 15-30 minutes before activity.

HOW SUPPLIED: MDI: 90mcg/inh (18g)

WARNINGS/PRECAUTIONS: D/C if paradoxical bronchospasm or cardiovascular events occur. Avoid excessive use. Caution with coronary insufficiency, arrhythmias, HTN, DM, hyperthyroidism, seizures, sensitivity to sympathomimetics. Hypersensitivity reactions may occur. May cause transient hypokalemia.

ADVERSE REACTIONS: Throat irritation, viral respiratory infections, upper respiratory inflammation, cough, musculoskeletal pain.

INTERACTIONS: Avoid other short-acting sympathomimetic bronchodilators; caution with oral sympathomimetics. Extreme caution with MAOIs, TCAs during or within 2 weeks of discontinuation. May cause severe bronchospasm with β-blockers. Decreases digoxin levels. ECG changes and/or hypokalemia with nonpotassium-sparing diuretics.

PREGNANCY: Category C, not for use in nursing.

Veramyst
fluticasone furoate (GlaxoSmithKline)   RX

THERAPEUTIC CLASS: Corticosteroid

INDICATIONS: Treatment of the symptoms of seasonal and perennial allergic rhinitis in patients ≥2 yrs.

DOSAGE: *Adults:* Initial: 2 sprays per nostril qd. Maint: 1 spray per nostril qd.
Pediatrics: ≥12 yrs: Initial: 2 sprays per nostril qd. Maint: 1 spray per nostril qd. 2-11 yrs: Initial: 1 spray per nostril qd. Titrate: If inadequate response, may increase to 2 sprays per nostril.

HOW SUPPLIED: Spray: 27.5mcg/spray (10g)

WARNINGS/PRECAUTIONS: Excessive use may cause hypercorticism and adrenal suppression. Risk of adrenal insufficiency and withdrawal symptoms when replacing systemic corticosteroids with topical corticosteroids. Caution with active or quiescent TB, ocular herpes simplex, or untreated bacterial, fungal, and systemic viral infections. Risk for more severe/fatal course of infections (eg, chickenpox, measles); avoid exposure in patients who have not had disease or have not been properly immunized. Epistaxis and nasal ulcerations may occur. Candida infection of nose reported. Avoid with recent nasal trauma, ulcers, or surgery. May result in glaucoma and cataracts. Potential for growth velocity reduction in pediatrics.

ADVERSE REACTIONS: Headache, epistaxis, nasopharyngitis, pyrexia, pharynolaryngeal pain, cough, nasal ulceration, back pain.

INTERACTIONS: Ketoconazole or other potent CYP3A4 inhibitors may increase serum fluticasone levels; co-administer with caution. Increased levels with ritonavir; avoid use.

PREGNANCY: Category C, caution in nursing.

Verdeso
desonide (Stiefel)   RX

THERAPEUTIC CLASS: Corticosteroid

INDICATIONS: Mild-to-moderate atopic dermatitis.

DOSAGE: *Adults:* Apply thin layer to affected area bid. Max Duration: 4 consecutive weeks. Not to dispense directly on face; use hands to gently massage. Avoid occlusive dressings.
Pediatrics: ≥3 months: Apply thin layer to affected area bid. Max Duration: 4 consecutive weeks. Not to dispense directly on face; use hands to gently massage. Avoid occlusive dressings.

HOW SUPPLIED: Foam: 0.05% (50g, 100g)

WARNINGS/PRECAUTIONS: May produce reversible HPA axis suppression, manifestations of Cushing's syndrome, hyperglycemia, and glucosuria. Discontinue if irritation occurs. Caution when applied to large surface areas. Pediatrics may be more susceptible to systemic toxicity. Use an appropriate antifungal or antibacterial with concomitatnt skin infections; discontinue if infection does not clear.

ADVERSE REACTIONS: Application site burning, upper respiratory tract infection, cough.

PREGNANCY: Category C, caution in nursing.

Versed Injection
midazolam HCl (Roche Labs)   CIV

> Associated with respiratory depression and respiratory arrest especially when used for sedation in non-critical care settings. Do not administer by rapid injection to neonates. Continuous monitoring required.

THERAPEUTIC CLASS: Benzodiazepine

VERSED SYRUP

INDICATIONS: For sedation, anxiolysis, and amnesia induction pre-op, prior to or during diagnostic, therapeutic, or endoscopic procedures, either alone or in combination with other CNS depressants. For induction of general anesthesia. For sedation of intubated and ventilated patients.

DOSAGE: *Adults:* IV: Sedation/Anxiolysis/Amnesia Induction: <60 yrs: Initial: 1-2.5mg IV over 2 min. Max: 5mg. Titrate: In small increments at 2 min intervals if needed. Concomitant Narcotics/Other CNS Depressants: Reduce by 30%. ≥60 yrs/Debilitated/Chronically Ill: Initial: 1-1.5mg IV over 2 min. Max: 3.5mg. Titrate: In small increments at 2 min intervals if needed. Concomitant Narcotics/Other CNS Depressants. Reduce by 50%. Maint: 25% of sedation dose by slow titration. IM: Preoperative Sedation/Anxiolysis/Amnesia: <60 yrs: 0.07-0.08mg/kg IM up to 1 hr before surgery. ≥60 yrs/Debilitated: 1-3mg IM. Anesthesia Induction: Unpremedicated: <55 yrs: Initially: 0.3-0.35mg/kg IV over 20-30 seconds. May give additional doses of 25% of initial dose to complete induction. ≥55 yrs: Initial: 0.3mg/kg IV. Debilitated: Initial: 0.15-0.25mg/kg IV. Premedicated: <55 yrs: Initial: 0.25mg/kg IV over 20-30 seconds. ≥55 yrs: Initial: 0.2mg/kg IV. Debilitated: 0.15mg/kg IV. Maintenance Sedation: LD: 0.01-0.05mg/kg IV. May repeat dose at 10-15 min intervals until adequate sedation. Maint: 0.02-0.1mg/kg/hr. Titrate to desired level of sedation using 25-50% adjustments. Infusion rate should be decreased 10-25% every few hrs to find minimum effective infusion rate.

Pediatrics: Sedation/Anxiolysis/Amnesia Induction: IV: <6 months: Limited information; titrate with small increments and monitor. 6 months-5 yrs: Initial: 0.05-0.1mg/kg IV over 2-3 min, up to 0.6mg/kg if needed. Max: 6mg. 6-12 yrs: Initial: 0.025-0.05mg/kg IV over 2-3 min, up to 0.4mg/kg if needed. Max: 10mg. 12-16 yrs: 1-2.5mg IV over 2 min. Titrate: In small increments at 2 min intervals if needed. Max: 10mg. IM: 0.1-0.15mg/kg IM, up to 0.5mg/kg if needed. Max: 10mg. Sedation: LD: 0.05-0.2mg/kg IV infusion over 2-3 min. Maint: 0.06-0.12mg/kg/hr IV infusion. May adjust dose by 25%. Sedation in Critical Care: Neonatal Dose: <32 weeks: Initial: 0.03mg/kg/hr IV infusion. >32 weeks: Initial: 0.06mg/kg/hr IV infusion. Adjust to lowest effective dose.

HOW SUPPLIED: Inj: 1mg/mL, 5mg/mL

CONTRAINDICATIONS: Acute narrow-angle glaucoma, untreated open-angle glaucoma, intrathecal or epidural use.

WARNINGS/PRECAUTIONS: Agitation, involuntary movements, hyperactivity, and combativeness reported. Caution with CHF, chronic renal failure, pulmonary disease, uncompensated acute illnesses (eg, severe fluid or electrolyte disturbances), elderly or debilitated. Avoid use with shock or coma, or in acute alcohol intoxication with depression of vital signs. Contains benzyl alcohol.

ADVERSE REACTIONS: Decreased tidal volume and/or respiratory rate, BP/HR variations, apnea, hypotension, pain and local reactions at injection site, hiccoughs, nausea, vomiting, desaturation.

INTERACTIONS: Prolonged sedation with CYP450 3A4 inhibitors (eg, erythromycin, diltiazem, verapamil, ketoconazole, itraconazole, saquinavir, cimetidine). Increased sedative effects with morphine, meperidine, fentanyl, secobarbital, droperidol or other CNS depressants. Avoid use with acute alcohol intoxication. Decreases concentration of halothane and thiopental required for anesthesia. May cause severe hypotension with concomitant use of fentanyl in neonates.

PREGNANCY: Category D, caution in nursing.

VERSED SYRUP
midazolam HCl (Roche Labs)

CIV

> Associated with respiratory depression and respiratory arrest especially when used for sedation in non-critical care settings. Reports of airway obstruction, desaturation, hypoxia, and apnea especially with other CNS depressants. Continuous monitoring required.

THERAPEUTIC CLASS: Benzodiazepine

INDICATIONS: Use in pediatric patients for sedation, anxiolysis and amnesia prior to diagnostic procedures or before induction of anesthesia.

DOSAGE: *Pediatrics:* 0.25-1mg/kg single dose. Max: 20mg.

HOW SUPPLIED: Syrup: 2mg/mL (118mL)

CONTRAINDICATIONS: Acute narrow-angle glaucoma.

WARNINGS/PRECAUTIONS: Monitor for respiratory adverse events and paradoxical reactions.

ADVERSE REACTIONS: Emesis, nausea, agitation, hypoxia, laryngospasm, bradycardia, prolonged sedation, rash.

INTERACTIONS: Decreased levels with CYP3A4 inducers (eg, rifampin, carbamazepine, phenytoin). Increased levels with CYP3A4 inhibitors (eg, azole antimycotics, protease inhibitors, calcium channel blockers, macrolide antibiotics, cimetidine). Increased sedative and respiratory effects with narcotics, propofol, ketamine, nitrous oxide, droperidol, barbiturates, alcohol and other CNS depressants. Caution with anesthetics.

PREGNANCY: Category D, caution in nursing.

Vesanoid RX
tretinoin (Roche Labs)

> Administer under strict supervision of experienced physician and institution. Risk of retinoic acid-APL syndrome and leukocytosis. High risk of teratogenic effects.

THERAPEUTIC CLASS: Retinoid

INDICATIONS: Induction of remission in acute promyelocytic leukemia (APL) in those resistant to anthracycline therapy or those where anthracycline-based therapy is contraindicated.

DOSAGE: *Adults:* 45mg/m^2/day in 2 divided doses. D/C 30 days after achieving complete remission or after 90 days of therapy, whichever occurs 1st.
Pediatrics: 45mg/m^2/day in 2 divided doses. D/C 30 days after achieving complete remission or after 90 days of therapy, whichever occurs 1st.

HOW SUPPLIED: Cap: 10mg

CONTRAINDICATIONS: Sensitivity to parabens.

WARNINGS/PRECAUTIONS: May cause abortion or fetal abnormalities. Females should use contraception during and 1 month after therapy. Confirm APL diagnosis. Pseudotumor cerebri reported, especially in pediatrics. Reversible hypercholesterolemia, hypertriglyceridemia reported. Elevated LFTs reported; d/c if >5x ULN. Monitor for signs of respiratory compromise or leukocytosis. Check hematologic profile, coagulation profile, LFTs, and cholesterol frequently.

ADVERSE REACTIONS: Malaise, shivering, hemorrhage, infections, peripheral edema, pain, chest discomfort, edema, disseminated intravascular coagulation, weight change, injection site reactions, dyspnea, pleural effusion, respiratory insufficiency, pneumonia.

INTERACTIONS: Possible interactions with drugs that affect CYP450 system. Aggravated symptoms of hypervitaminosis A with vitamin A. Cases of fatal thrombotic complications with antifibrinolytic agents (eg, tranexamic acid, aminocaproic acid).

PREGNANCY: Category D, not for use in nursing.

Vibramycin RX
doxycycline hyclate (Pfizer)

OTHER BRAND NAMES: Vibra-Tabs (Pfizer)

THERAPEUTIC CLASS: Tetracycline derivative

INDICATIONS: Treatment of susceptible infections including respiratory, urinary, skin and skin structure, lymphogranuloma, psittacosis, trachoma, uncomplicated urethral/endocervical/rectal, nongonococcal urethritis, rickettsiae, chancroid, plague, cholera, brucellosis, anthrax. When penicillin is contraindicated, treatment of uncomplicated gonorrhea, syphilis, listeriosis, *Clostridium* species, and others. Adjunct therapy for amebiasis and severe acne. Prophylaxis of malaria.

DOSAGE: *Adults:* Usual: 100mg q12h on day 1, then 100mg qd or 50mg q12h. Severe Infection: 100mg q12h. Treat for 10 days with strep infection. Uncomplicated Gonococcal Infection (Except Anorectal in Men): 100mg bid for 7 days or 300mg followed by 300mg in 1 hour. Uncomplicated Urethral/Endocervical/Rectal Infection and

Vibramycin IV

Nongonococcal Urethritis: 100mg bid for 7 days. Syphilis: 100mg bid for 2 weeks. Syphilis for >1 yr: 100mg bid for 4 weeks. Acute Epididymo-orchitis: 100mg bid for at least 10 days. Inhalation Anthrax (Post-Exposure): 100mg bid for 60 days. Malaria Prophylaxis: 100mg qd. Begin 1-2 days before travel and continue for 4 weeks after leaving malarious area.

Pediatrics: >8 yrs: ≤100 lbs: 1mg/lb bid on day 1, then 1mg/lb qd or 0.5mg/lb bid. Severe Infections: Maint: 2mg/lb. >100lbs: Usual: 100mg q12h on day 1, then 100mg qd or 50mg q12h. Severe Infection: 100mg q12h. Treat for 10 days with strep infection. Inhalation Anthrax (Post-Exposure): <100lbs: 1mg/lb bid for 60 days. ≥100lbs: 100mg bid for 60 days. Malaria Prophylaxis: 2mg/kg qd. Max: 100mg/day. Begin 1-2 days before travel and continue for 4 weeks after leaving malarious area.

HOW SUPPLIED: Cap: (Doxycycline Hyclate) 50mg, 100mg; Syr: (Doxycycline Calcium) 50mg/5mL; Sus: (Doxycycline Monohydrate) 25mg/5mL (60mL); Tab: (Vibra-Tabs) 100mg

WARNINGS/PRECAUTIONS: May cause fetal harm with pregnancy. Permanent tooth discoloration during tooth development (last half of pregnancy and children <8 yrs) reported. May increase BUN. Photosensitivity, enamel hypoplasia reported. Superinfection with prolonged use. Syrup contains sodium metabisulfite. Bulging fontanels in infants and benign intracranial HTN in adults reported. Monitor renal/hepatic and hematopoietic function with long-term use. Take adequate fluids with caps or tabs to reduce esophageal irritation. Take with food or milk if GI irritation occurs.

ADVERSE REACTIONS: GI effects, photosensitivity, increased BUN, hypersensitivity reactions, blood dyscrasias.

INTERACTIONS: May decrease PT, adjust anticoagulants. May interfere with bactericidal agents (eg, penicillin). May decrease effects of oral contraceptives. Aluminum-, calcium-, iron- and magnesium-containing products and bismuth subsalicylate impair absorption. Decreased half-life with barbiturates, carbamazepine, and phenytoin. Fatal renal toxicity with methoxyflurane.

PREGNANCY: Category D, not for use in nursing.

Vibramycin IV   RX
doxycycline hyclate (Pfizer)

THERAPEUTIC CLASS: Tetracycline derivative

INDICATIONS: Treatment of rickettsiae, *Mycoplasma pneumoniae*, psittacosis, ornithosis, lymphogranuloma venereum, granuloma inguinale, relapsing fever, chancroid, *Pasteurella pestis*, *Pasturella tularensis*, *Bartonella bacilliformis*, *Bacteroides* species, *Vibrio comma*, *Vibrio fetus*, *Brucella* species, *E.coli*, *Enterobacter aerogenes*, *Shigella* species, *Mima* species, *Herellea* species, *Haemophilus influenzae*, *Klebsiella* species, *Streptococcus* species, *Diplococcus pneumoniae*, *Staphylococcus aureus*, anthrax, and trachoma. When PCN is contraindicated; treatment of *Neisseria gonorrhoeae*, *N.meningitidis*, syphilis, yaws, *Listeria monocytogenes*, *Clostridium* species, *Fusobacterium fusiforme* and *Actinomyces* species. Adjunct therapy for amebiasis.

DOSAGE: *Adults:* Usual: 200mg IV divided qd-bid on Day 1 then 100-200mg/day IV depending on severity, with 200mg administered in 1 or 2 infusions. Primary/Secondary Syphilis: 300mg/day IV for at least 10 days. Inhalational Anthrax (Post-Exposure): 100mg IV bid. Institute oral therapy as soon as possible and continue therapy for a total of 60 days.

Pediatrics: >8 yrs: >100 lbs: Usual: 200mg IV divided qd-bid on Day 1 then 100-200mg/day IV depending on severity, with 200mg administered in 1 or 2 infusions. ≤100 lbs: 2mg/lb IV divided qd-bid on Day 1 then 1-2mg/lb/day IV divided qd-bid depending on severity. Inhalational Anthrax (Post-Exposure): <100 lbs: 1 mg/lb IV bid. Institute oral therapy as soon as possible and continue therapy for a total of 60 days.

HOW SUPPLIED: Inj: 100mg, 200mg

WARNINGS/PRECAUTIONS: May cause fetal harm during pregnancy. Permanent tooth discoloration during tooth development (last half of pregnancy and children <8 yrs) reported; avoid use in this age group except for anthrax treatment. Decreased bone growth in premature infants reported. May increase BUN. Photosensitivity, enamel hypoplasia reported. Superinfection with prolonged use. Monitor hematopoietic, renal and hepatic values periodically with long term therapy. Bulging fontanels in infants and benign intracranial HTN in adults reported.

VICOPROFEN
ibuprofen - hydrocodone bitartrate (Abbott)

CIII

OTHER BRAND NAME: Reprexain (Watson)

THERAPEUTIC CLASS: Opioid analgesic

INDICATIONS: Short-term (generally <10 days) management of acute pain.

DOSAGE: *Adults:* Usual: 1 tab q4-6h prn. Max: 5 tabs/day. Elderly: Use lowest dose or longest interval.
Pediatrics: ≥16 yrs: Usual: 1 tab q4-6h prn. Max: 5 tabs/day.

HOW SUPPLIED: (Hydrocodone-Ibuprofen) Tab: (Vicoprofen) 7.5mg-200mg; (Reprexain) 5mg-200mg* *scored

CONTRAINDICATIONS: ASA or other NSAID allergy that precipitates asthma, urticaria, or other allergic reaction.

WARNINGS/PRECAUTIONS: May produce dose-related respiratory depression. May obscure acute abdominal conditions or head injuries. Avoid with ASA triad, late pregnancy, advanced renal disease, ASA-sensitive asthma. Caution in elderly, debilitated, dehydration, renal disease, intrinsic coagulation defects, severe hepatic dysfunction, asthma, hypothyroidism, Addison's disease, prostatic hypertrophy, urethral stricture, heart failure, HTN, ulcer disease, pulmonary disease, postoperative use. May be habit-forming. Suppresses cough reflex. Risk of GI ulceration, bleeding, perforation. Anemia, fluid retention, edema, severe hepatic reactions reported. Possible risk of aseptic meningitis, especially in SLE patients. Increased risk of serious cardiovascular thrombotic events, MI and stroke. Fluid retention and edema observed. Skin reactions (eg, exfoliative dermatitis, TEN, SJS) can occur.

ADVERSE REACTIONS: Headache, somnolence, dizziness, constipation, dyspepsia, nausea, vomiting, infection, edema, nervousness, anxiety, pruritus, diarrhea, asthenia, abdominal pain, insomnia, dry mouth, sweating.

INTERACTIONS: Additive CNS depression with other narcotics, antihistamines, antipsychotics, antianxiety agents, alcohol, CNS depressants. Increased effect of antidepressant or hydrocodone with MAOIs or TCAs. May produce paralytic ileus with anticholinergics. May decrease effects of furosemide and thiazide diuretics, ACE-inhibitors. Avoid ASA. Risk of serious GI bleeding with warfarin. May enhance methotrexate toxicity. Monitor for lithium toxicity.

PREGNANCY: Category C, not for use in nursing.

VIDEX
didanosine (Bristol-Myers Squibb)

RX

> Fatal/nonfatal pancreatitis, lactic acidosis, and severe hepatomegaly with steatosis reported. Suspend therapy if suspect pancreatitis and discontinue if pancreatitis confirmed. Fatal lactic acidosis reported in pregnant women receiving concomitant stavudine.

OTHER BRAND NAME: Videx EC (Bristol-Myers Squibb)

THERAPEUTIC CLASS: Nucleoside analogue

INDICATIONS: Treatment of HIV-1 infection in combination with other antiretrovirals (use Videx EC when management requires once daily dosing or alternative didanosine formulation).

DOSAGE: *Adults:* ≥60kg: (Cap) 400mg qd; (Sol) 200mg bid or 400mg qd. <60kg: (Cap) 250mg qd; (Sol) 125mg bid or 250mg qd. CrCl 30-59mL/min: ≥60kg: (Cap) 200mg qd; (Sol) 200mg qd or 100mg qd. <60kg: (Cap) 125mg qd; (Sol) 150mg qd or 75mg bid. CrCl 10-29mL/min: ≥60kg: (Cap) 125mg qd; (Sol) 150mg qd. <60kg: (Cap) 125mg qd; (Sol) 100mg qd. CrCl <10mL/min: ≥60kg: (Cap) 125mg qd; (Sol) 100mg qd. <60kg:

(Sol) 75mg qd. Concomitant Viread: CrCl ≥60mL/min :≥60kg: 250mg qd; <60kg: 200mg qd. Take on empty stomach at least 30 minutes before or 2 hrs after meals. Swallow caps whole.

Pediatrics: 2 weeks-8 months: (Sol) 100mg/m^2 bid. >8 months: 120mg/m^2 bid.

HOW SUPPLIED: Sol: 2g, 4g (120mL, 240mL); Cap, Delayed Release: (Videx EC) 125mg, 200mg, 250mg, 400mg

WARNINGS/PRECAUTIONS: Risk of toxicity with CrCl <60mL/min; reduce dose. Retinal changes and optic neuritis reported; perform periodic retinal exams. Peripheral neuropathy reported. Caution with hepatic dysfunction. May cause asymptomatic hyperuricemia. Twice daily dosing is preferred over once daily dosing. Chewable tabs contain phenylalanine. Caution with sodium restricted diets; buffered powder solution contains 1380mg sodium. Monitor for lactic acidosis in pregnancy if used with stavudine. Possible redistribution or accumulation of fat. Immune reconstitution syndrome has been reported in patients treated with combination antiretroviral therapy. Fatal and non-fatal pancreatitis reported; increased risk in combination with stavudine, with or without hydroxyurea.

ADVERSE REACTIONS: Pancreatitis, lactic acidosis, hepatomegaly, visual changes, diarrhea, neuropathy, abdominal pain, headache, nausea, vomiting, rash, elevated LFTs.

INTERACTIONS: Extreme caution with drugs that may cause pancreatitis. Increase risk of peripheral neuropathy with neurotoxic agents (eg, stavudine). Aluminum- and magnesium-containing antacids may potentiate adverse events. Space dose by 2 hrs of drugs whose absorption can be affected by stomach acidity (eg, ketoconazole, itraconazole). Increased serum levels with oral ganciclovir. Space dose by 2 hrs after or 6 hrs before ciprofloxacin. Avoid allopurinol. Decreased serum levels with methadone. Caution with tenofovir or ribavirin; monitor closely for didanosine-related toxicities and suspend therapy if signs of pancreatitis, symptomatic hyperlactatemia, or lactic acidosis develop.

PREGNANCY: Category B, not for use in nursing.

VIGAMOX   RX
moxifloxacin HCl (Alcon)

THERAPEUTIC CLASS: Fluoroquinolone

INDICATIONS: Treatment of bacterial conjunctivitis.

DOSAGE: *Adults:* 1 drop tid for 7 days.

Pediatrics: ≥1 yr: 1 drop tid for 7 days.

HOW SUPPLIED: Sol: 0.5% (3mL)

WARNINGS/PRECAUTIONS: Not for injection. Do not inject subconjunctivally or into the anterior chamber of the eye. Superinfection may result with prolonged use. Fatal hypersensitivity reactions reported after first dose of systemic quinolone therapy. Avoid contact lenses when symptoms are present.

ADVERSE REACTIONS: Conjunctivitis, decreased visual acuity, dry eye, keratitis, ocular discomfort/hyperemia, ocular pain/pruritus, subconjunctival hemorrhage, tearing.

PREGNANCY: Category C, caution in nursing.

VINBLASTINE   RX
vinblastine sulfate (Various)

> For IV use only; fatal if given intrathecally. Considerable irritation if leakage occurs into surrounding tissue. If this occurs, discontinue and restart in another vein. Heat and hyaluronidase minimize discomfort and cellulitis.

THERAPEUTIC CLASS: Vinca alkaloid

INDICATIONS: Palliative treatment of generalized Hodgkin's disease (Stages III and IV), lymphocytic lymphoma, histiocytic lymphoma, advanced mycosis fungoides, advanced testis carcinoma, Kaposi's sarcoma, Letterer-Siwe disease, and resistant choriocarcinoma and unresponsive breast carcinoma.

VINCRISTINE SULFATE

DOSAGE: *Adults:* Dose at intervals of ≤7 days. 1st Dose: 3.7mg/m^2. 2nd Dose: 5.5mg/m^2. 3rd Dose: 7.4mg/m^2. 4th Dose: 9.25mg/m^2. 5th Dose: 11.1mg/m^2. Max: 18.5mg/m^2. Do not increase dose after that dose which reduces WBC to 3000 cells/mm^3. Maint: Use dose of 1 increment smaller than this dose at weekly intervals. Reduce to 50% dose if direct serum bilirubin >3mg/100mL. Only dose if WBC ≥4000cells/mm^3.

Pediatrics: Dose at intervals of ≤7 days. 1st Dose: 2.5mg/m^2. 2nd Dose: 3.75mg/m^2. 3rd Dose: 5mg/m^2. 4th Dose: 6.25mg/m^2. 5th Dose: 7.5mg/m^2. Max: 12.5mg/m^2. Do not increase dose after that dose which reduces WBC to 3000 cells/mm^3. Maint: Use dose of 1 increment smaller than this dose at weekly intervals. Reduce to 50% dose if direct serum bilirubin >3mg/100mL. Only dose if WBC ≥4000cells/mm^3.

HOW SUPPLIED: Inj: 1mg/mL, 10mg

CONTRAINDICATIONS: Significant granulocytopenia (unless result of disease being treated), bacterial infections.

WARNINGS/PRECAUTIONS: Avoid pregnancy. Acute shortness of breath, severe bronchospasm, aspermia, stomatitis, neurologic toxicity reported. Increased toxicity with hepatic insufficiency. Monitor for infection with WBC <2000cells/mm^3. Avoid with malignant-cell infiltration of bone marrow, or in older persons with cachexia or ulcerated skin. Small daily amounts for long periods is not advised. Avoid eye contamination. Monitor WBCs. May cause fetal harm during pregnancy.

ADVERSE REACTIONS: Leukopenia (granulocytopenia), anemia, thrombocytopenia, alopecia, constipation, anorexia, nausea, vomiting, abdominal pain, diarrhea, HTN, paresthesis.

INTERACTIONS: May increase phenytoin metabolism/elimination, or decrease phenytoin absorption. Caution with CYP3A inhibitors (eg, erythromycin, doxorubicin, etoposide), or with hepatic dysfunction; may cause earlier onset and/or an increased severity of side effects. Increased risk of acute shortness of breath and severe bronchospasm with mitomycin-C.

PREGNANCY: Category D, not for use in nursing.

VINCRISTINE SULFATE RX
vincristine sulfate (Pharmacia & Upjohn)

> Properly position IV needle or catheter before injection; considerable irritation with extravasation. Use hyaluronidase and heat to minimize discomfort and cellulitis with extravasation. Fatal with intrathecal use. For IV use only.

THERAPEUTIC CLASS: Vinca alkaloid

INDICATIONS: For treatment of acute leukemia. As an adjunct in the treatment of Hodgkin's disease, non-Hodgkin's malignant lymphomas, rhabdomyosarcoma, neuroblastoma, and Wilms' tumor.

DOSAGE: *Adults:* Usual: 1.4mg/m^2 IV at weekly intervals. Bilirubin >3mg/dL: 50% dose reduction.

Pediatrics: Usual: 2mg/m^2 IV at weekly intervals. ≤10kg: Initial: 0.05mg/kg IV once weekly. Bilirubin >3mg/dL: 50% dose reduction.

HOW SUPPLIED: Inj: 1mg/mL

CONTRAINDICATIONS: Demyelinating form of Charcot-Marie-Tooth syndrome.

WARNINGS/PRECAUTIONS: Acute uric acid nephropathy may occur. May require additional agents with CNS leukemia. Neurotoxicity is dose-limiting toxicity. Perform CBC before each dose. Determine serum uric acid levels frequently during 1st 3-4 weeks. Acute shortness of breath, severe bronchospasm reported. Monitor with pre-existing neuromuscular disease. Avoid eye contamination. May cause fetal harm during pregnancy.

ADVERSE REACTIONS: Alopecia, abdominal cramps, weight loss, nausea, vomiting, diarrhea, constipation, paralytic ileus, HTN, hypotension, polyuria, dysuria, urinary retention, sensory impairment, paresthesia, neuritic pain, motor difficulties, rash, fever.

INTERACTIONS: Reduced levels of phenytoin and increased seizures reported. Increased risk of acute shortness of breath and severe bronchospasm with mitomycin-C. Monitor with other neurotoxic agents. Discontinue drugs known to cause urinary retention for 1st few days after administration. Give 12-24 hrs before L-asparaginase therapy to minimize toxicity. Do not give with radiation therapy through ports that include the liver. Do not dilute in solutions that raise or lower the pH outside the range of 3.5-5.5.

PREGNANCY: Category D, not for use in nursing.

VIOKASE
lipase - amylase - protease (Axcan Scandipharm)

RX

THERAPEUTIC CLASS: Pancreatic enzyme supplement

INDICATIONS: Treatment of pancreatic exocrine insufficiency (eg, cystic fibrosis, chronic pancreatitis, pancreatectomy, and pancreatic ductal obstruction).

DOSAGE: *Adults:* (Powder) Cystic Fibrosis: 0.7g (1/2 tsp) with meals. (Tab) Cystic Fibrosis/Pancreatitis: 8,000-32,000 U Lipase with meals. Pancreatectomy/Pancreatic Duct Obstruction: 8,000-16,000 U Lipase q2h.

Pediatrics: (Powder) Cystic Fibrosis: 0.7g (1/2 tsp) with meals. (Tab) Cystic Fibrosis/Pancreatitis: 8,000-32,000 U Lipase with meals. Pancreatectomy/Pancreatic Duct Obstruction: 8,000-16,000 U Lipase q2h.

HOW SUPPLIED: (Amylase-Lipase-Protease) Powder: 70,000 U-16,800 U-70,000 U/0.7g (240g); Tab: (Viokase 8) 30,000 U-8,000 U-30,000 U; (Viokase 16) 60,000 U-16,000 U-60,000 U

CONTRAINDICATIONS: Pork protein hypersensitivity.

WARNINGS/PRECAUTIONS: May have allergic reactions if previously sensitized to trypsin, pancreatin or pancrelipase. Irritating to oral mucosa if held in mouth. Inhalation of powder can cause an asthma attack. High doses can cause hyperuricemia and hyperuricosuria.

ADVERSE REACTIONS: Irritation to nasal mucosa and respiratory tract with inhaled powder.

PREGNANCY: Category C, caution in nursing.

VIRA-A
vidarabine (King)

RX

THERAPEUTIC CLASS: Purine nucleoside antiviral

INDICATIONS: Treatment of acute keratoconjunctivitis and recurrent epithelial keratitis due to HSV1 and HSV2. Effective in superficial keratitis due to HSV unresponsive to or intolerant to idoxuridine.

DOSAGE: *Adults:* Apply 1/2 inch 5 times daily at 3-hr intervals. Discontinue, if no improvement after 7 days or incomplete re-epithelialization by 21 days. Continue for 7 more days at a reduced dose (eg, bid) after re-epithelialization.

Pediatrics: ≥2 yrs: Apply 1/2 inch 5 times daily at 3 hr intervals. Discontinue, if no improvement after 7 days or incomplete re-epithelialization by 21 days. Continue for 7 more days at a reduced dose (eg, bid) after re-epithelialization.

HOW SUPPLIED: Oint: 3% (3.5g)

WARNINGS/PRECAUTIONS: May produce temporary visual haze. Establish diagnosis of keratoconjunctivitis due to HSV before starting therapy. Not for RNA virus, adenoviral ocular infection, bacterial, fungal or chlamydial infections.

ADVERSE REACTIONS: Lacrimation, foreign body sensation, conjunctival injection, burning, irritation, superficial punctate keratitis, pain, photophobia, punctal occlusion.

PREGNANCY: Category C, not for use in nursing.

VIRACEPT
nelfinavir mesylate (Pfizer)

RX

THERAPEUTIC CLASS: Protease inhibitor

INDICATIONS: Treatment of HIV infection in combination with other antiretrovirals.

DOSAGE: *Adults:* 1250mg bid or 750mg tid. Concomitant rifabutin: Reduce rifabutin dose by one-half and nelfinavir 1250mg bid is preferred dose. Take with a meal or light snack. May crush or dissolve whole tab in water or mix in food and consume immediately. May store mixture under refrigeration up to 6 hrs.

Pediatrics: 2-13 yrs: 20-30mg/kg tid. Take with a meal or light snack. May mix powder with non-acidic liquid (eg, water, milk, formula, etc.); consume immediately. May store up to 6 hrs under refrigeration.

HOW SUPPLIED: Sus: (powder) 50mg/g (144g); Tab: 250mg, 625mg

CONTRAINDICATIONS: Concomitant pimozide, triazolam, midazolam, ergot derivatives, amiodarone or quinidine.

WARNINGS/PRECAUTIONS: Powder contains phenylalanine. New-onset DM, exacerbation of DM and hyperglycemia reported. Register pregnant patients (800-258-4263). Caution with hepatic dysfunction. Increased bleeding reported. Possible redistribution or accumulation of fat.

ADVERSE REACTIONS: Diarrhea, nausea, flatulence, rash, redistribution of body fat, jaundice, hypersensitivity reactions, bilirubinemia, hyperglycemia, metabolic acidosis.

INTERACTIONS: See Contraindications. Avoid pimozide, triazolam, midazolam, ergot derivatives, amiodarone or quinidine; potential for life-threatening adverse events. Avoid rifampin. Avoid lovastatin or simvastatin; caution with other HMG-CoA reductase inhibitors. May increase sildenafil levels and adverse effects. Avoid St. John's wort; may decrease levels of nelfinavir. May increase levels of drugs metabolized by CYP450 3A (eg, dihydropyridine calcium channel blockers, immunosuppressants, etc). Use alternative or additional contraception with oral contraceptives. May increase levels of cyclosporine, tacrolimus, sirolimus, atorvastatin, cerivastatin, fluticasone, azithromycin. Carbamazepine, phenobarbital may decrease levels of nelfinavir. May decrease levels of phenytoin, methadone. Give didanosine 1 hr before or 2 hrs after nelfinavir. Omeprazole decreases levels of nelfinavir; concomitant use with proton pump inhibitors may lead to loss of virologic response and development of resistance.

PREGNANCY: Category B, not for use in nursing.

VIRAMUNE
nevirapine (Boehringer Ingelheim) — RX

> Severe, life-threatening, in some cases fatal, hepatotoxicity and skin reactions (eg, Stevens-Johnson syndrome, toxic epidermal necrolysis, hypersensitivity) reported. Women, including pregnant women, and/or patients with higher CD4 counts are at higher risk of hepatotoxicity. Permanently discontinue following severe hepatitic, skin or hypersensitivity reactions.

THERAPEUTIC CLASS: Non-nucleoside reverse transcriptase inhibitor

INDICATIONS: Treatment of HIV-1 infection in combination with other antiretrovirals.

DOSAGE: *Adults:* 200mg qd for 14 days (lead-in period), then 200mg bid. Do not increase dose if rash occurs, until it resolves. Retitrate if interrupt >7 days.

Pediatrics: 2 months-8 yrs: 4mg/kg qd for 14 days, then 7mg/kg bid. Max: 400mg/day. ≥8 yrs: 4mg/kg qd for 14 days, then 4mg/kg bid. Max: 400mg/day. Do not increase dose if rash occurs, until it resolves. Retitrate if interrupt >7 days.

HOW SUPPLIED: Sus: 50mg/5mL (240mL); Tab: 200mg* *scored

WARNINGS/PRECAUTIONS: Avoid with severe hepatic impairment. Caution with moderate impairment and dialysis. Perform laboratory tests (eg, LFTs) at baseline and during first 18 weeks of therapy. Possible redistribution or accumulation of body fat.

ADVERSE REACTIONS: Headache, fever, severe rash, GI effects, fatigue, thrombocytopenia, fatigue, hepatotoxicity, granulocytopenia (pediatrics).

INTERACTIONS: Avoid use of prednisone for prevention of therapy-associated rash. Decreased levels of clarithromycin; consider alternative. Decreased levels of efavirenz, indinavir, nelfinavir, saquinavir. May decrease effectiveness of oral contraceptives and other hormonal contraceptives; use alternate or additional method of contraception. Increased levels with fluconazole. Avoid with ketoconazole, St. John's wort, rifampin. Decreased levels of lopinavir; adjust lopinavir/ritonavir doses. May decrease levels of methadone; monitor for signs of withdrawal. Increased levels of rifabutin. Possible

VIRAZOLE

decreased levels with antiarrhythmics (eg, amiodarone, disopyramide, lidocaine), anticonvulsants (eg, carbamazepine, clonazepam, ethosuximide), itraconazole, calcium channel blockers (eg, diltiazem, nifedipine, verapamil), cyclophosphamide, ergotamine, immunosuppressants (eg, cyclosporine, tacrolimus, sirolimus), cisapride, fentanyl. Monitor with warfarin.

PREGNANCY: Category C, not for use in nursing.

Virazole
ribavirin (Valeant)

RX

> Sudden deterioration of respiratory function associated with initiation in infants. Monitor respiratory function carefully. Not for use in adults. Use with mechanical ventilator assistance with staff familiar with mode of administration and specific type of ventilator.

THERAPEUTIC CLASS: Nucleoside analogue

INDICATIONS: Treatment of hospitalized infants and young children with severe lower respiratory tract infections due to respiratory syncytial virus.

DOSAGE: *Pediatrics:* Continuous aerosol administration of 20mg/mL in the drug reservoir of the SPAG-2 unit for 12-18 hrs/day for 3-7 days.

HOW SUPPLIED: Sol, Inhalation: 6g

CONTRAINDICATIONS: Women who are or may become pregnant during exposure to drug.

WARNINGS/PRECAUTIONS: Monitor respiratory function and fluid status according to SPAG-2 manual. Accumulation of drug precipitate can result in mechanical ventilator dysfunction and associated increased pulmonary pressures.

ADVERSE REACTIONS: Worsening of respiratory status, bronchospasm, pulmonary edema, hypoventilation, cyanosis, dyspnea, bacterial pneumonia, pneumothorax, apnea, atelectasis, ventilator dependence, cardiac arrest, hypotension, bradycardia.

INTERACTIONS: Digoxin toxicity reported.

PREGNANCY: Category X, safety in nursing not known.

Viroptic
trifluridine (King)

RX

THERAPEUTIC CLASS: Fluorinated pyrimidine nucleoside antiviral

INDICATIONS: Treatment of primary keratoconjunctivitis and recurrent epithelial keratitis due to herpes simplex virus, types 1 and 2.

DOSAGE: *Adults:* 1 drop q2h while awake until re-epithelialization. Max: 9 drops/day. Following Re-epithelialization: 1 drop q4h while awake for 7 days; minimum of 5 drops/day. If no improvement after 7 days or if complete re-epithelialization has not occurred after 14 days, consider other therapy. Avoid using >21 days.

Pediatrics: ≥6 yrs: 1 drop q2h while awake until re-epithelialization. Max: 9 drops/day. Following Re-epithelialization: 1 drop q4h while awake for 7 days; minimum of 5 drops/day. If no improvement after 7 days or if complete re-epithelialization has not occurred after 14 days, consider other therapy. Avoid using >21 days.

HOW SUPPLIED: Sol: 1% (7.5mL)

WARNINGS/PRECAUTIONS: Only use with a clinical diagnosis of herpetic keratitis. May cause transient, mild local irritation of the conjunctiva and cornea when instilled.

ADVERSE REACTIONS: Burning, stinging, palpebral edema, superficial punctate keratopathy, epithelial keratopathy, hypersensitivity reaction, stromal edema, irritation, keratitis sicca, hyperemia, increased IOP.

PREGNANCY: Category C, caution in nursing.

Visine A.C.
zinc sulfate - tetrahydrozoline HCl (McNeil)

OTC

THERAPEUTIC CLASS: Decongestant/astringent

INDICATIONS: Temporary relief of discomfort and redness of the eyes due to minor eye irritations.

DOSAGE: *Adults:* 1-2 drops in affected eye up to qid.
Pediatrics: ≥6 yrs: 1-2 drops in affected eye up to qid.
HOW SUPPLIED: Sol: (Tetrahydrozoline-Zinc) 0.05%-0.25% (15mL, 30mL)
WARNINGS/PRECAUTIONS: May temporarily enlarge pupils. Overuse may cause more redness. Remove contact lenses before use. Do not touch container tip to any surface to avoid contamination. D/C if eye pain or vision changes occur, if redness or irritation continues, or if condition worsens or continues >72 hrs. Supervision required with glaucoma.
ADVERSE REACTIONS: Brief tingling sensation.
PREGNANCY: Safety in pregnancy and nursing not known.

VISINE ADVANCED RELIEF OTC
povidone - dextran 70 - polyethylene glycol 400 - tetrahydrozoline HCl (McNeil)

THERAPEUTIC CLASS: Decongestant/lubricant
INDICATIONS: Relief of eye redness due to minor eye irritations. Use as a protectant against further irritation or to relieve eye dryness.
DOSAGE: *Adults:* 1-2 drops in affected eye up to qid.
Pediatrics: ≥6 yrs: 1-2 drops in affected eye up to qid.
HOW SUPPLIED: Sol: (Dextran 70-Polyethylene Glycol 400-Povidone, Tetrahydrozoline) 0.05%-0.1%-1%-1%-0.05% (15mL, 30mL)
WARNINGS/PRECAUTIONS: May temporarily enlarge pupils. Overuse may cause more redness. Remove contact lenses before use. Do not touch container tip to any surface to avoid contamination. D/C if eye pain or vision changes occur, if redness or irritation continues, or if condition worsens or continues >72 hrs. Supervision required with glaucoma.
PREGNANCY: Safety in pregnancy and nursing not known.

VISINE FOR CONTACTS OTC
glycerin - hydroxypropyl methylcellulose (McNeil)

THERAPEUTIC CLASS: Lubricant
INDICATIONS: To moisten daily wear soft lenses while on the eyes during the day. To moisten extended wear soft lenses upon awakening, prior to retiring at night, and as needed during the day.
DOSAGE: *Adults:* Use prn throughout the day. Minor Irritation/Discomfort/Blurring With Lenses: Instill 1-2 drops on eye and blink 2-3 times. If discomfort continues; remove lenses.
Pediatrics: Use prn throughout the day. Minor Irritation/Discomfort/Blurring With Lenses: Instill 1-2 drops on eye and blink 2-3 times. If discomfort continues; remove lenses.
HOW SUPPLIED: Sol: (15mL, 30mL)
WARNINGS/PRECAUTIONS: Eye problems including corneal ulcers can occur; remove contacts if eye discomfort, excessive tearing, vision changes or eye redness occur. Do not touch container tip to any surface to avoid contamination.
ADVERSE REACTIONS: Eye irritation, excessive tearing, unusual eye secretions, eye redness, reduced visual acuity, blurred vision, photophobia, dry eyes.
PREGNANCY: Safety in pregnancy and nursing not known.

VISINE L.R. OTC
oxymetazoline HCl (McNeil)

THERAPEUTIC CLASS: Decongestant
INDICATIONS: Relief of eye redness due to minor eye irritations.

VISINE ORIGINAL

DOSAGE: *Adults:* 1-2 drops in affected eye q6h prn.
Pediatrics: ≥6 yrs: 1-2 drops in affected eye q6h prn.
HOW SUPPLIED: Sol: 0.025% (15mL, 30mL)
WARNINGS/PRECAUTIONS: Overuse may cause more redness. Remove contact lenses before use. Do not touch container tip to any surface to avoid contamination. D/C if eye pain or vision changes occur, if redness or irritation continues, or if condition worsens or continues >72 hrs. Supervision required with glaucoma.
PREGNANCY: Safety in pregnancy and nursing not known.

VISINE ORIGINAL OTC
tetrahydrozoline HCl (McNeil)

THERAPEUTIC CLASS: Decongestant
INDICATIONS: Relief of eye redness due to minor eye irritations.
DOSAGE: *Adults:* 1-2 drops in affected eye up to qid.
Pediatrics: ≥6 yrs: 1-2 drops in affected eye up to qid.
HOW SUPPLIED: Sol: 0.05% (15mL, 30mL)
WARNINGS/PRECAUTIONS: May temporarily enlarge pupils. Overuse may cause more redness. Remove contact lenses before use. Do not touch container tip to any surface to avoid contamination. D/C if eye pain or vision changes occur, if redness or irritation continues, or if condition worsens or continues >72 hrs. Supervision required with glaucoma.
PREGNANCY: Safety in pregnancy and nursing not known.

VISINE TEARS OTC
glycerin - polyethylene glycol 400 - hydroxypropyl methylcellulose (McNeil)

THERAPEUTIC CLASS: Lubricant
INDICATIONS: Temporary relief of burning and irritation due to dryness of the eye and protection against further irritation.
DOSAGE: *Adults:* 1-2 drops prn.
Pediatrics: ≥6 yrs: 1-2 drops prn.
HOW SUPPLIED: Sol: (Glycerin-Hydroxypropyl Methylcellulose-Polyethylene Glycol 400) 0.2%-0.2%-1% (15mL, 30mL)
WARNINGS/PRECAUTIONS: Remove contact lenses before use. Do not touch container tip to any surface to avoid contamination. D/C if eye pain or vision changes occur, if redness or irritation continues, or if condition worsens or continues >72 hrs.
PREGNANCY: Safety in pregnancy and nursing not known.

VISINE-A OTC
naphazoline HCl - pheniramine maleate (McNeil)

THERAPEUTIC CLASS: Decongestant/antihistamine
INDICATIONS: Temporary relief of itchy, red eyes due to pollen, ragweed, grass, animal hair, and dander.
DOSAGE: *Adults:* 1-2 drops in affected eye up to qid.
Pediatrics: ≥6 yrs: 1-2 drops in affected eye up to qid.
HOW SUPPLIED: Sol: (Naphazoline-Pheniramine) 0.025%-0.3% (15mL)
WARNINGS/PRECAUTIONS: May temporarily enlarge pupils. Overuse may cause more redness. Remove contact lenses before use. Do not touch container tip to any surface to avoid contamination. D/C if eye pain or vision changes occur, if redness or irritation continues, or if condition worsens or continues >72 hrs. Supervision required with glaucoma.
ADVERSE REACTIONS: Brief tingling sensation.
PREGNANCY: Safety in pregnancy and nursing not known.

VITRASERT
ganciclovir (Bausch & Lomb)

RX

THERAPEUTIC CLASS: Nucleoside analogue antiviral

INDICATIONS: Treatment of cytomegalovirus (CMV) retinitis in AIDS patients.

DOSAGE: *Adults:* Each implant releases 4.5mg over 5-8 months. Remove and replace when there is evidence of progression of retinitis.
Pediatrics: ≥9 yrs: Each implant releases 4.5mg over 5-8 months. Remove and replace when there is evidence of progression of retinitis.

HOW SUPPLIED: Implant: 4.5mg

CONTRAINDICATIONS: Hypersensitivity to acyclovir, patients with contraindication for intraocular surgery (eg, external infection, severe thrombocytopenia).

WARNINGS/PRECAUTIONS: For intravitreal implantation only. Monitor for extraocular CMV disease. Implant does not treat systemic CMV. Complications from surgery include vitreous loss or hemorrhage, cataract formation, retinal detachment, uveitis, endophthalmitis, decrease in visual acuity. Immediate decrease in visual acuity will last 2-4 weeks postop. Maintain sterility of the surgical field, implant. Handle implant by suture tab to avoid damage to polymer coating. Handling and disposal of the implant should follow guidelines for antineoplastics.

ADVERSE REACTIONS: Visual acuity loss, vitreous hemorrhage, retinal detachments, cataract formation/lens opacities, macular abnormalities, IOP spikes, optic disk/nerve changes, uveitis, hyphemas.

PREGNANCY: Category C, not for use in nursing.

VIVACTIL
protriptyline HCl (Odyssey)

RX

> Antidepressants increased the risk of suicidal thinking and behavior (suicidality) in short-term studies in children and adolescents with Major Depressive Disorder (MDD) and other psychiatric disorders. Protriptyline is not approved for use in pediatric patients.

THERAPEUTIC CLASS: Tricyclic antidepressant

INDICATIONS: Treatment of symptoms of depression in those under close medical supervision.

DOSAGE: *Adults:* Usual: 15-40mg/day taken tid-qid. Titrate: May increase to 60mg/day. Max: 60mg/day. Elderly: Initial: 5mg tid. Titrate: Increase gradually if needed. Monitor cardiovascular system with doses >20mg/day.
Pediatrics: Adolescents: Initial: 5mg tid. Titrate: Increase gradually if needed.

HOW SUPPLIED: Tab: 5mg, 10mg

CONTRAINDICATIONS: Within 14 days of MAOI therapy, cisapride, acute recovery period following MI.

WARNINGS/PRECAUTIONS: Caution with history of seizures, urinary retention, increased IOP, cardiovascular disorders, hyperthyroidism, elderly. May aggravate psychotic symptoms in schizophrenia, manic symptoms in manic-depressive psychosis, and anxiety/agitation in overactive/agitated patients. D/C several days before elective surgery.

ADVERSE REACTIONS: Tachycardia, hypotension, confusion, anxiety, insomnia, nightmares, seizures, EPS, dizziness, headache, anticholinergic effects, rash, photosensitivity, blood dyscrasias, GI effects, impotence, decreased libido, flushing.

INTERACTIONS: Risk of hyperpyrexia with anticholinergics and neuroleptics. Reduced hepatic metabolism with cimetidine. Enhanced seizure risk with tramadol. Enhanced response to alcohol, barbiturates, other CNS depressants. Use with CYP2D6 enzyme inhibitors (eg, quinidine, cimetidine, other antidepressants, phenothiazines, propafenone, flecainide, SSRIs) require lower doses for either TCA or other drug. Hyperpyretic crises, severe convulsions, and deaths reported with MAOIs. May block antihypertensive effect of guanethidine, or similarly acting compounds.

PREGNANCY: Safety in pregnancy and nursing not known.

VoSoL HC
acetic acid - hydrocortisone (Wallace)
RX

OTHER BRAND NAME: Acetasol HC (Alpharma)

THERAPEUTIC CLASS: Antibacterial/corticosteroid combination

INDICATIONS: Treatment of superficial infections of the external auditory canal complicated by inflammation.

DOSAGE: *Adults:* Remove cerumen and debris. Insert cotton wick into ear canal; saturate cotton before or after insertion. Add 3-5 drops q4-6h to keep moist. Remove after 24 hrs; continue with 5 drops tid-qid as long as indicated.

Pediatrics: ≥3 yrs: Remove cerumen and debris. Insert cotton wick into ear canal; saturate cotton before or after insertion. Add 3-4 drops q4-6h to keep moist. Remove after 24 hrs; continue with 3-4 drops tid-qid as long as indicated.

HOW SUPPLIED: Sol: (Acetic Acid-Hydrocortisone) 2%-1% (10mL)

CONTRAINDICATIONS: Herpes simplex, vaccinia, varicella, perforated tympanic membrane.

WARNINGS/PRECAUTIONS: Discontinue promptly if sensitization occurs.

ADVERSE REACTIONS: Transient stinging, burning.

PREGNANCY: Safety in pregnancy and nursing not known.

VoSpire ER
albuterol sulfate (Odyssey)
RX

THERAPEUTIC CLASS: Beta$_2$ agonist

INDICATIONS: Treatment of bronchospasm in reversible obstructive airway disease.

DOSAGE: *Adults:* Usual: 4-8mg q12h. Low Body Weight: Initial: 4mg q12h. Titrate: May increase to 8mg q12h. Max: 32mg/day in divided doses. Swallow whole with liquids; do not chew or crush.

Pediatrics: >12 yrs: Usual: 4-8mg q12h. Low Body Weight: Initial: 4mg q12h. Titrate: May increase to 8mg q12h. Max: 32mg/day in divided doses. 6-12 yrs: Usual: 4mg q12h. Max: 24mg/day in divided doses. Swallow whole with liquids; do not chew or crush.

HOW SUPPLIED: Tab, Extended Release: 4mg, 8mg

WARNINGS/PRECAUTIONS: Hypersensitivity reactions reported. Caution with cardiovascular disorders, especially coronary insufficiency, arrhythmias and HTN. Increased doses may signify need for concomitant corticosteroids. Can produce paradoxical bronchospasm. Caution with DM, hyperthyroidism, seizures. May produce transient hypokalemia. Erythema multiforme and Stevens-Johnson (rare) reported in children.

ADVERSE REACTIONS: Tremor, headache, nervousness, tachycardia, palpitations, nausea, vomiting, muscle cramps.

INTERACTIONS: Avoid oral sympathomimetic agents. Extreme caution within 14 days of MAOI or TCA therapy. Monitor digoxin. May worsen ECG changes and/or hypokalemia with nonpotassium-sparing diuretics. Antagonized by β-blockers.

PREGNANCY: Category C, not for use in nursing.

Vumon
teniposide (Bristol-Myers Squibb)
RX

> Cytotoxic. Severe myelosuppression, with resulting infection or bleeding, and/or hypersensitivity reactions may occur.

THERAPEUTIC CLASS: Type II topoisomerase inhibitor

INDICATIONS: With other anticancer agents, for induction therapy of refractory childhood acute lymphoblastic leukemia.

DOSAGE: *Pediatrics:* 165mg/m^2 with cytarabine 300mg/m^2 IV twice weekly for 8-9 doses; or 250mg/m^2 with vincristine 1.5mg/m^2 IV weekly for 4-8 weeks and prednisone 40mg/m^2 PO for 28 days.

HOW SUPPLIED: Inj: 10mg/mL

CONTRAINDICATIONS: Hypersensitivity to Cremophor EL (polyoxyethylated castor oil).

WARNINGS/PRECAUTIONS: Monitor CBC, hepatic and renal function before and during therapy. Avoid rapid IV infusion. May cause fetal harm. Dose-limiting bone marrow suppression. D/C if significant hypotension occurs. Hypersensitivity (HS) reactions manifested by chills, fever, urticaria, tachycardia, bronchospasm, dyspnea, HTN, and hypotension may occur. If re-treating patient with earlier HS reaction, pretreat with corticosteroid and antihistamine. Continuously observe for at least 60 minutes after infusion and frequently thereafter. Use gloves when handling or preparing solution. Reduce dose or d/c if severe reactions occur.

ADVERSE REACTIONS: Myelosuppression, leukopenia, neutropenia, thrombocytopenia, anemia, mucositis, diarrhea, nausea, vomiting, infection, alopecia, bleeding, hypersensitivity reactions, rash, fever.

INTERACTIONS: Risk of CNS depression with antiemetics and high dose teniposide. Tolbutamide, sodium salicylate, and sulfamethizole displace protein-bound teniposide; may potentiate toxicity. Increased plasma clearance of methotrexate.

PREGNANCY: Category D, not for use in nursing.

VYTONE
iodoquinol - hydrocortisone (Dermik)

RX

THERAPEUTIC CLASS: Corticosteroid/Anti-infective

INDICATIONS: "Possibly" Effective: Contact or atopic dermatitis, impetiginized eczema, nummular eczema, endogenous chronic infectious dermatitis, stasis dermatitis, pyoderma, nuchal eczema and chronic eczematoid otitis externa, acne urticata, localized or disseminated neurodermatitis, lichen simplex chronicus, anogenital pruritus (vulvae, scroti, ani), folliculitis, bacterial dermatoses, mycotic dermatoses such as tinea (capitis, cruris, corporis, pedis), monliasis, intertrigo.

DOSAGE: *Adults:* Apply to affected area(s) tid-qid.
Pediatrics: ≥12 yrs: Apply tid-qid.

HOW SUPPLIED: Cre: (Hydrocortisone-Iodoquinol) 1%-1% (30g)

WARNINGS/PRECAUTIONS: For external use only. Avoid eyes. Discontinue if irritation develops. May stain skin, hair, or fabrics. Risk of systemic absorption with treatment of extensive areas or use of occlusive dressings. Increased risk of systemic absorption in children. Iodoquinol may interfere with thyroid tests. False-positive phenylketonuria test reported.

ADVERSE REACTIONS: Burning, itching, irritation, dryness, folliculitis, hypertrichosis, acneiform eruptions, hypopigmentation, perioral dermatitis, allergic dermatitis, skin maceration, secondary infection, skin atrophy, striae, miliaria.

PREGNANCY: Category C, caution in nursing.

VYVANSE
lisdexamfetamine dimesylate (Shire)

CII

> High abuse potential; prolonged periods of administration may lead to dependence. Misuse of amphetamine may cause sudden death and serious cadiovascular events.

THERAPEUTIC CLASS: Sympathomimetic Amine

INDICATIONS: Treatment of attention deficit hyperactivity disorder (ADHD) in children 6 to 12 yrs old.

DOSAGE: *Pediatrics:* 6-12 yrs: Usual: 30mg qam. Titrate: If needed, increase at increments of 20mg/day at weekly intervals. Max: 70mg/day. Swallow caps or dissolve contents in glass of water; do not store once dissolved. Re-evaluate in long-term use.

HOW SUPPLIED: Cap: 30mg, 50mg, 70mg

CONTRAINDICATIONS: Advanced arteriosclerosis, symptomatic cardiovscular disease, moderate to severe HTN, hyperthyroidism, glaucoma, agitated states, history of drug abuse, during or within 14 days of MAOI use.

Westcort (continued)

WARNINGS/PRECAUTIONS: May exacerbate symptoms of behavior disturbance and thought disorder in psychotic patients. Caution with comorbid bipolar disorder; concern for possible induction of mixed/manic episode. Aggressive behavior or hostility reported. Monitor growth in children. Stimulants may lower the convulsive threshold; d/c in the presence of seizures. Difficulties with accommodation and blurring of vision reported. May exacerbate Tourette's syndrome and phonic or motor tics. Caution with HTN, heart failure, MI, or ventricular arrhythnmia; monitor BP and HR. Avoid use with structural cardiac abnormalities, cardiomyopathy, serious heart rhythm abnormalities, or other serious cardiac problems; sudden death reported. Treatment emergent psychotic or manic symptoms may occur (eg, hallucinations, delusional thinking, or mania, without prior history of psychotic illness); d/c treatment if needed.

ADVERSE REACTIONS: Decreased appetite, insomnia, upper abdominal pain, headache, weight loss, irritability, vomiting, nausea, dry mouth, dizziness, affect lability, rash.

INTERACTIONS: GI acidifying agents (eg, guanethidine, reserpine, glutamic acid, etc.) and urinary acidifying agents (eg, ammonium chloride, etc) decrease efficacy. MAOIs may cause hypertensive crisis. Potentiated effects of both agents with TCAs. May delay absorption of phenytoin, ethosuximide, phenobarbital. Potentiates meperidine, norepinephrine, phenobarbital, phenytoin. Antagonized by haloperidol, chlorpromazine, lithium. Inhibits adrenergic blockers, antihistamines, antihypertensives (veratrum alkaloids), methanamine therapy. Methenamine increases urinary excretion. Potentiated by propoxyphene overdose; fatal convulsions may occur.

PREGNANCY: Pregnancy C, not for use in nursing.

Westcort RX
hydrocortisone valerate (Westwood-Squibb)

THERAPEUTIC CLASS: Corticosteroid

INDICATIONS: Corticosteroid responsive dermatoses.

DOSAGE: *Adults:* Apply bid-tid. May use occlusive dressings for psoriasis or recalcitrant conditions; discontinue dressings if infection develops.
Pediatrics: Apply bid-tid. May use occlusive dressings for psoriasis or recalcitrant conditions; discontinue dressings if infection develops.

HOW SUPPLIED: Cre, Oint: 0.2% (15g, 45g, 60g)

WARNINGS/PRECAUTIONS: May produce reversible HPA axis suppression, manifestations of Cushing's syndrome, hyperglycemia, and glucosuria. Caution when applied to large surface areas or under occlusive dressings. Use appropriate antifungal or antibacterial agent with dermatological infections; discontinue if infection does not clear. Pediatrics may be more susceptible to systemic toxicity. Avoid eyes. Discontinue if irritation occurs.

ADVERSE REACTIONS: Burning, itching, dryness, irritation, folliculitis, hypertrichosis, acneiform eruptions, hypopigmentation, allergic contact dermatitis, skin maceration, secondary infection, skin atrophy, striae, miliaria.

PREGNANCY: Category C, caution in nursing.

WinRho SDF RX
rho (D) immune globulin (Baxter)

THERAPEUTIC CLASS: Immuneglobulin

INDICATIONS: Treatment of non-splenectomized, $Rh_o(D)$ positive children with chronic or acute immune thrombocytopenic purpura (ITP), adults with chronic ITP, or children and adults with ITP secondary to HIV infection. To prevent Rh immunization in Rh_o (D) negative mothers who had not been previously sensitized to Rh_o (D) factor. To suppress Rh isoimmunization in non-sensitized, $Rh_o(D)$ negative women within 72 hours after spontaneous or induced abortions, amniocentesis, chorionic villus sampling, ruptured tubal pregnancy, abdominal trauma or transplacental hemorrhage or in the normal course of pregnancy, unless fetus or father is known to be $Rh_o(D)$ negative. To suppress Rh isoimmunization in $Rh_o(D)$ negative female children and adults transfused with $Rh_o(D)$ positive blood products.

DOSAGE: Adults: ITP: Initial: 50mcg/kg IV as a single dose or in 2 divided doses on separate days. Hgb <10g/dL: 25-40mcg/kg. Subsequent/Maint: 25-60mcg/kg. Hgb 8-10g/dL: 25-40mcg/kg. Hgb >10g/dL: 50-60mcg/kg. Hgb <8g/dL: Use caution. Rh Suppression: Pregnancy: Give as IM or IV. 28 Weeks Gestation: 300mcg. If early in pregnancy, give at 12 week intervals. Postpartum: With Rh Positive Baby: 120mcg at birth, but no later than 72 hours after. Rh Status of Baby Unknown at 72 Hours: Administer to mother at 72 hours after birth. May give up to 28 days after birth. Abortion/Amniocentesis or Other Manipulation After 34 Weeks Gestation: 120mcg dose within 72 hours. Amniocentesis Before 34 Weeks Gestation/Post Chorionic Villus Sampling: 300mcg dose immediately after procedure. Repeat every 12 weeks. Threatened Abortion: 300mcg as soon as possible. Transfusion: Exposure to $Rh_o(D)$ Positive Blood: 9mcg/mL blood given as 600mcg q8h IV or 12mcg/mL blood given as 1200mcg q12h IM. Exposure to $Rh_o(D)$ Positive RBCs: 18mcg/mL cells given as 600mcg q8h IV or 24mcg/mL cells given as 1200mcg q12h IM.

Pediatrics: ITP: Initial: 50mcg/kg IV as a single dose or in 2 divided doses on separate days. Hgb <10g/dL: 25-40mcg/kg. Subsequent/Maint: 25-60mcg/kg. Hgb 8-10g/dL: 25-40mcg/kg. Hgb >10g/dL: 50-60mcg/kg. Hgb <8g/dL: Use caution. Transfusion: Exposure to $Rh_o(D)$ Positive Blood: 9mcg/mL blood given as 600mcg q8h IV or 12mcg/mL blood given as 1200mcg q12h IM. Exposure to $Rh_o(D)$ Positive RBCs: 18mcg/mL cells given as 600mcg q8h IV or 24mcg/mL cells given as 1200mcg q12h IM.

HOW SUPPLIED: Inj: 120mcg (600 IU), 300mcg (1500 IU), 1000mcg (5000 IU)

CONTRAINDICATIONS: When used to prevent Rh alloimmunization, should not be adminstered to $Rh_o(D)$ positive individuals including babies; $Rh_o(D)$ negative women who are Rh immunized as evidenced by standard manual Rh antibody screening test; individuals with a history of anaphylactic or other severe systemic reaction to immune globulins. When used to treat patients with ITP, should not be administered to $Rh_o(D)$ negative individuals; splenectomized individuals; individuals with known hypersensitivity to plasma products.

WARNINGS/PRECAUTIONS: May transmit disease. Avoid use in $Rh_o(D)$ negative, $Rh_o(D)$ negative who are Rh immunized, or spelenectomized patients. Not for replacement therapy for immuneglobulin deficiency syndromes. Caution with IgA deficiency; anaphylactic reactions may occur. (ITP): Monitor for intravascular hemolysis, clinically compromising anemia, renal insufficiency. If transfused, use $Rh_o(D)$ negative RBCs. Caution if platelets from $Rh_o(D)$ positive donors are transfused.

ADVERSE REACTIONS: Headache, chills, fever, decreased Hgb, back pain, intravascular hemolysis.

INTERACTIONS: May interfere with response to live vaccines; delay immunization for 3 months.

PREGNANCY: Category C, safety in nursing not known.

XENICAL
orlistat (Roche Labs)

RX

THERAPEUTIC CLASS: Lipase inhibitor

INDICATIONS: For weight loss and weight maintenance and to reduce the risk of weight regain after weight loss in obese patients with an initial BMI $\geq 30kg/m^2$ or $\geq 27kg/m^2$ in the presence of other risk factors.

DOSAGE: *Adults:* 120mg tid with each main meal containing fat. Take during or up to 1 hr after meals. Use with reduced calorie diet with about 30% of calories from fat. Omit dose if meal is missed or contains no fat. Separate multivitamin (containing fat-soluble vitamins) by at least 2 hrs.

Pediatrics: ≥ 12 yrs: 120mg tid with each main meal containing fat. Take during or up to 1 hr after meals. Use with reduced calorie diet with about 30% of calories from fat. Omit dose if meal is missed or contains no fat. Separate multivitamin (containing fat-soluble vitamins) by at least 2 hrs.

HOW SUPPLIED: Cap: 120mg

CONTRAINDICATIONS: Chronic malabsorption syndrome, cholestasis.

WARNINGS/PRECAUTIONS: Exclude organic causes of obesity. Caution with history of hyperoxaluria or calcium oxalate nephrolithiasis. Gastrointestinal effects may increase

XIFAXAN

with a diet high in fat (>30%). Weight loss may improve metabolic control; monitor dosage of antidiabetic agents. Increased risk of cholelithiasis due to substantial weight loss.

ADVERSE REACTIONS: Oily spotting, flatus with discharge, fecal urgency, fatty/oily stool, oily evacuation, increased defecation, fecal incontinence.

INTERACTIONS: Monitor warfarin and cyclosporine (separate cyclosporine dose by 2 hrs). May decrease absorption of fat soluble vitamins and beta carotene; supplement with fat-soluble multivitamin.

PREGNANCY: Category B, not for use in nursing.

XIFAXAN RX
rifaximin (Salix)

THERAPEUTIC CLASS: Semi-synthetic rifampin analog

INDICATIONS: Traveler's diarrhea caused by noninvasive strains of E.coli

DOSAGE: Adults: 1 tab tid for 3 days.
Pediatrics: ≥12 yrs: 1 tab tid for 3 days.

HOW SUPPLIED: Tab: 200mg

WARNINGS/PRECAUTIONS: Avoid in diarrhea complicated by fever or blood in the stool or diarrhea due to pathogens other than E.coli. Discontinue if diarrhea symptoms worsen or persist >24-48 hrs; consider alternative antibiotic therapy. Pseudomembranous colitis reported.

ADVERSE REACTIONS: Flatulence, headache, abdominal pain, rectal tenesmus, defecation urgency, nausea, constipation, pyrexia.

PREGNANCY: Category C; not for use in nursing.

XOLAIR RX
omalizumab (Genentech)

THERAPEUTIC CLASS: Monoclonal antibody/IgE-blocker

INDICATIONS: Moderate-severe persistent asthma in those who have a positive skin test or in vitro reactivity to a perennial aeroallergen and whose symptoms are inadequately controlled with inhaled corticosteroids.

DOSAGE: Adults: 150-375mg SQ every 2 or 4 weeks based on body weight and pre-treatment serum total IgE level. Max: 150mg/site. 30-90kg & IgE ≥30-100 IU/mL: 150mg q4 weeks; >90-150kg & IgE ≥30-100 IU/mL OR 30-90kg & IgE >100-200 IU/mL OR 30-60kg & IgE >200-300 IU/mL: 300mg q4 weeks; >90-150kg & IgE >100-200 IU/mL OR >60-90kg & IgE >200-300 IU/mL OR 30-70kg & IgE >300-400 IU/mL: 225mg q2 weeks; >90-150kg & IgE >200-300 IU/mL OR >70-90kg & IgE >300-400 IU/mL OR 30-70kg & IgE >400-500 IU/mL OR 30-60kg & IgE >500-600 IU/mL: 300mg q2 weeks; >70-90kg & IgE >400-500 IU/mL OR >60-70kg & IgE >500-600 IU/mL OR 30-60kg & IgE >600-700 IU/mL: 375mg q2 weeks.

Pediatrics: ≥12 yrs: 150-375mg SQ every 2 or 4 weeks based on body weight and pre-treatment serum total IgE level. Max injection = 150mg/site. 30-90kg & IgE ≥30-100 IU/mL: 150mg q4 weeks; >90-150kg & IgE ≥30-100 IU/mL OR 30-90kg & IgE >100-200 IU/mL OR 30-60kg & IgE >200-300 IU/mL: 300mg q4 weeks; >90-150kg & IgE >100-200 IU/mL OR >60-90kg & IgE >200-300 IU/mL OR 30-70kg & IgE >300-400 IU/mL: 225mg q2 weeks; >90-150kg and IgE >200-300 IU/mL OR >70-90kg & IgE >300-400 IU/mL OR 30-70kg & IgE >400-500 IU/mL OR 30-60kg & IgE >500-600 IU/mL: 300mg q2 weeks; >70-90kg & IgE >400-500 IU/mL OR >60-70kg & IgE >500-600 IU/mL OR 30-60kg & IgE >600-700 IU/mL: 375mg q2 weeks.

HOW SUPPLIED: Inj.: 150mg (5mL)

WARNINGS/PRECAUTIONS: Malignant neoplasms reported. Serious life-threatening anaphylaxis reported usually within 2 hrs of dose; monitor closely. Not for use in treatment of acute bronchospasm or status asthmaticus. Systemic or inhaled corticosteroids should not be abruptly discontinued when initiating therapy. Malignant neoplasms and anaphylaxis reported. Not for use in treatment of acute bronchospasm or status asthmaticus. Systemic or inhaled corticosteroids should not be abruptly discontinued when initiating therapy.

ADVERSE REACTIONS: Injection site reactions, viral infections, upper respiratory infection, sinusitis, headache, pharyngitis, pain, arthralgia, leg pain.

PREGNANCY: Category B, caution in nursing.

XOPENEX
levalbuterol HCl (Sepracor)
RX

THERAPEUTIC CLASS: Beta$_2$ agonist

INDICATIONS: Prevention and treatment of bronchospasm with reversible obstructive airway disease.

DOSAGE: *Adults:* Initial: 0.63mg tid, q6-8h. Severe Asthma: 1.25mg tid, q6-8h. Administer by nebulizer.
Pediatrics: ≥12 yrs: Initial: 0.63mg tid, q6-8h. Severe Asthma: 1.25mg tid, q6-8h. 6-11 yrs: 0.31mg tid. Max: 0.63mg tid. Administer by nebulizer.

HOW SUPPLIED: Sol: 0.31mg/3mL, 0.63mg/3mL, 1.25mg/3mL (3mL, 24's)

WARNINGS/PRECAUTIONS: Hypersensitivity reactions reported. Discontinue immediately if paradoxical bronchospasm occurs. May produce ECG changes; caution with cardiovascular disorders, coronary insufficiency, arrhythmias, and HTN. Caution with convulsive disorders, hyperthyroidism, and diabetes. May produce transient hypokalemia.

ADVERSE REACTIONS: Tachycardia, migraine, dyspepsia, leg cramps, nervousness, dizziness, tremor, rhinitis, increased cough, chest pain, HTN, hypotention, diarrhea, dry mouth, anxiety, insomnia, paresthesia, wheezing.

INTERACTIONS: Avoid other sympathomimetic agents. Extreme caution with MAOIs and TCAs. Monitor digoxin. ECG changes and/or hypokalemia with nonpotassium-sparing diuretics. Antagonized by β-blockers.

PREGNANCY: Category C, not for use in nursing.

XOPENEX HFA
levalbuterol tartrate (Sepracor)
RX

THERAPEUTIC CLASS: Beta$_2$ agonist

INDICATIONS: Prevention and treatment of bronchospasm with reversible obstructive airway disease.

DOSAGE: *Adults:* 2 inh (90mcg) q4-6hrs or 1 inh (45mcg) q4hrs may be sufficient.
Pediatrics: ≥4 yrs: 2 inh (90mcg) q4-6hrs or 1 inh (45mcg) q4hrs may be sufficient.

HOW SUPPLIED: MDI: 45mcg/inh (15g)

WARNINGS/PRECAUTIONS: Discontinue immediately if paradoxical bronchospasm occurs. May produce ECG changes; caution with cardiovascular disorders, coronary insufficiency, arrhythmias, and HTN. Caution with convulsive disorders, hyperthyroidism, and diabetes. May produce transient hypokalemia.

ADVERSE REACTIONS: Asthma, pharyngitis, rhinitis, pain, vomiting.

INTERACTIONS: Avoid other sympathomimetic agents. Extreme caution with MAOIs and TCAs. Monitor digoxin. ECG changes and/or hypokalemia with nonpotassium-sparing diuretics. Antagonized by β-blockers.

PREGNANCY: Category C, not for use in nursing.

XYLOCAINE INJECTION
lidocaine HCl (Abraxis)
RX

OTHER BRAND NAME: Xylocaine-MPF (Abraxis)

THERAPEUTIC CLASS: Local anesthetic

INDICATIONS: For production of local or regional anesthesia by infiltration techniques such as percutaneous injection and IV regional anesthesia by peripheral nerve block techniques such as brachial plexus and intercostal and by central neural techniques such as lumbar and caudal epidural blocks.

XYLOCAINE JELLY

DOSAGE: *Adults:* Dosage varies depending on procedure, depth and duration of anesthesia, degree of muscular relaxation, and patient physical condition. Max: 4.5mg/kg or total dose of 300mg. Epidural/Caudal Anesthesia: Max: Intervals not less than 90 minutes. Paracervical Block: Max: 200mg/90 minutes. Regional Anesthesia: IV: Max: 4mg/kg. Children/Elderly/Debilitated/Cardiac or Liver Disease: Reduce dose.
Pediatrics: >3 yrs: Max: 1.5-2mg/lb. Regional Anesthesia: IV: Max: 3mg/kg.

HOW SUPPLIED: Inj: 0.5%, 1%, 2%; (MPF) 0.5%, 1%, 1.5%, 2%

WARNINGS/PRECAUTIONS: Acidosis, cardiac arrest, death reported from delay in toxicity management. Local anesthetic solutions containing antimicrobial preservatives should not be used for epidural or spinal anesthesia. Use lowest effective dose. During epidural anesthesia, administer initial test dose and monitor for CNS and cardiovascular toxicity as well as for signs of unintended intrathecal administration. Reduce dose with debilitated, elderly, acutely ill, and children. Extreme caution when using lumbar and caudal epidural anesthesia with existing neurological disease, spinal deformities, septicemia, and severe HTN. Monitor cardiovascular and respiratory vital signs and state of consciousness after each injection. Caution with hepatic disease, cardiovascular disorders. Monitor circulation and respiration with injections into head and neck area.

ADVERSE REACTIONS: Lightheadedness, nervousness, euphoria, confusion, dizziness, drowsiness, tinnitus, blurred vision, vomiting, heat/cold sensations, twitching, tremors, convulsions, respiratory depression, bradycardia, hypotension, urticaria, edema, anaphylactoid reactions.

PREGNANCY: Category B, caution in nursing.

XYLOCAINE JELLY   RX
lidocaine HCl (Abraxis)

THERAPEUTIC CLASS: Acetamide local anesthetic

INDICATIONS: Prevention and control of pain in procedures involving the male and female urethra. Topical treatment of painful urethritis. Anesthetic lubricant for endotracheal intubation.

DOSAGE: *Adults:* Max: 600mg/12 hrs. Surface Anesthesia of Male Urethra: Instill about 15mL (300mg). Instill an additional dose of not more than 15mL if needed. Prior to Sounding or Cystoscopy: A total dose of 30mL (600mg) is usually required. Prior to Catheterization: 5-10mL usually adequate. Surface Anesthesia of Female Urethra: Instill 3-5mL. Elderly/Debilitated: Reduce dose.
Pediatrics: Determine dose by age and weight. Max: 4.5mg/kg.

HOW SUPPLIED: Jelly: 2% (Tube: 5mL, 30mL; Syringe: 10mL, 20mL)

WARNINGS/PRECAUTIONS: Avoid excessive dosage or frequent administration; may result in serious adverse effects requiring resuscitative measures. Caution with heart block and severe shock. Extreme caution if mucosa traumatized or sepsis is present in the area of application; risk of rapid systemic absorption.

ADVERSE REACTIONS: Lightheadedness, nervousness, confusion, euphoria, dizziness, drowsiness, blurred vision, tremors, convulsions, respiratory depression, bradycardia, hypotension, urticaria, edema, anaphylactoid reactions.

PREGNANCY: Category B, caution in nursing.

XYLOCAINE VISCOUS   RX
lidocaine HCl (Abraxis)

THERAPEUTIC CLASS: Acetamide local anesthetic

INDICATIONS: Topical anesthesia of irritated or inflamed mucous membranes of the mouth and pharynx. To reduce gagging during X-ray or dental procedures.

DOSAGE: *Adults:* Irritated/Inflamed Mucous Membranes: Usual: 15mL undiluted. (Mouth) Swish and spit out. (Pharynx) Gargle and may swallow. Do not administer in <3 hr intervals. Max: 8 doses/24hr; (Single Dose) 4.5mg/kg or total of 300mg.

Pediatrics: >3 yrs: Max: Determine by age and weight. Infants <3 yrs: Apply 1.25mL with cotton-tipped applicator to immediate area. Do not administer in <3 hour intervals. Max: 8 doses/24hr.

HOW SUPPLIED: Sol: 2% (100mL, 450mL)

WARNINGS/PRECAUTIONS: Reduce dose in elderly, debilitated, acutely ill and children. Caution with heart block and severe shock. Excessive dosage or too frequent administration may result in high plasma levels and serious adverse effects requiring resuscitative measures. Extreme caution if mucosa traumatized; risk of rapid systemic absorption. Overdose reported in pediatrics due to inappropriate dosing.

ADVERSE REACTIONS: Lightheadedness, nervousness, confusion, euphoria, dizziness, drowsiness, blurred vision, tremors, convulsions, respiratory depression, bradycardia, hypotension, urticaria, edema, anaphylactoid reactions.

PREGNANCY: Category B, caution in nursing.

XYLOCAINE WITH EPINEPHRINE RX
epinephrine - lidocaine HCl (Abraxis)

OTHER BRAND NAME: Xylocaine-MPF with Epinephrine (Abraxis)

THERAPEUTIC CLASS: Local anesthetic

INDICATIONS: For production of local or regional anesthesia by infiltration techniques such as percutaneous injection and IV regional anesthesia by peripheral nerve block techniques such as brachial plexus and intercostal and by central neural techniques such as lumbar and caudal epidural blocks.

DOSAGE: *Adults:* Dosage varies depending on procedure, depth and duration of anesthesia, degree of muscular relaxation, and patient physical condition. Max: 7mg/kg or total dose of 500mg. Epidural/Caudal Anesthesia: Max: Intervals not less than 90 minutes. Paracervical Block: Max: 200mg/90 minutes. Regional Anesthesia: IV: Max: 4mg/kg. Children/Elderly/Debilitated/Cardiac or Liver Disease: Reduce dose.

Pediatrics: >3 yrs: Max: 1.5-2mg/lb. Regional Anesthesia: IV: Max: 3mg/kg.

HOW SUPPLIED: Inj: (Lidocaine-Epinephrine) 0.5%/1:200,000, 1%/1:100,000, 2%/1:100,000; (MPF) 1%/1:200,000, 1.5%/1:200,000, 2%/1:200,000

WARNINGS/PRECAUTIONS: Acidosis, cardiac arrest, death reported from delay in toxicity management. Local anesthetic solutions containing antimicrobial preservatives should not be used for epidural or spinal anesthesia. Xylocaine with epinephrine solutions contain sodium metabisulfite which may cause allergic-type reactions in susceptible people. Use lowest effective dose. During epidural anesthesia, administer initial test dose and monitor for CNS and cardiovascular toxicity as well as for signs of unintended intrathecal administration. Reduce dose with debilitated, elderly, acutely ill, and children. Extreme caution when using lumbar and caudal epidural anesthesia with existing neurological disease, spinal deformities, septicemia, and severe HTN. Caution when local anesthetic injections containing a vasoconstrictor are used in areas of the body supplied by end arteries or having otherwise compromised blood supply; ischemic injury or necrosis may result with peripheral or hypertensive vascular disease due to exaggerated vasoconstrictor response. Monitor cardiovascular and respiratory vital signs and state of consciousness after each injection. Caution with hepatic disease, cardiovascular disorders. Monitor circulation and respiration with injections into head and neck area.

ADVERSE REACTIONS: Lightheadedness, nervousness, euphoria, confusion, dizziness, drowsiness, tinnitus, blurred vision, vomiting, heat/cold sensations, twitching, tremors, convulsions, respiratory depression, bradycardia, hypotension, urticaria, edema, anaphylactoid reactions.

INTERACTIONS: Anesthetic solutions containing epinephrine or norepinephrine with MAOIs or TCAs may produce severe, prolonged HTN; avoid concurrent use or monitor closely if concurrent use is essential. Phenothiazines and butyrophenones may reduce or reverse pressor effect of epinephrine; avoid concurrent use or monitor closely if concurrent use is essential. Vasopressors, ergot-type oxytocic drugs may cause severe, persistent HTN or CVA.

PREGNANCY: Category B, caution in nursing.

XYREM
sodium oxybate (Orphan Medical)

> Sodium oxybate is GHB (gamma hydroxybutyrate), a known drug of abuse. Do not use with alcohol or other CNS depressants. Associated with confusion, depression, and other neuropsychiatric events. Available only through the Xyrem Success Program, call 1-866-XYREM88.

THERAPEUTIC CLASS: CNS Depressant

INDICATIONS: Treatment of excessive daytime sleepiness and cataplexy in patients with narcolepsy.

DOSAGE: *Adults:* Initial: 2.25g qhs, then take 2.25g 2.5-4 hrs later. Titrate: Increase by 0.75g/dose every 1-2 weeks. Range: 6-9g/night. Max: 9g/night. Hepatic Insufficiency: Initial: Decrease by 50%. Titrate dose increments to effect. Take 1st dose at bedtime while in bed and the 2nd dose while sitting in bed. Dilute each dose with 2 ounces of water.

Pediatrics: ≥16 yrs: Initial: 2.25g qhs, then take 2.25g 2.5-4 hrs later. Titrate: Increase by 0.75g/dose every 1-2 weeks. Range: 6-9g/night. Max: 9g/night. Hepatic Insufficiency: Initial: Decrease by 50%. Titrate dose increments to effect. Take 1st dose at bedtime while in bed and the 2nd dose while sitting in bed. Dilute each dose with 2 ounces of water.

HOW SUPPLIED: Sol: 500mg/mL (180mL)

CONTRAINDICATIONS: Sedative hypnotic agents, succinic semialdehyde dehydrogenase deficiency.

WARNINGS/PRECAUTIONS: Rapid onset of CNS depressant effects; ingest only at bedtime and while in bed. Avoid engaging in activities requiring mental alertness for 6 hrs after ingestion. Daily sodium intake ranges from 0.5g (with 3g dose) to 1.6g (with 9g dose); caution in heart failure, HTN, or renal impairment. Caution with compromised respiratory function, hepatic insufficiency, history of depressive illness or suicide attempts, elderly. Evaluate patients who develop through disorders or behavior abnormalities. Sleepwalking reported. Rule out worsening sleep apnea or nocturnal seizures if incontinence develops.

ADVERSE REACTIONS: Headache, nausea, dizziness, pain, somnolence, pharyngitis, infection, flu syndrome, diarrhea, urinary incontinence, vomiting, rhinitis, asthenia, sinusitis, nervousness, back pain, confusion, sleepwalking, depression, dyspepsia, abdominal pain, abnormal dreams, insomnia.

INTERACTIONS: Avoid alcohol, sedative hypnotics, or other CNS depressants. Food decreases bioavailability.

PREGNANCY: Category B, caution in nursing.

XYZAL
levocetirizine dihydrochloride (UCB)

RX

THERAPEUTIC CLASS: H_1 antagonist

INDICATIONS: Seasonal and perennial allergic rhinitis. Chronic idiopathic urticaria.

DOSAGE: *Adults:* 5mg qd in evening. Adjust dose with decreased renal function.

Pediatrics: ≥12 yrs: 5mg qd in evening. Adjust dose with decreased renal function. 6-11 yrs: 2.5mg (1/2 tab) qd in evening.

HOW SUPPLIED: Tab: 5mg* *scored

CONTRAINDICATIONS: End stage renal disease (CrCl <10mL/min) or hemodialysis. Pediatrics 6-11 yrs with renal impairment.

WARNINGS/PRECAUTIONS: May impair mental/physical abilities.

ADVERSE REACTIONS: Somnolence, fatigue, dry mouth, headache, pharyngitis, abdominal pain, cough, epistaxis.

INTERACTIONS: Avoid alcohol and CNS depressants. Possible decreased clearance with large doses of theophylline.

PREGNANCY: Category B, not for use in nursing.

YAZ
drospirenone - ethinyl estradiol (Berlex)

RX

THERAPEUTIC CLASS: Estrogen/progestogen combination

INDICATIONS: Prevention of pregnancy. Treatment of symptoms of premenstrual dysphoric disorder (PMDD). Treatment of moderate acne vulgaris in women 14 yrs and older.

DOSAGE: *Adults:* 1 tab qd for 28 days (24 active plus 4 inert pills), then repeat. Start 1st Sunday after menses begin or 1st day of menses.

Pediatrics: ≥14 yrs: Acne: 1 tab qd for 28 days (24 active plus 4 inert pills), then repeat. Start 1st Sunday after menses begin or 1st day of menses.

HOW SUPPLIED: Tab: (Ethinyl Estradiol-Drospirenone) 0.02mg-3mg

CONTRAINDICATIONS: Renal or adrenal insufficiency, hepatic dysfunction, thrombophlebitis, thromboembolic disorders, history of deep vein thrombophlebitis, valvular heart disease with thrombogenic complications, severe HTN, DM with vascular involvement, HA with focal neurological symptoms, major surgery with prolonged immobilization, cerebrovascular or CAD, breast carcinoma, endometrial carcinoma, estrogen-dependent neoplasia, undiagnosed abnormal genital bleeding, cholestatic jaundice of pregnancy or jaundice with prior pill use, liver tumor, active liver disease, pregnancy, heavy smoking (>15 cigarettes daily) and >35 yrs.

WARNINGS/PRECAUTIONS: Cigarette smoking increases risk of serious CV side effects. Risk increases with age (especially >35 yrs) and with heavy smoking. Increased risk of MI, thromboembolism, thrombotic disease, cerebrovascular events, and gallbladder disease. Monitor K^+ levels during first cycle with conditions predisposing to hyperkalemia. Retinal thrombosis, hepatic neoplasia, carcinoma of breast and reproductive organs reported. May cause glucose intolerance. May increase BP, elevate LDL levels or cause other lipid changes, fluid retention, breakthrough bleeding and spotting. May cause or exacerbate migraine. May develop visual changes with contact lens. Increased risk of MI with HTN, hyperlipidemia, obesity and DM. D/C if jaundice, significant depression or ophthalmic irregularities develop. Use before menarche is not indicated.

ADVERSE REACTIONS: Nausea, vomiting, breakthrough bleeding, spotting, amenorrhea, migraine, mental depression, vaginal candidiasis, edema, weight changes, depression decrease in serum folate levels, aggravation of varicose veins, uritcaria, angioedema, severe reactions with respiratory and circulatory symptoms, dysmenorrhea.

INTERACTIONS: Reduced effects, increased breakthrough bleeding, and menstrual irregularities with rifampin, phenobarbital, phenytoin, carbamazepine, possibly with griseofulvin, ampicillin, tetracycline, St. John's wort, and phenylbutazone. Increased levels with atorvastatin, ascorbic acid and APAP. Risk of hyperkalemia with ACE inhibitors, angiotensin-II receptor antagonists, potassium-sparing diuretics, heparin, aldosterone antagonists, and NSAIDs; monitor K^+ levels during 1st cycle. Increased levels of cyclosporine, prednisolone, and theophylline. May decrease APAP levels and increase clearance of temazepam, salicylic acid, morphine, and clofibric acid.

PREGNANCY: Category X, not for use in nursing.

YF-VAX
yellow fever vaccine (Sanofi Pasteur)

RX

THERAPEUTIC CLASS: Vaccine

INDICATIONS: Active immunization of persons ≥9 months living or traveling to endemic areas or for international travel when required or laboratory personnel who might be exposed to virulent yellow fever virus.

DOSAGE: *Adults:* Primary Vaccination: 0.5mL (4.74 $\log_{10}$ PFU) SQ. Booster: 0.5mL (4.74 $\log_{10}$ PFU) every 10 yrs. Desensitization: 0.05mL of 1:10 dilution, then 0.05mL of full strength, then 0.10mL of full strength, then 0.15mL of full strength, then 0.20mL of full strength SQ at 15-20 minute intervals.

ZADITOR

Pediatrics: ≥9 months: Primary Vaccination: 0.5mL (4.74 $\log_{10}$ PFU) SQ. Booster: 0.5mL (4.74 $\log_{10}$ PFU) every 10 years. Desensitization: 0.05mL of 1:10 dilution, then 0.05mL of full strength, then 0.10mL of full strength, then 0.15mL of full strength, then 0.20mL of full strength SQ at 15-20 minute intervals.

HOW SUPPLIED: Inj: 4.74 $\log_{10}$ PFU/0.5mL

CONTRAINDICATIONS: Hypersensitivity to eggs or egg products. Immunosuppressed patients due to illness (eg, HIV infection, leukemia, lymphoma, thymoma, generalized malignancy) or drug therapy (eg, corticosteriods, alkylating drugs, or antimetabolites) or radiation.

WARNINGS/PRECAUTIONS: Epinephrine (1:1000) should be immediately available. Vaccine-associated viscerotropic disease (rare) and vaccine-associated neurotropic disease (rare).

ADVERSE REACTIONS: Systemic: Headache, myalgia, low-grade fevers. Local: Edema, hypersensitivity, pain or mass at injection site.

INTERACTIONS: Prednisone and other corticosteroids may decrease immunogenicity and increase risk of adverse events.

PREGNANCY: Category C, not for use in nursing.

ZADITOR
ketotifen fumarate (Novartis Ophthalmics)
OTC

THERAPEUTIC CLASS: H_1 antagonist and mast cell stabilizer

INDICATIONS: Temporary prevention of itching of the eye due to allergic conjunctivitis.

DOSAGE: *Adults:* 1 drop q8-12h.

Pediatrics: ≥3 yrs: 1 drop q8-12h.

HOW SUPPLIED: Sol: 0.025% (5mL)

WARNINGS/PRECAUTIONS: Not for contact lens irritation. Do not wear a contact lens if eye is red. If eyes are not red, wait 10 minutes after instillation before inserting contacts. Soft contact lens can absorb benzalkonium chloride.

ADVERSE REACTIONS: Rhinitis, allergic reactions, burning, stinging, conjunctivitis, dry eye, eye pain, eyelid disorder, itching, keratitis, lacrimation disorder, mydriasis, photophobia, headache, rash.

PREGNANCY: Category C, caution in nursing.

ZANTAC
ranitidine HCl (GlaxoSmithKline)
RX

THERAPEUTIC CLASS: H_2 blocker

INDICATIONS: (PO) Short-term treatment of active duodenal (DU) and benign gastric ulcers (GU). Maintenance therapy for duodenal and gastric ulcers. Treatment of pathological hypersecretory conditions (eg, Zollinger-Ellison) and GERD. Treatment and maintenance of erosive esophagitis. (Inj) Hospitalized patients with pathological hypersecretory conditions or intractable duodenal ulcer. Short term alternate to oral therapy.

DOSAGE: *Adults:* (PO) DU/GU: 150mg bid or (DU) 300mg after evening meal or qhs. Maint: 150mg qhs. GERD: 150mg bid. Erosive Esophagitis: 150mg qid. Maint: 150mg bid. Hypersecretory Conditions: 150mg bid. May give up to 6g/day with severe disease. (Inj) Usual: 50mg IV/IM q6-8 hrs or 6.25mg/hr continuous IV. Max: 400mg/day. Zollinger-Ellison: Initial: 1mg/kg/hr. Titrate: May increase after 4 hrs by 0.5mg/kg/hr increments. Max: 2.5mg/kg/hr or 220mg/hr. CrCl <50mL/min: 50mg IV q18-24 hrs or 150mg PO q24h. Give more frequent (q12h) if necessary. Hemodialysis: Give dose at end of treatment. Dissolve each 150mg effervescent tab in 6-8oz of water before administration.

Pediatrics: 1 month-16 yrs: (PO) DU/GU: 2-4mg/kg bid. Max: 300mg/day. Maint: 2-4mg/kg qd. Max: 150mg/day. GERD/Erosive Esophagitis: 2.5-5mg/kg bid. (Inj) DU:

2-4mg/kg/day IV given q6-8 hrs. Max: 50mg q6-8 hrs. CrCl <50mL/min: 50mg IV q18-24 hrs or 150mg PO q24h. Give more frequent (q12h) if necessary. Hemodialysis: Give dose at end of treatment. Dissolve each 25mg effervescent tab in 5mL of water before administration.

HOW SUPPLIED: Inj: 1mg/mL, 25mg/mL; Syrup: 15mg/mL; Tab: 150mg, 300mg; Tab, Effervescent: 25mg, 150mg

WARNINGS/PRECAUTIONS: Do not exceed recommended infusion rates; bradycardia reported with rapid infusion. Caution with liver and renal dysfunction. Monitor SGPT if on IV therapy for ≥5 days at dose >100mg qid. Avoid use with history of acute porphyria. Symptomatic response does not preclude the presence of gastric malignancy. May cause false (+) urine protein test. Granules and effervescent tablets contain phenylalanine.

ADVERSE REACTIONS: Headache, constipation, diarrhea, nausea, abdominal discomfort, vomiting, hepatitis, blood dyscrasias, rash, injection site reactions (IV/IM).

INTERACTIONS: Increases plasma levels of triazolam. Monitor anticoagulants.

PREGNANCY: Category B, caution with nursing.

ZANTAC OTC
ranitidine HCl (McNeil)

OTC

OTHER BRAND NAMES: Zantac 75 (McNeil) - Zantac 150 (McNeil)

THERAPEUTIC CLASS: H_2 blocker

INDICATIONS: For prevention and relief of heartburn associated with acid indigestion and sour stomach brought on by certain foods and beverages.

DOSAGE: *Adults:* Treatment/Relief of Heartburn: 75-150mg with water. Heartburn Prevention: 75-150mg 30-60 minutes before eating food or drinking beverages that cause heartburn. Max: 150mg/24 hrs.

Pediatrics: ≥12 yrs: Treatment/Relief of Heartburn: 75-150mg with water. Heartburn Prevention: 75-150mg 30-60 minutes before eating food or drinking beverages that cause heartburn. Max: 150mg/24 hrs.

HOW SUPPLIED: Tab: 75mg, 150mg

CONTRAINDICATIONS: Trouble or pain swallowing food, vomiting with blood, or bloody or black stools.

WARNINGS/PRECAUTIONS: Trouble swallowing or persistent abdominal pain may indicate a more serious condition.

INTERACTIONS: Avoid other acid reducers.

PREGNANCY: Safety in pregnancy and nursing not known.

ZARONTIN
ethosuximide (Parke-Davis)

RX

THERAPEUTIC CLASS: Succinimide

INDICATIONS: Control of absence (petit mal) epilepsy.

DOSAGE: *Adults:* 500mg qd. Titrate: May increase daily dose by 250mg every 4-7 days. Max: 1.5g/day.

Pediatrics: Initial: 3-6 yrs: 250mg qd. ≥6 yrs: 500mg qd. Titrate: May increase daily dose by 250mg every 4-7 days. Usual: 20mg/kg/day. Max: 1.5g/day.

HOW SUPPLIED: Cap: 250mg; Syrup: 250mg/5mL

WARNINGS/PRECAUTIONS: Extreme caution in liver and renal dysfunction. Monitor blood counts, liver and renal function periodically. SLE, blood dyscrasias reported. Adjust dose slowly and avoid abrupt withdrawal. May increase grand mal seizures in mixed types of epilepsy when used alone. Caution with mental/physical activities.

ADVERSE REACTIONS: Anorexia, nausea, vomiting, abdominal pain, blood dyscrasias, drowsiness, headache, urticaria, SLE, myopia.

INTERACTIONS: May increase phenytoin levels. Valproic acid may alter levels.

PREGNANCY: Safety in pregnancy and nursing not known.

Zemplar IV
paricalcitol (Abbott) — RX

THERAPEUTIC CLASS: Vitamin D analog

INDICATIONS: Prevention and treatment of secondary hyperparathyroidism associated with chronic renal failure.

DOSAGE: *Adults:* Initial: 0.04-0.1mcg/kg bolus no more frequently than every other day during dialysis. Max: 0.24mcg/kg (16.8mcg). Titrate: May increase by 2-4mcg at 2-4 week intervals. Monitor serum Ca and phosphorus more frequently during dose adjustments. Reduce or interrupt dose if elevated Ca level or Ca x P product >75, may reinitiate at lower dose once normalized. May need dose decrease as PTH levels decrease (see labeling).

Pediatrics: ≥5 yrs: (Inj) Initial: 0.04-0.1mcg/kg bolus no more frequently than every other day during dialysis. Max: 0.24mcg/kg (16.8mcg). Titrate: May increase by 2-4mcg at 2-4 week intervals. Monitor serum Ca and phosphorus more frequently during dose adjustments. Reduce or interrupt dose if elevated Ca level or Ca x P product >75, may reinitiate at lower dose once normalized. May need dose decrease as PTH levels decrease (see labeling).

HOW SUPPLIED: Inj: 2mcg/mL, 5mcg/mL

CONTRAINDICATIONS: Vitamin D toxicity, hypercalcemia.

WARNINGS/PRECAUTIONS: Overdose may cause progressive hypercalcemia. Should supplement wiht calcium and restrict phosphorus. May need phosphate-binding compounds to control serum phosphorus levels.

ADVERSE REACTIONS: Nausea, vomiting, edema, chills, flu, GI bleeding, lightheadness, pneumonia, pain, allergic reaction, headache, HTN, diarrhea, arthritis, rash.

INTERACTIONS: Digitalis toxicity potentiated by hypercalcemia. Avoid excessive use of aluminum containing compounds.

PREGNANCY: Category C, caution in nursing.

Zemuron
rocuronium bromide (Organon USA) — RX

THERAPEUTIC CLASS: Skeletal muscle relaxant (nondepolarizing)

INDICATIONS: Adjunct to general anesthesia to facilitate both rapid sequence and routine tracheal intubation, and to provide skeletal muscle relaxation during surgery or mechanical ventilation

DOSAGE: *Adults:* Individualize dose. Rapid Sequence Intubation: 0.6-1.2mg/kg; Tracheal Intubation: Initial: 0.6mg/kg. Maint: 0.1, 0.15, or 0.2mg/kg. Continous Infusion: Initial: 10-12mcg/kg/min. Range: 4-16mcg/kg/min.

Pediatrics: 3 months-14 yrs: Individualize dose. Initial: 0.6mg/kg.

HOW SUPPLIED: Inj: 10mg/mL

WARNINGS/PRECAUTIONS: Employ peripheral nerve stimulator to monitor drug response. May have profound effects with myasthenia gravis or myasthenic (Eaton-Lambert) syndrome; use small test dose and monitor closely. Do not mix with alkaline solutions (eg, barbiturate solutions) in the same syringe or administer simultaneously during IV infusion through the same needle. Anaphylactic reactions reported. Tolerance may develop during chronic administration. Not recommended for rapid sequence induction in Cesarean section. Caution with clinically significant hepatic disease. Conditions associated with slower circulation time (eg, cardiovascular disease or advanced age) may delay onset time. Electrolyte imbalances may enhance neuromuscular blockade.

ADVERSE REACTIONS: Arrhythmia, abnormal ECG, tachycardia, nausea, vomiting, asthma, hiccup, rash, injection site edema, pruritus.

INTERACTIONS: Use of inhalation anesthetics has been shown to enhance the activity of other neuromuscular blocking agents. Resistance observed with chronic anticonvulsant therapy. Certain antibiotics (eg, aminoglycosides, vancomycin; tetracyclines, bacitracin, polymyxins, colistin, and sodium colistimethate) may cause prolongation of neuromuscular block. Quinidine injection during recovery from use of other muscle relaxants suggests that recurrent paralysis may occur. Magnesium salts may enhance neuromuscular blockade.

PREGNANCY: Category C, safety in nursing not known.

ZENAPAX   RX
daclizumab (Roche Labs)

THERAPEUTIC CLASS: Immunosuppressive agent

INDICATIONS: For prophylaxis of acute organ rejection in renal transplants, in combination with cyclosporine and corticosteroids.

DOSAGE: *Adults:* 1mg/kg IV over 15 minutes for 5 doses. Administer 1st dose no more than 24 hrs prior to transplant and remaining 4 doses at 14-day intervals.
Pediatrics: ≥11 months: 1mg/kg IV over 15 minutes for 5 doses. Administer 1st dose no more than 24 hrs prior to transplant and remaining 4 doses at 14-day intervals.

HOW SUPPLIED: Inj: 25mg/5mL

WARNINGS/PRECAUTIONS: Increased risk of lymphoproliferative disorder and opportunistic infections. Anaphylactic reactions reported. Caution in elderly. Re-administration after initial course of therapy has not been studied in humans.

ADVERSE REACTIONS: Constipation, nausea, vomiting, diarrhea, abdominal pain, pyrosis, dyspepsia, abdominal distention, epigastric pain.

PREGNANCY: Category C, not for use in nursing.

ZERIT   RX
stavudine (Bristol-Myers Squibb)

> Lactic acidosis and severe, fatal hepatomegaly reported. Fatal and non-fatal pancreatitis reported with didanosine.

THERAPEUTIC CLASS: Synthetic thymidine nucleoside analogue

INDICATIONS: Treatment of HIV-1 infection in combination with other antiretrovirals.

DOSAGE: *Adults:* ≥60kg: 40mg q12h. <60kg: 30mg q12h. Interrupt therapy if develop peripheral neuropathy, resume at 1/2 dose when neuropathy resolves. D/C permanently if neuropathy recurs after resumption. Suspend therapy if lactic acidosis or hepatotoxicity occurs. CrCl 26-50mL/min: ≥60kg: 20mg q12h. <60kg: 15mg q12h. CrCl 10-25mL/min: ≥60kg: 20mg q24h. <60kg: 15mg q24h.
Pediatrics: ≥60kg: 40mg q12h. 30-59 kg: 30mg q12h. ≥14 days and <30kg: 1mg/kg q12h. Birth-13 days: 0.5mg/kg q12h. Interrupt therapy if develop peripheral neuropathy, resume with 1/2 dose when neuropathy resolves. D/C permanently if neuropathy recurs after resumption. Suspend therapy if lactic acidosis or hepatotoxicity occurs. Renal Impairment: Reduce dose and/or increase interval.

HOW SUPPLIED: Cap: 15mg, 20mg, 30mg, 40mg; Sus: 1mg/mL (200mL)

WARNINGS/PRECAUTIONS: Obesity and prolonged nucleoside exposure may increase risk to lactic acidosis and hepatomegaly. Caution with risk factors for hepatic disease. Peripheral neuropathy reported. Monitor for lactic acidosis in pregnancy if used with didanosine. D/C if motor weakness develops.

ADVERSE REACTIONS: Peripheral neuropathy, rash, elevated LFTs and amylase, headache, diarrhea, nausea, vomiting.

INTERACTIONS: Avoid zidovudine. Increased risk of neuropathy with neurotoxic drugs (eg, didanosine). Increased risk of hepatotoxicity with didanosine and hydroxyurea. Motor weakness reported with other antiretrovirals.

PREGNANCY: Category C, not for use in nursing.

ZETACET   RX
sulfur - sulfacetamide sodium (Stiefel)

THERAPEUTIC CLASS: Sulfonamide/sulfur combination

INDICATIONS: Topical treatment of acne vulgaris, acne rosacea, and seborrheic dermatitis.

ZIAGEN

DOSAGE: *Adults:* Apply a thin layer qd-tid. Shake well before use.
Pediatrics: ≥12 yrs: Apply a thin layer qd-tid. Shake well before use.
HOW SUPPLIED: Lot: (Sulfacetamide-Sulfur) 10%-5% (25g)
CONTRAINDICATIONS: Kidney disease.
WARNINGS/PRECAUTIONS: Caution with denuded or abraded skin. Caution in patients prone to hypersensitivity to topical sulfonamides. Discontinue if irritation occurs. For external use only; avoid eye contact. Can cause reddening and scaling of epidermis.
ADVERSE REACTIONS: Local irritation.
PREGNANCY: Category C, caution in nursing.

ZIAGEN
abacavir sulfate (GlaxoSmithKline)

RX

> Fatal hypersensitivity reactions, lactic acidosis, severe hepatomegaly with steatosis, including fatal cases reported. Discontinue if hypersensitivity reaction is suspected and do not restart.

THERAPEUTIC CLASS: Synthetic carbocyclic nucleoside analogue
INDICATIONS: Treatment of HIV-1 infection in combination with other antiretrovirals.
DOSAGE: *Adults:* >16 yrs: 300mg bid or 600mg qd.
Pediatrics: 3 months-16 yrs: 8mg/kg bid. Max: 300mg bid.
HOW SUPPLIED: Sol: 20mg/mL (240mL); Tab: 300mg
WARNINGS/PRECAUTIONS: Register abacavir hypersensitive patients at 800-270-0425. Caution with liver disease; lactic acidosis and severe hepatomegaly with steatosis, including fatal cases, have been reported. Not for monotherapy when antiretroviral regimens are changed. Immune reconstitution syndrome reported. Should not be coadministered with Epzicom or Trizivir.
ADVERSE REACTIONS: Hypersensitivity reactions (eg, fever, rash, fatigue, GI symptoms), nausea, vomiting, diarrhea, loss of appetite, insomnia, chills, headache, fatigue.
INTERACTIONS: Decreased elimination with ethanol.
PREGNANCY: Category C, not for use in nursing.

ZIANA
tretinoin - clindamycin phosphate (Medicis)

RX

THERAPEUTIC CLASS: Lincosamide derivative/retinoid
INDICATIONS: Topical treatment of acne vulgaris.
DOSAGE: *Adults:* Apply pea-sized amount to entire face qd at bedtime. Avoid eyes, mouth, angles of nose, or mucous membranes. Not for oral, ophthalmic, or intravaginal use.
Pediatrics: ≥12 yrs: Apply pea-sized amount to entire face qd at bedtime. Avoid eyes, mouth, angles of nose, or mucous membranes. Not for oral, ophthalmic, or intravaginal use.
HOW SUPPLIED: Gel: (Clindamycin-Tretinoin) 1.2%-0.025% (2g, 30g, 60g)
CONTRAINDICATIONS: Regional enteritis, ulcerative colitis, or history of antibiotic-associated colitis.
WARNINGS/PRECAUTIONS: May cause severe colitis; d/c if significant diarrhea occurs. Avoid exposure to sunlight and sunlamps; wear sunscreen daily.
ADVERSE REACTIONS: Nasopharyngitis, erythema, scaling, itching, burning.
INTERACTIONS: Caution with concomitant topical medications, medicated/abrasive soaps and cleansers, soaps/cosmetics with strong drying effect, products with high concentrations of alcohol, astringents, spices, or lime. Avoid with erythromycin-containing products. Caution with neuromuscular blocking agents.
PREGNANCY: Category C, not for use in nursing.

ZITHROMAX
azithromycin (Pfizer)

RX

THERAPEUTIC CLASS: Macrolide antibiotic

INDICATIONS: (PO) Treatment of acute bacterial exacerbations of COPD, acute bacterial sinusitis (ABS), community acquired pneumonia (CAP), pharyngitis/tonsillitis, uncomplicated skin and skin structure, urethritis/cervicitis, genital ulcer disease (men), acute otitis media, prevention of disseminated *Mycobacterium avium* complex (MAC) disease in advanced HIV infection. (IV) Treatment of CAP and pelvic inflammatory disease (PID).

DOSAGE: *Adults:* (PO) COPD/CAP/Pharyngitis/Tonsillitis (second line therapy)/SSSI: ≥16 yrs: 500mg on day 1, then 250mg qd on days 2-5. COPD: 500mg qd for 3 days. ABS: 500mg qd for 3 days. Genital Ulcer Disease and Non-Gonococcal Urethritis/Cervicitis: 1g single dose. Urethritis/Cervicitis due to *N.gonorrhea:* 2g single dose. MAC Prophylaxis: 1200mg once weekly. MAC Treatment: 600mg qd with ethambutol 15mg/kg/day. (IV) ≥16 yrs: CAP: 500mg qd for at least 2 days, then 500mg PO to complete 7-10 day course. PID: 500mg qd for 1-2 days, then 250mg PO to complete 7 day course.

Pediatrics: (Sus) Otitis Media: ≥6 months: 30mg/kg single dose; 10mg/kg qd for 3 days; or 10mg/kg qd on day 1, then 5mg/kg qd on days 2-5. ABS: ≥6 months: 10mg/kg qd for 3 days. CAP: ≥6 months: 10mg/kg qd on day 1, then 5mg/kg qd on days 2-5. (Sus, Tab) Pharyngitis/Tonsillitis: ≥2 yrs: 12mg/kg qd for 5 days. 1g sus not for pediatric use.

HOW SUPPLIED: Inj: 500mg; Sus: 100mg/5mL (15mL), 200mg/5mL (15mL, 22.5mL, 30mL), 1g/pkt (3^s 10^s); Tab: 250mg (Z-PAK, 6 tabs), 500mg (TRI-PAK, 3 tabs), 600mg

WARNINGS/PRECAUTIONS: D/C if allergic reaction occurs. Oral therapy is only for community acquired pneumonia of mild severity. Hypersensitivity reactions may recur after initial successful symptomatic treatment. Monitor for pseudomembranous colitis. Caution with renal/hepatic dysfunction. 1g sus not for pediatric use.

ADVERSE REACTIONS: Diarrhea/loose stools, nausea, abdominal pain.

INTERACTIONS: Monitor theophylline, terfenadine, cyclosporine, hexobarbital, phenytoin, warfarin. May increase digoxin, carbamazepine levels. Potentiates triazolam. Aluminum- and magnesium-containing antacids reduce oral levels. Acute ergot toxicity may occur with ergotamine or dihydroergotamine. Monitor for azithromycin side effects (eg, liver enzyme abnormalities, hearing impairment) with nelfinavir.

PREGNANCY: Category B, caution in nursing.

Zocor
simvastatin (Merck)

RX

THERAPEUTIC CLASS: HMG-CoA reductase inhibitor

INDICATIONS: May initiate with diet in patients with, or at high risk for, coronary heart disease (CHD). In high risk patients with CHD, diabetes, peripheral vessel disease, history of stroke or other cerebrovascular disease to reduce risk of total mortality by reducing CHD deaths, risk of non-fatal MI and stroke, need for revascularization procedures. To reduce elevated total-C, LDL-C, Apo B, TG, and increase HDL-C in primary hypercholesterolemia (heterozygous familial and nonfamilial) and mixed dyslipidemia (Types IIa and IIb). To treat hypertriglyceridemia (Type IV) and primary dysbetalipoproteinemia (Type III). To reduce total-C, LDL-C in homozygous familial hypercholesterolemia as adjunct to other lipid-lowering agents or if such treatments are unavailable. To reduce total-C, LDL-C, Apo B in adolescents 10-17 yrs old, at least 1yr post-menarche, with heterozygous familial hypercholesterolemia. To reduce elevated LDL-C, TG in Type IIb hyperlipidemia.

DOSAGE: *Adults:* Initial: 20-40mg qpm. Usual: 5-80mg/day. Titrate: Adjust at ≥4-week intervals. High Risk for CHD Events: Initial: 40mg/day. Homozygous Familial Hypercholesterolemia: 40mg qpm or 80mg/day given as 20mg bid plus 40mg qpm. Concomitant Cyclosporine: Initial: 5mg/day. Max: 10mg/day. Concomitant Gemfibrozil (try to avoid): Max: 10mg/day. Concomitant Amiodarone/Verapamil: Max: 20mg/day. Severe Renal Insufficiency: 5mg/day; monitor closely.

Pediatrics: Heterozygous Familial Hypercholesterolemia: 10-17 yrs (at least 1yr postmenarchal): Initial: 10mg qpm. Usual: 10-40mg/day. Titrate: Adjust at ≥4-week intervals. Max: 40mg/day.

HOW SUPPLIED: Tab: 5mg, 10mg, 20mg, 40mg, 80mg

CONTRAINDICATIONS: Active liver disease, unexplained persistent elevations of serum transaminases, pregnancy, nursing mothers.

ZOFRAN

WARNINGS/PRECAUTIONS: Caution with heavy alcohol use, severe renal insufficiency or history of hepatic disease. Monitor LFT's prior to therapy, periodically thereafter for 1st year, or until 1 year after last dose elevation (additional test at 3 months for 80mg dose). D/C if AST or ALT ≥3X ULN persist, if myopathy is suspected or diagnosed, a few days prior to major surgery. Rhabdomyolysis (rare), myopathy reported.

ADVERSE REACTIONS: Abdominal pain, headache, CK and transaminase elevations.

INTERACTIONS: Avoid use with concomitant itraconazole, ketoconazole, erythromycin, clarithromycin, telithromycin, HIV protease inhibitors, nefazodone, grapefruit juice (>1 quart/day); increased risk of myopathy/rhabdomyolysis. Max 10mg/day with gemfibrozil, cyclosporin, danazol. Max 20mg/day with amiodarone, verapamil. Caution with other fibrates, ≥1g/day of niacin. Monitor digoxin, warfarin.

PREGNANCY: Category X, not for use in nursing.

ZOFRAN   RX
ondansetron (GlaxoSmithKline)

THERAPEUTIC CLASS: 5-HT$_3$ antagonist

INDICATIONS: (Inj) Prevention of nausea and vomiting associated with initial and repeat courses of emetogenic cancer chemotherapy, including high-dose cisplatin. Prevention of postoperative nausea and/or vomiting. (Sol/Tab) Prevention of nausea and vomiting associated with: highly emetogenic cancer chemotherapy, including cisplatin ≥50mg/m^2; initial and repeat courses of moderately emetogenic cancer chemotherapy; and radiotherapy in patients receiving either total body irradiation, single high-dose fraction to the abdomen, or daily fractions to the abdomen. Prevention of postoperative nausea and/or vomiting.

DOSAGE: *Adults:* Prevention of Chemotherapy-Induced Nausea/Vomiting: (Inj) 32mg single dose or three 0.15mg/kg doses, 1st dose 30 minutes before chemotherapy, then 4 and 8 hours after the 1st dose. Prevention of Nausea/Vomiting Associated With Highly Emetogenic Cancer Chemotherapy: (Tab) 24mg single dose tab 30 minutes before chemotherapy. Prevention of Nausea/Vomiting Associated With Moderately Emetogenic Cancer Chemotherapy: (Sol/Tab) 8mg bid, 1st dose 30 minutes before chemotherapy, then 8 hrs later, then bid for 1-2 days after chemotherapy. Prevention of Post-Op Nausea/Vomiting: (Inj) 4mg IM/IV immediately before anesthesia or post-op after surgery if nausea or vomiting occurs. (Sol/Tab) 16mg 1 hr before anesthesia. Prevention of Nausea/Vomiting Associated with Radiation Therapy: (Sol/Tab) Usual: 8mg tid. Total Body Irradiation: 8mg 1-2 hrs before therapy daily. Single High-Dose Therapy To Abdomen: 8mg 1-2 hrs before therapy then q8h after 1st dose for 1-2 days after completion of therapy. Daily Fractionated Therapy To Abdomen: 8mg 1-2 hrs before therapy then q8h after 1st dose. Severe Hepatic Dysfunction (Child-Pugh^2 ≥10): Max: 8mg/day IV single dose infused over 15 minutes, start 30 minutes before chemotherapy or 8mg/day PO.

Pediatrics: Prevention of Chemotherapy-Induced Nausea/Vomiting: (Inj) 6 months-18 yrs: Three 0.15mg/kg doses, 1st dose 30 minutes before chemotherapy, then 4 and 8 hrs after the 1st dose. (Sol/Tab) Prevention of Nausea/Vomiting Associated With Moderately Emetogenic Cancer Chemotherapy: ≥12 yrs: 8mg bid, 1st dose 30 minutes before chemotherapy, then 8mg 8 hrs later, then bid for 1-2 days. 4-11 yrs: 4mg tid, 1st dose 30 minutes before chemotherapy, then 4 and 8 hrs after 1st dose, then tid for 1-2 days. Prevention of Post-Op Nausea/Vomiting: (Inj) >12 yrs: 4mg IM/IV immediately before anesthesia or post-op after surgery if nausea or vomiting occurs. 1 month-12 yrs: ≤40kg: 0.1mg/kg single dose. >40kg: 4mg single dose. Severe Hepatic Dysfunction: Max: 8mg/day IV single dose infused over 15 minutes, start 30 minutes before chemotherapy or 8mg/day PO.

HOW SUPPLIED: Inj: 2mg/mL, 32mg/50mL; Sol: 4mg/5mL (50mL); Tab: 4mg, 8mg, 24mg; Tab, Disintegrating: 4mg, 8mg

ZOLOFT

WARNINGS/PRECAUTIONS: Hypersensitivity reactions have been reported in those hypersensitive to other 5-HT$_3$ receptor antagonists. Transient ECG changes including QT interval prolongation have been reported with IV administration. May mask a progressive ileus or gastric distension. Orally disintegrating tablets contain phenylalanine; caution in phenylketonurics.

ADVERSE REACTIONS: Headache, diarrhea, dizziness, drowsiness, malaise/fatigue, constipation, LFT abnormalities.

INTERACTIONS: Ondansetron is metabolized by CYP450 enzymes; inducers or inhibitors of these enzymes may change the clearance and half-life of ondansetron.

PREGNANCY: Category B, caution in nursing.

ZOLOFT
sertraline HCl (Pfizer)

RX

> Antidepressants increased the risk of suicidal thinking and behavior (suicidality) in short-term studies in children and adolescents with Major Depressive Disorder (MDD) and other psychiatric disorders. Sertraline HCl is not approved for use in pediatric patients except for patients with obsessive compulsive disorder (OCD).

THERAPEUTIC CLASS: Selective serotonin reuptake inhibitor

INDICATIONS: Treatment of MDD, social anxiety disorder (SAD), OCD, panic disorder with or without agoraphobia, premenstrual dysphoric disorder (PMDD) and posttraumatic stress disorder (PTSD).

DOSAGE: *Adults:* MDD/OCD: 50mg qd. Titrate: Adjust dose at 1 week intervals. Max: 200mg/day. Panic Disorder/PTSD/SAD: Initial: 25mg qd. Titrate: Increase to 50mg qd after 1 week. Adjust dose at 1 week intervals. Max: 200mg/day. PMDD: Initial: 50mg qd continuous or limited to luteal phase of cycle. Titrate: Increase 50mg/cycle if needed up to 150mg/day for continuous or 100mg/day for luteal phase dosing. If 100mg/day is established for luteal phase dosing, a 50mg/day titration step for 3 days should take place at the beginning of each luteal phase dosing period. Hepatic Impairment: Use lower or less frequent doses. Dilute solution with 4oz of water, ginger ale, lemon/lime soda, lemonade or orange juice. Take immediately after mixing.

Pediatrics: OCD: Initial: 6-12 yrs: 25mg qd. 13-17 yrs: 50mg qd. Titrate: Adjust dose at 1 week intervals. Max: 200mg/day. Hepatic Impairment: Use lower or less frequent doses. Dilute solution with 4oz of water, ginger ale, lemon/lime soda, lemonade or orange juice. Take immediately after mixing.

HOW SUPPLIED: Sol: 20mg/mL (60mL); Tab: 25mg*, 50mg*, 100mg* *scored

CONTRAINDICATIONS: Concomitant use with MAOIs or pimozide. Concomitant disulfiram with solution.

WARNINGS/PRECAUTIONS: Activation of mania/hypomania reported. Monitor weight loss. Caution with conditions that could affect metabolism or hemodynamic responses, seizure disorder. Dose adjust with liver dysfunction. Altered platelet function and hyponatremia reported. Weak uricosuric effects reported. Caution with latex sensitivity; solution dropper dispenser contains rubber. Monitor for clinical worsening and/or suicidality, especially at initiation of therapy or dose changes. Avoid abrupt withdrawal. Monitor for discontinuation symptoms.

ADVERSE REACTIONS: Ejaculation failure, dry mouth, increased sweating, somnolence, tremor, anorexia, dizziness, headache, vomiting, diarrhea, dyspepsia, nausea, agitation, insomnia, nervousness, abnormal vision.

INTERACTIONS: See Contraindications. Increased levels with cimetidine. Avoid with alcohol, pimozide or MAOIs. Decreases clearance of tolbutamide. Rare reports of weakness, hyperreflexia, incoordination with an SSRI and sumatriptan. May potentiate drugs metabolized by CYP2D6 (eg, TCAs, Type 1C antiarrhythmics). Caution with CNS drugs (eg, diazepam). Monitor lithium. Caution with TCAs; may need dose adjustment. May shift concentrations with plasma protein-bound drugs (eg, warfarin, digitoxin). Monitor PT with warfarin. Caution with OTC products. May induce metabolism of cisapride. Caution with drugs that interfere with hemostasis (eg, non-selective NSAIDs, aspirin, warfarin) due to increased risk of bleeding.

PREGNANCY: Category C, caution in nursing.

ZONEGRAN
zonisamide (Eisai)

RX

THERAPEUTIC CLASS: Sulfonamide anticonvulsant

INDICATIONS: Adjunctive therapy in the treatment of partial seizures.

DOSAGE: *Adults:* Initial: 100mg qd for 2 weeks. Titrate: Increase to 200mg/day for 2 weeks, then increase to 300mg/day, then to 400mg/day at 2 week intervals. Max: 400mg/day.

Pediatrics: ≥16 yrs: Initial: 100mg qd for 2 weeks. Titrate: Increase to 200mg/day for 2 weeks, then increase to 300mg/day, then to 400mg/day at 2 week intervals. Max: 400mg/day.

HOW SUPPLIED: Cap: 25mg, 50mg, 100mg

CONTRAINDICATIONS: Sulfonamide hypersensitivity.

WARNINGS/PRECAUTIONS: Sulfonamide hypersensitivity reactions (eg, Stevens-Johnson syndrome, toxic epidermal necrolysis, fulminant hepatic necrosis, blood dyscrasias), cognitive/neuropsychiatric effects, kidney stones, sudden death reported. Discontinue with unexplained rash. Increased risk of oligohydrosis and hyperthermia in pediatrics; monitor for decreased sweating and increased body temperature. Advise females to use contraceptives to prevent pregnancy. Caution with renal/hepatic impairment. Avoid abrupt withdrawal.

ADVERSE REACTIONS: Somnolence, anorexia, dizziness, tremor, convulsion, dry mouth, incoordination, amblyopia, tinnitus, GI effects, flu syndrome, ataxia, nystagmus, pruritus.

INTERACTIONS: Enzyme inducers increase metabolism and clearance. Caution with drugs that predispose patients to heat-related disorders (eg, carbonic anhydrase inhibitors, anticholinergic drugs).

PREGNANCY: Category C, not for use in nursing.

ZOVIRAX
acyclovir (GlaxoSmithKline)

RX

THERAPEUTIC CLASS: Nucleoside analogue

INDICATIONS: Acute treatment of herpes zoster (shingles). Treatment of initial and recurrent episodes of genital herpes. Treatment of chickenpox (varicella).

DOSAGE: *Adults:* Herpes Zoster: 800mg q4h, 5x/day for 7-10 days. Start within 72 hrs after onset of rash. Genital Herpes: Initial: 200mg q4h, 5x/day for 10 days. Chronic Therapy: 400mg bid or 200mg 3-5x/day up to 12 months, then re-evaluate. Intermittent Therapy: 200mg q4h, 5x/day for 5 days. Start with 1st sign/symptom of recurrence. Chickenpox: 800mg qid for 5 days. CrCl 10-25mL/min: For a dose of 800mg q4h, give 800mg q8h. CrCl 0-10mL/min: For a dose of 200mg q4h, give 200mg q12h. For a dose of 400mg q12h, give 200mg q12h. For a dose of 800mg q4h, give 800mg q12h. Elderly: Reduce dose.

Pediatrics: ≥2 yrs: ≤40kg: Chickenpox: 20mg/kg qid for 5 days. >40kg: 800mg qid for 5 days.

HOW SUPPLIED: Cap: 200mg; Sus: 200mg/5mL; Tab: 400mg, 800mg

CONTRAINDICATIONS: Hypersensitivity to valacyclovir.

WARNINGS/PRECAUTIONS: Adust dose in renal impairment, elderly. Renal failure and death reported. Thrombotic thrombocytopenic purpura/hemolytic uremic syndrome in immunocompromised patients reported.

ADVERSE REACTIONS: Nausea, vomiting, diarrhea, headache, malaise, renal dysfunction.

INTERACTIONS: Probenecid increased levels of IV formulation. Caution with potentially nephrotoxic agents.

PREGNANCY: Category B, caution in nursing.

ZOVIRAX CREAM
acyclovir (Biovail)

RX

THERAPEUTIC CLASS: Nucleoside analogue antiviral

INDICATIONS: Treatment of recurrent herpes labialis (cold sores).

DOSAGE: *Adults:* Apply 5x/day for 4 days. Initiate with 1st sign/symptom.
Pediatrics: ≥12 yrs: Apply 5x/day for 4 days. Initiate with 1st sign/symptom.
HOW SUPPLIED: Cre: 5% (2g)
WARNINGS/PRECAUTIONS: Cutaneous use only; not for use in the eye, mouth or nose.
ADVERSE REACTIONS: Dry lips, desquamation, dryness of skin, cracked lips, burning skin, pruritus, flakiness of skin, stinging on skin.
PREGNANCY: Category B, caution in nursing.

Zyflo CR
zileuton (Critical Therapeutics)

RX

OTHER BRAND NAME: Zyflo (Critical Therapeutics)
THERAPEUTIC CLASS: Leukotriene inhibitor
INDICATIONS: Prophylaxis and chronic treatment of asthma.
DOSAGE: *Adults:* 600mg qid, with meals and at bedtime. (Tab, Extended-Release) 1200mg bid within 1 hr after am and pm meals. Max: 2400mg/day.
Pediatrics: ≥12 yrs: 600mg qid, with meals and at bedtime. (Tab, Extended-Release) 1200mg bid within 1 hr after am and pm meals. Max: 2400mg/day.
HOW SUPPLIED: Tab, Extended-Release: 600mg; Tab: 600mg* *scored
CONTRAINDICATIONS: Active liver disease or transaminase elevations (≥3X ULN).
WARNINGS/PRECAUTIONS: Not for treatment of acute attacks. Evaluate liver function prior to therapy and periodically thereafter. D/C if signs of liver disease occur.
ADVERSE REACTIONS: (Zyflo, Zyflo CR) Headache, ALT elevation, dyspepsia, pain, nausea, asthenia, myalgia. (Zyflo CR) Sinusitis, pharyngolaryngeal pain.
INTERACTIONS: Monitor drugs metabolized by CYP450 3A4. Increases theophylline levels; reduce theophylline by 50% and monitor levels. Potentiates warfarin, propranolol. (Zyflo) Potentiates terfenadine.
PREGNANCY: Category C, not for use in nursing.

Zyloprim
allopurinol (Prometheus)

RX

THERAPEUTIC CLASS: Xanthine oxidase inhibitor
INDICATIONS: Management of symptoms of primary and secondary gout. Management of hyperuricosuria and hyperuricemia due to chemotherapy. Management of recurrent calcium oxalate calculi in those with hyperuricosuria (uric acid excretion >800mg/day in males and >750mg/day in females).
DOSAGE: *Adults:* Gout: Initial: 100mg/day. Titrate: Increase by 100mg/week until serum uric acid level is ≤6mg/dL. Mild Gout: 200-300mg/day. Moderately Severe Gout: Usual: 400-600mg/day. Max: 800mg/day. Recurrent Calcium Oxalate Stones: Usual: 200-300mg/day. Prevention of Uric Acid Nephropathy with Chemotherapy: Usual: 600-800mg/day for 2-3 days with high fluid intake. CrCl 10-20mL/min: 200mg/day. CrCl <10mL/min: Max: 100mg/day. CrCl <3mL/min: Also increase dosing intervals. Take after meals. Divide dose if >300mg.
Pediatrics: Hyperuricemia with Malignancies: 6-10 yrs: 300mg/day. <6 yrs: 150mg/day. Evaluate response after 48 hrs. Take after meals.
HOW SUPPLIED: Tab: 100mg*, 300mg* *scored
WARNINGS/PRECAUTIONS: Discontinue if skin rash occurs. Severe hypersensitivity reactions, hepatotoxicity, and bone marrow depression reported. Monitor LFTs during early stages of therapy with liver disease. Caution with activities that require alertness. Caution with renal impairment. Renal failure reported with hyperuricemia secondary to neoplastic diseases. Fluid intake should yield ≥2 liters of urinary output/day. Maintain neutral or slightly alkaline urine. Acute gout attacks increase during early stages of therapy; give colchicine.
ADVERSE REACTIONS: Acute gout attacks, rash, diarrhea, SGOT/SGPT increase, alkaline phosphatase increase, nausea.

INTERACTIONS: Increased toxicity with thiazide diuretics or renal impairment; monitor renal function. Reduce mercaptopurine or azathioprine to 1/3 or 1/4 of usual dose. Potentiates dicumarol, chlorpropamide and cyclosporine. Decreased effects with uricosurics. Increased skin rash with ampicillin, amoxicillin. Enhanced bone marrow suppression with cytotoxic agents (eg, cyclophosphamide). Caution with sulfinpyrazone.

PREGNANCY: Category C, caution in nursing.

ZYMAR
gatifloxacin (Allergan)
RX

THERAPEUTIC CLASS: Fluoroquinolone

INDICATIONS: Treatment of bacterial conjunctivitis.

DOSAGE: *Adults:* 1 drop q2h while awake, up to 8x/day for 2 days; then 1 drop up to qid while awake for 5 days.
Pediatrics: ≥1 yr: 1 drop q2h while awake, up to 8x/day for 2 days; then 1 drop up to qid while awake for 5 days.

HOW SUPPLIED: Sol: 0.3% (5mL)

WARNINGS/PRECAUTIONS: Not for injection. Do not inject subconjunctivally or into the anterior chamber of the eye. Superinfection may result with prolonged use. Fatal hypersensitivity reactions reported after 1st dose of systemic quinolone therapy. Avoid contact lenses when symptoms are present.

ADVERSE REACTIONS: Conjunctival irritation, increased lacrimation, keratitis, papillary conjunctivitis, chemosis, conjunctival hemorrhage, dry eye, eye discharge/irritation/pain, red eye, eyelid edema, headache, reduced visual acuity, taste disturbance.

INTERACTIONS: Systemic quinolone therapy may increase theophylline levels, interfere with caffeine metabolism, enhance warfarin effects, and elevate serum creatinine with cyclosporine.

PREGNANCY: Category C, caution in nursing.

ZYMASE
lipase - amylase - protease (Organon)
RX

THERAPEUTIC CLASS: Pancreatic enzyme supplement

INDICATIONS: Treatment of conditions with pancreatic enzyme deficiency with resultant inadequate fat digestion (eg, chronic pancreatitis, pancreatectomy, cystic fibrosis, steatorrhea).

DOSAGE: *Adults:* 1-2 caps with each meal or snack. Contents of cap may be mixed with liquids or soft foods that do not require chewing.
Pediatrics: 1-2 caps with each meal or snack. Contents of cap may be mixed with liquids or soft foods that do not require chewing.

HOW SUPPLIED: Cap, Delayed Release: (Amylase-Lipase-Protease) 24,000U-12,000U-24,000U

CONTRAINDICATIONS: Pork protein hypersensitivity.

WARNINGS/PRECAUTIONS: Do not chew or crush contents of capsules. High doses can cause hyperuricemia and hyperuricosuria.

PREGNANCY: Safety in pregnancy and nursing not known.

ZYRTEC
cetirizine HCl (Pfizer)
RX

THERAPEUTIC CLASS: H₁ antagonist

INDICATIONS: Seasonal or perennial allergic rhinitis. Chronic idiopathic urticaria.

DOSAGE: *Adults:* 5-10mg qd. Hepatic Impairment/Hemodialysis/CrCl <31mL/min: 5mg qd.
Pediatrics: ≥12 yrs: 5-10mg qd. 6-11 yrs: 5-10mg qd. 2-5 yrs: 2.5mg qd. Max: 5mg qd or 2.5mg q12h. Perennial Allergic Rhinitis/Urticaria: 6 months-23 months: 2.5mg qd. 12

months-23 months: May increase to max 5mg/day given as 2.5mL q12h. Hepatic Impairment/Hemodialysis/CrCl <31mL/min: ≥12 yrs: 5mg qd. 6-11 yrs: Use lower the recommended dose. <6 yrs: Not recommended.

HOW SUPPLIED: Syrup: 1mg/mL (120mL, 480mL); Tab: 5mg, 10mg; Tab, Chewable: 5mg, 10mg

CONTRAINDICATIONS: Hydroxyzine hypersensitivity.

WARNINGS/PRECAUTIONS: Adjust dose with hepatic or renal impairment. May impair mental/physical abilities.

ADVERSE REACTIONS: Somnolence, fatigue, dry mouth, headache, pharyngitis, abdominal pain, cough, epistaxis, diarrhea, bronchospasm.

INTERACTIONS: Avoid alcohol and CNS depressants. Possible decreased clearance with large doses of theophylline.

PREGNANCY: Category B, not for use in nursing.

ZYRTEC-D
cetirizine HCl - pseudoephedrine HCl (Pfizer)

RX

THERAPEUTIC CLASS: Antihistamine/decongestant

INDICATIONS: Relief of nasal and non-nasal symptoms associated with seasonal or perennial allergic rhinitis.

DOSAGE: *Adults:* 1 tab bid. Hepatic Impairment/Renal Dysfunction (CrCl <31mL/min): 1 tab qd. Swallow tabs whole.

Pediatrics: ≥12 yrs: 1 tab bid. Hepatic Impairment/Renal Dysfunction (CrCl <31mL/min): 1 tab qd. Swallow tabs whole.

HOW SUPPLIED: Tab, Extended Release: (Cetirizine-Pseudoephedrine) 5mg-120mg

CONTRAINDICATIONS: Narrow angle glaucoma, urinary retention, MAOIs during or within 14 days of use, severe HTN, severe CAD, hypersensitivity to adrenergics.

WARNINGS/PRECAUTIONS: Caution with HTN, DM, ischemic heart disease, increased IOP, hyperthyroidism, renal impairment, or prostatic hypertrophy. May produce CNS stimulation with convulsions or cardiovascular collapse.

ADVERSE REACTIONS: Insomnia, dry mouth, fatigue, somnolence.

INTERACTIONS: Avoid MAOIs during or within 14 days of use.

PREGNANCY: Category C, not for use in nursing.

ZYVOX
linezolid (Pfizer)

RX

THERAPEUTIC CLASS: Oxazolidinone class antibacterial

INDICATIONS: Vancomycin resistant *Enterococcus faecium* (VRE) infections, nosocomial pneumonia caused by *Staphylococcus aureus* (methicillin-susceptible and -resistant strains) or *Streptococcus pneumoniae* (including multi-drug resistant strains (MDRSP)), complicated skin and skin structure infections (SSSI) including diabetic foot infections without concomitant osteomyelitis caused by *Staphylococcus aureus* (methicillin-susceptible and -resistant strains), *Streptococcus pyogenes*, or *Streptococcus agalactiae*, uncomplicated SSSI caused by *Staphylococcus aureus* (methicillin-susceptible only) or *Streptococcus pyogenes*, community-acquired pneumonia (CAP) caused by *Streptococcus pneumoniae* (MDRSP), including concurrent bacteremia, or *Staphylococcus aureus* (methicillin-susceptible strains only).

DOSAGE: *Adults:* Complicated SSSI/CAP/Nosocomial Pneumonia: 600mg IV/PO q12h for 10-14 days. VRE: 600mg IV/PO q12h for 14-28 days. Uncomplicated SSSI: 400mg PO q12h for 10-14 days.

Pediatrics: Complicated SSSI/CAP/Nosocomial Pneumonia: Treat for 10-14 days. ≥12 yrs: 600mg IV/PO q12h. Birth-11yrs: 10mg/kg IV/PO q8h. VRE: Treat for 14-28 days: ≥12 yrs: 600mg IV/PO q12h; Birth-11 yrs: 10mg/kg IV/PO q8h. Uncomplicated SSSI: Treat for 10-14 days: ≥12 yrs: 600mg PO q12h; 5-11 yrs: 10mg/kg PO q12h; <5 yrs: 10mg/kg PO

ZYVOX

q8h. Neonates <7 days should be initiated with dosing regimen of 10mg/kg q12h; may increase to 10mg/kg q8h if sub-optimal response. All neonatal patients should receive 10mg/kg q8h by 7 days of life.

HOW SUPPLIED: Inj: 2mg/mL (100mL, 200mL, 300mL); Sus: 100mg/5mL; Tab: 400mg, 600mg

WARNINGS/PRECAUTIONS: Myelosuppression including anemia, thrombocytopenia, pancytopenia, and leukopenia reported; monitor CBC weekly. Superinfection and pseudomembranous colitis may occur. May permit overgrowth of clostridia. Oral suspension contains phenylalanine. Peripheral and optic neuropathy have been reported; monitor visual function if on for extended periods (=3 months). Lactic acidosis reported.

ADVERSE REACTIONS: Diarrhea, headache, nausea, vomiting.

INTERACTIONS: Potential interaction with adrenergic and serotonergic agents. May enhance pressor response to sympathomimetics, vasopressors, and dopaminergic agents; caution with dopamine, epinephrine, pseudoephedrine, and phenylpropanolamine. Serotonin syndrome may occur with SSRIs and other antidepressants. Avoid large quantities of tyramine-containing foods or beverages.

PREGNANCY: Category C, caution in nursing.

NeoFax® Drug Monographs

NeoFax Key

Monograph Name

Dose & Administration
Evidence-based dosage and administration information for neonates.

Uses
Includes evidence-based indications.

Monitoring
Important monitoring parameters.

Adverse Effects/Precautions
Details harmful conditions and adverse reactions related to the use of the drug.

Pharmacology
Summary of the pharmacological characteristics of the product.

Special Considerations
Brief description of how to prepare medicine for administration. It also highlights the medication's compatibilities and incompatibilities.

Selected References
- Citations for evidence-based information.

Acetaminophen

DOSE & ADMINISTRATION: Oral Loading dose: 20 to 25 mg/kg. Maintenance: 12 to 15 mg/kg per dose. **Rectal Loading dose:** 30 mg/kg. Maintenance: 12 to 18 mg/kg per dose. **Maintenance intervals:** Term infants: Q6 hours Preterm infants ≥ 32 weeks GA: Q8 hours; Preterm infants < 32 weeks GA: Q12 hours

USES: Fever reduction and treatment of mild to moderate pain.

MONITORING: Assess for signs of pain. Monitor temperature. Assess liver function. Serum acetaminophen concentration is obtained only to assess toxicity.

ADVERSE EFFECTS/PRECAUTIONS: Liver toxicity occurs with excessive doses or after prolonged administration (>48 hours) of therapeutic doses. Rash, fever, thrombocytopenia, leukopenia, and neutropenia have been reported in children.

PHARMACOLOGY: Acetaminophen is a nonnarcotic analgesic and antipyretic. Peak serum concentration occurs approximately 60 minutes after an oral dose. Absorption after rectal administration is variable and prolonged. Extensively metabolized in the liver, primarily by sulfation with a small amount by glucuronidation. Metabolites and unchanged drug are excreted by the kidney. Elimination half-life is approximately 3 hours in term neonates, 5 hours in preterm neonates > 32 weeks gestation, and up to 11 hours in more immature neonates. Elimination is prolonged in patients with liver dysfunction.

SPECIAL CONSIDERATIONS/PREPARATION: Dosage forms: Drops: 100 mg/mL, 48 mg/mL (alcohol-free). Elixir: 16 mg/mL, 24 mg/mL, 32 mg/mL. Liquid: 32 mg/mL (alcohol-free). Liquid: 33.33 mg/mL (7% alcohol). Suppositories: 80, 120, 325, 600, and 650 mg. Inaccurate dosing may occur with rectal administration because of unequal distribution of acetaminophen in the suppositories. **Treatment of Serious Acetaminophen Toxicity:** N-acetylcysteine, 150 mg/kg, in 5% dextrose given IV over 30 minutes (loading dose), followed by 50 mg/kg over 4 hours, then 100 mg/kg per 24 hours until the International Normalized Prothrombin (INR) normalizes.

SELECTED REFERENCES

- Anderson BJ, van Lingen RA, Hansen TG, et al: Acetaminophen developmental pharmacokinetics in premature neonates and infants. *Anesthesiology* 2002;96:1336-45.
- Isbister GK, Bucens IK, Whyte IM: Paracetamol overdose in a preterm neonate. *Arch Dis Child Fetal Neonatal Ed* 2001;85:F70-F72.
- Arana A, Morton NS, Hansen TG: Treatment with paracetamol in infants. *Acta Anaesthesiol Scand* 2001;45:20-29.
- Levy G, Khanna NN, Soda DM, et al: Pharmacokinetics of acetaminophen in the human neonate: Formation of acetaminophen glucuronide and sulfate in relation to plasma bilirubin concentration and D-glucaric acid excretion. *Pediatrics* 1975;55:818.

Acyclovir

DOSE & ADMINISTRATION: 20 mg/kg per dose Q8 hours IV infusion by syringe pump over 1 hour. Prolong the dosing interval in premature infants <34 weeks PMA, or in patients with significant renal impairment or hepatic failure. Treat localized herpes simplex infections for 14 days, disseminated or CNS infections for 21 days. **Chronic suppression:** 75 mg/kg per dose PO Q12 hours.

USES: Treatment of neonatal herpes simplex infections, varicella zoster infections with CNS and pulmonary involvement, and herpes simplex encephalitis.

MONITORING: Periodic CBC. Serum concentrations two hours after a dose should be approximately 2 mcg/mL. Follow renal and hepatic function. Monitor IV site for phlebitis—if noted, make infusion solution more dilute.

ADVERSE EFFECTS/PRECAUTIONS: Neutropenia occurs in approximately 20% of patients - decrease dose or treat with GCSF if ANC remains less than 500/mm^3. Phlebitis may occur at IV site due to alkaline pH of 10. Risk of transient renal dysfunction and crystalluria is minimized by slow infusion rates and adequate patient hydration. Resistant viral strains may emerge during long-term therapy; these patients are at high risk for progressive life-threatening disease.

PHARMACOLOGY: Acyclovir is an antiviral drug that is preferentially taken up by infected cells; inhibits viral DNA synthesis. CSF concentrations are 30 to 50% of serum concentrations. Oral absorption is 15 to 30%. Most of administered dose is excreted

Adenosine

unchanged in urine, primarily via glomerular filtration. Protein binding and metabolism are minimal. Serum half-life is 3 to 4 hours in patients with normal renal and hepatic function.

SPECIAL CONSIDERATIONS/PREPARATION: Available in 500-mg and 1-g vials. Prepared by dissolving contents of 500-mg vial in 10 mL sterile water for injection. Reconstituted solution is stable at room temperature for 12 hours. **Do not refrigerate. Infusion solution concentration should be no greater than 7 mg/mL.** A 5-mg/mL dilution may be made by adding 1 mL of 50 mg/mL concentration to 9 mL of preservative-free normal saline. Dilution is stable for 24 hours at room temperature. Oral suspension available in 200 mg/5 mL concentration. Store at room temperature. Shake well before administration.

Solution Compatibility: D_5W, $D_{10}W$, and NS.

Solution Incompatibility: Dex/AA.

Terminal Injection Site Compatibility: Amikacin, ampicillin, aminophylline, cefazolin, cefotaxime, cefoxitin, ceftazidime, ceftriaxone, chloramphenicol, cimetidine, clindamycin, dexamethasone, erythromycin lactobionate, famotidine, fluconazole, gentamicin, heparin, hydrocortisone succinate, imipenem/cilastatin, linezolid, lorazepam, meropenem, metoclopramide, metronidazole, milrinone, morphine, nafcillin, oxacillin, penicillin G, pentobarbital, piperacillin, potassium chloride, propofol, ranitidine, remifentanil, sodium bicarbonate, theophylline, ticarcillin/clavulanate, tobramycin, trimethoprim-sulfamethoxazole, vancomycin, and zidovudine.

Incompatibility: Fat emulsion. Aztreonam, caffeine citrate, cefepime, dobutamine, dopamine, and piperacillin-tazobactam.

SELECTED REFERENCES

- Tiffany KF, Benjamin DK Jr, Palasanthiran P, et al: Improved neurodevelopmental outcomes following long-term high-dose acyclovir therapy in infants with central nervous system and disseminated herpes simplex disease. J Perinatol 2005;25:156-161.
- Kimberlin DW, Lin C-Y, Jacobs RF, et al: Safety and efficacy of high-dose intravenous acyclovir in the management of neonatal herpes simplex infections. Pediatrics 2001;108:230-238.
- American Academy of Pediatrics. Herpes simplex. In: Pickering LK, ed. 2006 Red Book: Report of the Committee on Infectious Diseases. 27th ed. Elk Grove Village, IL: American Academy of Pediatrics;2006:361.
- Rudd R, Rivadeneira ED, Gutman LT: Dosing considerations for oral acyclovir following neonatal herpes disease. Acta Paediatr 1994;83:1237-43.
- Whitley R, Arvin A, Prober C, et al: A controlled trial comparing vidarabine with acyclovir in neonatal herpes simplex virus infection. N Engl J Med 1991;324:444.
- Englund JA, Zimmerman BS, Swierkosz EM, et al: Herpes simplex virus resistant to acyclovir: A study in a tertiary care center. Ann Intern Med 1990;112:416.
- McDonald L, Tartaglione TA, Mendelman PM, et al: Lack of toxicity in two cases of neonatal acyclovir overdose. Pediatr Infect Dis J 1989;8:529.
- Sullender WM, Arvin AM, Diaz PS, et al: Pharmacokinetics of acyclovir suspension in infants and children. Antimicrob Agents Chemother 1987;31:1722.
- Hintz M, Connor JD, Spector SA, et al: Neonatal acyclovir pharmacokinetics in patients with herpes virus infections. Am J Med 1982;73(suppl):210.

Adenosine

DOSE & ADMINISTRATION: Starting dose: 50 mcg/kg rapid IV push (1 to 2 seconds). Increase dose in 50 mcg/kg increments Q2 minutes until return of sinus rhythm. Usual maximum dose: 250 mcg/kg. Infuse as close to IV site as possible. Flush IV with saline immediately. Intraosseous administration has also been reported to be successful.

USES: Acute treatment of sustained paroxysmal supraventricular tachycardia. It may also be useful in establishing the cause of the SVT.

MONITORING: Continuous EKG and blood pressure monitoring.

ADVERSE EFFECTS/PRECAUTIONS: Flushing, dyspnea, and irritability occur frequently, but usually resolve within 1 minute. Transient (duration <1 minute) arrhythmias may occur between termination of SVT and onset of normal sinus rhythm. Apnea has been reported in one preterm infant. Recurrence of SVT occurs in approximately 30% of treated patients. Aminophylline/Theophylline and caffeine diminish adenosine's effect by competitive antagonism.

PHARMACOLOGY: Adenosine is the pharmacologically active metabolite of ATP. It acts by depressing sinus node automaticity and A-V node conduction. It does **not** have negative inotropic effects. Response should occur within 2 minutes of the dose. Estimated serum half-life is 10 seconds.

SPECIAL CONSIDERATIONS/PREPARATION: Supplied in 2 mL vials containing 6 mg adenosine dissolved in NS. Contains no preservative. Store at room temperature. **Do not refrigerate;** crystallization will occur. Solution must be clear at the time of use. Dilutions can be made with NS for doses <0.2 mL (600 mcg). Use 1 mL (3000 mcg) with 9 mL NS to make a solution with a final concentration of 300 mcg/mL.

Solution Compatibility: D_5W and NS

SELECTED REFERENCES

- Paret G, Steinmetz D, Kuint J et al: Adenosine for the treatment of paroxysmal supraventricular tachycardia in fullterm and preterm newborn infants. Am J Perinatol 1996;13:343-46.
- Friedman FD: Intraosseous adenosine for the termination of supraventricular tachycardia in an infant. Ann Emerg Med 1996;28:356-58.
- Crosson JE, Etheridge SP, Milstein S et al: Therapeutic and diagnostic utility of adenosine during tachycardia evaluation in children. Am J Cardiol 1994;74:155-60.
- Till J, Shinebourne EA, Rigby ML, et al: Efficacy and safety of adenosine in the treatment of supraventricular tachycardia in infants and children. Br Heart J 1989;62:204.
- Overholt ED, Rhuban KS, Gutgesell HP, et al: Usefulness of adenosine for arrhythmias in infants and children. Am J Cardiol 1988;61:336.

ALBUTEROL

DOSE & ADMINISTRATION: Bronchodilation: 0.1 to 0.5 mg/kg per dose Q2 to 6 hours via nebulizer. 1 MDI actuation per dose (approx. 0.1 mg or 100 mcg) Q2 to 6 hours. **Oral:** 0.1 to 0.3 mg/kg per dose Q6 to 8 hours PO. **Treatment of hyperkalemia:** 0.4 mg/kg per dose Q2 hours via nebulizer.

USES: Bronchodilator. Treatment of hyperkalemia.

MONITORING: Assess degree of bronchospasm. Continuous EKG monitoring. **Consider not administering when heart rate is greater than 180 beats per minute.** Serum potassium.

ADVERSE EFFECTS/PRECAUTIONS: Tachycardia, arrhythmias, tremor, hypokalemia, and irritable behavior.

PHARMACOLOGY: Albuterol is a specific β_2-adrenergic agonist. Minimal cardiovascular effects unless used concurrently with aminophylline. Stimulates production of intracellular cyclic AMP, enhancing the binding of intracellular calcium to the cell membrane and endoplasmic reticulum, resulting in bronchodilation. Enhances mucociliary clearance. Drives potassium intracellular. Studies in vitro indicate that approximately 5% of a MDI dose administered using an in-line holding chamber/spacer device, versus less than 1% of a nebulizer dose, is delivered to the lung. Optimal aerosol dose in neonates is uncertain due to differences in aerosol drug delivery techniques. The therapeutic margin appears to be wide. Well absorbed when administered PO. Onset of action is 30 minutes; duration is 4 to 8 hours. Serum half-life is approximately 6 hours (adults). Time to peak serum concentration is 3 to 4 hours. Tolerance may develop.

SPECIAL CONSIDERATIONS/PREPARATION: Oral dosage form: Syrup, 2 mg/5 mL. **Inhalation solution:** Available as either 5 mg/mL or 0.83 mg/mL. A 0.1 mg/mL dilution for inhalation may be made by adding 3 mL of 0.83 mg/mL albuterol concentration to 22 mL of preservative-free normal saline. Label for inhalation use only. Stable for 7 days refrigerated. **MDI:** Available in a pressurized hydrofluoroalkane metered dose inhaler (contains no chlorofluorocarbons (CFC)). Proventil® HFA 100 mcg albuterol per actuation.

SELECTED REFERENCES

- Singh BS, Sadiq HF, Noguchi A, Keenan WJ: Efficacy of albuterol inhalation in treatment of hyperkalemia in premature neonates. J Pediatr 2002;141:16-20.
- Lugo RA, Kenney JK, Keenan J: Albuterol delivery in a neonatal ventilated lung model: nebulization versus chlorofluorocarbon- and, hydrofluoroalkane- pressurized metered dose inhalers. Pediatr Pulmonol 2001;31:247-254.
- Stefano JL, Bhutani VK, Fox WW: A randomized placebo-controlled study to evaluate the effects of oral albuterol on pulmonary mechanics in ventilator-dependent infants at risk of developing BPD. Pediatr Pulmonol 1991;10:183-90.
- Wong CS, Pavord ID, Williams J, et al: Bronchodilator, cardiovascular, and hypokalemic effects of fenoterol, salbutamol, and terbutaline in asthma. Lancet 1990;336:1396.

ALPROSTADIL (PROSTAGLANDIN E₁)

- Morgan DJ, Paull JD, Richmond BH, et al: Pharmacokinetics of intravenous and oral salbutamol and its sulphate conjugate. *Br J Clin Pharmacol* 1986;22:587.
- Beck R, Robertson C, Galdes-Sebaldt M, Levison H: Combined salbutamol and ipratropium bromide by inhalation in the treatment of severe acute asthma. *J Pediatr* 1985;107:605.

ALPROSTADIL (PROSTAGLANDIN E₁)

DOSE & ADMINISTRATION: Initial dose: 0.05 to 0.1 mcg/kg per minute by continuous IV infusion. Titrate to infant's response—oxygenation *versus* adverse effects. **Maintenance dose:** May be as low as 0.01 mcg/kg per minute. Higher initial doses are usually no more effective and have a high incidence of adverse effects. May also be given via UAC positioned near ductus arteriosus.

Sample Dilution and Infusion Rate: Mix 1 ampule (500 mcg) in 49 mL of compatible solution (e.g.,D5W) yielding a concentration of 10 mcg/mL. Infuse at a rate of 0.6 mL/kg per hour to provide a dose of 0.1 mcg/kg per minute.

USES: To promote dilation of ductus arteriosus in infants with congenital heart disease dependent on ductal shunting for oxygenation/perfusion.

MONITORING: Closely monitor respiratory and cardiovascular status. Assess for improvement in oxygenation. Closely monitor infant's temperature. Ensure reliable IV access: duration of effect is short.

ADVERSE EFFECTS/PRECAUTIONS: Be prepared to intubate/resuscitate. Common (6% to 15%): Apnea (consider treating with aminophylline), fever, leukocytosis, cutaneous flushing, and bradycardia. Gastric outlet obstruction and reversible cortical proliferation of the long bones after prolonged treatment (>120 hours). **Uncommon (1% to 5%):** Seizures, hypoventilation, hypotension, tachycardia, cardiac arrest, edema, sepsis, diarrhea, and disseminated intravascular coagulation. **Rare (<1%):** Urticaria, bronchospasm, hemorrhage, hypoglycemia, and hypocalcemia. **Musculoskeletal changes:** Widened fontanels, pretibial and soft tissue swelling, and swelling of the extremities may occur after 9 days of therapy. Cortical hyperostosis and periostitis may occur with long-term (>3 months) therapy. These changes resolve over weeks after discontinuation of therapy.

PHARMACOLOGY: Vasodilation of **all** arterioles. Inhibition of platelet aggregation. Stimulation of uterine and intestinal smooth muscle. Maximal drug effect usually seen within 30 minutes in cyanotic lesion; may take several hours in acyanotic lesions.

SPECIAL CONSIDERATIONS/PREPARATION: Supplied in 1 mL (500 mcg) ampules that must be refrigerated. **Dilute before administration to a concentration less than 20 mcg/mL.** Prepare fresh infusion solutions every 24 hours. Osmolality of undiluted (500 mcg/mL) is 23,250 mOsm/kg. Extravasation may cause tissue sloughing and necrosis. **Sample Dilution and Infusion Rate:** Mix 1 ampul (500 mcg) in 49 mL of compatible solution (e.g. D_5W) yielding a concentration of 10 mcg/mL. Infuse at a rate of 0.6 mL/kg per hour to provide a dose of 0.1 mcg/kg per minute.

Solution Compatibility: D_5W and NS. No data are currently available on Dex/AA.

Terminal Injection Site Compatibility: Aminophylline, atropine, caffeine citrate, calcium chloride, cefazolin, cimetidine, clindamycin, dexamethasone, digoxin, dopamine, epinephrine, furosemide, gentamicin, glycopyrrolate, heparin, hydralazine, hydrocortisone succinate, isoproterenol, lidocaine, metoclopramide, metronidazole, midazolam, morphine, nitroglycerin, nitroprusside, pancuronium, phenobarbital, potassium chloride, penicillin G, and ranitidine.

SELECTED REFERENCES

- Lim DS, Kulik TJ, Kim CW: Aminophylline for the prevention of apnea during prostaglandin E₁ infusion. *Pediatrics* 2003;112:e27-e29.
- Arav-Boger R, Baggett HC, Spevak PJ, Willoughby RE: Leukocytosis caused by prostaglandin E₁ in neonates. *J Pediatr* 2001;138:263-265.
- Kaufman MB, El-Chaar GM: Bone and tissue changes following prostaglandin therapy in neonates. *Ann Pharmacother* 1996;30:269.
- Peled N, Dagan O, Babyn P, et al: Gastric-outlet obstruction induced by prostaglandin therapy in neonates. *N Engl J Med* 1992;327:505.
- Gannaway WI, et al: Chemical stability of alprostadil (PGE-1) in combination with common injectable medications (abstract #P-152E). *American Society of Hospital Pharmacists Midyear Clinical Meeting Abstracts* 1989;24:75A.
- Roberts RJ: *Drug Therapy in Infants*. Philadelphia: WB Saunders Co, 1984, p 250.
- Lewis AB, Freed MD, Heymann MA, et al: Side effects of therapy with prostaglandin E₁ in infants with congenital heart disease. *Circulation* 1981;64:893.
- Heymann MA: Pharmacologic use of prostaglandin E₁ in infants with congenital heart disease. *Am Heart J* 1981;101:837.

Alteplase

Tissue Plasminogen Activator (t-PA)

DOSE & ADMINISTRATION: Restoration of function to central venous catheter: Instill into dysfunctional catheter at a concentration of 1 mg/mL. Use 110% of the internal lumen volume of the catheter, not to exceed 2 mg in 2 mL. If catheter function is not restored in 120 minutes after 1 dose, a second dose may be instilled. **Dissolution of intravascular thrombi:** 200 mcg/kg per hour (0.2 mg/kg per hour). Duration of therapy is 6 to 48 hours. If administering directly into the thrombus, dose may be increased after 6 hours to a maximum of 500 mcg/kg per hour. If localized bleeding occurs, stop infusion for 1 hour and restart using 100 mcg/kg per hour. Discontinue heparin several hours prior to initiation of therapy. **Note:** Reports in the literature are a collection of cases gathered over several years. Some authors used loading doses, others did not. Infused doses ranged from 20 to 500 mcg/kg per hour. Complications were most often linked with higher doses and longer duration of therapy. Call 1-800-NOCLOTS for case reporting and treatment guidance.

USES: Dissolution of intravascular thrombi of recent onset that are either intraarterial or life-threatening. Adjuvant treatment of infective endocarditis vegetations.

MONITORING: Follow coagulation studies (PT, aPTT, fibrinogen, fibrin split products) prior to therapy and at least daily during treatment. Maintain fibrinogen levels greater than 100 mg/dL and platelets > 50,000/mm^3. Echocardiography to assess clot lysis at least every 12 hours (every 6 hours optimal). Cranial ultrasound to assess for hemorrhage prior to therapy.

ADVERSE EFFECTS/PRECAUTIONS: Intracranial hemorrhage may occur, especially in premature infants treated for prolonged periods. Bleeding from venipuncture sites occurs in approximately half of treated patients. The risk of complications increases at doses above 450 mcg/kg per hour.

PHARMACOLOGY: Alteplase binds strongly and specifically to fibrin in a thrombus and converts the entrapped plasminogen to plasmin. This initiates local fibrinolysis with limited systemic proteolysis. Alteplase has a shorter half-life than streptokinase and does not cause anaphylactic reactions. It is cleared rapidly from the plasma, primarily via the liver.

SPECIAL CONSIDERATIONS/PREPARATION: Cathflo™ Activase® is supplied as lyophilized powder in 2 mg vials. Reconstitute by adding 2.2 mL Sterile Water for Injection to a final concentration of 1 mg/mL. Mix by gently swirling until the contents are completely dissolved. DO NOT SHAKE. Use reconstituted solution within 8 hours of mixing. Reconstituted solution may be stored refrigerated or at room temperature.

Solution Compatibility: NS, and D_5W

Terminal Injection Site Compatibility: Lidocaine, morphine, nitroglycerin, and propranolol.

Incompatibility: Dobutamine, dopamine, and heparin.

SELECTED REFERENCES

- Manco-Johnson M, Nuss R: Neonatal thrombotic disorders. *NeoReviews* 2000;1:e201.
- Hartmann J, Hussein A, Trowitzsch E, et al: Treatment of neonatal thrombus formation with recombinant tissue plasminogen activator: six years experience and review of the literature. *Arch Dis Child Fetal Neonatal Ed* 2001;85:F18-F22.
- Marks KA, Zucker N, Kapelushnik J, et al: Infective endocarditis successfully treated in extremely low birth weight infants with recombinant tissue plasminogen activator. *Pediatrics* 2002;109:153-158.
- Weiner GM, Castle VP, DiPietro MA, Faix RG: Successful treatment of neonatal arterial thromboses with recombinant tissue plasminogen activator. *J Pediatr* 1998;133:133-136.
- Product Information, Genentech, Inc., 2002.

Amikacin

DOSE & ADMINISTRATION: IV infusion by syringe pump over 30 minutes. Administer as a separate infusion from penicillin-containing compounds. IM injection is associated with variable absorption, especially in the very small infant. To use the dosing chart, please refer to explanatory note in "How to Use This Book."

AMIKACIN

Dosing Chart

PMA (weeks)	Postnatal (days)	Dose (mg/kg)	Interval (hours)
≤29*	0 to 7	18	48
	8 to 28	15	36
	≥29	15	24
30 to 34	0 to 7	18	36
	≥8	15	24
≥35	ALL	15	24

* or significant asphyxia, PDA, or treatment with indomethacin

USES: Restricted to treatment of infections caused by gram-negative bacilli that are resistant to other aminoglycosides. Usually used in combination with a β-lactam antibiotic.

MONITORING: Measure serum concentrations when treating for more than 48 hours. Obtain peak concentration 30 minutes after end of infusion, and trough concentration just prior to the next dose. When treating patients with serious infections or significantly changing fluid or renal status consider measuring the serum concentration 24 hours after a dose, and use the chart below for the suggested dosing interval. Blood samples obtained to monitor serum drug concentrations should be spun and refrigerated or frozen as soon as possible. Therapeutic serum concentrations: **Peak:** 20 to 30 mcg/mL (or C_{max}/MIC ratio greater than 8:1) (Draw 30 minutes after end of infusion, 1 hour after IM injection.) **Trough:** 2 to 5 mcg/mL

Suggested Dosing Intervals

Level at 24 hrs (mcg/mL)	Half-life (hours)	Suggested Dosing Interval (hours)
≤5.0	≈9	24
5.1 to 8.0	≈12	36
8.1 to 10.5	≈16	48
≥10.6		Measure level in 24 hours

ADVERSE EFFECTS/PRECAUTIONS: Transient and reversible renal tubular dysfunction may occur, resulting in increased urinary losses of sodium, calcium, and magnesium. Vestibular and auditory ototoxicity. The addition of other nephrotoxic and/or ototoxic medications (e.g. furosemide, vancomycin) may increase these adverse effects. Increased neuromuscular blockade (i.e. neuromuscular weakness and respiratory failure) may occur when used with pancuronium or other neuromuscular blocking agents and in patients with hypermagnesemia.

PHARMACOLOGY: Dosing recommendations for Amikacin are based on: (1) Higher peak concentrations increase concentration-dependent bacterial killing; (2) There is a post-antibiotic effect on bacterial killing, especially when treating concurrently with a β-lactam antibiotic: (3) There may be less toxicity with less frequent dosing, due to less renal drug accumulation. Volume of distribution is increased and clearance is decreased in patients with PDA. Serum half-life is prolonged in premature and asphyxiated newborns. Inactivation of amikacin by penicillin-containing compounds appears to be a time-, temperature-, and concentration-dependent process. This is probably clinically significant only when penicillin-containing compounds are mixed in IV solutions or when the blood is at room temperature for several hours before the assay is performed.

SPECIAL CONSIDERATIONS/PREPARATION: Available in concentrations of 50 and 250 mg/mL. For IV use, dilute with a compatible solution to a concentration of 5 mg/mL.

Solution Compatibility: D_5W, $D_{10}W$, $D_{20}W$, and NS.

Terminal Injection Site Compatibility: Dex/AA solutions. Acyclovir, aminophylline, amiodarone, aztreonam, caffeine citrate, calcium chloride, calcium gluconate, cefazolin, cefepime, cefotaxime, cefoxitin, ceftazidime, ceftriaxone, chloramphenicol, cimetidine, clindamycin, dexamethasone, enalaprilat, epinephrine, esmolol, fluconazole, furosemide, heparin (concentrations ≤1 U/mL), hydrocortisone succinate, hyaluronidase, linezolid, lorazepam, metronidazole, midazolam, milrinone, morphine, nicardipine, pentobarbital, phenobarbital, potassium chloride, ranitidine, remifentanil, sodium bicarbonate, vancomycin, vitamin K_1, and zidovudine.

Incompatibility: Fat emulsion. Amphotericin B, ampicillin, azithromycin, carbenicillin, heparin (concentrations >1 U/mL), imipenem/cilastatin, methicillin, mezlocillin, nafcillin, oxacillin, penicillin G, phenytoin, propofol, thiopental, and ticarcillin/clavulanate.

SELECTED REFERENCES

- Contopoulos-Ioannidis DG, Giotis ND, Baliatsa DV, Ioannidis JPA: Extended-interval aminoglycoside administration for children: a meta-analysis. *Pediatrics* 2004;114;e111-e118.
- Langhendries JP, Battisti O, Bertrand JM, et al: Adaptation in neonatology of the once-daily concept of aminoglycoside administration: Evaluation of a dosing chart for amikacin in an intensive care unit. *Biol Neonate* 1998;74:351-362.

AMINOPHYLLINE

DOSE & ADMINISTRATION: Loading dose: 8 mg/kg IV infusion over 30 minutes, or PO. **Maintenance:** 1.5 to 3 mg/kg per dose PO, or IV slow push Q8 to 12 hours (start maintenance dose 8 to 12 hours after the loading dose). In older infants (greater than 55 weeks PMA), dosage may need to be increased to 25 to 30 mg/kg per day in divided doses Q4 to 8 hours. If changing from IV to PO aminophylline: increase dose 20%. If changing from IV aminophylline to PO theophylline: no adjustment.

USES: Treatment of neonatal apnea, including post-extubation, post-anesthesia, and prostaglandin E_1-induced. Bronchodilator. May improve respiratory function.

MONITORING: Monitor heart rate and check blood glucose periodically with reagent strips. Assess for agitation and feeding intolerance. **Consider withholding next dose if heart rate is greater than 180 beats per minute.** When indicated by lack of efficacy or clinical signs of toxicity, serum trough concentration should be obtained. Therapeutic ranges are: 1) Apnea of prematurity: 7 to 12 mcg/mL. 2) Bronchospasm: 10 to 20 mcg/mL (older infants with bronchospasm may need these higher levels because of increased protein binding).

ADVERSE EFFECTS/PRECAUTIONS: GI irritation. Hyperglycemia. CNS irritability and sleeplessness. May be associated with renal calcifications when used concurrently with furosemide and/or dexamethasone. **Signs of toxicity:** Sinus tachycardia, failure to gain weight, vomiting, jitteriness, hyperreflexia, and seizures.

Treatment of Serious Theophylline Toxicity: Activated charcoal, 1 g/kg as a slurry by gavage tube Q2 to 4 hours. Avoid sorbitol-containing preparations: They may cause osmotic diarrhea.

PHARMACOLOGY: Aminophylline stimulates central respiratory drive and peripheral chemoreceptor activity. May increase diaphragmatic contractility. Cerebral blood flow is acutely decreased following IV bolus dose. Renal effects include diuresis and increased urinary calcium excretion. Stimulates gastric acid secretion and may cause GE reflux. Cardiac output is increased due to higher sensitivity to catecholamines. Elimination in preterm infants is primarily as unchanged drug, although significant interconversion to caffeine occurs. In the very immature neonate, the serum half-life of theophylline is prolonged (20 to 30 hours). Theophylline metabolism and clearance mature to adult values by 55 weeks postmenstrual age. Aminophylline salt is 78.9% theophylline. Theophylline administered orally is approximately 80% bioavailable; therefore, no dosage adjustment is necessary when changing from IV aminophylline to PO theophylline.

SPECIAL CONSIDERATIONS/PREPARATION: Available as aminophylline for IV use (25 mg/mL) in 10- and 20-mL vials. Dilute 1 mL (25 mg) with 4 mL NS or D_5W to yield a final concentration of 5 mg/mL. Stable for 4 days refrigerated. Aminophylline oral solution is available in a concentration of 21 mg/mL. Dilute with sterile water to a final concentration of 2 to 4 mg/mL for oral use. Theophylline oral solution is available as an alcohol- and dye-free preparation in a concentration of 5.33 mg/mL.

Solution Compatibility: D_5W, $D_{10}W$, and NS.

Terminal Injection Site Compatibility: Dex/AA (white precipitate forms within 2 hours) solutions, fat emulsion. Acyclovir, ampicillin, amikacin, aztreonam, caffeine citrate, calcium gluconate, cefazolin, ceftazidime, chloramphenicol, cimetidine, dexamethasone, dopamine, enalaprilat, erythromycin lactobionate, esmolol, famotidine, fluconazole, flumazenil, furosemide, heparin, hydrocortisone succinate, isoproterenol, lidocaine, linezolid, meropenem, methicillin, metoclopramide, metronidazole, midazolam, morphine, nafcillin, netilmicin, nicardipine, nitroglycerin, nitroprusside, pancuronium bromide, pentobarbital, phenobarbital, piperacillin, piperacillin-tazobactam, potassium chloride, propofol, prostaglandin E_1, ranitidine, remifentanil, sodium bicarbonate, ticarcillin/clavulanate, tobramycin, vancomycin, and vecuronium.

Incompatibility: Amiodarone, cefepime, cefotaxime, ceftriaxone, ciprofloxacin, clindamycin, dobutamine, epinephrine, hydralazine, insulin, methadone, methylprednisolone, penicillin G, and phenytoin.

SELECTED REFERENCES

- Lim DS, Kulik TJ, Kim DW: Aminophylline for the prevention of apnea during prostaglandin E_1 infusion. Pediatrics 2003;112:e27-e29.
- Hochwald C, Kennedy K, Chang J, Moya F: A randomized, controlled, double-blind trial comparing two loading doses of aminophylline. J Perinatol 2002;22:275-278.
- Carnielli VP, Verlato G, Benini F, et al: Metabolic and respiratory effects of theophylline in the preterm infant. Arch Dis Child Fetal Neonatal Ed 2000;83:F39-F43.
- Zanardo V, Dani C, Trevisanuto D: Methylxanthines increase renal calcium excretion in preterm infants. Biol Neonate 1995;68:169-74.
- Reese J, Prentice G, Yu VYH: Dose conversion from aminophylline to theophylline in preterm infants. Arch Dis Child 1994;71:F51-F52.
- Kraus DM, Fischer JH, Reitz SJ, et al: Alterations in theophylline metabolism during the first year of life. Clin Pharmacol Ther 1993;54:351-59.
- Shannon M, Amitai Y, Lovejoy FH: Multiple dose activated charcoal for theophylline poisoning in young infants. Pediatrics 1987;80:368.
- Gal P, Boer HR, Toback J, et al: Effect of asphyxia on theophylline clearance in newborns. South Med J 1982;75:836.
- Srinivasan G, Pildes RS, Jaspan JB, et al: Metabolic effects of theophylline in preterm infants. J Pediatr 1981;98:815.
- Aranda JV, Sitar DS, Parsons WD, et al: Pharmacokinetic aspects of theophylline in premature newborns. N Engl J Med 1976;295:413.

AMIODARONE

DOSE & ADMINISTRATION: IV Loading dose: 5 mg/kg IV infusion given over 30 to 60 minutes, preferably in a central vein. **Maintenance infusion:** 7 to 15 mcg/kg per minute (10 to 20 mg/kg per 24 hours). Begin at 7 mcg/kg per minute and titrate by monitoring effects. **Prepare fresh drug Q24 hours due to degradation of amiodarone in solution. Consider switching to oral therapy within 24 to 48 hours. PO:** 5 to 10 mg/kg per dose every 12 hours.

USES: Treatment of life-threatening or drug-resistant refractory supraventricular (SVT), ventricular tachyarrhythmias (VT), and postoperative junctional ectopic tachycardia (JET) - see Adverse Effects.

MONITORING: Continuous EKG and blood pressure (for IV). Follow AST and ALT. Monitor T_3, T_4, and TSH. Observe IV site for extravasation.

ADVERSE EFFECTS/PRECAUTIONS: Short term toxicity: Bradycardia and hypotension (possibly associated with rapid rates of infusion). Polymorphic ventricular tachycardia. Irritating to the peripheral vessels (concentrations > 2 mg/mL). Administer through central vein preferred. **Long term toxicity:** Hyperthyroidism (due to inhibition of T_4 to T_3) and hypothyroidism (due to high concentration of inorganic iodine). Contains 2% benzyl alcohol (20mg/mL). Hepatitis and cholestatic hepatitis (rare). Photosensitivity (10%), nausea and vomiting (10%), optic neuritis (4 to 9%), and pulmonary fibrosis (4 to 9%) have been reported with prolonged oral use in adults.

PHARMACOLOGY: Class III antiarrhythmic agent that is an iodinated benzofuran compound. Electrophysiologic activity is accomplished by prolonging the duration of the action potential and increasing the effective refractory period. Increases cardiac blood flow and decreases cardiac work and myocardial oxygen consumption. Highly protein bound (95%) in adults. Extensively metabolized to an active metabolite by the cytochrome CYP3A4 isoenzyme system (limited in preterm infants). Drug-drug interaction potentially occur when given in combination with drugs that inhibit cytochrome CYP3A4: phenytoin, fosphenytoin, clarithromycin, erythromycin, azole antifungals (e.g. fluconazole, ketoconazole, itraconazole), protease inhibitors (e.g. indinavir, ritonavir), class IA and class III antiarrhythmics (e.g. quinidine, procainamide, sotalol) and cimetidine (amiodarone levels increase). Amiodarone prevents the elimination of digoxin resulting in high digoxin levels. Half-life reported to be 26 to 107 days in adults. No data in preterm infants. Accumulates in tissues; serum levels can be detected for months. Contains 37.3% iodine by weight. Adheres to PVC tubing: low infusion rates in neonates may lead to reduced drug delivery during continuous infusions. Oral absorption is variable with approximately 50% bioavailability.

SPECIAL CONSIDERATIONS/PREPARATION: IV: Available as 50 mg/mL concentration in 3 mL ampules. Contains 2% (20 mg/mL) of benzyl alcohol and 10% (100 mg/mL) polysorbate (Tween) 80 as a preservative. Store at room temperature and protect from light. **Infusions greater than 1 hour, amiodarone IV concentrations should not exceed 2 mg/mL unless using a central line. PO:** Supplied in 200 mg tablets. An oral suspension with a final concentration of 5 mg/mL may be made as follows: crush a 200 mg tablet, slowly mix in 20 mL of 1% methylcellulose, then add in 20 mL of simple syrup to make a total volume of 40 mL. Stable for six weeks at room temperature and three months refrigerated when stored in glass or plastic.

Solution Compatibility: D_5W, and NS.

Solution Incompatibility: No data available for Dex/AA solutions.

Terminal Injection Site Compatibility: Amikacin, amphotericin B, atropine, calcium chloride, calcium gluconate, ciprofloxacin, ceftizoxime, ceftriaxone, cefuroxime, clindamycin, dobutamine, dopamine, epinephrine, famotidine, fentanyl, fluconazole, furosemide, esmolol, erythromycin, gentamicin, insulin, isoproterenol, lidocaine, lorazepam, metronidazole, midazolam, milrinone, morphine, nitroglycerin, norepinephrine, penicillin G, phentolamine, potassium chloride, procainamide, tobramycin, vancomycin, and vecuronium.

Incompatibility: Aminophylline, ampicillin, ceftazidime, cefazolin, digoxin, heparin, imipenem-cilastatin, mezlocillin, piperacillin, piperacillin-tazobactam, sodium bicarbonate, and sodium nitroprusside. No data available for Dex/AA solutions.

SELECTED REFERENCES

- Etheridge SP, Craig JE, Compton SJ. Amiodarone is safe and highly effective therapy for supraventricular tachycardia in infants. *Am Heart J* 2001;141:105-110.
- Yap SC, Hoomtje T, Sreeram N: Polymorphic ventricular tachycardia after use of intravenous amiodarone for postoperative junctional ectopic tachycardia. *Internat J Cardiol* 2000;76:245-247.
- Drago F, Mazza A, Guccione P, et al: Amiodarone used alone or in combination with propranolol: A very effective therapy for tachyarrhythmias in infants and children. *Pediatr Cardiol* 1998;19:445-449.
- Grandy J, Wonko N, Kantoch MJ, et al: Risks of intravenous amiodarone in neonates. *Can J Cardiol* 1998;14:855-858.
- Bowers PN, Fields J, Schwartz D, et al: Amiodarone induced pulmonary fibrosis in infancy. *PACE* 1998;21:1665-1667.
- Nahata MC, Morosco RS, Hipple TF: Stability of amiodarone in extemporaneously oral suspension prepared from commonly available vehicles. *J Pediatr Pharm Pract* 1999;4:186-189.
- Pramar YV: Chemical stability of amiodarone hydrocortisone in intravenous fluids. *Int J Pharm Comp* 1997;1:347-348.
- Perry JC, Fenrich AL, Hulse JE, et al: Pediatric use of intravenous amiodarone: Efficacy and safety in critically ill patients from a multicenter protocol. *J Am Coll Cardiol* 1996;27:1246-1250.
- Soult JA, Munoz M, Lopez JD, et al: Efficacy and safety of intravenous amiodarone for short-term treatment of paroxysmal supraventricular tachycardia in children. *Pediatr Cardiol* 1995;16:16-19.
- Figa FH, Gow RW, Hamilton RM, et al: Clinical efficacy and safety of intravenous amiodarone in infants and children. *Am J Cardiol* 1994;74:573-577.

AMPHOTERICIN B

DOSE & ADMINISTRATION: 0.5 to 1 mg/kg Q24 hours IV infusion over 2 to 6 hours. Dosage modification for renal dysfunction is only necessary if serum creatinine increases >0.4 mg/dL during therapy - hold dose for 2 to 5 days.

USES: Treatment of systemic fungal infections and severe superficial mycoses.

MONITORING: Monitor CBC, electrolytes, urine output, BUN, and serum creatinine at least every other day. Observe IV site for irritation—phlebitis is common. Serum amphotericin concentrations are not routinely followed.

ADVERSE EFFECTS/PRECAUTIONS: Decreases renal blood flow and GFR by 20% to 60%. Injures tubular epithelium with resultant urinary loss of potassium and magnesium, decreased reabsorption of sodium, and renal tubular acidosis. Sodium intake > 4 mEq/kg per day may prevent or decrease nephrotoxicity. Anemia, thrombocytopenia,

Amphotericin B Lipid Complex

hypokalemia, nausea/vomiting, and fever/chills. Consider analgesia before beginning infusion. Cardiac arrest has occurred in patients who received 10 times the recommended dose.

PHARMACOLOGY: Amphotericin B binds to ergosterol in the membrane of sensitive fungi and may be fungicidal or fungistatic. The therapeutic concentration range is not well-defined. Highly protein-bound (greater than 90%). Elimination half-life is approximately 15 days. Drug may accumulate in tissues to a significant concentration and be excreted renally for months.

SPECIAL CONSIDERATIONS/PREPARATION: Available as powder for injection in 50-mg vials. Reconstitute using D_5W to a concentration of 5 mg/mL, then dilute further using D_5W to a concentration no greater than 0.1 mg/mL for infusion. **Do not flush IV or mix amphotericin with saline solution**— precipitation will occur. May filter if necessary using a 0.45 micron filter. **Protect from light.**

Solution Compatibility: D_5W, $D_{10}W$, $D_{15}W$, and $D_{20}W$.

Solution Incompatibility: Dex/AA solutions and NS.

Terminal Injection Site Compatibility: Amiodarone, heparin, hydrocortisone, sodium bicarbonate, and zidovudine.

Incompatibility: Fat emulsion. Amikacin, aztreonam, calcium chloride, calcium gluconate, cefepime, cimetidine, ciprofloxacin, dopamine, enalaprilat, fluconazole, gentamicin, linezolid, magnesium sulfate, meropenem, netilmicin, penicillin G, piperacillin-tazobactam, potassium chloride, propofol, ranitidine, remifentanil, and tobramycin.

SELECTED REFERENCES

- Holler B, Omar SA, Farid MD, Patterson MJ: Effects of fluid and electrolyte management on amphotericin B-induced nephrotoxicity among extremely low birth weight infants. *Pediatrics* 2004;113:e608-e616.
- Chapman RL: *Candida* infections in the neonate. *Curr Opin Pediatr* 2003;15:97-102.
- Bliss JM, Wellington M, Gigliotti F: Antifungal pharmacotherapy for neonatal candidiasis. *Semin Perinatol* 2003;27:365-374.
- Lyman CA, Walsh TJ: Systemically administered antifungal agents: A review of their clinical pharmacology and therapeutic applications. *Drugs* 1992;44:9.
- Baley JE, Meyers C, Kliegman RM, et al: Pharmacokinetics, outcome of treatment, and toxic effects of amphotericin B and 5-fluorocytosine in neonates. *J Pediatr* 1990;116:791.
- Starke JR, Mason EL, Kramer WG, Kaplan SL: Pharmacokinetics of amphotericin B in infants and children. *J Infect Dis* 1987;155:766.
- Dodds Ashley ES, Lewis R, Lewis JS, et al: Pharmacology of systemic antifungal agents. *Clin Infect Dis* 2006;43:S29-39.

Amphotericin B Lipid Complex

DOSE & ADMINISTRATION: 5 mg/kg per dose Q24 hours IV infusion by syringe pump over 2 hours.

USES: Treatment of systemic fungal infections resistant to conventional amphotericin B therapy or in patients with renal or hepatic dysfunction.

MONITORING: Serum amphotericin B concentrations are not routinely followed. Monitor urine output. Periodic CBC for thrombocytopenia, electrolytes for hypokalemia, BUN, serum creatinine, and hepatic transaminases.

ADVERSE EFFECTS/PRECAUTIONS: Anemia, thrombocytopenia, hypokalemia, nausea/vomiting, and fever/chills.

PHARMACOLOGY: ABELCET® consists of amphotericin B complexed with two phospholipids in a 1:1 drug-to-lipid ratio. Acts by binding to the sterol component of a cell membrane leading to alterations in the cell wall permeability and death. Penetrates the cell wall of susceptible fungi. Concentrates in the liver and spleen. Less nephrotoxic than conventional amphotericin B. Mean serum half-life in adults 24 to 38 hours. The pharmacokinetics of amphotericin B lipid complex is nonlinear.

SPECIAL CONSIDERATIONS/PREPARATION: Available as a ready-to-use admixture containing 50- and 100-mg ABELCET® in 10- and 20-mL suspension (5 mg/mL) respectively. Shake the vial gently until there is no evidence of any yellow sediment on the bottom. Withdraw the appropriate dose into a syringe using an 18 gauge needle. Remove the needle and replace with the supplied 5 micron filter needle. Inject the drug into a different syringe containing a measured amount of D_5W so that the **final infusion concentration is 1 to 2 mg/mL**. Shake until thoroughly mixed. Check for complete dispersion. The diluted admixture is stable for 48 hours refrigerated and an additional 6 hours at room temperature. **Do not freeze. Protect from light. Do not flush IV or mix ABELCET® with saline solutions - precipitation will occur.**

Solution Compatibility: D_5W at 1 to 2 mg/mL, $D_{10}W$ and $D_{15}W$ at 1 mg/mL dilution.

Solution Incompatibility: Dex/AA and NS.

Terminal Injection Site Compatibility: No available data.

SELECTED REFERENCES

- Adler-Shohet F, Waskin H, Lieberman J M: Amphotericin B lipid complex for neonatal invasive candidiasis . *Arch Dis Child Fetal Neonatal Ed* 2001;84:F131-F133.
- Walsh TJ, Seibel NL, Arndt C, et al: Amphotericin B lipid complex in pediatric patients with invasive fungal infections. *Pediatr Infect Dis J* 1999;18:702-708.
- Wong-Beringer A, Jacobs RA, Guglielmo BJ: Lipid formulations of amphotericin B: Clinical efficacy and toxicities. *Clin Infect Dis* 1998;27:603-618.
- Dodds Ashley ES, Lewis R, Lewis JS, et al. Pharmacology of systemic antifungal agents. *Clin Infect Dis* 2006;43:S29-39.
- Product Information, Enzon, Inc. and Personal Communication, Enzon, Inc.

AMPHOTERICIN B LIPOSOME

DOSE & ADMINISTRATION: 5 to 7 mg/kg per dose Q24 hours IV infusion by syringe pump over 2 hours.

USES: Treatment of systemic fungal infections resistant to conventional amphotericin B therapy or in patients with renal or hepatic dysfunction.

MONITORING: Serum amphotericin B concentrations are not routinely followed. Monitor urine output. Periodic CBC for thrombocytopenia, electrolytes for hypokalemia, BUN, serum creatinine, and hepatic transaminases.

ADVERSE EFFECTS/PRECAUTIONS: Anemia, thrombocytopenia, hypokalemia, nausea/vomiting, and fever/chills.

PHARMACOLOGY: AmBisome® consists of amphotericin B intercalated within a single bilayer liposomal drug delivery system. Acts by binding to the sterol component of a cell membrane leading to alterations in the cell wall permeability and death. Penetrates the cell wall of susceptible fungi. Concentrates in the liver and spleen but penetrates the CNS less than conventional amphotericin B. Less nephrotoxic than conventional amphotericin B. Mean serum half-life in adults 24 to 38 hours. The pharmacokinetics of amphotericin B liposome is nonlinear.

SPECIAL CONSIDERATIONS/PREPARATION: Available as powder for injection in 50 mg vials. Reconstitute by adding 12 mL of sterile water for injection to a yield a concentration of 4 mg/mL. Immediately shake vial vigorously for 30 seconds. Check for complete dispersion. Reconstituted suspension stable for 24 hours refrigerated. **Do not freeze. Protect from light**. Before administration, AmBisome® must be diluted with D_5W to a final concentration less than 2 mg/mL. A 1 mg/mL dilution may be made by filtering (using 5 micron filter) 1 mL of reconstituted solution into 3 mL of D_5W. Use one filter per vial of AmBisome®. Use dilution immediately. **Do not flush IV or mix Ambisome® with saline solutions**-precipitation will occur.

Solution Compatibility: D_5W.

Solution Incompatibility: Dex/AA and NS.

Terminal Injection Site Compatibility: No available data.

SELECTED REFERENCES

- Juster-Reicher A, Flidel-Rimon O, Amitay M, et al: High dose liposomal amphotericin B in the therapy of systemic candidiasis in neonates. *Eur J Clin Microbiol Infect Dis* 2003;22:603-07.
- Scarcella A, Pasquariello MB, Giugliano B, et al: Liposomal amphotericin B treatment for neonatal fungal infections. *Pediatr Infect Dis J* 1998;17:146-148.
- Evdoridou J, Roilides E, Bibashi E, Kremenopoulos G: Multifocal osteoarthritis due to Candida albicans in a neonate: Serum level monitoring of liposomal amphotericin B and literature review. *Infection* 1997;25:112.
- Weitkamp JH, Poets CF, Sievers R, et al: Candida infection in very low birthweight infants: Outcome and nephrotoxicity of treatment with liposomal amphotericin B (AmBisome®). *Infection* 1998;26:11-15.
- Dodds Ashley ES, Lewis R, Lewis JS, et al. Pharmacology of systemic antifungal agents. *Clin Infect Dis* 2006;43:S29-39.

Ampicillin

DOSE & ADMINISTRATION: 25 to 50 mg/kg per dose by IV slow push, or IM. Some experts recommend 100 mg/kg/per dose when treating meningitis and severe group B streptococcal sepsis. To use dosing chart, please refer to explanatory note in "How to Use This Book."

Dosing Interval Chart

PMA (weeks)	PostNatal (days)	Interval (hours)
≤29	0 to 28 >28	12 8
30 to 36	0 to 14 >14	12 8
37 to 44	0 to 7 >7	12 8
≥45	ALL	6

USES: Broad-spectrum antibiotic useful against group B *streptococcus*, *Listeria monocytogenes*, and susceptible *E coli* species.

MONITORING: Serum concentration can be measured but is not usually necessary.

ADVERSE EFFECTS/PRECAUTIONS: Very large doses may result in CNS excitation or seizure activity. Hypersensitivity reactions (maculopapular rash, urticarial rash, or fever) are rare in neonates.

PHARMACOLOGY: Ampicillin is a semisynthetic penicillin that is bactericidal. Clearance is primarily by the renal route and is inversely related to postnatal age. Serum half-life in term infants younger than 7 days is approximately 4 hours.

SPECIAL CONSIDERATIONS/PREPARATION: Available as powder for injection in 125-, 250-, 500-mg, 1-g, and 2-g vials. Reconstitute using sterile water for injection. Maximum concentration for IV infusion is 100 mg/mL. Mix to a final concentration of 250 mg/mL for IM administration. Reconstituted solution must be used within 1 hour of mixing because of loss of potency.

Solution Compatibility: D_5W, $D_{10}W$, and NS.

Solution Incompatibility: Dex/AA.

Terminal Injection Site Compatibility: Fat emulsion. Acyclovir, aminophylline, aztreonam, calcium gluconate, cefepime, chloramphenicol, cimetidine, clindamycin, dopamine, enalaprilat, epinephrine, famotidine, furosemide, heparin, hydrocortisone succinate, insulin, lidocaine, linezolid, metronidazole, milrinone, morphine, phytonadione, potassium chloride, propofol, ranitidine, remifentanil, sodium bicarbonate, and vancomycin.

Incompatibility: Amikacin, amiodarone, erythromycin lactobionate, fluconazole, gentamicin, hydralazine, metoclopramide, midazolam, nicardipine, and tobramycin.

SELECTED REFERENCES

- Shaffer CL, Davey AM, Ransom JL, et al: Ampicillin-induced neurotoxicity in very-low-birth-weight neonates. *Ann Pharmacother* 1998;32:482-484.
- Prober CG, Stevenson DK, Benitz WE: The use of antibiotics in neonates weighing less than 1200 grams. *Pediatr Infect Dis J* 1990;9:111.
- Kaplan JM, McCracken GH, Horton LJ, et al: Pharmacologic studies in neonates given large dosages of ampicillin. *J Pediatr* 1974;84:571.
- Boe RW, Williams CPS, Bennett JV, Oliver TK Jr: Serum levels of methicillin and ampicillin in newborn and premature infants in relation to postnatal age. *Pediatrics* 1967;39:194.
- Axline SG, Yaffe SJ, Simon HJ: Clinical pharmacology of antimicrobials in premature infants: II. Ampicillin, methicillin, oxacillin, neomycin, and colistin. *Pediatrics* 1967;39:97.

Atropine

DOSE & ADMINISTRATION: IV: 0.01 to 0.03 mg/kg per dose IV over 1 minute, or IM. Dose can be repeated Q10 to 15 minutes to achieve desired effect, with a maximum total dose of 0.04 mg/kg. **ET:** 0.01 to 0.03 mg/kg per dose immediately followed by 1 mL NS. **PO:** Begin with 0.02 mg/kg per dose given Q4 to 6 hours. May increase gradually to 0.09 mg/kg per dose.

USES: Reversal of severe sinus bradycardia, particularly when parasympathetic influences on the heart (digoxin, beta-blocker drugs, hyperactive carotid sinus reflex) predominate. Also used to reduce the muscarinic effects of neostigmine when reversing neuromuscular blockade.

MONITORING: Heart rate.

ADVERSE EFFECTS/PRECAUTIONS: Cardiac arrhythmias can occur, particularly during the first 2 minutes following IV administration; usually a simple A-V dissociation, more often caused by smaller rather than larger doses. Fever, especially in brain-damaged infants. Abdominal distention with decreased bowel activity. Esophageal reflux. Mydriasis and cycloplegia.

PHARMACOLOGY: Anticholinergic. Increases heart rate by decreasing the effects of the parasympathetic system while increasing the effects of the sympathetic system. Peak tachycardia is 12 to 16 minutes after dose is given. Relaxes bronchial smooth muscle, thus reducing airway resistance and increasing dead space by 30%. Motor activity in the stomach and small and large intestines is reduced. Esophageal sphincter tone is reduced. Salivary secretion is inhibited. Duration of action is 6 hours. Primarily excreted renally unchanged.

SPECIAL CONSIDERATIONS/PREPARATION: Supplied in multiple concentrations (0.05-, 0.1-, 0.3-, 0.4-, 0.5-, 0.8-, and 1-mg/mL) for injection. Give IV dosage form PO. Prepare IV or PO dilution by mixing 1 mL of injectable atropine (0.4 mg/mL) in 7 mL of sterile water for injection to yield final concentration of 0.05 mg/mL. Stable for 28 days refrigerated.

Solution Compatibility: D_5W, $D_{10}W$, and NS.

Solution Incompatibility:

Terminal Injection Site Compatibility: Dex/AA. Amiodarone, cimetidine, dobutamine, famotidine, fentanyl, furosemide, glycopyrrolate, heparin, hydrocortisone succinate, meropenem, metoclopramide, midazolam, milrinone, morphine, nafcillin, netilmicin, pentobarbital, potassium chloride, propofol, prostaglandin E_1, ranitidine, and sodium bicarbonate.

Incompatibility: No data are currently available.

SELECTED REFERENCES

- Miller BR, Friesen RH: Oral atropine premedication in infants attenuates cardiovascular depression during Halothane anesthesia. *Anesth Analg* 1988;67:180.
- Roberts RJ: *Drug Therapy in Infants.* Philadelphia: WB Saunders Co, 1984, p 284.
- Adams RG, Verma P, Jackson AJ, Miller RL: Plasma pharmacokinetics of intravenously administered atropine in normal human subjects. *J Clin Pharmacol* 1982;22:477.
- Kattwinkel J, Fanaroff AA, Klaus M: Bradycardia in preterm infants: Indications and hazards of atropine therapy. *Pediatrics* 1976;58:494.
- Unna KR, Glaser K, Lipton E, Patterson PR: Dosage of drugs in infants and children: I. Atropine. *Pediatrics* 1950;6:197.

AZITHROMYCIN

DOSE & ADMINISTRATION: Treatment of Pertussis infections: 10 mg/kg per dose orally, once daily for 5 days. **Treatment of Chlamydia trachomatis conjunctivitis and pneumonitis:** 20 mg/kg per dose orally, once daily for 3 days. Intravenous treatment is limited to those who cannot be treated orally. To date no clinical studies have been conducted to evaluate the safety or efficacy of IV azithromycin in the pediatric population. Suggested IV dose: 5 mg/kg per dose once daily.

USES: Treatment and postexposure prophylaxis against *Bordetella pertussis*. As a substitute for penicillin in situations of significant allergic intolerance.

MONITORING: Assess gastrointestinal tolerance.

ADVERSE EFFECTS/PRECAUTIONS: Limited data in neonates. Diarrhea and/or vomiting occur in 5 to 12% of patients. Irritability, rash, and blood in stool have also been reported. There is one new case report of pyloric stenosis in 2 of 3 triplets treated with azithromycin for pertussis.

PHARMACOLOGY: Azithromycin is classified as an azalide, a subclass of macrolide antibiotics. In vitro activity has been demonstrated against *Bordetella pertussis*, as well as Streptococci (Groups C, F, G and Viridans), *Ureaplasma urealyticum*, and Peptostreptococcus species. Eradication of *B. pertussis* in unimmunized individuals (e.g., neonates) takes longer and requires higher doses than immunized individuals. Oral bioavailability is 38% in adults and children and is not affected by food. Primarily excreted

Aztreonam

unchanged in the bile, with some hepatic metabolism to inactive metabolites. The prolonged terminal half-life (approximately 80 hours) is thought to be due to extensive uptake and subsequent release of drug from tissues.

SPECIAL CONSIDERATIONS/PREPARATION: Oral suspension is available in 300, 600, 900, and 1,200 mg bottles. Reconstitute 300 mg bottle with 9 mL of water to provide a final concentration of 100 mg per 5 mL (20 mg/mL). Shake well before administration. Do not refrigerate. Use within 10 days once bottle has been opened. Zithromax® for intravenous injection is supplied in single use vials containing 500 mg lyophilized powder. Reconstitute by adding 4.8 mL Sterile Water for Injection, then shake the vial until all the drug is dissolved. The concentration of the reconstituted solution is 100 mg/mL. It is stable at room temperature for 24 hours. **Dilute prior to administration** using a compatible solution to a final concentration of 1 to 2 mg/mL. Do not use higher concentrations due to local IV site reactions. **Infuse over at least 60 minutes.**

Solution Compatibility: D_5W, NS, 5% Dextrose in 0.45% NaCl with 20 mEq/L KCl, and Lactated Ringer's.

Terminal Injection Site Compatibility: Do not infuse other drugs through the same IV line.

Incompatibility: Amikacin, aztreonam, cefotaxime, ceftazidime, ceftriaxone, cefuroxime, clindamycin, famotidine, fentanyl, furosemide, gentamicin, imipenem-cilastatin, morphine, piperacillin-tazobactam, potassium chloride, ticarcillin-clavulanate, and tobramycin.

SELECTED REFERENCES

- American Academy of Pediatrics. Chlamydia trachomatis, and Pertussis. In: Pickering LK, Baker CJ, Long SS, McMillan JA, eds. *Red Book: 2006 Report of the Committee on Infectious Diseases.* 27th ed. Elk Grove Village, IL: American Academy of Pediatrics; 2006: pp 255, and 500-502.
- Centers for Disease Control and Prevention. Recommended antimicrobial agents for the treatment and postexposure prophylaxis of pertussis. 2005 CDC guidelines. *MMWR* 2005;54(No. RR-14):pp. 4, 10.
- Friedman DS, Curtis CR, Schauer SL, et al. Surveillance for transmission and antibiotic adverse events among neonates and adults exposed to a healthcare worker with pertussis. *Infect Control Hosp Epidemiol* 2004;25:967-73.
- Langley JM, Halperin SA, Boucher FD, et al. Azithromycin is as effective and better tolerated than erythromycin estolate for the treatment of pertussis. *Pediatrics* 2004;114:96-101.
- Jacobs RF, Maples HD, Aranda JV, et al. Pharmacokinetics of intravenously administered azithromycin in pediatric patients. *Pediatr Infect Dis J* 2005;24:34-39.
- Morrison W. Infantile hypertrophic pyloric stenosis in infants treated with azithromycin. *Pediatr Infect Dis J* 2007;26:186-188
- Product Information, Pfizer, Inc., 2006.

Aztreonam

DOSE & ADMINISTRATION: 30 mg/kg per dose IV slow push over 5 to 10 minutes, or IM. To use dosing chart, please refer to explanatory note in "How to Use This Book."

Dosing Interval Chart

PMA (weeks)	PostNatal (days)	Interval (hours)
≤29	0 to 28 >28	12 8
30 to 36	0 to 14 >14	12 8
37 to 44	0 to 7 >7	12 8
≥45	ALL	6

USES: Treatment of neonatal sepsis caused by susceptible gram-negative organisms (e.g. *E coli, H influenzae, Klebsiella, Pseudomonas,* and *Serratia*). Generally used in combination with ampicillin (empirical treatment of sepsis) or an aminoglycoside (for synergism against *Pseudomonas* and *Enterobacteriaceae*).

MONITORING: Check serum glucose one hour after administration. Measuring serum concentration is not usually necessary. Periodic CBC, AST, ALT.

ADVERSE EFFECTS/PRECAUTIONS: Aztreonam contains 780 mg L-arginine per gram of drug (23.4 mg/kg body weight per dose). Adequate amounts of glucose must be provided to prevent hypoglycemia. Side effects are rare but include eosinophilia, elevation of serum transaminases, and phlebitis at the injection site.

PHARMACOLOGY: Aztreonam is a synthetically-produced monocyclic β-lactam antibiotic. Although bactericidal against aerobic gram-negative bacteria, it has virtually no activity against aerobic gram-positive and anaerobic bacteria, thereby producing little alteration of bowel flora. Good tissue and fluid penetration has been demonstrated in adults, along with protein-binding of 50 to 65%. Eliminated renally, primarily as unchanged drug. Serum half-life in neonates is 3 to 9 hours. Aztreonam does not interfere with bilirubin-albumin binding.

SPECIAL CONSIDERATIONS/PREPARATION: Available as powder for injection in 500-mg, 1-g, and 2-g vials. Reconstitute 500-mg vial with 10 mL of either sterile water for injection or NS (50 mg/mL). **Shake immediately and vigorously.** Reconstituted solution stable for 48 hours at room temperature, 7 days refrigerated.

Solution Compatibility: D_5W, $D_{10}W$, and NS.

Terminal Injection Site Compatibility: Dex/AA and fat emulsion. Amikacin, aminophylline, ampicillin, bumetanide, calcium gluconate, cefazolin, cefepime, cefotaxime, cefoxitin, ceftazidime, ceftriaxone, cimetidine, clindamycin, dexamethasone, dobutamine, dopamine, enalaprilat, famotidine, fluconazole, furosemide, gentamicin, heparin, hydrocortisone succinate, imipenem, insulin, linezolid, metoclopramide, mezlocillin, morphine, netilmicin, nicardipine, piperacillin, piperacillin/tazobactam, potassium chloride, propofol, quinupristin/dalfopristin, ranitidine, remifentanil, sodium bicarbonate, ticarcillin/clavulanate, tobramycin, vancomycin, and zidovudine.

Incompatibility: Acyclovir, amphotericin B, azithromycin, ganciclovir, lorazepam, metronidazole, and nafcillin.

SELECTED REFERENCES

- Uauy R, Mize C, Argyle C, McCracken GH: Metabolic tolerance to arginine: Implications for the safe use of arginine salt-aztreonam combination in the neonatal period. *J Pediatr* 1991;118:965.
- Cuzzolin L, Fanos V, Zambreri D, et al: Pharmacokinetics and renal tolerance of aztreonam in premature infants. *Antimicrob Agents Chemother* 1991;35:1726.
- Prober CG, Stevenson DK, Benitz WE: The use of antibiotics in neonates weighing less than 1200 grams. *Pediatr Infect Dis J* 1990;9:111.
- Likitnukul S, McCracken GH, Threlkeld N, et al: Pharmacokinetics and plasma bactericidal activity of aztreonam in low-birth-weight infants. *Antimicrob Agents Chemother* 1987;31:81.

BUMETANIDE

DOSE & ADMINISTRATION: 0.005 to 0.05 mg/kg per dose Q6 hours IV slow push, IM, or PO.

USES: Diuretic used in patients with renal insufficiency, congestive heart failure, or significant edema that is refractory to furosemide.

MONITORING: Serum electrolytes and urine output. Assess patients receiving digoxin concurrently for potassium depletion. Follow weight changes.

ADVERSE EFFECTS/PRECAUTIONS: Water and electrolyte imbalances occur frequently, especially hyponatremia, hypokalemia, and hypochloremic alkalosis. Potentially ototoxic, but less so than furosemide. May displace bilirubin from albumin binding sites when given in high doses or for prolonged periods.

PHARMACOLOGY: Bumetanide is 40 times more potent than furosemide with a similar mechanism of action. Inhibits chloride reabsorption in the ascending limb of Henle's loop and inhibits tubular sodium transport, causing major loss of sodium and chloride. Increases urinary losses of potassium, calcium, and bicarbonate. Urine sodium losses are lower with bumetanide than furosemide, but urine calcium losses are higher. Decreases CSF production by weak carbonic anhydrase inhibition. Decreases pulmonary transvascular fluid filtration. Increases renal blood flow and prostaglandin secretion. Highly protein bound (>97%). Data from adults indicate excellent oral bioavailability and significant hepatic metabolism (40%) via the cytochrome CYP pathway. Serum half-life is 2 to 6 hours in neonates.

SPECIAL CONSIDERATIONS/PREPARATION: Supplied as 2-mL ampules and 2-, 4-, and 10-mL vials (0.25-mg/mL solution). Contains 1% (10 mg/mL) benzyl alcohol; pH adjusted to 6.8 to 7.8. A 0.125 mg/mL dilution may be made by adding 3 mL of 0.25 mg/mL injectable solution to 3 mL preservative-free normal saline for injection. Refrigerated dilution is stable for 24 hours. Discolors when exposed to light.

Solution Compatibility: D_5W and NS. No data are available on Dex/AA.

Terminal Injection Site Compatibility: Fat emulsion. Aztreonam, cefepime, furosemide, lorazepam, milrinone, morphine, piperacillin-tazobactam, and propofol.

Incompatibility: Dobutamine and midazolam. No other data are available.

SELECTED REFERENCES

- Sullivan JE, Witte MK, Yamashita TS, Myers CM, Blumer JL: Dose-ranging evaluation of bumetanide pharmacodynamics in critically ill infants. *Clin Pharmacol Ther* 1996;60:424. (2 other related articles by same authors in same issue).
- Shankaran S, Liang K-C, Ilagan N, Fleischmann L: Mineral excretion following furosemide compared with bumetanide therapy in premature infants. *Pediatr Nephrol* 1995;9:159-62.
- Wittner M, Stefano AD, Wangemann P, Greger R: How do loop diuretics act? *Drugs* 1991;41(suppl 3):1.
- Brater DC: Clinical pharmacology of loop diuretics. *Drugs* 1991;41(suppl 3):14.

CAFFEINE CITRATE

DOSE & ADMINISTRATION: Loading dose: 20 to 40 mg/kg of caffeine citrate IV over 30 minutes or PO. (Equivalent to 10 to 20 mg/kg caffeine base). **Maintenance dose:** 5 to 8 mg/kg per dose of caffeine citrate IV slow push or PO Q24 hours. (Equivalent to 2.5 to 4 mg/kg caffeine base). Maintenance dose should be started 24 hours after the loading dose. (Please note that emphasis has changed to caffeine citrate due to commercially available product. This product (Cafcit®) may be administered both intravenously and orally).

USES: Treatment of neonatal apnea, including post-extubation and post-anesthesia. (More favorable therapeutic index than aminophylline).

MONITORING: Therapeutic trough serum concentration is 5 to 25 mcg/mL. Concentrations greater than 40 to 50 mcg/mL are toxic. Monitoring of serum drug concentration should be based on a trough level determined on approximately day 5 of therapy. Assess for agitation. Monitor heart rate; **consider withholding dose if greater than 180 beats per minute.**

ADVERSE EFFECTS/PRECAUTIONS: Adverse effects are usually mild, and include restlessness, vomiting, and functional cardiac symptoms. There has been a suggested association with NEC, but causality has never been proven. Loading doses of 25 mg/kg caffeine (50 mg/kg caffeine citrate) have been reported to decrease cerebral and intestinal blood flow velocity.

PHARMACOLOGY: The pharmacological effects of caffeine are mediated by its antagonism of the actions of adenosine at cell surface receptors. It is rapidly distributed in the brain, with CNS levels approximating plasma levels. Caffeine increases the respiratory center output, chemoreceptor sensitivity to CO_2, smooth muscle relaxation, and cardiac output. Oxygen consumption may be increased and weight gain may be reduced. Renal effects include diuresis and increased urinary calcium excretion. Orally administered caffeine citrate is rapidly and completely absorbed. There is almost no first-pass metabolism. In neonates, approximately 86% is excreted unchanged in the urine, with the remainder metabolized via the CYP1A2 enzyme system. The serum half-life of caffeine ranges from 40 to 230 hours, decreasing with advancing postmenstrual age until 60 weeks PMA. Half-life is prolonged in infants with cholestatic hepatitis.

SPECIAL CONSIDERATIONS/PREPARATION: Both Cafcit® Oral Solution and Cafcit® Injection for intravenous administration (Mead Johnson) are preservative free and available in 3-mL single use vials. Each mL of Cafcit® contains 20 mg of caffeine citrate (equivalent to 10 mg caffeine base). The osmolality is 160 mOsm/kg. Store at room temperature. Alternatively, an oral solution may be prepared by dissolving 2.5 g of caffeine anhydrous powder in 250 mL of water, yielding a final concentration of 10 mg/mL. Solution is stable for 4 weeks refrigerated. Crystals form when stored at low temperature but dissolve at room temperature without loss of potency. **Do not freeze.**

Solution Compatibility: D_5W, $D_{50}W$, and NS.

Terminal Injection Site Compatibility: Dex/AA solutions, fat emulsion. Amikacin, aminophylline, calcium gluconate, cefotaxime, cimetidine, clindamycin, fentanyl, dexamethasone, dobutamine, dopamine, doxapram, epinephrine, fentanyl, gentamicin, heparin (concentration < 1 Unit/mL), isoproterenol, lidocaine, metoclopramide, morphine, nitroprusside, pancuronium, penicillin G, phenobarbital, sodium bicarbonate, and vancomycin.

Incompatibility: Acyclovir, furosemide, lorazepam, oxacillin, and nitroglycerin.

SELECTED REFERENCES

- Comer AM, Perry CM, Figgitt DP: Caffeine citrate: A review of its use in apnoea of prematurity. *Paediatr Drugs* 2001;3:61-70.
- Bauer J, Maier K, Linderkamp O, Hentschel R: Effect of caffeine on oxygen consumption and metabolic rate in very low birth weight infants with idiopathic apnea. *Pediatrics* 2001;107:660-663.
- Erenberg A, Leff RD, Haack DG, et al: Caffeine citrate for the treatment of apnea of prematurity: A double-blind, placebo-controlled study. *Pharmacotherapy* 2000;20:644-652.
- Anderson BJ, Gunn TR, Holford NHG, et al: Caffeine overdose in a premature infant: Clinical course and pharmacokinetics. *Anaesth Intensive Care* 1999;27:307-311.
- Lane AJP, Coombs RC, Evans DH, et al: Effect of caffeine on neonatal splanchnic blood flow. *Arch Dis Child Fetal Neonatal Ed* 1999;80:F-128-F129.
- Lee TC, Charles B, Steer P: Population pharmacokinetics of intravenous caffeine in neonates with apnea of prematurity. *Clin Pharmacol Ther* 1997;61:628-640.
- Falcao AC, Fernandez de Gatta MM, Delgado Iribarnegaray MF, et al: Population pharmacokinetics of caffeine in premature neonates. *Eur J Clin Pharmacol* 1997;52:211-217.
- Zanardo V, Dani C, Trevisanuto D: Methylxanthines increase renal calcium excretion in preterm infants. *Biol Neonate* 1995;68:169-74.

CALCIUM CARBONATE

SPECIAL CONSIDERATIONS/PREPARATION: Calcium carbonate suspension (1250 mg/5 mL) yields 100 mg/mL elemental calcium.

CALCIUM CHLORIDE 10%

DOSE & ADMINISTRATION: Symptomatic hypocalcemia - acute treatment: 35 to 70 mg/kg per dose (0.35 to 0.7 mL/kg per dose, equivalent to 10 to 20 mg/kg elemental calcium). Dilute in appropriate fluid, then infuse IV over 10 to 30 minutes while monitoring for bradycardia. Stop infusion if heart rate is less than 100 beats per minute. **Do not give intra-arterially. Maintenance treatment:** 75 to 300 mg/kg per day (0.75 to 3 mL/kg per day, equivalent to 20 to 80 mg/kg elemental calcium). Administer by continuous IV infusion. Treat for 3 to 5 days, and follow serum concentrations periodically. **Exchange transfusion:** 33 mg per 100 mL citrated blood exchanged (equals 0.33 mL per 100 mL blood exchanged). Infuse IV over 10 minutes.

USES: Treatment and prevention of hypocalcemia, usually defined as a serum ionized calcium concentration less than approximately 4 mg/dL (or total serum calcium less than approximately 8 mg/dL).

MONITORING: If possible, measure ionized calcium directly. Avoid hypercalcemia during treatment. Correct hypomagnesemia if present. Observe IV infusion site closely for extravasation. Observe IV tubing for precipitates. Monitor continuously for bradycardia when giving bolus doses.

ADVERSE EFFECTS/PRECAUTIONS: Rapid administration is associated with bradycardia or cardiac standstill. Cutaneous necrosis or calcium deposition occurs with extravasation. Bolus infusions by UAC have been associated with intestinal bleeding and lower-extremity tissue necrosis.

PHARMACOLOGY: Calcium chloride may be more bioavailable than calcium gluconate, but it also is more likely to cause metabolic acidosis. Administration by continuous infusion is more efficacious than intermittent bolus dosing due to less renal calcium loss. Ionized calcium is the physiologically active fraction, accounting for approximately 50% of total blood calcium. The remainder is bound to albumin (40%) or complexed (10%) with citrate, phosphate, and bicarbonate. Early hypocalcemia is common in asphyxiated infants, premature infants, and infants of diabetic mothers. Significant decreases in ionized calcium may occur during acute alkalosis and following exchange transfusions with citrated blood. Clinical signs suggestive of hypocalcemia in neonates include muscle twitching, jitteriness, generalized seizures, and QTc above 0.4 second.

SPECIAL CONSIDERATIONS/PREPARATION: Calcium chloride 10% injection yields 27 mg/mL elemental calcium (1.36 mEq/mL). Osmolarity is 2040 mOsm/L. Injectable calcium salts should be stored at room temperature and are stable indefinitely.

Solution Compatibility: D_5W, $D_{10}W$, and NS.

Calcium Glubionate 6.5%

Terminal Injection Site Compatibility: Dex/AA solutions, fat emulsion. Amikacin, amiodarone, chloramphenicol, dobutamine, dopamine, epinephrine, esmolol, hydrocortisone, isoproterenol, lidocaine, methicillin, milrinone, morphine, penicillin G, pentobarbital, phenobarbital, potassium chloride, prostaglandin E_1, and sodium nitroprusside.

Incompatibility: Amphotericin B, methylprednisolone, metoclopramide, sodium bicarbonate, and phosphate and magnesium salts when mixed directly.

SELECTED REFERENCES

- Rigo J, DeCurtis M: Disorders of calcium, phosphorus, and magnesium metabolism. In: Martin RJ, Fanaroff AA, Walsh MC (eds): *Neonatal-Perinatal Medicine: Diseases of the Fetus and Newborn*, ed 8. St. Louis: Mosby, 2005, pp 1508-1514.
- Mimouni F, Tsang RC: Neonatal hypocalcemia: to treat or not to treat? (A review). *J Am Coll Nutr* 1994;13:408-15.
- Broner CW, Stidham GL, Westernkirchner DF, Watson DC: A prospective, randomized, double-blind comparison of calcium chloride and calcium gluconate therapies for hypocalcemia in critically ill children. *J Pediatr* 1990;117:986.
- Scott SM, Ladenson JH, Aguanna JJ, et al: Effect of calcium therapy in sick premature infats with early neonatal hypocalcemia. *J Pediatr* 1984;104:747.
- Roberts RJ: *Drug Therapy in Infants*. Philadelphia: WB Saunders Co, 1984, p 294.

Calcium Glubionate 6.5%

DOSE & ADMINISTRATION: Maintenance treatment: 360 to 1260 mg/kg per day (1 to 3.5 mL/kg/day). Administer PO in 4 divided doses after diluting in feeding.

ADVERSE EFFECTS/PRECAUTIONS: Gastric irritation and diarrhea may occur during oral therapy; NEC has been related to oral administration of hyperosmolar preparations such as Calcium glubionate. Calcium gluconate 10% may also be given orally if infant can tolerate the drug volume.

SPECIAL CONSIDERATIONS/PREPARATION: Calcium glubionate 6.5% syrup yields 23 mg/mL elemental calcium (1.16 mEq/mL). Osmolarity is 2500 mOsm/L.

Calcium Gluconate 10%

DOSE & ADMINISTRATION: Symptomatic hypocalcemia - acute treatment: 100 to 200 mg/kg per dose (1 to 2 mL/kg per dose, equivalent to 10 to 20 mg/kg elemental calcium). Dilute in appropriate fluid, then infuse in IV over 10 to 30 minutes while monitoring for bradycardia. Stop infusion if heart rate is less than 100 beats per minute. **Do not give intra-arterially. Maintenance treatment:** 200 to 800 mg/kg per day (2 to 8 mL/kg per day, equivalent to 20 to 80 mg/kg elemental calcium). Administer by continuous IV infusion. Treat for 3 to 5 days, and follow serum concentrations periodically. **May also be give orally in the same dose. Exchange transfusion:** 100 mg per 100 mL citrated blood exchanged (equals 1 mL per 100 mL blood exhanged). Infuse IV over 10 minutes.

USES: Treatment and prevention of hypocalcemia, usually defined as a serum ionized calcium concentration less than approximately 4 mg/dL (or total serum calcium less than approximately 8 mg/dL). Treatment of asymptomatic infants is controversial.

MONITORING: If possible, measure ionized calcium directly. Avoid hypercalcemia during treatment. Correct hypomagnesemia if present. Observe IV infusion site closely for extravasation. Observe IV tubing for precipitates. Monitor continuously for bradycardia when giving bolus doses. Assess for GI intolerance when treating PO.

PHARMACOLOGY: Ionized calcium is the physiologically active fraction, accounting for approximately 50% of total blood calcium. The remainder is bound to albumin (40%) or complexed (10%) with citrate, phosphate, and bicarbonate. Early hypocalcemia is common in asphyxiated infants, premature infants, and infants of diabetic mothers. Significant decreases in ionized calcium may occur during acute alkalosis and following exchange transfusions with citrated blood. Clinical signs suggestive of hypocalcemia in neonates include muscle twitching, jitteriness, generalized seizures, and QT_c above 0.40 second. Calcium chloride may be more bioavailable than calcium gluconate, but it also is more likely to cause metabolic acidosis. Administration by continuous infusion is more efficacious than intermittent bolus dosing due to less renal calcium loss.

SPECIAL CONSIDERATIONS/PREPARATION: Calcium gluconate 10% injection yields 9.3 mg/mL elemental calcium (0.46 mEq/mL). Osmolarity is 700 mOsm/L. Injectable calcium salts should be stored at room temperature and are stable indefinitely.

Solution Compatibility: D_5W, $D_{10}W$, and NS.

Terminal Injection Site Compatibility: Dex/AA solutions, fat emulsion. Amikacin, aminophylline, amiodarone, ampicillin, aztreonam, caffeine citrate, cefazolin, cefepime, chloramphenicol, dobutamine, enalaprilat, epinephrine, famotidine, furosemide, heparin, hydrocortisone, isoproterenol, lidocaine, linezolid, meropenem, methicillin, midazolam, milrinone, netilmicin, nicardipine, penicillin G, phenobarbital, piperacillin-tazobactam, potassium chloride, propofol, remifentanil, tobramycin, and vancomycin.

Incompatibility: Amphotericin B, clindamycin, esmolol, fluconazole, indomethacin, methylprednisolone, metoclopramide, sodium bicarbonate, and phosphate and magnesium salts when mixed directly.

SELECTED REFERENCES

- Rigo J, DeCurtis M: Disorders of calcium, phosphorus, and magnesium metabolism. In: Martin RJ, Fanaroff AA, Walsh MC (eds): *Neonatal-Perinatal Medicine: Diseases of the Fetus and Newborn*, ed 8. St. Louis: Mosby, 2005, pp 1508-1514.
- Porcelli PJ, Oh W: Effects of single dose calcium gluconate infusion in hypocalcemic preterm infants. *Am J Perinatol* 1995;12:18-21.
- Mimouni F, Tsang RC: Neonatal hypocalcemia: to treat or not to treat? (A review). *J Am Coll Nutr* 1994;13:408-15.
- Broner CW, Stidham GL, Westernkirchner DF, Watson DC: A prospective, randomized, double-blind comparison of calcium chloride and calcium gluconate therapies for hypocalcemia in critically ill children. *J Pediatr* 1990;117:986.
- Scott SM, Ladenson JH, Aguanna JJ, et al: Effect of calcium therapy in sick premature infats with early neonatal hypocalcemia. *J Pediatr* 1984;104:747.
- Roberts RJ: *Drug Therapy in Infants*. Philadelphia: WB Saunders Co, 1984, p 294.

Calcium - Oral

DOSE & ADMINISTRATION: 20 to 80 mg/kg elemental calcium per day PO in divided doses. **Calcium gluconate** 10% (IV formulation): 2 to 8 mL/kg per day. **Calcium carbonate** suspension, 250 mg/mL: 0.2 to 0.8 mL/kg per day. **Calcium glubionate** 6.5% syrup: 1 to 3.5 mL/kg per day.

USES: Treatment of non-acute hypocalcemia in babies able to tolerate oral medications.

MONITORING: Periodically measure serum calcium concentrations. Assess GI tolerance. Assess serum phosphorus and vitamin D levels when indicated.

ADVERSE EFFECTS/PRECAUTIONS: Oral calcium preparations are hypertonic, especially calcium glubionate syrup. Gastric irritation and diarrhea occur often. Use with caution in infants who are at risk for necrotising enterocolitis.

PHARMACOLOGY: Absorption of calcium administered orally is approximately 50%. Absorption takes place throughout the small intestine, and is primarily regulated by 1,25-dihydroxy vitamin D. Calcium carbonate significantly interferes with the absorption of levothyroxine. The osmolarity of calcium glubionate syrup is 2500 mOsm/L, and of calcium gluconate is 700 mOsm/L.

SPECIAL CONSIDERATIONS/PREPARATION: Calcium carbonate (Roxane) is available as a 250 mg/mL suspension (equivalent to 100 mg/mL elemental calcium) in 5-mL unit dose cups. Calcium glubionate 6.5% syrup (Rugby/Watson) yields 23 mg/mL elemental calcium (1.16 mEq/mL) and is available in 480 mL bottles. Osmolarity is 2500 mOsm/L.

SELECTED REFERENCES

- Hsu SC, Levine MA: Perinatal calcium metabolism: physiology and pathophysiology. *Semin Neonat* 2004;9:23-36.
- Singh N, Weisler SL, Hershman JM: The acute effect of calcium carbonate on the intestinal absorption of levothyroxine. *Thyroid* 2001;11:967-71.
- Product information, Roxane, 1996.

Captopril

DOSE & ADMINISTRATION: Initial dose: 0.01 to 0.05 mg/kg per dose PO Q8 to 12 hours. Adjust dose and interval based on response. Administer 1 hour before feeding.

CAPTOPRIL

USES: Treatment of moderate to severe hypertension. Afterload reduction in patients with congestive heart failure.

MONITORING: Frequent assessment of blood pressure, particularly after the first dose. Periodic assessment of renal function and serum potassium.

ADVERSE EFFECTS/PRECAUTIONS: Neonates are more sensitive to the effects of captopril than are older infants and children. Significant decreases in cerebral and renal blood flow have occurred in premature infants with chronic hypertension who received higher doses (0.15 to 0.30 mg/kg per dose) than those recommended above. These episodes occurred unpredictably during chronic therapy, and some were associated with neurologic (seizures, apnea, lethargy) and renal (oliguria) complications. **The use of captopril is contraindicated in** patients with bilateral renovascular disease or with unilateral renal artery stenosis in a solitary kidney, as the loss of adequate renal perfusion could precipitate acute renal failure. Hyperkalemia occurs primarily in patients receiving potassium-sparing diuretics or potassium supplements.

PHARMACOLOGY: Captopril is an angiotensin-converting enzyme (ACE) inhibitor that blocks the conversion of angiotensin I to angiotensin II, a potent vasoconstrictor. It thereby decreases plasma and tissue concentrations of angiotensin II and aldosterone, and increases plasma and tissue renin activity. Captopril also prevents the breakdown of bradykinin, a potent vasodilator. Vascular resistance is reduced without reflex tachycardia. Beneficial effects are thought to be caused by a combination of afterload reduction and long-term inhibition of salt and water retention. Bioavailability is good in neonates, although food will decrease absorption. Onset of action is 15 minutes after a dose, with peak effects seen in 30 to 90 minutes. Duration of action is usually 2 to 6 hours, but may be significantly longer (>24 hours).

SPECIAL CONSIDERATIONS/PREPARATION: Captopril oral suspension can be made by dissolving 6.25 mg (one-half of a scored 12.5 mg tablet) in 10 mL of sterile water, adding 1000 mg of sodium ascorbate for injection (4 mL of 250 mg/mL solution) to decrease oxidation, then adding sufficient water to make a final volume of 200 mL. The final concentration is 0.03 mg/mL captopril and 5 mg/mL sodium ascorbate. Solution is stable for 14 days at room temperature, 56 days refrigerated. Some undissolved excipients will remain visible.

SELECTED REFERENCES

- Nahata MC, Morosco RS, Hipple TF: Stability of captopril in liquid containing ascorbic acid or sodium ascorbate. *Am J Hosp Pharm* 1994;1707-1708.
- Perlman JM, Volpe JJ: Neurologic complications of captopril treatment of neonatal hypertension. *Pediatrics* 1989;83:47.
- O'Dea RF, Mirkin BL, Alward CT: Treatment of neonatal hypertension with captopril. *J Pediatr* 1988;113:403.

CASPOFUNGIN

DOSE & ADMINISTRATION: 1 to 2 mg/kg per dose Q24h IV infusion via syringe pump over at least 1 hour. The above dosage is based on a small number of case reports in neonates, as there are no pharmacokinetic data in neonates available at this time. Pharmacokinetic studies in children suggest that a larger dose (50 mg/m^2) may be required to obtain serum concentrations similar to adults. Adults with moderate hepatic insufficiency require dosage reductions.

USES: Treatment of patients with refractory Candidemia, intra-abdominal abscesses, peritonitis and pleural space infections, and those patients intolerant of amphotericin B. Treatment of invasive Aspergillosis in patients who are refractory to or intolerant of other therapies. There are case reports, but not controlled clinical trials, treating endocarditis, osteomyelitis, and meningitis due to *Candida*.

MONITORING: Assess IV site for signs of irritation. Periodic measurement of serum potassium, calcium, and hepatic transaminases.

ADVERSE EFFECTS/PRECAUTIONS: Adverse effects reported in neonates (small number of patients): thrombophlebitis, hypercalcemia, hypokalemia, elevated liver enzymes, and isolated direct hyperbilirubinemia. In adult studies the primary adverse effects are fever, headache, vomiting, diarrhea, signs of histamine release and irritation at the injection site. These occurred less frequently than with amphotericin B or with AmBisome®.

PHARMACOLOGY: Caspofungin is the first of a new class of antifungal agents (echinocandins) that inhibit the synthesis of β-(1,3)-D-glucan, an integral component of the fungal cell wall. It is fungicidal against *Candida* species, but fungistatic against

Aspergillus. The echinocandins are excreted primarily by the liver, presumably metabolized through an O-methyltransferase. They are not metabolized through the CYP enzyme system, and therefore, have significantly fewer drug-drug interactions than the azoles. Dexamethasone, phenytoin, carbamazepine, nevirapine, and rifampin all induce caspofungin drug clearance, lowering serum concentrations.

SPECIAL CONSIDERATIONS/PREPARATION: Cancidas® is supplied as a white to off-white powder cake in single use vials, containing either 50- or 70 mg. To prepare the 50 mg Cancidas infusion: 1) Equilibrate the refrigerated vial to room temperature. 2) Aseptically add 10.5 mL Normal Saline or Sterile Water for Injection to the vial. The powder cake will dissolve completely with gentle mixing. This reconstituted solution can be stored at room temperature for up to one hour. Visually inspect the reconstituted solution for particulate matter or discoloration. Do not use if the solution is cloudy or has precipitated. 3) Aseptically transfer 10 mL of the reconstituted solution to a 250 mL bag or bottle of 0.9%, 0.45%, or 0.225% Sodium Chloride Injection, or Lactated Ringer's Injection. This final patient infusion solution has a concentration of 0.2 mg/mL caspofungin, and can be stored for up to 24 hours at room temperature or up to 48 hours refrigerated. **Do not use diluents containing dextrose.**

Solution Compatibility: Normal Saline, Lactated Ringer's.

Solution Incompatibility: All solutions containing dextrose.

Terminal Injection Site Compatibility: Do not co-infuse with any other medications. (No data).

SELECTED REFERENCES
- Smith PB, Steinbach WJ, Cotton CM, et al. Caspofungin for the treatment of azole resistant candidemia in a premature infant. *J Perinatol* 2007;27:127-129.
- Manzar S, Kamat M, Pyati S. Caspofungin for refractory candidemia in neonates. *Pediatr Infect Dis J* 2006;25:282-283.
- Odio CM, Araya R, Pinto Le, et al. Caspofungin therapy of neonates with invasive candidiasis. *Pediatr Infect Dis J* 2004;23:1093-1097.
- Steinbach WJ, Benjamin DK. New agents under development in children and neonates. *Curr Opin Infect Dis* 2005;18:484-489.
- Pannaraj PS, Walsh TJ, Baker CJ. Advances in antifungal therapy. *Pediatr Infect Dis J* 2005;10:921-923.
- Walsh TJ, Adamson PC, Seibel NL, et al. Pharmacokinetics, safety, and tolerability of caspofungin in children and adolescents. *Antimicrob Agents Chemother* 2005;49:4536-4545.
- Dodds Ashley ES, Lewis R, Lewis JS, et al. Pharmacology of systemic antifungal agents. *Clin Infect Dis* 2006;43:S29-39.
- Product Information, Merck & Co., 2005.

CEFAZOLIN

DOSE & ADMINISTRATION: 25 mg/kg per dose IV slow push, or IM.

DOSING INTERVAL CHART

PMA (weeks)	PostNatal (days)	Interval (hours)
≤29	0 to 28 >28	12 8
30 to 36	0 to 14 >14	12 8
37 to 44	0 to 7 >7	12 8
≥45	ALL	6

USES: Use in neonates is generally limited to perioperative infection prophylaxis and treatment of urinary tract and soft tissue infections caused by susceptible organisms, e.g. penicillin-resistant *Staph. aureus*, *Klebsiella*, and *Proteus*.

MONITORING: Serum concentrations are not routinely monitored.

ADVERSE EFFECTS/PRECAUTIONS: Adverse effects are rare, but include phlebitis and eosinophilia.

PHARMACOLOGY: Cefazolin is a first generation cephalosporin that is bactericidal against many gram-positive and a few gram-negative organisms. Inactivated by β-lactamase producing organisms. Poor CNS penetration. Renally excreted as unchanged drug. Half-life in neonates is 3 to 5 hours.

CEFEPIME

SPECIAL CONSIDERATIONS/PREPARATION: Available as powder for injection in 500-mg, and 1000-mg vials. Reconstitute using NS or sterile water for injection to a concentration of 225 mg/mL. A 20 mg/mL dilution may be made by adding 1-mL of reconstituted solution to 10 mL sterile water for injection, or D_5W.

Solution Compatibility: D_5W, $D_{10}W$, and NS.

Terminal Injection Site Compatibility: Dex/AA and fat emulsion. Acyclovir, amikacin, aminophylline, aztreonam, calcium gluconate, clindamycin, enalaprilat, esmolol, famotidine, fluconazole, heparin, insulin, lidocaine, linezolid, midazolam, milrinone, morphine, metronidazole, multivitamins, nicardipine, pancuronium bromide, propofol, prostaglandin E_1, ranitidine, remifentanil, and vecuronium.

Incompatibility: Amiodarone, cimetidine, pentobarbital, and vancomycin. No data are currently available for potassium chloride.

SELECTED REFERENCES

- Saez-Llorens X, McCracken GH: Clinical pharmacology of antibacterial agents. In: Remington JS, Klein JO (eds): *Infectious Diseases of the Fetus and Newborn Infant*, ed 5. Philadelphia: WB Saunders Co, 2001.
- Pickering LK, O'Connor DM, Anderson D, et al: Clinical and pharmacologic evaluation of cefazolin in children. *J Infect Dis* 1973;128:S407.

CEFEPIME

DOSE & ADMINISTRATION: Term and preterm infants >14 days of age: 50 mg/kg per dose Q12 hr. **Term and preterm infants ≤14 days of age**: 30 mg/kg per dose Q12 hr. **Meningitis and severe infections** due to *Pseudomonas aeruginosa* or *Enterobacter* spp.: Doses above administered Q8 hours Administer via IV infusion by syringe pump over 30 minutes, or IM. To reduce pain at IM injection site, cefepime may be mixed with 1% lidocaine without epinephrine.

USES: Treatment of serious infections caused by susceptible gram-negative organisms (e.g. *E coli, H influenzae, Enterobacter, Klebsiella, Morganella, Neisseria, Serratia*, and *Proteus* species), especially *Pseudomonas aeruginosa* that are resistant to 3rd generation cephalosporins. Treatment of serious infections caused by susceptible Gram-positive organisms (e.g. *Strep pneumoniae, Strep. pyogenes, Strep. agalactiae,* and *Staph. aureus*).

MONITORING: Measuring serum concentration is not usually necessary.

ADVERSE EFFECTS/PRECAUTIONS: Safety has been documented to be the same as commonly used second- and third-generation cephalosporins. Reported adverse effects are uncommon but include rash, diarrhea, elevated hepatic transaminases, eosinophilia, and positive Coombs' test.

PHARMACOLOGY: Cefepime is a fourth-generation cephalosporin with treatment efficacy equivalent to third-generation cephalosporins. Potential advantages include: more rapid penetration through the cell wall of Gram-negative pathogens; enhanced stability to hydrolysis by β-lactamases; and enhanced affinity for penicillin-binding proteins. The drug distributes widely in body tissues and fluids (i.e. CSF, bile, bronchial secretions, lung tissue, ascitic fluid, middle ear). Protein binding is low (~ 20%), and it is primarily excreted unchanged in the urine. Serum half-life in infants older than 2 months of age is approximately 2 hours.

SPECIAL CONSIDERATIONS/PREPARATION: Available as powder for injection in 500-mg and 1-g, and 2-g vials. Reconstitute 500-mg vial with 5 mL of sterile water for injection to a concentration of 100 mg/mL. Maximum concentration for IV administration is 160 mg/mL, and for IM administration 280 mg/mL. Reconstituted solution stable for 24 hours at room temperature, 7 days refrigerated.

Solution Compatibility: D_5W, $D_{10}W$, D_5LR, and NS.

Terminal Injection Site Compatibility: Dex/AA solutions. Amikacin, ampicillin, aztreonam, bumetanide, calcium gluconate, clindamycin, dexamethasone, fluconazole, furosemide, heparin, hydrocortisone succinate, imipenem/cilastatin, lorazepam, methylprednisolone, metronidazole, milrinone, piperacillin-tazobactam, potassium chloride, ranitidine, sodium bicarbonate, ticarcillin/clavulanate, trimethoprim/sulfamethoxazole, and zidovudine.

Incompatibility: Aminophylline, acyclovir, amphotericin B, cimetidine, diazepam, dobutamine, dopamine, enalaprilat, famotidine, ganciclovir, gentamicin, magnesium sulfate, metoclopramide, morphine, netilmicin, tobramycin, and vancomycin.

SELECTED REFERENCES

- Capparelli E, Hochwald C, Rasmussen M, et al: Population pharmacokinetics of cefepime in the neonate. *Antimicrob Agents Chemother* 2005;49:2760-2766.
- Gutierrez K: Newer antibiotics: cefepime. *NeoReviews* 2004;5:e382-386.
- Blumer JL, Reed MD, Knupp C: Review of the pharmacokinetics of cefepime in children. *Pediatr Infect Dis J* 2001;20:337-342.
- Bradley JS, Arrieta A: Empiric use of cefepime in the treatment of lower respiratory tract infections in children. *Pediatr Infect Dis J* 2001;20:343-349.
- Saez-Llorens XO, O'Ryan M: Cefepime in the empiric treatment of meningitis in children. *Pediatr Infect Dis J* 2001;20:356-361.
- Kessler RE: Cefepime microbiologic profile and update. *Pediatr Infect Dis J* 2001; 20:331-336.

CEFOTAXIME

DOSE & ADMINISTRATION: 50 mg/kg per dose IV infusion by syringe pump over 30 minutes, or IM. **Gonococcal infections:** 25 mg/kg per dose IV over 30 minutes, or IM. To use dosing chart, please refer to explanatory note in "How to Use This Book."

DOSING INTERVAL CHART

PMA (weeks)	PostNatal (days)	Interval (hours)
≤29	0 to 28 >28	12 8
30 to 36	0 to 14 >14	12 8
37 to 44	0 to 7 >7	12 8
≥45	ALL	6

Gonococcal ophthalmia prophylaxis in newborns whose mothers have gonorrhea at the time of delivery: 100 mg/kg IV over 30 minutes or IM, single dose. (Note: topical antibiotic therapy alone is inadequate and is unnecessary if systemic treatment is administered.)

USES: Treatment of neonatal meningitis and sepsis caused by susceptible gram-negative organisms (e.g. *E coli, H influenzae, Klebsiella,* and *Pseudomonas*). Treatment of disseminated gonococcal infections.

MONITORING: Measuring serum concentration is not usually necessary. Periodic CBC.

ADVERSE EFFECTS/PRECAUTIONS: Side effects are rare but include rash, phlebitis, diarrhea, leukopenia, granulocytopenia, and eosinophilia.

PHARMACOLOGY: Cefotaxime is one of many third-generation cephalosporin antibiotics. The mechanism of action appears to be by bacterial cell wall disruption. Metabolized in the liver to an active compound, desacetylcefotaxime. The drug distributes widely (i.e. CSF, bile, bronchial secretions, lung tissue, ascitic fluid, middle ear). Excreted renally. Serum half-life in the premature infant is approximately 3 to 6 hours.

SPECIAL CONSIDERATIONS/PREPARATION: Available as powder for injection in 500-mg, 1-g, and 2-g vials. The 500-mg vial is reconstituted with 4.9 mL sterile water for injection to yield a concentration of 100 mg/mL. Reconstituted solution stable for 24 hours at room temperature, 5 days refrigerated.

Solution Compatibility: D_5W, $D_{10}W$, and NS.

Terminal Injection Site Compatibility: Dex/AA solutions, fat emulsion. Acyclovir, amikacin, aztreonam, caffeine citrate, clindamycin, famotidine, heparin, lorazepam, metronidazole, midazolam, milrinone, morphine, potassium chloride, and propofol, and remifentanil.

Incompatibility: Aminophylline, azithromycin, fluconazole, sodium bicarbonate, and vancomycin.

SELECTED REFERENCES

- Centers for Disease Control and Prevention: Sexually transmitted diseases treatment guidelines 2006. *MMWR* 2006;55(No. RR-11):47-48.
- Prober CG, Stevenson DK, Benitz WE: The use of antibiotics in neonates weighing less than 1200 grams. *Pediatr Infect Dis J* 1990;9:111.

CEFOXITIN

- Kearns GL, Jacobs RF, Thomas BR, et al: Cefotaxime and desacetylcefotaxime pharmacokinetics in very low birth weight neonates. *J Pediatr* 1989;114:461.
- de Louvois J, Mulhall A, Hurley R: The safety and pharmacokinetics of cefotaxime in the treatment of neonates. *Pediatr Pharmacol* 1982;2:275.
- Kafetzis DA, Brater DC, Kapiki AN: Treatment of severe neonatal infections with cefotaxime: Efficacy and pharmacokinetics. *J Pediatr* 1982;100:483.

CEFOXITIN

DOSE & ADMINISTRATION: 25 to 33 mg/kg per dose IV infusion by syringe pump over 30 minutes, or IM. To use dosing chart, please refer to explanatory note in "How to Use This Book."

DOSING INTERVAL CHART

PMA (weeks)	PostNatal (days)	Interval (hours)
≤29	0 to 28	12
	>28	8
30 to 36	0 to 14	12
	>14	8
37 to 44	0 to 7	12
	>7	8
≥45	ALL	6

USES: Use in neonates is generally limited to treatment of skin, intra-abdominal and urinary tract infections caused by susceptible bacteria - anaerobes (e.g. *Bacteroides fragilis*), gram positives (e.g. *Staphylococcus aureus*, *Streptococcus pneumoniae*, and other streptococci except enterococcus) and gram negatives (e.g. *Haemophilus influenzae*, *Klebsiella* sp., *E. coli*, *Proteus vulgaris*, and *Neisseria gonorrhoeae*).

MONITORING: Serum concentrations are not routinely monitored.

ADVERSE EFFECTS/PRECAUTIONS: Adverse effects are rare. Transient eosinophilia and elevation of hepatic transaminases have been reported in < 3% of treated patients. Severe overdose can cause tachypnea, pallor, hypotonia, and metabolic acidosis.

PHARMACOLOGY: Cefoxitin is a broad spectrum bactericidal second generation cephalosporin that has enhanced activity against anaerobic bacteria. Inhibits bacterial cell wall synthesis by binding to one or more penicillin-binding proteins. Not inactivated by β-lactamase. Poor CNS penetration. Highly protein bound. Renally excreted as unchanged drug (85 to 90%). Half-life in term neonates is approximately 1.4 hours, and 2.3 hours in preterm neonates —considerably longer than children (0.6 hours) and adults (0.8 hours).

SPECIAL CONSIDERATIONS/PREPARATION: Available as powder for injection in 1-g, and 2-g vials. **IV administration:** Reconstitute 1-g vial with 9.5 mL sterile water for injection to a concentration of 100 mg/mL. A 40 mg/ml dilution may be made by adding 4 mL of reconstituted solution to 6 mL sterile water for injection, or D_5W. Stable for 24 hours at room temperature or 7 days refrigerated. **IM administration:** Reconstitute 1-g vial with 4.5 mL of 0.5% Lidocaine solution without epinephrine to a concentration of 200 mg/mL.

Solution Compatibility: D_5W, $D_{10}W$, and NS.

Terminal Injection Site Compatibility: Dex/AA and fat emulsion. Acyclovir, amikacin, aztreonam, cimetidine, clindamycin, famotidine, fluconazole, gentamicin, heparin, insulin, lidocaine, linezolid, magnesium sulfate, metronidazole, morphine, multivitamins, potassium chloride, propofol, ranitidine, remifentanil, sodium bicarbonate, tobramycin and vecuronium.

Incompatibility: Vancomycin

SELECTED REFERENCES

- Regazzi MB, Chirico G, Cristiani D, et al: Cefoxitin in newborn infants. *Eur J Clin Pharmacol* 1983;25:507-509.
- Yogev R, Delaplane D, Wiringa K: Cefoxitin in a neonate. *Ped Infect Dis J* 1983;2:342-343.
- Farmer K: Use of cefoxitin in the newborn. *New Zealand Med J* 1982;95:398.
- Marget W: Tenfold overdose of cefoxitin in a newborn. *Infection* 1982;10:243.
- Brogden RN, Heel RC, Speight TM, et al: Cefoxitin: A review of its antibacterial activity, pharmacological properties and therapeutic use. *Drugs* 1979;17:1-37.
- Feldman WE, Moffitt S, Sprow N: Clinical and pharmacokinetic evaluation of parenteral cefoxitin in infants and children. *Antimicrob Agents Chemother* 1980;17:669-674.

CEFTAZIDIME

DOSE & ADMINISTRATION: 30 mg/kg per dose IV infusion by syringe pump over 30 minutes, or IM. To reduce pain at IM injection site, ceftazidime may be mixed with 1% lidocaine without epinephrine. To use dosing chart, please refer to explanatory note in "How to Use This Book."

DOSING INTERVAL CHART

PMA (weeks)	PostNatal (days)	Interval (hours)
≤29	0 to 28 >28	12 8
30 to 36	0 to 14 >14	12 8
37 to 44	0 to 7 >7	12 8
≥45	ALL	8

USES: Treatment of neonatal meningitis and sepsis caused by susceptible gram-negative organisms (e.g., *E. coli, H. influenzae, Neisseria, Klebsiella,* and *Proteus* species), especially *Pseudomonas aeruginosa*. Resistance among strains of *Serratia* and *Enterobacteriaceae* is increasing.

MONITORING: Measuring serum concentration is not usually necessary.

ADVERSE EFFECTS/PRECAUTIONS: Reported adverse effects are uncommon but include rash, diarrhea, elevated hepatic transaminases, eosinophilia, and positive Coombs' test.

PHARMACOLOGY: Ceftazidime is one of many third-generation cephalosporins. The drug distributes widely in body tissues and fluids (i.e. CSF, bile, bronchial secretions, lung tissue, ascitic fluid, middle ear). Protein binding is low, and it is excreted unchanged in the urine. Ceftazidime is synergistic with aminoglycosides. Serum half-life in neonates is 3 to 12 hours.

SPECIAL CONSIDERATIONS/PREPARATION: Available as powder for injection in 500-mg and 1-g, 2-g, and 6-g vials. **Intravenous solution:** Reconstitute 500-mg vial with 10 mL of sterile water for injection to make a concentration of 50 mg/mL. Reconstituted solution stable for 24 hours at room temperature, 7 days refrigerated. **Intramuscular solution:** Prepared by reconstituting 500-mg vial with 2.2 mL of 1% lidocaine without epinephrine to a concentration of 200 mg/mL. Solution is stable for 24 hours at room temperature, 3 days refrigerated. Ceftazdime mixtures with L-arginine are not approved for pediatric use. All dosage forms approved for pediatric use contain sodium carbonate; when reconstituted, carbon dioxide bubbles will form. Using a vented needle may help reduce spraying and leaking.

Solution Compatibility: D_5W, $D_{10}W$, and NS.

Terminal Injection Site Compatibility: Dex/AA solutions, fat emulsion. Acyclovir, aminophylline, amikacin, aztreonam, cimetidine, ciprofloxacin, clindamycin, enalaprilat, esmolol, famotidine, furosemide, gentamicin, heparin, linezolid, metronidazole, milrinone, morphine, potassium chloride, propofol, ranitidine, remifentanil, sodium bicarbonate, tobramycin, and zidovudine.

Incompatibility: Amiodarone, azithromycin, erythromycin lactobionate, fluconazole, midazolam, nicardipine, and vancomycin.

SELECTED REFERENCES

- Prober CG, Stevenson DK, Benitz WE: The use of antibiotics in neonates weighing less than 1200 grams. *Pediatr Infect Dis J* 1990;9:111.
- Tessin I, Thiringer K, Trollfors B, Brorson JE: Comparison of serum concentrations of ceftazidime and tobramycin in newborn infants. *Eur J Pediatr* 1988;147:405.
- Odio CM, Umana MA, Saenz A, et al: Comparative efficacy of ceftazidime vs. carbenicillin and amikacin for treatment of neonatal septicemia. *Pediatr Infect Dis* 1987;6:371.
- McCracken GH, Threlkeld N, Thomas ML: Pharmacokinetics of ceftazidime in newborn infants. *Antimicrob Agents Chemother* 1984;26:583.

CEFTRIAXONE

DOSE & ADMINISTRATION: Sepsis and disseminated gonococcal infection: 50 mg/kg Q24 hours. **Meningitis:** 100 mg/kg loading dose, then 80 mg/kg Q24 hours. **Uncomplicated gonococcal ophthalmia:** 50 mg/kg (maximum 125 mg) single dose. (Note: topical antibiotic therapy alone is inadequate and is unnecessary if systemic treatment is administered.) **IV administration:** Infusion by syringe pump over 30 minutes. **IM administration:** To reduce pain at the injection site, reconstitute with 1% lidocaine without epinephrine.

USES: Treatment of neonatal sepsis and meningitis caused by susceptible gram-negative organisms (e.g., *E. coli, Pseudomonas, Klebsiella, H. influenzae*). Treatment of gonococcal infections.

MONITORING: CBC for eosinophilia, thrombocytosis, leukopenia. Serum electrolytes, BUN, creatinine. AST, ALT, bilirubin. Consider abdominal ultrasonography.

ADVERSE EFFECTS/PRECAUTIONS: Not recommended for use in neonates with hyperbilirubinemia. Displaces bilirubin from albumin binding sites, resulting in higher free bilirubin serum concentrations. Eosinophilia, thrombocytosis, leukopenia. Increase in bleeding time. Diarrhea. Increase in BUN and serum creatinine. Increase in AST and ALT. Skin rash. Transient gallbladder precipitations occasionally associated with colicky abdominal pain, nausea, and vomiting.

PHARMACOLOGY: Ceftriaxone is one of many third-generation cephalosporin antibiotics. The drug distributes widely (i.e., CSF, bile, bronchial secretions, lung tissue, ascitic fluid, middle ear). It is eliminated unchanged by both biliary (40%) and renal mechanisms. Serum half-life in premature infants is 5 to 16 hours. Dosage adjustment is necessary only for patients with combined hepatic and renal failure.

SPECIAL CONSIDERATIONS/PREPARATION: Intravenous solution: Available as a powder for injection in 250-mg, 500-mg, 1-g, and 2-g vials. Prepared by reconstituting powder with compatible solution (sterile water for injection, D_5W, or $D_{10}W$) to a concentration of 40 mg/mL. Reconstituted solution is stable for 3 days at room temperature, 10 days refrigerated. A dark color may appear after reconstitution; however, potency is retained. To make 40-mg/mL solution add 6.2 mL to the 250-mg vial. **Intramuscular solution:** Prepared by reconstituting 250-mg vial with 0.9 mL of 1% lidocaine without epinephrine to a concentration of 250 mg/mL. Solution is stable for 24 hours at room temperature, 3 days refrigerated.

Solution Compatibility: D_5W, $D_{10}W$, and NS.

Terminal Injection Site Compatibility: Dex/AA solutions, fat emulsion. Acyclovir, amikacin, amiodarone, aztreonam, clindamycin, famotidine, gentamicin, heparin, lidocaine, linezolid, metronidazole, morphine, potassium chloride, propofol, remifentanil, sodium bicarbonate, and zidovudine.

Incompatibility: Aminophylline, azithromycin, fluconazole and vancomycin.

SELECTED REFERENCES

- Centers for Disease Control and Prevention: Sexually transmitted diseases treatment guidelines 2006. *MMWR* 2006;55(No. RR-11):47-48.
- Prober CG, Stevenson DK, Benitz WE: The use of antibiotics in neonates weighing less than 1200 grams. *Pediatr Infect Dis J* 1990;9:111.
- Schaad UB, Suter S, Gianella-Borradori A, et al: A comparison of ceftriaxone and cefuroxime for the treatment of bacterial meningitis in children. *N Engl J Med* 1990;332:141.
- Fink S, Karp W, Roberson A: Ceftriaxone effect on bilirubin-albumin binding. *Pediatrics* 1987;80:873.
- Laga M, Naamara W, Brunham RC, et al: Single-dose therapy of gonococcal ophthalmia neonatorum with ceftriaxone. *N Engl J Med* 1986;315:1382.
- Yogev R, Shulman ST, Chadwick E, et al: Once daily ceftriaxone for central nervous system infections and other serious pediatric infections. *Pediatr Infect Dis J* 1986;5:298.
- Martin E, Koup JR, Paravicini U, Stoeckel K: Pharmacokinetics of ceftriaxone in neonates and infants with meningitis. *J Pediatr* 1984;105:475.
- Schaad UB, Stoeckel K: Single-dose pharmacokinetics of ceftriaxone in infants and young children. *Antimicrob Agents Chemother* 1982;21:248.

Chloral Hydrate

DOSE & ADMINISTRATION: 25 to 75 mg/kg per dose PO or PR. Oral preparation should be diluted or administered after a feeding to reduce gastric irritation.

USES: Sedative/hypnotic for short-term use only. Chloral hydrate has no analgesic properties; excitement may occur in patients with pain.

MONITORING: Assess level of sedation.

ADVERSE EFFECTS/PRECAUTIONS: Episodes of bradycardia are more frequent for up to 24 hours after a single dose in former premature infants. Gastric irritation and paradoxical excitement may also occur after a single dose. Other toxic effects have generally been reported in patients who received either repeated doses at regular intervals or acute overdoses. These effects may persist for days and include CNS, respiratory, and myocardial depression; cardiac arrhythmias; and ileus and bladder atony. Indirect hyperbilirubinemia may occur because TCE and bilirubin compete for hepatic conjugation. **Do not use in patients with significant hepatic and/or renal disease.**

PHARMACOLOGY: Chloral hydrate is a well absorbed from the oral route, with the onset of action in 10 to 15 minutes. Chloral hydrate is rapidly converted by alcohol dehydrogenase to the active and potentially toxic metabolite trichloroethanol (TCEt), which is excreted renally after glucuronidation in the liver. It is also metabolized to trichloroacetic acid (TCA), which is carcinogenic in mice when given in very high doses. Both TCEt (8 to 64 hours) and TCA (days) have long serum half-lives in neonates and accumulate with repeated doses.

SPECIAL CONSIDERATIONS/PREPARATION: Chloral hydrate is available in syrup as 50-mg/mL and 100-mg/mL concentrations. Osmolality is 3285 mOsm/kg of water. **The preparations are light-sensitive: Store in a dark container.** Also available as 324- and 648-mg suppositories. Inaccurate dosing may occur with rectal administration because of unequal distribution of chloral hydrate in the suppositories.

SELECTED REFERENCES

- Allegaert K, Daniels H, Naulaers G, et al: Pharmacodynamics of chloral hydrate in former premature infants. *Eur J Pediatr* 2005;164:403-407.
- American Academy of Pediatrics, Committee on Drugs and Committee on Environmental Health: Use of chloral hydrate for sedation in children. *Pediatrics* 1993;92:471.
- Mayers DJ, Hindmarsh KW, Gorecki DKJ, Sankaran K: Sedative/hypnotic effects of chloral hydrate in the neonate: Trichloroethanol or parent drug? *Dev Pharmacol Ther* 1992;19:141.
- Anyebuno MA, Rosenfeld CR: Chloral hydrate toxicity in a term infant. *Dev Pharmacol Ther* 1991;17:116.
- Mayers DJ, Hindmarsh KW, Sankaran K, et al: Chloral hydrate disposition following single-dose administration to critically ill neonates and children. *Dev Pharmacol Ther* 1991;16:71.
- Reimche LD, Sankaran K, Hindmarsh KW, et al: Chloral hydrate sedation in neonates and infants: Clinical and pharmacologic considerations. *Dev Pharmacol Ther* 1989;12:57.

Chloramphenicol

DOSE & ADMINISTRATION: Loading dose: 20 mg/kg IV infusion by syringe pump over 30 minutes. **Maintenance dose:** (Begin 12 hours after loading dose.) Premature infants under 1 month of age: 2.5 mg/kg per dose Q6 hours. Fullterm infants under 1 week of age and premature infants over 1 month of age: 5 mg/kg per dose Q6 hours. Fullterm infants over 1 week of age: 12.5 mg/kg per dose Q6 hours. (Absorption of oral chloramphenicol palmitate is erratic in newborns.)

USES: A wide-spectrum antimicrobial bacteriostatic agent. May be bactericidal to species such as *H. influenzae* and *Neisseria meningitidis*.

MONITORING: Close monitoring of serum concentration is mandatory. Small changes in dose and interval can lead to disproportionately large changes in serum concentration. Therapeutic peak serum concentration: 10 to 25 mcg/mL. Monitor CBC and reticulocyte counts. Assess hepatic and renal function.

Chlorothiazide (continued from Chloramphenicol)

ADVERSE EFFECTS/PRECAUTIONS: Reversible bone marrow suppression, irreversible aplastic anemia. Serum concentration greater than 50 mcg/mL has been associated with the "gray baby" syndrome (i.e. abdominal distention, pallid cyanosis, vasomotor collapse; may lead to death within hours of onset). Fungal overgrowth.

PHARMACOLOGY: Both esters of chloramphenicol (succinate and palmitate) are biologically inactive prodrugs. Hydrolysis to the active compound is erratic in newborns. Metabolized by hepatic glucuronyl transferase. Hepatically and renally eliminated. Inhibits metabolism of phenobarbital, phenytoin, and other agents.

SPECIAL CONSIDERATIONS/PREPARATION: Chloramphenicol succinate is available as powder for injection in a 1-g vial. Reconstitute with 10 mL sterile water for injection, or D_5W to a concentration of 100 mg/mL. Reconstituted solution stable for 4 days refrigerated.

Solution Compatibility: D_5W, $D_{10}W$, and NS.

Terminal Injection Site Compatibility: Dex/AA solutions, fat emulsion. Acyclovir, amikacin, aminophylline, ampicillin, calcium chloride, calcium gluconate, dopamine, enalaprilat, erythromycin lactobionate, esmolol, heparin, hydrocortisone succinate, lidocaine, magnesium sulfate, methicillin, metronidazole, morphine, nafcillin, nicardipine, oxacillin, penicillin G, pentobarbital, potassium chloride, ranitidine, sodium bicarbonate, and vitamin K_1.

Incompatibility: Fluconazole, metoclopramide, phenytoin, and vancomycin.

SELECTED REFERENCES

- Roberts RJ: *Drug Therapy in Infants*. Philadelphia: WB Saunders Co, 1984, p 70.
- Rajchgot P, Prober CG, Soldin S: Initiation of chloramphenicol therapy in the newborn infant. *J Pediatr* 1982;101:1018.
- Glazer JP, Danish MA, Plotkin SA, Yaffe SJ: Disposition of chloramphenicol in low birth weight infants. *Pediatrics* 1980;66:573.

Chlorothiazide

DOSE & ADMINISTRATION: Diuresis: 10 to 20 mg/kg per dose Q12 hours PO. **Adjuvant treatment of central diabetes insipidus:** 5 mg/kg per dose Q12 hours PO. Administer with food (improves absorption). IV administration not recommended because of a lack of data. **Note: Do not confuse with hydrochlorothiazide.**

USES: Diuretic used in treating both mild to moderate edema and mild to moderate hypertension. Effects increased when used in combination with furosemide or spironolactone. May improve pulmonary function in patients with BPD. Adjuvant treatment of central diabetes insipidus.

MONITORING: Serum electrolytes, calcium, phosphorus, and glucose; urine output and blood pressure.

ADVERSE EFFECTS/PRECAUTIONS: Hypokalemia and other electrolyte abnormalities. Hyperglycemia. Hyperuricemia. **Do not use in patients with significant impairment of renal or hepatic function.**

PHARMACOLOGY: Limited data in neonates. Variable absorption from GI tract. Onset of action within 1 hour. Elimination half-life depends on GFR, and is approximately 5 hours. Major diuretic effect results from inhibition of sodium reabsorption in the distal nephron. Increases urinary losses of sodium, potassium, magnesium, chloride, bicarbonate, and phosphorus. Decreases renal excretion of calcium. Inhibits pancreatic release of insulin. Displaces bilirubin from albumin binding sites.

SPECIAL CONSIDERATIONS/PREPARATION: Available as a 250 mg/5mL suspension for oral use.

SELECTED REFERENCES

- Pogacar PR, Mahnke S, Rivkees SA: Management of central diabetes insipidus in infancy with low renal solute load formula and chlorothiazide. *Curr Opin Pediatr* 2000;12:405-411.
- Wells TG: The pharmacology and therapeutics of diuretics in the pediatric patient. *Pediatr Clin North Am* 1990;37:463.
- Albersheim SG, Solimano AJ, Sharma AK, et al: Randomized, double-blind, controlled trial of long-term diuretic therapy for bronchopulmonary dysplasia. *J Pediatr* 1989;115:615.
- Roberts RJ: *Drug Therapy in Infants*. Philadelphia: WB Saunders Co, 1984, p 244.

- Kao LC, Warburton D, Cheng MH, et al: Effect of oral diuretics on pulmonary mechanics in infants with chronic bronchopulmonary dysplasia: Results of a double-blind crossover sequential trial. *Pediatrics* 1984;74:37.

CIMETIDINE

DOSE & ADMINISTRATION: 2.5 to 5 mg/kg per dose Q6 to 12 hours PO or IV infusion over 15 to 30 minutes.

USES: Prevention and treatment of stress ulcers and GI hemorrhage aggravated by gastric acid secretion.

MONITORING: Gastric pH may be measured to assess efficacy. Observe for impaired consciousness and reduced spontaneous movements.

ADVERSE EFFECTS/PRECAUTIONS: Known adverse effects of cimetidine in adults include mental confusion, seizures, renal dysfunction, hepatic dysfunction, flushing and transpiration, neutropenia, diarrhea, hypothalamic-pituitary-gonadal dysfunction, and muscular pain. Cimetidine has been reported to increase the serum level and potentiate toxicity of other drugs such as aminophylline, carbamazepine, diazepam, lidocaine, morphine, phenytoin, procainamide, propranolol, quinidine, theophylline, and warfarin. **Contraindicated** in patients receiving cisapride due to precipitation of life-threatening arrhythmias.

PHARMACOLOGY: Inhibits gastric acid secretion by histamine H_2-receptor antagonism. Peak inhibition occurs in 15 to 60 minutes after both oral and IV administration. Metabolized in the liver via sulfation and hydroxylation to inactive compounds that are 90% renally eliminated. Half-life in neonates is 1.1 to 3.4 hours, and is prolonged in patients with renal or hepatic insufficiency. The sulfoxide metabolite may accumulate in the CNS and cause toxicity. Antacids interfere with absorption; therefore, concomitant administration is not recommended.

SPECIAL CONSIDERATIONS/PREPARATION: Available as a 150-mg/mL injectable solution in 2-mL single-use vials and 8-mL multidose vials. A 15-mg/mL dilution may be made by adding 1 mL of 150 mg/mL concentration to 9 mL of preservative-free normal saline. Dilution stable for 48 hours. Manufacturer's oral solution (60 mg/mL) contains 2.8% alcohol. A 2.4 mg/mL oral dilution may be prepared by adding 1 mL (60 mg) of manufacturer's oral solution to 24 mL of sterile water. Stable for 14 days refrigerated. Also available in 300-, 400-, and 800-mg tablets.

Solution Compatibility: D_5W, $D_{10}W$, and NS.

Terminal Injection Site Compatibility: Dex/AA solutions, fat emulsion. Acetazolamide, acyclovir, amikacin, aminophylline, ampicillin, atropine, aztreonam, caffeine citrate, cefoxitin, ceftazidime, clindamycin, dexamethasone, diazepam, digoxin, enalaprilat, epinephrine, erythromycin lactobionate, esmolol, fentanyl, fluconazole, flumazenil, furosemide, gentamicin, glycopyrrolate, heparin, insulin, isoproterenol, lidocaine, linezolid, lorazepam, meperidine, meropenem, metoclopramide, midazolam, milrinone, morphine, nafcillin, nicardipine, nitroprusside, pancuronium, penicillin G, piperacillin-tazobactam, potassium chloride, propofol, prostaglandin E_1, protamine, remifentanil, sodium bicarbonate, vancomycin, vecuronium, vitamin K_1, and zidovudine.

Incompatibility: Amphotericin B (Immediate precipitation occurs), cefazolin, cefepime, indomethacin, pentobarbital, phenobarbital, and secobarbital.

SELECTED REFERENCES

- Vandenplas Y, Sacre L: The use of cimetidine in newborns. *Am J Perinatol* 1987;4:131.
- Lloyd CW, Martin WJ, Taylor BD: The pharmacokinetics of cimetidine and metabolites in a neonate. *Drug Intell Clin Pharm* 1985;19:203.
- Ziemniak JA, Wynn RJ, Aranda JV, et al: The pharmacokinetics and metabolism of cimetidine in neonates. *Dev Pharmacol Ther* 1984;7:30.
- Aranda JV, Outerbridge EW, Shentag JJ: Pharmacodynamics and kinetics of cimetidine in a premature newborn. *Am J Dis Child* 1983;137:1207.

Clindamycin

DOSE & ADMINISTRATION: 5 to 7.5 mg/kg per dose IV infusion by syringe pump over 30 minutes, or PO. To use dosing chart, please refer to explanatory note in "How to Use This Book."

Dosing Interval Chart

PMA (weeks)	PostNatal (days)	Interval (hours)
≤29	0 to 28 >28	12 8
30 to 36	0 to 14 >14	12 8
37 to 44	0 to 7 >7	12 8
≥45	ALL	6

Increase dosing interval in patients with significant liver dysfunction.

USES: Bacteriostatic antibiotic used for the treatment of bacteremia and pulmonary and deep tissue infections caused by anaerobic bacteria and some gram-positive cocci. Clindamycin should not be used in the treatment of meningitis.

MONITORING: Assess liver function. Monitor GI status closely. Therapeutic serum concentration ranges from 2 to 10 mcg/mL (bioassay yields variable results).

ADVERSE EFFECTS/PRECAUTIONS: The most serious adverse effect is pseudomembranous colitis, characterized by bloody diarrhea, abdominal pain, and fever. Discontinue clindamycin if any of these signs or symptoms occur, begin bowel rest and TPN, and consider treatment with oral metronidazole.

PHARMACOLOGY: Clindamycin inhibits bacterial protein synthesis and is primarily bacteriostatic at therapeutically attainable concentrations. Widely distributed into most tissues, especially the lung. Poor CSF penetration. Oral clindamycin is completely absorbed from the GI tract. Highly protein bound. Almost complete metabolism in the liver, with excretion via bile and feces. Available data in neonates suggest extremely variable clearance, especially in premature infants. No data are available regarding conversion of ester to active drug.

SPECIAL CONSIDERATIONS/PREPARATION: Oral preparation (clindamycin palmitate) is reconstituted with sterile water for injection, yielding a 75 mg per 5 mL solution. **Do not refrigerate.** Stable at room temperature for 2 weeks. IV preparation (clindamycin phosphate) is available as a 150 mg/mL solution in 2-mL, 4-mL, and 6-mL vials containing 9.45 mg/mL benzyl alcohol. It should be diluted using D_5W, NS, or LR to a concentration of 6 mg/mL, and infused at a rate no greater than 5 mL/min (30 mg/min).

Solution Compatibility: D_5W, $D_{10}W$, and NS.

Terminal Injection Site Compatibility: Dex/AA solutions, fat emulsion. Acyclovir, amikacin, amiodarone, ampicillin, aztreonam, caffeine citrate, cefazolin, cefepime, cefotaxime, cefoxitin, ceftazidime, ceftriaxone, cimetidine, enalaprilat, esmolol, gentamicin, heparin, hydrocortisone succinate, linezolid, magnesium sulfate, metoclopramide, metronidazole, midazolam, milrinone, morphine, netilmicin, nicardipine, penicillin G, piperacillin, piperacillin/tazobactam, potassium chloride, propofol, prostaglandin E_1, ranitidine, remifentanil, sodium bicarbonate, tobramycin, and zidovudine.

Incompatibility: Aminophylline, azithromycin, barbiturates, calcium gluconate, ciprofloxacin, fluconazole, and phenytoin.

SELECTED REFERENCES

- Koren G, Zarfin Y, Maresky D, et al: Pharmacokinetics of intravenous clindamycin in newborn infants. *Pediatr Pharmacol* 1986;5:287.
- Bell MJ, Shackelford P, Smith R, Schroeder K: Pharmacokinetics of clindamycin phosphate in the first year of life. *J Pediatr* 1984;105:482.
- Feigin RD, Pickering LK, Anderson D, et al: Clindamycin treatment of osteomyelitis and septic arthritis in children. *Pediatrics* 1975;55:213.
- Lwin N, Collipp PJ: Absorption and tolerance of clindamycin 2-palmitate in infants below 6 months of age. *Curr Ther Res Clin Exp* 1970;12:648.

Curosurf®

(Poractant Alfa) Intratracheal Suspension

DOSE & ADMINISTRATION: Initial dose is 2.5 mL/kg per dose intratracheally, divided into 2 aliquots followed by up to two subsequent doses of 1.25 mL/kg per dose administered at 12-hour intervals if needed. Clear the trachea of secretions. Shorten a 5F end-hole catheter so the tip of the catheter will protrude just beyond end of ET tube above infant's carina. Slowly withdraw entire contents of vial into a plastic syringe through a large (greater than 20 gauge) needle. **Do not filter or shake.** Attach shortened catheter to syringe. Fill catheter with surfactant. Discard excess through catheter so only total dose to be given remains in syringe. Administer in two to four aliquots with the infant in different positions to enhance distribution in the lungs. The catheter can be inserted into the infant's endotracheal tube without interrupting ventilation by passing the catheter through a neonatal suction valve attached to the endotracheal tube. Alternatively, surfactant can be instilled through the catheter by briefly disconnecting the endotracheal tube from the ventilator. After administration of each aliquot, the dosing catheter is removed from the ET tube and the infant is ventilated for at least 30 seconds until stable.

PHARMACOLOGY: Pulmonary lung surfactants are essential for effective ventilation by modifying alveolar surface tension thereby stabilizing the alveoli. Curosurf® is a modified porcine-derived minced lung extract containing phospholipids, neutral lipids, fatty acids, and surfactant-associated proteins B and C. Each mL of surfactant contains 80 mg of total phospholipids (54 mg of phosphatidylcholine of which 30.5 mg dipalmitoyl phosphatidylcholine) and 1 mg of protein including 0.3 mg of SP-B.

SPECIAL CONSIDERATIONS/PREPARATION: Available in 1.5 mL (120 mg phospholipid) and 3 mL (240 mg phospholipid) vials. Refrigerate (2 °C to 8 °C (36 °F to 46 °F)) and protect from light. Inspect Curosurf® for discoloration; normal color is creamy white. If settling occurs during storage, gently turn vial upside-down in order to uniformly suspend. **Do not shake.** Used vials with residual drug should be discarded. Unopened vials that have been warmed to room temperature one time may be refrigerated within 24 hours and stored for future use.

SELECTED REFERENCES

- Collaborative European Multicenter Study Group: Surfactant replacement therapy for severe neonatal respiratory distress syndrome: A international randomized clinical trial. *Pediatrics* 1988;82:683-691.
- Bevilacqua G, Parmigiani S, Robertson B: Prophylaxis of respiratory distress syndrome by treatment with modified porcine surfactant at birth: a multicentre prospective randomized trial. *J Perinat Med* 1996;24:609-620.
- Egberts J, de Winter JP, Sedin G, et al: Comparison of prophylaxis and rescue treatment with Curosurf® in neonates less than 30 weeks' gestation: A randomized trial. *Pediatrics* 1993;92:768-774.
- Halliday HL, Tarnow-Mordi WO, Corcoran JD, et al: Multicentre randomised trial comparing high and low dose surfactant regimens for the treatment of respiratory distress syndrome (the Curosurf® 4 trials). *Arch Dis Child* 1993;69:276-280.

Cyclopentolate (Ophthalmic)

DOSE & ADMINISTRATION: 1 or 2 drops instilled in the eye 10 to 30 minutes prior to funduscopy. Use solutions containing concentrations of 0.5% or less in neonates. May be used in conjunction with 1 drop of phenylephrine 2.5% ophthalmic solution. Apply pressure to the lacrimal sac during and for 2 minutes after instillation to minimize systemic absorption.

USES: Induction of mydriasis and cycloplegia for diagnostic and therapeutic ophthalmic procedures.

MONITORING: Monitor heart rate and assess for signs of ileus prior to feeding.

ADVERSE EFFECTS/PRECAUTIONS: Feedings should be withheld for 4 hours following procedure. Systemic effects are those of anticholinergic drugs: Fever, tachycardia, vasodilatation, dry mouth, restlessness, delayed gastric emptying and decreased gastrointestinal motility, and urinary retention. The use of solutions with concentrations of 1% or greater have caused systemic toxicity in infants.

PHARMACOLOGY: Ophthalmic cyclopentolate is an anticholinergic drug that produces pupillary dilation by inhibiting the sphincter pupillae muscle, and paralysis of accommodation. Maximal mydriasis occurs 30 to 60 minutes following administration. Recov-

DEXAMETHASONE

ery of accommodation occurs in 6 to 24 hours. Without lacrimal sac occlusion, approximately 80% of each drop may pass through the nasolacrimal system and be available for rapid systemic absorption by the nasal mucosa.

SPECIAL CONSIDERATIONS/PREPARATION: Supplied as ophthalmic solution in 0.5%, 1% and 2% concentrations in 2- to 15-mL bottles. Store away from heat. **Do not refrigerate.** A preparation containing cyclopentolate 0.2% and phenylephrine 1% (Cyclomydril®) is commercially available in 2- and 8-mL Drop-tainers. A combination eye drop solution ("Caputo drops") may be prepared in a 15-mL bottle with 3.75 mL of cyclopentolate 2%, 7.5 mL of tropicamide 1%, and 3.75 mL of phenylephrine 10%. The final solution contains cyclopentolate 0.5%, tropicamide 0.5%, and phenylephrine 2.5%.

SELECTED REFERENCES

- Bonthala S, Sparks JW, Musgrove KH, Berseth CL: Mydriatics slow gastric emptying in preterm infants. *J Pediatr* 2000;137:327-30.
- Wallace DK, Steinkuller PG: Ocular medications in children. *Clin Pediatr* 1998;37:645.
- Laws DE, Morton C, Weindling M, Clark D: Systemic effects of screening for retinopathy of prematurity. *Br J Ophthalmol* 1996;80:425-428.
- McGregor MLK: Anticholinergic agents, in Mauger TF, Craig EL (eds): *Havener's Ocular Pharmacology*, ed 6. St. Louis: Mosby-YearBook, 1994, pp 148-155.
- Caputo AR, Schnitzer RE, Lindquist TD, Sun S: Dilation in neonates: a protocol. *Pediatrics* 1982;69:77-80.
- Isenberg S, Everett S: Cardiovascular effects of mydriatics in low-birth-weight infants. *J Pediatr* 1984;105:111-112.

DEXAMETHASONE

DOSE & ADMINISTRATION: Physiologic replacement dose: 0.022 to 0.045 mg/kg per day, IV push or PO. **Stress dose:** 0.07 to 0.15 mg/kg per day. The February 2002 AAP and CPS statement strongly discourages routine use of dexamethasone. If dexamethasone is used for CLD risk reduction, 1) Treat only those infants at highest risk; 2) Use lower than traditional pharmacologic doses; 3) Begin treatment after Day 7 but before Day 14 of life; 4) Do not give concurrently with indomethacin; 5) Use preservative-free drug wherever possible.

USES: Anti-inflammatory glucocorticoid used to facilitate extubation and improve lung function in infants at high risk for developing chronic lung disease.

MONITORING: Assess for hyperglycemia and hyperlipidemia. Monitor blood pressure. Guaiac gastric aspirates. Echocardiogram if treating longer than 7 days.

ADVERSE EFFECTS/PRECAUTIONS: Data regarding neurodevelopmental outcome are increasingly worrisome, with 3 studies and a meta-analysis reporting an increased risk of cerebral palsy. Most evidence suggests no increase in the incidence of ROP or the need for cryotherapy. Gastrointestinal perforation and GI hemorrhage occur more frequently in patients treated beginning on Day 1 and in those also being treated concurrently with indomethacin. Hyperglycemia and glycosuria occur frequently after the first few doses, and one case of diabetic ketoacidosis has been reported. Blood pressure increases are common, and hypertension occurs occasionally. Cardiac effects noted by Day 14 of therapy include increased left ventricular wall thickness with outflow tract obstruction and transient impairment of left ventricular filling, systolic anterior motion of the mitral valve, and ST-segment depression. Other potential short-term adverse effects include sodium and water retention, hypokalemia, hypocalcemia, hypertriglyceridemia, increased risk of sepsis, renal stones (in patients receiving furosemide), osteopenia, and inhibition of growth. Adrenal insufficiency may occur secondary to pituitary suppression.

PHARMACOLOGY: Dexamethasone stabilizes lysosomal and cell membranes, inhibits complement-induced granulocyte aggregation, improves integrity of alveolar-capillary barrier, inhibits prostaglandin and leukotriene production, rightward shifts oxygen-hemoglobin dissociation curve, increases surfactant production, decreases pulmonary edema, relaxes bronchospasm. Hyperglycemia is caused by inhibition of glucose uptake into cells and decreased glucokinase activity. Increased triglyceride synthesis is due to hyperinsulinemia and increased acetyl-CoA carboxylase activity. Blood pressure is increased due to increased responsiveness to endogenous catecholamines. Increases protein catabolism with potential loss of muscle tissue, increases urinary calcium excretion because of bone resorption, and suppresses pituitary ACTH secretion. Biologic half-life is 36 to 54 hours.

SPECIAL CONSIDERATIONS/PREPARATION: Dexamethasone phosphate for injection has been available in limited supply, especially preservative-free preparations. Sulfite preservative concentrations are approximately 1 mg/mL and are potentially toxic. A 0.2 mg/mL dilution may be made by adding 1 mL of the 4 mg/mL concentration to 19 mL preservative-free sterile water for injection. Dilution is stable for 4 days refrigerated and may be used for PO administration.

Solution Compatibility: D_5W, $D_{10}W$, and NS.

Terminal Injection Site Compatibility: Dex/AA solutions, fat emulsion. Acyclovir, amikacin, aminophylline, aztreonam, caffeine citrate, cefepime, cimetidine, famotidine, fentanyl, fluconazole, furosemide, heparin, hydrocortisone succinate, lidocaine, linezolid, lorazepam, meropenem, metoclopramide, milrinone, morphine, nafcillin, netilmicin, piperacillin-tazobactam, potassium chloride, propofol, prostaglandin E_1, ranitidine, remifentanil, sodium bicarbonate, and zidovudine.

Incompatibility: Ciprofloxacin, glycopyrrolate, midazolam and vancomycin.

SELECTED REFERENCES

REVIEWS

- American Academy of Pediatrics, Canadian Paediatric Society: Postnatal corticosteroids to treat or prevent chronic lung disease in preterm infants. *Pediatrics* 2002;109:330.
- Kennedy KA: Controversies in the use of postnatal steroids. *Semin Perinatol* 2001;25:397-405.
- Halliday HL, Ehrenkranz RA, Doyle LW: Moderately early (7-14 days) postnatal corticosteroids for preventing chronic lung disease in preterm infants. (Cochrane Review). In: *The Cochrane Library*, Issue 1, 2003. Oxford: Update Software.
- Arias-Camison JM, Lau J, Cole CH, Frantz ID: Meta-analysis of dexamethasone therapy started in the first 15 days of life for prevention of chronic lung disease in premature infants. *Pediatr Pulmonol* 1999;28:167-174.

ADVERSE EFFECTS

- Stark AR, Carlo W, Tyson JE, et al: Adverse effects of early dexamethasone treatment extremely low birth weight infants. *N Engl J Med* 2001;344:95-101.
- Stoll BJ, Temprosa MS, Tyson JE, et al: Dexamethasone therapy increases infection in very low birth weight infants. *Pediatrics* 1999;104(5). URL:http://www.pediatrics.org/cgi/content/full/104(5)/e63.
- Amin SB Sinkin RA, McDermott MP, Kendig JW: Lipid intolerance in neonates receiving dexamethasone for bronchopulmonary dysplasia. *Arch Pediatr Adolesc Med* 1999;153:795-800.
- Bensky AS, Kothadia JM, Covitz, W: Cardiac effects of dexamethasone In very low birth weight infants. *Pediatrics* 1996;97:818.
- Wright K, Wright SP: Lack of association of glucocorticoid therapy and retinopathy of prematurity. *Arch Pediatr Adolesc Med* 1994;148:848.
- Ng PC: The effectiveness and side effects of dexamethasone in preterm infants with bronchopulmonary dysplasia. *Arch Dis Child* 1993;68:330.

DEVELOPMENTAL FOLLOWUP

- O'Shea TM, Kothadia JM, Klinepeter KL, et al: Randomized placebo-controlled trial of a 42-day tapering course of dexamethasone to reduce the duration of ventilator dependency in very low birth weight infants: Outcome of study participants at 1 year adjusted age. *Pediatrics* 1999;104:15-21.
- Shinwell ES, Karplus M, Reich D, et al: Early postnatal dexamethasone therapy and increased incidence of cerebral palsy. *Arch Dis Child Fetal Neonatal Ed* 2000; 83:F177-181.
- Yeh TF, Lin YJ, Huang CC et al.Earlypostnatal(<12 hrs) dexamethasone therapy for prevention of BPD in preterm infants with RDS: a two-year follow-up study. *Pediatrics* 1998; 101(5). URL: http://www.pediatrics.org/cgi/content/full/101/5/e7.

DIAZOXIDE

DOSE & ADMINISTRATION: 2 to 5 mg/kg per dose PO given Q8 hours. Begin therapy at the higher dosage and taper by response.

USES: Treatment of persistent (more than a few days) or severe hypoglycemia due to hyperinsulinism. Positive responses are usually seen within 48 to 72 hours, and occur in less than 50% of neonates.

MONITORING: Periodic CBC and serum uric acid concentrations if treating long term.

ADVERSE EFFECTS/PRECAUTIONS: Sodium and fluid retention is common—consider concurrent treatment with chlorothiazide (which may also potentiate the hyperglycemic action of diazoxide). Hyperuricemia, leukopenia, and neutropenia are rare complications. Excessive hair growth and coarse facial features develop with long term use. Ketoacidosis may occur during times of intercurrent illness.

PHARMACOLOGY: Diazoxide inhibits insulin release by acting as a specific ATP-sensitive potassium channel agonist in normal pancreatic beta cells. It also reduces insulin release and counters the peripheral actions of insulin via catecholamine stimulation. The serum half-life is 10 to 24 hours in infants. Diazoxide is more than 90% protein-bound in adults, and is excreted entirely by the kidneys.

SPECIAL CONSIDERATIONS/PREPARATION: Proglycem® is available as an oral suspension, 50 mg/mL concentration. Alcohol content is 7.25%. Shake well before use. Protect from light. Store at 2 to 36 °C (36 to 80 °F).

SELECTED REFERENCES
- Hoe FM, Thornton PS, Wanner LA, et al. Clinical features and insulin regulation in infants with a syndrome of prolonged neonatal hyperinsulinism. *J Pediatr* 2006;148:207-212.
- Schwitzgebel VM, Gitelman SE: Neonatal hyperinsulinism. *Clin Perinatol* 1998;25:1015-1038.
- Kane C, Lindley KJ, Johnson PRV, et al: Therapy for persistent hyperinsulinemic hypoglycemia of infancy: understanding the responsiveness of beta cells to diazoxide and somatostatin. *J Clin Investig* 1997;100:1888-1893.
- Stanley CA: Hyperinsulinism in infants and children. *Pediatr Clin North Am* 1997;44:363-374.

DIGOXIN

DOSE & ADMINISTRATION: Loading doses ("Digitalization") is generally used only when treating arrhythmias and acute congestive heart failure. Give over 24 hours as 3 divided doses. Administer IV slow push over 5 to 10 minutes. Oral doses should be 25% greater than IV doses. Do not administer IM.

TOTAL LOADING DOSE

PMA weeks	IV mcg/kg	PO mcg/kg
≤29	15	20
30 to 36	20	25
37 to 48	30	40
≥49	40	50
Divide into 3 doses over 24 hours		

MAINTENANCE DOSES

PMA weeks	IV mcg/kg	PO mcg/kg	Interval hours
≤29	4	5	24
30 to 36	5	6	24
37 to 48	4	5	12
≥49	5	6	12
Titrate based on clinical response			

Note: These beginning doses are based primarily on studies that measured echocardiographic changes and EKG signs of toxicity and take into account renal maturation. We recommend titrating dosage based on clinical response. Decrease dose proportional to the reduction in creatinine clearance.

USES: Treatment of heart failure caused by diminished myocardial contractility. Treatment of SVT, atrial flutter, and atrial fibrillation.

MONITORING: Follow heart rate and rhythm closely. Periodic EKGs to assess both desired effects and signs of toxicity. Follow closely (especially in patients receiving diuretics or amphotericin B) for decreased serum potassium and magnesium, or increased calcium and magnesium, all of which predispose to digoxin toxicity. Assess renal function. Be aware of drug interactions. May follow serum drug concentrations if assay is available that excludes endogenous digoxin-like substances. Therapeutic serum concentration is 1 to 2 ng/mL.

ADVERSE EFFECTS/PRECAUTIONS:

Toxic Cardiac Effects:
- PR interval prolongation
- Sinus bradycardia or SA block
- Atrial or nodal ectopic beats
- Ventricular arrhythmias

Nontoxic Cardiac Effects:
- QTc interval shortening
- ST segment sagging
- T-wave amplitude dampening
- Heart rate slowing

Other Effects: Feeding intolerance, vomiting, diarrhea, and lethargy.

Treatment of Life-Threatening Digoxin Toxicity: Digibind® Digoxin Immune Fab, IV over 30 minutes through 0.22 micron filter.

$$\text{Dose (\# of vials)} = \frac{\text{(weight (kg)} \times \text{(serum digoxin concentration)}}{100}$$

Each vial of digibind contains 38 mg (enough to bind 0.5 mg Digoxin).

PHARMACOLOGY: Digitalis glycoside with positive inotropic and negative chronotropic actions. Increases myocardial catecholamine levels (low doses) and inhibits sarcolemmal sodium-potassium-ATPase (higher doses) to enhance contractility by increasing systolic intracellular calcium-ion concentrations. Indirectly increases vagal activity, thereby slowing S-A node firing and A-V node conduction. Other effects include peripheral, splanchnic, and perhaps, pulmonary vasoconstriction, and reduced CSF production. Serum concentration peaks 30 to 90 minutes after an oral dose, with myocardial peak occurring in 4 to 6 hours. Large volume of distribution that increases with age during infancy. Rapid absorption of oral dose from small intestine; reduced by antacids and rapid transit times. 20% protein bound. Probably not significantly metabolized. Glomerular filtration and tubular secretion account for most of the total body clearance of digoxin, although significant nonrenal elimination has been proposed.

SPECIAL CONSIDERATIONS/PREPARATION: Pediatric dosage forms: Injectable (100 mcg/mL) and elixir (50 mcg/mL). Store at room temperature and protect from light. Dilute injectable as follows: 1) Draw up digoxin into syringe. 2) Inject desired amount of drug into second syringe containing a fourfold or greater volume of solution-compatible diluent. Use diluted product immediately.

Drug Interactions: Amiodarone, indomethacin, spironolactone, quinidine, and verapamil decrease digoxin clearance. Cisapride and metoclopramide decrease digoxin absorption. Spironolactone interferes with radioimmunoassay. Erythromycin may increase digoxin absorption.

Solution Compatibility: (only when diluted fourfold or greater): D_5W, $D_{10}W$, NS, and sterile water for injection.

Terminal Injection Site Compatibility: Dex/AA solutions, fat emulsion. Cimetidine, ciprofloxacin, famotidine, furosemide, heparin, hydrocortisone succinate, insulin, lidocaine, linezolid, meropenem, midazolam, milrinone, morphine, potassium chloride, propofol, prostaglandin E_1, ranitidine, and remifentanil.

Incompatibility: Amiodarone, dobutamine and fluconazole.

SELECTED REFERENCES

- Product Information, GlaxoSmithKline, 2002.
- Smith TW: Digitalis: Mechanisms of action and clinical use. *N Engl J Med* 1988;318:358.
- Roberts RJ: *Drug Therapy in Infants*. Philadelphia: WB Saunders Co, 1984, p 138.
- Johnson GL, Desai NS, Pauly TH, Cunningham MD: Complications associated with digoxin in low-birth-weight infants. *Pediatrics* 1982;69:463.
- Nyberg L, Wettrell G: Pharmacokinetics and dosage of digoxin in neonates and infants. *Eur J Clin Pharmacol* 1980;18:69.
- Pinsky WW, Jacobsen JR, Gillette PC, et al: Dosage of digoxin in premature infants. *J Pediatr* 1979;96:639.

DOBUTAMINE

DOSE & ADMINISTRATION: 2 to 25 mcg/kg per minute continuous IV infusion. Begin at a low dose and titrate by monitoring effects. Use a large vein for IV.

USES: Treatment of hypoperfusion and hypotension, especially if related to myocardial dysfunction.

MONITORING: Continuous heart rate and intra-arterial blood pressure monitoring preferable. Observe IV site for signs of extravasation.

ADVERSE EFFECTS/PRECAUTIONS: May cause hypotension if patient is hypovolemic. Volume loading is recommended bmarily β_1-adrenergic activity. Inotropic vasopressor. Increases myocardial contractility, cardiac index, oxygen delivery, and oxygen consumption. Decreases systemic and pulmonary vascular resistance (adults). Dobutamine has a more prominent effect on cardiac output than dopamine but less of an effect on blood pressure. Onset of action is 1 to 2 minutes after IV administration, with peak effect in 10 minutes. Must be administered by continuous IV infusion because of rapid metabolism of drug. Serum half-life is several minutes. Metabolized in the liver by sulfoconjugation to an inactive compound. There is wide interpatient variability in plasma clearance due to differences in metabolism and renal excretion.

DOBUTAMINE

SPECIAL CONSIDERATIONS/PREPARATION: Supplied as 250 mg per 20 mL vial (12.5 mg/mL). Reconstituted solution stable for 6 hours at room temperature and 48 hours refrigerated. Diluted solutions for infusion are stable for 24 hours. Slight discoloration does not indicate loss of potency.

Solution Compatibility: D_5W, D_5NS, D10W, LR, and NS.

Terminal Injection Site Compatibility: Dex/AA solutions. Atropine, amiodarone, aztreonam, cafeine citrate, calcium chloride, calcium gluconate, ciprofloxacin, dopamine, enclaprilat, epinephrine, famotidine, fentanyl, fluconazole, flumazenil, heparin, hydralazine, insulin, isoproterenol, lidocaine, linezolid, lorazepam, magnesium sulfate, meropenem, midazolam, milrinone, morphine, nicardipine, nitroglycerin, nitroprusside, pancuronium bromide, phentolamine, potassium chloride, procainamide, propofol, propranolol, phytonadione, ranitidine, remifentanil, vecuronium, and zidovudine.

Incompatibility: Acyclovir, alteplase, aminophylline, cefepime, bumetanide, diazepam, digoxin, furosemide, indomethacin, phenytoin, piperacillin-tazobactam, and sodium bicarbcnate.

DOBUTAMINE TITRATION CHART

Concentration (mcg/mL)	Dose (mcg/kg/min)	IV Rate (mL/kg/hour)
500	2.5 5 7.5 10	0.3 0.6 0.9 1.2
800	2.5 5 7.5 10	0.19 0.38 0.56 0.75
1000	2.5 5 7.5 10	0.15 0.3 0.45 0.6
1600	2.5 5 7.5 10	0.094 0.19 0.28 0.38
2000	2.5 5 7.5 10	0.075 0.15 0.23 0.3
3200	2.5 5 7.5 10	0.047 0.094 0.14 0.19
4000	2.5 5 7.5 10	0.038 0.075 0.11 0.15

Solution Preparation Calculations

To calculate the **AMOUNT** of drug needed per defined final fluid volume:
desired final concentration (mg/mL) x defined final fluid volume (mL) = amount of drug to add to final infusion solution (mg)

To calculate the **VOLUME** of drug needed per defined final fluid volume:

$$\frac{\text{*AMOUNT of drug to add (mg)}}{\text{drug (vial) concentration (mg/mL)}} = \text{VOLUME of drug to add (mL)}$$

Example (for Dobutamine:): Mix 30 mL of 800 mcg/mL solution using dobutamine concentration of 12.5 mg.mL.
800 mcg/mL = 0.8 mg/mL
0.8 mg/mL x 30 mL = 24 mg of dobutamine

$$\frac{*24 \text{ mg}}{12.5 \text{ mg/mL}} = 1.9 \text{ mL of dobutamine}$$

Add 1.9 mL of dobutamine (12.5 mg/mL) to 28.1 mL of compatible solution (eg, D$_5$W) to yield 30 mL of infusion solution with a concentration of 800 mcg/mL.

SELECTED REFERENCES

- Noori S, Friedlich P, Seri I: The use of dobutamine in the treatment of neonatal cardiovascular compromise. *NeoReviews* 2004;5:e22-e26.
- Berg RA, Donnerstein RL, Padbury JF: Dobutamine infusion in stable, critically ill children: pharmacokinetics and hemodynamic actions. *Crit Care Med* 1993;21:678-86.
- Martinez AM, Padbury JF, Thio S: Dobutamine pharmacokinetics and cardiovascular responses in critically ill neonates. *Pediatrics* 1992;89:47.
- Leier CV, Unverferth DV: Dobutamine. *Ann Intern Med* 1983;99:490.
- Perkin RM, Levin DL, Webb R, et al: Dobutamine: A hemodynamic evaluation in children with shock. *J Pediatr* 1982;100:977.

DOPAMINE

DOSE & ADMINISTRATION: 2 to 20 mcg/kg per minute continuous IV infusion. Begin at a low dose and titrate by monitoring effects. Use a large vein for IV.

USES: Treatment of hypotension.

MONITORING: Continuous heart rate and intra-arterial blood pressure monitoring is preferable. Assess urine output and peripheral perfusion frequently. Observe IV site closely for blanching and infiltration.

ADVERSE EFFECTS/PRECAUTIONS: Tachycardia and arrhythmias. May increase pulmonary artery pressure. Reversible suppression of prolactin and thyrotropin secretion. Tissue sloughing may occur with IV infiltration. **Suggested treatment:** Inject a 1 mg/mL solution of phentolamine into the affected area. The usual amount needed is 1 to 5 mL, depending on the size of the infiltrate.

PHARMACOLOGY: Catecholamine. Metabolized rapidly. Serum half-life is 2 to 5 minutes, but clearance is quite variable. Dopamine increases blood pressure primarily by increasing systemic vascular resistance via α-adrenergic effects. Effects on cardiac output vary with gestational age and baseline stroke volume. Selective renal vasodilation associated with increases in urine output has been noted in preterm neonates at doses of 2.5 to 7.5 mcg/kg/minute. No changes in mesenteric or cerebral blood flow were observed. Mechanism of action in neonates is controversial. Relative effects of dopamine at different doses are uncertain because of developmental differences in 1) endogenous norepinephrine stores, 2) α-adrenergic, β-adrenergic, and dopaminergic receptor functions, and 3) the ability of the neonatal heart to increase stroke volume. Responses tend to be individualized. Use higher doses with caution in patients with persistent pulmonary hypertension of the newborn.

SPECIAL CONSIDERATIONS/PREPARATION: Available in 40-mg/mL, 80-mg/mL, and 160-mg/mL vials for injection and premixed bags in concentrations of 800-, 1600-, and 3200-mcg/mL. Refrigerate open vial and use within 24 hours. **Admixtures exhibiting a color change should not be used.**

Solution Compatibility: D$_5$W, D5NS, D10W, LR, and NS.

Terminal Injection Site Compatibility: Dex/AA solutions. Aminophylline, ampicillin, amiodarone, aztreonam, caffeine citrate, calcium chloride, chloramphenicol, dobutamine, enalaprilat, epinephrine, esmolol, famotidine, fentanyl, flumazenil, fluconazole, gentamicin, heparin, hydrocortisone succinate, lidocaine, lorazepam, linezolid, meropenem, metronidazole, midazolam, milrinone, morphine, nicardipine, nitroglycerin, nitroprusside, oxacillin, pancuronium bromide, penicillin G, piperacillin-tazobactam, potassium chloride, propofol, prostaglandin E$_1$, ranitidine, tobramycin, vecuronium, and zidovudine.

Incompatibility: Fat emulsion. Acyclovir, alteplase, amphotericin B, cefepime, furosemide, indomethacin, insulin, and sodium bicarbonate.

DOPAMINE

DOPAMINE TITRATION CHART

Concentration (mcg/mL)	Dose (mcg/kg/min)	IV Rate (mL/kg/hour)
500	2.5 5 7.5 10	0.3 0.6 0.9 1.2
800	2.5 5 7.5 10	0.19 0.38 0.56 0.75
1000	2.5 5 7.5 10	0.15 0.3 0.45 0.6
1600	2.5 5 7.5 10	0.094 0.19 0.28 0.38
2000	2.5 5 7.5 10	0.075 0.15 0.23 0.3
3200	2.5 5 7.5 10	0.047 0.094 0.14 0.19

SOLUTION PREPARATION CALCULATIONS:

To calculate the **AMOUNT** of drug needed per defined fluid volume:
desired final concentration (mg/mL) x defined final fluid volume (mL) = amount of drug to add to final infusion solution (mg)

To calculate the **VOLUME** of drug needed per defined final fluid volume:

$$\frac{\text{*AMOUNT of drug to add (mg)}}{\text{drug (vial) concentration (mg/mL)}} = \text{VOLUME of drug to add (mL)}$$

Example (for Dopamine): Mix 30 mL of 800 mcg/mL solution using dopamine concentration of 40 mg/mL:

800 mcg/mL = 0.8 mg/mL
0.8 mg/mL x 30 mL = 24 mg of dopamine

$$\frac{\text{*24 mg}}{\text{40 mg/mL}} = 0.6 \text{ mL of dopamine}$$

Add 0.6 mL dopamine (40 mg/mL) to 29.4 mL of compatible solution (eg, D_5W) to yield 30 mL of infusion solution with a concentration of 800 mcg/mL.

SELECTED REFERENCES

- Valverde E, Pellicer A, Madero R, et al: Dopamine versus epinephrine for cardiovascular support in low birth weight infants: analysis of systemic effects and neonatal clinical outcomes. *Pediatrics* 2006;117:e1213-e1222.
- Seri I, Abbasi S, Wood DC, Gerdes JS: Regional hemodynamic effects of dopamine in the sick preterm neonate. *J Pediatr* 1998;133:728-734.
- Seri I: Cardiovascular, renal, and endocrine actions of dopamine in neonates and children. *J Pediatr* 1995;126:333.
- Filippi L, Pezzati M, Cecchi A, et al: Dopamine infusion and anterior pituitary gland function in very low birth weight infants. *Biol Neonate* 2006;89:274-280.
- Van den Berghe G, de Zegher F, Lauwers P: Dopamine suppresses pituitary function in infants and children. *Crit Care Med* 1994;22:1747.
- Roze JC, Tohier C, Maingueneau C, et al : Response to dobutamine and dopamine in the hypotensive very preterm infant. *Arch Dis Child* 1993;69:59-63.

DT Vaccine

(Diphtheria and Tetanus Toxoids for Pediatric Use)

DOSE & ADMINISTRATION: 0.5 mL IM in the anterolateral thigh. Immunize premature infants according to their postnatal age. Please refer to most recent AAP/ACIP immunization schedule. **When giving multiple vaccines, use a separate syringe for each and give at different sites.** Care should be taken to draw back on the plunger of the syringe before injection to be certain the needle is not in a blood vessel.

USES: Immunoprophylaxis against diphtheria and tetanus for infants who have a contraindication for pertussis vaccine.

MONITORING: Observe injection site for erythema, induration (common), palpable nodule (uncommon), or sterile abscess (rare). Fever (common) may be treated with acetaminophen. Other common, self-limited, systemic effects are drowsiness, frettulness, and anorexia. Rare anaphylactic reactions (i.e. hives, swelling of the mouth, hypotension, breathing difficulty, and shock) have been reported.

ADVERSE EFFECTS/PRECAUTIONS: Infants with stable neurologic conditions, including well-controlled seizures, may be vaccinated. Infants who have had prior seizures are at increased risk for seizures following DT vaccination; acetaminophen should be used to prevent postvaccination fever.

PHARMACOLOGY: Diphtheria and tetanus toxoids are prepared by formaldehyde treatment of the respective toxins. DT vaccine is an aluminum-salt-adsorbed preparation.

SPECIAL CONSIDERATIONS/PREPARATION: DT vaccine (for pediatric use) is available from several manufacturers in 0.5-mL Tubex® and 5-mL vials. Store refrigerated. Do not freeze. Shake vial well before withdrawing each dose. Do not use if product contains clumps that cannot be resuspended with vigorous shaking. Normal appearance is a turbid whitish suspension.

SELECTED REFERENCES

- American Academy of Pediatrics. Tetanus. In: Pickering LK, ed. *2006 Red Book: Report of the Committee on Infectious Diseases.* 27th ed. Elk Grove Village, IL: American Academy of Pediatrics; 2006: pp 67-71.
- Advisory Committee on Immunization Practices: Recommendations of the ACIP. Most recent updates available on the National Immunization Program website: http://www.cdc.gov/nip/publications/acip-list.htm.

DTaP Vaccine

(Diptheria and Tetanus Toxoids and Acellular Pertussis Vaccine Adsorbed)

DOSE & ADMINISTRATION: 0.5 mL IM in the anterolateral thigh. Shake vial vigorously before withdrawing each dose. Immunize premature infants according to their postnatal age. Please refer to the most recent AAP/ACIP immunization schedule. **When giving multiple vaccines, use a separate syringe for each and give at different sites.** Care should be taken to draw back on the plunger of the syringe before injection to be certain the needle is not in a blood vessel.

USES: Preferred immunoprophylaxis against diphtheria, tetanus, and pertussis.

MONITORING: Minor reactions, such as drowsiness, irritability, fever, anorexia, and pain/erythema/induration at the injection site are similar to those observed with DTwP vaccine, but are significantly less frequent. Moderate to severe reactions are also less frequent. Refer to Precautions section for more information.

ADVERSE EFFECTS/PRECAUTIONS: It is prudent to delay the initial dose of DTaP vaccine in infants with neurologic disorders until further observation and study have clarified their neurologic status and the effect of treatment. Those infants with stable neurologic conditions, including well-controlled seizures, may be vaccinated. Infants who have had prior seizures are at increased risk for seizures following DTP vaccination; acetaminophen should be used to prevent postvaccination fever. **Precautions to further DTaP vaccination** (the benefits of administering DTaP may exceed risks in areas with a high incidence of pertussis; otherwise administer DT vaccine): 1) Temperature of ≥ 40.5 °C

DTaP-HepB-IPV Combination Vaccine

(105 °F) within 48 hours with no other cause. (Frequency approximately 1 per 3000 doses) 2) Hypotonic-hyporesponsive collapse or shock-like state within 48 hours. (Frequency approximately 1 per 10,000 doses) 3) Inconsolable crying (≥ 3 hours) occurring within 48 hours. (Frequency approximately 1 per 2000 doses) 4) Convulsions with or without fever occurring within 3 days. (Frequency approximately 1 per 14,000 doses)

Contraindications to further DTaP vaccination: In children who develop encephalopathy within 7 days following any DTP vaccination, DT vaccine should be substituted for the remaining doses. In children who develop an immediate anaphylactic reaction, further immunization with any of the three antigens should be deferred.

PHARMACOLOGY: DTaP vaccines are aluminum-salt-adsorbed preparations. All acellular pertussis vaccines contain inactivated pertussis toxoid, but vary in the inclusion and concentration of four other pertussis antigens. Diphtheria and tetanus toxoids are prepared by formaldehyde treatment of the respective toxins. Daptacel™, Infanrix® and Tripedia® are thimerosal-free. Each dose of Daptacel™ contains 15 Lf diphtheria toxoid, 5 Lf tetanus toxoid, 5 mcg fimbriae types 2 and 3, 5 mcg FHA, and 3 mcg pertactin, with 3.3 mg 2-phenoxyetntains 25 Lf diphtheria toxoid, 10 Lf tetanus toxoid, 25 mcg inactivated toxin, 25 mcg FHA, and 8 mcg pertactin, with 2.5 mg 2-phenoxyethanol as a preservative. Each dose of Tripedia® contains 6.7 Lf diphtheria toxoid, 5 Lf tetanus toxoid, 23.4 mcg inactivated toxin, and 23.4 mcg FHA.

SPECIAL CONSIDERATIONS/PREPARATION: FDA-licensed DTaP vaccines as of March 2003: Infanrix® (GlaxoSmithKline Beecham), available in single dose vials, Daptacel™ (Aventis Pasteur), available in single dose vials, and Tripedia® (Aventis Pasteur), available in single dose vials and in a 15-dose (7.5 mL) vial. Store refrigerated at 2 °C to 8 °C (36 °F to 46 °F). **Do not freeze.** SHAKE VIAL WELL before withdrawing dose. Do not use if product contains clumps that cannot be resuspended with vigorous shaking. Normal appearance is a turbid whitish suspension.

SELECTED REFERENCES

- American Academy of Pediatrics. Pertussis. In: Pickering LK, Baker CJ, Long SS, McMillan JA, eds. *Red Book: 2006 Report of the Committee on Infectious Diseases.* 27th ed. Elk Grove Village, IL: American Academy of Pediatrics; 2006: pp 505-513.
- American Academy of Pediatrics, Committee on Infectious Diseases : Acellular pertussis vaccine: recommendations for use as the initial series in infants and children. *Pediatrics* 1997;99:282.
- Advisory Committee on Immunization Practices: Recommendations of the ACIP. Most recent updates available on the National Immunization Program website: http://www.cdc.gov/nip/publications/acip-list.htm
- Product information, GlaxoSmithKline, 2004.
- Product information, Aventis Pasteur, 2004.

DTaP-HepB-IPV Combination Vaccine

(Diphtheria and Tetanus Toxoids and Acellular Pertussis Adsorbed, Hepatitis B (Recombinant) and Inactivated, Polio Virus Vaccine Combined)

DOSE & ADMINISTRATION: 0.5 mL IM in the anterolateral thigh. Shake vial vigorously before withdrawing dose. PEDIARIX™ should not be administered to any infant before the age of 6 weeks. Only monovalent hepatitis B vaccine can be used for the birth dose. Please refer to the most recent AAP/ACIP immunization schedule. It is recommended that premature infants should be immunized according to their postnatal age; however, inadequate seroconversion against hepatitis B may occur in chronically ill premature infants.

USES: Immunoprophylaxis against diphtheria, tetanus, pertussis, hepatitis B, and polio. Using PEDIARIX™ to complete the hepatitis B vaccination series in infants who were born of HBsAg-positive mothers and who received monovalent Hepatitis B vaccine (Recombinant) has not been studied.

MONITORING: Cardiorespiratory monitoring and pulse oximetry are recommended for premature infants who remain hospitalized at the time of vaccination.

ADVERSE EFFECTS/PRECAUTIONS: Fever is more common (~20%) after PEDIARIX™ than with the individual component vaccines administered separately. Other local and systemic adverse events occur at similar rates. Apnea, bradycardia, and desaturation events are common in premature infants for 48 hours after vaccination.

PHARMACOLOGY: Each dose of PEDIARIX™ contains the type and amount of diphtheria and tetanus toxoids and pertussis antigens as INFANRIX®, and hepatitis B virus antigens as Engerix-B®. The poliovirus component of DTaP-HepB-IPV contains the same strains and quantity of inactivated poliovirus Types 1, 2, and 3 as IPV from a different manufacturer (IPOL®, Aventis Pasteur, South Africa). The immunologic responses following 3 doses of DTaP-HepB-IPV were generally similar to those following 3 doses of the individual vaccines administered separately.

SPECIAL CONSIDERATIONS/PREPARATION: PEDIARIX™ is supplied as a turbid white suspension in single dose (0.5 mL) vials, and in disposable prefilled Tip-Lock syringes. Shake well prior to administration. Do not use if resuspension does not occur after vigorous shaking. Store refrigerated at 2° to 8°C (36°F to 46°F). **Do not freeze**. Discard if the vaccine has been frozen.

SELECTED REFERENCES

- Advisory Committee on Immunization Practices: Recommendations of the ACIP. Most recent updates available on the National Immunization Program website: http://www.cdc.gov/nip/publications/acip-list.htm
- Centers for Disease Control and Prevention: FDA licensure of diphtheria and tetanus toxoids and acellular pertussis adsorbed, hepatitis B (recombinant), and poliovirus vaccine combined, (PEDIARIX™) for use in infants. *MMWR* 2003;52(RR-10):202-203.
- Pfister RE, Aeschbach V, Niksic-Stuber V, et al: Safety of DTaP-based combined immunization in very-low-birth-weight premature infants: frequent but mostly benign cardiorespiratory events. *J Pediatr* 2004;145:58-66.
- Product information, GlaxoSmithKline Biologicals, 2003.

EMLA

(Eutectic Mixture of Local Anesthetics)

DOSE & ADMINISTRATION: Apply 1 to 2 gm to distal half of the penis, then wrap with occlusive dressing. Allow dressing to remain intact for 60 to 90 minutes, remove and clean treated area completely prior to circumcision to avoid systemic absorption.

USES: Topical analgesia for circumcision. Not effective for heel lancing.

MONITORING: Blood methemoglobin concentration if concerned about toxicity.

ADVERSE EFFECTS/PRECAUTIONS: Blanching and redness resolve without treatment. When measured, blood levels of methemoglobin in neonates after the application of 1 g of EMLA cream have been well below toxic levels. Two cases of methemoglobinemia in infants occurred after >3 g of EMLA cream was applied; in 1 of these cases, the infant also was receiving sulfamethoxazole. EMLA cream should not be used in neonates who are receiving other drugs known to induce methemoglobinemia: sulfonamides, acetaminophen, nitrates, nitroglycerin, nitroprusside, phenobarbital, and phenytoin.

PHARMACOLOGY: EMLA cream, containing 2.5% lidocaine and 2.5% prilocaine, attenuates the pain response to circumcision when applied 60 to 90 minutes before the procedure. The analgesic effect is limited during the phases associated with extensive tissue trauma such as during lysis of adhesions and tightening of the clamp. Stabilizes the neuronal membranes by inhibiting the ionic fluxes required for conduction and initiation of nerve impulses. There is a theoretic concern about the potential for neonates to develop methemoglobinemia after the application of EMLA cream, because a metabolite of prilocaine can oxidize hemoglobin to methemoglobin. Neonates are deficient in methemoglobin NADH cytochrome b_5 reductase. Lidocaine is metabolized rapidly by the liver to a number of active metabolites and then excreted renally.

SPECIAL CONSIDERATIONS/PREPARATION: Available in 5-gm and 30-gm tubes with Tegaderm dressing and in a 1-gm Anesthetic Disc, boxes of 2 and 10. Each gram of EMLA contains lidocaine 25 mg and prilocaine 25 mg in a eutectic mixture. pH of the product is 9. Contains no preservatives.

SELECTED REFERENCES

- American Academy of Pediatrics, Task Force on Circumcision. Circumcision policy statement. *Pediatrics* 1999;103:686-693.
- Taddio A, Ohlsson A, Einarson TR, et al: A systematic review of lidocaine-prilocaine cream (EMLA) in the treatment of acute pain in neonates. *Pediatrics* 1998;101:1-9.
- Lander J, Brady-Fryer B, Metcalfe JB, et al: Comparison of ringblock, dorsal penile nerve block, and topical anesthesia for neonatal circumcision: A randomized controlled trial. *JAMA* 1997;278:2157-2162.
- Taddio A, Stevens B, Craig K, et al: Efficacy and safety of lidocaine-prilocaine cream for pain during circumcision. *N Engl J Med* 1997;336:1197-1201.
- Product information, AstraZeneca, 2004.

ENALAPRIL MALEATE

DOSE & ADMINISTRATION: Begin with 40 mcg/kg per dose (0.04 mg/kg per dose) given PO Q24 hours. Usual maximum dose 150 mcg/kg per dose (0.15 mg/kg per dose), as frequently as Q6 hours. Titrate subsequent doses and interval based on amount and duration of response. Deed to be increased every few days.

USES: Treatment of moderate to severe hypertension. Afterload reduction in patients with congestive heart failure.

MONITORING: Frequent assessment of blood pressure, particularly after the first dose. Periodic assessment of renal function and serum potassium.

ADVERSE EFFECTS/PRECAUTIONS: Use with extreme caution in patients with impaired renal function: oliguria and increased serum creatinine occur frequently. Hypotension occurs primarily in patients who are volume-depleted. Hyperkalemia occurs primarily in patients receiving potassium-sparing diuretics or potassium supplements. Cough has been reported frequently in adults.

PHARMACOLOGY: Enalapril is a prodrug that is hydrolyzed in the liver to form the active angiotensin-converting enzyme (ACE) inhibitor enalaprilat, which blocks the conversion of angiotensin I to angiotensin II, a potent vasoconstrictor. It thereby decreases plasma and tissue concentrations of angiotensin II and aldosterone, and increases plasma and tissue renin activity. Enalaprilat also prevents the breakdown of bradykinin, a potent vasodilator. Vascular resistance is reduced without reflex tachycardia. Beneficial effects are thought to be caused by a combination of afterload reduction and long-term inhibition of salt and water retention. Bioavailability of oral dosage form is uncertain in neonates, but is significantly less than the 60% reported in adults. Onset of action after oral dose is 1 to 2 hours. Duration of action is quite variable in neonates, ranging from 8 to 24 hours.

SPECIAL CONSIDERATIONS/PREPARATION: Supplied in 2.5-mg, 5-mg, 10-mg, and 20-mg tablets. Enalapril maleate oral suspension can be prepared by crushing a 2.5 mg tablet and adding to 25 mL of isotonic citrate buffer, yielding a final concentration of 100 mcg/mL (0.1 mg/mL). Suspension is stable for 30 days refrigerated.

SELECTED REFERENCES

- Schilder JLAM, Van den Anker JN: Use of enalapril in neonatal hypertension. *Acta Paediatr* 1995;84:1426.
- Nahata MC, Morosco RS, Hipple TF: Stability of enalapril maleate in three extemporaneously prepared oral liquids. *Am J Health Syst Pharm* 1998;55:1155-1157.
- Mason T, Polak MJ, Pyles L, et al: Treatment of neonatal renovascular hypertension with intravenous enalapril. *Am J Perinatol* 1992;9:254.
- Rasoulpour M, Marinelli KA: Systemic hypertension. *Clin Perinatol* 1992;19:121.
- Wells TG, Bunchman TE, Kearns GL: Treatment of neonatal hypertension with enalaprilat. *J Pediatr* 1990;117:665.
- Frenneaux M, Stewart RAH, Newman CMH, Hallidie-Smith KA: Enalapril for severe heart failure in infancy. *Arch Dis Child* 1989;64:219.

ENALAPRILAT

DOSE & ADMINISTRATION: Begin with 10 mcg/kg per dose (0.01 mg/kg per dose) IV over 5 minutes Q24 hours. Titrate subsequent doses and interval based on amount and duration of response. Dosage may need to be increased every few days.

USES: Treatment of moderate to severe hypertension. Afterload reduction in patients with congestive heart failure.

MONITORING: Frequent assessment of blood pressure, particularly after the first dose. Periodic assessment of renal function and serum potassium.

ADVERSE EFFECTS/PRECAUTIONS: Use with extreme caution in patients with impaired renal function: oliguria and increased serum creatinine occur frequently. Hypotension occurs primarily in patients who are volume-depleted. Hyperkalemia occurs primarily in patients receiving potassium-sparing diuretics or potassium supplements. Cough has been reported frequently in adults.

PHARMACOLOGY: Enalaprilat is an ACE inhibitor which blocks the production of the potent vasoconstrictor angiotensin II. It thereby decreases plasma and tissue concentrations of angiotensin II and aldosterone, and increases plasma and tissue renin activity. Enalaprilat also prevents the breakdown of bradykinin, a potent vasodilator.

Vascular resistance is reduced without reflex tachycardia. Beneficial effects are thought to be caused by a combination of afterload reduction and long-term inhibition of salt and water retention. Duration of action is quite variable in neonates, ranging from 8 to 24 hours.

SPECIAL CONSIDERATIONS/PREPARATION: Enalaprilat is supplied as a 1.25 mg/mL solution for injection in 1 mL and 2 mL vials. Benzyl alcohol content is 9 mg/mL. To make a dilution for IV use, take 1 mL (1.25 mg) of solution and add 49 mL NS to make a final concentration of 25 mcg/mL (0.025 mg/mL).

Solution Compatibility: D_5W, D_5NS, and NS.

Terminal Injection Site Compatibility: Fat emulsion. Amikacin, aminophylline, ampicillin, aztreonam, calcium gluconate, cefazolin, ceftazidime, chloramphenicol, cimetidine, clindamycin, dobutamine, dopamine, erythromycin lactobionate, esmolol, famotidine, fentanyl, gentamicin, heparin, hydrocortisone succinate, lidocaine, linezolid, magnesium sulfate, meropenem, metronidazole, morphine, nafcillin, nicardipine, nitroprusside, penicillin G, phenobarbital, piperacillin, piperacillin-tazobactam, potassium chloride, propofol, ranitidine, remifentanil, tobramycin, trimethoprim-sulfamethoxazole, and vancomycin.

Incompatibility: Amphotericin B, cefepime, and phenytoin.

SELECTED REFERENCES
- Schilder JLAM, Van den Anker JN: Use of enalapril in neonatal hypertension. *Acta Paediatr* 1995;84:1426.
- Mason T, Polak MJ, Pyles L, et al: Treatment of neonatal renovascular hypertension with intravenous enalapril. *Am J Perinatol* 1992;9:254.
- Rasoulpour M, Marinelli KA: Systemic hypertension. *Clin Perinatol* 1992;19:121.
- Wells TG, Bunchman TE, Kearns GL: Treatment of neonatal hypertension with enalaprilat. *J Pediatr* 1990;117:665.
- Frenneaux M, Stewart RAH, Newman CMH, Hallidie-Smith KA: Enalapril for severe heart failure in infancy. *Arch Dis Child* 1989;64:219.

ENOXAPARIN

(Low Molecular Weight Heparin)

DOSE & ADMINISTRATION: Initial treatment of thrombosis: 1.5 mg/kg per dose subQ every 12 hours. Adjust dosage to maintain anti-factor X_a level between 0.5 and 1.0 units/mL. It will usually take several days to attain levels in the target range. Preterm infants may require a higher dose to maintain target anti-factor X_a levels: Mean 2 mg/kg every 12 hours, range 0.8 to 3 mg/kg. Infants older than 3 months of age: 1 mg/kg per dose subQ every 12 hours. Call 1-800-NOCLOTS for case reporting and treatment guidance. **Low-risk prophylaxis:** 0.75 mg/kg per dose subQ every 12 hours. Infants older than 3 months of age: 0.5 mg/kg per dose subQ every 12 hours. Adjust dosage to maintain anti-factor X_a level between 0.1 and 0.4 units/mL. Administration may be aided by using a small plastic subcutaneous catheter (Insuflon, Viggo, Lynge, Denmark).

USES: Anticoagulation. Advantages over standard unfractionated heparin: (1) may be given subcutaneously, (2) more predictable pharmacokinetics, (3) dosing every 8 to 12 hours, (4) less frequent bleeding complications.

MONITORING: Measure anti-factor X_a concentrations 4 hours after a dose (See above for desired range). Preterm infants are likely to require several dosage adjustments to achieve the target levels. After attaining target levels, dosage adjustments will be necessary once or twice a month, perhaps more often in preterm infants and infants with hepatic or renal dysfunction. Assess for signs of bleeding and thrombosis.

ADVERSE EFFECTS/PRECAUTIONS: In the prospective cohort study (Streif, et al) 4 of 62 patients developed serious bleeding and 4 of 62 developed minor bleeding.

PHARMACOLOGY: Enoxaparin is a low-molecular weight heparin that has considerably less activity against thrombin than does standard heparin. Efficacy in neonates is decreased due to low antithrombin plasma concentrations. It is also much less likely to interfere with platelet function or cause osteoporosis. It activates antithrombin III, which progressively inactivates both thrombin and factor X_a, key proteolytic enzymes in the formation of fibrinogen and activation of prothrombin. Bioavailability is almost 100% after subcutaneous administration, with peak activity 2.5 to 4 hours later. The apparent half-life of anti-X_a activity is 4 to 5 hours. Clearance in neonates is more rapid than in older infants, children or adults.

EPINEPHRINE

SPECIAL CONSIDERATIONS/PREPARATION: Available as 100 mg/mL concentration preservative-free supplied in prefilled syringes and ampules.

Solution Compatibility: NS and sterile water.

Terminal Injection Site Compatibility: No data are currently available.

SELECTED REFERENCES

- Streif W, Goebel G, Chan AKC, Massicotte MP: Use of low molecular mass heparin (enoxaparin) in newborn infants: a prospective cohort study of 62 newborn infants. *Arch Dis Child Fetal Neonatal Ed* 2003;88:F365-F370.
- Fareed J, Hoppensteadt D, Walenga J, et al: Pharmacodynamic and pharmacokinetic properties of enoxaparin. *Clin Pharmacokinet* 2003;42:1043-57.
- Monagle P, Michelson AD, Bovill E, Andrew M: Antithrombotic therapy in children. *Chest* 2001;119:344-370S.
- Edstrom CS, Christensen RD: Evaluation and treatment of thrombosis in the neonatal intensive care unit. *Clin Perinatol* 2000;27:623-41.
- Dunaway KK, Gal P, Ransom JL: Use of enoxaparin in a preterm infant. *Ann Pharmacother* 2000;34:1410-3.
- Klinger G, Hellmann J, Daneman A: Severe aortic thrombosis in the neonate - successful treatment with low-molecular-weight heparin: Two case reports and review of the literature. *Am J Perinatol* 2000;17:151-8.
- Massicotte P, Adams M, Marzinotto V, et al: Low-molecular-weight heparin in pediatric patients with thrombotic disease: A dose finding study. *J Pediatr* 1996;128:313-8.

EPINEPHRINE

DOSE & ADMINISTRATION: Severe bradycardia and hypotension: 0.1 to 0.3 mL/kg 1:10,000 concentration; equal to 0.01 to 0.03 mg/kg (10 to 30 mcg/kg). IV push, or IC. May be given ET, immediately followed by 1 mL NS. **IV continuous infusion:** Start at 0.1 mcg/kg per minute and adjust to desired response, to a maximum of 1 mcg/kg per minute. If possible, correct acidosis before administration of epinephrine to enhance the effectiveness of the drug.

USES: Acute cardiovascular collapse. Short-term use for cardiac failure resistant to other drug management. In older infants, may be used subcutaneously for relief of bronchospasm.

MONITORING: Monitor heart rate and blood pressure continuously. Observe IV site for signs of infiltration.

ADVERSE EFFECTS/PRECAUTIONS: Cardiac arrhythmias (PVCs and ventricular tachycardia). Renal vascular ischemia. Severe hypertension with intracranial hemorrhage. Increases myocardial oxygen requirements. Therapeutic doses may cause hypokalemia. IV infiltration may cause tissue ischemia and necrosis.

PHARMACOLOGY: Stimulates alpha and beta adrenergic receptors—increases heart rate; increases myocardial contractility, automaticity, and conduction velocity; increases systemic vascular resistance (via constriction of arterioles); increases blood flow to skeletal muscle, brain, liver, and myocardium; decreases renal blood flow by 40%.

SPECIAL CONSIDERATIONS/PREPARATION: Always use as a 1:10,000 concentration (0.1 mg/mL) for individual doses. Use 1:1000 (1 mg/mL) concentration to prepare continuous infusion solution. Protect from light.

Solution Compatibility: D_5W, $D_{10}W$, and NS.

Terminal Injection Site Compatibility: Dex/AA. Amikacin, amiodarone, ampicillin, caffeine citrate, calcium chloride, calcium gluconate, cimetidine, dobutamine, dopamine, famotidine, fentanyl, furosemide, heparin, hydrocortisone succinate, lorazepam, midazolam, milrinone, morphine, nicardipine, nitroglycerin, nitroprusside, pancuronium bromide, potassium chloride, propofol, prostaglandin E_1, ranitidine, remifentanil, vecuronium, and vitamin K_1.

Incompatibility: Aminophylline, hyaluronidase, and sodium bicarbonate.

Administration Calculations

To calculate the **AMOUNT** of drug needed per **50 mL** infusion solution:

$$3 \times \frac{\text{desired dose } (mcg/kg/min)}{\text{desired fluid rate } (mL/hr)} \times \text{weight } (kg) = \text{mg of epinephrine}$$

To calculate the **VOLUME** of drug needed per **50 mL** infusion solution:

$$\frac{\text{mg of drug (found using equation above)}}{\text{concentration of drug } (mg/mL)} = \text{mL of epinephrine}$$

Example: 2-kg infant to receive epinephrine 0.1 mcg/kg per minute at infusion rate of 0.5 mL per hour. Concentration of the 1:1000 epinephrine solution is 1 mg/mL.

$$3 \times \frac{0.1 \text{ mcg/kg/min}}{0.5 \text{ mL/hr}} \times 2 \text{ kg} = 1.2 \text{ mg of epinephrine in 50 mL of infusion solution}$$

$$\frac{1.2 \text{ mg of epinephrine}}{1 \text{ mg/mL}} = 1.2 \text{ mL of epinephrine in 50 mL of infusion solution}$$

Add 1.2 mL epinephrine (1:1000) to 48.8 mL of compatible solution (e.g. D_5W) to yield 50 mL of epinephrine infusion with a concentration of 24 mcg/mL.

Maximum concentration is 64 mcg/mL.

SELECTED REFERENCES

- Kattwinkel J, Niermeyer S, Nadkarni V, et al: ILCOR advisory statement: Resuscitation of the newly born infant. *Pediatrics* 1999;103(4).
- URL: http://www.pediatrics.org/cgi/content/full/103/4/e56.
- Burchfield DJ: Medication use in neonatal resuscitation. *Clin Perinatol* 1999;26:683-691.
- Bloom RS, Cropley C: *Textbook of Neonatal Resuscitation*. American Heart Association, 1994, p 6-9.
- Zaritsky A, Chernow B: Use of catecholamines in pediatrics. *J Pediatr* 1984;105:341.

EPOETIN ALFA

DOSE & ADMINISTRATION: 200 to 400 units/kg/dose, 3 to 5 times per week, for 2 to 6 weeks. Total dose **per week** is 600 to 1400 units per kg. **Short course:** 300 units/kg per dose daily for 10 days. Administer subQ, or IV over at least 4 hours (even continuously in TPN). Supplemental iron therapy should be initiated concurrently.

USES: To stimulate erythropoiesis and decrease the need for erythrocyte transfusions in high-risk preterm infants. Those most likely to benefit are infants with birth weights < 800 g and phlebotomy losses > 30 mL/kg.

MONITORING: Weekly CBC to check for neutropenia and monitor RBC response.

ADVERSE EFFECTS/PRECAUTIONS: The only adverse effect in premature neonates is neutropenia, which occurs rarely and resolves with discontinuation of the drug.

PHARMACOLOGY: Epoetin alfa is a 165-amino acid glycoprotein manufactured by recombinant DNA technology that has the same biological effects as endogenous erythropoietin. It acts on mature erythroid progenitors, CFU-E, by binding to cell surface receptors and stimulating differentiation and cell division. Noticeable effects on hematocrit and reticulocyte counts occur within 2 weeks. Adequate iron and protein intake is necessary for epoetin to be effective (additional Vitamin E intake may be necessary as well). Subcutaneously administered drug appears to be pharmacodynamically as effective as IV, despite only 40% bioavailability. Half-life of r-HuEPO in preterm infants is approximately 12 hours. Doses reported in the literature are all stated as Units/kg **per week**. Efficacy may be dose dependent in the range of 500 to 1500 Units/kg per week (see meta-analysis by Garcia et al), but no differences were observed in the randomized trial (Maier et al).

SPECIAL CONSIDERATIONS/PREPARATION: Available in preservative-free, single-use, 1-mL vials containing 2000, 3000, 4000, or 10,000 Units formulated in an isotonic, sodium chloride/sodium citrate buffered solution with 2.5 mg human albumin. **Do not shake.** Undiluted epoetin is stable in plastic syringes for 2 weeks. For IV infusions, dilute epoetin in 2 mL of solutions containing at least 0.05% protein and infuse over 4 hours- these dilutions are stable for 24 hours. Product support for use in neonates is handled by Ortho Biotech, Inc. (Procrit®). A multidose 2-mL vial is also available from both Ortho Biotech (Procrit®) and Amgen (Epogen®) containing 20,000 Units in a 1% (10 mg/mL) benzyl alcohol solution with 2.5-mg albumin per mL.

ERYTHROMYCIN

SELECTED REFERENCES

- Reiter PD, Rosenberg AA, Valuck R, Novak K: Effect of short-term erythropoietin therapy in anemic premature infants. J Perinatol 2005;25:125-129.
- Ohls R: Human recombinant erythropoietin in the prevention and treatment of anemia of prematurity. Paediatr Drugs 2002;4:111-121.
- Garcia MG, Hutson AD, Christensen RD: Effect of recombinant erythropoietin on "late" transfusions in the neonatal intensive care unit: A meta-analysis. J Perinatol 2002;22:108-111.
- Donato H, Vain N, Rendo P, et al: Effect of early versus late administration of human recombinant human erythropoietin on transfusion requirements in premature infants: Results of a randomized, placebo-controlled, multicenter trial Pediatrics 2000;105:1066.
- Maier RF, Obladen M, Kattner E, et al: High- versus low-dose erythropoietin in extremely low birth weight infants. J Pediatr 1998;132:866-870.
- Ohls RK, Christensen RD: Stability of recombinant human epoetin alfa in commonly used neonatal intravenous solutions. Ann Pharmacother 1996;30:466.
- Shannon KM, Keith JF, Mentzer WC, et al: Recombinant human erythropoietin stimulates erythropoiesis and reduces erythrocyte transfusions in very low birth weight preterm infants. Pediatrics 1995;95:1.
- Ohls RK, Osborne KA, Christensen RD: Efficacy and cost analysis of treating very low birth weight infants with erythropoietin during their first two weeks of life: A randomized placebo controlled trial. J Pediatr 1995;126:421.
- Meyer MP, Meyer JH, Commerford A, et al: Recombinant erythropoietin in the treatment of the anemia of prematurity: Results of a double-blind, placebo-controlled study. Pediatrics 1994;93:918.

ERYTHROMYCIN

DOSE & ADMINISTRATION: Treatment of pneumonitis and conjunctivitis due to *Chlamydia trachomatis*: 12.5 mg/kg per dose PO Q6 hours for 14 days. **Other infections and prophylaxis:** 10 mg/kg per dose PO Q6 hours. Oral treatment with E. ethylsuccinate (e.g., E. E. S.®, EryPed®). Administer with infant formula to enhance absorption of the ethylsuccinate and reduce possible GI side effects. **Severe infections when PO route unavailable:** 5 to 10 mg/kg per dose IV infusion by syringe pump over at least 60 minutes Q6 hours. **Do not administer IM. Prophylaxis of ophthalmia neonatorum:** Ribbon of 0.5% ointment instilled in each conjunctival sac. **Treatment of feeding intolerance due to dysmotility:** 10 mg/kg per dose PO every 6 hours for 2 days, followed by 4 mg/kg per dose PO every 6 hours for 5 days.

USES: Treatment of infections caused by *Chlamydia*, *Mycoplasma*, and *Ureaplasma*. Treatment for and prophylaxis against *Bordetella pertussis*. As a substitute for penicillin in situations of significant allergic intolerance. As a prokinetic agent in cases of feeding intolerance.

MONITORING: Watch for diarrhea and signs of abdominal discomfort. CBC for eosinophilia. **Monitor heart rate and blood pressure closely during IV administration.** Observe IV site for signs of infiltration.

ADVERSE EFFECTS/PRECAUTIONS: The risk of hypertrophic pyloric stenosis is increased 10-fold in neonates under 2 weeks of age who receive oral erythromycin for pertussis prophylaxis (1 additional case per every 42 infants treated). No studies of premature infants with feeding intolerance have been large enough to assess safety. Two reported cases of severe bradycardia and hypotension occurring during IV administration of erythromycin lactobionate. Intrahepatic cholestasis. Loose stools occur infrequently. Bilateral sensorineural hearing loss has been reported rarely in adults, usually associated with intravenous administration and renal or hepatic dysfunction. The hearing loss occurred after the first few doses and was reversible after discontinuing the drug. Venous irritation is common while using the IV dosage form.

PHARMACOLOGY: Erythromycin may be bacteriostatic or bactericidal depending on the tissue concentration of drug and the microorganism involved. IV administration of E. lactobionate to preterm infants, using doses of 6.25 to 10 mg/kg, yielded peak serum concentrations of 1.9 to 3.7 mcg/mL and a half-life of 2 hours. The drug penetrates poorly into the CNS, is concentrated in the liver and bile, and is excreted via the bowel. It is a motilin receptor agonist and induces stomach and small intestine motor activity. Plasma clearance of midazolam is reduced by 50%. Digoxin, midazolam, theophylline and carbamazepine serum concentrations may be significantly increased because of prolongation of their half-life.

SPECIAL CONSIDERATIONS/PREPARATION: E. ethylsuccinate oral suspension is available in concentrations of 200 mg- and 400 mg per 5 mL. Refrigeration not required except to preserve taste. Shake suspension well before administering. Available as powder for injection in 500-mg and 1-g vials. Reconstitute 500-mg vial with 10 mL of sterile water for injection to concentration of 50 mg/mL. After reconstitution, dilute to a concentration of 1 to 5 mg/mL for infusion. To make a 5-mg/mL dilution, add 1 mL of reconstituted solution to 9 mL sterile water for injection. Use diluted drug within 8 hours. Filter before administration to reduce venous irritation. Use only preservative-free IV erythromycin.

Solution Compatibility: NS and sterile water for injection.

Solution Incompatibility: D_5W and $D_{10}W$ (unless buffered with 4% sodium bicarbonate to maintain stability).

Terminal Injection Site Compatibility: Dex/AA solutions, fat emulsion. Acyclovir, aminophylline, amiodarone, chloramphenicol, cimetidine, enalaprilat, esmolol, famotidine, heparin, hydrocortisone succinate, lidocaine, lorazepam, magnesium sulfate, methicillin, midazolam, morphine, nicardipine, penicillin G, pentobarbital, potassium chloride, ranitidine, sodium bicarbonate, and zidovudine.

Incompatibility: Ampicillin, ceftazidime, fluconazole, furosemide, linezolid, and metoclopramide.

SELECTED REFERENCES

- American Academy of Pediatrics. Chlamydia trachomatis. In: Pickering LK, Baker CJ, Long SS, McMillan JA, eds. *Red Book: 2006 Report of the Committee on Infectious Diseases.* 27th ed. Elk Grove Village, IL: American Academy of Pediatrics; 2006: p255.
- Centers for Disease Control and Prevention: Sexually transmitted diseases treatment guidelines 2006. *MMWR* 2006;55(No. RR-11).
- Nuntnarumit P, Kiatchoosakun P, Tantiprapa W, Boonkasidecha S: Efficacy of oral erythromycin for treatment of feeding intolerance in preterm infants. *J Pediatr* 2006;148:600-605.
- Patole S, Rao S, Doherty D: Erythromycin as a prokinetic agent in preterm neonates: a systematic review. *Arch Dis Child Fetal Neonatal Ed* 2005;90:F301-F306.
- Oei J, Lui K: A placebo-controlled trial of low-dose erythromycin to promote feed tolerance in preterm infants. *Acta Paediatr* 2001;90:904-908.
- Pai MP, Graci DM, Amsden GW: Macrolide drug interactions: an update. *Ann Pharmacother* 2000;34:495-513.
- Honein MA, Paulozzi LJ, Himelright IM, et al: Infantile hypertrophic pyloric stenosis after pertussis prophylaxis with erythromycin: a case review and cohort study. *Lancet* 1999;354:2101-2105.
- Waites KB, Sims PJ, Crouse DT, et al: Serum concentrations of erythromycin after intravenous infusion in preterm neonates treated for *Ureaplasma* urealyticum infection. *Pediatr Infect Dis J* 1994;13:287.
- Farrar HC, Walsh-Sukys MC, Kyllonen K, Blumer JL: Cardiac toxicity associated with intravenous erythromycin lactobionate: Two case reports and a review of the literature. *Pediatr Infect Dis J* 1993;12:688.
- Ginsburg CM: Pharmacology of erythromycin in infants and children. *Pediatr Infect Dis* 1986;5:124.
- Eichenwald H: Adverse reactions to erythromycin. *Pediatr Infect Dis* 1986;5:147.

ESMOLOL

DOSE & ADMINISTRATION: Starting IV doses: Supraventricular tachycardia (SVT): 100 mcg/kg per minute continuous infusion. Increase in increments of 50 to 100 mcg/kg per minute every 5 minutes until control of the ventricular rate is achieved. **Acute managment of postoperative hypertension:** 50 mcg/kg per minute continuous infusion. Increase in increments of 25 to 50 mcg/kg per minute every 5 minutes until desired blood pressure is achieved. **Usual maximum dosage:** 200 mcg/kg per minute. Doses greater than 300 mcg/kg per minute are likely to cause hypotension.

USES: Short term treatment of postoperative hypertension, supraventricular tachycardia (SVT), and ventricular tachycardia (VT).

MONITORING: Continuous EKG monitoring during acute treatment of arrhythmias. Measure systemic blood pressure and heart rate frequently.

ADVERSE EFFECTS/PRECAUTIONS: May cause hypotension in high doses. Adverse effects reversable with discontinuation of drug. Monitor IV site closely for vein irrication and phlebitis, especially at high concentrations (> 10 mg/mL).

PHARMACOLOGY: Esmolol is a potent cardio-selective beta-blocking agent with a uniquely short half-life (2.8 to 4.5 minutes) and a brief (10 to 15 minute) duration of action. There appears to be no correlation between age and pharmacodynamic response or pharmacokinetic profile. Esmolol is cleared primarily by red blood cell esterases. Renal or hepatic failure does not effect elimination.

SPECIAL CONSIDERATIONS/PREPARATION: Esmolol is supplied in preservative-free 10 mL (10 mg/mL) and a 5-mL (ready-to-use) vials (20 mg/mL). Maximum infusion concentration should not exceed 10 mg/mL. The pH is approximately 3.5-5.5. Osmolarity is 312 mOsm/L. Store at room temperature.

Exosurf®

Solution Compatibility: D_5W and NS.

Terminal Injection Site Compatibility: Amikacin, aminophylline, atracurium, calcium chloride, cefazolin, ceftazidime, chloramphenicol, cimetidine, clindamycin, digoxin, dopamine, enalaprilat, erythromycin lactobionate, famoditine, fentanyl, gentamicin, heparin, hydrocortisone, insulin, lidocaine, linezolid, magnesium sulfate, metronidazole, midazolam, morphine, nafcillin, nicardipine, nitroglycerin, norepinephrine, pancuronium, penicillin G, phenytoin, piperacillin, potassium chloride, propofol, ranitidine, remifentanil, sodium nitroprusside, tobramycin, trimethoprim-sulfamethoxazole, vancomycin, and vecuronium.

Incompatibility: Amphotericin B, diazepam, furosemide, and procainamide.

SELECTED REFERENCES

- Wiest DB, Garner SS, Uber WE, et al: Esmolol for the management of pediatric hypertension after cardiac operations. *J Thoracic Cardiov Surg* 1998;115:890-897.
- Cuneo B, Zales VR, Blahunka PC, et al: Pharmacodynamics and pharmacokinetics of esmolol, a short-acting β-blocking agent, in children. *Pediatr Cardiol* 1994;15:296-301.
- Trippel MD, Wiest DB, Gillette PC: Cardiovascular and antiarrhythmic effects of esmolol in children. *J Pediatr* 1991;119:142-147.
- Wiest DB, Trippel MD, Gillette PC, et al: Pharmacokinetics of esmolol in children. *Clin Pharmacol Ther* 1991;49:618-623.
- Product information, Baxter, 2006.

Exosurf®

(Synthetic Surfactant)

DOSE & ADMINISTRATION: 5 mL/kg per dose ET. **Prophylaxis** (for neonates less than 29 weeks gestation): The first dose is given as soon as possible after birth. Two additional doses are given at 12 and 24 hours if indicated. **Rescue treatment of RDS:** Two doses 12 hours apart; the first dose given as soon as possible after intubation for respiratory deterioration.

After ET suctioning, administer in two 2.5-mL/kg aliquots using the sideport on the supplied ET tube adapter without interrupting mechanical ventilation. Each half-dose is instilled over 1 to 2 minutes in small bursts timed with inspiration, with the infant's head in the midline position. After each half dose, the head and torso are turned 45° to the side for 30 seconds to improve distribution. After dosing, frequent assessments of oxygenation and ventilation should be performed to prevent postdose hyperoxia and hypocarbia. Suctioning should not be performed for 2 hours following administration, except when dictated by clinical necessity.

ADVERSE EFFECTS/PRECAUTIONS: Reflux of Exosurf® up the ET tube and falls in oxygenation occur frequently. If the infant becomes dusky or agitated, heart rate slows, oxygen saturation falls more than 15%, or Exosurf® backs up in the ET tube, dosing should be slowed or halted. If necessary, ventilator settings and/or FiO_2 should be turned up. Pulmonary hemorrhage occurs in 2% to 4% of treated infants, primarily the smallest patients with untreated PDA possibly the result of hemorrhagic pulmonary edema caused by the rapid fall in pulmonary vascular resistance and resulting increased pulmonary blood flow.

PHARMACOLOGY: Exosurf® is a synthetic, protein-free surfactant, supplied as a sterile lyophilized powder. After reconstitution, each mL of Exosurf® suspension contains 13.5 mg colfosceril palmitate (DPPC, the major lipid component of natural surfactant), 1.5 mg cetyl alcohol (a spreading agent), and 1 mg tyloxapol (a nonionic surfactant that disperses the DPPC and cetyl alcohol).

SPECIAL CONSIDERATIONS/PREPARATION: Reconstitute immediately before administration using only preservative-free sterile water for injection (supplied). 1) Fill a 10-mL or 12-mL syringe with 8 mL of sterile water. 2) Allow vacuum in the Exosurf® vial to draw sterile water into vial. 3) Aspirate as much as possible out of vial back into syringe (while maintaining vacuum), then suddenly release syringe plunger. 4) Step 3 should be repeated 3 or 4 times to assure adequate mixing. 5) Draw appropriate dosage volume into syringe **from below froth** in vial. Each vial yields 7.5 to 8 mL of Exosurf® suspension (enough to treat an infant weighing up to ~1600 g. The suspension appears milky white, has a pH of 5 to 7, and an osmolality of 185 mOsm/L. The reconstituted suspension is stable for 12 hours when stored at 2 °C to 30 °C (36 °F to 86 °F).

FAMOTIDINE

DOSE & ADMINISTRATION: IV: 0.25 to 0.5 mg/kg per dose Q24 hours, IV slow push; Continuous infusion of the daily dose in adults provides better gastric acid suppression than intermittent dosing. **PO:** 0.5 to 1 mg/kg per dose Q24 hours orally.

USES: Prevention and treatment of stress ulcers and GI hemorrhage aggravated by gastric acid secretion.

MONITORING: Gastric pH may be measured to assess efficacy (>4.0).

ADVERSE EFFECTS/PRECAUTIONS: No adverse events have been reported in infants and children, although data are limited to a few small studies. The most common (<5% of patients) adverse effects noted in adults were headache, dizziness, constipation, and diarrhea.

PHARMACOLOGY: Inhibits gastric acid secretion by histamine H_2-receptor antagonism. Elimination half-life is dependent on renal function, and decreases with age from 11 hours (range 5 to 22) in neonates to 8 hours (range 4 to 12) by 3 months of age. Oral bioavailability is 42 to 50%.

SPECIAL CONSIDERATIONS/PREPARATION: Available as 10-mg/mL solution for intravenous use in 2-mL preservative-free single-dose vials, and 4-mL multidose vials containing 0.9% (9 mg/mL) benzyl alcohol as a preservative. Although diluted PEPCID Injection has been shown to be physically and chemically stable for 7 days at room temperature, there are no data on the maintenance of sterility after dilution. Therefore, it is recommended that if not used immediately after preparation, diluted solutions of PEPCID Injection should be refrigerated and used within 48 hours. PEPCID for oral suspension is supplied as a powder containing 400 mg famotidine. Constitute by slowly adding 46 mL Purified Water and shaking vigorously for 5-10 seconds. Stable at room temperature for 30 days. Shake bottle before each use. A 1-mg/mL dilution may be made by adding 1 mL of the 10 mg/mL concentrated solution to 9 mL of sterile water for injection. Dilution stable for 14 days refrigerated.

Solution Compatibility: D_5W, $D_{10}W$, NS. Dex/AA solutions, fat emulsion.

Terminal Injection Site Compatibility: Acyclovir, aminophylline, amiodarone, ampicillin, atropine, aztreonam, calcium gluconate, cefazolin, cefotaxime, cefoxitin, ceftazidime, ceftriaxone, dexamethasone, digoxin, dobutamine, dopamine, enalaprilat, epinephrine, erythromycin lactobionate, esmolol, fluconazole, flumazenil, furosemide, gentamicin, heparin, hydrocortisone succinate, imipenem/cilastatin, insulin, isoproterenol, lidocaine, linezolid, lorazepam, magnesium sulfate, metoclopramide, mezlocillin, midazolam, morphine, nafcillin, nicardipine, nitroglycerin, oxacillin, phenytoin, piperacillin, potassium chloride, procainamide, propofol, remifentanil, sodium bicarbonate, sodium nitroprusside, ticarcillin/clavulanate, vancomycin, and vitamin K_1.

Incompatibility: Azithromycin, cefepime and piperacillin-tazobactam.

SELECTED REFERENCES

- Wenning LA, Murphy MG, James LP, et al: Pharmacokinetics of famotidine in infants. *Clin Pharmacokinet* 2005;44:395-406.
- James LP, Marotti T, Stowe CD, et al: Pharmacokinetics and pharmacodynamics of famotidine in infants. *J Clin Pharmacol* 1998;38:1089-1095.
- James LP, Marshall JD, Heulitt MJ, et al: Pharmacokinetics and pharmacodynamics of famotidine in children. *J Clin Pharmacol* 1996;21:48-54.
- Bullock L, Fitzgerald JF, Glick MR: Stability of famotidine 20 and 50 mg/L in total nutrient admixtures. *Am J Hosp Pharm* 1989;46:2326-29.
- Product information, Merck Inc., 2004.

FENTANYL

DOSE & ADMINISTRATION: Sedation and analgesia: 1 to 4 mcg/kg per dose IV slow push. Repeat as required (usually Q2 to 4 hours). **Infusion rate:** 1 to 5 mcg/kg per hour. Tolerance may develop rapidly following constant infusion. **Anesthesia:** 5 to 50 mcg/kg per dose.

FERROUS SULFATE

USES: Analgesia. Sedation. Anesthesia.

MONITORING: Monitor respiratory and cardiovascular status closely. Observe for abdominal distention, loss of bowel sounds, and muscle rigidity.

ADVERSE EFFECTS/PRECAUTIONS: Respiratory depression occurs when anesthetic doses (>5 mcg/kg) are used and may also occur unexpectedly because of redistribution. Chest wall rigidity has occurred in 4% of neonates who received 2.2 to 6.5 mcg/kg per dose, occasionally associated with laryngospasm. This was reversible with administration of naloxone. Urinary retention may occur when using continuous infusions. Tolerance may develop to analgesic doses with prolonged use. Significant withdrawal symptoms have been reported in patients treated with continuous infusion for 5 days or longer.

PHARMACOLOGY: Fentanyl is a synthetic opioid narcotic analgesic that is 50 to 100 times more potent than morphine on a weight basis. Extremely lipid soluble. Penetrates the CNS rapidly. Transient rebound in fentanyl serum concentration may reflect sequestration and subsequent release of fentanyl from body fat. Metabolized extensively in the liver by CYP 3A4 enzyme system and then excreted by the kidney. Serum half-life is prolonged in patients with liver failure. Highly protein bound. Wide variability in apparent volume of distribution (10 to 30 L/kg) and serum half-life (1 to 15 hours).

SPECIAL CONSIDERATIONS/PREPARATION: Naloxone should be readily available to reverse adverse effects. Available in 2-, 5-, 10-, and 20-mL ampules in a concentration of 50 mcg/mL. A 10 mcg/mL dilution may be made by adding 1 mL of the 50 mcg/mL concentration to 4 mL preservative-free normal saline. Stable for 24 hours refrigerated. Protect from light.

Solution Compatibility: D_5W, $D_{10}W$, and NS.

Terminal Injection Site Compatibility: Dex/AA solutions, fat emulsion. Amiodarone, atropine, caffeine citrate, cimetidine, dexamethasone, dobutamine, dopamine, enalaprilat, epinephrine, esmolol, furosemide, heparin, hydrocortisone succinate, lidocaine, linezolid, lorazepam, metoclopramide, midazolam, milrinone, mivacurium, morphine, nafcillin, nicardipine, pancuronium bromide, potassium chloride, propofol, ranitidine, remifentanil, sodium bicarbonate, and vecuronium.

Incompatibility: Azithromycin, pentobarbital and phenytoin.

SELECTED REFERENCES

- Fahnenstich H, Steffan J, Kau N, Bartmann P: Fentanyl-induced chest wall rigidity and laryngospasm in preterm and term infants. *Crit Care Med* 2000;28:836-839.
- Saarenmaa E, Neuvonen PJ, Fellman V: Gestational age and birth weight effects on plasma clearance of fentanyl in newborn infants. *J Pediatr* 2000;136:767-770.
- Muller P and Vogtmann C: Three cases with different presentation of fentanyl-induced muscle rigidity-A rare problem in intensive care of neonates. *Am J Perinatol* 2000;17:23-26.
- Santeiro ML, Christie J, Stromquist C, et al: Pharmacokinetics of continuous infusion fentanyl in newborns. *J Perinatol* 1997;17:135-139.
- Arnold JH, Truog RD, Orav EJ, et al: Tolerance and dependence in neonates sedated with fentanyl during extracorporeal membrane oxygenation. *Anesthesiology* 1990;73:1136.
- Koehntop DE, Rodman JH, Brundage DM, et al: Pharmacokinetics of fentanyl in neonates. *Anesth Analg* 1986;65:227.
- Johnson KL, Erickson JP, Holley FO, Scott JC: Fentanyl pharmacokinetics in the pediatric population. *Anesthesiology* 1984;61:A441.
- Reilly CS, Wood AJ, Wood M: Variability of fentanyl pharmacokinetics in man. *Anaesthesia* 1984;40:837.
- Mather LE: Clinical pharmacokinetics of fentanyl and its newer derivatives. *Clin Pharmacokinet* 1983;8:422.

FERROUS SULFATE

DOSE & ADMINISTRATION: 2 mg/kg per day of elemental iron for growing premature infants. (Maximum of 15 mg/day). Begin therapy after 2 weeks of age. Infants with birthweights less than 1000 grams may need 4 mg/kg per day. 6 mg/kg per day of elemental iron for patients receiving erythropoietin. Administer PO in 1 or 2 divided doses, preferably diluted in formula.

USES: Iron supplementation for prevention and treatment of anemia.

MONITORING: Monitor hemoglobin and reticulocyte counts during therapy. Observe stools, check for constipation.

ADVERSE EFFECTS/PRECAUTIONS: In growing premature infants, iron supplementation should not be started until adequate vitamin E is supplied in the diet; otherwise, iron may increase hemolysis. Nausea, constipation, black stools, lethargy, hypotension, and erosion of gastric mucosa.

PHARMACOLOGY: Well absorbed from stomach.

SPECIAL CONSIDERATIONS/PREPARATION: Drops: Contain 15 mg elemental iron per 0.6 mL (0.2% alcohol). **Elixir:** Contains 44 mg elemental iron per 5 mL (some with 5% alcohol).

SELECTED REFERENCES

- Rao R, Georgieff M: Microminerals, In: Tsang R, Uauy R, Koletzko B, Zlotkin S. *Nutrition of the Preterm Infant. Scientific Basis and Practical Guidelines.* Cincinnati, Ohio: Digital Publishing Inc; 2005: pp 277-288.
- Rao R, Georgieff MK: Neonatal iron nutrition. *Semin Neonatol* 2001;6:425-35.
- Siimes MA, Järvenpää A-L: Prevention of anemia and iron deficiency in very low-birth-weight infants. *J Pediatr* 1982;101:277-280.
- Oski FA: Iron requirements of the premature infant, in Tsang R (ed): *Vitamin and Mineral Requirements in Preterm Infants.* New York: Marcel Dekker, 1985, p 18.

FLECAINIDE

DOSE & ADMINISTRATION: Begin at 2 mg/kg per dose Q12 hours PO. Adjust dose based on response and serum concentrations to a maximum of 4 mg/kg per dose Q12 hours. Correct preexisting hypokalemia or hyperkalemia before administration. Optimal effect may take 2 to 3 days of therapy to achieve, and steady-state plasma levels may not be reached until 3 to 5 days at a given dosage in patients with normal renal and hepatic function. Therefore, do not increase dosage more frequently than approximately once every 4 days.

USES: Treatment of supraventricular arrhythmias not responsive to conventional therapies. Contraindicated in patients with structurally abnormal hearts.

MONITORING: Continuous EKG during initiation of therapy, as this is the most common time to see drug-induced arrhythmias. Follow trough serum concentrations closely at initiation, 3 to 5 days after any dose change, and with any significant change in clinical status or diet. Therapeutic trough levels are 200 to 800 nanograms/mL.

ADVERSE EFFECTS/PRECAUTIONS: Flecainide can cause new or worsened arrhythmias, including AV block, bradycardia, ventricular tachycardia, torsades de pointes. There is also a negative inotropic effect. Dizziness, blurred vision, and headache have been reported in children.

PHARMACOLOGY: Flecainide is a Class I-C antiarrhythmic that produces a dose-related decrease in intracardiac conduction in all parts of the heart, thereby increasing PR, QRS and QT intervals. Effects upon atrioventricular (AV) nodal conduction time and intra-atrial conduction times are less pronounced than those on the ventricle. Peak serum concentrations occur 2 to 3 hours after an oral dose. Infant formula and milk products interfere with drug absorption. Plasma protein binding is about 40% in adults and is independent of plasma drug level. Children under 1 year of age have elimination half-life values of 11 to 12 hours. Elimination half-life in newborns after maternal administration is as long as 29 hours.

SPECIAL CONSIDERATIONS/PREPARATION: Supplied in 50-mg, 100-mg, and 150-mg tablets. An oral suspension with a final concentration of 5 mg/mL can be made as follows: crush 6 (six) 100-mg tablets, slowly mix in 20 mL of a 1:1 mixture of Ora-Sweet® and Ora-Plus®, or cherry syrup (cherry syrup concentrate diluted 1:4 with simple syrup) to form a uniform paste, then add to this mixture enough vehicle to make a final volume of 120 mL. Shake well and protect from light. Stable for 45 days refrigerated and at room temperature when stored in amber glass or plastic.

SELECTED REFERENCES

- O'Sullivan JJ, Gardiner HM, Wren C: Digoxin or flecainide for prophylaxis of supraventricular tachycardia in infants? *J Am Coll Cardiol* 1995;26:991-994.
- Luedtke SA, Kuhn RJ, McCaffrey FM: Pharmacologic management of supraventricular tachycardia in children. *Ann Pharmacother* 1997;31:1227-43.
- Perry JC, Garson A: Flecainide acetate for treatment of tachyarrhythmias in children: Review of world literature on efficacy, safety, and dosing. *Am Heart J* 1992;124:1614-21.
- Wiest DB, Garner SS, Pagacz LR, et al: Stability of flecainide acetate in an extemporaneously compounded oral suspension. *Am J Hosp Pharm* 1992;49:1467-70.

FLUCONAZOLE

DOSE & ADMINISTRATION: Systemic infections, including meningitis: 12 mg/kg loading dose, then 6 mg/kg per dose IV infusion by syringe pump over 30 minutes, or PO. To use dosing chart, please refer to explanatory note in "How to Use This Book."

SYSTEMIC INFECTIONS DOSING INTERVAL CHART

PMA (weeks)	PostNatal (days)	Interval (hours)
≤29	0 to 14 >14	72 48
30 to 36	0 to 14 >14	48 24
37 to 44	0 to 7 >7	48 24
≥45	ALL	24

Prophylaxis: 3 mg/kg per dose via IV infusion twice weekly. (Consider only in ELBW infants cared for in NICUs with high rates of invasive fungal disease). **Thrush:** 6 mg/kg on Day 1, then 3 mg/kg per dose Q24 hours PO.

USES: Treatment of systemic infections, meningitis, and severe superficial mycoses caused by Candida species. Resistance has been reported with C glabrata and C krusei and in patients receiving long-term suppressive therapy.

MONITORING: Serum fluconazole concentrations are not routinely followed. Assess renal function. Follow AST, ALT, and CBC for eosinophilia.

ADVERSE EFFECTS/PRECAUTIONS: Data in neonates are limited. Reversible elevations of transaminases have occurred in 12% of children. A retrospective study using historical controls reports direct hyperbilirubinemia in the absence elevated transaminases in some infants treated prophylactically for 6 weeks. Interferes with metabolism of barbiturates and phenytoin. May also interfere with metabolism of aminophylline, caffeine, theophylline, and midazolam. **Contraindicated** in patients receiving **cisapride** due to precipitation of life-threatening arrhythmias.

PHARMACOLOGY: Fluconazole is a water-soluble triazole antifungal agent. Inhibits cytochrome P-450-dependent ergosterol synthesis. Well absorbed after oral administration, with peak serum concentrations reached within 1 to 2 hours. Less than 12% protein binding. Good penetration into CSF after both oral and IV administration. Serum half-life is 30 to 180 hours in severely ill VLBW infants in the first 2 weeks of life and approximately 17 hours in children. Primarily excreted unchanged in the urine.

SPECIAL CONSIDERATIONS/PREPARATION: Available as a premixed solution for IV injection in concentrations of 200 mg/100 mL and 400 mg/200 mL in Viaflex® bags (2 mg/mL). Oral dosage form is available as powder for suspension in concentrations of 10 mg/mL and 40 mg/mL. Prepare both concentrations by adding 24 mL distilled water to bottle of powder and shaking vigorously. Suspension is stable at room temperature for 2 weeks. Do not freeze.

Solution Compatibility: D_5W and $D_{10}W$.

Terminal Injection Site Compatibility: Dex/AA solutions, fat emulsion. Acyclovir, amikacin, aminophylline, amiodarone, aztreonam, cefazolin, cefepime, cefoxitin, cimetidine, dexamethasone, dobutamine, dopamine, famotidine, gentamicin, heparin, hydrocortisone succinate, intravenous immune globulin (human), linezolid, lorazepam, meropenem, metoclopramide, metronidazole, midazolam, morphine, nafcillin, nitroglycerin, oxacillin, pancuronium bromide, penicillin G, phenytoin, piperacillin/tazobactam, potassium chloride, propofol, quinupristin/dalfopristin, ranitidine, remifentanil, ticarcillin/clavulanate, tobramycin, vancomycin, vecuronium, and zidovudine.

Incompatibility: Amphotericin B, ampicillin, calcium gluconate, cefotaxime, ceftazidime, ceftriaxone, chloramphenicol, clindamycin, digoxin, erythromycin lactobionate, furosemide, imipenem, piperacillin, ticarcillin, and trimethoprim-sulfamethoxazole.

SELECTED REFERENCES

- Kaufman D, Boyle R, Hazen KC, et al: Twice weekly fluconazole prophylaxis for prevention of invasive Candida infection in high-risk infants of <1000 grams birth weight. *J Pediatr* 2005;147:172-179.
- Aghai ZH, Mudduluru M, Nakhla TA, et al. Fluconazole prophylaxis in extremely low birth weight infants: association with cholestasis. *J Perinatol* 2006;26:550-555.
- Huttova M, Hartmanova I, Kralinsky K, et al: Candida fungemia in neonates treated with fluconazole: report of forty cases, including eight with meningitis. *Pediatr Infect Dis J* 1998;17:1012-1015.
- Driessen M, Ellis JB, Cooper PA, et al: Fluconazole vs. amphotericin B for the treatment of neonatal fungal septicemia: a prospective randomized trial. *Pediatr Infect Dis J* 1996;15:1107.
- Flynn PM, Cunningham CK, Kerkering T, et al: Oropharyngeal candidiasis in immuno-compromised children: a randomized, multicenter study of orally administered fluconazole suspension versus nystatin. The Multicenter Fluconazole Study Group. *J Pediatr* 1995;127:322.
- Fasano C, O'Keefe J, Gibbs D: Fluconazole treatment of neonates and infants with severe fungal infections not treatable with conventional agents. *Eur J Clin Microbiol Infect Dis* 1994;13:351.
- Saxen H, Hoppu K, Pohjavuori M: Pharmacokinetics of fluconazole in very low birth weight infants during the first two weeks of life. *Clin Pharmacol Ther* 1993;54:269.
- Dodds Ashley ES, Lewis R, Lewis JS, et al. Pharmacology of systemic antifungal agents. *Clin Infect Dis* 2006;43:S29-39.
- Product information, Roerig Division of Pfizer, Inc., 2004.

FLUCYTOSINE

DOSE & ADMINISTRATION: 12.5 to 37.5 mg/kg per dose Q6 hours PO. Increase dosing interval if renal dysfunction is present.

USES: Antifungal agent used in combination with amphotericin B or fluconazole for treatment of infections caused by *Candida, Cryptococcus,* and other sensitive fungi.

MONITORING: Desired peak serum concentration ranges from 50 to 80 mcg/mL. Assess renal function. Follow GI status closely. Twice-weekly CBC and platelet counts. Periodic AST, ALT.

ADVERSE EFFECTS/PRECAUTIONS: Toxicities are related to serum concentration above 100 mcg/mL, and are usually reversible if the drug is stopped or the dose is reduced. Fatal bone marrow depression (related to fluorouracil production), hepatitis, severe diarrhea, rash. Amphotericin B may increase toxicity by decreasing renal excretion.

PHARMACOLOGY: Well absorbed orally. Transformed within cell to fluorouracil, which interferes with RNA synthesis. Excellent penetration into CSF and body tissues. 90% renal elimination of unchanged drug, proportional to GFR. Serum half-life in adults is 3 to 5 hours if renal function is normal, but 30 to 250 hours if renal impairment is present. Limited pharmacokinetic data in premature infants. Resistance develops frequently if used alone. Synergistic with amphotericin even if treating resistant strain.

SPECIAL CONSIDERATIONS/PREPARATION: Flucytosine is available only in 250 and 500-mg capsules. A pediatric suspension (10 mg/mL) may be prepared using distilled water; adjust pH from 5 to 7 with dilute sodium hydroxide. The capsule contains talc, which forms large-particle precipitates of inactive compound. The remaining suspension, containing the active drug, may be decanted. Shake well before use. The suspension is stable for 7 days at room temperature.

SELECTED REFERENCES

- Marr B, Gross S, Cunningham C, et al: Candidal sepsis and meningitis in a very-low-birth-weight infant successfully treated with fluconazole and flucytosine. *Clin Infect Dis* 1994;19:795.
- Smego RA, Perfect JR, Durack DT: Combined therapy with amphotericin B and 5-fluorocytosine for Candida meningitis. *Rev Infect Dis* 1984;6:791.
- Johnson DE, Thompson TR, Green TP, Ferrieri P: Systemic candidiasis in very low-birth-weight infants (< 1500 grams). *Pediatrics* 1984;73:138.
- Koldin MH, Medoff G: Antifungal chemotherapy. *Pediatr Clin North Am* 1983;30:49.

FLUMAZENIL

DOSE & ADMINISTRATION: IV: 5 to 10 mcg/kg per dose IV over 15 seconds. May repeat every 45 seconds until the patient is awake. Maximum reported dose should not exceed 50 mcg/kg (0.05 mg/kg) or 1 mg in infants, which ever is smaller. No reported maximum dose in neonates has been tested. Administer intravenously through a freely running large vein to minimize pain upon injection. **Intranasal:** 40 mcg/kg per dose divided equally between both nostrils. Administer via TB syringe for accurate equal dosing. **Rectal:** 15 to 30 mcg/kg per dose, may repeat if sedation not reversed within 15 to 20 minutes.

FOSPHENYTOIN

USES: Reversal of sedative effect from benzodiazepines, in cases of suspected benzodiazepines overdose, and in neonatal apnea secondary to prenatal benzodiazepine exposure.

MONITORING: Monitor for the return of sedation and respiratory depression. Continuous EKG and blood pressure.

ADVERSE EFFECTS/PRECAUTIONS: The reported experience in neonates is very limited. Use with caution in neonates with pre-existing seizure disorders. Hypotension has been reported in the adults following rapid administration. Resedation has been reported in 10% of treated pediatric patients, occuring 19 to 50 minutes after initial dosing. May cause pain on injection. Observe IV site for extravasation.

PHARMACOLOGY: Flumazenil is an imidazobenzodiazepine that is a benzodiazepine receptor antagonist. Competitively inhibits the activity at the benzodiazepine recognition site on the GABA/benzodiazepine receptor. Eliminated rapidly by hepatic metabolism to three inactive metabolites. Highly lipid soluble and penetrates the brain rapidly. Elimination half-life in children 20 to 75 minutes. Peak concentration reached in 3 minutes when delivered intravenously (children). Limited pharmacokinetic data in neonates.

SPECIAL CONSIDERATIONS/PREPARATION: Available in an injectable form as a 0.1 mg/mL concentration in 5- and 10-mL multi-dose vials. Discard opened vials within 24 hours. Store at room temperature.
  Solution Compatibility: D_5W, LR, and NS.
  Terminal Injection Site Compatibility: Aminophylline, cimetidine, dobutamine, dopamine, famotidine, heparin, lidocaine, procainamide, and ranitidine.

SELECTED REFERENCES

- Phelps SJ, Hak EB: *Pediatric Injectable Drugs.* Maryland: American Society of Health System Pharmacists, 2004, p176.
- Zaw W, Knoppert DC, da Silva O: Flumazenil's reversal of myoclonic-like movements associated with midazolam in term newborns. *Pharmacotherapy* 2001;21:642-6.
- Carbajal R, Simon N, Blanc P, et al: Rectal flumazenil to reverse midazolam sedation in children. *Anest Analog* 1996;82:895.
- Richard P, Autret E, Bardol J, et al: The use of flumazenil in a neonate. *Clin Toxicol* 1991;29:137-40.
- Brogden RN, Goa KL: Flumazenil. A review of its benzodiazepine antagonist properties, intrinsic activity and therapeutic use. *Drugs* 1988;35:448-67.
- Product information, Hoffman-La Roche, 2004.

FOSPHENYTOIN

DOSE & ADMINISTRATION: Note: Fosphenytoin dosing is expressed in phenytoin equivalents (PE). (Fosphenytoin 1 mg PE = phenytoin 1 mg) **Loading dose:** 15 to 20 mg PE/kg IM or IV infusion over at least 10 minutes. **Maintenance dose:** 4 to 8 mg PE/kg Q24 hours IM or IV slow push. Begin maintenance 24 hours after loading dose. Maximum rate of infusion 1.5 mg PE/kg per minute. May be administered more rapidly than phenytoin due to less infusion-related toxicity. Flush IV with saline before and after administration. Term infants older than 1 week of age may require up to 8 mg PE/kg per dose Q8 to 12 hours.

USES: Anticonvulsant. Generally used to treat seizures that are refractory to phenobarbital. Can be administered with lorazepam for rapid onset of seizure control.

MONITORING: Monitor blood pressure closely during infusion. Measure trough serum phenytoin (**not** fosphenytoin) concentration; obtain 48 hours after IV loading dose. Therapeutic serum phenytoin concentration: Probably 6 to 15 mcg/mL (up to 10 to 20 mcg/mL). Collect blood samples in EDTA tubes to minimize fosphenytoin to phenytoin conversion in the tube.

ADVERSE EFFECTS/PRECAUTIONS: Clinical signs of toxicity, such as drowsiness, are difficult to identify in infants, but are dose and infusion rate dependent. Minor venous irritation upon IV administration. Fosphenytoin drug interactions are similar to phenytoin (i.e., carbamazepine, cimetidine, corticosteroids, digoxin, furosemide, phenobarbital, and valproate). Use with caution in neonates with hyperbilirubinemia: both fosphenytoin and bilirubin displace phenytoin from protein-binding sites, resulting in increased serum free phenytoin concentration.

PHARMACOLOGY: Fosphenytoin is a water-soluble prodrug of phenytoin rapidly converted by phosphatases in blood and tissue. It has no known intrinsic pharmacologic activity before conversion to phenytoin. Each 1.5 mg of fosphenytoin is metabolically converted to 1 mg phenytoin. Conversion half-life of fosphenytoin administered intravenously to young pediatric patients is approximately 7 minutes. Data obtained using spiked blood samples from term and preterm neonates demonstrated similar conversion rates. No drugs have been identified to interfere with the conversion of fosphenytoin to phenytoin. Fosphenytoin is highly protein bound (adults 95% to 99%) and does not penetrate the blood-brain barrier. Serum half-life reflects that of phenytoin (18 to 60 hours) due to rapid conversion. The conversion of fosphenytoin to phenytoin yields very small amounts of formaldehyde and phosphate. This is only significant in cases of large overdosage. Phenytoin serum concentrations measured up to two hours after IV and four hours after IM dose may be falsely elevated due to fosphenytoin interaction with immunoanalytic methods (e.g., TDx fluorescence polarization).

SPECIAL CONSIDERATIONS/PREPARATION: Available as an injectable solution in a concentration equivalent to 50 mg PE/mL, in 2- and 10-mL vials. Administer IM undiluted. Administer IV after diluting in NS or D_5W to a concentration of 1.5 to 25 mg PE/mL. The pH is 8.6 to 9.0. **Store refrigerated.** Stable for 48 hours at room temperature. Do not use vials containing particulate matter.

Solution Compatibility: D_5W, $D_{10}W$ and NS.

Terminal Injection Site Compatibility: Lorazepam, phenobarbital, and potassium chloride.

Incompatibility: Midazolam.

SELECTED REFERENCES

- Fischer JH, Patel TV, Fischer PA: Fosphenytoin: Clinical pharmacokinetics and comparative advantages in the acute treatment of seizures. *Clin Pharmacokinet* 2003;42:33-58.
- Takeoka M, Krishnamoorthy KS, Soman TB, et al: Fosphenytoin in infants. *J Child Neurol* 1998;13:537-540.
- Morton LD: Clinical experience with fosphenytoin in children. *J Child Neurol* 1998;13(Suppl 1): S19-S22.
- Hatzopoulus FK, Carlos MA, Fischer JH: Safety and pharmacokinetics of intramuscular fosphenytoin in neonates. *Pediatr Res* 1998;43:60A.
- Fischer JH, Cwik MJ, Luer RS, et al: Stability of fosphenytoin sodium with intravenous solutions in glass bottles, polyvinyl chloride bags, and polypropylene syringes. *Ann Pharmacother* 1997;31:553-559.
- English BA, Riggs RM, Webster AA, Benner KW: Y-site stability of fosphenytoin and sodium phenobarbital. *Int J Pharm Compound* 1999;3:64-66.
- Riggs RM, English BA, Webster AA, et al: Fosphenytoin Y-site stability studies with lorazepam and midazolam hydrochloride. *Int J Pharm Compound* 1999;3:235-238.

FUROSEMIDE

DOSE & ADMINISTRATION: Initial dose: 1 mg/kg IV slow push, IM, or PO. May increase to a maximum of 2 mg/kg per dose IV or 6 mg/kg per dose PO. **Initial intervals:** Premature infant: Q24 hours. Fullterm infant: Q12 hours. Fullterm infant older than 1 month: Q6 to 8 hours. Consider alternate-day therapy for long-term use.

USES: Diuretic that may also improve pulmonary function.

MONITORING: Follow urine output and serum electrolytes and phosphorus. Assess closely for potassium depletion in patients receiving digoxin concurrently. Follow weight changes.

ADVERSE EFFECTS/PRECAUTIONS: Water and electrolyte imbalances occur frequently, especially hyponatremia, hypokalemia, and hypochloremic alkalosis. Hypercalciuria and development of renal calculi occur with long-term therapy. Potentially ototoxic, especially in patients also receiving aminoglycosides. Cholelithiasis has been reported in patients with BPD or congenital heart disease who received long-term TPN and furosemide therapy.

PHARMACOLOGY: The diuretic actions of furosemide are primarily at the ascending limb of Henle's loop, and are directly related to renal tubular drug concentration. Furosemide causes major urinary losses of sodium, potassium, and chloride. Urinary calcium and magnesium excretion, and urine pH are also increased. Prostaglandin production is stimulated, with increases in renal blood flow and renin secretion. Free water clearance is increased and CSF production is decreased by weak carbonic anhydrase inhibition. Nondiuretic effects include decreased pulmonary transvascular fluid filtration and improved pulmonary function. Protein binding is extensive, but bilirubin displacement is negligible when using normal doses. Oral bioavailability is good. Time to peak effect when given IV is 1 to 3 hours; duration of effect is approximately 6 hours, although half-life may be as long as 67 hours in the most immature neonates.

Ganciclovir

SPECIAL CONSIDERATIONS/PREPARATION: Furosemide oral solution is available in a 10-mg/mL concentration with only 0.02% alcohol (Roxane). The injectable solution may also be used for oral administration. Furosemide for injection is available as a 10-mg/mL concentration in 2-, 4-, and 10-mL ampules, and single use vials. A 2-mg/mL dilution may be made by adding 2 mL of the 10 mg/mL injectable solution to 8 mL preservative-free normal saline for injection. Dilution should be used within 24 hours. Protect from light and do not refrigerate.

Solution Compatibility: NS and sterile water for injection. Acidic solutions (pH <5.5) such as D_5W, $D_{10}W$, and Dex/AA cause furosemide to degrade when they are mixed together for several hours.

Terminal Injection Site Compatibility: Fat emulsion. Amikacin, aminophylline, amiodarone, ampicillin, atropine, aztreonam, bumetanide, calcium gluconate, cefepime, ceftazidime, cimetidine, dexamethasone, digoxin, epinephrine, famotidine, fentanyl, heparin, hydrocortisone succinate, indomethacin, lidocaine, lorazepam, linezolid, meropenem, morphine, nitroglycerin, penicillin G, piperacillin-tazobactam, potassium chloride, propofol, prostaglandin E_1, ranitidine, remifentanil, sodium bicarbonate, sodium nitroprusside, and tobramycin.

Incompatibility: Azithromycin, ciprofloxacin, dobutamine, dopamine, erythromycin lactobionate, esmolol, fluconazole, gentamicin, hydralazine, isoproterenol, metoclopramide, midazolam, milrinone, netilmicin, nicardipine, and vecuronium.

SELECTED REFERENCES

- Stefano JL, Bhutani VK: Role of furosemide after booster-packed erythrocyte transfusions in infants with bronchopulmonary dysplasia. *J Pediatr* 1990;117:965.
- Rush MG, Engelhardt B, Parker RA, Hazinski TA: Double-blind, placebo-controlled trial of alternate-day furosemide therapy in infants with chronic bronchopulmonary dysplasia. *J Pediatr* 1990;117:112.
- Mirochnick MH, Miceli JJ, Kramer PA, et al: Furosemide pharmacokinetics in very low birth weight infants. *J Pediatr* 1988;112:653.
- Green TP: The pharmacologic basis of diuretic therapy in the newborn. *Clin Perinatol* 1987;14:951.
- Hufnagle KG, Khan SN, Penn D: Renal calcifications: A complication of longterm furosemide therapy in preterm infants. *Pediatrics* 1982;70:360.
- Ross BS, Pollak A, Oh W: The pharmacological effects of furosemide therapy in the low-birth-weight infant. *J Pediatr* 1978;92:149.
- Ghanekar AG, Das Gupta V, Gibbs CW Jr: Stability of furosemide in aqueous systems. *J Pharm Sci* 1978;67:808.

Ganciclovir

DOSE & ADMINISTRATION: 6 mg/kg per dose Q12 hours IV infusion by syringe pump over 1 hour. Treat for a minimum of 6 weeks if possible. Reduce the dose by half for significant neutropenia (<500 cells/mm^3). **Chronic oral suppression:** 30 to 40 mg/kg per dose Q8 hours PO.

USES: Prevention of progressive hearing loss in babies with symptomatic congenital CMV infection.

MONITORING: CBC every 2 to 3 days during first 3 weeks of therapy, weekly thereafter if stable.

ADVERSE EFFECTS/PRECAUTIONS: Significant neutropenia will occur in the majority of treated patients. Discontinue treatment if the neutropenia does not resolve after reducing the dosage by half. Anemia and thrombocytopenia may also occur.

PHARMACOLOGY: Ganciclovir is an acyclic nucleoside analog of guanine that inhibits replication of herpes viruses in vivo. There is large interpatient variability in pharmacokinetic parameters. Mean half-life in infants less than 49 days postnatal age is 2.4 hours. Metabolism is minimal; almost all drug is excreted unchanged in the urine via glomerular filtration and active tubular secretion.

SPECIAL CONSIDERATIONS/PREPARATION: Cytovene® is supplied as lyophilized powder for injection, 500 mg per vial. Reconstitute by injecting 10 mL of Sterile Water for Injection into the vial. Do not use bacteriostatic water for injection containing parabens; it is incompatible with ganciclovir and may cause precipitation. Shake the vial to dissolve the drug. Visually inspect the reconstituted solution for particulate matter and discoloration prior to proceeding with infusion solution. Discard the vial if particulate matter or discoloration is observed. Reconstituted solution in the vial is stable at room temperature for 12 hours. Do not refrigerate, may cause precipitation. The pH is approximately 11: use caution when handling. Osmolarity is 320 mOsm/kg. Based on patient weight, remove the appropriate volume of the reconstituted solution (ganciclovir concentration 50 mg/mL) from the vial and add to a compatible diluent fluid to make a final infusion concentration less than 10 mg/mL. Although stable for 14 days, the infusion solution must be used within 24 hours of dilution to reduce the risk of bacterial contamination. Refrigerate the infusion solution. Do not freeze. Available as 250-mg and 500-mg capsules. Do not open or crush ganciclovir capsules. Prepare oral suspension in a vertical-flow laminar hood. Oral suspension (100 mg/mL) may be prepared by emptying eighty (80) 250-mg capsules into a glass mortar wetted and triturated with Oral-Sweet® to a smooth paste. Add 50-mL of Oral-Sweet® to the paste, mix, and transfer contents to an amber polyethylene terephthalate bottle. Rinse the mortar with another 50 mL of Oral-Sweet® and transfer contents to the bottle. Add enough Oral-Sweet® to make a final volume of 200 mL. Stable for 123 days when stored at 23° to 25° C. Protect from light.

Solution Compatibility: NS, D_5W, and LR.

Solution Incompatibility: Dex/AA.

Terminal Injection Site Compatibility: Enalaprilat, fluconazole, linezolid, propofol, and remifentanil.

Incompatibility: Aztreonam, cefepime, and piperacillin-tazobactam.

SELECTED REFERENCES

- Kimberlin DW, Lin C-Y, Sanchez PJ, et al: Effect of ganciclovir therapy on hearing in symptomatic congenital cytomegalovirus disease involving the central nervous system: a randomized, controlled trial. *J Pediatr* 2003;143:16-25.
- Michaels MG, Greenberg DP, Sabo DL, Wald ER: Treatment of children with cytomegalovirus infection with ganciclovir. *Pediatr Infect Dis J* 2003;22:504-08.
- Frenkel LM, Capparelli EV, Dankner WM, et al: Oral ganciclovir in children: pharmacokinetics, safety, tolerance, and antiviral effects. *J Infect Dis* 2000;182:1616-24.
- Anaizi NH, Swenson CF, and Dentinger PJ: Stability of ganciclovir in extemporaneously compounded oral liquids. *Am J Health Syst Pharm* 1999;56:1738-41.

Gentamicin

DOSE & ADMINISTRATION: IV infusion by syringe pump over 30 minutes. Administer as a separate infusion from penicillin-containing compounds. IM injection is associated with variable absorption, especially in the very small infant. To use dosing chart, please refer to explanatory note in "How to Use This Book."

Dosing Chart

PMA (weeks)	Postnatal (days)	Dose (mg/kg)	Interval (hours)
≤29*	0 to 7	5	48
	8 to 28	4	36
	≥29	4	24
30 to 34	0 to 7	4.5	36
	≥8	4	24
≥35	ALL	4	24
* or significant asphyxia, PDA, or treatment with indomethacin			

USES: Treatment of infections caused by aerobic gram-negative bacilli (e.g., *Pseudomonas, Klebsiella, E. coli*). Usually used in combination with a β-lactam antibiotic.

MONITORING: Measure serum concentrations when treating for more than 48 hours. Obtain peak concentration 30 minutes after end of infusion, and trough concentration just prior to the next dose. When treating patients with serious infections or significantly changing fluid or renal status consider measuring the serum concentration 24 hours after a dose, and use the chart below for the suggested dosing interval. Blood samples obtained to monitor serum drug concentrations should be spun and refrigerated or frozen as soon as possible. Therapeutic serum concentrations: **Peak:** 5 to 12 mcg/mL (or C_{max}/MIC ratio greater than 8:1) **Trough:** 0.5 to 1 mcg/mL

Suggested Dosing Intervals

Level at 24 hours (mcg/mL)	Half-life (hours)	Suggested Dosing Interval (hours)
≤1	≈8	24
1.1 to 2.3	≈12	36
2.4 to 3.2	≈15	48
≥3.3		Measure level in 24 hours

ADVERSE EFFECTS/PRECAUTIONS: Transient and reversible renal tubular dysfunction may occur, resulting in increased urinary losses of sodium, calcium, and magnesium. Vestibular and auditory ototoxicity. The addition of other nephrotoxic and/or ototoxic medications (e.g., furosemide, vancomycin) may increase these adverse effects. Increased neuromuscular blockade (i.e., neuromuscular weakness and respiratory failure) may occur when used with pancuronium or other neuromuscular blocking agents and in patients with hypermagnesemia.

PHARMACOLOGY: Dosing recommendations for gentamicin are based on: (1) Higher peak concentrations increase concentration-dependent bacterial killing; (2) There is a post-antibiotic effect on bacterial killing, especially when treating concurrently with a β-lactam antibiotic; (3) There may be less toxicity with less frequent dosing, due to less renal drug accumulation. Volume of distribution is increased and clearance is decreased in patients with PDA. Serum half-life is prolonged in premature and asphyxiated newborns. Inactivation of gentamicin by penicillin-containing compounds appears to be a time-, temperature-, and concentration-dependent process. This is probably clinically significant only when penicillin-containing compounds are mixed in IV solutions or when the blood is at room temperature for several hours before the assay is performed.

SPECIAL CONSIDERATIONS/PREPARATION: Pediatric injectable solution available in a concentration of 10 mg/mL.

Solution Compatibility: D_5W, $D_{10}W$, and NS.

Terminal Injection Site Compatibility: Dex/AA solutions, fat emulsion. Acyclovir, amiodarone, aztreonam, caffeine citrate, cefoxitin, ceftazidime, ceftriaxone, cimetidine, clindamycin, dopamine, enalaprilat, esmolol, famotidine, fluconazole, insulin, lorazepam, heparin (concentrations >1 unit/mL), linezolid, magnesium sulfate, meropenem, metronidazole, midazolam, milrinone, morphine, nicardipine, pancuronium bromide, prostaglandin E_1, ranitidine, remifentanil, vecuronium, and zidovudine.

Incompatibility: Amphotericin B, ampicillin, azithromycin, cefepime, furosemide, imipenem/cilastatin, heparin (concentrations >1 U/mL), indomethacin, methicillin, mezlocillin, nafcillin, oxacillin, penicillin G, propofol, and ticarcillin/clavulanate.

SELECTED REFERENCES

- Contopoulos-Ioannidis DG, Giotis ND, Baliatsa DV, Ioannidis JPA: Extended-interval aminoglycoside administration for children: a meta-analysis. Pediatrics 2004;114:e111-e118.
- Stolk LML, Degraeuwe PLJ, Nieman FHM, et al: Population pharmacokinetics and relationship between demographic and clinical variables and pharmacokinetics of gentamicin in neonates. Ther Drug Monit 2002;24:527-31.
- Avent ML, Kinney JS, Istre GR, Whitfield JM: Gentamicin and tobramycin in neonates: comparison of a new extended dosing regimen with a traditional multiple daily dosing regimen. Am J Perinatol 2002;8:413-19.
- Giapros VI, Andronikou S, Cholevas VI, Papadopoulou ZL: Renal function in premature infants during aminoglycoside therapy. Pediatr Nephrol 1995;9:163.
- Daly JS, Dodge RA, Glew RH, et al: Effect of time and temperature on inactivation of aminoglycosides by ampicillin at neonatal dosages. J Perinatol 1997;17:42-45.
- Williams BS, Ransom JL, Gal P, et al: Gentamicin pharmacokinetics in neonates with patent ductus arteriosus. Crit Care Med 1997;25:273-75.

GLUCAGON

DOSE & ADMINISTRATION: 200 mcg/kg per dose (0.2 mg/kg per dose) IV push, IM, or SC. **Maximum dose:** 1 mg. **Continuous infusion:** Begin with 10 to 20 mcg/kg per hour (0.5 to 1 mg per day). Rise in blood glucose should occur with one hour of starting infusion.

USES: Treatment of hypoglycemia refractory to intravenous dextrose infusions, or when dextrose infusion is unavailable, or in cases of documented glucagon deficiency.

MONITORING: Follow blood glucose concentration closely. Watch for rebound hypoglycemia. Rise in blood glucose will last approximately 2 hours.

ADVERSE EFFECTS/PRECAUTIONS: Nausea and vomiting, tachycardia, and ileus. Hyponatremia and thrombocytopenia have also been reported.

PHARMACOLOGY: Glucagon stimulates synthesis of cyclic AMP, especially in liver and adipose tissue. Stimulates gluconeogenesis. In high doses, glucagon has a cardiac inotropic effect. Inhibits small-bowel motility and gastric-acid secretion.

SPECIAL CONSIDERATIONS/PREPARATION: Supplied in 1-mg single-dose vials. Dissolve the lyophilized product in the supplied diluent. Precipitates in chloride solutions. One unit (1 U) of glucagon and 1 mg of glucagon are equivalent. Use immediately after reconstitution.

Solution Compatibility: No data are currently available on Dex/AA and other intravenous solutions.

Terminal Injection Site Compatibility: No data are currently available.

SELECTED REFERENCES
- Charsha DS, McKinley PS, Whitfield JM: Glucagon infusion for treatment of hypoglycemia: efficacy and safety in sick, preterm neonates. *Pediatrics* 2003;111:220-1.
- Miralles RE, Lodha A, Perlman M, Moore AM: Experience with intravenous glucagon infusions as a treatment for resistant neonatal hypoglycemia. *Arch Pediatr Adolesc Med* 2002;156:99-1004.
- Hawdon JM, Aynsley-Green A, Ward Platt MP: Neonatal blood glucose concentrations: metabolic effect of intravenous glucagon and intragastric medium chain triglyceride. *Arch Dis Child* 1993;68:255.
- Mehta A, Wootton R, Cheng KN, et al: Effect of diazoxide or glucagon on hepatic production rate during extreme neonatal hypoglycemia. *Arch Dis Child* 1987;62:924.
- Davis SN, Granner DK: Insulin and oral hypoglycemic agents and the pharmacology of the endocrine pancreas, in Hardman JG, Limbird LE, Gilman AG (eds): *The Pharmacological Basis of Therapeutics*, ed 10. New York: Macmillan Co, 2001, pp 1707-08.

HAEMOPHILUS B (HIB) CONJUGATE VACCINE

DOSE & ADMINISTRATION: 0.5 mL IM in the anterolateral thigh. Please refer to the most recent AAP/ACIP immunization schedule. It is recommended that premature infants should be immunized according to their postnatal age; however, inadequate seroconversion may occur in chronically ill premature infants. For HbOC and PRP-T, second and third doses are given at 2-month intervals, followed by a fourth dose given at age 15 months. For PRP-OMP, only the second dose is given after a 2-month interval; the third dose is given at age 15 months. **When giving multiple vaccines, use a separate syringe for each and give at different sites.** Care should be taken to draw back on the plunger of the syringe before injection to be certain the needle is not in a blood vessel.

USES: Immunoprophylaxis against invasive disease caused by *Haemophilus influenzae* type b.

MONITORING: Observe injection site for local reactions.

ADVERSE EFFECTS/PRECAUTIONS: Soreness at the injection site with local erythema, swelling, tenderness, and fever.

PHARMACOLOGY: Three conjugate vaccines are currently approved for use in infants older than 2 months of age. These vaccines are derived from *H influenzae* type b capsular polysaccharide, polyribosylribitol phosphate (PRP), which is linked to a T-cell-dependent protein antigen to enhance immunogenicity.

SPECIAL CONSIDERATIONS/PREPARATION:

PRODUCTS

Manufacturer	Abbreviation	Trade Name	Carrier Protein
Wyeth-Lederle Pharmaceuticals	HbOC	HibTITER®	CRM_{197} (a nontoxic mutant diphtheria toxin)
Sanofi Pasteur	PRP-T	ActHIB®	Tetanus toxoid
Merck & Co, Inc	PRP-OMP Liquid	PedvaxHIB®	OMP (an outer membrane protein complex of N meningitidis)

Heparin

HibTITER® is a clear, colorless solution supplied in single dose (preservative-free) and multidose (thimerosal-containing) vials. Discard if discolored or turbid. Store refrigerated at 2 °C to 8 °C (36 °F to 46 °F). **Do not freeze.** ActHIB® is supplied as lyophilized powder. Store the lyophilized vaccine and diluent refrigerated at 2 °C to 8 °C (36 °F to 46 °F). **Do not freeze.** Reconstitute using only the 0.4% saline diluent provided in prefilled single-use 0.6-mL syringe and use immediately. Reconstituted vaccine is a clear, colorless solution. Liquid PedvaxHIB® is supplied in single dose vials. It is a slightly opaque white suspension. Shake well before withdrawal and use. Store refrigerated at 2 °C to 8 °C (36 °F to 46 °F). **Do not freeze.**

SELECTED REFERENCES

- American Academy of Pediatrics. *Haemophilus Influenzae* Infections. In: Pickering LK, Baker CJ, Long SS, McMillan JA, eds. Red Book: 2006 Report of the Committee on Infectious Diseases. 27th ed. Elk Grove Village, IL: American Academy of Pediatrics; 2006: pp 315-317.
- Advisory Committee on Immunization Practices: Recommendations of the ACIP. Most recent updates available on the National Immunization Program website: http://www.cdc.gov/nip/publications/acip-list.htm
- Washburn LK, O'Shea TM, Gillis DC, et al: Response to *Haemophilus influenzae* type b conjugate vaccine in chronically ill premature infants. *J Pediatr* 1993;123:791.
- Product information, Wyeth-Lederle Pharmaceuticals, 2004.
- Product information, Merck & Co, 2004.
- Product information, Sanofi Pasteur, 2005.

Heparin

DOSE & ADMINISTRATION: Maintaining patency of peripheral and central vascular catheters: 0.5 to 1 units/mL of IV fluid. **Treatment of thrombosis:** 75 units/kg bolus, followed by 28 units/kg per hour continuous infusion. Four hours after initiating therapy, measure aPTT, then adjust dose to achieve an aPTT that corresponds to an anti-factor X_a level of 0.3 to 0.7 (this is usually equivalent to an aPTT of 60 to 85 seconds). Treatment should be limited to 10 to 14 days. **Make certain correct concentration is used.**

USES: See above. Only continuous infusions (rather than intermittent flushes) have been demonstrated to maintain catheter patency. Treatment of renal vein thromboses is limited to those that are bilateral or extend into the IVC. Although data are limited, enoxaparin may be preferable to heparin for treatment of thromboses. Call 1-800-NOCLOTS for case reporting and treatment guidance.

MONITORING: Follow platelet counts every 2 to 3 days. When treating thromboses, maintain a prolonged aPTT in a range corresponding to an anti-factor X_a level of 0.3 to 0.7 units/mL. Assess for signs of bleeding and thrombosis.

ADVERSE EFFECTS/PRECAUTIONS: Data are insufficient to make specific recommendations regarding anticoagulation therapy. Heparin-induced thrombocytopenia (HIT) has been reported to occur in approximately 1% of newborns exposed to heparin. Heparin-associated antiplatelet antibodies were found in half of the newborns who were both thrombocytopenic and heparin-exposed. Although the thrombocytopenia resolved spontaneously in most patients upon stopping the heparin, a high incidence of ultrasonographic-documented aortic thrombosis was seen. Contraindicated in infants with evidence of intracranial or GI bleeding or thrombocytopenia (below 50,000/mm^3). Long term use of therapeutic doses of heparin can lead to osteoporosis.

PHARMACOLOGY: Activates antithrombin III, which progressively inactivates both thrombin and factor X_a, key proteolytic enzymes in the formation of fibrinogen and activation of prothrombin. Efficacy in neonates is decreased due to low antithrombin plasma concentrations. Metabolized by liver. Renal excretion should occur within 6 hours, but may be delayed. Clearance in neonates is more rapid than in children or adults. Half-life is dose-dependent, but averages 1 to 3 hours.

SPECIAL CONSIDERATIONS/PREPARATION: Keep protamine sulfate on hand to manage hemorrhage (1 mg for each 100 U of heparin given in last 4 hours). Available in 10 units/mL (for IV reservoirs); 100 units/mL; 1000 units/mL (for central catheters); and 10,000 units/mL.

Solution Compatibility: D_5W, $D_{10}W$, and NS.

Terminal Injection Site Compatibility: Dex/AA solutions, fat emulsion. Acyclovir, aminophylline, ampicillin, amphotericin B, atropine, aztreonam, caffeine citrate, calcium gluconate, cefazolin, cefepime, cefotaxime, cefoxitin, ceftazidime, ceftriaxone, chloramphenicol, cimetidine, clindamycin, dexamethasone, digoxin, dobutamine, dopamine, enalaprilat, epinephrine, erythromycin lactobionate, esmolol, famotidine, fentanyl, fluconazole, flumazenil, furosemide, hydralazine, hydrocortisone succinate, insulin, isoproterenol, lidocaine, linezolid, lorazepam, meropenem, methicillin, metoclopramide, metronidazole, mezlocillin, midazolam, milrinone, morphine, nafcillin, naloxone, netilmicin, neostigmine, nitroglycerin, oxacillin, pancuronium bromide, penicillin G, phenobarbital, phytonadione, piperacillin, piperacillin-tazobactam, potassium chloride, procainamide, propofol, propranolol, prostaglandin E_1, ranitidine, remifentanil, sodium bicarbonate, sodium nitroprusside, ticarcillin/clavulanate, trimethoprim-sulfamethoxazole, vecuronium, and zidovudine.

Incompatibility: Alteplase, amikacin, amiodarone, ciprofloxacin, diazepam, gentamicin, hyaluronidase, methadone, phenytoin, tobramycin, and vancomycin.

SELECTED REFERENCES

- Schmugge M, Risch L, Huber AR, et al: Heparin-induced thrombocytopenia-associated thrombosis in pediatric intensive care patients. *Pediatrics* 2002;109(1). URL:http://www.pediatrics.org/cgi/content/full/109/1/e10.
- Monagle P, Michelson AD, Bovill E, Andrew M : Antithrombotic therapy in children. *Chest* 2001;119:344-370S.
- Edstrom CS, Christensen RD: Evaluation and treatment of thrombosis in the neonatal intensive care unit. *Clin Perinatol* 2000;27:623-41.
- Sutor AH, Massicotte P, Leaker M, Andrew M: Heparin therapy in pediatric patients. *Semin Thromb Hemostas* 1997;23:303-19.
- Chang GY, Leuder FL, DiMichele DM, et al: Heparin and the risk of intraventricular hemorrhage in premature infants. *J Pediatr* 1997;131:362-66.
- Paisley MK, Stamper M, Brown J, et al: The use of heparin and normal saline flushes in neonatal intravenous catheters. *Pediatr Nurs* 1997;23:521-27.
- Kotter RW: Heparin vs saline for intermittent intravenous device maintenance in neonates. *Neonat Network* 1996;15:43-47.
- Moclair A, Bates I: The efficacy of heparin in maintaining peripheral infusions in neonates. *Eur J Pediatr* 1995;154:567-70.
- Spadone D, Clark F, James E, et al: Heparin-induced thrombocytopenia in the newborn. *J Vasc Surg* 1992;15:306.

HEPATITIS B IMMUNE GLOBULIN (HUMAN)

DOSE & ADMINISTRATION: 0.5 mL IM in the anterolateral thigh. Term and preterm newborns with BW more than 2000 g: Give as soon as it is determined that the mother is HBsAg-positive, within 7 days of birth. Preterm newborns <2000 g BW: Give within 12 hours of birth. **When given at the same time as the first dose of hepatitis B vaccine, use a separate syringe and a different site.** Care should be taken to draw back on the plunger of the syringe before injection to be certain the needle is not in a blood vessel.

USES: Passive immunization of newborns whose mothers have acute hepatitis B infection at the time of delivery, or who are HBsAg-positive. Infants born to mothers who are HBeAg-positive have the highest risk.

MONITORING: No specific monitoring required.

ADVERSE EFFECTS/PRECAUTIONS: Local pain and tenderness may occur at the injection site. **Do not administer IV** because of the risk of serious systemic reactions. Serious complications of IM injections are rare. Universal precautions should be used with neonates born to HBsAg-positive mothers until they have been bathed carefully to remove maternal blood and secretions.

PHARMACOLOGY: Hepatitis B Immune Globulin (human) is a hyperimmune globulin solution prepared from pooled plasma of individuals with high titers of antibody to hepatitis B surface antigen (anti-HBsAg). All donors are HBsAg-negative and HIV-antibody negative. Nabi-HB™ (Nabi) and BayHep B™ (Bayer) are solvent detergent treated and thimerosal free hepatitis B immune globulin preparations.

SPECIAL CONSIDERATIONS/PREPARATION: Refrigerate. Supplied in 1-mL and 5-mL single-dose vials and 0.5-mL unit-dose syringes.

SELECTED REFERENCES

- American Academy of Pediatrics. Hepatitis B. In: Pickering LK, Baker CJ, Long SS, McMillan JA, eds. *Red Book: 2006 Report of the Committee on Infectious Diseases.* 27th ed. Elk Grove Village, IL: American Academy of Pediatrics; 2006: pp 341-343.
- Crumpacker CS: Hepatitis, in Remington JS, Klein JO (eds): *Infectious Diseases of the Fetus and Newborn Infant*, ed 5. Philadelphia: WB Saunders Co, 2001, pp 932-33.

Hepatitis B Vaccine (Recombinant)

DOSE & ADMINISTRATION: Engerix-B® 10 mcg (0.5 mL) or Recombivax HB® 5 mcg (0.5 mL) IM. **Maternal HBsAg-Positive:** Administer first dose before 12 hours of age regardless of gestational age (administer HBIG also). Infants with BW <2000 g should receive 3 additional doses, beginning at 1 month of age. **Maternal HBsAg Unknown:** Administer first dose before 12 hours of age regardless of gestational age. If preterm or BW <2000 g, also administer HBIG before 12 hours of age. Administration of HBIG to term newborns should depend on results of serologic screening of the mother, which should be done as soon as possible, but not later than 7 days after birth. **Maternal HBsAg Negative:** Administer first dose shortly after birth, before hospital discharge. If preterm or BW <2000 g and medically stable, administer first dose as early as 30 days of age or at time of hospital discharge. Please refer to the most recent AAP/ACIP immunization schedule for subsequent doses. Engerix-B® also has an alternative four-dose schedule: Birth, 1, 2, and 12 to 18 months of age.

USES: Immunoprophylaxis against hepatitis B. Safe for use in infants born to HIV-positive mothers, although it may be less effective.

MONITORING: Testing for immunity 3 months after completion of the vaccination series is recommended for infants born to HBsAg-positive mothers and, perhaps, for premature infants who received an early first dose.

ADVERSE EFFECTS/PRECAUTIONS: The only common side effect is soreness at the injection site. Fever greater than 37.7 °C occurs in 1 to 6%.

PHARMACOLOGY: Recombinant hepatitis B vaccines are produced by *Saccharomyces cerevisiae* (common baker's yeast) that has been genetically modified to synthesize HBsAg. Both vaccines are inactivated (noninfective) products that contain HBsAg protein adsorbed to aluminum hydroxide, and may be interchanged with comparable efficacy.

SPECIAL CONSIDERATIONS/PREPARATION: Recombivax HB® for infant use is supplied in 0.5 mL single-dose vials containing 5 mcg. Engerix-B® is supplied in 0.5 mL single-dose vials and 0.5 mL single-dose prefilled disposable syringes containing 10 mcg per 0.5 mL. Preservative free. The vaccine should be used as supplied; do not dilute. **Shake well before withdrawal and use.** Store refrigerated at **2 °C to 8 °C (36 °F to 46 °F)**. **Do not freeze**-destroys potency.

SELECTED REFERENCES

- American Academy of Pediatrics. Hepatitis B. In: Pickering LK, Baker CJ, Long SS, McMillan JA, eds. *Red Book: 2006 Report of the Committee on Infectious Diseases.* 27th ed. Elk Grove Village, IL: American Academy of Pediatrics; 2006: pp 341-343.
- Centers for Disease Control and Prevention: A comprehensive immunization strategy to eliminate transmission of hepatitis B virus in the United States. Recommendations of the Advisory Committee on Immunization Practices (ACIP) part 1: immunization of infants, children and adolescents. *MMWR Recomm Rep* 2005;54 (RR-16):1-23.
- Saari TN, Committee on Infectious Diseases: Immunization of preterm and low birth weight infants. *Pediatrics* 2003;112:193-98.

Hib Conjugate - Hepatitis B Combination Vaccine

DOSE & ADMINISTRATION: 0.5 mL IM in the anterolateral thigh. Please refer to the most recent AAP/ACIP immunization schedule. It is recommended that premature infants should be immunized according to their postnatal age; some data, however, suggest delaying the first dose in chronically ill premature infants due to inadequate seroconversion against *H. influenzae*. **When giving multiple vaccines, use a separate syringe for each and give at different sites.** Care should be taken to draw back on the plunger of the syringe before injection to be certain the needle is not in a blood vessel.

USES: COMVAX™ is indicated for vaccination against invasive disease caused by Haemophilus influenzae type b and against infection caused by all known subtypes of hepatitis B virus in infants 6 weeks to 15 months of age born to HBsAg-negative mothers. COMVAX™ should not be used in infants younger than 6 weeks of age.

MONITORING: Observe injection site for local reactions.

ADVERSE EFFECTS/PRECAUTIONS: Local pain and tenderness may occur at the injection site.

PHARMACOLOGY: COMVAX™ (preservative-free) combines the antigenic components of Recombivax HB® and PedvaxHIB®. Each 0.5 mL dose contains 5 mcg HBsAg and 7.5 mcg *Haemophilus b* -PRP.

SPECIAL CONSIDERATIONS/PREPARATION: Supplied in 0.5-mL single-dose vial. Store refrigerated. Do not freeze.

SELECTED REFERENCES

- American Academy of Pediatrics. Hepatitis B. In: Pickering LK, Baker CJ, Long SS, McMillan JA, eds. Red Book: 2006 Report of the Committee on Infectious Diseases. 27th ed. Elk Grove Village, IL: American Academy of Pediatrics; 2006: pp 341-343.
- Product information, Merck & Co, 2004.

HYALURONIDASE

DOSE & ADMINISTRATION: Inject 1 mL (150 units) as 5 separate 0.2-mL subcutaneous injections around the periphery of the extravasation site. Use 25- or 26-gauge needle and change after each injection. The chances of therapeutic success may be increased by: 1) Initiating treatment within 1 hour of extravasation; 2) Subcutaneously flushing the affected area with up to 500 mL of normal saline after the hyaluronidase treatment; 3) Covering with a hydrogel dressing for 48 hours.

USES: Prevention of tissue injury caused by IV extravasation. Suggested indications (some anecdotal) are for extravasations involving drugs that are irritating to veins because of hyperosmolarity or extreme pH (e.g., aminophylline, amphotericin B, calcium, diazepam, erythromycin, gentamicin, methicillin, nafcillin, oxacillin, phenytoin, potassium chloride, rifampin, sodium bicarbonate, tromethamine, vancomycin, and TPN, and concentrated IV solutions). Hyaluronidase is **not** indicated for treatment of extravasations of vasoconstrictive agents (e.g., dopamine, epinephrine, and norepinephrine).

MONITORING: No specific monitoring required.

ADVERSE EFFECTS/PRECAUTIONS: Not recommended for IV use.

PHARMACOLOGY: Hyaluronidase is a mucolytic enzyme that disrupts the normal intercellular barrier and allows rapid dispersion of extravasated fluids through tissues.

SPECIAL CONSIDERATIONS/PREPARATION: Amphadase™ is supplied sterile as 150 USP units/mL in 2 mL glass vials. Store refrigerated. Do not freeze.

Terminal Injection Site Compatibility: Amikacin, pentobarbital, and sodium bicarbonate.

Incompatibility: Epinephrine, heparin, and phenytoin.

SELECTED REFERENCES

- Ramasethu J: Prevention and management of extravasation injuries in neonates. *NeoReviews* 2004;5:e491-e497.
- Casanova D, Bardot J, Magalon G: Emergency treatment of accidental infusion leakage in the newborn: report of 14 cases. *Br J Plast Surg* 2001;545:396-399.
- Davies J, Gault D, Buchdahl: Preventing the scars of neonatal intensive care. *Arch Dis Child* 1994;70:F50-F51.
- Raszka WV, Kueser TK, Smith FR, Bass JW: The use of hyaluronidase in the treatment of intravenous extravasation injuries. *J Perinatol* 1990;10:146.
- Lehr VT, Lulic-Botica M, Lindblad WJ, et al: Management of infiltration injury in neonates using duoderm hydroactive gel. *Am J Perinatol* 2004;21:409-414.
- Product information, Amphastar Pharmaceuticals, Inc.

HYDRALAZINE

DOSE & ADMINISTRATION: IV (if available): Begin with 0.1 to 0.5 mg/kg per dose Q6 to 8 hours. Dose may be gradually increased as required for blood pressure control to a maximum of 2 mg/kg per dose Q6 hours. **PO:** 0.25 to 1 mg/kg per dose Q6 to 8 hours, or approximately twice the required IV dose. Administer with food to enhance absorption. **Note:** Use with a beta-blocking agent is often recommended to enhance the

Hydrochlorothiazide

antihypertensive effect and decrease the magnitude of the reflex tachycardia. This is expected to reduce hydralazine IV dosage requirements to less than 0.15 mg/kg per dose.

USES: Treatment of mild to moderate neonatal hypertension by vasodilation. Afterload reduction in patients with congestive heart failure.

MONITORING: Frequent assessment of blood pressure and heart rate. Guaiac stools. Periodic CBC during long-term use.

ADVERSE EFFECTS/PRECAUTIONS: Diarrhea, emesis, and temporary agranulocytosis have been reported in neonates. Tachycardia, postural hypotension, headache, nausea, and a lupus-like syndrome occur in 10% to 20% of adults. Uncommon reactions in adults include GI irritation and bleeding, drug fever, rash, conjunctivitis, and bone marrow suppression.

PHARMACOLOGY: Causes direct relaxation of smooth muscle in the arteriolar resistance vessels. Major hemodynamic effects: Decrease in systemic vascular resistance and a resultant increase in cardiac output. Increases renal, coronary, cerebral, and splanchnic blood flow. When administered orally, hydralazine has low bioavailability because of extensive first-pass metabolism by the liver and intestines. The rate of enzymatic metabolism is genetically determined by the acetylator phenotype—slow acetylators have higher plasma concentrations and a higher incidence of adverse effects.

SPECIAL CONSIDERATIONS/PREPARATION: Hydralazine hydrochloride injection for IV use (20 mg/mL) is available in 1 mL vial from SoloPak Laboratories. A 1 mg/mL dilution may be made by diluting 0.5 mL of the 20 mg/mL concentrate with 9.5 mL of preservative-free normal saline for injection. Dilution is stable for 24 hours. Only 10-, 25-, 50-, and 100-mg tablets are manufactured for oral use. Oral formulations using simple syrups containing dextrose, fructose, or sucrose are unstable. To prepare an oral suspension, crush a 50 mg tablet and dissolve in 4 mL of 5% mannitol, then add 46 mL of sterile water to make a final concentration of 1 mg/mL. Protect from light. Stable for 7 days refrigerated.

Solution Compatibility: D_5W, $D_{10}W$, and NS.

Terminal Injection Site Compatibility: Dex/AA. Dobutamine, heparin, hydrocortisone succinate, potassium chloride, and prostaglandin E_1.

Incompatibility: Aminophylline, ampicillin, diazoxide, furosemide, and phenobarbital.

SELECTED REFERENCES

- Artman M, Graham TP Jr: Guidelines for vasodilator therapy of congestive heart failure in infants and children. *Am Heart J* 1987;113:995.
- Gupta VD, Stewart KR, Bethea C: Stability of hydralazine hydrochloride in aqueous vehicles. *J Clin Hosp Pharm* 1986;11:215.
- Beekman RH, Rocchini AP, Rosenthal A: Hemodynamic effects of hydralazine in infants with a large ventricular septal defect. *Circulation* 1982;65:523.
- Fried R, Steinherz LJ, Levin AR, et al: Use of hydralazine for intractable cardiac failure in childhood. *J Pediatr* 1980;97:1009.

Hydrochlorothiazide

DOSE & ADMINISTRATION: 1 to 2 mg/kg per dose Q12 hours PO. Administer with food (improves absorption). **Note: Do not confuse with chlorothiazide.**

USES: Diuretic used in treating both mild to moderate edema and mild to moderate hypertension. Effects increased when used in combination with furosemide or spironolactone. May improve pulmonary function in patients with BPD.

MONITORING: Serum electrolytes, calcium, phosphorus, and glucose; urine output and blood pressure.

ADVERSE EFFECTS/PRECAUTIONS: Hypokalemia and other electrolyte abnormalities. Hyperglycemia. Hyperuricemia. **Do not use in patients with significant impairment of renal or hepatic function.**

PHARMACOLOGY: Limited data in neonates. Rapidly absorbed from GI tract. Onset of action is within 1 hour. Elimination half-life depends on GFR and is longer than that of chlorothiazide. Major diuretic effect results from inhibition of sodium reabsorption in the distal nephron. Increases urinary losses of sodium, potassium, magnesium, chloride, phosphorus, and bicarbonate. Decreases renal excretion of calcium. Inhibits pancreatic release of insulin. Displaces bilirubin from albumin.

SPECIAL CONSIDERATIONS/PREPARATION: Supplied as a 50-mg/5mL oral solution.

SELECTED REFERENCES

- Albersheim SG, Solimano AJ, Sharma AK, et al: Randomized, double-blind, controlled trial of long-term diuretic therapy for bronchopulmonary dysplasia. *J Pediatr* 1989;115:615.
- Roberts RJ: *Drug Therapy in Infants*. Philadelphia: WB Saunders Co, 1984, p 244.

HYDROCORTISONE

DOSE & ADMINISTRATION: Physiologic replacement: 7 to 9 mg/m^2 per day IV or PO, in 2 or 3 doses. **Treatment of pressor- and volume-resistant hypotension (Stress doses):** 20 to 30 mg/m^2 per day IV, in 2 or 3 doses, or approximately 1 mg/kg per dose every 8 hours.

BODY SURFACE AREA

Weight (kg)	Surface Area* (sq meters)
0.6	0.08
1	0.1
1.4	0.12
2	0.15
3	0.2
4	0.25

*BSA (m^2) = (0.05 x kg) + 0.05

Treatment of chorioamnionitis-exposed ELBW infants to decrease risk of CLD: Initial dose: 0.5 mg/kg/dose IV Q12 hours for 9 days, followed by 0.25 mg/kg IV Q 12 hours for 3 days.

USES: Treatment of cortisol deficiency. Treatment of pressor-resistant hypotension. Adjunctive therapy for persistent hypoglycemia. May improve survival and decrease CLD in ELBW infants exposed to chorioamnionitis.

MONITORING: Measure blood pressure and blood glucose frequently during acute illness.

ADVERSE EFFECTS/PRECAUTIONS: Hyperglycemia, hypertension, salt and water retention. There is an increased risk of GI perforations when treating concurrently with indomethacin. There is also an increased risk of disseminated *Candida* infections. Developmental followup data from the study of Watterberg, et al, should be available in late 2005.

PHARMACOLOGY: Hydrocortisone is the main adrenal corticosteroid, with primarily glucocorticoid effects. It increases the expression of adrenergic receptors in the vascular wall, thereby enhancing vascular reactivity to other vasoactive substances, such as norepinephrine and angiotensin II. Hypotensive babies who are cortisol deficient (< 15 mcg/dL) are most likely to respond, and blood pressure will increase within 2 hours of the first dose. Hydrocortisone also stimulates the liver to form glucose from amino acids and glycerol, and stimulates the deposition of glucose as glycogen. Peripheral glucose utilization is diminished, protein breakdown is increased, and lipolysis is activated. The net result is an increase in blood glucose levels. Renal effects include increased calcium excretion. The apparent half-life in premature infants is 9 hours.

SPECIAL CONSIDERATIONS/PREPARATION: Hydrocortisone sodium succinate is available as powder for injection in 2-mL vials containing 100 mg. Reconstitute using preservative-free sterile water for injection to 50 mg/mL (reconstituted solution contains 9 mg/mL benzyl alcohol). Also available in 2-, 4-, and 8-mL vials with a concentration of 125 mg/mL after reconstitution. Dilute with preservative-free normal saline or D$_5$W to a final concentration of 1 mg/mL. Dilution stable for 3 days refrigerated. Hydrocortisone sodium phosphate powder for injection is available in 2- and 10-mL vials with a concentration of 50 mg/mL reconstituted. Dilute with preservative-free normal saline or D$_5$W to a final concentration of 1 mg/mL. Dilution stable for 3 days refrigerated. Hydrocortisone acetate is not suitable for IV or IM administration.

Hydrocortisone phophate

Solution Compatibility: D$_5$W and NS.

Terminal Injection Site Compatibility: Fat emulsion. Amikacin, amphotericin B, aztreonam, fluconazole, metoclopramide, and sodium bicarbonate.

Hydrocortisone succinate

Solution Compatibility: D$_5$W, D$_{10}$W, and NS.

Ibuprofen Lysine

Terminal Injection Site Compatibility: Dex/AA solutions, fat emulsion. Acyclovir, amikacin, aminophylline, amphotericin B, ampicillin, atropine, aztreonam, calcium chloride, calcium gluconate, cefepime, chloramphenicol, clindamycin, dexamethasone, digoxin, dopamine, enalaprilat, epinephrine, erythromycin lactobionate, esmolol, famotidine, fentanyl, furosemide, heparin, hydralazine, insulin, isoproterenol, lidocaine, linezolid, lorazepam, magnesium, methicillin, metoclopramide, metronidazole, morphine, neostigmine, netilmicin, nicardipine, oxacillin, pancuronium, penicillin G, piperacillin, piperacillin-tazobactam, potassium chloride, procainamide, propofol, propranolol, prostaglandin E_1, remifentanil, sodium bicarbonate, vecuronium and vitamin K_1.

Incompatibility: Hydrocortisone succinate: Ciprofloxacin, midazolam, nafcillin, pentobarbital, phenobarbital, and phenytoin.

SELECTED REFERENCES

- Ng PC, Lee CH, Bnur FL, et al: A double-blind, randomized, controlled study of a "stress dose" of hydrocortisone for rescue treatment of refractory hypotension in preterm infants. *Pediatrics* 2006;117:367-375.
- Watterberg KL, Gerdes JS, Cole CH, et al: Prophylaxis of early adrenal insufficiency to prevent bronchopulmonary dysplasia: a multicenter trial. *Pediatrics* 2004;114:1649-1657.
- Fernandez E, Schrader R, Watterberg K: Prevalence of low cortisol values in term and near-term infants with vasopressor-resistant hypotension. *J Perinatol* 2004;25:114-118.
- Seri I, Tan R, Evans J: Cardiovascular effects of hydrocortisone in preterm infants with pressor-resistant hypotension. *Pediatrics* 2001;107:1070-1074.
- Botas CM, Kurlat I, Young SM, Sola A: Disseminated candidal infections and intravenous hydrocortisone in preterm infants. *Pediatrics* 1995;95:883.
- Briars GL, Bailey BJ: Surface area estimation: pocket calculator versus nomogram. *Arch Dis Child* 1994;70:246-247.

Ibuprofen Lysine

DOSE & ADMINISTRATION: First dose: 10 mg/kg. **Second and third** doses: 5 mg/kg. Administer IV by syringe pump over 15 minutes at 24 hour intervals.

USES: Closure of Patent Ductus Arteriosus. Not indicated for IVH prophylaxis.

MONITORING: Assess for ductal closure. Monitor urine output. Assess for signs of bleeding.

ADVERSE EFFECTS/PRECAUTIONS: NeoProfen® is contraindicated in preterm neonates with 1) infection, 2) active bleeding, 3) thrombocytopenia or coagulation defects, 4) NEC, 5) significant renal dysfunction, and 6) congenital heart disease with ductal-dependent systemic blood flow. Decreased urine output is less severe and occurs less frequently than with indomethacin. Although the available (and few) data suggest that the displacement of bilirubin from albumin is minimal with an ibuprofen dosing regimen of 10-5-5 mg /kg (q24hr), a more significant increase in unbound bilirubin can be expected in those infants with a high unconjugated bilirubin/albumin ratio and those in whom high ibuprofen concentrations are achieved. There is one recent case report of pulmonary hypertension in a 32 week gestation infant in Italy who received ibuprofen lysine (not NeoProfen) for treatment of PDA. Several studies have demonstrated an increased risk of oxygen dependency at 28 days postnatal age, but not 36 weeks PMA. Ibuprofen, like other nonsteroidal anti-inflammatory drugs, can inhibit platelet aggregation.

PHARMACOLOGY: NeoProfen® is a lysine salt solution of racemic ibuprofen, an inhibitor of prostaglandin synthesis. In adults (no data in neonates) metabolism is primarily via hydroxylation by hepatic CYP 2C9 and 2C8, with renal elimination of unchanged drug (10-15%) and metabolites. The mean half-life in premature neonates is approximately 43 hours, with large interpatient variability. Clearance increases rapidly with postnatal age and PDA closure.

SPECIAL CONSIDERATIONS/PREPARATION: Supplied as a 10 mg/mL sterile solution for injection in 2 mL single use vials. May be diluted prior to administration. Contains no preservatives and is not buffered. Administer within 30 minutes of preparation. The pH is adjusted to 7.0. Store at room temperature. **Protect from light**.

Solution Compatibility: NS, 0.45% NS, D5W, D10W, and LR.

Terminal Injection Site Compatibility: No data available.

SELECTED REFERENCES

- Aranda JV, et al. Multicentre randomized double-blind placebo controlled trial of ibuprofen L-lysine intravenous solution (IV ibuprofen) in premature infants for the early treatment of patent ductus arteriosus (PDA). Late-breaker Abstract presented at the Pediatric Academic Societies Annual Meeting, 2005.
- Capparelli EV, et al. Population pharmacokinetics of ibuprofen L-lysine during early treatment of patent ductus arteriosus in premature infants. Abstract 2863.253, Pediatric Academic Societies Annual Meeting, 2006.
- Ohlsson A, Walia R, Shah S. Ibuprofen for the treatment of patent ductus arteriosus in preterm and/or low birth weight infants. The Cochrane Database of Systematic Reviews 2005, Issue 4. Art. No.: CD003481. DOI: 10.1002/14651858.CD003481.pub2.
- Thomas RL, Parker GC, Van Overmeire B, Aranda JV. A meta-analysis of ibuprofen versus indomethacin for closure of patent ductus arteriosus. Eur J Pediatr 2005;164:135-140.
- Desfrere L, Zohar S, Morville P, et al. Dose-finding study of ibuprofen in patent ductus arteriosus using the continual reassessment method. J Clin Pharm Ther 2005;30:121-132.
- Van Overmeire B, Touw D, Schepens PJC, et al. Ibuprofen pharmacokinetics in preterm infants with patent ductus arteriosus. Clin Pharmacol Ther 2001;70:336-343.
- Bellini C, Campone F, Serra G. Pulmonary hypertension following L-lysine ibuprofen therapy in a preterm infant with patent ductus arteriosus. CMAJ 2006;174:1843-44.

IMIPENEM / CILASTATIN

DOSE & ADMINISTRATION: 20 to 25 mg/kg per dose Q12 hours IV infusion over 30 minutes.

USES: Restricted to treatment of non-CNS infections caused by bacteria, primarily Enterobacteriaceae and anaerobes, resistant to other antibiotics.

MONITORING: Periodic CBC and hepatic transaminases. Assess IV site for signs of phlebitis.

ADVERSE EFFECTS/PRECAUTIONS: Seizures occur frequently in patients with meningitis, preexisting CNS pathology, and severe renal dysfunction. Local reactions at the injection site and increased platelet counts are the most frequent adverse effects. Others including eosinophilia, elevated hepatic transaminases, and diarrhea also occur in more than 5% of patients.

PHARMACOLOGY: Imipenem is a broad-spectrum carbapenem antibiotic combined in a 1:1 ratio with cilastatin, a renal dipeptidase inhibitor with no intrinsic antibacterial activity. Bactericidal activity is due to inhibition of cell wall synthesis. Clearance is directly related to renal function. Serum half-life of imipenem in neonates is 2.5 hours; the half-life of cilastatin is 9 hours.

SPECIAL CONSIDERATIONS/PREPARATION: Available as powder for injection in 250-mg, and 500-mg vials. Reconstitute with 100 mL of compatible diluent. Maximum concentration 5 mg/mL. When reconstituted with NS, solution is stable for 10 hours at room temperature, 48 hours refrigerated. When reconstituted with other compatible diluents, solution is stable for 4 hours at room temperature or 24 hours refrigerated.

Solution Compatibility: D_5W, $D_{10}W$, and NS.

Terminal Injection Site Compatibility: Fat emulsion. Acyclovir, aztreonam, cefepime, famotidine, insulin, linezolid, midazolam, propofol, remifentanil, and zidovudine.

Incompatibility: Amikacin, amiodarone, azithromycin, fluconazole, gentamicin, lorazepam, milrinone, sodium bicarbonate, and tobramycin.

SELECTED REFERENCES

- Garges HP, Alexander KA: Newer antibiotics: imipenem/cilastatin and meropenem. NeoReviews 2003;4:e364-68.
- Stuart RL, Turnidge J, Grayson ML: Safety of imipenem in neonates. Pediatr Infect Dis J 1995;14:804.
- Reed MD, Kliegman RM, Yamashita TS, et al: Clinical pharmacology of imipenem and cilastatin in premature infants during the first week of life. Antimicrob Agents Chemother 1990;34:1172.
- Ahonkhai VI, Cyhan GM, Wilson SE, Brown KR: Imipenem-cilastatin in pediatric patients: and overview of safety and efficacy in studies conducted in the United States. Pediatr Infect Dis J 1989;8:740.
- Nalin DR, Jacobsen CA: Imipenem/cilastatin therapy for serious infections in neonates and infants. Scand J Infect Dis 1987;Suppl.2:46.

INDOMETHACIN

DOSE & ADMINISTRATION: IV infusion by syringe pump over at least 30 minutes to minimize adverse effects on cerebral, GI, and renal blood flow velocities. Usually three

INDOMETHACIN

doses per course, maximum two courses. Give at 12- to 24-hour intervals with close monitoring of urine output. If anuria or severe oliguria occurs, subsequent doses should be delayed. Longer treatment courses may be used: 0.2 mg/kg Q24 hours for a total of 5 to 7 days. **Prevention of IVH:** 0.1 mg/kg Q24 hours for 3 doses, beginning at 6 to 12 hours of age.

PDA Closure Dose (mg/kg)

Age at 1st dose	1st	2nd	3rd
< 48 h	0.2	0.1	0.1
2 to 7 d	0.2	0.2	0.2
> 7 d	0.2	0.25	0.25

USES: Closure of ductus arteriosus. Prevention of intraventricular hemorrhage.

MONITORING: Monitor urine output, serum electrolytes, glucose, creatinine and BUN, and platelet counts. Assess murmur, pulse pressure. Assess for GI bleeding by guaiacing stools and gastric aspirate. Observe for prolonged bleeding from puncture sites.

ADVERSE EFFECTS/PRECAUTIONS: If oliguria occurs, observe for hyponatremia and hypokalemia, and consider prolonging the dosing interval of renally excreted drugs (e.g. gentamicin). Consider withholding feedings. Hypoglycemia is common, usually preventable by increasing the glucose infusion rate by 2 mg/kg per minute. Causes platelet dysfunction. Contraindicated in active bleeding, significant thrombocytopenia or coagulation defects, necrotizing enterocolitis, and/or significantly impaired renal function. Rapid (<5-minute) infusions are associated with reductions in organ blood flow. Gastrointestinal perforations occur frequently if used concurrently with corticosteroids.

PHARMACOLOGY: Inhibitor of prostaglandin synthesis. Decreases cerebral, renal and GI blood flow. Metabolized in the liver to inactive compounds and excreted in the urine and feces. Serum half-life is approximately 30 hours, with a range of 15 to 50 hours, partially dependent on postnatal age. In most studies, the response of the ductus and adverse effects of indomethacin are only weakly correlated with plasma concentration.

SPECIAL CONSIDERATIONS/PREPARATION: Supplied as a lyophilized powder in 1-mg single dose vials. Indomethacin sodium trihydrate salt is not buffered, and is insoluble in solutions with pH <6.0; the manufacturer therefore recommends against continuous infusion in typical IV solutions. Reconstitute using 1 to 2 mL of preservative-free NS or sterile water for injection. Reconstituted indomethacin is stable in polypropylene syringes and glass vials for 12 days when stored at room temperature or refrigerated. Observe for precipitation.

Solution Compatibility: Sterile water for injection. (No visual precipitation in 24 hours): $D_{2.5}W$, D_5W, and NS.

Terminal Injection Site Compatibility: Furosemide, insulin, nitroprusside, potassium chloride, and sodium bicarbonate.

Incompatibility: $D_{7.5}W$, $D_{10}W$, Dex/AA. Calcium gluconate, cimetidine, dobutamine, dopamine, gentamicin, and, tobramycin.

SELECTED REFERENCES

- Fowlie PW, Davis PG: Prophylactic indomethacin for preterm infants: a systematic review and meta-analysis. Arch Dis Child Fetal Neonatal Ed 2003;88:F464-66.
- Itabashi K, Ohno T, Nishida H: Indomethacin responsiveness of patent ductus arteriosus and renal abnormalities in preterm infants treated with indomethacin. J Pediatr 2003;143:203-7.
- Clyman RI: Recommendations for the postnatal use of indomethacin: an analysis of four separate treatment strategies. J Pediatr 1996;128:601.
- Hammerman C, Aramburo MJ: Prolonged indomethacin therapy for the prevention of recurrences of patent ductus arteriosus. J Pediatr 1990;117:771.
- Hosono S, Ohono T, Kimoto H: Preventative management of hypoglycemia in very low-birthweight infants following indomethacin therapy for patent ductus arteriosus. Pediatr Internat 2001;43:465-468.
- Coombs RC, Morgan MEI, Durbin GM, et al: Gut blood flow velocities in the newborn: Effects of patent ductus arteriosus and parenteral indomethacin. Arch Dis Child 1990;65:1067.
- Colditz P, Murphy D, Rolfe P, Wilkinson AR: Effect of infusion rate of indomethacin on cerebrovascular responses in preterm infants. Arch Dis Child 1989;64:8.
- Walker SE, Gray S, Schmidt B: Stability of reconstituted indomethacin sodium trihydrate in original vials and polypropylene syringes. Am J Health-Syst Pharm 1998;15:154.

- Ishisaka DY, Van Vleet J, Marquardt E: Visual compatibility of indomethacin sodium trihydrate with drugs given to neonates by continuous infusion. *Am J Hosp Pharm* 1991;48:2442.
- Gersony WM, Peckham GJ, Ellison RC, et al: Effects of indomethacin in premature infants with patent ductus arteriosus: Results of a national collaborative study. *J Pediatr* 1983;102:895.
- Brash AR, Hickey DE, Graham TP, et al: Pharmacokinetics of indomethacin in the neonate: Relation of plasma indomethacin levels to response of the ductus arteriosus. *N Engl J Med* 1981;305:67.
- Yaffe SJ, Friedmann WF, Rogers D, et al: The disposition of indomethacin in preterm babies. *J Pediatr* 1980;97:1001.
- Schmidt B, Davis P, Moddeman D, et al: Long-term effects of indomethacin prophylaxis in extremely-low-birth-weight infants. *N Engl J Med* 2001; 344:1966-1972.
- Ment LR, Oh W, Ehrenkranz RA, et al: Low-dose indomethacin and prevention of intraventricular hemorrhage: A multicenter randomized trial. *Pediatrics* 1994;93:543.

INFASURF®

(Calfactant) Intratracheal Suspension

DOSE & ADMINISTRATION: Initial dose is 3 mL/kg per dose intratracheally, divided into 2 aliquots followed by up to three subsequent doses of 3 mL/kg per dose administered at 12-hour intervals if needed. Clear the trachea of secretions. Shorten a 5F end-hole catheter so the tip of the catheter will protrude just beyond end of ET tube above infant's carina. Slowly withdraw entire contents of vial into a plastic syringe through a large (greater than 20 gauge) needle. **Do not filter or shake.** Attach shortened catheter to syringe. Fill catheter with surfactant. Discard excess through catheter so only total dose to be given remains in syringe. Administer in two to four aliquots with the infant in different positions to enhance distribution in the lungs. The catheter can be inserted into the infant's endotracheal tube without interrupting ventilation by passing the catheter through a neonatal suction valve attached to the endotracheal tube. Alternatively, surfactant can be instilled through the catheter by briefly disconnecting the endotracheal tube from the ventilator. After administration of each aliquot, the dosing catheter is removed from the ET tube and the infant is ventilated for at least 30 seconds until stable.

PHARMACOLOGY: Pulmonary lung surfactants are essential for effective ventilation by modifying alveolar surface tension thereby stabilizing the alveoli. Infasurf® is a sterile, non-pyrogenic natural surfactant extracted from calf lungs containing phospholipids, neutral lipids, fatty acids, and surfactant-associated proteins B and C. Preservative free. Each mL of Infasurf® contains 35 mg of total phospholipids (26 mg of phosphatidylcholine of which 16 mg is disaturated phosphatidylcholine) and 0.65 mg of proteins including 0.26 mg of SP-B.

SPECIAL CONSIDERATIONS/PREPARATION: Available in 3-mL and 6-mL single-use vials. Refrigerate (2 °C to 8 °C (36 °F to 46 °F)) and protect from light. Inspect Infasurf® for discoloration; normal color is off-white. If settling occurs during storage, gently swirl vial in order to uniformly suspend. **Do not shake.** Used vials with residual drug should be discarded. Unopened vials that have been warmed to room temperature one time may be refrigerated within 24 hours and stored for future use.

SELECTED REFERENCES

- Bloom BT, Kattwinkel J, Hall RT, et al: Comparison of Infasurf® (calf lung surfactant extract) to Survanta (beractant) in the treatment and prevention of respiratory distress syndrome. *Pediatrics* 1997;100:31-38.
- Hudak ML, Farrell EE, Rosenberg AA, et al: A multicenter randomized, masked comparison trial of natural versus synthetic surfactant for the treatment of respiratory distress syndrome. *J Pediatr* 1996;128:396-406.
- Kendig JW, Ryan RM, Sinkin RA, et al: Comparison of two strategies for surfactant prophylaxis in very premature infants: A multicenter randomized trial. *Pediatrics* 1998;101:1006-1012.

INFUVITE™ PEDIATRIC

Infuvite™ *Pediatric*, Multiple Vitamins of Infusion

DOSE & ADMINISTRATION: IV administration: Infuvite® *Pediatric* is a sterile product consisting of two vials: a 4 mL vial labeled **Vial 1** and a 1 mL vial labeled **Vial 2**. The daily dose is a function of infant weight as indicated in the following table. **Do not exceed this daily dose.**

INSULIN

WEIGHT OF INFANT

	< 1 kg	≥ 1 kg and < 3 kg	≥ 3 kg
Vial 1	1.2 mL	2.6 mL	4 mL
Vial 2	0.3 mL	0.65 mL	1 mL

PHARMACOLOGY:

INFUVITE™ PEDIATRIC

Vial 1 (4 mL)	Amount*
Vitamin A** (as palmitate)	2300 IU (0.7 mg)
Vitamin D** (IU) (cholecalciferol)	400 IU (10 mcg)
Ascorbic Acid (vitamin C)	80 mg
Vitamin E** (dl-alpha tocopheryl acetate)	7 IU (7 mg)
Thiamine (as hydrochloride) B_1	1.2 mg
Riboflavin (as phosphate) B_2	1.4 mg
Niacinamide B_3	17 mg
Pyridoxine hydrochloride B_6	1 mg
d-Panthenol	5 mg
Vitamin K_1**	0.2 mg
Vial 2 (1 mL)	
Biotin	20 mcg
Folic Acid	140 mcg
Vitamin B_{12} (cyanocobalamin)	1 mcg

* Amounts based upon guidelines published by the American Medical. Association Department of Foods and Nutrition, JPEN 3(4);25862:1979.
Vial 1 (4 mL) Inactive ingredients: 50 mg polysorbate 80, sodium hydroxide and/or hydrochloric acid for pH adjustment and water for injection.
** Polysorbate 80 is used to water solubilize the oil-soluble vitamins A, D, E, and K.
Vial 2 (1 mL) Inactive ingredients: 75 mg mannitol, citric acid and/or sodium citrate for pH adjustment and water for injection.

ADVERSE EFFECTS/PRECAUTIONS: Warnings: INFUVITE™ Pediatric is administered in intravenous solutions, which may contain aluminum that may be toxic. Aluminum may reach toxic levels with prolonged parenteral administration if kidney function is impaired. Premature neonates are particularly at risk because their kidneys are immature, and they require large amounts of calcium and phosphate solution, which contain aluminum. Research indicates that patients with impaired kidney function, including premature neonates who receive parenteral levels of aluminum at greater than 4 to 5 mcg/kg per day accumulate aluminum at levels associated with central nervous system and bone toxicity. Tissue loading may occur at even lower rates of administration.

SPECIAL CONSIDERATIONS/PREPARATION: After INFUVITE™ Pediatric is diluted in an intravenous infusion, the resulting solution is ready for immediate use. Inspect visually for particulate matter and discoloration prior to administration, whenever solution and container permit. Exposure to light should be minimized. Discard any unused portion. **Store between 2-8 °C (36-46 °F).**

Incompatibility: Alkaline solutions or moderately alkaline drugs: acetazolamide, aminophylline, ampicillin, and chlorothiazide. Direct addition to intravenous fat emulsions is not recommended.

SELECTED REFERENCES
- Product Information, Baxter Clinitec 2001

INSULIN

DOSE & ADMINISTRATION: Continuous IV infusion: 0.01 to 0.1 Unit/kg per hour. (Only regular insulin for injection may be administered intravenously.) To saturate plastic tubing binding sites, fill IV tubing with insulin solution and wait for at least 20 minutes before infusing. The use of higher insulin concentrations and longer wait times will shorten the time to steady-state. Titrate using blood glucose concentration/reagent strips. **Intermittent dose:** 0.1 to 0.2 Unit/kg Q6 to 12 hours subQ.

USES: Treatment of VLBW hyperglycemic infants with persistent glucose intolerance. Adjuvant therapy for hyperkalemia.

MONITORING: Follow blood glucose concentration frequently (Q15 to 30 minutes) after starting insulin infusion and after changes in infusion rate.

ADVERSE EFFECTS/PRECAUTIONS: May rapidly induce hypoglycemia. Insulin resistance may develop, causing a larger dose requirement. Euglycemic hyperinsulinemia due to exogenous insulin administration may cause metabolic acidosis.

PHARMACOLOGY: Insulin is degraded in liver and kidney. Enhances cellular uptake of glucose, conversion of glucose to glycogen, amino acid uptake by muscle tissue, synthesis of fat, and cellular uptake of potassium. Inhibits lipolysis and conversion of protein to glucose. Plasma half-life in adults is 9 minutes.

SPECIAL CONSIDERATIONS/PREPARATION: Regular human insulin (rDNA origin) is available as 100 Unit/mL concentration in 10-mL vials. For subcutaneous administration, dilute with sterile water or NS to a concentration of 0.5 or 1 Unit/mL. For IV administration, make a 10 Unit/mL dilution with sterile water, then further dilute in compatible solution to a concentration of 0.05 to 0.2 Unit/mL. **Keep refrigerated.**

Solution Compatibility: D_5W, and $D_{10}W$, and NS.

Terminal Injection Site Compatibility: Dex/AA solutions, fat emulsion. Amiodarone, ampicillin, aztreonam, cefazolin, cefoxitin, cimetidine, digoxin, dobutamine, esmolol, famotidine, gentamicin, heparin, hydrocortisone succinate, imipenem, indomethacin, lidocaine, meropenem, metoclopramide, midazolam, milrinone, morphine, nitroglycerin, pentobarbital, potassium chloride, propofol, ranitidine, sodium bicarbonate, sodium nitroprusside, ticarcillin/clavulanate, tobramycin, and vancomycin.

Incompatibility: Aminophylline, dopamine, nafcillin, phenobarbital, and phenytoin.

SELECTED REFERENCES

- Mena P, Llanos A, Uauy R: Insulin homeostasis in the extremely low birth weight infant. *Semin Perinatol* 2001;25:436-446.
- Fuloria M, Friedberg MA, DuRant RH, Aschner JL: Effect of flow rate and insulin priming on the recovery of insulin from microbore infusion tubing. *Pediatrics* 1998;102:1401-1406.
- Poindexter BB, Karn CA, Denne SC: Exogenous insulin reduces proteolysis and protein synthesis in extremely low birth weight infants. *J Pediatr* 1998;132:948-953.
- Ostertag SG, Jovanovic L, Lewis B, Auld PAM: Insulin pump therapy in the very low birth weight infant. *Pediatrics* 1986;78:625.

INTRAVENOUS IMMUNE GLOBULIN (HUMAN)

DOSE & ADMINISTRATION: Usual dosage: 500 to 750 mg/kg per dose over 2 to 6 hours. For neonatal alloimmune thrombocytopenia, doses have ranged from 400 mg/kg to 1 gram/kg. Most studies have used a single dose, although additional doses have been given at 24 hour intervals. See *Special Considerations/Preparation* for product-specific information.

USES: Adjuvant treatment of fulminant neonatal sepsis, hemolytic jaundice, and neonatal alloimmune thrombocytopenia.

MONITORING: Frequent monitoring of heart rate and blood pressure. Check IV site for signs of phlebitis.

ADVERSE EFFECTS/PRECAUTIONS: Rare cases of hypoglycemia, transient tachycardia, and hypotension that resolved after stopping the infusion have been reported. No short-term or long-term adverse effects have been reported in neonates. Animal studies have demonstrated reticuloendothelial system blockade when higher doses (>1 g/kg) have been used. All donor units are nonreactive to HBsAg and HIV. The manufacturing process of these products now includes a solvent/detergent treatment to inactivate hepatitis C and other membrane-enveloped viruses.

PHARMACOLOGY: IVIG is a plasma-derived, concentrated form of IgG antibodies present in the donor population. Significant lot-to-lot variation of specific antibodies may occur with all products. No significant differences in clinical outcomes using the different products have been seen. All preparations are reported to contain more than 92% IgG monomers and a normal distribution of IgG subclasses. Total IgG titers in treated, septic neonates remain elevated for approximately 10 days.

SPECIAL CONSIDERATIONS/PREPARATION: Reconstitute lyophilized products with supplied diluent. All products are preservative-free. Shelf life varies, but is at least 2 years when stored properly.

IVIG Preparations

Brand	Form	Storage	Preparation*
Gamunex (Bayer)	10% solution, pH 4.25	Refrigerate Do not freeze	Allow to come to room temperature.
Flebogamma 5% (Grifols)	10, 50, 100, and 200 mL vials 50 mg/mL, 5% solution	Room temperature	Rotate gently. Preservative-free.
Octagam (Octapharma)	1, 2.5, 5, and 10 g vials 5% solution	Room temperature	5% solution. Do not shake.
Gammar®-P (Sanofi-Aventis)	1, 2.5, 5, and 10 g vials 5% sucrose, pH 6.8	Room temperature Do not freeze	5% solution. Preservative-free.
Panglobulin® (American Red Cross)	12 g vial sucrose, pH 6.8	Room temperature	5% solution. Preservative-free.
Carimune NF (ZLB Bioplasma)	1, 3, 6, and 12 g vials	Refrigerate	Preservative-free.
Polygam®, S/D (American Red Cross)	2.5, 5, and 10 g vials 5% glucose, pH 6.8	Room temperature	5% and 10% solution. Preservative-free.
Panglobulin NF (American Red Cross)	1, 3, 6, and 12 g vials	Refrigerate	Preservative-free.

* Reconstitute lyophilized products with supplied diluent. All products are preservative free. Shelf life varies, but is at least 2 years, when stored properly.

Solution Compatibility: D_5W, $D_{15}W$, and Dex/AA.

Terminal Injection Site Compatibility: Fluconazole.

SELECTED REFERENCES

- Sandberg K, Fasth A, Berger A, et al: Preterm infants with low immunoglobulin G levels have increased risk for neonatal sepsis but do not benefit from prophylactic immunoglobulin G. J Pediatr 2000;137:623-628.
- Jensen HB, Pollock BH: Meta-analyses of the effectiveness of intravenous immune globulin for prevention and treatment of neonatal sepsis. Pediatrics 1997;99(2):e2.
- Blanchette VS, Rand ML: Platelet disorders in newborn infants: diagnosis and management. Semin Perinatol 1997;21:53-62.
- Weisman LE, Stoll BJ, Kueser TJ: Intravenous immunoglobulin therapy for early-onset sepsis in premature neonates. J Pediatr 1992;121:434.
- Christensen RD, Brown MS, Hall DC, et al: Effect on neutrophil kinetics and serum opsonic capacity of intravenous administration of immune globulin to neonates with clinical signs of early-onset sepsis. J Pediatr 1991;118:606.
- Gottstein R, Cooke RWI: Systematic review of intravenous immunoglobulin in haemolytic disease of the newborn. Arch Dis Child Fetal Neonatal Ed 2003;88:F6-F10.
- Tanyer G, Suklar Z, Dallar Y, et al: Multiple dose IVIG treatment of neonatal immune hemolytic jaundice. J Trop Pediatr 2001:47:50-53.

IPRATROPIUM

DOSE & ADMINISTRATION: Administer Q6 to 8 hours as nebulized solution. Doses studied in intubated neonates range from 36 to 72 mcg via metered dose inhaler (MDI) with spacer, and 75 to 175 mcg via jet nebulizer. Studies in adults indicate that approximately 10% of an MDI dose, versus 1 to 2% of a nebulizer dose, is delivered to the lung. MDI devices are not recommended for use in infants with tidal volumes less than 100 mL because of safety concerns: Potentially hypoxic mixture of ventilator gas and propellant, and unknown hazards of exposure to chlorofluorocarbons. Optimal dose in neonates has yet to be determined due to differences in aerosol drug delivery techniques, although the therapeutic margin appears to be wide.

USES: Anticholinergic bronchodilator for primary treatment of chronic obstructive pulmonary diseases and adjunctive treatment of acute bronchospasm. Ipratropium is not useful in the treatment of bronchiolitis.

MONITORING: Assess degree of bronchospasm.

ADVERSE EFFECTS/PRECAUTIONS: Temporary blurring of vision, precipitation of narrow-angle glaucoma, or eye pain may occur if solution comes into direct contact with the eyes.

PHARMACOLOGY: Ipratropium bromide is a quaternary ammonium derivative of atropine. It produces primarily large airway bronchodilation by antagonizing the action of acetylcholine at its receptor site. It is relatively bronchospecific when administered by inhalation because of limited absorption through lung tissue. Peak effect occurs 1 to 2 hours after administration. Duration of effect is 4 to 6 hours in children. The combination of ipratropium with a beta-agonist produces more bronchodilation than either drug individually.

SPECIAL CONSIDERATIONS/PREPARATION: Inhalation solution is supplied in 2.5-mL vials, containing ipratropium bromide 0.02% (200 mcg/mL) in a sterile, preservative-free, isotonic saline solution that is pH-adjusted to 3.4 with hydrochloric acid. It may be mixed with albuterol if used within 1 hour. Compatibility data are not currently available with other drugs. Store at room temperature in foil pouch provided. Protect from light.

SELECTED REFERENCES

- Lee H, Arnon S, Silverman M: Bronchodilator aerosol administered by metered dose inhaler and spacer in subacute neonatal respiratory distress syndrome. *Arch Dis Child* 1994;70:F218.
- Consensus Conference in Aerosol Delivery: Aerosol Consensus Statement. *Respir Care* 1991;36:916.
- Brundage KL, Mohsini KJ Froese AB, Fisher JT: Bronchodilator response to ipratropium bromide in infants with bronchopulmonary dysplasia. *Am Rev Respir Dis* 1990;142:1137.
- Gross NJ: Ipratropium bromide. *N Engl J Med* 1988;319:486.

IRON DEXTRAN

DOSE & ADMINISTRATION: 0.4 to 1 mg/kg (400 to 1000 mcg/kg) per day IV continuous infusion in Dex/AA solutions containing at least 2% amino acids.

USES: Iron supplementation in patients unable to tolerate oral iron, especially those also being treated with erythropoietin.

MONITORING: Periodic CBC and reticulocyte count. Observe Dex/AA solution for rust-colored precipitates.

ADVERSE EFFECTS/PRECAUTIONS: No adverse effects have been observed in patients who have received low doses infused continuously. Large (50 mg) intramuscular doses administered to infants were associated with increased risk of infection. Retrospective reviews of adult patients who received larger doses injected over a few minutes report a 0.7% risk of immediate serious allergic reactions, and a 5% risk of delayed such as myalgia, arthralgia, phlebitis, and lymphadenopathy.

PHARMACOLOGY: Iron dextran for intravenous use is a complex of ferric hydroxide and low molecular mass dextran. The dextran serves as a protective lipophilic colloid. Radiolabeled iron dextran injected into adult subjects localized to the liver and spleen before being incorporated into RBC hemoglobin. Complete clearance occurred by 3 days. Approximately 40% of the labeled iron was bound to transferrin within 11 hours. The addition of iron dextran to Dex/AA solutions inhibits the spontaneous generation of peroxides.

SPECIAL CONSIDERATIONS/PREPARATION: Available as a 50 mg/mL concentration in 2-mL single-dose vials. Store at room temperature. ***Mix only in Dex/AA solutions containing at least 2% amino acids.**

SELECTED REFERENCES

- Mayhew SL, Quick MW: Compatibility of iron dextran with neonatal parenteral nutrition solutions. *Am J Health-Syst Pharm* 1997;54:570-1.
- Lavoie J-C, Chessex P: Bound iron admixture prevents the spontaneous generation of peroxides in total parenteral nutrition solutions. *J Pediatr Gastroenterol Nutr* 1997;25:307-11.
- Friel JK, Andrews WL, Hall MS, et al: Intravenous iron administration to very-low-birth-weight newborns receiving total and partial parenteral nutrition. *JPEN* 1995;19:114-18.
- Burns DL, Mascioli EA, Bistrian BR: Parenteral iron dextran therapy: a review. *Nutrition* 1995;11:163-68.
- Kanakakorn K, Cavill I, Jacobs A: The metabolism of intravenously administered iron-dextran. *Br J Haematol* 1973;25:637-43.

ISOPROTERENOL

DOSE & ADMINISTRATION: 0.05 to 0.5 mcg/kg per minute continuous IV infusion. Maximum dose 2 mcg/kg per minute. Dosage often titrated according to heart rate. Acidosis should be corrected before infusion.

USES: Increases cardiac output in patients with cardiovascular shock. Pulmonary vasodilator (older infants).

MONITORING: Continuous vital signs, intra-arterial blood pressure, CVP monitoring preferable. Periodic blood glucose reagent strips.

ADVERSE EFFECTS/PRECAUTIONS: Cardiac arrhythmias. Tachycardia severe enough to cause CHF. Decreases venous return to heart. Systemic vasodilation. May cause hypoxemia by increasing intrapulmonary shunt. Hypoglycemia.

PHARMACOLOGY: β-receptor stimulant, sympathomimetic. Increases cardiac output by 1) increasing rate (major) and 2) increasing strength of contractions (minor). Insulin secretion is stimulated. Afterload reduction via $β_2$ effects on arterioles.

SPECIAL CONSIDERATIONS/PREPARATION: Supplied as 0.2-mg/mL (1:5000) solution in 1-mL and 5-mL vials.

Solution Compatibility: D_5W, $D_{10}W$, and NS.

Terminal Injection Site Compatibility: Dex/AA solutions, fat emulsion. Aminophylline, amiodarone, caffeine citrate, calcium chloride, calcium gluceptate, calcium gluconate, cimetidine, dobutamine, famotidine, heparin, hydrocortisone succinate, milrinone, netilmicin, nitroprusside, pancuronium bromide, potassium chloride, propofol, prostaglandin E_1, ranitidine, remifentanil, and vecuronium.

Incompatibility: Furosemide and sodium bicarbonate.

Administration Calculations

To calculate the **AMOUNT** of drug needed per **50 mL** infusion solution:

$$3 \times \frac{\text{desired dose } (mcg/kg/min)}{\text{desired fluid rate } (mL/hr)} \times \text{weight } (kg) = \text{mg of isoproterenol}$$

To calculate the **VOLUME** of drug needed per **50 mL** infusion solution:

$$\frac{\text{mg of drug (found using equation above)}}{\text{concentration of drug } (mg/mL)} = \text{mL of isoproterenol}$$

Example: 2-kg infant to receive isoproterenol 0.1 mcg/kg per minute at infusion rate of 1 mL per hour. Concentration of isoproterenol solution is 0.2 mg/mL.

$$3 \times \frac{0.1 \text{ mcg/kg/min}}{1 \text{ mL/hr}} \times 2 \text{ kg} = 0.6 \text{ mg of isoproterenol in 50 mL of infusion solution}$$

$$\frac{0.6 \text{ mg of isoproterenol}}{0.2 \text{ mg/mL}} = 3 \text{ mL of isoproterenol in 50 mL of infusion solution}$$

Add 3 mL isoproterenol (0.2 mg/mL) to 47 mL of compatible solution (e.g. D_5W) to yield 50 mL of isoproterenol infusion with a concentration of 12 mcg/mL.

Maximum concentration is 20 mcg/mL.

SELECTED REFERENCES

- Cabal LA, Devaskar U, Siassi B, et al: Cardiogenic shock associated with perinatal asphyxia in preterm infants. *J Pediatr* 1980;96:705.
- Daoud FS, Reeves JT, Kelly DB: Isoproterenol as a potential pulmonary vasodilator in primary pulmonary hypertension. *Am J Cardiol* 1978;42:817.

LAMIVUDINE (3TC)

DOSE & ADMINISTRATION: PO: 2 mg/kg per dose Q12 hours for one week following birth.

USES: Used **only** in combination with zidovudine in the treatment of neonates born to HIV-infected women who have had no therapy during pregnancy. (Mother receives oral ZDV and 3TC during labor.) Dosing guidelines above are for prophylactic treatment of neonates born to HIV-infected women. Treatment of infected infants using drug combination regimens should be done in consultation with pediatric infectious disease experts.

MONITORING: Specific monitoring unnecessary due to short treatment course.

ADVERSE EFFECTS/PRECAUTIONS: Generally well tolerated - limited data in neonates.

PHARMACOLOGY: Lamivudine (3TC) is a synthetic nucleoside analog "prodrug" that inhibits HIV replication by interfering with viral reverse transcriptase. It is intracellularly converted in several steps to the active compound, then renally excreted. Poor CNS penetration, CSF:plasma ratio is 1:100. The oral solution is well-absorbed, with 66% bioavailability in children. The serum half-life in preterm infants less than 33 weeks gestation is approximately 14 hours. Viral resistance develops rapidly to monotherapy with lamivudine (3TC). TMP-SMX increases lamivudine blood levels (significance unknown).

SPECIAL CONSIDERATIONS/PREPARATION: Available as an oral solution in concentrations of 5 mg/mL (Epivir-HBV®) and 10 mg/mL (Epivir®). Store at room temperature and protected from light.

SELECTED REFERENCES

- Perinatal HIV Guidelines Working Group. Public Health Service Task Force Recommendations for Use of Antiretroviral Drugs in Pregnant HIV-1 Infected Women for Maternal Health and Interventions to Reduce Perinatal HIV-1 Transmission in the United States. October 12, 2006. Available at http://aidsinfo.nih.gov/ContentFiles/PerinatalGL.pdf.
- Mueller BU, Lewis LL, Yuen GJ, et al: Serum and cerebrospinal fluid pharmacokinetics of intravenous and oral lamivudine in human immunodeficiency virus-infected children. *Antimicrob Agents Chemother* 1998;42:3187-3192.
- Moodley J, Moodley D, Pillay K, et al: Pharmacokinetics and antiretroviral activity of lamivudine alone or when coadministered with zidovudine in human immunodeficiency virus type 1-infected pregnant women and their offspring. *J Infect Dis* 1998;178:1327-1333.
- Paediatric European Network for Treatment of AIDS: A randomized double-blind trial of the addition of lamivudine or matching placebo to current nucleoside analogue reverse transcriptase inhibitor therapy in HIV-infected children: the PENTA-4 trial. *AIDS* 1998;12:F151-F160.
- Horneff G, Adams O, Wahn V: Pilot study of zidovudine-lamivudine combination therapy in vertically HIV-infected antiretroviral-naive children. *AIDS* 1998;12:489-494.

LANSOPRAZOLE

DOSE & ADMINISTRATION: 0.73 to 1.66 mg/kg per dose PO, once a day. See Special Considerations/Preparation for preparation.

USES: Treatment of reflux esophagitis.

MONITORING: Observe for symptomatic improvement within 3 days. Consider intraesophageal pH monitoring to assess for efficacy (pH >4.0). Measure AST and ALT if duration of therapy is greater than 8 weeks.

ADVERSE EFFECTS/PRECAUTIONS: Hypergastrinemia and mild transaminase elevations are the only Adverse Effects reported in children who received lansoprazole for extended periods of time. Available data are limited to small studies of infants and children.

PHARMACOLOGY: Lansoprazole inhibits gastric acid secretion by inhibition of hydrogen-potassium ATPase, the enzyme responsible for the final step in the secretion of hydrochloric acid by the gastric parietal cell ("proton pump"). Extensively metabolized in the liver by CYP 2C19 and 3A4. Onset of action is within one hour of administration, maximal effect is at approximately 1.5 hours. Average elimination half-life is 1.5 hours. Inhibition of acid secretion is about 50% of maximum at 24 hours and the duration of action is approximately 72 hours. The absorption of weakly acidic drugs (e.g., digoxin, furosemide) is enhanced. The absorption of weakly basic drugs (e.g., ketoconazole) is inhibited.

Levothyroxine (T₄)

SPECIAL CONSIDERATIONS/PREPARATION: Prevacid® is supplied in packets for oral suspension containing either 15 mg or 30 mg lansoprazole as enteric-coated granules, and delayed-release capsules. For patients able to drink, prepare the oral suspension as follows: empty the packet contents into a container containing 30 mL of water. Stir well. Draw up the patient-specific dose and administer immediately after mixing. Do not administer the oral suspension via enteral tubes. For administration via nasogastric tube, use the capsules. Open the capsule and mix thoroughly in 30 mL of apple juice. Do not use other liquids. Immediately draw up the patient-specific dose and inject through the NG tube into the stomach. After administering the granules, flush the NG tube with additional apple juice to clear the tube.

Incompatibility: Procainamide.

SELECTED REFERENCES

- Gibbons TE, Gold BD: The use of proton pump inhibitors in children: a comprehensive review. *Paediatr Drugs* 2003;5:25-40.
- Scott LJ: Lansoprazole in the management of gastroesophageal reflux disease in children. *Paediatr Drugs* 2003;5:57-61.
- Tran A, Rey E, Pons G, Pariente-Khayat A, et al: Pharmacokinetic-pharmacodynamic study of oral lansoprazole in children. *Clin Pharmacol Ther* 2002;71:359-67.
- Franco M, Salvia G, Terrin G, Spadaro R, et al: Lansoprazole in the treatment of gastro-oesophageal reflux disease in childhood. *Dig Liver Dis* 2000;32:660-6.
- Product information, TAP Pharmaceuticals, 2004.

Levothyroxine (T₄)

DOSE & ADMINISTRATION: Initial oral dose: 10 to 14 mcg/kg per dose PO Q24 hours. (37.5 to 50 mcg/dose for an average term infant). Dosage is adjusted in 12.5-mcg increments. Always round upward. **Initial IV dose:** 5 to 8 mcg/kg per dose Q24 hours.

USES: Treatment of hypothyroidism.

MONITORING: After 2 weeks of treatment, serum levothyroxine (T_4) concentration should be in the high normal range—10 to 16 mcg/dL—and should be maintained in this range for the first year of life. Serum triiodothyronine (T_3) concentration should be normal (70 to 220 ng/dL), and TSH should have declined from initial value. After 12 weeks of treatment, serum TSH concentration should be in the normal range, less than 15 mU/L. Serum T_4 and TSH concentrations should be measured at two weeks of age, then every 1 to 2 months, or 2 weeks after any change in dosage. Assess for signs of hypothyroidism: Lethargy, poor feeding, constipation, intermittent cyanosis, and prolonged neonatal jaundice. Assess for signs of thyrotoxicosis: hyperreactivity, altered sleep pattern, tachycardia, tachypnea, fever, exophthalmos, and goiter. Periodically assess growth, development, and bone-age advancement.

ADVERSE EFFECTS/PRECAUTIONS: Prolonged overtreatment can produce premature craniosynostosis and acceleration of bone age.

PHARMACOLOGY: Tissue deiodination converts T_4 to T_3, the active metabolite. Elimination of both T_4 and T_3 is equally in the urine and feces. Clinical effects will persist for 1 week after discontinuation of the drug. Levothyroxine prepared as an oral suspension is 50% to 80% bioavailable. Oral dosing produces effects within 3 to 5 days, while IV dosing produces effects in 6 to 8 hours.

SPECIAL CONSIDERATIONS/PREPARATION: Oral suspension is not commercially available. Available as scored tablets ranging from 25 to 300 mcg per tablet. Prepare oral dosage form by crushing tablet(s) and suspending in a small amount of sterile water, breast milk, or non-soy formula. **Use immediately.** Monitor patients closely when switching brand of drug, due to some differences in bioavailability. **The injectable form should not be given orally,** as it crystallizes when exposed to acid. Injectable form is available as lyophilized powder in vials containing 200 or 500 mcg. **Use only NS for reconstitution.** Manufacturer's suggested final concentrations are 40 mcg/mL or 100 mcg/mL; however, we suggest diluting to a final concentration of 20 mcg/mL. **Use immediately. Do not add to any other IV solution.**

SELECTED REFERENCES

- Selva KA, Mandel SH, Rien L, et al: Initial treatment of L-thyroxine in congenital hypothyroidism. *J Pediatr* 2002;141:786-92.
- AAP Section on Endocrinology and Committee on Genetics, and Committee on Public Health, American Thyroid Association: Newborn screening for congenital hypothyroidism: Recommended guidelines. *Pediatrics* 1993;91:1203-1209.
- Germak JA, Foley TP: Longitudinal assessment of L-thyroxine therapy for congenital hypothyroidism. *J Pediatr* 1990;117:211.

LIDOCAINE - ANTIARRHYTHMIC

DOSE & ADMINISTRATION: Initial bolus dose: 0.5 to 1 mg/kg IV push over 5 minutes. Repeat Q10 minutes as necessary to control arrhythmia. Maximum total bolus dose should not exceed 5 mg/kg. **Maintenance IV infusion:** 10 to 50 mcg/kg per minute. Premature neonates should receive lowest dosage.

USES: Short-term control of ventricular arrhythmias, including ventricular tachycardia, premature ventricular contractions, and arrhythmias resulting from digitalis intoxication.

MONITORING: Continuous monitoring of EKG, heart rate, and blood pressure. Assess level of consciousness. Observe for seizure activity. Therapeutic total lidocaine serum concentrations are 1 to 5 mcg/mL.

ADVERSE EFFECTS/PRECAUTIONS: Early signs of CNS toxicity are drowsiness, agitation, vomiting, and muscle twitching. Later signs include seizures, loss of consciousness, respiratory depression, and apnea. Cardiac toxicity is associated with excessive doses and includes bradycardia, hypotension, heart block, and cardiovascular collapse. **Contraindicated in infants with cardiac failure and heart block.** Serum lidocaine concentrations increase when using either cimetidine or propranolol in combination.

PHARMACOLOGY: Lidocaine is a Type 1b antiarrhythmic agent used intravenously. Onset of action is 1 to 2 minutes after bolus administration. Plasma half-life in neonates is 3 hours. Free drug fraction in both term and premature neonates is approximately twice that found in older children because of significantly reduced protein binding by α_1-acid glycoprotein. Transformed in the liver to metabolites with antiarrhythmic activity; approximately 30% is excreted unchanged in neonates.

SPECIAL CONSIDERATIONS/PREPARATION: Use only preservative-free lidocaine without epinephrine. Available in multiple concentrations ranging from 1% to 20%. To make a dilution for bolus dosing, dilute 10 mg lidocaine (0.5 mL of 2% solution) in 9.5 mL NS or D_5W, yielding a 1 mg/mL final concentration.

Solution Compatibility: D_5W, $D_{10}W$, and NS.

Terminal Injection Site Compatibility: Dex/AA solutions, fat emulsion. Alteplase, aminophylline, amiodarone, ampicillin, caffeine citrate, calcium chloride, calcium gluconate, cefazolin, cefoxitin, ceftriaxone, chloramphenicol, cimetidine, dexamethasone, digoxin, dobutamine, dopamine, enalaprilat, erythromycin lactobionate, esmolol, famotidine, fentanyl, flumazenil, furosemide, glycopyrrolate, heparin, hydrocortisone succinate, insulin, linezolid, methicillin, metoclopramide, morphine, nafcillin, nicardipine, nitroglycerin, penicillin G, pentobarbital, potassium chloride, procainamide, prostaglandin E_1, ranitidine, sodium bicarbonate, and sodium nitroprusside.

Incompatibility: Phenytoin.

Administration Calculations

To calculate the **AMOUNT** of drug needed per **50 mL** infusion solution:

$$3 \times \frac{\text{desired dose } (mcg/kg/min)}{\text{desired fluid rate } (mL/hr)} \times \text{weight } (kg) = \text{mg of lidocaine}$$

To calculate the **VOLUME** of drug needed per **50 mL** infusion solution:

$$\frac{\text{mg of drug (found using equation above)}}{\text{concentration of drug } (mg/mL)} = \text{mL of lidocaine}$$

Example: 2-kg infant to receive lidocaine 10 mcg/kg per minute at infusion rate of 0.5 mL per hour. Concentration of the 2% lidocaine solution is 20 mg/mL.

$$3 \times \frac{10 \text{ mcg/kg/min}}{0.5 \text{ mL/hr}} \times 2 \text{ kg} = \text{120 mg of lidocaine in 50 mL of infusion solution}$$

$$\frac{120 \text{ mg of lidocaine}}{20 \text{ mg/mL}} = \text{6 mL of lidocaine in 50 mL of infusion solution}$$

Add 6 mL lidocaine (20 mg/mL) to 44 mL of compatible solution (e.g. D_5W) to yield 50 mL of infusion with a concentration of 2.4 mcg/mL.

Maximum infusion concentration is 4 mg/mL.

LIDOCAINE - ANTICONVULSANT

SELECTED REFERENCES

- Lerman J, Strong A, LeDez KM, et al: Effects of age on the serum concentration of α_1-acid glycoprotein and the binding of lidocaine in pediatric patients. Clin Pharmacol Ther 1989;46:219.
- Mihaly GW, Moore RG, Thomas J: The pharmacokinetics and metabolism of the anilide local anesthetics in neonates. I. Lignocaine. Eur J Clin Pharmacol 1978;13:143.
- Gelband H, Rosen MR: Pharmacologic basis for the treatment of cardiac arrhythmias. Pediatrics 1975;55:59.

LIDOCAINE - ANTICONVULSANT

DOSE & ADMINISTRATION: Loading dose: 2 mg/kg IV over 10 minutes, followed immediately by a **Maintenance infusion**: 6 mg/kg per hour. Begin to taper infusion after 12 to 24 hours, as drug accumulation will occur.

USES: Treatment of severe recurrent or prolonged seizures that do not respond to first-line therapies.

MONITORING: Continuous monitoring of EKG, heart rate, and blood pressure. Observe for worsening of seizure activity. Measuring blood concentrations is not clinically useful except when accumulation is suspected.

ADVERSE EFFECTS/PRECAUTIONS: Do not use concurrently with phenytoin due to cardiac effects. Stop infusion immediately if significant cardiac arrhythmia occurs. Arrhythmias and significant bradycardia have occurred in 5% of reported cases. Slowing of the heart rate is common.

PHARMACOLOGY: The mode of action for lidocaine as an anticonvulsant drug is unknown. Lidocaine is metabolized in the liver into 2 active metabolites: monoethylglycinexylidide (MEGX) and glycinxylidide (GX). Approximately 30% is excreted unchanged in the urine. The half-life in neonates is at least 3 hours, and clearance is dose-dependent. The clinically effective dose of 6 mg/kg/hr will lead to accumulation of both lidocaine and metabolites within several hours. Free drug fraction in both term and premature neonates is approximately twice that found in older children because of significantly reduced protein binding by alpha 1-acid glycoprotein.

SPECIAL CONSIDERATIONS/PREPARATION: Use only preservative-free lidocaine without epinephrine. Available in multiple concentrations ranging from 1% to 20%. To make a dilution for bolus dosing, dilute 10 mg lidocaine (0.5 mL of 2% solution) in 9.5 mL NS or D_5W, yielding a 1 mg/mL final concentration.

Solution Compatibility: D_5W, $D_{10}W$, and NS.

Terminal Injection Site Compatibility: Dex/AA solutions, fat emulsion. Alteplase, aminophylline, amiodarone, ampicillin, caffeine citrate, calcium chloride, calcium gluconate, cefazolin, cefoxitin, ceftriaxone, chloramphenicol, cimetidine, dexamethasone, digoxin, dobutamine, dopamine, enalaprilat, erythromycin lactobionate, famotidine, fentanyl, flumazenil, furosemide, glycopyrrolate, heparin, hydrocortisone succinate, insulin, linezolid, methicillin, metoclopramide, morphine, nafcillin, nicardipine, nitroglycerin, penicillin G, pentobarbital, potassium chloride, procainamide, prostaglandin E1, ranitidine, sodium bicarbonate, and sodium nitroprusside.

Incompatibility: Phenytoin.

SELECTED REFERENCES

- Van Rooij LGM, Toet MC, Rademaker KMA, et al: Cardiac arrhythmias in neonates receiving lidocaine as anticonvulsive treatment. Eur J Pediatr 2004;163:637-641.
- Hellstrom-Westas L, Svenningsen NW, Westgren U, et al: Lidocaine for treatment of severe seizures in newborn infants. II. Blood concentrations of lidocaine and metabolites during intravenous infusion. Acta Paediatr 1992;81:35-39.
- Hellstrom-Westas L, Westgren U, Rosen I, Svenningsen NW: Lidocaine for treatment of severe seizures in newborn infants. I. Clinical effects and cerebral electrical activity monitoring. Acta Paediatr Scand 1988;77:79-84.
- Rey E, Radvanyi-Bouvet MF, Bodiou C, et al: Intravenous lidocaine in the treatment of convulsions in the neonatal period: Monitoring plasma levels. Ther Drug Monit 1990;12:316-320.

LINEZOLID

DOSE & ADMINISTRATION: 10 mg/kg per dose Q8 hours by IV infusion over 30 to 120 minutes. Preterm newborns < 1 week of age: 10 mg/kg per dose Q12 hours. Oral dosing is the same as IV.

LINEZOLID

USES: Limited to treatment of non-CNS infections, including endocarditis, caused by gram positive organisms resistant to other antibiotics, e.g. methicillin-resistant *Staph. aureus*, penicillin-resistant *Strep. pneumoniae*, and vancomycin-resistant *Enterococcus faecium*. Treatment of VRE endocarditis that has failed conventional therapy. Do not use as empiric treatment or in any patient with infections caused by gram-negative organisms.

MONITORING: Weekly CBC, AST, ALT. Blood pressure if receiving sympathomimetics.

ADVERSE EFFECTS/PRECAUTIONS: Elevated transaminases and diarrhea occur in 6 to 10% of treated patients; thrombocytopenia, anemia, and rash occur in 1 to 2%. The FDA issued an alert regarding Zyvox (linezolid) on March 16, 2007. Patients in an open-label, randomized trial comparing linezolid to vancomycin, oxacillin, or dicloxacillin in the treatment of seriously ill patients with intravascular catheter-related bloodstream infections had a higher chance of death than did patients treated with any comparator antibiotic, and the chance of death was related to the type of organism causing the infection. Patients with Gram positive infections had no difference in mortality according to their antibiotic treatment. In contrast, mortality was higher in patients treated with linezolid who were infected with Gram negative organisms alone, with both Gram positive and Gram negative organisms, or who had no infection when they entered the study. See <http://www.fda.gov/cder/drug/InfoSheets/HCP/linezolidHCP.htm>.

PHARMACOLOGY: Linezolid is an oxazolidinone agent that has a unique mechanism of inhibition of bacterial protein synthesis. It is usually bacteriostatic, although it may be bactericidal against *S. pneumoniae*, *B. fragilis*, and *C. perfringens*. Rapidly penetrates osteoarticular tissues and synovial fluid. CSF concentrations were 70% of plasma concentrations in older patients with non-inflamed meninges. Completely and rapidly absorbed when administered orally to adults and children. Metabolized by oxidation without cytochrome CYP induction. Excreted in the urine as unchanged drug (30%) and two inactive metabolites. Serum half-life in most neonates is 2 to 3 hours, with the exception of preterm neonates less than one week of age, who have a serum half-life of 5 to 6 hours.

SPECIAL CONSIDERATIONS/PREPARATION: (Zyvox®) IV injection is supplied as a 2 mg/mL solution in single-use, ready-to-use 100-mL, 200-mL, and 300-mL plastic infusion bags in a foil laminate overwrap. Keep in the overwrap until use. Store at room temperature. Protect from freezing. IV injection may exhibit a yellow color that can intensify over time without affecting potency. An oral suspension is available, 100 mg per 5 mL. Store at room temperature. Use within 21 days after reconstitution. Protect from light.

Solution Compatibility: D_5W, NS, Lactated Ringers.

Terminal Injection Site Compatibility: Dex/AA. Acyclovir, amikacin, aminophylline, ampicillin, aztreonam, calcium gluconate, cefazolin, cefoxitin, ceftazidime, ceftriaxone, cefuroxime, cimetidine, clindamycin, dexamethasone, digoxin, dobutamine, dopamine, enalaprilat, esmolol, famotidine, fentanyl, fluconazole, furosemide, ganciclovir, gentamicin, heparin, hydrocortisone succinate, imipenem/cilastatin, lidocaine, lorazepam, magnesium, meropenem, methylprednisolone, metoclopramide, metronidazole, mezlocillin, midazolam, morphine, naloxone, netilmicin, nicardipine, nitroglycerin, pentobarbital, phenobarbital, piperacillin, piperacillin-tazobactam, potassium chloride, propranolol, ranitidine, remifentanil, sodium bicarbonate, theophylline, ticarcillin, tobramycin, trimethoprim-sulfamethoxazole, vancomycin, vecuronium, and zidovudine.

Incompatibility: Amphotericin B, diazepam, erythromycin lactobionate, and phenytoin.

SELECTED REFERENCES

- Tan TQ: Update on the use of linezolid: a pediatric perspective. *Pediatr Infect Dis J* 2004;23:955-956.
- Jungbluth GL, Welshman IR, Hopkins NK: Linezolid pharmacokinetics in pediatric patients: an overview. *Pediatr Infect Dis J* 2003;23:S153-157.
- Kearns GL, Jungbluth GL, Abdel-Rahman SM, et al: Impact of ontogeny on linezolid disposition in neonates and infants. *Clin Pharmacol Ther* 2003;74:413-22.
- DeVille JG, Adler S, Azimi PH: Linezolid versus vancomycin in the treament of known or suspected resistant Gram-positive infections in neonates. *Pediatr Infect Dis J* 2003;22:S158-63.
- Saiman L, Goldfarb J, Kaplan SA, et al: Safety and tolerability of linezolid in children. *Pediatr Infect Dis J* 2003;22:S193-200.
- Garges HP, Alexander KA: Newer antibiotics: Linezolid. *NeoReviews* 2003;4:e128-32.

LORAZEPAM

- Trissel LA, Williams KY, Gilbert DL: Compatibility screening of linezolid injection during simulated Y-site administration with other drugs and infusion solutions. *J Amer Pharm Assoc* 2000;40:515-519.
- Product information, Pfizer (Pharmacia & UpJohn), 2005.

LORAZEPAM

DOSE & ADMINISTRATION: 0.05 to 0.1 mg/kg per dose IV slow push. Repeat doses based on clinical response.

USES: Anticonvulsant—acute management of patients with seizures refractory to conventional therapy.

MONITORING: Monitor respiratory status closely. Observe IV site for signs of phlebitis or extravasation.

ADVERSE EFFECTS/PRECAUTIONS: Respiratory depression. Rhythmic myoclonic jerking has occurred in premature neonates receiving lorazepam for sedation.

PHARMACOLOGY: Lorazepam has been associated with dose-dependent CNS depression. Onset of action within 5 minutes; peak serum concentration within 45 minutes. Duration of action is 3 to 24 hours. Mean half-life in term neonates is 40 hours. Metabolized to an inactive glucuronide, which is excreted by the kidneys. Highly lipid-soluble. Phenobarbital serum concentrations may increase after lorazepam administration.

SPECIAL CONSIDERATIONS/PREPARATION: Limited data are available for neonates. Available in 2-mg/mL and 4-mg/mL concentrations. Preparation contains 2% (20 mg/mL) benzyl alcohol and 18% polyethylene glycol 400 in propylene glycol. A dilution of 0.4 mg/mL may be prepared by adding 1 mL of 4 mg/mL concentration in 9 mL of preservative-free sterile water for injection. This will make it easier to measure the dose and decrease the benzyl alcohol content to 0.5 mg/kg per dose. Solutions should not be used if they are discolored or contain a precipitate.

Solution Compatibility: D_5W, NS, and sterile water for injection.

Terminal Injection Site Compatibility: Dex/AA solutions. Acyclovir, amikacin, amiodarone, bumetanide, cefepime, cefotaxime, cimetidine, dexamethasone, dobutamine, dopamine, epinephrine, erythromycin lactobionate, famotidine, fentanyl, fluconazole, fosphenytoin, furosemide, gentamicin, heparin, hydrocortisone succinate, labetalol, linezolid, metronidazole, midazolam, milrinone, morphine, nicardipine, nitroglycerin, pancuronium bromide, piperacillin, piperacillin-tazobactam, potassium chloride, propofol, ranitidine, remifentanil, trimethoprim-sulfamethoxazole, vancomycin, vecuronium, and zidovudine.

Incompatibility: Fat emulsion. Aztreonam, caffeine citrate, imipenem/cilastatin, and omeprazole.

SELECTED REFERENCES

- Sexson WR, Thigpen J, Stajich GV: Stereotypic movements after lorazepam administration in premature neonates: a series and review of the literature. *J Perinatol* 1995;15:146-49.
- McDermott CA, Kowalczyk AL, Schnitzler ER, et al: Pharmacokinetics of lorazepam in critically ill neonates with seizures. *J Pediatr* 1992;120:479.
- Deshmukh A, Wittert W, Schnitzler E, Mangurten HH: Lorazepam in the treatment of refractory neonatal seizures. *Am J Dis Child* 1986;140:1042.

MEROPENEM

DOSE & ADMINISTRATION: Sepsis: 20 mg/kg per dose Q12 hours IV infusion over 30 minutes. **Meningitis and infections caused by Pseudomonas species:** 40 mg/kg per dose Q8 hours IV infusion over 30 minutes.

USES: Limited to treatment of pneumococcal meningitis and other serious infections caused by susceptible gram-negative organisms resistant to other antibiotics, especially extended-spectrum beta-lactamase producing *Klebsiella pneumoniae*.

MONITORING: Periodic CBC (for thrombocytosis and eosinophilia) and hepatic transaminases. Assess IV site for signs of inflammation.

ADVERSE EFFECTS/PRECAUTIONS: Diarrhea (4%), nausea/vomiting (1%) and rash (2%). May cause inflammation at the injection site. The use of carbapenem antibiotics can result in the development of cephalosporin resistance in *Enterobacter*, *Pseudomonas*, *Serratia*, *Proteus*, *Citrobacter*, and *Acinetobacter* species. The risks of pseudomembranous colitis and fungal infections are also increased.

PHARMACOLOGY: Meropenem is a broad-spectrum carbapenem antibiotic that penetrates well into the CSF and most body tissues. It is relatively stable to inactivation by human renal dehydropeptidase. Plasma protein binding is minimal. Clearance is directly related to renal function, and 70% of a dose is recovered intact in the urine. Hepatic function does not affect pharmacokinetics. Serum half-life of meropenem is 3 hours in preterm and 2 hours in full term neonates.

SPECIAL CONSIDERATIONS/PREPARATION: Available (USA) as powder for injection in 500-mg, and 1000-mg vials. Reconstitute with 100 mL of compatible diluent. Maximum concentration 50 mg/mL. Freshly prepared solutions should be used whenever possible. When reconstituted with NS, solution is stable in the vial for 2 hours at room temperature, 12 hours refrigerated. When reconstituted with D_5W, solution in the vial is stable for 1 hour at room temperature or 8 hours refrigerated.

Solution Compatibility: D_5W, $D_{10}W$, and NS.

Terminal Injection Site Compatibility: Dex/AA and fat emulsion. Acyclovir, aminophylline, atropine, calcium gluconate, cimetidine, dexamethasone, digoxin, dobutamine, dopamine, enalaprilat, fluconazole, furosemide, gentamicin, heparin, insulin, linezolid, metoclopramide, milrinone, morphine, norepinephrine, phenobarbital, ranitidine, sodium bicarbonate, vancomycin, and zidovudine.

Incompatibility: Amphotericin B and metronidazole.

SELECTED REFERENCES

- Garges HP, Alexander KA: Newer antibiotics: imipenem/cilastatin and meropenem. *NeoReviews* 2003;4:e364-68.
- Bradley JS: Meropenem: a new, extremely broad spectrum β-lactam antibiotic for serious infections in pediatrics. *Pediatr Infect Dis J* 1997;16:263-68.
- Blumer JL: Pharmacokinetic determinants of carbapenem therapy in neonates and children. *Pediatr Infect Dis J* 1996;15:733-37.
- Piyush PR: Compatibility of meropenem with commonly used injectable drugs. *Am J Health-Syst Pharm* 1996;53:2853-55.
- Blumer JL, Reed MD, Kearns GL, et al: Sequential, single-dose pharmacokinetic evaluation of meropenem in hospitalized infants and children. *Antimicrob Agents Chemother* 1995;39:1721-25.
- Hurst M, Lamb HM: Meropenem: a review of its use in patients in intensive care. *Drugs* 2000;59:653-680.

METHADONE

DOSE & ADMINISTRATION: Initial dose: 0.05 to 0.2 mg/kg per dose Q12 to 24 hours PO. Reduce dose by 10 to 20% per week over 4 to 6 weeks. Adjust weaning schedule based on signs and symptoms of withdrawal.

USES: Treatment of opiate withdrawal.

MONITORING: Monitor respiratory and cardiac status closely. Assess for gastric residuals, abdominal distention, and loss of bowel sounds.

ADVERSE EFFECTS/PRECAUTIONS: Respiratory depression in excessive doses. Ileus and delayed gastric emptying.

PHARMACOLOGY: Methadone is a long-acting narcotic analgesic. Oral bioavailability is 50%, with peak plasma levels obtained in 2 to 4 hours. Metabolized extensively via hepatic N-demethylation. Highly protein bound (90% adults). Serum half-life ranges from 16 to 25 hours in neonates and is prolonged in patients with renal failure. Rifampin and phenytoin accelerate the metabolism of methadone and can precipitate withdrawal symptoms.

SPECIAL CONSIDERATIONS/PREPARATION: Available as oral solutions in 1- and 2-mg/mL concentrations containing 8% alcohol, and a 10-mg/mL alcohol-free solution. May dilute 1 mL of the 10-mg/mL concentrated solution with 19 mL of sterile water to provide an oral dilution with a final concentration of 0.5 mg/mL. Stable for 24 hours refrigerated. Also available as 5- and 10-mg tablets.

SELECTED REFERENCES

- Guo J, Greenberg M, Finer NN, Heldt GP: Methadone is a superior detoxification agent compared to tincture opium for treatment of neonatal narcotic abstinence syndrome (NAS). Abstract 4850.230, 2006 Pediatric Academic Societies Annual Meeting.
- Tobias JD, Schleien CL, Haun SE: Methadone as treatment for iatrogenic narcotic dependency in pediatric intensive care unit patients. *Crit Care Med* 1990;18:1292.
- Koren G, Maurice L: Pediatric uses of opioids. *Ped Clin North Am* 1989;36:1141.
- Rosen TS, Pippenger CE: Pharmacologic observations on the neonatal withdrawal syndrome. *J Pediatr* 1976;88:1044.

Metoclopramide

DOSE & ADMINISTRATION: 0.033 to 0.1 mg/kg per dose PO or IV slow push Q8 hours.

USES: To facilitate gastric emptying and GI motility. May improve feeding intolerance. Use in GE reflux patients is controversial. (Also used to enhance lactation—10 mg Q8 hours.)

MONITORING: Measure gastric residuals. Observe for increased irritability or vomiting.

ADVERSE EFFECTS/PRECAUTIONS: Intended for short-term use (several weeks). Dystonic reactions and extrapyramidal symptoms are seen frequently at higher doses and with prolonged use; children are more susceptible than adults.

PHARMACOLOGY: Derivative of procainamide. Exact mode of action is unknown; however, metoclopramide has both dopamine-receptor blocking activity and peripheral cholinergic effects. Well absorbed from GI tract. Variable first-pass metabolism by liver. Significant fraction excreted unchanged in urine. Lipid-soluble, large volume of distribution. Serum half-life in adults is 4 hours; prolonged in patients with renal failure.

SPECIAL CONSIDERATIONS/PREPARATION: Available as a 5-mg/mL injectable solution (osmolarity 280 mOsm/kg) in 2-, 10-, 20-, and 30-mL vials. **Protect from light.** A 0.1 mg/mL dilution may be made by adding 0.4 mL of the 5-mg/mL concentration to 19.6 mL of preservative-free NS. Dilution is stable for 24 hours refrigerated. Oral preparation available in 1-mg/mL and 10-mg/mL concentrations. A 0.1 mg/mL oral dilution may be made by adding 1 mL of the 1 mg/mL concentration to 9 mL simple syrup. Stable for 4 weeks at room temperature.

Solution Compatibility: D_5W, and NS.

Terminal Injection Site Compatibility: Dex/AA solutions, fat emulsion. Acyclovir, aminophylline, atropine, aztreonam, caffeine citrate, cimetidine, ciprofloxacin, clindamycin, dexamethasone, famotidine, fentanyl, fluconazole, heparin, hydrocortisone, insulin, lidocaine, linezolid, meropenem, midazolam, morphine, multivitamins, piperacillin-tazobactam, potassium chloride, potassium phosphate, prostaglandin E_1, quinupristin-dalfopristin, ranitidine, remifentanil, and zidovudine.

Incompatibility: Ampicillin, calcium chloride, calcium gluconate, cefepime, chloramphenicol, erythromycin lactobionate, furosemide, penicillin G, propofol, and sodium bicarbonate.

SELECTED REFERENCES

- Meadow WL, Bui K, Strates E, et al: Metoclopramide promotes enteral feeding in preterm infants with feeding intolerance. *Dev Pharmacol Ther* 1989;13:38.
- Machida HM, Forbes DA, Gall DG, et al: Metoclopramide in gastroesophageal reflux of infancy. *J Pediatr* 1988;112:483.
- Ehrenkranz RA, Ackerman BA: Metoclopramide effect on faltering milk production by mothers of premature infants. *Pediatrics* 1986;78:614.
- Sankaran K, Yeboah E, Bingham WT, Ninan A: Use of metoclopramide in premature infants. *Dev Pharmacol Ther* 1982;5:114.

Metronidazole

DOSE & ADMINISTRATION: Loading dose: 15 mg/kg PO or IV infusion by syringe pump over 60 minutes. **Maintenance dose:** 7.5 mg/kg per dose PO or IV infusion over 60 minutes. Begin one dosing interval after initial dose. To use dosing chart, please refer to explanatory note in "How to Use This Book."

Dosing Interval Chart

PMA (weeks)	PostNatal (days)	Interval (hours)
≤29	0 to 28	48
	>28	24
30 to 36	0 to 14	24
	>14	12
37 to 44	0 to 7	24
	>7	12
≥45	ALL	8

USES: Reserved for treatment of meningitis, ventriculitis, and endocarditis caused by *Bacteroides fragilis* and other anaerobes resistant to penicillin; treatment of serious intra-abdominal infections; and treatment of infections caused by *Trichomonas vaginalis*. Treatment of *C. difficile* colitis.

MONITORING: Measure CSF drug concentrations when treating CNS infections. Trough drug concentration should be greater than minimum inhibitory concentration for organism.

ADVERSE EFFECTS/PRECAUTIONS: Metronidazole has been shown to be carcinogenic in mice and rats, and therefore, has not been approved for pediatric use. Seizures and sensory polyneuropathy have been reported in a few adult patients receiving high doses over a prolonged period. Drug metabolites may cause brownish discoloration of the urine.

PHARMACOLOGY: Metronidazole is bactericidal for many anaerobic organisms. It is well absorbed after oral administration, with peak serum concentrations attained in 1 to 3 hours. Distribution in all tissues throughout the body is excellent. It is less than 20% protein bound. Hydroxylation in the liver occurs in term infants and premature infants exposed to antenatal betamethasone. Unchanged drug and the active metabolite are excreted renally. Elimination half-life is strongly related to gestational age, ranging from 22 to 109 hours.

SPECIAL CONSIDERATIONS/PREPARATION: Available in 5 mg/mL concentration in 100 mL single-dose plastic ready-to-use solution containers. Store at controlled room temperature. **Do not refrigerate** (crystals form, but redissolve on warming to room temperature). Osmolarity is 310 mOsm/L, pH is 5 to 7. Each container contains 14 mEq of sodium. Supplied as 250 mg and 500 mg for oral administration. Suspension may be prepared by crushing five 250-mg tablets (1250 mg), dissolving powder in 10 mL purified water, then adding cherry syrup to make a total volume of 83 mL. Final concentration is 15 mg/mL. **Protect from light.** Shake well. Suspension is stable for 30 days refrigerated.

Solution Compatibility: D_5W, and NS.

Solution Incompatibility: Manufacturer recommends that if metronidazole is used with a primary IV fluid system, the primary solution should be discontinued during metronidazole infusion.

Terminal Injection Site Compatibility: Dex/AA solutions, fat emulsion. Acyclovir, amikacin, aminophylline, amiodarone, ampicillin, cefazolin, cefepime, cefotaxime, cefoxitin, ceftazidime, ceftriaxone, clindamycin, chloramphenicol, dopamine, enalaprilat, esmolol, fluconazole, gentamicin, heparin, hydrocortisone succinate, linezolid, lorazepam, magnesium sulfate, midazolam, milrinone, morphine, netilmicin, nicardipine, penicillin G, piperacillin-tazobactam, prostaglandin E_1, remifentanil, and tobramycin.

Incompatibility: Aztreonam and meropenem.

SELECTED REFERENCES

- Wenisch C, Parschalk B, Hasenhundl M, et al: Comparison of vancomycin, teicoplanin, metronidazole, and fusidic acid for the treatment of *Clostridium difficile* - associated diarrhea. *Clin Infect Dis* 1996;22:813.
- Allen LV, Errickson MA: Stability of ketoconazole, metolazone, metronidazole, procainamide hydrochloride, spironolactone in extemporaneously compounded oral liquids. *Am J Health Syst Pharm* 1996;53:2073-2078.
- Feder HM Jr: *Bacteroides fragilis* meningitis. *Rev Infect Dis* 1987;9:783.
- Roberts RJ: *Drug Therapy in Infants*. Philadelphia: WB Saunders Co, 1984, p 76.
- Hall P, Kaye CM, McIntosh N, Steele J: Intravenous metronidazole in the newborn. *Arch Dis Child* 1983;58:529.
- Oldenburg B, Speck WT: Metronidazole. *Pediatr Clin North Am* 1983;30:71.
- Jager-Roman E, Doyle PE, Baird-Lambert J, et al: Pharmacokinetics and tissue distribution of metronidazole in the newborn infant. *J Pediatr* 1982;100:651.

MIDAZOLAM

DOSE & ADMINISTRATION: IV: 0.05 to 0.15 mg/kg **over at least 5 minutes.** Repeat as required, usually Q2 to 4 hours. May also be given IM. Dosage requirements are decreased by concurrent use of narcotics. **Continuous IV infusion:** 0.01 to 0.06 mg/kg per hour (10 to 60 mcg/kg/hour). Dosage may need to be increased after several days of therapy because of development of tolerance and/or increased clearance. **Intra-

Midazolam

nasal: 0.2 to 0.3 mg/kg per dose using 5-mg/mL injectable form. **Sublingual:** 0.2 mg/kg per dose using 5-mg/mL injectable form mixed with a small amount of flavored syrup. **Oral:** 0.25 mg/kg per dose using Versed® oral syrup.

USES: Sedative/hypnotic. Anesthesia induction. Treatment of refractory seizures.

MONITORING: Follow respiratory status and blood pressure closely, especially when used concurrently with narcotics. Assess hepatic function. Observe for signs of withdrawal after discontinuation of prolonged therapy.

ADVERSE EFFECTS/PRECAUTIONS: Respiratory depression and hypotension are common when used in conjunction with narcotics, or following rapid bolus administration. Seizure-like myoclonus has been reported in 8% of premature infants receiving continuous infusions - this also may occur following rapid bolus administration and in patients with underlying CNS disorders. Nasal administration may be uncomfortable because of a burning sensation.

PHARMACOLOGY: Midazolam is a relatively short-acting benzodiazepine with rapid onset of action. Sedative and anticonvulsant properties related to GABA accumulation and occupation of benzodiazepine receptor. Antianxiety properties related to increasing the glycine inhibitory neurotransmitter. Metabolized by hepatic CYP 3A4 to a less active hydroxylated metabolite, then glucuronidated before excretion in urine. Drug accumulation may occur with repeated doses, prolonged infusion therapy, or concurrent administration of cimetidine, erythromycin or fluconazole. Highly protein bound. Duration of action is 2 to 6 hours. Elimination half-life is approximately 4 to 6 hours in term neonates, and quite variable, up to 22 hours, in premature babies and those with impaired hepatic function. Bioavailability is approximately 36% with oral administration and 50% with sublingual and intranasal administration. Midazolam is water soluble in acidic solutions and becomes lipid soluble at physiologic pH.

SPECIAL CONSIDERATIONS/PREPARATION: A preservative-free preparation is available as 1- and 5-mg/mL concentrations in 1-, 2-, and 5-mL vials (available from Bedford). Versed® is available in an injectable form as 1- and 5-mg/mL concentrations in 1-, 2-, 5-, and 10-mL vials. Contains 1% (10 mg/mL) benzyl alcohol as a preservative. To decrease benzyl alcohol content, a 0.5 mg/mL dilution may be made by adding 1 mL of the 5-mg/mL concentration to 9 mL preservative-free sterile water for injection. Dilution stable for 24 hours refrigerated. Versed® oral syrup is available in a 2 mg/mL concentration. Store at room temperature.

Solution Compatibility: D_5W, NS, and sterile water for injection.

Terminal Injection Site Compatibility: Dex/AA solutions. Amiodarone, amikacin, aminophylline, atropine, calcium gluconate, cefazolin, cefotaxime, cimetidine, clindamycin, digoxin, dobutamine, dopamine, epinephrine, erythromycin lactobionate, esmolol, famotidine, fentanyl, fluconazole, gentamicin, glycopyrrolate, heparin, imipenem/cilastatin, insulin, linezolid, lorazepam, methadone, metoclopramide, metronidazole, milrinone, mivacurium, morphine, nicardipine, nitroglycerin, nitroprusside, pancuronium bromide, piperacillin, potassium chloride, propofol, prostaglandin E_1, ranitidine, remifentanil, sodium nitroprusside, theophylline, tobramycin, vancomycin, and vecuronium.

Incompatibility: Fat emulsion. Albumin, ampicillin, bumetanide, ceftazidime, dexamethasone, fosphenytoin, furosemide, hydrocortisone succinate, nafcillin, omeprazole, pentobarbital, phenobarbital, and sodium bicarbonate.

SELECTED REFERENCES

- de Wildt SN, Kearns GL, Hop WCJ, et al: Pharmacokinetics and metabolism of intravenous midazolam in preterm infants. *Clin Pharmacol Ther* 2001;70:525-531.
- Coté CJ, Cohen IT, Suresh S, et al: A comparison of three doses of a commercially prepared oral midazolam syrup in children. *Anesth Analg* 2002;94:37-43.
- Sheth RD, Buckley DJ, Gutierrez AR: Midazolam in the treatment of refractory neonatal seizures. *Clin Neuropharmacol* 1996;2:165-70.
- Olkkola KT, Ahonen J, Neuvonen PJ: The effect of the systemic antimycotics, itraconazole and fluconazole, on the pharmacokinetics and pharmacodynamics of intravenous and oral midazolam. *Anesth Analg* 1996;82:511.
- Jacqz-Aigrain E, Daoud P, Burtin P, et al: Placebo-controlled trial of midazolam sedation in mechanically ventilated newborn babies. *Lancet* 1994;344:646-50.
- Magnyn JF, d'Allest AM, Nedelcoux H, et al: Midazolam and myoclonus in neonate. *Eur J Pediatr* 1994;153:389.
- Karl HW, Rosenberger JL, Larach MG, Ruffie JM: Transmucosal administration of midazolam for premedication of pediatric patients: Comparison of the nasal and sublingual routes. *Anesthesiology* 1993;78:885.

- Jacqz-Aigrain E, Daoud P, Burtin P, et al: Pharmacokinetics of midazolam during continuous infusion in critically ill neonates. *Eur J Clin Pharmacol* 1992;42:329.
- van Straaten HLM, Rademaker CMA, de Vries LS: Comparison of the effect of midazolam or vecuronium on blood pressure and cerebral blood flow velocity in the premature newborn. *Dev Pharmacol Ther* 1992;19:191.

MILRINONE

DOSE & ADMINISTRATION: Loading dose: 75 mcg/kg IV infused over 60 minutes, immediately followed by **Maintenance infusion:** 0.5 to 0.75 mcg/kg per minute. Note: Above doses are from studies of older infants and children. Adjust infusion rate based upon hemodynamic and clinical response. **Premature infants < 30 weeks GA: Loading dose:** 0.75 mcg/kg per minute for 3 hours, immediately followed by **Maintenance infusion:** 0.2 mcg/kg per minute. (Preliminary data from pilot study referenced below)

USES: Short term (<72 hours) treatment of acute low cardiac output after cardiac surgery or due to septic shock.

MONITORING: Continuous monitoring of blood pressure, heart rate and rhythm. Assess signs of cardiac output. Carefully monitor fluid and electrolyte changes and renal function during therapy. Monitor platelet counts.

ADVERSE EFFECTS/PRECAUTIONS: Assure adequate vascular volume prior to initiating therapy. Blood pressure will likely fall 5 to 9% after the loading dose, but should gradually return to baseline by 24 hours. Heart rate increases of 5 to 10% are also common. Thrombocytopenia was reported frequently in some studies and rarely in others. Arrhythmias occur occasionally.

PHARMACOLOGY: Milrinone improves cardiac output by enhancing myocardial contractility, enhancing myocardial diastolic relaxation and decreasing vascular resistance. It acts via selective phosphodiesterase III inhibition that leads to increased intracellular cyclic AMP, increased myocardial intracellular calcium, and increased reuptake of calcium after systole. Vasodilatation is related to increased levels of cyclic GMP in vascular smooth muscle. Unlike catecholamines, myocardial oxygen consumption is not increased. Elimination is primarily via renal mechanisms. Half-life is quite variable, ranging from approximately 10 hours in ELBW neonates to approximately 3 hours in older and more mature infants.

SPECIAL CONSIDERATIONS/PREPARATION: Available in 1 mg/mL solution for injection in 10-, 20-, and 50-mL single-dose vials. Dilute with compatible diluent prior to administration. Maximum concentration for infusion is 200 mcg/mL. Also available as premixed solution for injection, 200 mcg/mL in 5% Dextrose. pH of 3.2 to 4.

Solution Compatibility: D_5W, NS, and LR.

Terminal Injection Site Compatibility: Dex/AA. Acyclovir, amikacin, aminophylline, amiodarone, ampicillin, atracurium, atropine, bumetanide, calcium chloride, calcium gluconate, cefazolin, cefepime, cefotaxime, ceftazidime, cimetidine, clindamycin, dexamethasone, digoxin, dopamine, dobutamine, epinephrine, fentanyl, gentamicin, heparin, insulin, isoproterenol, lorazepam, meropenem, methylprednisolone, metronidazole, midazolam, morphine, nicardipine, nitroglycerin, norepinephrine, oxacillin, pancuronium, piperacillin, piperacillin-tazobactam, potassium chloride, propofol, propranolol, ranitidine, sodium bicarbonate, sodium nitroprusside, theophylline, ticarcillin, ticarcillin-clavulanate, tobramycin, vancomycin, and vecuronium.

Incompatibility: Furosemide, imipenem-cilastatin and procainamide.

SELECTED REFERENCES

- Paradisis M, Jiang X, McLachlan AJ, et al: Population pharmacokinetics and dosing regimen of milrinone for in preterm infants. *Arch Dis Child Fetal Neonatal Ed* 2007;92:F204-209.
- Hoffman TM, Wernovsky G, Atz AM, et al: Efficacy and safety of milrinone in preventing low cardiac output syndrome in infants and children after corrective surgery for congenital heart disease. *Circulation* 2003;107:996-1002.
- Lindsay CA, Barton P, Lawless S, et al: Pharmacokinetics and pharmacodynamics of milrinone in pediatric patients with septic shock. *J Pediatr* 1998;132:329-34.
- Chang AC, Atz AM, Wernovsky G, et al: Milrinone: Systemic and pulmonary hemodynamic effects in neonates after cardiac surgery. *Crit Care Med* 1995;23:1907-14.
- Veltri MA, Conner KG: Physical compatibility of milrinone lactate injection with intravenous drugs commonly used in the pediatric intensive care unit. *Am J Health-Syst Pharm* 2002;59: 452-54.
- Akkerman SR, Zhang H, Mullins RE, Vaughn K: Stability of milrinone lactate in the presence of 29 critical care drugs and 4 i.v. solutions. *Am J Health-Syst Pharm* 1999;56:63-68.
- Paradisis M, Evans N, Kluckow M, et al: Pilot study of milrinone for prevention of low systemic blood flow in very preterm infants. *J Pediatr* 2006;148:306-313.

Mivacurium

DOSE & ADMINISTRATION: 0.2 mg/kg IV push over 30 seconds.

USES: Skeletal muscle relaxation/paralysis in infants requiring endotracheal intubation.

MONITORING: Assess vital signs frequently, and blood pressure continuously if possible.

ADVERSE EFFECTS/PRECAUTIONS: Hypotension may occur, most likely caused by mast cell activation and histamine release. There are also occasional reports of bronchospasm in children with asthma. Inherited plasma cholinesterase deficiency may cause prolonged neuromuscular blockade. The mild form, affecting 1 in 25, results in ~50% prolongation which is unlikely to be clinically significant. The severe form, affecting 1 in 2500, results in prolongation of paralysis for several hours.

PHARMACOLOGY: Mivacurium is a short-acting, nondepolarizing skeletal muscle relaxant for IV administration. Competitive binding to cholinergic receptors occurs on the motor end-plate to antagonize the action of acetylcholine, resulting in a block of neuromuscular transmission. Onset of action is usually 80 to 120 seconds. Duration of action is usually 15 to 20 minutes. Data in neonates are limited. Skeletal relaxation/paralysis may be reversed by acetylcholinesterase inhibitors such as neostigmine. The drug is a mixture of isomers that are extensively metabolized by plasma cholinesterase. This process appears to be fully active in most neonates. Renal and biliary excretion of unchanged mivacurium are minor elimination pathways; urine and bile are important elimination pathways for the two relatively inactive metabolites. Sensation remains intact. Analgesia should be used for painful procedures.

SPECIAL CONSIDERATIONS/PREPARATION: Available in 5-and 10-mL single-use vials (2 mg/mL) in Water for Injection. pH 3.5 to 5. Protect from light.

Solution Compatibility: D_5W, NS, LR, and D_5NS.

Solution Incompatibility: No data.

Terminal Injection Site Compatibility: Fentanyl and midazolam.

Incompatibility: Alkaline solutions having a pH greater than 8.5, barbiturates, phenytoin, and sodium bicarbonate.

SELECTED REFERENCES

- McCluskey A, Meakin G: Dose-response and minimum time to satisfactory intubation conditions after mivacurium in children. *Anaesthesia* 1996;51:438-41.
- Cook DR, Gronert BJ, Woelfel SK: Comparison of the neuromuscular effects of mivacurium and suxamethonium in infants and children. *Acta Anaesthesiol Scand* 1995;39:Suppl 106:35-40.
- Meretoja OA, Taivainen T, Wirtavuori K: Pharmacodynamics of mivacurium in infants. *Br J Anaesth* 1994;73:490-93.

Morphine

DOSE & ADMINISTRATION: 0.05 to 0.2 mg/kg per dose IV over at least 5 minutes, IM, or SC. Repeat as required (usually Q4 hours). **Continuous infusion:** Give a loading dose of 100 to 150 mcg/kg over 1 hour followed by 10 to 20 mcg/kg per hour. **Treatment of opioid dependence:** Begin at most recent IV morphine dose equivalent. Taper 10 to 20% per day as tolerated. Oral dose is approximately 3 to 5 times IV dose. **Initial treatment of neonatal narcotic abstinence:** 0.03 to 0.1 mg/kg per dose PO Q3 to 4 hours. Wean dose by 10 to 20% every 2 to 3 days based on abstinence scoring. (The Finnegan score should be < 9). Use a 0.4-mg/mL dilution made from a concentrated oral morphine sulfate solution.

USES: Analgesia. Sedation. Treatment of opioid withdrawal and abstinence.

MONITORING: Monitor respiratory and cardiovascular status closely. Observe for abdominal distention and loss of bowel sounds. Consider urine retention if output is decreased.

ADVERSE EFFECTS/PRECAUTIONS: Naloxone should be readily available to reverse adverse effects. Marked respiratory depression (decreases the responsiveness of the respiratory center to CO_2 tension). Hypotension and bradycardia. Transient hypertonia. Ileus and delayed gastric emptying. Urine retention. Tolerance may develop after prolonged use—wean slowly. Seizures reported in two infants who received bolus plus infusion.

PHARMACOLOGY: Morphine is a narcotic analgesic that stimulates brain opioid receptors. Increases venous capacitance, caused by release of histamine and central suppression of adrenergic tone. GI secretions and motility decreased. Increases smooth muscle tone. Morphine is converted in the liver to two glucuronide metabolites (morphine-6-glucuronide and morphine-3-glucuronide) that are renally excreted. Morphine-6-glucuronide (M6G) is a potent respiratory-depressant and analgesic. Morphine-3-glucuronide (M3G) is an antagonist to the effects of morphine and morphine-6-glucuronide. Morphine is 20 to 40% bioavailable when administered orally. Pharmacokinetics are widely variable. Elimination half-life is approximately 9 hours for morphine and 18 hours for morphine-6-glucuronide. Steady state concentrations of morphine are reached by 24 to 48 hours.

SPECIAL CONSIDERATIONS/PREPARATION: Injectable solutions are available in dosage strengths ranging from 0.5- to 50-mg/mL. Oral morphine sulfate solutions are available in concentrations of 2, 4, and (alcohol-free) 20 mg/mL. A 0.4-mg/mL oral morphine dilution may be made by adding 1 mL of the 4-mg/mL injectable solution to 9 mL preservative-free normal saline. Stable for 7 days refrigerated. **Protect from light.**

Solution Compatibility: D_5W, $D_{10}W$, and NS. For continuous infusions of morphine **containing heparin:** Use only NS; maximum morphine concentration 5 mg/mL.

Terminal Injection Site Compatibility: Dex/AA solutions, fat emulsion. Acyclovir, alteplase, amikacin, aminophylline, amiodarone, ampicillin, atropine, aztreonam, bumetanide, caffeine citrate, calcium chloride, cefotaxime, cefoxitin, ceftazidime, ceftriaxone, chloramphenicol, cefazolin, cimetidine, clindamycin, dexamethasone, digoxin, dobutamine, dopamine, enalaprilat, epinephrine, erythromycin lactobionate, esmolol, famotidine, fentanyl, fluconazole, furosemide, gentamicin, glycopyrrolate, heparin, hydrocortisone succinate, insulin, lidocaine, linezolid, lorazepam, meropenem, metoclopramide, metronidazole, mezlocillin, midazolam, milrinone, nafcillin, nicardipine, nitroglycerin, oxacillin, pancuronium bromide, penicillin G, phenobarbital, piperacillin, piperacillin-tazobactam, potassium chloride, propofol, propranolol, prostaglandin E_1, ranitidine, remifentanil, sodium bicarbonate, sodium nitroprusside, ticarcillin/clavulanate, tobramycin, trimethoprim-sulfamethoxazole, vancomycin, vecuronium, and zidovudine.

Incompatibility: Azithromycin, cefepime, pentobarbital, and phenytoin.

SELECTED REFERENCES

- Langenfeld S, Birkenfeld L, Herkenrath P, et al: Therapy of the neonatal abstinence syndrome with tincture of opium or morphine drops. *Drug Alcohol Depend* 2005;77:31-36.
- Oei J, Lui K: Management of the newborn infant affected by maternal opiates and other drugs of dependency. *J Paediatr Child Health* 2007;43:9-18.
- Saarenmaa E, Neuvonen PJ, Rosenberg P, Fellman V: Morphine clearance and effects in newborn infants in relation to gestational age. *Clin Pharmacol Ther* 2000;68:160-166.
- American Academy of Pediatrics Committee on Drugs: Neonatal drug withdrawal. *Pediatrics* 1998;101:1079-1088.
- Yaster M, Kost-Byerly S, Berde C, Billet C: The management of opioid and benzodiazepine dependence in infants, children, and adolescents. *Pediatrics* 1996;98:135-40.
- Barrett DA, Barker DP, Rutter N, et al: Morphine, morphine-6-glucuronide and morphine-3-glucuronide pharmacokinetics in newborn infants receiving diamorphine infusions. *Br J Clin Pharmacol* 1996;41:531.
- Hartley R, Green M, Quinn M, Levene MI: Pharmacokinetics of morphine infusion in premature neonates. *Arch Dis Child* 1993;69:55.
- Chay PCW, Duffy BJ, Walker JS: Pharmacokinetic-pharmacodynamic relationships of morphine in neonates. *Clin Pharmacol Ther* 1992;51:334.
- Koren G, Butt W, Chinyanga H, et al: Postoperative morphine infusion in newborn infants: Assessment of disposition characteristics and safety. *J Pediatr* 1985;107:963.

MUPIROCIN

DOSE & ADMINISTRATION: Apply small amounts topically to affected areas 3 times daily.

USES: Topical use for skin infections caused by *Staphylococcus aureus*, *S. epidermidis*, *S. saprophyticus*, and *Streptococcus pyogenes*.

MONITORING: Assess affected area for continued infection.

ADVERSE EFFECTS/PRECAUTIONS: Use only on the skin. No adverse effects reported from topical administration. Routine use may lead to selective bacterial resistance.

PHARMACOLOGY: Mupirocin is a topical antibacterial produced by fermentation of the organism *Pseudomonas fluorescens*. Inhibits protein synthesis by bonding to bacterial

Nafcillin

isoleucyl-transfer-RNA synthetase. Highly protein bound. Not absorbed into the systemic circulation after topical administration (older infants and children). Metabolized in the skin to an inactive compound and excreted.

SPECIAL CONSIDERATIONS/PREPARATION: Available in unit-dose packets and 15 and 30-g tubes as a 2% ointment and cream (20 mg/g).

SELECTED REFERENCES

- Zakrzewska-Bode A, Muytjens HL, Liem KD, Hoogkamp-Korstanje JAA: Mupirocin resistance in coagulase-negative staphylococci, after topical prophylaxis for the reduction of colonization of central venous catheters. *J Hosp Infect* 1995;31:189.
- Pappa KA: The clinical development of mupirocin. *J Am Acad Dermatol* 1990;22:873.
- Leyden JJ: Mupirocin: A new topical antibiotic. *Semin Dermatol* 1987;6:48.
- Davies EA, Emmerson AM, Hogg GM, et al: An outbreak of infection with a methicillin-resistant *Staphylococcus aureus* in a special care baby unit: Value of topical mupirocin and of traditional methods of infection control. *J Hosp Infect* 1987;10:120.

Nafcillin

DOSE & ADMINISTRATION: Usual dosage: 25 mg/kg per dose IV over 15 minutes. **Meningitis:** 50 mg/kg per dose. To use dosing chart, please refer to explanatory note in "How to Use This Book."

Dosing Interval Chart

PMA (weeks)	PostNatal (days)	Interval (hours)
≤29	0 to 28 >28	12 8
30 to 36	0 to 14 >14	12 8
37 to 44	0 to 7 >7	12 8
≥45	ALL	6

USES: Treatment of infections caused by penicillinase-producing staphylococci, particularly if evidence of renal dysfunction.

MONITORING: Periodic CBC. Observe IV site for signs of extravasation.

ADVERSE EFFECTS/PRECAUTIONS: Increase dosing interval in patients with hepatic dysfunction. Irritating to veins—watch for phlebitis. Cases of granulocytopenia have been reported.

PHARMACOLOGY: Nafcillin inhibits synthesis of bacterial cell wall. Better penetration into CSF than methicillin. Excreted via hepatic clearance.

SPECIAL CONSIDERATIONS/PREPARATION: Available in 1 and 2-g vials. Reconstitute 1-g vial with 3.4 mL of sterile water for injection to provide a final volume of 4 mL and a concentration of 250 mg/mL. Also available in 1-g in 50-mL and 2-g in 100-mL frozen single-dose bags. Thaw bags at room temperature or under refrigeration. Do not force thaw by immersing into water baths or microwaving. pH of resulting solution 6 to 8.5. Reconstituted solution stable for 3 days at room temperature, 21 days refrigerated. Osmolality was determined to be 709 mOsm/kg of water.

Solution Compatibility: D_5W, $D_{10}W$, and NS.

Terminal Injection Site Compatibility: Dex/AA solutions, fat emulsion. Acyclovir, aminophylline, atropine, chloramphenicol, cimetidine, dexamethasone, enalaprilat, esmolol, famotidine, fentanyl, fluconazole, heparin, lidocaine, morphine, nicardipine, potassium chloride, propofol, sodium bicarbonate, zidovudine.

Incompatibility: Amikacin, aztreonam, gentamicin, hydrocortisone succinate, insulin, methylprednisolone, midazolam, netilmicin, tobramycin, and vancomycin.

SELECTED REFERENCES

- Prober CG, Stevenson DK, Benitz WE: The use of antibiotics in neonates weighing less than 1200 grams. *Pediatr Infect Dis J* 1990;9:111.
- Kitzing W, Nelson JD, Mohs E: Comparative toxicities of methicillin and nafcillin. *Am J Dis Child* 1981;135:52.
- Banner W, Gooch WM, Burckart G, Korones SB: Pharmacokinetics of nafcillin in infants with low birth weights. *Antimicrob Agents Chemother* 1980;17:691.

Naloxone

DOSE & ADMINISTRATION: 0.1 mg/kg IV push. May give IM if adequate perfusion. Tracheal administration is not recommended. Naloxone is not recommended as part of the initial resuscitation of newborns with respiratory depression in the delivery room. Before naloxone is given, providers should restore heart rate and color by supporting ventilation.

USES: Narcotic antagonist. Adjuvant therapy to customary resuscitation efforts for narcotic-induced respiratory (CNS) depression.

MONITORING: Assess respiratory effort and neurologic status.

ADVERSE EFFECTS/PRECAUTIONS: No short-term toxicity observed. One case report of seizures secondary to acute opioid withdrawal after administration to an infant born to an opioid abuser. Long-term safety has not been investigated.

PHARMACOLOGY: Naloxone reverses respiratory depression by competing for CNS narcotic receptor sites. Onset of action within 1 to 2 minutes after IV administration, within 15 minutes of IM administration. Metabolized by the liver and excreted in the urine. Increases circulating catecholamines.

SPECIAL CONSIDERATIONS/PREPARATION: Do not mix in an alkaline solution. Available in 1 mg/mL and 0.4 mg/mL concentrations. **Store at room temperature and protect from light.**

Solution Compatibility: No data are currently available on Dex/AA.

Terminal Injection Site Compatibility: Heparin, linezolid, and propofol. No data are currently available on potassium chloride and other medications.

SELECTED REFERENCES

- The International Committee on Resuscitation: The International Liaison Committee on Resuscitation (ILCOR) Consensus on Science With Treatment Recommendations for Pediatric and Neonatal Patients: Neonatal Resuscitation. *Pediatrics* 2006(5).
- URL: http://www.pediatrics.org/cgi/content/full/117/5/e978.
- Gibbs J, Newson T, Williams J, Davidson DC: Naloxone hazard in infant of opioid abuser. *Lancet* 1989;2:159.
- Gerhart T, Bancalari E, Cohen H, Rocha LF: Use of naloxone to reverse narcotic respiratory depression in the newborn infant. *J Pediatr* 1977;90:1009.
- Wiener PC, Hogg MIJ, Rosen M: Effects of naloxone on pethidine-induced neonatal depression. Part I: Intravenous naloxone. Part II: Intramuscular naloxone. *Br Med J* 1977;2:228.

Neostigmine

DOSE & ADMINISTRATION: Myasthenia gravis: 0.1 mg IM (give 30 minutes before feeding). 1 mg PO (give 2 hours before feeding). Dose may have to be increased and should be titrated. **Reversal of neuromuscular blockade:** 0.04 to 0.08 mg/kg IV, in addition to atropine 0.02 mg/kg.

USES: Neonatal transient myasthenia gravis. Neonatal persistent (congenital) myasthenia gravis. Reversing effects of neuromuscular blocking drugs.

MONITORING: Monitor respiratory and cardiovascular status closely.

ADVERSE EFFECTS/PRECAUTIONS: Contraindicated in presence of intestinal or urinary obstruction, bradycardia, or hypotension. Use cautiously in patients with bronchospasm or cardiac arrhythmia. Adverse effects include muscle weakness, tremors, bradycardia, hypotension, respiratory depression, bronchospasm, diarrhea, and excessive salivation.

PHARMACOLOGY: Neostigmine inhibits acetylcholinesterase at the neuromuscular junction, allowing accumulation of acetylcholine and thus restoring activity.

SPECIAL CONSIDERATIONS/PREPARATION: Available as injectable solution in 1-mL ampules and 10-mL vials in concentrations of 1:1000 (1 mg/mL), 1:2000 (0.5 mg/mL), and 1:4000 (0.25 mg/mL). **Protect from light.**

Solution Compatibility: No data.

Terminal Injection Site Compatibility: Glycopyrrolate, heparin, hydrocortisone succinate, netilmicin, pentobarbital and potassium chloride.

SELECTED REFERENCES

- Fisher DM, Cronnelly R, Miller RD, Sharma M: The neuromuscular pharmacology of neostigmine in infants and children. *Anesthesiology* 1983;59:220.
- Goudsouzian NG, Crone RK, Todres ID: Recovery from pancuronium blockade in the neonatal intensive care unit. *Br J Anaesth* 1981;53:1303.
- Sarnat HB: Neuromuscular disorders in the neonatal period, in Korobken R, Guillemenault C (eds): *Advances in Perinatal Neurology*. New York: Spectrum Publications, 1979, p 153.

NETILMICIN

DOSE & ADMINISTRATION: IV infusion by syringe pump over 30 minutes. Administer as a separate infusion from penicillin-containing compounds. IM injection is associated with variable absorption, especially in the very small infant. To use dosing chart, please refer to explanatory note in "How to Use This Book."

DOSING CHART

PMA (weeks)	Postnatal (days)	Dose (mg/kg)	Interval (hours)
≤29*	0 to 7	5	48
	8 to 28	4	36
	≥29	4	24
30 to 34	0 to 7	4.5	36
	≥8	4	24
≥35	ALL	4	24

* or significant asphyxia, PDA, or treatment with indomethacin

USES: Treatment of infections caused by aerobic gram-negative bacilli (e.g. *Pseudomonas, Klebsiella, E coli*). Usually used in combination with a β-lactam antibiotic.

MONITORING: Measure serum concentrations when treating for more than 48 hours. Obtain peak concentration 30 minutes after end of infusion, and trough concentration just prior to the next dose. When treating patients with serious infections or significantly changing fluid or renal status consider measuring the serum concentration 24 hours after a dose, and use the chart below for the suggested dosing interval. Blood samples obtained to monitor serum drug concentrations should be spun and refrigerated or frozen as soon as possible. Therapeutic serum concentrations: **Peak:** 5 to 12 mcg/mL (or C_{max}/MIC ratio greater than 8:1) **Trough:** 0.5 to 1 mcg/mL

SUGGESTED DOSING INTERVALS

Level at 24 hours (mcg/mL)	Half-life (hours)	Suggested Dosing Interval (hours)
≤1	~ 8	24
1.1 to 2.3	~ 12	36
2.4 to 3.2	~ 15	48
≥3.3		Measure level in 24 hours

ADVERSE EFFECTS/PRECAUTIONS: Transient and reversible renal tubular dysfunction may occur, resulting in increased urinary losses of sodium, calcium, and magnesium. Vestibular and auditory ototoxicity. The addition of other nephrotoxic and/or ototoxic medications (e.g. furosemide, vancomycin) may increase these adverse effects. Increased neuromuscular blockade (i.e., neuromuscular weakness and respiratory failure) may occur when used with pancuronium or other neuromuscular blocking agents and in patients with hypermagnesemia.

PHARMACOLOGY: Dosing recommendations for netilmicin are based on: (1) Higher peak concentrations increase concentration-dependent bacterial killing; (2) There is a post-antibiotic effect on bacterial killing, especially when treating concurrently with a β-lactam antibiotic; (3) There may be less toxicity with less frequent dosing, due to less renal drug accumulation. Volume of distribution is increased and clearance is decreased in patients with PDA. Serum half-life is prolonged in premature and asphyxiated newborns. Inactivation of netilmicin by penicillin-containing compounds appears to be a time-, temperature-, and concentration-dependent process. This is probably clinically significant only when penicillin-containing compounds are mixed in IV solutions or when the blood is at room temperature for several hours before the assay is performed.

SPECIAL CONSIDERATIONS/PREPARATION: Available in a concentration of 100 mg/mL in 1.5 mL vials. A 10 mg/mL dilution may be made by adding 1 mL of this solution to 9 mL of sterile water for injection. Dilution is stable for 72 hours refrigerated. Do not freeze.

Solution Compatibility: D_5W, $D_{10}W$, and NS.

Terminal Injection Site Compatibility: Dex/AA solutions, fat emulsion. Aminophylline, atropine, aztreonam, calcium gluconate, cefuroxime, clindamycin, dexamethasone, hydrocortisone succinate, heparin (concentrations ≤1 unit/mL), iron dextran, linezolid, isoproterenol, metronidazole, neostigmine, norepinephrine, pancuronium bromide, potassium chloride, procainamide, remifentanil, sodium bicarbonate, and vitamin K_1.

Incompatibility: Amphotericin B, ampicillin, cefepime, furosemide, heparin (concentrations >1 U/mL), methicillin, mezlocillin, nafcillin, oxacillin, penicillin G, propofol, and ticarcillin/clavulanate.

SELECTED REFERENCES

- Contopoulos-Ioannidis DG, Giotis ND, Baliatsa DV, Ioannidis JPA: Extended-interval aminoglycoside administration for children: a meta-analysis. Pediatrics 2004;114:e111-e118.
- Stolk LML, Degraeuwe PLJ, Nieman FHM, et al: Population pharmacokinetics and relationship between demographic and clinical variables and pharmacokinetics of gentamicin in neonates. Ther Drug Monit 2002;24:527-31.
- Avent ML, Kinney JS, Istre GR, Whitfield JM: Gentamicin and tobramycin in neonates: comparison of a new extended dosing regimen with a traditional multiple daily dosing regimen. Am J Perinatol 2002;8:413-19.
- Giapros VI, Andronikou S, Cholevas VI, Papadopoulou ZL: Renal function in premature infants during aminoglycoside therapy. Pediatr Nephrol 1995;9:163.
- Daly JS, Dodge RA, Glew RH, et al: Effect of time and temperature on inactivation of aminoglycosides by ampicillin at neonatal dosages. J Perinatol 1997;17:42-45.

NEVIRAPINE

DOSE & ADMINISTRATION: PO: 2 mg/kg single dose at 48 to 72 hours of age. If the mother received nevirapine less than one hour prior to delivery, administer 2 mg/kg as soon as possible after birth, and again at 48 to 72 hours.

USES: Used **only** in combination with zidovudine in the treatment of neonates born to HIV-infected women who have had no therapy during pregnancy. (Mother receives a single 200-mg oral dose of nevirapine during labor). Dosing guidelines above are for prophylactic treatment of neonates born to HIV-infected women. Treatment of infected infants using drug combination regimens should be done in consultation with pediatric infectious disease experts.

MONITORING: Specific monitoring unnecessary due to short treatment course.

ADVERSE EFFECTS/PRECAUTIONS: Limited data on toxicity—none reported in neonates.

PHARMACOLOGY: Nevirapine is a non-nucleoside antiretroviral agent that inhibits HIV-1 replication by selectively interfering with viral reverse transcriptase without requiring intracellular metabolism. It also inactivates cell-free virions in the genital tract and breast milk. Synergistic antiviral activity occurs when administered with zidovudine. Nevirapine is rapidly absorbed after oral administration to pregnant women and is highly lipophilic, resulting in therapeutic concentrations being readily transferred across the placenta to the fetus. Serum half-life in the neonates is approximately 44 hours. With the maternal/newborn regimen described above, serum concentrations are above 100 mcg/L throughout the first week of life. Nevirapine is extensively metabolized by, and an inducer of, hepatic CYP3A4 and CYP2B6 isoenzymes. Concomitant administration of phenobarbital or phenytoin, CYP3A inducers, may affect plasma concentrations.

NICARDIPINE

SPECIAL CONSIDERATIONS/PREPARATION: Available as an oral suspension in a concentration of 10 mg/mL. Store at room temperature and protect from light. Shake suspension gently prior to administration.

SELECTED REFERENCES
- Perinatal HIV Guidelines Working Group. Public Health Service Task Force Recommendations for Use of Antiretroviral Drugs in Pregnant HIV-1 Infected Women for Maternal Health and Interventions to Reduce Perinatal HIV-1 Transmission in the United States. October 12, 2006. Available at http://aidsinfo.nih.gov/ContentFiles/PerinatalGL.pdf.
- Mirochnick M, Dorenbaum A, Blanchard S, et al: Predose infant nevirapine concentration with the two-dose intrapartum neonatal nevirapine regimen: association with timing of maternal intrapartum nevirapine dose. *JAIDS* 2003;33:153-56.
- Mirochnick M, Clarke DF, Dorenbaum A: Nevirapine: pharmacokinetic considerations in children and pregnant women. *Drugs* 2000;39:281-293.

NICARDIPINE

DOSE & ADMINISTRATION: Initial dose: 0.5 mcg/kg per minute continuous IV infusion. Titrate dose to response. Blood pressure will begin to decrease within minutes of starting the infusion, reaching half of its ultimate decrease in approximately 45 minutes. Blood pressure equilibrium will not be achieved for approximately 50 hours (adult data). Maintenance doses are usually 0.5 to 2 mcg/kg per minute.

USES: Treatment of acute severe hypertension.

MONITORING: Continuous monitoring of blood pressure, heart rate and rhythm during initiation of therapy, and frequently thereafter. Observe IV site for signs of irritation.

ADVERSE EFFECTS/PRECAUTIONS: No adverse effects have been reported in neonates (small numbers). Hypotension and tachycardia are dose-dependent in adults. Headache, nausea, and vomiting were the other common effects reported.

PHARMACOLOGY: Nicardipine is a dihydropyridine calcium channel blocker that significantly decreases systemic vascular resistance. Unlike other calcium channel blockers, it has limited effects on the myocardium. It is extensively metabolized by the liver, and is highly protein bound. Following infusion in adults, nicardipine plasma concentrations decline tri-exponentially, with a rapid early distribution phase (alpha half-life of 2.7 minutes), an intermediate phase (beta half-life of 44.8 minutes), and a slow terminal phase (gamma half-life of 14.4 hours) that can only be detected after long-term infusions. Experience in neonates is limited, and there are no reported pharmacokinetic data.

SPECIAL CONSIDERATIONS/PREPARATION: Available as solution for injection, 2.5 mg/mL, in 10-mL ampuls. **Dilute prior to administration to a concentration of 0.1 mg/mL.** Dilution is stable at room temperature for 24 hours. Store ampuls at controlled room temperature. Freezing does not adversely affect the product, but exposure to elevated temperatures should be avoided. Protect from light. Store ampuls in carton until used.

Solution Compatibility: D_5W, NS, and D_5NS.

Solution Incompatibility: Lactated Ringers.

Terminal Injection Site Compatibility: No data available for Dex/AA solutions or fat emulsions. Amikacin, aminophylline, aztreonam, calcium gluconate, cefazolin, ceftizoxime, chloramphenicol, cimetidine, clindamycin, dobutamine, dopamine, enalaprilat, epinephrine, erythromycin lactobionate, esmolol, famotidine, fentanyl, gentamicin, heparin (concentrations ≤ 1 U/mL), hydrocortisone, lidocaine, linezolid, lorazepam, magnesium sulfate, metronidazole, midazolam, milrinone, morphine, nafcillin, nitroglycerin, norepinephrine, penicillin G potassium, piperacillin, potassium chloride, potassium phosphate, ranitidine, sodium acetate, sodium nitroprusside, tobramycin, trimethoprim-sulfamethoxazole, vancomycin, and vecuronium.

Incompatibility: Ampicillin, cefoperazone, ceftazidime, furosemide, heparin (concentrations > 1 U/mL), sodium bicarbonate and thiopental.

SELECTED REFERENCES
- McBride BF, White CM, Campbell M, Frey BM: Nicardipine to control neonatal hypertension during extracorporeal membrane oxygen support. *Ann Pharmacother* 2003;37:667-670.
- Tobias JD: Nicardipine to control mean arterial pressure after cardiothoracic surgery in infants and children. *Am J Ther* 2001;8:3-6.
- Milou C, Debuche-Benouachkou V, Semama DS et al: Intravenous nicardipine as a first-line antihypertensive drug in neonates. *Intensive Care Med* 2000;26:956-958.
- Gouyon JB, Geneste B, Semama, DS, et al: Intravenous nicardipine in hypertensive preterm infants. *Arch Dis Child Fetal Neonatal Ed* 1997;76:F126-127.
- Product Information, ESP Pharma, 2002.

Nitric Oxide

DOSE & ADMINISTRATION: Nitric oxide inhalation therapy (iNO) should be used only after mechanical ventilatory support has been optimized, including the use of surfactant. **Begin at 20 ppm.** If within 4 hours PaO_2 increases to at least 60 torr, decrease to 5 ppm. Continue at 5 ppm and wean fiO_2 as tolerated. When fiO_2 is less than 0.6 and ventilatory support has been decreased, wean iNO in 1 ppm increments at approximately 4 hour intervals as tolerated. Discontinue when stable on 1 ppm for 4 hours. The usual length of treatment is less than 4 days. Infants who cannot be weaned off after 4 days should undergo further diagnostic testing for other diseases. Administer via an FDA/EMEA approved delivery system designed to accurately deliver NO uninterrupted into the ventilator system in parts-per-million concentrations that are constant throughout the respiratory cycle, while limiting NO_2 production (e.g., INOvent™).

USES: Treatment of term and near-term infants (≥34 weeks GA) with hypoxic respiratory failure (Oxygenation Index > 25) associated with clinical or echocardiographic evidence of pulmonary hypertension. It is usually not effective in infants with congenital diaphragmatic hernia. Do not use in infants dependent on right-to-left cardiac blood flow.

MONITORING: Continuous monitoring of oxygenation, blood pressure and heart rate are mandatory. Measure blood methemoglobin concentration 4 hours after initiation of therapy and at 24 hour intervals thereafter. Monitoring of inspired gas must provide for continuous measurement of both NO and NO_2 concentrations, with a feedback mechanism that cuts off delivery if NO or NO_2 exceed acceptable limits.

ADVERSE EFFECTS/PRECAUTIONS: Abrupt discontinuation may result in worsening oxygenation and increased pulmonary artery pressures. The risks of methemoglobinemia and elevated NO_2 levels increase significantly at doses > 20 ppm. Methemoglobin has very high affinity for oxygen and has a profound effect on oxygen content. Small increases in methemoglobin cause significant decreases in available oxygen content. Normal methemoglobin levels are < 1%. In most neonatal studies methemoglobinemia was defined as levels of 5 to 7%. Cyanosis develops at levels of 10%, although the patients generally remain asymptomatic. At methemoglobin levels approaching 30%, patients begin to experience respiratory distress, and cardiac, gastrointestinal, and neurologic symptoms. A methemoglobin level greater than 50% is usually lethal. Avoid concomitant use of acetaminophen, metoclopramide, sulfa drugs, topical anesthetics (EMLA, benzocaine, lidocaine, prilocaine). Congenital deficiencies in the methemoglobin reductase enzyme system occur but are rare. The environmental exposure limit set by the Occupational Safety and Health Administration is 25 ppm for NO and 5 ppm for NO_2.

PHARMACOLOGY: Inhaled nitric oxide (iNO) is a selective pulmonary vasodilator that decreases extrapulmonary right-to-left shunting. It activates guanyl cyclase by binding to its heme component leading to production of cyclic GMP, with subsequent relaxation of pulmonary vascular smooth muscle. Oxygenation is also improved due to the redirecting of blood from poorly aerated to better aerated distal air spaces. In addition, iNO appears to have both anti-oxidant and anti-inflammatory activities.

SPECIAL CONSIDERATIONS/PREPARATION: Nitric oxide for inhalation is supplied in medical grade gas cylinders. Store vertically in well-ventilated areas at room temperature. All cylinders should be returned to the supplier for disposal. Hospital personnel should receive specific training in the administration of iNO.

SELECTED REFERENCES

- Finer NN, Barrington KJ: Nitric oxide for respiratory failure in infants born at term or near term (Cochrane Review). In: *The Cochrane Library*, Issue 2, 2002. Oxford. Update Software.
- Clark RH, Huckaby JL, Kueser TJ, et al. Low-dose nitric oxide therapy for persistent pulmonary hypertension: 1-year follow-up. *J Perinatol* 2003; 23(4):300-303.
- Lipkin PH, Davidson D, Spivak L, et al. Neurodevelopmental and medical outcomes of persistent pulmonary hypertension in term newborns treated with nitric oxide. *J Pediatr* 2002;140(3):306-310.
- Finer NN, Sun JW, Rich W, et al: Randomized, prospective study of low-dose versus high-dose inhaled nitric oxide in the neonate with hypoxic respiratory failure. *Pediatrics* 2001;108:948-55.
- Clark RH, Kueser TJ, Walker MW, et al: Low-dose nitric oxide therapy for persistent pulmonary hypertension of the newborn. *N Engl J Med* 2000;342:469-74.
- Kinsella JP, Abman SH: Clinical approach to inhaled nitric oxide therapy in the newborn with hypoxemia. *J Pediatr* 2000;136:717-26.

NIZATIDINE

- The Neonatal Inhaled Nitric Oxide Study Group: Inhaled nitric oxide in term and near-term infants: Neurodevelopmental follow-up of the The Neonatal Inhaled Nitric Oxide Study Group (NINOS). *J Pediatr* 2000;136:611-17.
- Davidson D, Barefield ES, Kattwinkel J, et al: Safety of withdrawing inhaled nitric oxide therapy in persistent pulmonary hypertension of the newborn. *Pediatrics* 1999;104:231-36.
- The Neonatal Inhaled Nitric Oxide Study Group: Inhaled nitric oxide in full-term and nearly full-term infants with hypoxic respiratory failure. *N Engl J Med* 1997;336:597-604.

NIZATIDINE

DOSE & ADMINISTRATION: PO: 2 to 5 mg/kg per dose Q12 hours orally.

USES: Prevention and treatment of stress ulcers and GI hemorrhage aggravated by gastric acid secretion.

MONITORING: Gastric pH may be measured to assess efficacy.

ADVERSE EFFECTS/PRECAUTIONS: Limited data in neonatal patients. One case report of thrombocytopenia. No other adverse effects have been reported in infants or children. Elevations in hepatic enzymes and asymptomatic ventricular tachycardia have been reported in adults.

PHARMACOLOGY: Inhibits gastric acid secretion by histamine H_2-receptor antagonism. Peak serum concentration occurs 0.5 to 3 hours after oral administration and is not influenced by food. Bioavailability is quite variable. Greater than 90% eliminated in the urine within 12 hours with 60% excreted unchanged. Elimination half-life in neonates is 3 to 7 hours, and is prolonged in preterm infants and patients with renal insufficiency.

SPECIAL CONSIDERATIONS/PREPARATION: Axid® alcohol-free oral solution (15 mg/mL) is supplied in 480 mL bottles. Store at room temperature.

SELECTED REFERENCES

- Orenstein SR, Gremse DA, Pantaleon CD, et al: Nizatidine for the treatment of pediatric gastroesophageal reflux symptoms: An open-label, multiple-dose, randomized, multicenter clinical trial in 210 children. *Clin Therapeutics* 2005;27:472-483.
- Hamamoto N, Hashimoto T, Adachi K, et al: Comparative study of nizatidine and famotidine for maintenance therapy of erosive esophagitis. *J Gastroenterol Hepatol* 2005;20:281-286.
- Abdel-Rahman SM, Johnson FK, Connor JD, et al: Developmental pharmacokinetics and pharmacodynamics of nizatidine. *JPGN* 2004;38:442-451.
- Abdel-Rahman SM, Johnson FK, Gauthier-Dubois G, et al: The bioequivalence of nizatidine (Axid®) in two extemporaneously and one commerically prepared oral liquid fomulations compared with capsule. *J Clin Pharmacol* 2003;43:148-153.
- Abdel-Rahman SM, Johnson FK, Manowitz N, et al: Single-dose pharmacokinetics of nizatidine (Axid®) in children. *J Clin Pharmacol* 2002;42:1089-1096.
- Product information, Braintree Laboratories, Inc., 2005.

NYSTATIN

DOSE & ADMINISTRATION: Topical: Apply ointment or cream to affected area Q6 hours. Continue treatment for 3 days after symptoms have subsided. **PO:** 1 mL (preterm) to 2 mL (term) of 100,000-units/mL suspension divided and applied with swab to each side of mouth Q6 hours. Continue treatment for 3 days after symptoms have subsided.

USES: Treatment of mucocutaneous candidal infections.

MONITORING: Assess response to drug.

ADVERSE EFFECTS/PRECAUTIONS: Possible skin rash caused by vehicle in ointment/cream.

PHARMACOLOGY: Nystatin is a polyene antifungal similar in structure to amphotericin B. May be fungicidal or fungistatic. Binds to the fungal cell membrane causing disruption of the cell structure. Not absorbed well from the GI tract, skin, or mucous membranes.

SPECIAL CONSIDERATIONS/PREPARATION: Topical ointment/cream: 100,000 units/g in 15- and 30-g tubes. Ointment dissolved in polyethylene and mineral-oil-gel base. **Oral suspension:** 100,000 units/mL in 5-, 60-, and 480-mL bottles. Shake well before applying to mouth. Appears to work best when not mixed with formula. Contains <1% alcohol, saccharin, and 50% sucrose.

SELECTED REFERENCES

- Hoppe JE: Treatment of oropharyngeal candidiasis and candidal diaper dermatitis in neonates and infants: review and reappraisal. *Ped Inf Dis J* 1997;16:885-94.

- Faix RG, Kovarik SM, Shaw TR, Johnson RV: Mucocutaneous and invasive candidiasis among very low birth weight (<1500 grams) infants in intensive care nurseries: A prospective study. *Pediatrics* 1989;83:101.
- Roberts RJ: *Drug Therapy in Infants*. Philadelphia: WB Saunders Co, 1984, p 81.
- Munz D, Powell KR, Pai CH: Treatment of candidal diaper dermatitis: A double-blind placebo-controlled comparison of topical nystatin with topical plus oral nystatin. *J Pediatr* 1982;101:1022.

OCTREOTIDE

DOSE & ADMINISTRATION: Treatment of hyperinsulinemic hypoglycemia: **Initial dose:** 1 mcg/kg per dose Q6h subQ or IV. Titrate upward to desired effect. Initial response should occur within 8 hours; tachyphylaxis may occur within several days. **Maximum dose:** 10 mcg/kg per dose Q6h. **Treatment of chylothorax:** Begin at 1 mcg/kg per hour continuous infusion, subQ or IV. Titrate upward as necessary; chyle production should significantly decrease within 24 hours. **Maximum dose:** 7 mcg/kg per hour.

USES: Treatment of refractory hyperinsulinemic hypoglycemia. Adjunctive treatment of congenital and post-operative chylothorax.

MONITORING: Monitor blood glucose closely.

ADVERSE EFFECTS/PRECAUTIONS: Vomiting, diarrhea, abdominal distention and steatorrhea may occur. Pulmonary hypertension has been reported in treated former premature infants with chronic lung disease. Hyperglycemia may occur in patients being treated for chylothorax.

PHARMACOLOGY: Octreotide is a long-acting analog of the natural hormone somatostatin. It is an even more potent inhibitor of growth hormone, glucagon, and insulin than somatostatin. Like somatostatin, it also suppresses LH response to GnRH, decreases splanchnic blood flow, and inhibits release of serotonin, gastrin, vasoactive intestinal peptide, secretin, motilin, and pancreatic polypeptide. After subcutaneous injection, octreotide is absorbed rapidly and completely from the injection site. The elimination half-life of octreotide from plasma is approximately 1.7 hours in adults, compared with 1 to 3 minutes for the natural hormone. Excreted unchanged into the urine.

SPECIAL CONSIDERATIONS/PREPARATION: Available in 1-mL single-dose ampules for injection containing 50-, 100-, or 500-mcg, and in 5-mL multiple-dose vials in concentrations of 200- and 1000-mcg/mL. pH 3.9 to 4.5. Osmolarity is 279 mOsm/kg. Refrigerate and protect from light. Do not warm artificially. After initial use, multiple dose vials should be discarded within 14 days. Ampuls should be opened just prior to administration and the unused portion discarded. For SC injection use undiluted drug unless dose volume is not accurately measurable. For continuous IV administration consider making a dilution of 10- to 25-mcg/mL using D_5W or NS.

Solution Compatibility: D_5W and NS.

Solution Incompatibility: Do not add directly to Dex/AA bag because of the formation of glycosyl octreotide conjugate.

Terminal Injection Site Compatibility: Dex/AA and heparin.

Incompatibility: Fat emulsion.

SELECTED REFERENCES

- Young S, Dalgleish S, Eccleston A, et al: Severe congenital chylothorax treated with octreotide. *J Perinatol* 2004;24:200-202.
- de Lonlay P, Touati G, Robert J-J, Saudubray J-M: Persistent hyperinsulinemic hypoglycaemia. *Semin Neonatol* 2002;7:95-100.
- Schwitzgebel VM, Gitelman SE: Neonatal hyperinsulinism. *Clin Perinatol* 1998;25:1015-38.
- Chung Y-F, Leung MP, Yip M-M: Octreotide for treatment of postoperative chylothorax. *J Pediatr* 2001;139:157-59.

OMEPRAZOLE

DOSE & ADMINISTRATION: 0.5 to 1.5 mg/kg per dose PO, once a day. See below for oral preparation.

USES: Short-term (less than 8 weeks) treatment of documented reflux esophagitis or duodenal ulcer refractory to conventional therapy.

MONITORING: Observe for symptomatic improvement within 3 days. Consider intraesophageal pH monitoring to assess for efficacy (pH >4.0). Measure AST and ALT if duration of therapy is greater than 8 weeks.

Oxacillin

ADVERSE EFFECTS/PRECAUTIONS: Hypergastrinemia and mild transaminase elevations are the only Adverse Effects reported in children who received omeprazole for extended periods of time. Available data are limited to small studies of infants and children.

PHARMACOLOGY: Omeprazole inhibits gastric acid secretion by inhibition of hydrogen-potassium ATPase, the enzyme responsible for the final step in the secretion of hydrochloric acid by the gastric parietal cell ("proton pump"). Onset of action is within one hour of administration, maximal effect is at approximately 2 hours. Inhibition of acid secretion is about 50% of maximum at 24 hours and the duration of action is approximately 72 hours.

SPECIAL CONSIDERATIONS/PREPARATION: Prilosec® is supplied in delayed-release capsules containing either 10, 20, and 40-mg omeprazole as enteric-coated granules. A 2 mg/mL oral liquid preparation can be prepared as follows: Empty the contents of five 20-mg omeprazole capsules into the barrel of a 60-mL syringe. Replace the plunger in the syringe and draw up 50 mL of 8.4% sodium bicarbonate injection. Replace the needle on the 60-mL syringe with a fluid-dispensing connector. Connect a second 60-mL syringe to the fluid-dispensing connector and gently transfer the contents of the syringes back and forth until the granules are completely dissolved. Transfer the entire 50-mL solution into one of the 60-mL syringes removing the fluid-dispensing connector. Attach a 19-gauge needle and transfer the contents to an empty vial. Stable for 30 days refrigerated. Protect from light.

SELECTED REFERENCES

- Alliet P, Raes M, Bruneel E, Gillis P: Omeprazole in infants with cimetidine-resistant peptic esophagitis. J Pediatr 1998;132:352-354.
- Quercia RA, Fan C, Liu X, et al: Stability of omeprazole in an extemporaneously prepared oral liquid. Am J Health-Syst Pharm 1997;54:1833-1836.
- Kato S, Ebina K, Fujii K, et al: Effect of omeprazole in the treatment of refractory acid-related diseases in childhood: endoscopic healing and twenty-four-hour intragastric acidity. J Pediatr 1996;128:415-421.
- Faure C, Michaud L, Shaghagi EK, Popon M, et al: Intravenous omeprazole in children: pharmacokinetics and effect on 24-hour intragastric pH. J Pediatr Gastroenterol Nutr 2001;33:144-8.
- Product information, AstraZeneca, LP, 2004.

Oxacillin

DOSE & ADMINISTRATION: Usual dosage: 25 mg/kg per dose IV over at least 10 minutes.
Meningitis: 50 mg/kg per dose. To use dosing chart, please refer to explanatory note in "How to Use This Book."

Dosing Interval Chart

PMA (weeks)	PostNatal (days)	Interval (hours)
≤29	0 to 28	12
	>28	8
30 to 36	0 to 14	12
	>14	8
37 to 44	0 to 7	12
	>7	8
≥45	ALL	6

USES: Treatment of infections caused by penicillinase-producing staphylococci.

MONITORING: Periodic CBC and urinalysis. AST, ALT. Irritating to veins—watch for phlebitis. Observe IV site for signs of extravasation.

ADVERSE EFFECTS/PRECAUTIONS: Interstitial nephritis associated with hematuria, albuminuria, and casts in urine. Bone marrow depression. Elevated AST and ALT. Hypersensitivity in the form of a rash. Tolerant strains of staphylococci have been reported.

PHARMACOLOGY: Oxacillin inhibits synthesis of bacterial cell wall. Rapidly excreted renally unchanged. Poor CSF penetration. Good penetration of pleural, pericardial, and synovial fluids.

SPECIAL CONSIDERATIONS/PREPARATION: Available as powder injection in 250-mg, 500-mg, 1-g, 2-g, and 10-g vials. Reconstitute 250 mg vial with 5 mL of sterile water for injection to make a concentration of 50 mg/mL. Reconstituted solution is stable for 3 days at room temperature, 7 days refrigerated. Dilute further using sterile water to a concentration less than 40 mg/mL. Dilution stable for 4 days refrigerated. Maximum concentration for IV infusion is 100 mg/mL.

Solution Compatibility: D_5W, $D_{10}W$, and NS.

Terminal Injection Site Compatibility: Dex/AA solutions, fat emulsion. Acyclovir, chloramphenicol, dopamine, famotidine, fluconazole, heparin, hydrocortisone succinate, milrinone, morphine, potassium chloride, and zidovudine.

Incompatibility: Amikacin, caffeine citrate, gentamicin, netilmicin, sodium bicarbonate, and tobramycin.

SELECTED REFERENCES

- Maraqa NF, Gomez MM, Rathore MH, Alvarez AM: Higher occurrence of hepatotoxicity and rash in patients treated with oxacillin, compared with those treated with nafcillin and other commonly used antimicrobials. Clin Infect Dis 2002;34:50-54.
- Prober CG, Stevenson DK, Benitz WE: The use of antibiotics in neonates weighing less than 1200 grams. Pediatr Infect Dis J 1990;9:111.
- Nahata MC, Debolt SL, Powell DA: Adverse effects of methicillin, nafcillin, and oxacillin in pediatric patients. Dev Pharmacol Ther 1982;4:117.
- Axline SG, Yaffe SJ, Simon HJ: Clinical pharmacology of antimicrobials in premature infants: II. Ampicillin, methicillin, oxacillin, neomycin, and colistin. Pediatrics 1967;39:97.

PALIVIZUMAB

DOSE & ADMINISTRATION: 15 mg/kg per dose IM, preferably in the anterolateral aspect of the thigh. Repeat monthly during RSV season.

USES: Immunoprophylaxis against severe RSV lower respiratory tract infections in high risk infants:
- up to 24 months of age, hemodynamically significant acyanotic and cyanotic congenital heart disease
- less than 24 months of age, chronic lung disease of prematurity (CLD) who have required medical therapy for CLD witin 6 months before the start of the RSV season
- up to 12 months of age, born at 28 weeks gestation or earlier
- up to 6 months of age, born at 29 to 32 weeks gestation
- less than 6 months of age, born between 32 and 35 weeks gestation with at least 2 additional risk factors

Risk factors include child care attendance, school-aged siblings, exposure to environmental air pollutants, congenital abnormalities of the airways, or severe neuromuscular disease. Once an infant qualifies for initiation of prophylaxis, it should continue throughout the RSV season. Palivizumab is not effective for treatment of established RSV disease.

MONITORING: Observe injection site for induration and swelling.

ADVERSE EFFECTS/PRECAUTIONS: In clinical trials, upper respiratory infection, otitis media, fever, and rhinitis occurred slightly more frequently in palivizumab recipients. Cyanosis and arrhythmia were also seen slightly more frequently in patients with CHD. There are rare reports (<1 per 100,000 patients) of anaphylaxis, and hypersensitivity reactions have been reported. Do not administer to patients with a history of a prior severe reaction.

PHARMACOLOGY: Synagis® is a humanized monoclonal antibody produced by recombinant DNA technology. This composite of human (95%) and murine (5%) antibody sequences inhibits RSV replication. The mean half-life of Synagis® is approximately 20 days. Adequate antibody titers are maintained in most infants for one month following a 15-mg/kg dose. Due to a faster matabolic rate, some hospitalized VLBW infants (<500 g) may not maintain optimal RSV titers for the entire initial month until after the second dose. Palivizumab does not interfere with the response to other vaccines and as such, they can be administered concurrently.

SPECIAL CONSIDERATIONS/PREPARATION: Synagis® is supplied as 50-mg and 100-mg single-dose vials. In the United States, beginning in the 2005-06 RSV season, the lyophilized powder form is being replaced with a ready-to-use, **NO RECONSTITUTION required**, liquid solution. Do not add any diluent to the liquid solution and use one dose per vial. Do not re-enter vial after initial withdrawal and discard any unused portions. Administer as soon as possible after withdrawal from the vial. **Do not FREEZE or SHAKE**. The lyophilized powder is reconstituted by slowly adding 0.6 mL sterile water for injection to the

PANCURONIUM

50-mg vial, and 1 mL sterile water for injection to the 100-mg vial. The vial should be tilted slightly and gently rotated to evenly wet the lyophilized powder. To avoid foaming, **DO NOT SHAKE OR AGITATE THE VIAL.** Let stand at room temperature for a minimum of 20 minutes until the solution clarifies. Use one dose per vial. Do not re-enter vial after initial withdrawal and discard any unused portions. Administer as soon as possible after withdrawal from the vial. Both the liquid solution and the un-reconstituted lyophilized powder should be stored **refrigerated between 2 to 8°C (36 to 46°F).** Synagis® contains no preservatives, thiomersol, or other mercury salts.

SELECTED REFERENCES

- American Academy of Pediatrics. Respiratory Syncytial Virus (RSV) Infections. In: Pickering LK, Baker CJ, Long SS, McMillan JA, eds. *Red Book: 2006 Report of the Committee on Infectious Diseases.* 27th ed. Elk Grove Village, IL: American Academy of Pediatrics; 2006:560-566.
- Meissner HC, Long SS, Committee on Infectious Diseases and Committee on Fetus and Newborn: Revised indications for the use of palivizumab and respiratory syncytial virus immune globulin intravenous for the prevention of respiratory syncytial virus infections. Policy Statement and Technical Report. *Pediatrics* 2003;122:1442-46 and 1447-52.
- Romero JR: Palivizumab prophylaxis of respiratory syncytial virus disease from 1998 to 2002: results from four years of palivizumab usage. *Pediatr Infect Dis J* 2003;22:S46-54.
- The Impact-RSV Study Group: Palivizumab, a humanized respiratory syncytial virus monoclonal antibody, reduces hospitalization from respiratory syncytial virus infection in high-risk infants. *Pediatrics* 1998;102:531-537.
- Groothuis JR: Safety and tolerance of palivizumab administration in a large northern hemisphere trial. *Pediatr Infect Dis J* 2001;20:628-629.
- Wu S-Y, Bonaparte J, Pyati S: Palivizumab use in very premature infants in the neonatal intensive care unit. *Pediatrics* 2004;114:e554-e556.
- Product Information, MedImmune, 2006.

PANCURONIUM

DOSE & ADMINISTRATION: 0.1 mg/kg (0.04 to 0.15 mg/kg) IV push, as needed for paralysis. Usual dosing interval is 1 to 2 hours. Adjust dose as needed based on duration of paralysis.

USES: Skeletal muscle relaxation/paralysis in infants requiring mechanical ventilation. Proposed desirable effects are improved oxygenation/ ventilation, reduced barotrauma, and reduced fluctuations in cerebral blood flow.

MONITORING: Monitor vital signs frequently, blood pressure continuously. Use some form of eye lubrication.

ADVERSE EFFECTS/PRECAUTIONS: Hypoxemia may occur because of inadequate mechanical ventilation and deterioration in pulmonary mechanics. Tachycardia and blood pressure changes (both hypotension and hypertension) occur frequently. Increased salivation.

PHARMACOLOGY: Pancuronium is a nondepolarizing muscle-relaxant that competitively antagonizes autonomic cholinergic receptors and also causes sympathetic stimulation. Partially hydroxylated by the liver, 40% excreted unchanged in urine. Onset of action is 1 to 2 minutes; duration varies with dose and age. Reversed by neostigmine and atropine. Factors affecting duration of neuromuscular blockade: **Potentiation:** Acidosis, hypothermia, neuromuscular disease, hepatic disease, renal failure, cardiovascular disease, younger age, aminoglycosides, hypermagnesemia, and hypokalemia. **Antagonism:** Alkalosis, epinephrine, and hyperkalemia. Sensation remains intact; analgesia should be used for painful procedures.

SPECIAL CONSIDERATIONS/PREPARATION: Available in concentrations of 1-mg/mL (10 mL vials) and 2-mg/mL (2-and 5-mL vials and ampules). Organon products contains 1% (10 mg/mL) benzyl alcohol. **Refrigerate.**

Solution Compatibility: D_5W and NS.

Terminal Injection Site Compatibility: Dex/AA. Aminophylline, caffeine citrate, cefazolin, cimetidine, dobutamine, dopamine, epinephrine, esmolol, fentanyl, fluconazole, gentamicin, heparin, hydrocortisone succinate, isoproterenol, lorazepam, midazolam, milrinone, morphine, netilmicin, nitroglycerin, nitroprusside, propofol, prostaglandin E_1, ranitidine, trimethoprim-sulfamethoxazole, and vancomycin.

Incompatibility: Pentobarbital and phenobarbital.

PAPAVERINE

DOSE & ADMINISTRATION: 30 mg per 250 mL of arterial catheter infusion solution.

USES: Prolongation of peripheral arterial catheter patency.

ADVERSE EFFECTS/PRECAUTIONS: Use with caution in VLBW infants in the first days after birth due to potential of developing or extending an intracranial hemorrhage. Chronic hepatitis, as evidenced by an increase in serum bilirubin and serum glutamic transaminase, has been reported in three adults following long-term papaverine therapy. One patient had jaundice, and another had abnormal liver function on biopsy.

PHARMACOLOGY: Papaverine directly relaxes the tonus of various smooth muscle, especially when it has been spasmodically contracted. It relaxes the smooth musculature of the larger blood vessels, especially coronary, systemic peripheral and pulmonary arteries. Vasodilation may be related to its ability to inhibit cyclic nucleotide phosphodiesterase, thus increasing levels of intracellular cyclic AMP. During administration, the muscle cell is not paralyzed and still responds to drugs and other stimuli causing contraction. Possibly because of its direct vasodilating action on cerebral blood vessels, papaverine increases cerebral blood flow and decreases cerebral vascular resistance in healthy subjects; oxygen consumption is unaltered. Papaverine is metabolized in the liver and excreted in the urine in an inactive form.

SPECIAL CONSIDERATIONS/PREPARATION: Supplied as 30 mg/mL solution for injection in 2 mL preservative-free vials and 10-mL multiple dose vials containing 0.5% chlorobutanol.

Solution Compatibility: NS, 0.45 NS, both with 1 Unit/mL heparin

Solution Incompatibility: Lactated Ringers (precipate forms)

Terminal Injection Site Compatibility: Phentolamine.

SELECTED REFERENCES

- Griffin MP, Siadaty MS: Papaverine prolongs patency of peripheral arterial catheters in neonates. *J Pediatr* 2005;146:62-65.
- Heulitt MJ, Farrington EA, O'Shea TM, et al: Double-blind randomized controlled trial of papaverine-containing solutions to prevent failure of arterial catheters in pediatric patients. *Crit Care Med* 1993;21:825-829.

PENICILLIN G

DOSE & ADMINISTRATION: "Use only aqueous crystalline penicillin G for IV administration" **Meningitis:** 75,000 to 100,000 units/kg per dose IV infusion over 30 minutes, or IM. **Bacteremia:** 25,000 to 50,000 units/kg per dose IV infusion over 15 minutes, or IM. To use dosing chart, please refer to explanatory note in "How to Use This Book."

DOSING INTERVAL CHART

PMA (weeks)	PostNatal (days)	Interval (hours)
≤29	0 to 28 >28	12 8
30 to 36	0 to 14 >14	12 8
37 to 44	0 to 7 >7	12 8
≥45	ALL	6

Group B streptococcal infections: Some experts recommend using 200,000 units/kg per day for bacteremia and 450,000 units/kg per day for meningitis, in divided doses at more frequent intervals than those listed above. Consider adding aminoglycoside if tolerance is suspected or confirmed. **Gonococcal infection (only with proven penicillin-**

susceptible isolate): Use higher doses listed for meningitis and bacteremia. **Congenital syphilis:** Aqueous crystalline penicillin G: 50,000 units/kg per dose IV over 15 minutes, given Q12 hours during the first 7 days of life, and Q8 hours thereafter, irrespective of gestational age; or Procaine penicillin G: 50,000 units/kg per dose IM, once daily. Treat for 10 to 14 days. **Procaine and benzathine penicillin G are for IM administration only.**

USES: Treatment of infections caused by susceptible organisms—congenital syphilis, gonococci, streptococci (non enterococcal).

MONITORING: Follow serum sodium and potassium when using high doses and in patients with renal failure. Observe IV site for signs of extravasation.

ADVERSE EFFECTS/PRECAUTIONS: Cardiac arrest has been reported in patients who received high doses infused rapidly. Significant CNS toxicity has been reported in adults with renal failure who developed CSF concentrations >10 mcg/mL. Bone marrow depression, granulocytopenia, and hepatitis are rare. Hypersensitivity has not been seen in neonates.

PHARMACOLOGY: Penicillin inhibits synthesis of bacterial cell wall. Excreted unchanged in the urine. CSF penetration is poor, except in inflamed meninges. Concentrates in joint fluid and urine.

SPECIAL CONSIDERATIONS/PREPARATION: Aqueous penicillin G is available as powder for injection in two salt forms: penicillin G potassium and penicillin G sodium. Penicillin G potassium contains 1.67 mEq (65.6 mg) potassium per 1 million units, and 0.3 mEq (6.8 mg) sodium per 1 million units. Penicillin G sodium contains 2 mEq (46 mg) sodium per 1 million units. Reconstitute the 5-million unit vial with 8 mL sterile water for injection to make a final concentration of 500,000 units /mL. Reconstituted solution good for 7 days refrigerated. A 100,000 unit/mL dilution may be made by adding 10 mL of reconstituted solution to 40 mL sterile water for injection. Dilution stable for 4 days refrigerated. Procaine and benzathine penicillin G for IM injection are available in multiple dosage strengths in vials and Tubex® syringes. **Note: Penicillin G is also known as benzylpenicillin - do not confuse with benzathine penicillin used for only for IM injections. 1 million units is the equivalent of 600 mg.**

Solution Compatibility: D_5W, $D_{10}W$, and NS.

Terminal Injection Site Compatibility: Dex/AA solutions, fat emulsion. Acyclovir, amiodarone, caffeine citrate, calcium chloride, calcium gluconate, chloramphenicol, cimetidine, clindamycin, dopamine, enalaprilat, erythromycin lactobionate, esmolol, fluconazole, furosemide, heparin, hydrocortisone succinate, lidocaine, methicillin, metronidazole, morphine, nicardipine, pentobarbital, potassium chloride, prostaglandin E_1, ranitidine and sodium bicarbonate.

Incompatibility: Amikacin, aminophylline, amphotericin B, gentamicin, metoclopramide, netilmicin, and tobramycin.

SELECTED REFERENCES

- American Academy of Pediatrics. Syphilis. In: Pickering LK, Baker CJ, Long SS, McMillan JA, eds. *Red Book: 2006 Report of the Committee on Infectious Diseases.* 27th ed. Elk Grove Village, IL: American Academy of Pediatrics; 2006: pp 637-638.
- Centers for Disease Control and Prevention: Sexually transmitted diseases treatment guidelines 2006. *MMWR* 2006;55(No. RR-11).
- Stoll BJ: Congenital syphilis: evaluation and management of neonates born to mothers with reactive serologic tests for syphilis. *Pediatr Infect Dis J* 1994;13;845.
- Prober CG, Stevenson DK, Benitz WE: The use of antibiotics in neonates weighing less than 1200 grams. *Pediatr Infect Dis J* 1990;9;111.
- Roberts RJ: *Drug Therapy in Infants.* Philadelphia: WB Saunders Co, 1984, p45.
- Pyati SP, Pildes RS, Jacobs NM, et al: Penicillin in infants weighing two kilograms or less with early onset group B streptococcal disease. *N Engl J Med* 1983;308:1383.
- McCracken GH Jr, Ginsburg C, Chrane DF, et al: Clinical pharmacology of penicillin in newborn infants. *J Pediatr* 1973;82:692.

PENTOBARBITAL

DOSE & ADMINISTRATION: 2 to 6 mg/kg IV slow push.

USES: Sedative/hypnotic, for short-term use.

MONITORING: Monitor respiratory status and blood pressure closely. Serum concentration for sedation: 0.5 to 3 mcg/mL.

ADVERSE EFFECTS/PRECAUTIONS: Respiratory depression. Tolerance, dependence, and cardiovascular depression occur with continued use. Enhances metabolism of phenytoin, sodium valproate, and corticosteroids by microsomal enzyme induction.

PHARMACOLOGY: Pentobarbital is a short-acting barbiturate. Pentobarbital has no analgesic effects. Serum half-life is dose-dependent (15 to 50 hours in adults) and unknown in neonates. Metabolized by hepatic microsomal enzyme system.

SPECIAL CONSIDERATIONS/PREPARATION: Available as a 50 mg/mL solution in 2 mL Tubex®. Solution contains propylene glycol 40%, and alcohol 10%. Irritating to veins—pH is 9.5. A 5 mg/mL dilution may be made by adding 1 mL of the 50 mg/mL solution to 9 mL of preservative-free normal saline. Use immediately.

Solution Compatibility: D_5W, $D_{10}W$, and NS. No data are currently available on Dex/AA.

Terminal Injection Site Compatibility: Acyclovir, amikacin, aminophylline, atropine, calcium chloride, chloramphenicol, erythromycin lactobionate, hyaluronidase, insulin, lidocaine, linezolid, neostigmine, penicillin G, propofol, and sodium bicarbonate.

Incompatibility: Fat emulsion. Cefazolin, cimetidine, clindamycin, fentanyl, hydrocortisone succinate, midazolam, mivacurium, morphine, pancuronium bromide, phenytoin, ranitidine, and vancomycin. No data are currently available on heparin and potassium chloride.

SELECTED REFERENCES

- Strain JD, Harvey LA, Foley LC, Campbell JB: Intravenously administered pentobarbital sodium for sedation in pediatric CT. *Radiology* 1986;161:105.

PHENOBARBITAL

DOSE & ADMINISTRATION: Loading dose: 20 mg/kg IV, given slowly over 10 to 15 minutes. Refractory seizures: Additional 5-mg/kg doses, up to a total of 40 mg/kg. **Maintenance:** 3 to 4 mg/kg **per day** beginning 12 to 24 hours after the load. **Frequency/Route:** Daily (Q12 hours probably unnecessary). IV slow push (most rapid control of seizures), IM, PO, or PR.

USES: Anticonvulsant. May improve outcomes in severely asphyxiated infants (40 mg/kg IV infusion over 1 hour, prior to onset of seizures). May enhance bile excretion in patients with cholestasis before ^{99}Tc-IDA scanning.

MONITORING: Phenobarbital monotherapy will control seizures in 43 to 85% of affected neonates - adding a second drug (phenytoin or lorazepam) is often needed. Therapeutic serum concentration is 15 to 40 mcg/mL. Drug accumulation may occur using recommended maintenance dose during the first two weeks of life. Altered (usually increased) serum concentrations may occur in patients also receiving phenytoin or valproate. Observe IV site for signs of extravasation and phlebitis.

ADVERSE EFFECTS/PRECAUTIONS: Sedation at serum concentrations above 40 mcg/mL. Respiratory depression at concentrations above 60 mcg/mL. Irritating to veins - pH is approximately 10 and osmolality is approximately 15,000 mOsm/kg H_2O.

PHARMACOLOGY: Phenobarbital limits the spread of seizure activity, possibly by increasing inhibitory neurotransmission. Approximately 30% protein bound. Primarily metabolized by liver, then excreted in the urine as p-hydroxyphenobarbital (no anticonvulsant activity). Serum half-life in neonates is 40 to 200 hours.

SPECIAL CONSIDERATIONS/PREPARATION: Injectable solution available in 1-mL Tubex® and vials, in concentrations of 30-, 60-, 65- and 130-mg/mL, all containing 10% (100 mg/mL) alcohol and 67.8% propylene glycol. Use within 30 minutes of opening. Oral elixirs are available in 15 mg/5 mL and 20 mg/5 mL concentrations. All contain 13.5% alcohol (135 mg/mL).

Solution Compatibility: D_5W, $D_{10}W$, and NS. No data are currently available on neonatal Dex/AA solutions.

Terminal Injection Site Compatibility: Amikacin, aminophylline, caffeine citrate, calcium chloride, calcium gluconate, enalaprilat, fentanyl, fosphenytoin, heparin, linezolid, meropenem, morphine, propofol, prostaglandin E_1, and sodium bicarbonate.

Incompatibility: Fat emulsion. Cimetidine, clindamycin, hydralazine, hydrocortisone succinate, insulin, methadone, midazolam, pancuronium, ranitidine, and vancomycin. No data available on potassium chloride.

PHENTOLAMINE

SELECTED REFERENCES

- Volpe JJ: *Neurology of the Newborn*, ed 4. Philadelphia: WB Saunders Co, 2001, p 203-204.
- Hall RT, Hall FK, Daily SK: High-dose phenobarbital therapy in term newborn infants with severe perinatal asphyxia: A randomized, prospective study with three-year follow-up. *J Pediatr* 1998;132:345-348.

PHENTOLAMINE

DOSE & ADMINISTRATION: Inject a 1-mg/mL solution of phentolamine subcutaneously into the affected area. Usual amount needed is 1 to 5 mL, depending on the size of the infiltrate. May be repeated if necessary.

USES: Prevention of dermal necrosis and sloughing caused by extravasation of vasoconstrictive agents, e.g. dopamine.

MONITORING: Assess affected area for reversal of ischemia. Monitor blood pressure.

ADVERSE EFFECTS/PRECAUTIONS: Hypotension could potentially occur if a very large dose is administered. Consider using topical 2% nitroglycerin ointment if affected extremity is significantly swollen.

PHARMACOLOGY: Alpha-adrenergic blocking agent that produces peripheral vasodilation, thereby reversing ischemia produced by vasopressor infiltration. The effect should be seen almost immediately. Biological half-life when injected subcutaneously is less than 20 minutes.

SPECIAL CONSIDERATIONS/PREPARATION: Available in 5-mg vial as a lyophilized powder. To prepare: 1) Reconstitute one vial with 1 mL of NS. 2) Dilute to a concentration of 1 mg/mL with 4 mL NS. Use immediately. **Do not use if solution is discolored or contains particulate contamination.**

Terminal Injection Site Compatibility: Amiodarone, dobutamine, and papaverine.

SELECTED REFERENCES

- Subhani M, Sridhar S, DeCristofaro JD: Phentolamine use in a neonate for the prevention of dermal necrosis caused by dopamine: A case report. *J Perinatol* 2001;21:324-326.
- Denkler KA, Cohen BE: Reversal of dopamine extravasation injury with topical nitroglycerin ointment. *Plast Reconstr Surg* 1989;84:811.
- Siwy BK, Sadove AM: Acute management of dopamine infiltration injury with Regitine. *Plast Reconstr Surg* 1987;80:610.

PHENYLEPHRINE (OPHTHALMIC)

DOSE & ADMINISTRATION: 1 drop instilled in the eye at least 10 minutes prior to funduscopic procedures. Use **only** the 2.5% ophthalmic solution in neonates. Apply pressure to the lacrimal sac during and for 2 minutes after instillation to minimize systemic absorption.

USES: Induction of mydriasis and cycloplegia for diagnostic and therapeutic ophthalmic procedures.

MONITORING: Monitor heart rate and oxygen saturation in babies with BPD.

ADVERSE EFFECTS/PRECAUTIONS: May cause decreased pulmonary compliance, tidal volume, and peak airflow in babies with BPD. Do not use in patients receiving beta-blocker medications (e.g. propranolol). The use of 10% solutions has caused systemic hypertension and tachycardia in infants.

PHARMACOLOGY: Ophthalmic phenylephrine is an alpha-adrenergic. Mydriasis begins within 5 minutes of instillation and lasts for 60 minutes. Without lacrimal sac occlusion, approximately 80% of each drop may pass through the nasolacrimal system and be available for rapid systemic absorption by the nasal mucosa.

SPECIAL CONSIDERATIONS/PREPARATION: Supplied as ophthalmic solution in 0.12%, 2.5%, and 10% concentrations in 2 to 15 mL quantities. Do not use solution that becomes discolored or contains precipitate. **Do not refrigerate.** A preparation containing cyclopentolate 0.2% and phenylephrine 1% (Cyclomydril®) is commercially available in 2- and 8-mL Drop-tainers. A combination eye drop solution ("Caputo drops") may be prepared in a 15-mL bottle with 3.75 mL of cyclopentolate 2%, 7.5 mL of tropicamide 1%, and 3.75 mL of phenylephrine 10%. The final solution contains cyclopentolate 0.5%, tropicamide 0.5%, and phenylephrine 2.5%. Use within 24 hours, as the solution contains no preservatives.

SELECTED REFERENCES

- Wallace DK, Steinkuller PG: Ocular medications in children. *Clin Pediatr* 1998;37:645-652.
- Laws DE, Morton C, Weindling M, Clark D: Systemic effects of screening for retinopathy of prematurity. *Br J Ophthalmol* 1996;80:425-428.
- McGregor MLK: Adrenergic agonists, in Mauger TF, Craig EL (eds): *Havener's Ocular Pharmacology*, ed 6. St. Louis: Mosby-YearBook, 1994, pp 70-72.
- Mirmanesh SJ, Abbasi S, Bhutani VK: Alpha-adrenergic bronchoprovocation in neonates with bronchopulmonary dysplasia. *J Pediatr* 1992;121:622-625.
- Isenberg S, Everett S: Cardiovascular effects of mydriatics in low-birth-weight infants. *J Pediatr* 1984;105:111-112
- Caputo AR, Schnitzer RE, Lindquist TD, Sun S: Dilation in neonates: a protocol. *Pediatrics* 1982;69:77-80.
- Borromeo-McGrall V, Bordiuk JM, Keitel H: Systemic hypertension following ocular administration of 10% phenylephrine in the neonate. *Pediatrics* 1973;51:1032-1036.

PHENYTOIN

DOSE & ADMINISTRATION: Loading dose: 15 to 20 mg/kg IV infusion over at least 30 minutes. **Maintenance dose:** 4 to 8 mg/kg Q24 hours IV slow push, or PO. (Up to 8 mg/kg per dose Q8 to 12 hours after 1 week of age). Maximum rate of infusion 0.5 mg/kg per minute. Flush IV with saline before and after administration. **Phenytoin is highly unstable in any IV solution. Avoid using in central lines because of the risk of precipitation. IM route not acceptable; drug crystallizes in muscle.** Oral absorption is erratic.

USES: Anticonvulsant often used to treat seizures refractory to phenobarbital.

MONITORING: Monitor for bradycardia, arrhythmias, and hypotension during infusion. Observe IV site for extravasation. Follow serum concentration closely: therapeutic range is 6 to 15 mcg/mL in the first weeks, then 10 to 20 mcg/mL due to changes in protein binding. Obtain initial trough level 48 hours after IV loading dose.

ADVERSE EFFECTS/PRECAUTIONS: Extravasation causes tissue inflammation and necrosis due to high pH and osmolality. High serum concentrations are associated with seizures. Drowsiness may be difficult to identify. Hypersensitivity reactions have been reported in infants. Toxicities with long-term therapy include cardiac arrhythmias, hypotension, gingivitis, nystagmus, rickets, hyperglycemia, and hypoinsulinemia. Phenytoin interacts with carbamazepine, cimetidine, corticosteroids, digoxin, furosemide, phenobarbital, and valproate.

PHARMACOLOGY: Hepatic metabolism capacity of Phenytoin is limited—saturation may occur within therapeutic range. Pharmacokinetics are dose-dependent. Elimination rate is increased during first few weeks of life. Serum half-life is 18 to 60 hours. 85% to 90% protein bound. Bilirubin displaces phenytoin from protein-binding sites, resulting in increased free drug.

SPECIAL CONSIDERATIONS/PREPARATION: Injectable solution available in a concentration of 50 mg/mL. Contains 40% propylene glycol and 10% alcohol (100 mg/mL). Oral suspension interacts with milk proteins in the stomach, resulting in subtherapeutic serum phenytoin concentrations.

Solution Compatibility: Phenytoin is highly unstable in any IV solution.

Solution Incompatibility: D_5W and $D_{10}W$.

Terminal Injection Site Compatibility: Esmolol, famotidine, fluconazole, sodium bicarbonate.

Incompatibility: Dex/AA solutions, fat emulsion. Amikacin, aminophylline, chloramphenicol, ciprofloxacin, clindamycin, dobutamine, enalaprilat, fentanyl, heparin, hyaluronidase, hydrocortisone succinate, insulin, lidocaine, linezolid, methadone, mivacurium, morphine, nitroglycerin, pentobarbital, potassium chloride, procainamide, propofol, ranitidine, and vitamin K_1.

SELECTED REFERENCES

- Volpe JJ: *Neurology of the Newborn*, ed 4. Philadelphia: WB Saunders Co, 2001, p 204-205.
- Wheless JW: Pediatric use of intravenous and intramuscular phenytoin: lessons learned. *J Child Neurol* 1998;13(Suppl 1): S11-14.

PIPERACILLIN

DOSE & ADMINISTRATION: 50 to 100 mg/kg per dose IV infusion by syringe pump over 30 minutes, or IM. To use dosing chart, please refer to explanatory note in "How to Use This Book."

DOSING INTERVAL CHART

PMA (weeks)	PostNatal (days)	Interval (hours)
≤29	0 to 28 >28	12 8
30 to 36	0 to 14 >14	12 8
37 to 44	0 to 7 >7	12 8
≥45	ALL	6

USES: Piperacillin is a semisynthetic penicillin with increased activity against *Pseudomonas aeruginosa* and many strains of *Klebsiella, Serratia, E coli, Enterobacter, Citrobacter,* and *Proteus*. Also effective against group B *Streptococcus*.

MONITORING: Desired peak serum concentration is approximately 150 mcg/mL. Desired trough concentration ranges from 15 to 50 mcg/mL (available as bioassay). Peak serum concentration is lower with IM administration. Observe IV site for signs of extravasation.

ADVERSE EFFECTS/PRECAUTIONS: Eosinophilia. Hyperbilirubinemia. Elevations in ALT, AST, BUN, and serum creatinine.

PHARMACOLOGY: Piperacillin is a potent, broad-spectrum, semi-synthetic, ureidopenicillin possessing high activity against gram-negative bacteria. Inactivation by beta-lactamase-producing bacteria. Synergistic with aminoglycosides. Good penetration into bone; CSF penetration similar to that of other penicillins. Serum half-life depends on gestational age and postnatal age. Primarily excreted renally unchanged.

SPECIAL CONSIDERATIONS/PREPARATION: Available as powder for injection in 2-g, 3-g, 4-g, and 40-g vials. Reconstitute 2-g vial with 10 mL of sterile water for injection to make a final concentration of 200 mg/mL. Reconstituted solution stable for 24 hours at room temperature, 2 days refrigerated. A 100 mg/mL dilution may be made by adding 2.5 mL of reconstituted solution to 7.5 mL sterile water for injection. Dilution stable for 7 days refrigerated. **IM Administration:** Use 400 mg/mL concentration.

Solution Compatibility: D_5W, $D_{10}W$, and NS.

Terminal Injection Site Compatibility: Dex/AA solutions, fat emulsion. Acyclovir, aminophylline, aztreonam, clindamycin, enalaprilat, esmolol, famotidine, heparin, hydrocortisone succinate, linezolid, lorazepam, midazolam, milrinone, morphine, nicardipine, potassium chloride, propofol, ranitidine, remifentanil, and zidovudine.

Incompatibility: Amikacin, amiodarone, gentamicin, netilmicin, fluconazole, tobramycin, and vancomycin.

SELECTED REFERENCES

- Kacet N, Roussel-Delvallez M, Gremillet C, et al: Pharmacokinetic study of piperacillin in newborns relating to gestational and postnatal age. *Pediatr Infect Dis J* 1992;11:365.
- Prober CG, Stevenson DK, Benitz WE: The use of antibiotics in neonates weighing less than 1200 grams. *Pediatr Infect Dis J* 1990;9:111.
- Reed MD, Myers CM, Yamashita TS, Blumer JL: Developmental pharmacology and therapeutics of piperacillin in gram-negative infections. *Dev Pharmacol Ther* 1986;9:102.
- Plazek M, Whitelaw A, Want S, et al: Piperacillin in early neonatal infection. *Arch Dis Child* 1983;58:1006.

PIPERACILLIN-TAZOBACTAM

DOSE & ADMINISTRATION: 50 to 100 mg/kg per dose (as piperacillin component) IV infusion by syringe pump over 30 minutes. To use dosing chart, please refer to explanatory note in "How to Use This Book."

Dosing Interval Chart

PMA (weeks)	PostNatal (days)	Interval (hours)
≤29	0 to 28 >28	12 8
30 to 36	0 to 14 >14	12 8
37 to 44	0 to 7 >7	12 8
≥45	ALL	8

USES: Treatment of non-CNS infections, caused by susceptible beta-lactamase producing bacteria, including many strains of *E. coli, Enterobacter, Klebsiella, Haemophilus influenzae, Proteus mirabilis, Pseudomonas spp.*, and *Staph. aureus*. Also effective against group B Streptococcus.

MONITORING: Observe IV site for signs of extravasation.

ADVERSE EFFECTS/PRECAUTIONS: Eosinophilia. Hyperbilirubinemia. Elevations in ALT, AST, BUN, and serum creatinine.

PHARMACOLOGY: Zosyn® combines the extended-spectrum antibiotic piperacillin with the beta-lactamase inhibitor tazobactam in an 8:1 ratio. Piperacillin is primarily eliminated unchanged by renal mechanisms, whereas tazobactam undergoes significant hepatic metabolism. The mean half-life of piperacillin and tazobactam in neonates is approximately 1.5 hours. CNS penetration is modest (limited data). Sodium content is 2.35 mEq per gram of piperacillin.

SPECIAL CONSIDERATIONS/PREPARATION: Available as powder for injection in 2-g, 3-g, 4-g, and 36-g preservative-free vials. Reconstitute 2-g vial with 10 mL of sterile water for injection to make a concentration of 200 mg/mL. Reconstituted solution stable for 24 hours at room temperature, 2 days refrigerated. pH 4.5 to 6.8. Contains 2.35 mEq (54 mg) of sodium per gram of piperacillin. Dilute reconstituted solution further to a final concentration of 50 mg/mL (some sources recommend 20 mg/mL) using compatible solution.

Solution Compatibility: D_5W, $D_{10}W$, and NS.

Terminal Injection Site Compatibility: Dex/AA solutions, fat emulsion. Aminophylline, aztreonam, bumetanide, calcium gluconate, cefepime, cimetidine, clindamycin, dexamethasone, dopamine, enalaprilat, esmolol, fluconazole, furosemide, heparin, hydrocortisone succinate, linezolid, lorazepam, metoclopramide, metronidazole, milrinone, morphine, potassium chloride, ranitidine, remifentanil, sodium bicarbonate, trimethoprim-sulfamethoxazole, and zidovudine.

Incompatibility: Acyclovir, amikacin, amiodarone, amphotericin B, azithromycin, dobutamine, famotidine, ganciclovir, gentamicin, netilmicin, tobramycin, and vancomycin.

SELECTED REFERENCES

- Pilley T, Pillay D, Adhikari M, Sturn A: Piperacillin/tazobactam in the treatment of Klebsiella pneumoniae infections in neonates. *Am J Perinatol* 1998;15:47-51.
- Reed MD, Goldfarb J, Yamashita TS, Blumer JL: Piperacillin and tazobactam in infants and children. *Antimicrob Agents Chemother* 1994;38:2817-26.
- Schoonover L, Occhipinti D, Rodvold K, et al: Piperacillin/tazobactam: A new beta-lactam/beta-lactamase inhibitor combination. *Ann Pharmacother* 1995;29:501-14.
- Prober CG, Stevenson DK, Benitz WE: The use of antibiotics in neonates weighing less than 1200 grams. *Pediatr Infect Dis J* 1990;9:111.

Pneumococcal 7-Valent Conjugate Vaccine

DOSE & ADMINISTRATION: 0.5 mL IM in the anterolateral thigh. Please refer to the most recent AAP/ACIP immunization schedule. Shake vial vigorously before withdrawing dose. **Do not mix with other vaccines. When giving multiple vaccines, use a separate syringe for each and give at different sites.** Care should be taken to draw back on the plunger of the syringe before injection to be certain the needle is not in a blood vessel.

Poliovirus Vaccine Enhanced-Inactivated

USES: Immunoprophylaxis against invasive disease caused by *S. pneumoniae*.

MONITORING: Observe injection site for erythema, induration (common), palpable nodule (uncommon), or sterile abscess (rare). Fever (common) may be treated with acetaminophen. Other common, self-limiting, systemic effects are drowsiness, fretfulness, and anorexia.

ADVERSE EFFECTS/PRECAUTIONS: Hypersensitivity to any component of the vaccine, including diphtheria toxoid, is a contraindication to the vaccine.

PHARMACOLOGY: Prevnar® is a sterile solution of saccharides of the capsular antigens of *Streptococcus pneumoniae* serotypes 4, 6B, 9V, 14, 18C, 19F, and 23F individually conjugated to diphtheria CRM_{197} protein. The seven serotypes account for over 80% of invasive pneumococcal disease in children in the United States. Eighty percent of penicillin-nonsusceptible strains in the United States are one of these 7 serotypes. Each dose contains 0.125 mg aluminum as aluminum phosphate adjuvant.

SPECIAL CONSIDERATIONS/PREPARATION: Prevnar® is supplied in 0.5-mL single-dose vials. After being shaken vigorously, it should appear as a homogeneous white suspension. The vaccine should not be used if it cannot be resuspended. Store refrigerated at 2 °C to 8 °C (36 °F to 46 °F). **Do not freeze.**

SELECTED REFERENCES

- American Academy of Pediatrics. Pneumococcal Infections. In: Pickering LK, Baker CJ, Long SS, McMillan JA, eds. *Red Book: 2006 Report of the Committee on Infectious Diseases*. 27th ed. Elk Grove Village, IL: American Academy of Pediatrics; 2006: pp 532-534.
- Advisory Committee on Immunization Practices: Recommendations of the ACIP. Most recent updates available on the National Immunization Program website: http://www.cdc.gov/nip/publications/acip-list.htm
- American Academy of Pediatrics, Committee on Infectious Diseases: Recommendations for the prevention of pneumococcal infections, including the use of pneumococcal conjugate vaccine (Prevnar®), pneumococcal polysaccharide vaccine, and antibiotic prophylaxis. *Pediatrics* 2000;106:362-366.
- Shinefield H, Black S, Ray P, et al: Efficacy, immunogenicity and safety of heptavalent pneumococcal conjugate vaccine in low birth weight and preterm infants. *Pediatr Infect Dis J* 2002;21:182-186.
- Product information, Wyeth Pharmaceuticals, 2004.

POLIOVIRUS VACCINE ENHANCED-INACTIVATED

DOSE & ADMINISTRATION: 0.5 mL injected **subcutaneously** in the midlateral thigh or IM in the anterolateral thigh. Immunize premature infants according to their postnatal age. Please refer to the most recent immunization schedule. **When giving multiple vaccines, use a separate syringe for each and give at different sites.** Care should be taken to draw back on the plunger of the syringe before injection to be certain the needle is not in a blood vessel.

USES: Inactivated poliovirus vaccine is now the only poliovirus vaccine available in the United States. Indications in other countries include hospitalized infants, and infants with contraindications for OPV (e.g. immunodeficiency, HIV-positive, those with immunodeficient contacts).

MONITORING: No specific monitoring required.

ADVERSE EFFECTS/PRECAUTIONS: Occasional reactions include erythema and tenderness at the injection site. Trace components may infrequently cause allergic reactions.

PHARMACOLOGY: Sterile suspension of types 1, 2, and 3 poliovirus inactivated with formaldehyde. The vaccine produced using a microcarrier culture technique of monkey kidney cells has enhanced potency. Contains traces of streptomycin, neomycin, and polymyxin B.

SPECIAL CONSIDERATIONS/PREPARATION: IPOL™ (Aventis Pasteur) is a clear, colorless solution, available in 0.5 mL single-dose syringes. Do not use if the vaccine is turbid or discolored. Refrigerate at 2 °C to 8 °C (36 °F to 46 °F). **Do not freeze.**

SELECTED REFERENCES

- American Academy of Pediatrics. Poliovirus Infections. In: Pickering LK, Baker CJ, Long SS, McMillan JA, eds. *Red Book: 2006 Report of the Committee on Infectious Diseases*. 27th ed. Elk Grove Village, IL: American Academy of Pediatrics; 2006: pp 544-545.
- Advisory Committee on Immunization Practices: Recommendations of the ACIP. Most recent updates available on the National Immunization Program website: http://www.cdc.gov/nip/publications/acip-list.htm

- American Academy of Pediatrics, Committee on Infectious Diseases: Poliomyelitis prevention: recommendations for use of inactivated poliovirus vaccine and live oral poliovirus vaccine. *Pediatrics* 1997;99:300.
- Product information, Aventis Pasteur: http://www.us.aventispasteur.com/PRODUCT/Default.cfm

POLY-VI-SOL® MVI DROPS

DOSE & ADMINISTRATION: 1 dropperful (1 mL) Q24 hours, or as directed by physician.

POLY-VI-SOL® MULTIVITAMIN DROPS

Nutrient amt	w/o Iron	with Iron
Vitamins		
A, IU	1500	1500
D, IU	400	400
C, mg	35	35
E, IU	5	5
Thiamine B_1, mg	0.5	0.5
Riboflavin B_2, mg	0.6	0.6
Niacin, mg	8	8
B_6, mg	0.4	0.4
B_{12}, mcg	2	0
Minerals		
Iron, mg	0	10

POTASSIUM CHLORIDE

DOSE & ADMINISTRATION: Initial oral replacement therapy: 0.5 to 1 mEq/kg per day divided and administered with feedings (small, more frequent aliquots preferred). Adjust dosage based on monitoring of serum potassium concentrations.

    1 g KCl = 13.4 mEq K^+ 1 mEq K^+ = 74.6 mg KCl

Acute treatment of symptomatic hypokalemia: Begin with 0.5 to 1 mEq/kg IV over 1 hour, then reassess. Maximum concentration: 40 mEq/L for peripheral, 80 mEq/L for central venous infusions.

MONITORING: Continuous EKG monitoring is mandatory if administering by the IV route, especially for central infusions. Observe IV site closely for signs of extravasation when using concentrated solutions. Monitor serum potassium concentration. Assess for GI intolerance.

ADVERSE EFFECTS/PRECAUTIONS: Rapid IV infusions, especially those through central lines, may cause arrhythmias including heart block and cardiac arrest. Peripheral IV administration of concentrated potassium solutions is associated with thrombophlebitis and pain at the injection site. GI irritation is common—most commonly diarrhea, vomiting, and bleeding— minimized by dividing oral doses and administering with feedings. Use with caution (if at all) in patients receiving potassium-sparing diuretics, e.g. spironolactone.

PHARMACOLOGY: Potassium is the major intracellular cation. Hypokalemia in critically ill neonates is usually the result of diuretic (furosemide, thiazides) therapy or diarrhea. Other causes include congenital adrenal hyperplasia and renal disorders. Alkalosis, as well as insulin infusions, will lower serum potassium concentrations by driving the ion intracellularly. Symptoms of hypokalemia include neuromuscular weakness and paralysis, ileus, urine retention, and EKG changes (ST segment depression, low-voltage T wave, and appearance of U wave). Hypokalemia increases digitalis toxicity. Oral potassium preparations are completely absorbed.

SPECIAL CONSIDERATIONS/PREPARATION: Potassium chloride for injection is supplied as 2-mEq/mL solution (equals 2000 mEq/L). **Always dilute before administration.** Hyperosmolar - 4355 mOsm/kg determined by freezing-point depression. pH ranges from 4 to 8 depending on buffering. Various oral solutions are available, with concentrations ranging from 10 to 40 mEq per 15 mL. Other oral forms available include powder packets, tablets, and sustained-release capsules.

PROCAINAMIDE

Solution Compatibility: Most standard IV solutions.

Terminal Injection Site Compatibility: Most drugs.

Incompatibility: Amphotericin B, diazepam, and phenytoin.

SELECTED REFERENCES

- Satlin LM, Schwartz GJ: Disorders of potassium metabolism, in Ichikawa I (ed): *Pediatric Textbook of Fluids and Electrolytes.* Baltimore: Williams & Wilkins, 1990, p 227.
- Morgan BC: Rapidly infused potassium chloride therapy in a child. *JAMA* 1981;245:2446.
- DeFronzo RA, Bia M: Intravenous potassium chloride therapy. *JAMA* 1981;245:2446.

PROCAINAMIDE

DOSE & ADMINISTRATION: Initial bolus dose: 7 to 10 mg/kg IV over 1 hour via syringe pump, followed by **Maintenance IV infusion:** 20 to 80 mcg/kg per minute. Premature neonates should receive the lowest dose.

USES: Acute treatment of supraventricular tachycardia (SVT) refractory to vagal maneuvers and adenosine. Acute treatment of ventricular tachycardia unresponsive to cardioversion and adenosine. Ectopic tachycardia, junctional ectopic tachycardia, and atrial flutter. Consider obtaining expert consultation before use.

MONITORING: Continuous monitoring of the EKG, blood pressure and heart rate. Measure procainamide and N-acetyl procainamide (NAPA) concentrations at 2, 12, and 24 hours after starting the loading dose infusion. **Therapeutic concentrations:** Procainamide: 4-10 mcg/mL, NAPA 6 to 20 mcg/mL. Sum of procainamide and NAPA: 10-30 mcg/mL.

ADVERSE EFFECTS/PRECAUTIONS: Severe hypotension with rapid infusion, bradycardia, AV block, and *V-fib* have been reported in adult patients. Normal procainamide concentrations widen the QRS complex due to slowing of conduction in the Purkinje system and ventricular muscle. The drug should be discontinued if the QRS duration increases by more than 35 to 50 percent to avoid serious toxicity. Adverse effects are reversible with discontinuation of drug.

PHARMACOLOGY: Procainamide is a class IA antiarrhythmic agent that increases the effective refractory period of the atria and the ventricles of the heart. Onset of action occurs within minutes of starting the loading dose. Half-life is a approximately 5 hours in the term neonate, and longer in preterms. Metabolized primarily (60%) in the liver to N-acetylprocainamide (NAPA), an active metabolite. The rate of acetylation is primarily genetically determined in adults and children. Preterm neonates have a higher NAPA:procainamide ratio than term infants presumably due to delayed excretion of NAPA. Renal function is a significant determinant of procainamide clearance. Cimetidine and amiodarone interact when given with procainamide, increasing procainamide serum levels.

SPECIAL CONSIDERATIONS/PREPARATION: Available in 10-mL vials providing 100 mg/mL or 2-mL vials and 2-mL syringe cartridges providing 500 mg/mL. Store at room temperature. **DO NOT FREEZE**. Dilute initial bolus dose to a final concentration of 20 mg/mL and administer over 1 hour. Maintenance infusion should be diluted to 2 mg/mL before administration.

Solution Compatibility: 0.45% NaCl and NS.

Solution Incompatibility: All dextrose containing solutions.

Terminal Injection Site Compatibility: Amiodarone, dobutamine, famotidine, flumazenil, heparin, hydrocortisone, lidocaine, netilmicin, ranitidine, and sodium nitroprusside.

Incompatibility: Esmolol, milrinone, and phenytoin.

SELECTED REFERENCES

- Moffett BS, Cannon BC, Friedman RA, Kertesz NJ: Therapeutic levels of intravenous procainamide in neonates: A retrospective assessment. *Pharmacotherapy* 2006;26:1687-1693.
- Wong KK, Potts JE, Ethridge SP, Sanatani S: Medications used to manage supraventricular tachycardia in the infant: a North American survey. *Pediatr Cardiol* 2006;27:199-203.
- Bryson SM, Leson CL, Irwin DB, et al: Therapeutic monitoring and pharmacokinetic evaluation of procainamide in neonates. *DICP* 1991;25:68-71.

PROPRANOLOL

DOSE & ADMINISTRATION: Starting oral dose: 0.25 mg/kg per dose Q6 hours. Increase as needed to maximum of 3.5 mg/kg per dose Q6 hours. **Starting IV dose:** 0.01 mg/kg Q6 hours over 10 minutes. Increase as needed to maximum of 0.15 mg/kg per dose Q6 hours. Effective dosage requirements will vary significantly.

USES: Treatment of tachyarrhythmias and hypertension. Preferred therapy for SVT if associated with Wolff-Parkinson-White syndrome. Palliation of tetralogy of Fallot and hypertrophic obstructive cardiomyopathy. Adjunctive treatment of neonatal thyrotoxicosis.

MONITORING: Continuous EKG monitoring during acute treatment of arrhythmias and during IV therapy. Measure systemic blood pressure frequently. Measure blood glucose during initiation of treatment and after dosage changes. Assess for increased airway resistance.

ADVERSE EFFECTS/PRECAUTIONS: Adverse effects are related to beta-receptor blockade: Bradycardia, bronchospasm, and hypoglycemia are most frequently reported. Hypotension occurs in patients with underlying myocardial dysfunction. Contraindicated in patients with reactive airway disease or diminished myocardial contractility. A withdrawal syndrome (nervousness, tachycardia, sweating, hypertension) has been associated with sudden cessation of the drug.

PHARMACOLOGY: Propranolol is the most widely used nonselective β-adrenergic-receptor blocking agent. Peak serum concentration is reached approximately 2 hours after an oral dose. Propranolol undergoes significant first-pass hepatic metabolism, resulting in 30% to 40% bioavailability. Protein binding is 70% in neonates. Serum half-life is prolonged in patients with liver disease. Elimination is by renal excretion of metabolites.

SPECIAL CONSIDERATIONS/PREPARATION: Oral solutions are available in concentrations of 4 mg/mL and 8 mg/mL and are stable for 6 months at room temperature. Injectable form is available in 1-mL ampules containing 1 mg. Make a 0.1 mg/mL dilution by adding 1 ampul to 9 mL preservative-free normal saline. **Protect from light.** Store at room temperature.

Solution Compatibility: D_5W and NS.

Terminal Injection Site Compatibility: Alteplase, dobutamine, heparin, hydrocortisone succinate, linezolid, milrinone, morphine, potassium chloride, and propofol.

SELECTED REFERENCES
- Schneeweiss A: Neonatal cardiovascular pharmacology, in Long WA (ed): *Fetal and Neonatal Cardiology*. Baltimore: WB Saunders Co, 1990, p 675.
- Pickoff AS, Zies L, Ferrer PL, et al: High-dose propranolol therapy in the management of supraventricular tachycardia. *J Pediatr* 1979;94:144.
- Gillette P, Garson A, Eterovic E, et al: Oral propranolol treatment in infants and children. *J Pediatr* 1978;92:141.

PROTAMINE

DOSE & ADMINISTRATION: 1 mg protamine sulfate/100 U of heparin given in last 4 hours. Slow IV push, or IM.

USES: Heparin antagonist.

MONITORING: Monitor vital signs, clotting functions, and blood pressure continuously. Observe for bleeding.

ADVERSE EFFECTS/PRECAUTIONS: Excessive doses can cause serious bleeding problems. Hypotension, bradycardia, dyspnea, and transitory flushing have been reported in adults.

PHARMACOLOGY: Anticoagulant when given alone. Combines ionically with heparin to form a stable complex devoid of anticoagulant activity. Rapid action after IV use (5 minutes).

SPECIAL CONSIDERATIONS/PREPARATION: Available as a 10-mg/mL concentration preservative-free in 5-, and 25-mL vials. **Keep refrigerated.**

Solution Compatibility: D_5W and NS. No data are currently available on Dex/AA.

Terminal Injection Site Compatibility: Cimetidine and ranitidine. No data are currently available on heparin, potassium chloride, or other medications.

SELECTED REFERENCES
- Roberts RJ: *Drug Therapy in Infants*. Philadelphia: WB Saunders Co, 1984, p 301.

PYRIDOXINE

DOSE & ADMINISTRATION: Initial diagnostic dose: 50 to 100 mg IV push, or IM. **Maintenance dose:** 50 to 100 mg PO Q24 hours. High doses may be required during periods of intercurrent illness.

USES: Diagnosis and treatment of pyridoxine-dependent seizures.

MONITORING: When possible, initial administration of pyridoxine should be accompanied by EEG monitoring.

ADVERSE EFFECTS/PRECAUTIONS: Risk of profound sedation. Ventilator support may be necessary.

PHARMACOLOGY: Pyridoxine-dependent seizures are a result of defective binding of pyridoxine in the formation of GABA (an inhibitory neurotransmitter). Administration of pharmacologic doses of pyridoxine will correct this GABA deficiency.

SPECIAL CONSIDERATIONS/PREPARATION: Injectable form available in concentration of 100 mg/mL in 1-mL vials. May use injectable form orally; mix in simple syrup if desired. **Protect from light.**

Solution Incompatibility: Alkaline solutions. No data are currently available on Dex/AA.

Terminal Injection Site Compatibility: Fat emulsion.

Incompatibility: Iron salts and oxidizing agents. No data are currently available on heparin and potassium chloride.

SELECTED REFERENCES

- Gospe SM: Current perspectives on pyridoxine-dependent seizures. *J Pediatr* 1998;132:919-923.
- Gordon N: Pyridoxine dependency: An update. *Dev Med Child Neurol* 1997;39:63.
- Mikati MA, Trevathan E, Krishnamoorthy KS, Lombroso CT: Pyridoxine-dependent epilepsy: Investigations and long-term followup. *Electroencephalogr Clin Neurophysiol* 1991;78:215
- Kroll JS: Pyridoxine for neonatal seizures: An unexpected danger. *Dev Med Child Neurol* 1985;27:369.
- Bankier A, Turner M, Hopkins IJ: Pyridoxine-dependent seizures: A wider clinical spectrum. *Arch Dis Child* 1983;58:415.

QUINUPRISTIN/DALFOPRISTIN

DOSE & ADMINISTRATION: >7.5 mg/kg/dose Q12 hours by IV infusion over 60 minutes. Administration via a central catheter is recommended.

USES: Limited to treatment of infections caused by gram positive organisms resistant to other antibiotics, e.g. methicillin-resistant *Staph. aureus* and vancomycin-resistant *Enterococcus faecium* (not *E faecalis*).

MONITORING: Periodic measurement of serum bilirubin and transaminases. Assess peripheral IV site for signs of inflammation.

ADVERSE EFFECTS/PRECAUTIONS: Myalgias and arthralgias occur frequently in adults with hepatic or renal failure. Elvations in serum bilirubin and transaminases are common. Diarrhea and rash occur infrequently.

PHARMACOLOGY: No data are available for infants. Synercid® is a new parenteral antimicrobial agent which consists of two streptogramin antibiotics (quinupristin and dalfopristin in a 30:70 ratio) that inhibit bacterial protein synthesis by binding to separate sites on the bacterial ribosome. Serum half-life of quinupristin in adults ranges from 1 to 3 hours, and of dalfopristin ranges from 5 to 9 hours. 75% is excreted via the biliary route.

SPECIAL CONSIDERATIONS/PREPARATION: Synercid® is supplied as a lyophilized powder in single-dose, 10-mL vials containing 500 mg. Store refrigerated. Reconstitute under aseptic conditions by adding 5 mL of Sterile Water for Injection or D_5W. Before administration, dilute with D_5W to a concentration not exceeding 2 mg/mL. Diluted solution is stable for 5 hours at room temperature, or 54 hours if stored under refrigeration.

Solution Compatibility: D_5W.

Solution Incompatibility: NS.

Terminal Injection Site Compatibility: Aztreonam, ciprofloxacin, fluconazole, metoclopramide, and potassium chloride.

SELECTED REFERENCES

- Loeffler AM, Drew RH, Perfect JR, et al: Safety and efficacy of quinupristin/dalfopristin for treatment of invasive Gram-positive infections in pediatric patients. *Pediatr Infect Dis J* 2002;21:950-56.
- Gray JW, Darbyshire PJ, Beath SV, et al: Experience with quinupristin/dalfopristin in treating infections with vancomycin-resistant *Enterococcus faecium* in children. *Pediatr Infect Dis J* 2000;19:234-238.
- Lamb HM, Figgitt DP, Faulds D: Quinupristin/Dalfopristin: A review of its use in the management of serious gram-positive infections. *Drugs* 1999;58:1061-1097.
- Product Information, Monarch Pharmaceuticals, 2004.

Ranitidine

DOSE & ADMINISTRATION: PO: 2 mg/kg per dose Q8 hours. **IV:** Term: 1.5 mg/kg per dose Q8 hours slow push. Preterm: 0.5 mg/kg per dose Q12 hours slow push. **Continuous IV infusion:** 0.0625 mg/kg per hour.

USES: Prevention and treatment of stress ulcers and GI hemorrhage aggravated by gastric acid secretion.

MONITORING: Gastric pH may be measured to assess efficacy.

ADVERSE EFFECTS/PRECAUTIONS: One case report of thrombocytopenia. No other adverse effects have been reported in infants or children. Elevations in hepatic enzymes, leukopenia, and bradycardia have been reported in adults.

PHARMACOLOGY: Inhibits gastric acid secretion by histamine H_2-receptor antagonism. Peak serum concentration occurs 1 to 3 hours after oral administration and is not influenced by food. Bioavailability is quite variable. Hepatic biotransformation predominates after oral absorption, with 30% excreted unchanged in the urine. In contrast, 70% of an IV dose is excreted unchanged in the urine. Elimination half-life in neonates is 3 to 7 hours, and is prolonged in preterm infants and patients with renal or hepatic insufficiency.

SPECIAL CONSIDERATIONS/PREPARATION: Available as a 1 mg/mL preservative-free solution for injection in 50 mL single-dose plastic containers, and a 25 mg/mL injectable solution in 2-, and 6-mL vials. A 2 mg/mL dilution may be made by adding 0.8 mL of the 25 mg/mL concentration to 9.2 mL preservative-free sterile water or normal saline for injection. Stable for 7 days refrigerated. May be given orally; absorption is equivalent to that of the oral solution. Manufacturer's oral solution (15 mg/mL) contains 7.5% alcohol. Also available as 150- and 300-mg tablets. May prepare oral solution by crushing a 150-mg tablet and dissolving in 30 mL of sterile water to yield a final concentration of 5 mg/mL. Stable for 28 days refrigerated.

Solution Compatibility: D_5W, $D_{10}W$, and NS.

Terminal Injection Site Compatibility: Dex/AA solutions, fat emulsion. Acyclovir, acetazolamide, amikacin, aminophylline, ampicillin, atropine, aztreonam, cefazolin, cefepime, cefoxitin, ceftazidime, chloramphenicol, clindamycin, dexamethasone, digoxin, dobutamine, dopamine, enalaprilat, epinephrine, erythromycin lactobionate, fentanyl, fluconazole, flumazenil, furosemide, gentamicin, glycopyrrolate, heparin, insulin, isoproterenol, lidocaine, linezolid, lorazepam, meropenem, metoclopramide, midazolam, milrinone, morphine, nicardipine, nitroprusside, pancuronium bromide, penicillin G, piperacillin, piperacillin-tazobactam, potassium chloride, propofol, prostaglandin E_1, protamine, remifentanil, tobramycin, vancomycin, vecuronium, vitamin K_1, and zidovudine.

Incompatibility: Amphotericin B, pentobarbital, phenobarbital, and phenytoin.

SELECTED REFERENCES

- Kuusela A-L: Long term gastric pH monitoring for determining optimal dose of ranitidine for critically ill preterm and term neonates. *Arch Dis Child Fetal Neonatal Ed* 1998;78:F151-F153.
- Kelly EJ, Chatfield SL, Brownlee KG, et al: The effect of intravenous ranitidine on the intragastric pH of preterm infants receiving dexamethasone. *Arch Dis Child* 1993;69:37.
- Fontana M, Massironi E, Rossi A, et al: Ranitidine pharmacokinetics in newborn infants. *Arch Dis Child* 1993;68:602.
- Sutphen JL, Dillard VL: Effect of ranitidine on twenty-four-hour gastric acidity in infants. *J Pediatr* 1989;114:472.
- Grant SM, Langtry HD, Brogden RN: Ranitidine: An updated review of its pharmacodynamic and pharmacokinetic properties and therapeutic use in peptic ulcer disease and other allied diseases. *Drugs* 1989;37:801.

Rifampin

DOSE & ADMINISTRATION: PO: 10 to 20 mg/kg per dose Q24 hours. May administer with feedings. **IV:** 5 to 10 mg/kg per dose Q12 hours, given via syringe pump over 30 minutes. **Do not administer IM or SC. Prophylaxis for high-risk contacts of invasive meningococcal disease:** 5 mg/kg per dose PO Q12 hours, for 2 days. **Prophylaxis for high-risk contacts of invasive H influenzae type b disease:** 10 mg/kg per dose PO Q24 hours, for 4 days.

USES: Used in combination with vancomycin or aminoglycosides for treatment of persistent staphylococcal infections. Prophylaxis against infections caused by *N. meningitidis* and *H. influenzae* type b.

MONITORING: Monitor hepatic transaminases and bilirubin. Periodic CBC for thrombocytopenia. Observe IV site for signs of extravasation.

ADVERSE EFFECTS/PRECAUTIONS: Causes orange/red discoloration of body secretions (e.g. sweat, urine, tears, sputum). Extravasation may cause local irritation and inflammation. Rifampin in a potent inducer of several cytochrome P450 enzymes. If administered concomitantly, the following drugs may have decreased pharmacologic effects due to increased metabolism: aminophylline, amiodarone, ecimetidine, corticosteroids, digoxin, enalapril, fluconazole, midazolam, morphine, phenobarbital, phenytoin, propranolol, and zidovudine.

PHARMACOLOGY: Rifampin is a semisynthetic antibiotic with a wide spectrum of antibacterial activity against staphylococci, most streptococci, *H. influenzae, Neisseria* sp., *Legionella, Listeria*, some *Bacteroides* species, Mycobacterium tuberculosis, and certain atypical mycobacterium. Enterococci and aerobic gram-negative bacilli are generally resistant. Not used as monotherapy because resistance may develop during therapy. Inhibits transcription of DNA to RNA by binding to the beta subunit of bacterial RNA-polymerase. Well absorbed orally. Rapidly deacetylated to desacetylrifampin (active metabolite) and undergoes enterohepatic circulation. Nearly all of the rifampin excreted into the bile is deacetylated within 6 hours. Serum half-life ranges from 1 to 3 hours.

SPECIAL CONSIDERATIONS/PREPARATION: Available as a lyophilized powder for injection in 600-mg vials. Reconstitute with 10 mL of sterile water for injection to make a final concentration of 60 mg/mL. Reconstituted solution is stable for 24 hours at room temperature. Further dilution is required - maximum concentration for infusion is 6 mg/mL. A 3 mg/mL dilution may be made by adding 0.5 mL of reconstituted solution to 9.5 mL of NS or D_5W. Dilution made with NS is stable for 24 hours at room temperature. Dilution made with D_5W is stable for 4 hours at room temperature. Do not use if solution precipitates. A neonatal suspension may be prepared by mixing 5 mL (300 mg) of the reconstituted IV solution with 25 mL of simple syrup to make a final concentration of 10 mg/mL. Shake well before use. Suspension is stable for 4 weeks at room temperature or refrigerated. Also available in 150- and 300-mg capsules. Preparation of oral suspension using capsules yields variable dosage bioavailability.

Solution Compatibility: D_5W and NS. No data available on Dex/AA or fat emulsion.

Terminal Injection Site Compatibility: No data available.

SELECTED REFERENCES

- Shama A, Patole SK, Whitehall JS: Intravenous rifampicin in neonates with persistent staphylococcal bacteraemia. *Acta Paediatr* 2002;91:670-673.
- Fernandez M, Rench MA, Albanyan EA, Edwards MS: Failure of rifampin to eradicate group B streptococcal colonization in infants. *Pediatr Infect Dis J* 2001;20:371-376.
- Tan TQ, Mason EO, Ou C-N, et al: Use of intravenous rifampin in neonates with persistent staphylococcal bacteremia. *Antimicrob Agents Chemother* 1993;37:2401.
- Koup JR, William-Warren J, Viswanathan CT, et al: Pharmacokinetics of rifampin in children. II. Oral bioavailability. *Ther Drug Monit* 1986;8:17.
- Koup JR, William-Warren J, Weber A, et al: Pharmacokinetics of rifampin in children. I. Multiple dose intravenous infusion. *Ther Drug Monit* 1986;8:11.
- McCracken GH, Ginsburg CM, Zweighaft TC, et al: Pharmacokinetics of rifampin in infants and children: relevance to prophylaxis against Haemophilus influenzae type B disease. *Pediatrics* 1980;66:17
- Nahata MC, Morosco RS, Hipple TF: Effect of preparation method and storage on rifampin concentration in suspensions. *Ann Pharmacother* 1994;28:182.

Rotavirus Vaccine

DOSE & ADMINISTRATION: 2 mL per dose. FOR ORAL USE ONLY. NOT FOR INJECTION. To administer the vaccine: 1) Tear open the pouch and remove the dosing tube. 2) Clear the fluid from the dispensing tip by holding tube vertically and tapping cap. 3) Puncture the dispensing tip by screwing cap *clockwise* unitl it becomes tight, then remove the cap by turning it *counterclockwise*. 4) Administer dose by gently squeezing liquid into infant's mouth toward the inner cheek until dosing tube is empty. If for any reason an incomplete dose is administered (e.g., infant spits or regurgitates the vaccine), a replacement dose is NOT recommended, since this was not studied in the clinical trials. The first dose should be given between 6 and 12 weeks of age, and the 2 subsequent doses at 4 to 10 weeks intervals. The third dose should be given at no later than 32 weeks of age due to lack of safety and efficacy data in infants after this age. Please refer to the most recent AAP/ACIP immunization schedule.

USES: Immunoprophylaxis against rotavirus gastroenteritis caused by serotypes G1, G2, G3, and G4.

ADVERSE EFFECTS/PRECAUTIONS: Data from the phase III efficacy trials (n = 71725) did not suggest an increased risk of intussusception relative to placebo. However, the Food and Drug Administration (FDA) notified health care providers and consumers on February 13, 2007 about 28 post-marketing reports of intussusception following administration of RotaTeq®. According to the FDA, approximately 3.5 million doses of RotaTeq® were distributed in the United States as of February 1, 2007. Intussusception can occur spontaneously in the absence of vaccination and its cause is usually unknown. Of the 28 reported cases of intussusception, it is not known how many, if any, were vaccine-related. However, the number of intussusception cases reported to date after RotaTeq® administration does not exceed the number expected based on background rates of 18-43 per 100,000 per year for an unvaccinated population of children ages 6 to 35 weeks. RotaTeq or placebo was administered to 2,070 pre-term infants (25 to 36 weeks gestational age, median 34 weeks) according to their age in weeks since birth. Safety and efficacy were similar as for full term infants.

PHARMACOLOGY: RotaTeq® is a bovine-based pentavalent vaccine containing 5 live reassortant rotaviruses. The rotavirus parent strains of the reassortants were isolated from human and bovine hosts. Four reassortant rotaviruses express 1 of the outer capsid proteins (G1, G2, G3, or G4) from the human rotavirus parent strain and the attachment protein (P7(5)) from the bovine rotavirus parent strain. The fifth reassortant virus expresses the attachment protein (P1A(8)) from the human rotavirus parent strain and the outer capsid protein G6 from the bovine rotavirus parent strain. The reassortants are suspended in a buffered stabilizer solution. Each vaccine dose contains sucrose, sodium citrate, sodium phosphate monobasic monohydrate, sodium hydroxide, polysorbate 80, cell-culture media, and trace amounts of fetal bovine serum. There are no preservatives or thimerosal. Fecal shedding of vaccine virus occurred in 32 (8.9%) of 360 subjects after dose 1, 0 (0%) of 249 subjects after dose 2, and 1 (0.3%) of 385 subjects after dose 3. In phase III studies, shedding was observed as early as 1 day and as late as 15 days after a dose. The potential for transmission of vaccine virus was not assessed through epidemiologic studies. RotaTeq® can be coadministered with other childhood vaccines. It has 98% efficacy for prevention of severe illness and 74% for prevention of rotavirus-induced diarrheal episodes.

SPECIAL CONSIDERATIONS/PREPARATION: RotaTeq is supplied as a suspension for oral use in individually pouched single-dose tubes. Each dosage tube contains 2 mL. It is a pale yellow clear liquid that may have a pink tint. Store and transport refrigerated. Protect from light. Administer as soon as possible after being removed from refrigeration. Discard in approved biological waste containers.

SELECTED REFERENCES

- American Academy of Pediatrics, Committee on Infectious Diseases. Prevention of rotavirus disease: guidelines for use of rotavirus vaccine. *Pediatrics* 2007;119:171-181.
- Centers for Disease Control and Prevention. Postmarketing monitoring of intussusception after RotaTeq® vaccination - United States, February 1, 2006 — February 15, 2007 *MMWR* 2007;56(10):218-222.
- Parashar UD, Alexander JP, Glass RI; Advisory Committee on Immunization Practices (ACIP), Centers for Disease Control and Prevention (CDC). Prevention of rotavirus gastroenteritis among infants and children: recommendations of the Advisory Committee on Immunization Practices. *MMWR Recomm Rep.* 2006;55(RR-12):1-13.
- Product information, Merck & Co., 2006.

RSV Immune Globulin

DOSE & ADMINISTRATION: >750 mg/kg per dose over approximately 3 hours. Begin infusion rate at 1.5 mL/kg/hr for first 15 minutes. If no change in clinical condition, increase to 3 mL/kg/hr for the next 15 minutes, then to a maximum of 6 mL/kg/hr for the remainder of the infusion. Repeat monthly during RSV season.

USES: Immunoprophylaxis against severe RSV lower respiratory tract infections in high risk infants: primarily those younger than 24 months of age with chronic lung disease, those younger than 12 months of age who were born at less than 28 weeks gestation, and those younger than 6 months of age who were born at less than 32 weeks gestation. RSV-IGIV is contraindicated in patients with severe congenital heart disease. It is not efficacious in the treatment of RSV respiratory infections.

MONITORING: Monitor vital signs and oxygen saturation frequently during infusion.

ADVERSE EFFECTS/PRECAUTIONS: Do not use in patients with cyanotic congenital heart disease. Do not use in patients with a history of a prior reaction to human immune globulin preparations, or those with selective IgA deficiency. Volume infused is 15 mL/kg: some patients will develop respiratory distress due to fluid overload; furosemide or bumetanide should be available for management. Fever occurs in 3%. Measles / mumps / rubella and varicella vaccines should be delayed until 9 months after the last dose.

PHARMACOLOGY: RespiGam® is purified from pooled adult human plasma selected for high titers of neutralizing antibody (IgG) against RSV. A solvent-detergent viral inactivation process is used to decrease the possibility of transmission of blood borne pathogens.

SPECIAL CONSIDERATIONS/PREPARATION: Available in 50 mL (2500 mg) and 20 mL (1000 mg) single-use vials. Refrigerate at 2 °C to 8 °C (36 °F to 46 °F). **Do not freeze. Do not shake.**

SELECTED REFERENCES

- Meissner HC, Long SS, Committee on Infectious Diseases and Committee on Fetus and Newborn: Revised indications for the use of palivizumab and respiratory syncytial virus immune globulin intravenous for the prevention of respiratory syncytial virus infections. Policy Statement and Technical Report. *Pediatrics* 2003;122:1442-46 and 1447-52.
- The PREVENT study group: Reduction of respiratory syncytial virus hospitalization among premature infants and infants with bronchopulmonary dysplasia using respiratory syncytial virus immune globulin prophylaxis. *Pediatrics* 1997;99:93.
- Rodriguez WJ, Gruber WC, Groothuis JR, et al: Respiratory syncytial virus immune globulin treatment of RSV lower respiratory tract infections in previously healthy children. *Pediatrics* 1997;100:937-42.
- Product information, MedImmune, 1996.

Sildenafil

DOSE & ADMINISTRATION: 0.3 to 1 mg/kg per dose via orogastric tube every 6 to 12 hours. Some authors have successfully used doses of 2 mg/kg.

USES: Limited to treatment of patients with persistent pulmonary hypertension refractory to inhaled nitric oxide and other conventional therapies, those who are persistently unable to be weaned off of inhaled nitric oxide, or in situations where nitric oxide is not available.

MONITORING: Continuous monitoring of blood pressure and oxygenation.

ADVERSE EFFECTS/PRECAUTIONS: Use in neonates should be restricted and considered experimental. Data in neonates are very limited. The most concerning short term adverse effects are worsening oxygenation and systemic hypotension. Use with caution in infants with sepsis. Sildenafil causes transient impairment of color discrimination in adults, and there is concern that it could increase the risk of severe retinopathy of prematurity.

PHARMACOLOGY: Sildenafil is a selective phosphodiesterase (PDE5) inhibitor. This inhibition leads to accumulation of cyclic GMP in pulmonary smooth muscle cells, causing pulmonary vascular relaxation. It may also potentiate the effect of inhaled nitric oxide. Oral absorption is rapid in adults with approximately 40% bioavailability; peak concentrations are reached in 30 to 120 minutes. It is metabolized primarily by hepatic CYP3A4 to an active metabolite (N-desmethyl sildenafil) that has PDE5 inhibitory activity. Both sildenafil and the metabolite have terminal half-lives of 4 hours in adults. Patients with significant hepatic or renal dysfunction have reduced clearance. Significant increases in sildenafil concentrations may occur when used concomitantly with drugs that are CYP3A4 inhibitors; e.g., erythromycin, amilodipine, and cimetidine.

SPECIAL CONSIDERATIONS/PREPARATION: Revatio™ is supplied as 20 mg tablets; Viagra® is supplied as 50 mg tablets. To prepare an oral suspension, thoroughly crush one tablet into a fine powder and add enough Ora-Plus to make a final concentration of 2 mg/mL. Suspension is stable for 1 month if refrigerated.

SELECTED REFERENCES

- Noori S, Friedlich P, Wong P, et al: Cardiovascular effects of sildenafil in neonates and infants with congenital diaphragmatic hernia and pulmonary hypertension. *Neonatology* 2007;91:92-100.
- Baquero H, Soliz A, Neira F, et al: Oral sildenafil in infants with persistent pulmonary hypertension of the newborn: a pilot randomized blinded study. *Pediatrics* 2006;117:1077-1083.
- Baquero H, Neira F, Venegas V, et al: Outcome at 18 months of age after sildenafil therapy for refractory neonatal hypoxemia. Poster at 2005 PAS Annual Meeting, Abstract 2119.
- Travadi JN, Patole SK: Phosphodiesterase inhibitors for persistent pulmonary hypertension of the newborn: a review. *Pediatr Pulmonol* 2003;36:529-535.
- Atz AM, Wessel DL: Sildenafil ameliorates effects of inhaled nitric oxide withdrawal. *Anesthesiology* 1999;91:307-310.

Sodium Bicarbonate

DOSE & ADMINISTRATION: Resuscitation: 1 to 2 mEq/kg IV over at least 30 minutes. **Correction of metabolic acidosis:** HCO_3 needed (mEq) = HCO_3 deficit (mEq/L) x (0.3 x body wt (kg)) Administer half of calculated dose, then assess need for remainder. **Maximum concentration used: 0.5 mEq/mL.** Dilute if desired. Can also be administered by continuous IV infusion or PO.

USES: Treatment of documented metabolic acidosis during prolonged resuscitation after establishment of effective ventilation. Treatment of bicarbonate deficit caused by renal or GI losses.

MONITORING: Follow acid/base status, ABGs.

ADVERSE EFFECTS/PRECAUTIONS: Rationale against use in resuscitation: 1) Rapid infusion of hypertonic solution is linked to IVH. 2) When administered during inadequate ventilation, PCO_2 increases, thereby decreasing pH. 3) Carbon dioxide diffuses more readily across cell membranes than bicarbonate, thereby decreasing intracellular pH. **Other adverse effects:** Local tissue necrosis, hypocalcemia, and hypernatremia.

PHARMACOLOGY: Rationale for use in prolonged resuscitation: 1) Decreases pulmonary vasculature resistance. 2) Improves myocardial function. 3) Increases response of myocardium to sympathomimetics.

SPECIAL CONSIDERATIONS/PREPARATION: Supplied by many manufacturers in multiple concentrations: 4% (0.48 mEq/mL), 4.2% (0.5 mEq/mL), 7.5% (0.9 mEq/mL) and 8.4% (1 mEq/mL). Maximum concentration used in neonates is 0.5 mEq/mL. May dilute with sterile water for injection. Do not infuse with calcium or phosphate containing solutions - precipitation will occur.

Osmolarity

Concentration (%)	Concentration (mEq/mL)	Approximate Osmolarity (mOsm/L)
8.4	1	1800
4.2	0.5	900
2.8	0.33	600
2.1	0.25	450

Solution Compatibility: D_5W, $D_{10}W$, and NS.

Terminal Injection Site Compatibility: Fat emulsion. Acyclovir, amikacin, aminophylline, amphotericin B, ampicillin, atropine, aztreonam, cefepime, cefoxitin, ceftazidime, ceftriaxone, chloramphenicol, cimetidine, clindamycin, dexamethasone, erythromycin lactobionate, esmolol, famotidine, fentanyl, furosemide, heparin, hyaluronidase, hydrocortisone succinate, indomethacin, insulin, lidocaine, linezolid, meropenem, milrinone, morphine, nafcillin, netilmicin, penicillin G, pentobarbital, phenobarbital,

SODIUM NITROPRUSSIDE

phenytoin, piperacillin-tazobactam, potassium chloride, propofol, remifentanil, vancomycin, and vitamin K_1.

Incompatibility: Dex/AA. Amiodarone, calcium chloride, calcium gluconate, cefotaxime, ciprofloxacin, dobutamine, dopamine, epinephrine, glycopyrrolate, imipenem/cilastatin, isoproterenol, magnesium sulfate, methadone, methicillin, metoclopramide, midazolam, mivacurium, nicardipine, norepinephrine, oxacillin, ticarcillin/clavulanate, and vecuronium.

SELECTED REFERENCES

- van Alfen-van der Velden AA, Hopman JC, Klaessens JH, et al: Effects of rapid versus slow infusion of sodium bicarbonate on cerebral hemodynamics and oxygenation in preterm infants. *Biol Neonate* 2006;90:122-127.
- Lokesh L, Kumar P, Murki S, Narang A. A randomized controlled trial of sodium bicarbonate in neonatal resuscitation - effect on immediate outcome *Resuscitation* 2004;60:219-23.
- Murki M, Kumar P, Lingappa L, Narang A. Effect of a single dose of sodium bicarbonate given during neonatal resuscitation at birth on the acid-base status on first day of life. *Journal of Perinatology* 2004;24:696-699.
- Ammari AN, Schulze KF: Uses and abuses of sodium bicarbonate in the neonatal intensive care unit. *Curr Opin Pediatr* 2002;14:151-156.
- Wyckoff MH, Perlman J, Niermeyer S: Medications during resuscitation - what is the evidence? *Semin Neonatal* 2001;6:251-259.
- Howell JH: Sodium bicarbonate in the perinatal setting—revisited. *Clin Perinatol* 1987;14:807.

SODIUM NITROPRUSSIDE

DOSE & ADMINISTRATION: Initial Dose: 0.25 to 0.5 mcg/kg per minute continuous IV infusion by syringe pump. Use a large vein for IV. Titrate dose upward Q20 minutes until desired response is attained. Usual **maintenance dose** is < 2 mcg/kg per minute. For hypertensive crisis, may use up to 10 mcg/kg per minute, but for no longer than 10 minutes. Consider administering in a 1:10 mixture with sodium thiosulfate to minimize cyanide accumulation.

USES: Acute treatment of hypertensive emergencies. Acute afterload reduction in patients with refractory congestive heart failure.

MONITORING: Continuous heart rate and intra-arterial blood pressure monitoring is mandatory. Daily measurement of RBC cyanide (should be less than 200 ng/mL) and serum thiocyanate (should be less than 50 mcg/mL) concentrations. Assess frequently for development of metabolic acidosis. Daily assessment of renal and hepatic function. Monitor IV site closely.

ADVERSE EFFECTS/PRECAUTIONS: Severe hypotension and tachycardia. Cyanide toxicity may occur with prolonged treatment (> 3 days) and high (>3 mcg/kg per minute) doses. Use with caution in liver and renal failure patients due to possible impairment of the metabolism of cyanide to thiocyanate. Extravasation can cause tissue sloughing and necrosis.

PHARMACOLOGY: Direct-acting nonselective (arterial and venous) vasodilator. Immediately interacts with RBC oxyhemoglobin, dissociating and forming methemoglobin with release of cyanide and nitric oxide. Rapid onset of action with a serum half-life of 3 to 4 minutes in adults. Further metabolized to thiocyanate in the liver and kidney. Thiocyanate is renally eliminated with a half-life of 4 to 7 days.

SPECIAL CONSIDERATIONS/PREPARATION: Available as powder for injection of 2 mL and 5 mL single-dose 50 mg vials. Reconstitute contents of vial with 2 to 3 mL of D_5W or NS. **Do not administer reconstituted drug directly from vial.** Dilute entire vial contents to a final concentration less than 200 mcg/mL (0.2 mg/mL) in D_5W or NS. Then prepare a 1:10 (by weight) solution of sodium nitroprusside and sodium thiosulfate. Use within 24 hours of preparation. Protect from light with aluminum foil or other opaque material. Blue, green or deep red discoloration indicates nitroprusside inactivation. Slight brownish discoloration is common and not significant. **Example:** Mix 50 mg (1 vial) of sodium nitroprusside in 250 mL D_5W. Add 500 mg sodium thiosulfate (5mL of 10% solution). Mixture is stable for 7 days. **Protect from light.**

Solution Compatibility: D_5W and NS only.

Terminal Injection Site Compatibility: Fat emulsion. Aminophylline, caffeine citrate, calcium chloride, cimetidine, dobutamine, dopamine, enalaprilat, epinephrine, esmolol, famotidine, furosemide, heparin, indomethacin, insulin, isoproterenol, lidocaine, magnesium, midazolam, milrinone, morphine, nicardipine, nitroglycerin, pancuronium, potassium chloride, procainamide, propofol, prostaglandin E_1, ranitidine, and vecuronium.

Incompatibility: Amiodarone.

SELECTED REFERENCES

- van Alfen-van der Velden AA, Hopman JC, Klaessens JH, et al: Effects of rapid versus slow infusion of sodium bicarbonate on cerebral hemodynamics and oxygenation in preterm infants. *Biol Neonate* 2006;90:122-127.
- Lokesh L, Kumar P, Murki S, Narang A. A randomized controlled trial of sodium bicarbonate in neonatal resuscitation - effect on immediate outcome. *Resuscitation* 2004;60:219-223.
- Seto W, Trope A, Carfrae L, et al: Visual compatibility of sodium nitroprusside with other injectable medications given to pediatric patients. *Am J Health-Syst Pharm* 2001;58:1422-6.
- Friederich JA, Butterworth JF: Sodium nitroprusside: Twenty years and counting. *Anesth Analg* 1995;81:152.
- Benitz WE, Malachowski N, Cohen RS, et al: Use of sodium nitroprusside in neonates: Efficacy and safety. *J Pediatr* 1985;106:102.
- Roberts RJ: *Drug Therapy in Infants*. Philadelphia: WB Saunders Co, 1984, p 184.
- Dillon TR, Janos GG, Meyer RA, et al: Vasodilator therapy for congestive heart failure. *J Pediatr* 1980;96:623.

SOTALOL

DOSE & ADMINISTRATION: Initial dose: 1 mg/kg per dose PO Q12 hours. Gradually increase as needed every 3 to 5 days until stable rhythm is maintained. **Maximum dose:** 4 mg/kg per dose PO Q12 hours.

USES: Treatment of refractory ventricular and supraventricular tachyarrhythmias.

MONITORING: Frequent EKG during initiation of therapy.

ADVERSE EFFECTS/PRECAUTIONS: Proarrhythmic effects occur in 10% of pediatric patients: sinoatrial block, A-V block, torsades de pointes and ventricular ectopic activity. These effects usually occur in the first few days of treatment. Prolongation of the QT interval is dose-dependent. Other adverse effects include fatigue, dyspnea, and hypotension.

PHARMACOLOGY: Sotalol is an antiarrhythmic agent that combines Class II beta-blocking properties with Class III prolongation of cardiac action potential duration. Betapace® is a racemic mixture of *d*- and *l*-sotalol. Oral bioavailability is good, but absorption is decreased by 20 to 30% by food, especially milk. Sotalol does not bind to plasma proteins, is not metabolized, and is renally excreted as unchanged drug. Limited pharmacokinetic data in infants show a half-life of 8 hours, increasing significantly in elderly patients and those with renal dysfunction.

SPECIAL CONSIDERATIONS/PREPARATION: Supplied in 80-mg, 120-mg, 160-mg, and 240-mg tablets. A 5 mg/mL oral suspension may be made as follows: crush 5 (five) 120-mg tablets, slowly mix in 84 mL of 1% methylcellulose, then add enough simple syrup to make a total volume of 120 mL. Stable for 60 days when kept refrigerated.

SELECTED REFERENCES

- Saul JP, Schaffer MS, Karpawich PP, et al: Single dose pharmacokinetics of sotalol in a pediatric population with supraventricular and/or ventricular tachyarrhythmia. *J Clin Pharmacol* 2001;41:35-43.
- Pfammatter JP, Paul T, Lehmann C, Kalifelz HC: Efficacy and proarrhythmia of oral sotalol in pediatric patients. *J Am Coll Cardiol* 1995;26:1002.
- Tanel RE, Walsh EP, Lulu JA, and Saul JP: Sotalol for refractory arrhythmias in pediatric and young adult patients: Initial efficacy and long-term outcome. *Am Heart J* 1995;130:791.
- Hohnloser SH, Woosley RL: Sotalol. *N Engl J Med* 1994;331:31.
- Nappi JM, McCollam PL: Sotalol: A breakthrough antiarrhythmic? *Ann Pharmacother* 1993;27:1359.
- Maragnes P, Tipple M, Fournier A: Effectiveness of oral sotalol for treatment of pediatric arrhythmias. *Am J Cardiol* 1992;69:751.

SPIRONOLACTONE

DOSE & ADMINISTRATION: 1 to 3 mg/kg per dose Q24 hours PO.

USES: Used in combination with other diuretics in the treatment of congestive heart failure and BPD (situations of increased aldosterone secretion).

MONITORING: Follow serum potassium closely during long-term therapy. Also, measuring urinary potassium is a useful indicator of effectiveness.

Sucrose

ADVERSE EFFECTS/PRECAUTIONS: Rashes, vomiting, diarrhea, paresthesias. Dose-dependent androgenic effects in females. Gynecomastia in males. Headaches, nausea, and drowsiness. Use with caution in patients with impaired renal function. May cause false positive ELISA screening tests for congenital adrenal hyperplasia.

PHARMACOLOGY: Competitive antagonist of mineralocorticoids (e.g. aldosterone). Metabolized to canrenone and 7-a-thiomethylspironolactone, active metabolites with extended elimination half-lives. Decreases excretion of potassium. Highly protein bound. Increases excretion of calcium, magnesium, sodium, and chloride (small effect). Serum half-life with long term use is 13 to 24 hours. Addition of spironolactone to thiazide diuretic therapy in patients with BPD may yield little, if any, additional benefit.

SPECIAL CONSIDERATIONS/PREPARATION: Available in 25-mg, 50-mg, and 100-mg tablets. A simple syrup suspension can be made by crushing eight 25-mg spironolactone tablets and suspending the powder in 50 mL of simple syrup. Final concentration is 4 mg/mL; solution is stable for 1 month refrigerated.

SELECTED REFERENCES

- Brion LP, Primhak RA, Ambrosio-Perz I: Diuretics acting on the distal renal tubule for preterm infants with (or developing) chronic lung disease (Cochrane Review). In: *The Cochrane Library* Issue 1, 2003. Oxford: Update Software.
- Hoffman DJ, Gerdes JS, Abbasi S: Pulmonary function and electrolyte balance following spironolactone treatment in preterm infants with chronic lung disease: a double-blind, placebo-controlled randomized trial. *J Perinatol* 2000;20:41-45.
- Terai I, Yamano K, Ichihara N, et al: Influence of spironolactone on neonatal screening for congenital adrenal hyperplasia. *Arch Dis Child Fetal Neonatal Ed* 1999;81:F179.
- Mathur LK, Wickman A: Stability of extemporaneously compounded spironolactone suspensions. *Am J Hosp Pharm* 1989;46:2040.
- Overdiek HW, Hermens WA, Merkus FW: New insights into the pharmacokinetics of spironolactone. *Clin Pharmacol Ther* 1985;38:469.
- Karim A: Spironolactone: Disposition, metabolism, pharmacodynamics, and bioavailability. *Drug Metab Rev* 1978;8:151.
- Loggie JMH, Kleinman LI, Van Maanen EF: Renal function and diuretic therapy in infants and children. Part II. *J Pediatr* 1975;86:657.

Sucrose

DOSE & ADMINISTRATION: Administer orally 2 minutes prior to the painful procedure by using a pacifier dipped in the sweet solution, up to a maximum of 2 mL. 0.5 mL of 24% sucrose is equivalent to 0.12 grams of sucrose. Other solutions containing 50% sucrose and artificial sweetener have also been shown to be effective.

USES: Mild analgesia and behavioral comforting.

MONITORING: Assess for signs of pain and discomfort.

ADVERSE EFFECTS/PRECAUTIONS: Sucrose 24% has an osmolarity of ~1000 mOsm/L. The adverse effects of repeated doses in premature infants are unknown.

SPECIAL CONSIDERATIONS/PREPARATION: Sweet-Ease™, a 24% sucrose and water solution, is aseptically packaged in an 11 mL cup with a peel off lid that is suitable for dipping a pacifier or for administration via a dropper.

SELECTED REFERENCES

- Stevens B, Yamada J, Ohlsson A: Sucrose for analgesia in newborn infants undergoing painful procedures (Cochrane Review). In: *The Cochrane Library*, Issue 1, 2003. Oxford Update Software.
- Abad F, Diaz-Gomez NM, Domenech E, et al: Oral sucrose compares favorably with lidocaine-prilocaine cream for pain relief during venepuncture in neonates. *Acta Paediatr* 2001;90:160-165.
- Blass EM, Watt LB: Suckling and sucrose-induced analgesia in human newborns. *Pain* 1999;83:611-623.
- Bucher H-U, Moser T, Von Siebenthal K, et al: Sucrose reduces pain reaction to heel lancing in preterm infants: A placebo-controlled, randomized and masked study. *Pediatr Res* 1995;38:332-335.

Surfactant (Natural, animal-derived)

USES: Prophylaxis of infants at high risk for RDS (those < 29 weeks gestation). **Rescue** treatment of infants with moderate to severe RDS. **Treatment of mature infants with respiratory failure** due to meconium aspiration syndrome, pneumonia, or persistent pulmonary hypertension.

MONITORING: Assess ET tube patency and position. Oxygen saturation, EKG, and blood pressure should be monitored continuously during dosing. Assess for impairment of gas

SURVANTA®

exchange caused by blockage of the airway. After dosing, frequent assessments of oxygenation and ventilation should be performed to prevent postdose hyperoxia, hypocarbia, and overventilation.

ADVERSE EFFECTS/PRECAUTIONS: Administration of exogenous surfactants should be restricted to highly supervised clinical settings, with immediate availability of clinicians experienced with intubation, ventilator management, and general care of premature infants. Reflux of exogenous surfactant up the ET tube and falls in oxygenation occur frequently. If the infant becomes dusky or agitated, heart rate slows, oxygen saturation falls more than 15%, or surfactant backs up in the ET tube, dosing should be slowed or halted. If necessary, ventilator settings and/or FiO_2 should be turned up. Pulmonary hemorrhage occurs in 2% to 4% of treated infants, primarily the smallest patients with untreated PDA. This may be due to hemorrhagic pulmonary edema caused by the rapid fall in pulmonary vascular resistance and resulting increased pulmonary blood flow.

PHARMACOLOGY: In infants with RDS, exogenous surfactant therapy reverses atelectasis and increases FRC, with rapid improvements in oxygenation. All preparations reduce mortality from RDS. Natural surfactants are more effective than synthetics in reducing pulmonary air leak. There are no significant differences between preparations in chronic lung disease or other long term outcomes. All commercially available preparations contain surfactant apoprotein C (SP-C), none contain SP-A. The lung-mince extracts Survanta® and Curosurf® contain less than 10% of the SP-B contained in the lung-wash extract Infasurf®.

SELECTED REFERENCES

REVIEW ARTICLES

- Suresh GK, Soll RF: Current surfactant use in premature infants. *Clin Perinatol* 2001;28:671-694.
- Rodriguez RJ, Martin RJ: Exogenous surfactant therapy in newborns. *Resp Care Clin North Am* 1999;5:595-616.
- Kattwinkel J: Surfactant: Evolving issues. *Clin Perinatol* 1998; 25:17-32.
- Morley CJ: Systematic review of prophylactic vs rescue surfactant. *Arch Dis Child* 1997;77:F70-F74.
- Halliday HL: Natural vs synthetic surfactants in neonatal respiratory distress syndrome. *Drugs* 1996;51:226-237.

SELECTED REFERENCES FOR NON-RDS INDICATIONS

- Lotze A, Mitchell BR, Bulas DI, et al: Multicenter study of surfactant (Beractant) use in the treatment of term infants with severe respiratory failure. *J Pediatr* 1998;132:40.
- Findlay RD, Taeusch HW, Walther FJ: Surfactant replacement therapy for meconium aspiration syndrome. *Pediatrics* 1996;97:48.

SURVANTA®

(Beractant) Intratracheal Suspension

DOSE & ADMINISTRATION: 4 mL/kg per dose intratracheally, divided into 4 aliquots. **Prophylaxis:** First dose is given as soon as possible after birth, with up to three additional doses in the first 48 hours of life, if indicated. **Rescue treatment of RDS:** Up to four doses in first 48 hours of life, no more frequently than Q6 hours. Before administration, allow to stand at room temperature for 20 minutes, or warm in the hand for at least 8 minutes. **Artificial warming methods should not be used.** Shorten a 5F end-hole catheter so tip of catheter will protrude just beyond end of ET tube above infant's carina. Slowly withdraw entire contents of vial into a plastic syringe through a large (greater than 20 gauge) needle. **Do not filter or shake.** Attach shortened catheter to syringe. Fill catheter with Survanta. Discard excess Survanta through catheter so only total dose to be given remains in syringe. Administer four quarter-doses with the infant in different positions to enhance distribution. The catheter can be inserted into the infant's endotracheal tube through a neonatal suction valve without interrupting ventilation. Alternatively, Survanta can be instilled through the catheter by briefly disconnecting the endotracheal tube from the ventilator. After administration of each quarter-dose, the dosing catheter is removed from the ET tube and the infant is ventilated for at least 30 seconds until stable.

THAM ACETATE

PHARMACOLOGY: Survanta® is a modified natural bovine lung extract containing phospholipids, neutral lipids, fatty acids, and surfactant-associated proteins B and C, to which colfosceril palmitate (DPPC), palmitic acid, and tripalmitin are added. Resulting drug provides 25 mg/mL phospholipids (including 11 to 15.5 mg/mL DPPC), 0.5 to 1.75 mg/mL triglycerides, 1.4 to 3.5 mg/mL fatty acids, and less than 1 mg/mL protein. Survanta® is suspended in NS and heat sterilized. Animal metabolism studies show that most of a dose becomes lung-associated within hours of administration, and lipids enter endogenous surfactant pathways of reuse and recycling.

SPECIAL CONSIDERATIONS/PREPARATION: Available in 4- and 8-mL single-use vials. Refrigerate (2 °C to 8 °C (36 °F to 46 °F)) and protect from light. Inspect Survanta for discoloration; normal color is off-white to light-brown. If settling occurs during storage, **swirl** vial gently. **Do not shake.** Vials should be entered only once. Used vials with residual drug should be discarded. Unopened vials that have been warmed to room temperature one time may be refrigerated within 24 hours and stored for future use.

SELECTED REFERENCES

- Zola EM, Overbach AM, Gunkel JH, et al: Treatment investigational new drug experience with Survanta (beractant). *Pediatrics* 1993;91:546.
- Hoekstra RE, Jackson JC, Myers TF, et al: Improved neonatal survival following multiple doses of bovine surfactant in very premature neonates at risk for respiratory distress syndrome. *Pediatrics* 1991;88:10.
- Liechty EA, Donovan E, Purohit D, et al: Reduction of neonatal mortality after multiple doses of bovine surfactant in low birth weight neonates with respiratory distress syndrome. *Pediatrics* 1991;88:19.

THAM ACETATE

(Tromethamine)

DOSE & ADMINISTRATION: 1 to 2 mmol/kg (3.3 to 6.6 mL/kg) per dose IV. Infuse in a large vein over at least 30 minutes. Dose (of the 0.3 M solution) may be calculated from the following formula: **Dose (mL) = Weight (kg) x Base deficit (mEq/L)** Maximum dose in neonates with normal renal function is approximately 5 to 7 mmol/kg per 24 hours. Clinical studies support only short term use.

USES: Treatment of metabolic acidosis, primarily in mechanically ventilated patients with significant hypercarbia or hypernatremia. **Do not use in patients who are anuric or uremic.** THAM is not indicated for treatment of metabolic acidosis caused by bicarbonate deficiency.

MONITORING: Observe IV site closely for signs of extravasation. Follow blood-gas results to assess therapeutic efficacy. Follow urine output. Monitor for respiratory depression, hypoglycemia, and hyperkalemia when using several doses.

ADVERSE EFFECTS/PRECAUTIONS: Most reports of toxicity in neonates (hypoglycemia, hyperkalemia, liver necrosis) were related to rapid umbilical venous infusion of high doses of THAM base solutions that were more alkaline and hypertonic than the THAM acetate solution currently available from Abbott (pH 8.6; osmolarity 380 mOsm/L). **Irritating to veins**.

PHARMACOLOGY: THAM (Tris-Hydroxymethyl Aminomethane) is a proton acceptor that generates NH_3^+ and HCO_3^- without generating CO_2. The protonated $R-NH_3^+$ is eliminated by the kidneys. Unlike bicarbonate, THAM does not require an open system for CO_2 elimination in order to exert its buffering effect.

SPECIAL CONSIDERATIONS/PREPARATION: Supplied as a 0.3-M solution (1 mmol = 3.3 mL) in a 500-mL single-dose container with no bacteriostatic agent. Use within 24 hours of opening. **Compatibilities:** No data are currently available on solutions and additives.

SELECTED REFERENCES

- Holmdahl MH, Wiklund L, Wetterberg T, et al: The place of THAM in the management of acidemia in clinical practice. *Acta Anaethesiol Scand* 2000;44:524-527.
- Nahas GG, Sutin KM, Fermon C, et al: Guidelines for the treatment of acidemia with THAM. *Drugs* 1998;55:191-224. (Errata published 1998;55:517).

- Baum JD, Robertson NRC: Immediate effects of alkaline infusion in infants with respiratory distress syndrome. *J Pediatr* 1975;87:255.
- Strauss J: Tris (hydroxymethyl amino-methane (THAM)): A pediatric evaluation. *Pediatrics* 1968;41:667.
- Gupta JM, Dahlenburg GW, Davis JW: Changes in blood gas tensions following administration of amine buffer THAM to infants with respiratory distress syndrome. *Arch Dis Child* 1967;42:416-427.

TICARCILLIN/CLAVULANATE

DOSE & ADMINISTRATION: >75 to 100 mg/kg per dose IV infusion by syringe pump over 30 minutes. To use dosing chart, please refer to explanatory note in "How to Use This Book."

DOSING INTERVAL CHART

PMA (weeks)	PostNatal (days)	Interval (hours)
≤29	0 to 28 >28	12 8
30 to 36	0 to 14 >14	12 8
37 to 44	0 to 7 >7	12 8
≥45	ALL	6

USES: Treatment of non-CNS infections, caused by susceptible β-lactamase producing bacteria, including many strains of *E. coli, Enterobacter, Klebsiella, Haemophilus influenzae, Proteus mirabilis, Pseudomonas spp.*, and *Staph. aureus*.

MONITORING: Serum concentrations are not routinely monitored. Assess renal function prior to therapy. Measure serum sodium concentrations and hepatic transaminases periodically. Observe IV site for signs of extravasation.

ADVERSE EFFECTS/PRECAUTIONS: Eosinophilia. Hyperbilirubinemia. Elevations in ALT, AST, BUN, and serum creatinine. Hypernatremia may be exacerbated in ELBW patients.

PHARMACOLOGY: Timentin® combines the extended-spectrum antibiotic ticarcillin with the β-lactamase inhibitor clavulanic acid in a 30:1 ratio. Ticarcillin is primarily eliminated unchanged by renal mechanisms, whereas clavulanate undergoes significant hepatic metabolism. As a result, the mean half-life of ticarcillin in neonates is 4.2 hours compared to a mean half-life of 2 hours for clavulanate. CNS penetration is modest (limited data). Sodium content is 4.75 mEq per gram; therefore, each dose will contain 0.35 to 0.48 mEq per kg body weight.

SPECIAL CONSIDERATIONS/PREPARATION: Available as powder for injection in 3.1-g vials. Reconstitute vial by adding 13.1 mL of sterile water for injection. Dilute further with a compatible solution to a concentration between 10 and 100 mg/mL. Dilutions are stable for 24 hours at room temperature, 3 days refrigerated, and 7 days frozen.

Solution Compatibility: D$_5$W, LR, and NS.

Terminal Injection Site Compatibility: Dex/AA solutions, fat emulsion. Acyclovir, aminophylline, aztreonam, cefepime, famotidine, fluconazole, heparin, insulin, milrinone, morphine, propofol, remifentanil, and theophylline.

Incompatibility: Amikacin, azithromycin, gentamicin, netilmicin, sodium bicarbonate, tobramycin, and vancomycin.

SELECTED REFERENCES

- Rubino CM, Gal P, Ransom JL: A review of the pharmacokinetic and pharmacodynamic characteristics of β-lactam/β-lactamase inhibitor combination antibiotics in premature infants. *Pediatr Infect Dis J* 1998;17:1200-1210.
- Reed MD: A reassessment of ticarcillin/clavulanic acid dose recommendations for infants, children, and adults. *Pediatr Infect Dis J* 1998;17:1195-1199.

TOBRAMYCIN

DOSE & ADMINISTRATION: IV infusion by syringe pump over 30 minutes. Administer as a separate infusion from penicillin-containing compounds. IM injection is associated with variable absorption, especially in the very small infant. To use dosing chart, please refer to explanatory note in "How to Use This Book."

TOBRAMYCIN

DOSING CHART

PMA (weeks)	Postnatal (days)	Dose (mg/kg)	Interval (hours)
≤29*	0 to 7 8 to 28 ≥29	5 4 4	48 36 24
30 to 34	0 to 7 ≥8	4.5 4	36 24
≥35	ALL	4	24

* or significant asphyxia, PDA, or treatment with indomethacin

USES: Treatment of infections caused by aerobic gram-negative bacilli (e.g. *Pseudomonas, Klebsiella, E. coli*). Usually used in combination with a β-lactam antibiotic.

MONITORING: Measure serum concentrations when treating for more than 48 hours. Obtain peak concentration 30 minutes after end of infusion, and trough concentration just prior to the next dose. When treating patients with serious infections or significantly changing fluid or renal status consider measuring the serum concentration 24 hours after a dose, and use the chart below for the suggested dosing interval. Blood samples obtained to monitor serum drug concentrations should be spun and refrigerated or frozen as soon as possible. Therapeutic serum concentrations: **Peak:** 5 to 12 mcg/mL (or C_{max}/MIC ratio greater than 8:1) **Trough:** 0.5 to 1 mcg/mL

SUGGESTED DOSING INTERVALS

Level at 24 hours (mcg/mL)	Half-life (hours)	Suggested Dosing Interval (hours)
≤1	≈8	24
1.1 to 2.3	≈12	36
2.4 to 3.2	≈15	48
≥3.3		Measure level in 24 hours

ADVERSE EFFECTS/PRECAUTIONS: Transient and reversible renal tubular dysfunction may occur, resulting in increased urinary losses of sodium, calcium, and magnesium. Vestibular and auditory ototoxicity. The addition of other nephrotoxic and/or ototoxic medications (e.g. furosemide, vancomycin) may increase these adverse effects. Increased neuromuscular blockade (i.e. neuromuscular weakness and respiratory failure) may occur when used with pancuronium or other neuromuscular blocking agents and in patients with hypermagnesemia.

PHARMACOLOGY: Dosing recommendations for tobramycin are based on: (1) Higher peak concentrations increase concentration-dependent bacterial killing; (2) There is a post-antibiotic effect on bacterial killing, especially when treating concurrently with a β-lactam antibiotic; (3) There may be less toxicity with less frequent dosing, due to less renal drug accumulation. Volume of distribution is increased and clearance is decreased in patients with PDA. Serum half-life is prolonged in premature and asphyxiated newborns. Inactivation of tobramycin by penicillin-containing compounds appears to be a time-, temperature-, and concentration-dependent process. This is probably clinically significant only when penicillin-containing compounds are mixed in IV solutions or when the blood is at room temperature for several hours before the assay is performed.

SPECIAL CONSIDERATIONS/PREPARATION: Pediatric injectable solution available in a concentration of 10 mg/mL.

Solution Compatibility: D_5W, $D_{10}W$, and NS.

Terminal Injection Site Compatibility: Dex/AA solutions, fat emulsion. Acyclovir, aminophylline, amiodarone, aztreonam, calcium gluconate, cefoxitin, ceftazidime, ciprofloxacin, clindamycin, dopamine, enalaprilat, esmolol, fluconazole, furosemide, heparin (concentrations ≤1 Unit/mL), insulin, linezolid, metronidazole, midazolam, milrinone, morphine, nicardipine, ranitidine, remifentanil, theophylline, and zidovudine.

Incompatibility: Amphotericin B, ampicillin, azithromycin, cefepime, imipenem/cilastatin, indomethacin, heparin (concentrations >1 unit/mL), methicillin, mezlocillin, nafcillin, oxacillin, penicillin G, propofol, and ticarcillin/clavulanate.

SELECTED REFERENCES

- Contopoulos-Ioannidis DG, Giotis ND, Baliatsa DV, Ioannidis JPA: Extended-interval aminoglycoside administration for children: a meta-analysis. *Pediatrics* 2004;114:e111-e118.
- Avent ML, Kinney JS, Istre GR, Whitfield JM: Gentamicin and tobramycin in neonates: comparison of a new extended dosing regimen with a traditional multiple daily dosing regimen. *Am J Perinatol* 2002;8:413-19.
- de Hoog M, Schoemaker RC, Mouton JW, van den Anker JN: Tobramycin population pharmacokinetics in neonates. *Clin Pharmacol Ther* 1997;62:392-399.
- Giapros VI, Andronikou S, Cholevas VI, Papadopoulou ZL: Renal function in premature infants during aminoglycoside therapy. *Pediatr Nephrol* 1995;9:163.
- Daly JS, Dodge RA, Glew RH, et al: Effect of time and temperature on inactivation of aminoglycosides by ampicillin at neonatal dosages. *J Perinatol* 1997;17:42-45.
- Williams BS, Ransom JL, Gal P, et al: Gentamicin pharmacokinetics in neonates with patent ductus arteriosus. *Crit Care Med* 1997;25:273-275.

TRI-VI-SOL® MVI DROPS

DOSE & ADMINISTRATION: 1 dropperful (1 mL) Q24 hours, or as directed by physician.

TRI-VI-SOL® MULTIVITAMIN DROPS

Nutrient amt	w/o Iron	with Iron
Vitamins		
A, IU	1500	1500
D, IU	400	400
C, mg	35	35
E, (IU)	0	0
Thiamine B_1, mg	0	0
Riboflavin B_2, mg	0	0
Niacin, mg	0	0
B_6, mg	0	0
B_{12}, mcg	0	0
Minerals		
Iron, mg	0	10

TROPICAMIDE (OPHTHALMIC)

DOSE & ADMINISTRATION: 1 drop instilled in the eye at least 10 minutes prior to funduscopic procedures. Use **only** the 0.5% ophthalmic solution in neonates. Apply pressure to the lacrimal sac during and for 2 minutes after instillation to minimize systemic absorption.

USES: Induction of mydriasis and cycloplegia for diagnostic and therapeutic ophthalmic procedures.

MONITORING: Monitor heart rate and assess for signs of ileus prior to feeding.

ADVERSE EFFECTS/PRECAUTIONS: Feedings should be withheld for 4 hours following procedure. Systemic effects are those of anticholinergic drugs: Fever, tachycardia, vasocilatation, dry mouth, restlessness, decreased gastrointestinal motility, and urinary retention. The use of solutions with concentrations of 1% or greater have caused systemic toxicity in infants

PHARMACOLOGY: Ophthalmic tropicamide is an anticholinergic drug that produces pupillary dilation by inhibiting the sphincter pupillae muscle, and paralysis of accommodation. Mydriasis begins within 5 minutes of instillation, cycloplegia occurs in 20 to 40

URSODIOL

minutes. Recovery of accommodation occurs in 6 hours. Without lacrimal sac occlusion, approximately 80% of each drop may pass through the nasolacrimal system and be available for rapid systemic absorption by the nasal mucosa.

SPECIAL CONSIDERATIONS/PREPARATION: Supplied as ophthalmic solution in 0.5%, and 1% concentrations in 2- and 15-mL dropper bottles. Store away from heat. **Do not refrigerate.** A combination eye drop solution ("Caputo drops") may be prepared in a 15-mL bottle with 3.75 mL of cyclopentolate 2%, 7.5 mL of tropicamide 1%, and 3.75 mL of phenylephrine 10%. The final solution contains cyclopentolate 0.5%, tropicamide 0.5%, and phenylephrine 2.5%. Use within 24 hours, as the solution contains no preservatives.

SELECTED REFERENCES

- Wallace DK, Steinkuller PG: Ocular medications in children. *Clin Pediatr* 1998;37:645-652.
- Laws DE, Morton C, Weindling M, Clark D: Systemic effects of screening for retinopathy of prematurity. *Br J Ophthalmol* 1996;80:425-428.
- McGregor MLK: Anticholinergic agents, in Mauger TF, Craig EL (eds): *Havener's Ocular Pharmacology*, ed 6. St. Louis: Mosby-YearBook, 1994, pp 148-155.
- Caputo AR, Schnitzer RE, Lindquist TD, Sun S: Dilation in neonates: a protocol. *Pediatrics* 1982;69:77-80.

URSODIOL

(Ursodeoxycholic Acid)

DOSE & ADMINISTRATION: 10 to 15 mg/kg per dose Q 12 hours PO.

USES: Treatment of cholestasis associated with parenteral nutrition, biliary atresia, and cystic fibrosis. Also used to dissolve cholesterol gallstones.

MONITORING: Hepatic transaminases and direct bilirubin concentration.

ADVERSE EFFECTS/PRECAUTIONS: Nausea/vomiting, abdominal pain, constipation, and flatulence.

PHARMACOLOGY: Ursodiol is a hydrophobic bile acid that decreases both the secretion of cholesterol from the liver and its intestinal absorption. It is well absorbed orally. After conjugation with taurine or glycine, it then enters the enterohepatic circulation where it is excreted into the bile and intestine. It is hydrolyzed back to the unconjugated form or converted to lithocholic acid which is excreted in the feces. Serum half-life is 3 to 4 days in adults. Dissolution of gallstones may take several months. Aluminum-containing antacids bind ursodiol and inhibit absorption.

SPECIAL CONSIDERATIONS/PREPARATION: Available in 300-mg capsules. A liquid suspension may be made by opening ten (10) 300-mg capsules into a glass mortar. Mix this powder with 10 mL of glycerin and stir until smooth. Add 60 mL of Ora-Plus® to the mixture and stir. Transfer the contents of the mortar to a glass amber bottle and shake well. Add a small amount of Orange Syrup to the mortar and rinse. Pour the remaining contents into the amber glass bottle, then add enough simple syrup to make the final volume 120 mL, with a final concentration of 25 mg/mL. Shake vigorously. Mixture is stable for 60 days stored at room temperature or refrigerated.

SELECTED REFERENCES

- Chen C-Y, Tsao P-N, Chen H-L, et al: Ursodeoxycholic acid (UDCA) therapy in very-low-birth-weight infants with parenteral nutrition-associated cholestasis. *J Pediatr* 2004;145:317-321.
- Levine A, Maayan A, Shamir R, et al: Parenteral nutrition-associated cholestasis in preterm neonates: Evaluation of ursodeoxycholic acid treatment. *J Pediatr Endocrinol Metab* 1999;12:549-553.
- Balisteri WF: Bile acid therapy in pediatric hepatobiliary disease: the role of ursodeoxycholic acid. *J Pediatr Gastroenterol Nutr* 1997;24:573-89.
- Teitelbaum DH: Parenteral nutrition-associated cholestasis. *Curr Opin Pediatr* 1997;9:270-75.
- Mallett MS Hagan RL, Peters DA: Stability of ursodiol 25mg/mL in an extemporaneously prepared oral liquid. *Am J Health-Syst Pharm* 1997;54:1401.
- Spagnuolo MI, Iorio R, Vegnente A, Guarino A: Ursodeoxycholic acid for treatment of cholestasis in children. *Gastroenterol* 1996;111:716-719.
- Ward A, Brogden RN, Heel RC, et al: Ursodeoxycholic acid: A review of its pharmacological properties and therapeutic efficacy. *Drugs* 1984;27:95.

VANCOMYCIN

DOSE & ADMINISTRATION: IV infusion by syringe pump over 60 minutes. **Meningitis:** 15 mg/kg per dose **Bacteremia:** 10 mg/kg per dose To use dosing chart, please refer to explanatory note in "How to Use This Book."

Dosing Interval Chart

PMA (weeks)	PostNatal (days)	Interval (hours)
≤29	0 to 14 >14	18 12
30 to 36	0 to 14 >14	12 8
37 to 44	0 to 7 >7	12 8
≥45	ALL	6

USES: Drug of choice for serious infections caused by methicillin-resistant staphylococci (e.g. *S aureus* and *S epidermidis*) and penicillin-resistant pneumococci.

MONITORING: Serum trough concentrations should be followed in neonates because of changes in renal function related to maturation and severity of illness. Peak concentrations have not been clearly demonstrated to correlate with efficacy, but monitoring these has been recommended when treating meningitis. **Trough:** 5 to 10 mcg/mL **Peak:** 30 to 40 mcg/mL (when treating meningitis) (Draw 30 minutes after end of infusion.) Assess renal function. Observe IV site for signs of extravasation and phlebitis.

ADVERSE EFFECTS/PRECAUTIONS: Nephrotoxicity and ototoxicity: Enhanced by aminoglycoside therapy. **Rash and hypotension (red man syndrome):** Appears rapidly and resolves within minutes to hours. Lengthening infusion time usually eliminates risk for subsequent doses. **Neutropenia:** Reported after prolonged administration (more than 3 weeks). **Phlebitis:** May be minimized by slow infusion and dilution of the drug.

PHARMACOLOGY: Vancomycin is bactericidal; interferes with cell wall synthesis, inhibits RNA synthesis, and alters plasma membrane function. Diffuses readily and is widely distributed in most body fluids. CSF concentrations in premature infants ranged from 26 to 68% of serum concentrations. Small amount of hepatic metabolism.

SPECIAL CONSIDERATIONS/PREPARATION: Available as powder for injection in 500-mg and 1-g vials. Reconstitute 500-mg vial with 10 mL sterile water for injection to make a final concentration of 50 mg/mL. Reconstituted solution stable for 14 days refrigerated. Dilute prior to administration using D5W or NS to a maximum concentration of 5 mg/mL. Dilutions are stable for 24 hours at room temperature and 60 days refrigerated.

Solution Compatibility: D_5W, $D_{10}W$, and NS.

Terminal Injection Site Compatibility: Dex/AA solutions, fat emulsion. Acyclovir, amikacin, ampicillin, aminophylline, amiodarone, aztreonam, caffeine citrate, calcium gluconate, cimetidine, enalaprilat, esmolol, famotidine, fluconazole, heparin (concentrations ≤1 unit/mL), hydrocortisone succinate, insulin, linezolid, lorazepam, meropenem, midazolam, milrinone, morphine, nicardipine, pancuronium bromide, potassium chloride, propofol, ranitidine, remifentanil, sodium bicarbonate, vecuronium, and zidovudine.

Incompatibility: Cefazolin, cefepime, cefotaxime, cefoxitin, ceftazidime, ceftriaxone, chloramphenicol, dexamethasone, heparin (concentrations >1 unit/mL), methicillin, mezlocillin, nafcillin, pentobarbital, phenobarbital, piperacillin, piperacillin-tazobactam, ticarcillin, and ticarcillin/clavulanate.

SELECTED REFERENCES

- de Hoog M, Schoemaker RC, Mouton JW, van den Anker JN: Vancomycin population pharmacokinetics in neonates. *Clin Pharmacol Ther* 2000;67:360-367.
- Ahmed A: A critical evaluation of vancomycin for treatment of bacterial meningitis. *Pediatr Infect Dis J* 1997;16:895-903.
- Trissel LA, Gilbert DL, Martinez JF: Concentration dependency of vancomycin hydrochloride compatibility with β-lactam antibiotics during simulated y-site administration. *Hosp Pharm* 1998;33:1515-1520.
- Reiter PD, Doron MW: Vancomycin cerebrospinal fluid concentrations after intravenous administration in premature infants. *J Perinatol* 1996;16:331-335.
- Schilling CG, Watson DM, McCoy HG, Uden DL: Stability and delivery of vancomycin hydrochloride when admixed in a total parenteral nutrition solution. *JPEN* 1989;13:63.
- Lacouture PG, Epstein MF, Mitchell AA: Vancomycin-associated shock and rash in newborn infants. *J Pediatr* 1987;111:615.
- Schaible DH, Rocci ML, Alpert GA, et al: Vancomycin pharmacokinetics in infants: Relationships to indices of maturation. *Pediatr Infect Dis* 1986;5:304.

VECURONIUM

DOSE & ADMINISTRATION: 0.1 mg/kg (0.03 to 0.15 mg/kg) IV push, as needed for paralysis. Usual dosing interval is 1 to 2 hours. Adjust dose as needed based on duration of paralysis.

USES: Skeletal muscle relaxation/paralysis in infants requiring mechanical ventilation. Proposed desirable effects are improved oxygenation/ventilation, reduced barotrauma, and reduced fluctuations in cerebral blood flow.

MONITORING: Monitor vital signs frequently, blood pressure continuously. Use some form of eye lubrication.

ADVERSE EFFECTS/PRECAUTIONS: Hypoxemia may occur because of inadequate mechanical ventilation and deterioration in pulmonary mechanics. When used alone, cardiovascular side effects are minimal; however, decreases in heart rate and blood pressure have been observed when used concurrently with narcotics.

PHARMACOLOGY: Vecuronium is a nondepolarizing muscle-relaxant that competitively antagonizes autonomic cholinergic receptors. Sympathetic stimulation is minimal. Vecuronium is metabolized rapidly in the liver to 3-desacetyl-vecuronium, which is 50% to 70% active, and is excreted renally. Newborns, particularly premature infants, are especially sensitive to vecuronium; this sensitivity diminishes with age. Onset of action is 1 to 2 minutes; duration of effect is prolonged with higher doses and in premature infants. Skeletal relaxation/paralysis is reversed by neostigmine and atropine. **Factors affecting duration of neuromuscular blockade: Potentiation:** Acidosis, hypothermia, neuromuscular disease, hepatic disease, cardiovascular disease, aminoglycosides, hypokalemia, hypermagnesemia, renal failure, and younger age. **Antagonism:** Alkalosis, epinephrine, and hyperkalemia. Sensation remains intact; analgesia should be used for painful procedures.

SPECIAL CONSIDERATIONS/PREPARATION: Available as powder for injection in 10-mg and 20-mg vials. A 0.4-mg/mL dilution may be made by diluting 1 mL of 1-mg/mL concentration with 1.5 mL of preservative-free normal saline. Dilution is stable for 24 hours at room temperature.

Solution Compatibility: D_5W and NS.

Terminal Injection Site Compatibility: Dex/AA solutions. Aminophylline, amiodarone, cefazolin, cefoxitin, cimetidine, ciprofloxacin, dobutamine, dopamine, epinephrine, esmolol, fentanyl, fluconazole, gentamicin, heparin, hydrocortisone succinate, isoproterenol, linezolid, lorazepam, midazolam, milrinone, morphine, nicardipine, nitroglycerin, nitroprusside, propofol, ranitidine, trimethoprim-sulfamethoxazole, and vancomycin.

Incompatibility: Diazepam, furosemide, and sodium bicarbonate.

SELECTED REFERENCES

- Martin LD, Bratton SL, O'Rourke P: Clinical uses and controversies of neuromuscular blocking agents in infants and children. *Crit Care Med* 1999;27:1358-1368.
- Segredo V, Matthay MA, Sharma ML, et al: Prolonged neuromuscular blockage after long-term administration of vecuronium in two critically ill patients. *Anesthesiology* 1990;72:566.
- Bhutani VK, Abbasi S, Sivieri EM: Continuous skeletal muscle paralysis: Effect on neonatal pulmonary mechanics. *Pediatrics* 1988;81:419.
- Gravlee GP, Ramsey FM, Roy RC, et al: Rapid administration of a narcotic and neuromuscular blocker: A hemodynamic comparison of fentanyl, sufentanil, pancuronium, and vecuronium. *Anesth Analg* 1988;67:39.
- Meretoja OA, Wirtavuori K, Neuvonen PJ: Age-dependence of the dose-response curve of vecuronium in pediatric patients during balanced anesthesia. *Anesth Analg* 1988;67:21.
- Costarino AT, Polin RA: Neuromuscular relaxants in the neonate. *Clin Perinatol* 1987;14:965.

Vi-Daylin® Multivitamin Products

Vi-Daylin® ADC Drops

DOSE & ADMINISTRATION: 1 dropperful (1 mL) Q24 hours, or as directed by physician.

Vi-Daylin® ADC Drops

Nutrient amt	w/o Iron	with Iron
Vitamins		
A, IU	1350	1350
D, IU	400	400
C, mg	32	32
E, IU	0	0
Thiamine B_1, mg	0	0
Riboflavin B_2, mg	0	0
Niacin, mg	0	0
B_6, mg	0	0
B_{12}, mcg	0	0
Minerals		
Iron, mg	0	9

Vi-Daylin® Multivitamin Products

DOSE & ADMINISTRATION: 1 dropperful (1 mL) Q24 hours, or as directed by physician. Percentages of the Reference Daily Intakes (%RDIs) listed in the table below are for infants.

Vi-Daylin® Multivitamin Products

	Vi-Daylin® ADC Vitamin Drops		Vi-Daylin® ADC Vitamins + Iron Drops		Vi-Daylin® Multivitamin Drops		Vi-Daylin® Multivitamin + Iron Drops	
	Amt	(%RDI)	Amt	(%RDI)	Amt	(%RDI)	Amt	(%RDI)
Vitamins								
A (IU)	1350	(90)	1350	(90)	1350	(90)	1350	(90)
D (IU)	400	(100)	400	(100)	360	(90)	360	(90)
C (mg)	32	(90)	32	(90)	32	(90)	32	(90)
E (IU)					5	(90)	5	(90)
Thiamine (B_1) (mg)					0.4	(80)	0.5	(89)
Riboflavin (B_2) (mg)					0.5	(90)	0.5	(90)
Niacin (mg)					7	(90)	7	(90)
B_6 (mg)					0.4	(90)	0.4	(90)
B_{12} (mcg)					1.4	(68)		
Minerals								
Iron (mg)			9	60			9	(60)

Vi-Daylin® MVI Drops

DOSE & ADMINISTRATION: 1 dropperful (1 mL) Q24 hours, or as directed by physician.

Vi-Daylin® Multivitamin Drops

Nutrient amt	w/o Iron	with Iron
Vitamins		
A, IU	1350	1350
D, IU	360	360
C, mg	32	32
E, IU	5	5
Thiamine B_1, mg	0.4	0.5
Riboflavin B_2, mg	0.5	0.5
Niacin, mg	7	7
B_6, mg	0.4	0.4
B_{12}, mcg	1.4	0
Minerals		
Iron, mg	0	9

Vi-Sol® Multivitamin Products

DOSE & ADMINISTRATION: 1 dropperful (1 mL) Q24 hours, or as directed by physician. Percentages of the Reference Daily Intakes (%RDIs) listed in the table below are for infants.

Vi-Sol® Products

	Tri-Vi-Sol® Multivitamin Drops		Tri-Vi-Sol® Multivitamin with Iron Drops		Poly-Vi-Sol® Multivitamin Drops		Poly-Vi-Sol® Multivitamin with Iron Drops	
	Amt	(%RDI)	Amt	(%RDI)	Amt	(%RDI)	Amt	(%RDI)
Vitamins								
A (IU)	1500	(100)	1500	(100)	1500	(100)	1500	(100)
D (IU)	400	(100)	400	(100)	400	(100)	400	(100)
C (mg)	35	(100)	35	(100)	35	(100)	35	(100)
E (IU)					5	(100)	5	(100)
Thiamine (B_1) (mg)					0.5	(100)	0.5	(100)
Riboflavin (B_2) (mg)					0.6	(100)	0.6	(100)
Niacin (mg)					8	(100)	8	(100)
B_6 (mg)					0.4	(100)	0.4	(100)
B_{12} (mcg)					2	(100)	2	(100)
Minerals								
Iron (mg)			10	(67)			10	(67)

Vitamin A

(Retinyl Palmitate)

DOSE & ADMINISTRATION: Parenteral treatment of Vitamin A deficiency: 5000 IU IM 3 times weekly for 4 weeks. Administer using 29-g needle and insulin syringe. **DO NOT ADMINISTER IV.**

USES: To reduce the risk of Chronic Lung Disease in high risk premature neonates with Vitamin A deficiency. In the NICHD-sponsored trial, 14 infants needed to be treated to prevent 1 case of Chronic Lung Disease.

MONITORING: Assess regularly for signs of toxicity: full fontanel, lethargy, irritability, hepatomegaly, edema, mucocutaneous lesions, and bony tenderness. Consider measuring plasma retinol concentrations if available, especially if patient is also receiving glucocorticoid therapy. Desired concentrations are approximately 30 to 60 mcg/dL. Concentrations < 20 mcg/dL indicate deficiency, while those > 100 mcg/dL are potentially toxic.

ADVERSE EFFECTS/PRECAUTIONS: See Monitoring section. Coincident treatment with glucocorticoids should be avoided, as it significantly raises plasma vitamin A concentrations.

PHARMACOLOGY: The pulmonary histopathologic changes of BPD and vitamin A deficiency are remarkably similar. Vitamin A is the generic name for a group of fat soluble compounds which have the biological activity of the primary alcohol, retinol. Retinol metabolites exhibit potent and site-specific effects on gene expression and on lung growth and development. Retinol is supplied in the diet as retinyl esters.

SPECIAL CONSIDERATIONS/PREPARATION: Available as Aquasol A® Parenteral (water-miscible vitamin A palmitate) (AstraZeneca), 50,000 IU per mL, equivalent to 15 mg retinol per mL, in 2 mL vials. **Protect from light.** Store refrigerated at 36 to 46 °F (2 to 8 °C). Do not freeze.

SELECTED REFERENCES

- Tyson JE, Wright LL, Oh W, Kennedy K, et al: Vitamin A supplementation for extremely-low-birth-weight infants. N Engl J Med 1999;340:1962-68.
- Darlow BA, Graham PJ. Vitamin A supplementation for preventing morbidity and mortality in very low birthweight infants (Cochrane Review). In: *The Cochrane Library*, Issue 1, 2004. Chichester, UK: John Wiley & Sons, Ltd.
- Shenai JP: Vitamin A supplementation in very low birthweight neonates: rationale and evidence. *Pediatrics* 1999;104:1369-74.
- Product information, AstraZeneca, 2002.

Vitamin E

(DL-Alpha-Tocopherol Acetate)

DOSE & ADMINISTRATION: 5 to 25 IU per day PO. Dilute with feedings. Do not administer simultaneously with iron—iron absorption is impaired.

USES: Prevention of vitamin E deficiency. May be indicated in babies receiving erythropoietin and high iron dosages. Higher doses used to reduce oxidant-induced injury (ROP, BPD, IVH) remain controversial.

MONITORING: Assess feeding tolerance. Signs of vitamin E deficiency include hemolytic anemia and thrombocytosis. Physiologic serum vitamin E concentrations are between 0.8 and 3.5 mg/dL.

ADVERSE EFFECTS/PRECAUTIONS: Feeding intolerance may occur due to hyperosmolarity of preparation. Pharmacologic doses of alpha tocopherol have been associated with increased rates of sepsis (antioxidant effect of drug) and NEC (osmolarity of oral formulation).

PHARMACOLOGY: Alpha-tocopherol is the most active antioxidant of the group of tocopherols known as Vitamin E. The amount required by the body is primarily dependent upon the dietary intake of fat, especially polyunsaturated fatty acids (PUFA). Human milk and currently available infant formulas contain adequate vitamin E and have appropriate E:PUFA ratios to prevent hemolytic anemia. Infants receiving supplemental iron amounts above 2 mg/kg/day may also require additional vitamin E. Oral absorption of vitamin E is dependent upon hydrolysis that requires bile salts and pancreatic esterases. This can be quite variable in very immature infants and those with fat malabsorption. Free tocopherol is absorbed in the small intestine, taken via chylomi-

Vitamin K$_1$

crons into the gastrointestinal lymphatics, then carried via low-density lipoproteins to be incorporated into cell membranes. Significant tissue accumulation may occur with pharmacologic doses.

SPECIAL CONSIDERATIONS/PREPARATION: Available as liquid drops: Aquavit E® (Cypress Pharmaceutical), 15 IU (=15 mg) per 0.3 mL. Water solubilized with polysorbate 80. Also contains propylene glycol. Hyperosmolar (3620 mOsm/kg H$_2$O). Store at controlled room temperature.

SELECTED REFERENCES

- Gross SJ: Vitamin E. In Tsang RC, Lucas A, Uauy R, Zlotkin S (eds): *Nutritional Needs of the Preterm Infant: Scientific Basis and Practical Guidelines*. Pauling, New York: Caduceus Medical Publishers, 1993, pp 101-109.
- Roberts RJ, Knight ME: Pharmacology of vitamin E in the newborn. *Clin Perinatol* 1987;14:843-855.
- Raju TNK, Langenberg P, Bhutani V, Quinn GE: Vitamin E prophylaxis to reduce retinopathy of prematurity: A reappraisal of published trials. *J Pediatr* 1997;131:844-850.

Vitamin K$_1$

DOSE & ADMINISTRATION: Recommended Prophylaxis: 0.5 to 1 mg IM at birth. **Preterm infants <32 weeks gestation: BW >1000 grams:** 0.5 mg IM. **BW <1000 grams:** 0.3 mg/kg IM. **Alternate strategy for healthy, term, exclusively breast-fed infants:** 2 mg PO with the first feed, at 1 week, 4 weeks, and 8 weeks of age. ***Note:** there is no approved oral formulation in the United States. Oral prophylaxis is contraindicated in infants who are premature, ill, on antibiotics, have cholestasis, or have diarrhea. There has been an increased number of cases of hemorrhagic disease of the newborn in countries that have changed to oral prophylaxis, primarily in patients who received only a single oral dose. Also: Maternal daily intake of 5 mg/day of phylloquinone significantly increases Vitamin K concentrations in breastmilk and infant plasma. **Treatment of severe hemorrhagic disease:** 1 to 10 mg IV slow push. (See Adverse Effects/Precautions for rate of administration.)

USES: Prophylaxis and therapy of hemorrhagic disease of the newborn. Treatment of hypoprothrombinemia secondary to factors limiting absorption or synthesis of vitamin K$_1$.

MONITORING: Check prothrombin time when treating clotting abnormalities. (A minimum of 2 to 4 hours is needed for measurable improvement.)

ADVERSE EFFECTS/PRECAUTIONS: Severe reactions, including death, have been reported with IV administration in adults. These reactions are extremely rare, and have resembled anaphylaxis and included shock and cardiac/respiratory arrest. **With IV administration, give very slowly, not exceeding 1 mg per minute, with physician present.** Pain and swelling may occur at IM injection site. Efficacy of treatment with vitamin K$_1$ is decreased in patients with liver disease. The risk of childhood cancer is not increased by IM administration of vitamin K$_1$. **Note:** A box warning statement in the AquaMEPHYTON® product information states that intramuscular administration "should be restricted to those situations where the subcutaneous route is not feasible and the serious risk is considered justified". However, this does not apply to newborns, and the American Academy of Pediatrics recommends the single intramuscular dose at birth as above. The product information labeling reflects this recommended newborn dosing.

PHARMACOLOGY: Vitamin K$_1$ (phytonadione) promotes formation of the following clotting factors in the liver: active prothrombin (factor II), proconvertin (factor VII), plasma thromboplastin component (factor IX), and Stuart factor (factor X). Vitamin K$_1$ does **not** counteract the anticoagulant action of heparin.

SPECIAL CONSIDERATIONS/PREPARATION: Available as a 2 mg/mL aqueous dispersion in 0.5-mL ampules and 10 mg/mL aqueous dispersion in 1-mL ampules and 2.5- and 5-mL vials. Contains 0.9% (9 mg/mL) benzyl alcohol as a preservative. *** **Efficacy with giving this preparation orally is uncertain.** *** Protect from light.

Solution Compatibility: D$_5$W, D$_{10}$W, and NS.

Terminal Injection Site Compatibility: Dex/AA. Amikacin, ampicillin, dobutamine, chloramphenicol, cimetidine, epinephrine, famotidine, heparin, hydrocortisone succinate, netilmicin, potassium chloride, ranitidine, and sodium bicarbonate.

Incompatibility: Phenytoin.

SELECTED REFERENCES

- American Academy of Pediatrics Committee on Nutrition: Vitamins. In: *Pediatric Nutrition Handbook*. 5th ed. Elk Grove Village, Il: American Academy of Pediatrics 2004: pp 350-51.
- Costakos DT, Greer FR, Love LA, et al: Vitamin K prophylaxis for premature infants: 1 mg versus 0.5 mg. *Am J Perinatol* 2003;20:485-90.
- American Academy of Pediatrics, Committee on Fetus and Newborn: Controversies concerning vitamin K and the newborn. *Pediatrics* 2003;112:191-92.
- Kumar D, Greer FR, Super DM, et al: Vitamin K status of premature infants: implications for current recommendations. *Pediatrics* 2001;108:1117-1122.
- Fiore LD, Scola MA, Cantillon CE, Brophy MT: Anaphylactoid reactions to Vitamin K. *J Thromb Thrombolysis* 2001;11:175-188.
- Zipursky AL: Prevention of vitamin K deficiency bleeding in newborns. *Br J Haematol* 1999;104:430-437.
- Greer FR: Vitamin K deficiency and hemorrhage in infancy. *Clin Perinatol* 1995;22:759.
- Greer FR, Marshall SP, Foley AL, Suttie JW: Improving the vitamin K status of breastfeeding infants with maternal vitamin K supplements. *Pediatrics* 1997;99:88.
- Product information, Merck & Co, Inc, 2004.

ZIDOVUDINE (ZDV, AZT)

DOSE & ADMINISTRATION: IV: 1.5 mg/kg per dose, given via infusion pump over 1 hour. **PO:** 2 mg/kg per dose. **Do not administer IM.** May administer with food, although manufacturer recommends administration 30 minutes before or 1 hour after a meal. To use dosing chart, please refer to explanatory note in "How to Use This Book."

DOSING INTERVAL CHART

Gestational Age (weeks)	Postnatal Age (days)	Interval (hours)
≤29	0 to 28	12
	>28	8
30 to 34	0 to 14	12
	>14	8
≥35	ALL	6

Begin treatment within 6 to 12 hours of birth, and continue for 6 weeks. Initiation of post-exposure prophylaxis after the age of 2 days is not likely to be effective. Subsequent treatment is based on HIV culture results.

USES: Dosing guidelines above are for prophylactic treatment of neonates born to HIV-infected women. Treatment of infected infants using drug combination regimens should be done in consultation with pediatric infectious disease experts.

MONITORING: CBC at the beginning of therapy, then every other week to assess for anemia, thrombocytopenia, and neutropenia.

ADVERSE EFFECTS/PRECAUTIONS: Anemia and neutropenia occur frequently, and are associated with serum concentrations greater than 3 micromol/L. Mild cases usually respond to a reduction in dose. Severe cases may require cessation of treatment and/or transfusion. Bone marrow toxicity may be increased by concomitant administration of acyclovir, ganciclovir, and TMP-SMX. Lactic acidemia is common in infants exposed to in utero highly active antiretroviral therapy. Concomitant treatment with fluconazole or methadone significantly reduces zidovudine metabolism - dosing interval should be prolonged.

PHARMACOLOGY: Zidovudine is a nucleoside analog that inhibits HIV replication by interfering with viral reverse transcriptase. It is converted intracellularly in several steps to a triphosphate derivative, metabolized via hepatic glucuronidation, then renally excreted. Protein binding is approximately 25%. Zidovudine distributes into cells by passive diffusion and is relatively lipophilic. The CSF: plasma ratio is 0.24. The relationship between serum concentration and clinical efficacy is unclear. The oral syrup is well-absorbed, but only 65% bioavailable due to significant first-pass metabolism. The serum half-life in term newborns is 3 hours, declining to 2 hours after 2 weeks of age. In preterm infants less than 33 weeks gestation, half-life during the first two weeks of life ranges from 5 to 10 hours, decreasing to 2 to 6 hours afterward.

SPECIAL CONSIDERATIONS/PREPARATION: Available as a syrup for oral use in a concentration of 10 mg/mL. The IV form is supplied in a concentration of 10 mg/mL in a 20 mL single-use vial. **Dilute before IV administration to a concentration not exceeding 4**

ZIDOVUDINE (ZDV, AZT)

mg/mL. A dilution of 4 mg/mL may be prepared by adding 4 mL of the 10-mg/mL concentration to 6 mL D_5W. After dilution the drug is stable at room temperature for 24 hours. Both forms should be stored at room temperature and protected from light.

Solution Compatibility: D_5W and NS.

Terminal Injection Site Compatibility: Dex/AA solutions, fat emulsion. Acyclovir, amikacin, amphotericin B, aztreonam, cefepime, ceftazidime, ceftriaxone, cimetidine, clindamycin, dexamethasone, dobutamine, dopamine, erythromycin lactobionate, fluconazole, gentamicin, heparin, imipenem, linezolid, lorazepam, meropenem, metoclopramide, morphine, nafcillin, oxacillin, piperacillin, piperacillin-tazobactam, potassium chloride, ranitidine, remifentanil, tobramycin, trimethoprim-sulfamethoxazole, and vancomycin.

Incompatibility: Blood products and protein solutions.

SELECTED REFERENCES

- American Academy of Pediatrics. Human Immunodeficiency Virus Infection. In: Pickering LK, Baker CJ, Long SS, McMillan JA, eds. *Red Book: 2006 Report of the Committee on Infectious Diseases.* 27th ed. Elk Grove Village, IL: American Academy of Pediatrics; 2006: pp 393-394.
- Perinatal HIV Guidelines Working Group. Public Health Service Task Force Recommendations for Use of Antiretroviral Drugs in Pregnant HIV-1 Infected Women for Maternal Health and Interventions to Reduce Perinatal HIV-1 Transmission in the United States. October 12, 2006. Available at http://aidsinfo.nih.gov/ContentFiles/PerinatalGL.pdf.
- Capparelli EV, Mirochnick MH, Danker WM: Pharmacokinetics and tolerance of zidovudine in preterm infants. *J Pediatr* 2003;142:47-52.
- Alimenti A, Burdge DR, Ogilvie GS, et al: Lactic acidemia in human immunodeficiency virus-uninfected infants exposed to antiretroviral therapy. *Pediatr Infect Dis J* 2003;22:782-8.
- Mirochnick MH, Capparelli EV, Conner J: Pharmacokinetics of zidovudine in infants: A population analysis across studies. *Clin Pharmacol Ther* 1999;66:16-24.
- Acosta EP, Page LM, Fletcher CV: Clinical pharmacokinetics of zidovudine. *Drugs* 1996;30:251.
- Conner EM, Sperling RS, Gelber R, et al: Reduction of maternal-infant transmission of human immunodeficiency virus type 1 with zidovudine treatment. *N Engl J Med* 1994;331:1173.
- Boucher FD, Modlin JF, Weller S: Phase I evaluation of zidovudine administered to infants exposed at birth to the human immunodeficiency virus. *J Pediatr* 1993;122:137.
- Product Information, GlaxoSmithKline, 2003.

Appendix: Reference Tables

ABBREVIATIONS, MEASUREMENTS AND CALCULATIONS
Abbreviations, Acronyms and Symbols A1
Calculations and Formulas A7

DRUG INFORMATION AND POISON CONTROL
Drug Information Centers A15
Poison Antidote Chart A23
Poison Control Centers A29

OTC DRUG COMPARISON CHARTS

Dermatology
Acne Products A35
Antiseborrheal Products A39
Contact Dermatitis Products A43
Dandruff Products A45
Diaper Rash Products A47
Dry Skin Products A49
Psoriasis Products A57
Wound Care Products A59

Gastrointestinal
Antacid and Heartburn Products A61
Antidiarrheal Products A65
Antiflatulant Products A67
Laxative Products A69

Respiratory
Allergic Rhinitis Products A73
Is it a Cold, Flu, or an Allergy? A77
Cough-Cold-Flu Products A78
Nasal Decongestant/Moisturizing Products .A91

Miscellaneous
Analgesic Products A93
Antipyretic Products A99

RX DRUG COMPARISON CHARTS
Acne Management: Topical Therapies A103
Acne Management: Systemic Therapies ...A105
Antibiotic Sensitivity Chart
  Aminoglycosides A106
  Carbapenems/Monobactams A110
  Cephalosporins A114
  Fluoroquinolones A119
  Macrolides and Clindamycin A123
  Penicillins A127
  Sulfonamides A131
  Tetracyclines A131
  Miscellaneous A135
Antibiotics: Oral A139
Antibiotics: Neonatal Recommended
  Concentrations for Administration A141
Antibiotics: Systemic A142
Asthma Management A177
Asthma Treatment Plan A179
HIV/AIDS Pharmacotherapy A181
Insulin Formulations A185
Oral Contraceptives A187
Topical Corticosteroids A189

IMMUNIZATION CHARTS
Recommended Immunization Schedule
  for Persons Aged 0-6 Years A191
Recommended Immunization Schedule
  for Persons Aged 7-18 Years A193
Catch-up Immunization Schedule for
  Persons Aged 4 Months–18 Years Who
  Start Late or Who Are More Than
  1 Month Behind A195
Recommended Adult Immunization
  Schedule, by Vaccine and Age Group ...A197
Recommended Adult Immunization
  Schedule, by Vaccine and Medical
  and Other Indications A201

MISCELLANEOUS
Drugs Excreted in Breast Milk A205
Use-in-Pregnancy Ratings A207
Vitamin Comparison Table A214

CDC GROWTH CHARTS
Boys Length-for-age and
  Weight-for-age, Birth to 36 months
  (5th-95th percentile) A219
Boys Head Circumference-for-age and
  Weight-for-length, Birth to 36 months
  (5th-95th percentile) A221
Girls Length-for-age and
  Weight-for-age, Birth to 36 months
  (5th-95th percentile) A223
Girls Head Circumference-for-age and
  Weight-for-length, Birth to 36 months
  (5th-95th percentile) A225
Boys Stature-for-age and
  Weight-for-age, Children 2 to 20 years
  (5th-95th percentile) A227
Boys BMI-for-age, Children 2 to 20 years
  (5th-95th percentile) A229
Girls Stature-for-age and Weight-for-age,
  Children 2 to 20 years
  (5th-95th percentile) A231
Girls BMI-for-age, Children 2 to 20 years
  (5th-95th percentile) A233
Boys Weight-for-stature,
  (5th-95th percentile) A235
Girls Weight-for-stature,
  (5th-95th percentile) A237
Boys Length-for-age and Weight-for-age,
  Birth to 36 months
  (3rd-97th percentile) A239

Boys Head Circumference-for-age and Weight-for-length, Birth to 36 months (3rd-97th percentile) A241
Girls Length-for-age and Weight-for-age, Birth to 36 months (3rd-97th percentile) A243
Girls Head Circumference-for-age and Weight-for-length, Birth to 36 months (3rd-97th percentile) A245
Boys Stature-for-age and Weight-for-age, Children 2 to 20 years (3rd-97th percentile) A247
Boys BMI-for-age, Children 2 to 20 years (3rd-97th percentile) A249
Girls Stature-for-age and Weight-for-age, Children 2 to 20 years (3rd-97th percentile) A251
Girls BMI-for-age, Children 2 to 20 years (3rd-97th percentile) A253
Boys Weight-for-stature (3rd-97th percentile) A255
Girls Weight-for-stature (3rd-97th percentile) A257

ABBREVIATIONS, ACRONYMS AND SYMBOLS

ABBREVIATIONS	DESCRIPTIONS
- (eg, 6-8)	to (eg, 6 to 8)
/	per
<	less than
>	greater than
≤	less than or equal to
≥	greater than or equal to
5-FU	5-fluorouracil
5-HT	5-hydroxytryptamine (serotonin)
ABECB	acute bacterial exacerbation of chronic bronchitis
aa	of each
ACTH	adrenocorticotrophic hormone
ad	right ear
ADHD	attention-deficit/hyperactivity disorder
A-fib	atrial fibrillation
A-flutter	atrial flutter
AIDS	acquired immunodeficiency syndrome
ALT	alanine transaminase (SGPT)
am	morning
AMI	acute myocardial infarction
AMP	adenosine monophosphate
ANA	antinuclear antibodies
ANC	absolute neutrophil count
APAP	acetaminophen
APTT	activated partial thromboplastin time
as	left ear
ASA	aspirin
AST	aspartate transaminase (SGOT)
ATP	adenosine triphosphate
ATPase	adenosine triphophatase
au	each ear
AUC	area under the curve
AV	atrioventricular
bid	twice daily
BMI	body mass index
BP	blood pressure
BPD	bronchopulmonary dysplasia
BPH	benign prostatic hypertrophy
bpm	beats per minute
BSA	body surface area
BUN	blood urea nitrogen
CABG	coronary artery bypass graft
CAD	coronary artery disease
Cap	capsule
CAP	community-acquired pneumonia
CBC	complete blood count
CF	cystic fibrosis
CHF	congestive heart failure
cm	centimeter
CMV	cytomegalovirus
C_{max}	maximum (peak) concentration
CNS	central nervous system

(Continued)

ABBREVIATIONS, ACRONYMS AND SYMBOLS

ABBREVIATIONS	DESCRIPTIONS
COPD	chronic obstructive pulmonary disease
CrCl	creatinine clearance
CRF	chronic renal failure
CSF	cerebrospinal fluid
CVA	cerebrovascular accident
CVD	cardiovascular disease
CYP450	cytochrome P450
D_5NS	5% dextrose in normal saline solution
D_5W	5% dextrose in water solution
$D_{10}W$	10% dextrose in water solution
$D_{15}W$	15% dextrose in water solution
$D_{20}W$	20% dextrose in water solution
d/c	discontinue
DIC	disseminated intravascular coagulation
DM	diabetes mellitus
DNA	deoxyribonucleic acid
DPPC	dipalmitoyl phosphatidylcholine
DT	diphtheria, tetanus (vaccine)
DTP	diphtheria, tetanus, pertussis (vaccine)
DVT	deep vein thrombosis
ECG	electrocardiogram
EEG	electroencephalogram
EKG	electrocardiogram
eg	for example
EPS	extrapyramidal symptom
ESRD	end-stage renal disease
ET	endotracheal
FiO_2	fractional inspired oxygen concentration
FRC	functional residual capacity
g	gram
GABA	gamma-aminobutyric acid
GAD	general anxiety disorder
GCSF	granulocyte colony stimulating factor
GE	gastroesophageal
GERD	gastroesophageal reflux disease
GFR	glomerular filtration rate
GI	gastrointestinal
GVHD	graft versus host disease
HBeAg	hepatitis B e antigen
HBIG	hepatitis B immune globulin
HBsAg	hepatitis B surface antigen
HCG	human chorionic gonadotropin
Hct	hematocrit
HCTZ	hydrochlorothiazide
HDL	high density lipoprotein
Hgb	hemoglobin
Hib	Haemophilus influenzae b
HIV	human immunodeficiency virus
HMG-CoA	3-hydroxy-3-methylglutaryl-coenzyme A
HR	heart rate
hr or hrs	hour or hours
hs	bedtime
HSV	herpes simplex virus
HTN	hypertension

(Continued)

ABBREVIATIONS, ACRONYMS AND SYMBOLS

ABBREVIATIONS	DESCRIPTIONS
IBD	inflammatory bowel disease
IBS	irritable bowel syndrome
IC	intracardiac
ICH	intracranial hemorrhage
IgG	immunoglobulin G
IM	intramuscular
INH	isoniazid
Inj	injection
IOP	intraocular pressure
IU	international unit
IV	intravenous/intravenously
IVH	intraventricular hemorrhage
IVIG	intravenous immune globulin (human)
K^+	potassium
kg	kilogram
KIU	kallikrein inhibitor unit
L	liter
lbs	pounds
LD	loading dose
LDL	low density lipoprotein
Lf	potency of a given weight of an internationally accepted standard
LFT	liver function test
Lot	lotion
Loz	lozenge
LR	lactated Ringer's solution
LVH	left ventricular hypertrophy
M	molar
MAC	mycobacterium avium complex
Maint	maintenance
MAOI	monoamine oxidase inhibitor
Max	maximum
mcg	microgram
mEq	milli-equivalent
mg	milligram
MI	myocardial infarction
min	minute (usually as mL/min)
mL	milliliter
mm	millimeter
mM	millimolar
MRI	magnetic resonance imaging
MS	multiple sclerosis
msec	millisecond
MTX	methotrexate
Na^+	sodium
NaCl	sodium chloride
NG	nasogastric
NKA	no known allergies
NMS	neuroleptic malignant syndrome
npo	nothing by mouth
NS	normal saline solution (0.9% sodium chloride)
NSAID	nonsteroidal anti-inflammatory drug
NV	nausea and vomiting

(Continued)

ABBREVIATIONS, ACRONYMS AND SYMBOLS

ABBREVIATIONS	DESCRIPTIONS
OA	osteoarthritis
OCD	obsessive-compulsive disorder
od	right eye
Oint	ointment
OPV	oral polio vaccine
os	left eye
ou	each eye
PAT	paroxysmal atrial tachycardia
pc	after meals
PCO_2	partial pressure of carbon dioxide in the blood
PD	Parkinson's disease
PDA	patent ductus arteriosus
PID	pelvic inflammatory disease
pm	evening
PMA	postmenstrual age
PO_2	partial pressure of oxygen in the blood
po	orally
PONV	postoperative nausea and vomiting
ppm	parts per million
pr	rectally
prn	as needed
PSA	prostate-specific antigen
PSVT	paroxysmal supraventricular tachycardia
pta	prior to admission
PT/INR	prothrombin time/international normalized ratio
PTSD	post-traumatic stress disorder
PTT	partial thromboplastin time
PTU	propylthiouracil
PUD	peptic ulcer disease
PVD	peripheral vascular disease
q4h, q6h, q8h…	every four hours, every six hours, every eight hours…
qd	once daily
qh	every hour
qid	four times daily
qod	every other day
qs	a sufficient quantity
qs ad	a sufficient quantity up to
RA	rheumatoid arthritis
RBC	red blood cells
RDIs	reference daily intakes
RDS	respiratory distress syndrome
REM	rapid eye movement
RNA	ribonucleic acid
ROP	retinopathy of prematurity
SA	sinoatrial node
SAH	subarachnoid hemorrhage
SBP	systolic blood pressure
SGA	small for gestational age
SGOT	serum glutamic-oxaloacetic transaminase (AST)

(Continued)

Abbreviations, Acronyms and Symbols

ABBREVIATIONS	DESCRIPTIONS
SGPT	serum glutamic-pyruvic transaminase (ALT)
SIADH	syndrome of inappropriate antidiuretic hormone secretion
SLE	systemic lupus erythematosus
SOB	shortness of breath
Sol	solution
SQ	subcutaneous
SrCr	serum creatinine
SSRI	selective serotonin reuptake inhibitor
SSSI	skin and skin structure infection
STD	sexually transmitted disease
subQ	subcutaneously
Sup	suppository
Sus	suspension
SVT	supraventricular tachycardia
^{99}Tc-IDA	technetium 99m-image display and analysis
$t_{1/2}$	half-life
Tab	tablet
Tab, SL	sublingual tablet
TB	tuberculosis
TBG	thyroxine binding globulin
tbl	tablespoon
TCA	tricyclic antidepressant
TD	tardive dyskinesia
TFT	thyroid function test
TG	triglyceride
tid	three times daily
T_{max}	time to maximum concentration
TNF	tumor necrosis factor
TPN	total parenteral nutrition
TSH	thyroid stimulating hormone
tsp	teaspoonful
TTP	thrombotic thrombocytopenic purpura
U	unit
UAC	umbilical artery catheter
ud	as directed
ULN	upper limit of normal
URI	upper respiratory infection
UTI	urinary tract infection
UV	ultraviolet
WBC	white blood cell count
Vd	volume of distribution
VLBW	very low birth weight
VTE	venous thromboembolism
X	times (eg, >2X ULN)
yr or yrs	year or years

Calculations and Formulas

WEIGHTS AND MEASURES

METRIC MEASURES

1 kilogram (kg)	1000 g
1 gram (g)	1000 mg
1 milligram (mg)	0.001 g
1 microgram (mcg or μg)	0.001 mg; 1×10^{-6} g
1 liter (L)	1000 mL
1 milliliter (mL)	0.001 L; 1 cc (cubic centimeter)

APOTHECARY MEASURES (AP)

1 scruple	20 grains (gr)
1 drachm	3 scruples; 60 gr
1 ounce (oz)	8 drachms; 24 scruples; 480 gr
1 pound (lb)	12 oz; 96 drachms; 288 scruples; 5760 gr

U.S. FLUID MEASURES

1 fluidrachm	60 minim
1 fluidounce	8 fluidrachm; 480 minim
1 pint (pt)	16 fl oz; 7680 minim
1 quart (qt)	2 pt; 32 fl oz
1 gallon (gal)	4 qt; 128 fl oz

AVOIRDUPOIS WEIGHT (AV)

1 ounce	437.5 gr
1 pound	16 oz

CONVERSION FACTORS

1 gram	15.4 gr
1 grain	64.8 mg
1 ounce (Av)	28.35 g; 437.5 gr
1 ounce (Ap)	31.1 g; 480 gr
1 pound (Av)	453.6 g; 2.68 lb (Ap); 2.20 lb (Av)
1 fluidounce	29.57 mL
1 fluidrachm	3.697 mL
1 minim	0.06 mL

COMMON MEASURES

1 teaspoonful	5 mL; 1/6 fl oz
1 tablespoonful	15 mL; 1/2 fl oz
1 wineglassful	60 mL; 2 fl oz
1 teacupful	120 mL; 4 fl oz
1 gallon	3800 mL; 128 fl oz
1 quart	960 mL; 32 fl oz
1 pint	480 mL; 16 fl oz (exactly 473.2 mL)
8 fluid ounces	240 mL
4 fluid ounces	120 mL
2.2 lb	1 kg

DOSE EQUIVALENTS

WEIGHT (METRIC)	WEIGHT (APOTHECARY)
30 g	1 ounce
15 g	4 drams
10 g	2 1/2 drams
7.5 g	2 drams
6 g	90 grains
5 g	75 grains
4 g	60 grains; 1 dram
3 g	45 grains
2 g	30 grains; 1/2 dram
1.5 g	22 grains
1 g	15 grains
750 mg	12 grains
600 mg	10 grains
500 mg	7 1/2 grains
400 mg	6 grains
300 mg	5 grains
250 mg	4 grains

(Continued)

CALCULATIONS AND FORMULAS

DOSE EQUIVALENTS (Continued)

WEIGHT (METRIC)	WEIGHT (APOTHECARY)
200 mg	3 grains
150 mg	2 1/2 grains
125 mg	2 grains
100 mg	1 1/2 grains
75 mg	1 1/4 grains
60 mg	1 grain
50 mg	3/4 grain
40 mg	2/3 grain
30 mg	3/8 grain
25 mg	3/8 grain
20 mg	1/3 grain
15 mg	1/6 grain
12 mg	1/5 grain
10 mg	1/6 grain
8 mg	1/8 grain
6 mg	1/10 grain
5 mg	1/12 grain
4 mg	1/15 grain
3 mg	1/20 grain
2 mg	1/30 grain
1.5 mg	1/40 grain
1.2 mg	1/50 grain
1 mg	1/60 grain

LIQUID MEASURES (METRIC)	LIQUID MEASURES (APOTHECARY)
1000 mL	1 quart
750 mL	1 1/2 pints
500 mL	1 pint
230 mL	8 fluid ounces
200 mL	7 fluid ounces
100 mL	3 1/2 fluid ounces
50 mL	1 3/4 fluid ounces
30 mL	1 fluid ounces
15 mL	4 fluid drams
10 mL	2 1/2 fluid drams
8 mL	2 fluid drams
5 mL	1 1/4 fluid drams
4 mL	1 fluid dram
3 mL	45 minims
2 mL	30 minims
1 mL	15 minims
0.75 mL	12 minims
0.6 mL	10 minims
0.5 mL	8 minims
0.3 mL	5 minims
0.25 mL	4 minims
0.2 mL	3 minims
0.1 mL	1 1/2 minims
0.06 mL	1 minim
0.05 mL	3/4 minim
0.03 mL	1/2 minim

MILLIEQUIVALENT (mEq) AND MILLIMOLE (mmol)

CALCULATIONS

$$\text{moles} = \frac{\text{weight of a substance (grams)}}{\text{molecular weight of that substance (grams)}} \quad \text{OR} \quad = \frac{\text{equivalent}}{\text{valence of ion}}$$

$$\text{millimoles} = \frac{\text{weight of a substance (milligrams)}}{\text{molecular weight of that substance (milligrams)}} \quad \text{OR} \quad = \frac{\text{milliequivalents}}{\text{valence of ion}} \quad \text{OR} \quad = \text{moles} \times 1000$$

equivalents = moles x valence of ion

milliequivalents = millimoles x valence of ion   OR   = equivalents x 1000

(Continued)

CALCULATIONS AND FORMULAS

CONVERSIONS

mg/100mL to mEq/L	mEq/L = $\dfrac{(mg/100mL) \times 10 \times valence}{atomic\ weight}$
mEq/L to mg/100mL	mg/100mL = $\dfrac{(mEq/L) \times atomic\ weight}{10 \times valence}$
mEq/L to volume percent of a gas	volume % = $\dfrac{(mEq/L) \times 22.4}{10}$

ACID-BASE ASSESSMENT

DEFINITIONS

PIO_2	Oxygen partial pressure of inspired gas (mmHg); 150 mmHg in room air at sea level
FiO_2	Fractional pressure of oxygen in inspired gas (0.21 in room air)
PAO_2	Alveolar oxygen partial pressure
$PACO_2$	Alveolar carbon dioxide partial pressure
PaO_2	Arterial oxygen partial pressure
$PaCO_2$	Arterial carbon dioxide partial pressure
R	Respiratory exchange quotient (typically 0.8, increases with high carbohydrate diet, decreases with high fat diet)

HENDERSON-HASSELBALCH EQUATION

pH = 6.1 + log [HCO_3^- / (0.03) (pCO_2)]

ALVEOLAR GAS EQUATION

PIO_2 = FiO_2 × (total atmospheric pressure - vapor pressure of H_2O at 37°C)
  = FiO_2 × (760 mmHg - 47 mmHg)

PaO_2 = PIO_2 - $PaCO_2$/R

ALVEOLAR/ARTERIAL OXYGEN GRADIENT

PAO_2 - PaO_2

ACID-BASE DISORDERS

Disorder	pH	HCO_3^-	PCO_2	Compensation
Metabolic acidosis	< 7.35	Primary decrease	Compensatory decrease	1.2-mmHg decrease in PCO_2 for every 1-mmol/L decrease in HCO_3^- **or** PCO_2 = (1.5 × HCO_3^-) + 8 (± 2) **or** PCO_2 = HCO_3^- + 15 **or** PCO_2 = last 2 digits of pH × 100
Metabolic alkalosis	> 7.45	Primary increase	Compensatory increase	0.6-0.75 mmHg increase in PCO_2 for every 1-mmol/L increase in HCO_3^-. PCO_2 should not rise above 60 mm Hg in compensation.
Respiratory acidosis	< 7.35	Compensatory increase	Primary increase	***Acute:*** 1-2 mmol decrease in HCO_3^-. for every 10-mmHg decrease in PCO_2. ***Chronic:*** 3-4 mmol increase in HCO_3^-. for every 10-mmHg increase in PCO_2.
Respiratory alkalosis	> 7.45	Compensatory decrease	Primary decrease	***Acute:*** 1-2 mmol increase in HCO_3^-. for every 10-mmHg increase in PCO_2. ***Chronic:*** 4-5 mmol decrease in HCO_3^-. for every 10-mmHg decrease in PCO_2.

ACID-BASE EQUATION

H^+ (in mEq/L) = (24 × $PaCO_2$) divided by HCO_3^-

(Continued)

CALCULATIONS AND FORMULAS

OTHER CALCULATIONS

ANION GAP

Anion gap = $Na^+ - (Cl^- + HCO_3^-$ measured)

AA GRADIENT

Aa gradient [(713) (FiO_2 - ($PaCO_2$ divided by 0.8))] - PaO_2

OSMOLALITY

Definition:
Osmolality is a measure of the total number of particles in a solution.

U.S. units (sodium as mEq/L, BUN (blood urea nitrogen) and glucose as (mg/dL)
  Plasma osmolality (mOsm/kg) = 2([Na^+] + [K^+]) + ([BUN]/2.8) + ([glucose]/18)
SI units (all variables in mmol/L):
  Plasma osmolality (mOsm/kg) = 2[Na^+] + [urea] + [glucose]
  Normal range plasma omolality: 280 - 303 mOsm/kg

Corrected Sodium
Corrected Na+ = measured Na^+ + [1.5 x (glucose - 150 divided by 100)]*
*Do not correct for glucose <150.

Total Serum Calcium Corrected for Albumin Level
[(Normal albumin - patient's albumin) x 0.8] + patient's measured total calcium

Water Deficit
Water deficit = 0.6 x body weight [1 - (140 divided by Na^+)]*
*Body weight is estimated weight in kg; Na^+ is serum or plasma sodium.

Bicarbonate Deficit
HCO_3^- deficit = [0.4 x weight (kg)] x (HCO_3^- desired - HCO_3^- measured)

CHILD-PUGH SCORE

The Child-Pugh classification used to assess the prognosis of chronic liver disease, mainly cirrhosis. Child-Pugh is also used to determine the required strength of treatment and the necessity of liver transplantation.

Score:
  The score employs five clinical measures of liver disease. Each measure is scored 1-3, with 3 indicating most severe derangement.

Measure	1 point	2 points	3 points	Units
Bilirubin (total)*	<34 (<2)	34-50 (2-3)	>50 (>3)	mol/L (mg/dL)
Serum albumin	>3	528-35	<28	mg/L
INR*	<1.7	1.71-2.20	> 2.20	no unit
Ascites	None	Suppressed with medication	Refractory	no unit
Hepatic encephalopathy	None	Grade I-II (or suppressed with medication)	Grade III-IV (or refractory)	no unit

* In primary sclerosing cholangitis and primary biliary cirrhosis, the bilirubin references are changed to reflect the fact that these diseases feature high conjugated bilirubin levels. The upper limit for 1 point is 68 mol/L (4 mg/dL) and the upper limit for 2 points is 170 mol/L (10 mg/dL).

** Some older reference works substitute PT prolongation for INR.

Interpretation:
  Chronic liver disease is classified into Child-Pugh class A to C, employing the added score from above.

Points	Class	One year survival	Two year survival
5-6	A	100%	85%
7-9	B	81%	57%
10-15	C	45%	35%

CREATININE CLEARANCE

Clinically, creatinine clearance is a useful measure for estimating the glomerular filtration rate (GFR) of the kidneys.

Factors	Abbreviations
Creatinine clearance	Cl_{Cr}
Plasma creatinine concentration	P_{Cr}
Serum creatinine concentration	S_{Cr}
Urine creatinine concentration	U_{Cr}
Urine flow rate	V
Plasma creatinine concentration	P_{Cr}

(Continued)

CREATININE CLEARANCE *(Continued)*

Calculations:

$$Cl_{Cr} = \frac{U_{Cr} \times V}{P_{Cr}}$$

Example:
Patient with P_{Cr} 1 mg/dL, U_{Cr} 60 mg/dL, and V of 0.5 dL/hr.

$$Cl_{Cr} = \frac{60 \text{ mg/dL} \times 0.5 \text{ dL/hr}}{1 \text{ mg/dL}} = 30 \text{ dL/hr}$$

Cockcroft-Gault formula: Estimates creatinine clearance (mL/min).

Male:

$$Cl_{Cr} = \frac{(140 - \text{age}) \times \text{mass (kg)}}{72 \times S_{Cr} \text{ (mg/dL)}}$$

Example:
Male patient, 67 years of age, weight 75 kg, and S_{Cr} 1 mg/dL.

$$Cl_{Cr} = \frac{(140 - 67) \times 75}{72 \times 1} = 76 \text{ mL/min}$$

Female:

$$Cl_{Cr} = \frac{(140 - \text{age}) \times \text{mass (kg)}}{72 \times S_{Cr} \text{ (mg/dL)}} \times 0.85 \text{ if female}$$

Example:
Female patient, 67 years of age, weight 75 kg, and S_{Cr} 1 mg/dL.

$$Cl_{Cr} = \frac{(140 - 67) \times 75}{72 \times 1} \times 0.85 = 64.6 \text{ mL/min}$$

Note: Using actual body weight (ABW) in obese patients can significantly overestimate creatinine clearance. Adjusted ideal body weight (IBW) can provide more approximate estimate. Adjusted IBW = IBW + 0.4 (ABW - IBW).

BASAL ENERGY EXPENDITURE (BEE)

Basal energy expenditure: the amount of energy required to maintain the body's normal metabolic activity (ie, respiration, maintenance of body temperature, etc).

H = height (cm), W = weight (kg), A = age (years)

Male:
BEE = 66.67 + 13.75W + 5H - 6.76A

Female:
BEE = 665.1 + 9.56W + 1.85H - 4.68A

BODY MASS INDEX (BMI)

$$BMI = \frac{\text{weight (kg)}}{[\text{height (m)}]^2}$$

BODY SURFACE AREA (BSA)

$$BSA \text{ (m}^2\text{)} = \sqrt{\frac{\text{height (in)} \times \text{weight (lb)}}{3131}} \quad \text{OR} \quad BSA \text{ (m}^2\text{)} = \sqrt{\frac{\text{height (cm)} \times \text{weight (kg)}}{3600}}$$

IDEAL BODY WEIGHT (IBW)

Adults (18 years and older; IBW is in kg):
IBW (male) = 50 + (2.3 x height [inches] over 5 feet)
IBW (female) = 45.5 + (2.3 x height [inches] over 5 feet)

Children (IBW is in kg; height is in cm):
1-18 years of age:

$$IBW = \frac{\text{height}^2 \times 1.65}{100}$$

5 feet and taller:
IBW (male) = 39 + (2.27 x height [inches] over 5 feet)
IBW (female) = 42.2 + (2.27 x height [inches] over 5 feet)

(Continued)

CALCULATIONS AND FORMULAS

POUNDS/KILOGRAM CONVERSION

1 pound = 0.45359 kilogram | | | | **1 kilogram = 2.2 pounds** | | |

lb	kg	lb	kg	lb	kg	lb	kg
1	0.45	105	47.63	210	95.25	315	142.88
5	2.27	110	49.89	215	97.52	320	145.15
10	4.54	115	52.16	220	99.79	325	147.42
15	6.80	120	54.43	225	102.06	330	149.68
20	9.07	125	56.70	230	104.33	335	151.95
25	11.34	130	58.97	235	106.59	340	154.22
30	13.61	135	61.23	240	108.86	345	156.49
35	15.88	140	63.50	245	111.13	350	158.76
40	18.14	145	65.77	250	113.40	355	161.02
45	20.41	150	68.04	255	115.67	360	163.29
50	22.68	155	70.31	260	117.93	365	165.56
55	24.95	160	72.57	265	120.20	370	167.83
60	27.22	165	74.84	270	122.47	375	170.10
65	29.48	170	77.11	275	124.74	380	172.36
70	31.75	175	79.38	280	127.01	385	174.63
75	34.02	180	81.65	285	129.27	390	176.90
80	36.29	185	83.91	290	131.54	395	179.17
85	38.56	190	86.18	295	133.81	400	181.44
90	40.82	195	88.45	300	136.08	405	183.70
95	43.09	200	90.72	305	138.34	405	183.70
100	45.36	205	92.99	310	140.61	415	188.24

TEMPERATURE CONVERSION

Fahrenheit to Celsius = (°F - 32) x 5/9 = °C | | | | **Celsius to Fahrenheit = (°C x 9/5) + 32 = °F** | | |

°F	°C	°F	°C	°C	°F	°C	°F
0.0	-17.8	92.0	33.3	0.0	32.0	49.0	120.2
5.0	-15.0	93.0	33.9	5.0	41.0	50.0	122.0
10.0	-12.2	94.0	34.4	10.0	50.0	51.0	123.8
15.0	-9.4	95.0	35.0	15.0	59.0	85.0	185.0
20.0	-6.7	96.0	35.6	20.0	68.0	52.0	125.6
25.0	-3.9	97.0	36.1	25.0	77.0	53.0	127.4
30.0	-1.1	98.0	36.7	30.0	86.0	54.0	129.2
35.0	1.7	98.6	37.0	35.0	95.0	55.0	131.0
40.0	4.4	99.0	37.2	36.0	96.8	56.0	132.8
45.0	7.2	100.0	37.8	37.0	98.6	57.0	134.6
50.0	10.0	101.0	38.3	38.0	100.4	58.0	136.4
55.0	12.8	102.0	38.9	39.0	102.2	59.0	138.2
60.0	15.6	103.0	39.4	40.0	104.0	60.0	140.0
65.0	18.3	104.0	40.0	41.0	105.8	65.0	149.0
70.0	21.1	105.0	40.6	42.0	107.6	70.0	158.0
75.0	23.9	106.0	41.1	43.0	109.4	75.0	167.0
80.0	26.7	107.0	41.7	44.0	111.2	80.0	176.0
85.0	29.4	108.0	42.2	45.0	113.0	90.0	194.0
90.0	32.2	109.0	42.8	46.0	114.8	95.0	203.0
91.0	32.8	110.0	43.3	47.0	116.6	100.0	212.0
				48.0	118.4	105.0	221.0

(Continued)

PEDIATRIC DOSAGE ESTIMATION FORMULAS

The following formulas can be used to estimate the approximate pediatric dosage of a medication. These formulas are based on the adult dose and either the child's age or weight. These formulas should be used with caution as the response to any drug is not always directly proportional to the age or weight of the child relative to the usual adult dose. Dosage will also vary based on the formula used. Care should be taken when using any of these methods to calculate the child's dosage. Some products have FDA approved pediatric indications and dosages, always refer to full prescribing information first before calculating a pediatric dosage.

BASED ON WEIGHT

Augsberger's Rule:

$[(1.5 \times \text{weight [kg]}) + 10] / 100 \times \text{adult dose} = \text{approximate child's dose}$

Example: If the child's weight is 15 kg (33 lb) and the adult dose is 50 mg then the child's dose is 16.25 mg.
$[(1.5 \times 15 \text{ kg}) + 10] / 100 \times 50 \text{ mg} = 0.325 \times 50 \text{ mg} = 16.25 \text{ mg}$

Clark's Rule:

(weight [lb]/150) × adult dose = approximate child's dose

Example: If the child's weight is 15 kg (33 lb) and the adult dose is 50 mg then the child's dose is 11 mg.
(33/150) × 50 mg = 0.22 × 50 mg = 11 mg

Based on Age

Augsberger's Rule:

$[(4 \times \text{age [years]}) + 20] / 100 \times \text{adult dose} = \text{approximate child's dose}$

Example: If the child's age is 8 years and the adult dose is 50 mg then the child's dose is 26 mg.
$[(4 \times 8) + 20)/100] \times 50 \text{ mg} = 0.52 \times 50 \text{ mg} = 26 \text{ mg}$

Dilling's Rule:

(age [years]/20) × adult dose = approximate child's dose

Example: If the child's age is 8 years and the adult dose is 50 mg then the child's dose is 20 mg.
(8/20) × 50 mg = 0.40 × 50 mg = 20 mg

Cowling's Rule:

[age at next birthday (years)] / 24 × adult dose = approximate child's dose

Example: If the child is going to turn 8 years old in few months and the adult dose is 50 mg then the child's dose is 16.7 mg. (8/24) × 50 mg = 0.33 × 50 mg = 16.7 mg

Younge's Rule:

[age (years)] / (age + 12) × adult dose = approximate child's dose

Example: If the child's age is 8 years and the adult dose is 50 mg then the child's dose is 20 mg.
[8/(8+12)] × 50 mg = 0.4 × 50 mg = 20 mg

Fried's Rule (younger than 1 year):

[age (months)] / 150 × adult dose = approximate infant's dose

Example: If the child's age is 10 months and the adult dose is 50 mg then the child's dose is 3.33 mg.
(10/150) × 50 mg = 0.067 × 50 mg = 3.33 mg

Drug Information Centers

ALABAMA

BIRMINGHAM

Drug Information Service
University of Alabama
UAB Hospital Pharmacy

Drug Information-JT1720
619 S. 19th St.
Birmingham, AL 35249-6860
Mon.-Fri. 8 AM-5 PM
 205-934-2162
www.health.uab.edu/pharmacy

**Global Drug
Information Service
Samford University
McWhorter School
of Pharmacy**

800 Lakeshore Dr.
Birmingham, AL 35229-7027
Mon.-Wed. 8 AM-9 PM
Thurs.-Fri. 8 AM-4:30 PM
 205-726-2519 or 2891
www.samford.edu/schools/
pharmacy/dic/index.html

HUNTSVILLE

Huntsville Hospital Drug Information Center

101 Sivley Rd.
Huntsville, AL 35801
Mon.-Fri. 7 AM-3:30 PM
 256-265-8284

ARIZONA

TUCSON

**Arizona Poison and Drug
Information Center
Arizona Health
Sciences Center
University Medical Center**

1501 N. Campbell Ave.
Room 1156
Tucson, AZ 85724
7 days/week, 24 hours
 520-626-6016
 800-222-1222 **(Emergency)**
www.pharmacy.arizona.edu

ARKANSAS

LITTLE ROCK

Arkansas Drug Information Center

4301 W. Markham St.
Slot 522-2
Little Rock, AR 72205
Mon.-Fri. 8:30 AM-5 PM
 501-686-5072
 (Little Rock area only - **for healthcare professionals only**)
 800-228-1233
 (AR only - **for healthcare professionals only**)

CALIFORNIA

LOS ANGELES

**Los Angeles Regional
Drug Information Center
LAC & USC Medical Center**

1200 N. State St.
Trailer 25
Los Angeles, CA 90033
Mon.-Fri. 8 AM-4 PM
Closed 12 PM to 1 PM
 323-226-7741

SAN DIEGO

**Drug Information Service
University of California
San Diego Medical Center**

200 West Arbor Dr.
MC 8925
San Diego, CA 92103-8925
Mon.-Fri. 9 AM-5 PM
 619-543-6971
 (for healthcare professionals only)

SAN FRANCISCO

**Drug Information Analysis Service
University of California,
San Francisco**

533 Parnassus Ave.
Room U12
San Francisco, CA 94143-0622
Mon.-Fri. 8:30 AM-4:30 PM
 415-502-9540
 (for healthcare professionals only)

STANFORD

**Drug Information Center
University of California
Stanford Hospital and Clinics**

300 Pasteur Dr.
Room H-0301
Stanford, CA 94305
Mon.-Fri. 8 AM-4 PM
 650-723-6422

COLORADO

DENVER

**Rocky Mountain Poison
and Drug Center**

990 Bannock St.
(Physical address)
777 Bannock St.
(Mailing address)
Denver, CO 80264
 303-739-1123
 800-222-1222 **(Emergency)**
www.rmpdc.org

CONNECTICUT

FARMINGTON

**Drug Information Service
University of Connecticut Health
Center**

263 Farmington Ave.
Farmington, CT 06030
Mon.-Fri. 7:30 AM-4 PM
 860-679-2783

HARTFORD

Drug Information Center Hartford Hospital

P.O. Box 5037
80 Seymour St.
Hartford, CT 06102
Mon.-Fri. 8:30 AM-5 PM
 860-545-2221
 860-545-2961 (After 5 PM)
www.hartfordhospital.org

NEW HAVEN

**Drug Information Center
Yale-New Haven Hospital**

20 York St.
New Haven, CT 06540-3202
Mon.-Fri. 8:30 AM-5 PM
 203-688-2248
www.ynhh.org

DISTRICT OF COLUMBIA

**Drug Information Service
Howard University Hospital**

Room BB06
2041 Georgia Ave. NW
Washington, DC 20060
Mon.-Fri. 8:30 AM-4 PM
 202-865-1325
 800-222-1222 **(Emergency)**
www.huhosp.org/patientpublic/
pharmacy.htm

FLORIDA

FT. LAUDERDALE

**Nova Southeastern University
College of Pharmacy
Drug Information Center**

3200 S. University Dr.
Ft. Lauderdale, FL 33328
Mon.-Fri. 9 AM-5 PM
 954-262-3103
http://pharmacy.nova.edu

Drug Information Centers

GAINESVILLE

Drug Information & Pharmacy Resource Center Shands Hospital at University of Florida

P.O. Box 100316
Gainesville, FL 32610-0316
Mon.-Fri. 9 AM-5 PM
352-265-0408
(for healthcare professionals only)
http://shands.org/professional/drugs

JACKSONVILLE

Drug Information Service Shands Jacksonville

655 W. 8th St.
Jacksonville, FL 32209
Mon.-Fri. 8:30 AM-5 PM
904-244-4185
(for healthcare professionals only)
904-244-4700
(for consumers, Mon.-Fri. 9:30 AM-4 PM)

ORLANDO

Orlando Regional Drug Information Service Orlando Regional Healthcare System

1414 Kuhl Ave., MP 192
Orlando, FL 32806
Mon.-Fri. 8 AM-4 PM
321-841-8717

TALLAHASSEE

Drug Information Education Center Florida Agricultural and Mechanical University College of Pharmacy and Pharmaceutical Sciences

Tallahassee, FL 32307
Mon.-Fri. 9 AM-5 PM
850-488-5239

WEST PALM BEACH

Drug Information Center Nova Southeastern University, West Palm Beach

3970 RCA Blvd., Suite 7006A
Palm Beach Gardens, FL 33410
Mon.-Fri. 9 AM-5 PM
561-622-0658
(for healthcare professionals only)

GEORGIA

ATLANTA

Emory University Hospital Dept. of Pharmaceutical Services-Drug Information

1364 Clifton Rd. NE
Atlanta, GA 30322
Mon.-Fri. 8 AM-1 PM
404-712-4644
(for healthcare professionals only)

Drug Information Service Northside Hospital

1000 Johnson Ferry Rd. NE
Atlanta, GA 30342
Mon.-Fri. 9 AM-5 PM
404-851-8676 (GA only)

AUGUSTA

Drug Information Center Medical College of Georgia Hospital and Clinic

BI2101
1120 15th St.
Augusta, GA 30912
Mon.-Fri. 8:30 AM-5 PM
706-721-2887

COLUMBUS

Columbus Regional Drug Information Center

710 Center St.
Columbus, GA 31902
Mon.-Fri. 8 AM-5 PM
706-571-1934
(for healthcare professionals only)

IDAHO

POCATELLO

Drug Information Center Idaho State University School of Pharmacy

970 S. 5th St.
Campus Box 8092
Pocatello, ID 83209
Mon.-Thur. 8:30 AM-5 PM
Fri. 8:30 AM-3 PM
208-282-4689
800-334-7139 (ID only)
http://pharmacy.isu.edu

ILLINOIS

CHICAGO

Drug Information Center Northwestern Memorial Hospital

Feinberg Pavilion, LC 700
251 E. Huron St.
Chicago, IL 60611
Mon.-Fri. 8:30 AM-5 PM
312-926-7573

Drug Information Services University of Chicago Hospitals

5841 S. Maryland Ave.
MC 0010
Chicago, IL 60637-1470
Mon.-Fri. 9 AM-5 PM
773-702-1388

Drug Information Center University of Illinois at Chicago

833 S. Wood St.
MC 886
Chicago, IL 60612-7231
Mon.-Fri. 8 AM-4 PM
312-996-5332
(for healthcare professionals only)
312-996-3682
(for consumers, Mon.-Fri. 9 AM-12 PM)
www.uic.edu/pharmacy/services/di/index.html

HARVEY

Drug Information Center Ingalls Memorial Hospital

1 Ingalls Dr.
Harvey, IL 60426
Mon.-Fri. 8 AM-4:30 PM
708-333-2300

HINES

Drug Information Service Hines Veterans Administration Hospital

2100 S. 5th Ave.
Pharmacy Services
MC119
P.O. Box 5000
Hines, IL 60141-5000
Mon.-Fri. 8 AM-4:30 PM
708-202-8387, ext. 23780

PARK RIDGE

Drug Information Center Advocate Lutheran General Hospital

1775 Dempster St.
Park Ridge, IL 60068
Mon.-Fri. 7:30 AM-4 PM
847-723-8128
(for healthcare professionals only)

DRUG INFORMATION CENTERS

INDIANA

INDIANAPOLIS

**Drug Information Center
St. Vincent Hospital
and Health Services**

2001 W. 86th St.
Indianapolis, IN 46260
Mon.-Fri. 8 AM-4 PM
317-338-3200
(for healthcare
professionals only)

**Drug Information Service
Clarian Health Partners**

Pharmacy Department I-65
at 21st St.
Room CG04
Indianapolis, IN 46202
Mon.-Fri. 8 AM-4:30 PM
317-962-1750

MUNCIE

**Drug Information Center
Ball Memorial Hospital**

2401 University Ave.
Muncie, IN 47303
Mon.-Fri. 8 AM-4:30 PM
765-747-3035

IOWA

DES MOINES

**Regional Drug Information Center
Mercy Medical Center-Des Moines**

1111 Sixth Ave.
Des Moines, IA 50314
Mon.-Fri. 8 AM-4:30 PM
(regional service; in-house
service answered 7 days/week,
24 hours)
515-247-3286

IOWA CITY

**Drug Information Center
University of Iowa
Hospitals and Clinics**

200 Hawkins Dr.
Iowa City, IA 52242
Mon.-Fri. 8 AM-4:30 PM
319-356-2600

KANSAS

KANSAS CITY

**Drug Information Center
University of Kansas
Medical Center**

3901 Rainbow Blvd.
Kansas City, KS 66160
Mon.-Fri. 8:30 AM-4:30 PM
913-588-2328
(for healthcare
professionals only)

KENTUCKY

LEXINGTON

**University of Kentucky
Central Pharmacy
Chandler Medical Center**

800 Rose St., C-114
Lexington, KY 40536-0293
7 days/week, 24 hours
859-323-5642

LOUISIANA

MONROE

**Louisiana Drug and Poison
Information Center
University of Louisiana at Monroe
College of Pharmacy**

Sugar Hall
Monroe, LA 71209-6430
Mon.-Fri. 8 AM-4:30 PM
318-342-1710

NEW ORLEANS

**Xavier University Drug Information
Center Tulane University Hospital
and Clinic**

1440 Canal St.
Suite 808
New Orleans, LA 70112
Mon.-Fri. 9 AM-5 PM
504-588-5670

MARYLAND

ANDREWS AFB

Drug Information Services

79 MDSS/SGQP
1050 W. Perimeter Rd.
Suite D1-119
Andrews AFB, MD 20762-6660
Mon.-Fri. 7:30 AM-5 PM
240-857-4565

BALTIMORE

**Drug Information Service
Johns Hopkins Hospital**

600 N. Wolfe St.
Carnegie 180
Baltimore, MD 21287-6180
Mon.-Fri. 8:30 AM-5 PM
410-955-6348

**Drug Information Service
University of Maryland
School of Pharmacy**

Pharmacy Hall Room 760
20 North Pine St.
Baltimore, MD 21201
Mon.-Fri. 8:30 AM-5 PM
410-706-7568
(for consumers only)
410-706-0898
(for healthcare
professionals only)
www.pharmacy.umaryland.
edu/umdi

EASTON

**Drug Information
Pharmacy Dept.
Memorial Hospital**

219 S. Washington St.
Easton, MD 21601
7 days/week, 7 AM-5:30 PM
410-822-1000, ext. 5645

MASSACHUSETTS

BOSTON

**Drug Information Services
Brigham and Women's Hospital**

75 Francis St.
Boston, MA 02115
Mon.-Fri. 7 AM-3 PM
617-732-7166

WORCESTER

**Drug Information Pharmacy
UMass Memorial
Medical Center
Healthcare Hospital**

55 Lake Ave. North
Worcester, MA 01655
Mon.-Fri. 8:30 AM-5 PM
508-856-3456
508-856-2775 (24-hour)

MICHIGAN

ANN ARBOR

**Drug Information Service Dept. of
Pharmacy Services
University of Michigan
Health System**

1500 East Medical Center Dr.
UH B2D301
Box 0008
Ann Arbor, MI 48109-0008
Mon.-Fri. 8 AM-5 PM
734-936-8200

DETROIT

**Drug Information Center
Department of Pharmacy Services
Detroit Receiving Hospital and
University Health Center**

4201 St. Antoine Blvd.
Detroit, MI 48201
Mon.-Fri. 9 AM-5 PM
313-745-4556
www.dmcpharmacy.org

LANSING

**Drug Information Services
Sparrow Hospital**

1215 East Michigan Ave.
Lansing, MI 48912
7 days/week, 24 hours
517-364-2444

A17

Drug Information Centers

PONTIAC

Drug Information Center
St. Joseph Mercy Oakland

44405 Woodward Ave.
Pontiac, MI 48341
Mon.-Fri. 8 AM-4:30 PM
248-858-3055

ROYAL OAK

Drug Information Services
William Beaumont Hospital

3601 West 13 Mile Rd.
Royal Oak, MI 48073-6769
Mon.-Fri. 8 AM-4:30 PM
248-898-4077

SOUTHFIELD

Drug Information Service
Providence Hospital

16001 West 9 Mile Rd.
Southfield, MI 48075
Mon.-Fri. 8 AM-4 PM
248-849-3125

MISSISSIPPI

JACKSON

Drug Information Center
University of Mississippi Medical Center

2500 N. State St.
Jackson, MS 39216
Mon.-Fri. 8 AM-4:30 PM
601-984-2060

MISSOURI

KANSAS CITY

University of Missouri-Kansas City
Drug Information Center

2411 Holmes St., MG-200
Kansas City, MO 64108
Mon.-Fri. 9 AM-4 PM
816-235-5490
http://druginfo.umkc.edu/

SPRINGFIELD

Drug Information Center
St. John's Hospital

1235 E. Cherokee St.
Springfield, MO 65804
Mon.-Fri. 8 AM-4:30 PM
417-820-3488

ST. JOSEPH

Regional Medical Center Pharmacy

5325 Faraon St.
St. Joseph, MO 64506
7 days/week, 24 hours
816-271-6141

MONTANA

MISSOULA

Drug Information Service
University of Montana School of Pharmacy and Allied Health Sciences

32 Campus Dr.
1522 Skaggs Bldg.
Missoula, MT 59812-1522
Mon.-Fri. 8 AM-5 PM
406-243-5254
800-501-5491
www.umt.edu/druginfo

NEBRASKA

OMAHA

Drug Informatics Service
School of Pharmacy
Creighton University

2500 California Plaza
Health Science Library
Room 204
Omaha, NE 68178
Mon.-Fri. 8:30 AM-4:30 PM
402-280-5101
http://druginfo.creighton.edu

NEW JERSEY

NEWARK

New Jersey Poison Information and Education System

65 Bergen St.
Newark, NJ 07107
Mon.-Fri. 8 AM- 5 PM
973-972-9280
800-222-1222 **(Emergency)**
www.njpies.org

NEW BRUNSWICK

Drug Information Service
Robert Wood Johnson University Hospital

Pharmacy Department
1 Robert Wood Johnson Pl.
New Brunswick, NJ 08901
Mon.-Fri. 8:30 AM-4:30 PM
732-937-8842

NEW MEXICO

ALBUQUERQUE

New Mexico Poison Center
University of New Mexico
Health Sciences Center

MSC09 5080
1 University of New Mexico
Albuquerque, NM 87131
7 days/week, 24 hours
505-272-4261
800-222-1222 **(Emergency)**
http://hsc.unm.edu/pharmacy/poison

NEW YORK

BROOKLYN

International Drug Information Center
Long Island University
Arnold & Marie Schwartz College of Pharmacy &
Health Sciences

75 DeKalb Ave.
RM-HS509
Brooklyn, NY 11201
Mon.-Fri. 9 AM-5 PM
718-488-1064
www.liu.edu

NEW HYDE PARK

Drug Information Center
St. John's University at Long Island Jewish Medical Center

270-05 76th Ave.
New Hyde Park, NY 11040
Mon.-Fri. 8 AM-3 PM
718-470-DRUG (3784)

NEW YORK CITY

Drug Information Center
Memorial Sloan-Kettering Cancer Center

1275 York Ave.
RM S-702
New York, NY 10021
Mon.-Fri. 9 AM-5 PM
212-639-7552

Drug Information Center
Mount Sinai Medical Center

1 Gustave Levy Pl.
New York, NY 10029
Mon.-Fri. 9 AM-5 PM
212-241-6619
(for in-house healthcare professionals only)

Drug Information Service
New York Presbyterian Hospital

Room K04
525 E. 68th St.
New York, NY 10021
Mon.-Fri. 9 AM-5 PM
212-746-0741

ROCHESTER

Finger Lakes Poison and Drug Information Center University of Rochester

601 Elmwood Ave.
Rochester, NY 14642
Mon.-Fri. 8 AM-5 PM
585-275-3718

DRUG INFORMATION CENTERS

ROCKVILLE CENTER

Drug Information Center
Mercy Medical Center

1000 North Village Ave.
Rockville Center, NY 11571-9024
Mon.-Fri. 8 AM-4 PM
    516-705-1053

NORTH CAROLINA

BUIES CREEK

Drug Information Center School of Pharmacy Campbell University

P.O. Box 1090
Buies Creek, NC 27506
Mon.-Fri. 8:30 AM-4:30 PM
    910-893-1200, ext. 2701
    800-760-9697 (Toll free)
        ext. 2701
    800-327-5467 (NC only)

CHAPEL HILL

University of North Carolina Hospitals Drug Information Center Dept. of Pharmacy

101 Manning Dr.
Chapel Hill, NC 27514
Mon.-Fri. 8 AM-4:30 PM
    919-966-2373

DURHAM

Drug Information Center Duke University Health Systems

DUMC Box 3089
Durham, NC 27710
Mon.-Fri. 8 AM-5 PM
    919-684-5125

GREENVILLE

Eastern Carolina Drug Information Center Pitt County Memorial Hospital Dept. of Pharmacy Service

P.O. Box 6028
2100 Stantonsburg Rd.
Greenville, NC 27835
Mon.-Fri. 8 AM-5 PM
    252-847-4257

WINSTON-SALEM

Drug Information Service Center Wake-Forest University Baptist Medical Center

Medical Center Blvd.
Winston-Salem, NC 27157
Mon.-Fri. 8 AM-5 PM
    336-716-2037
    (for healthcare
    professionals only)

OHIO

ADA

Drug Information Center Raabe College of Pharmacy Ohio Northern University

Ada, OH 45810
Mon.-Thurs. 8:30 AM-5 PM,
   7-10 PM
Fri. 8:30 AM- 4 PM;
Sun. 2 PM-10 PM
    419-772-2307
www.onu.edu/pharmacy/druginfo

CINCINNATI

Drug and Poison Information Center Children's Hospital Medical Center

3333 Burnet Ave. VP-3
Cincinnati, OH 45229
Mon.-Fri. 9 AM-5 PM
    513-636-5054
    (Administration)
    513-636-5111
    (7 days/week, 24 hours)

CLEVELAND

Drug Information Service Cleveland Clinic Foundation

9500 Euclid Ave.
Cleveland, OH 44195
Mon.-Fri. 8:30 AM-4:30 PM
    216-444-6456
    (for healthcare
    professionals only)

COLUMBUS

Drug Information Center Ohio State University Hospital Dept. of Pharmacy

Doan Hall 368
410 W. 10th Ave.
Columbus, OH 43210-1228
7 days/week, 24 hours
    614-293-8679
    (for in-house healthcare
    professionals only)

Drug Information Center Riverside Methodist Hospital

3535 Olentangy River Road
Columbus, OH 43214
7 days/week, 24 hours
    614-566-5425

TOLEDO

Drug Information Services St. Vincent Mercy Medical Center

2213 Cherry St.
Toledo, Ohio 43608-2691
Mon.-Fri. 7 AM-5 PM
    419-251-4227
www.rx.medctr.ohio-state.edu

OKLAHOMA

OKLAHOMA CITY

Drug Information Service Integris Health

3300 Northwest Expressway
Oklahoma City, OK 73112
Mon.-Fri. 8 AM-4:30 PM
    405-949-3660

Drug Information Center OU Medical Center Presbyterian Tower

700 NE 13th St.
Oklahoma City, OK 73104
Mon.-Fri. 8 AM-4:30 PM
    405-271-6226
Fax: 405-271-6281

TULSA

Drug Information Center Saint Francis Hospital

6161 S. Yale Ave.
Tulsa, OK 74136
Mon.-Fri. 8 AM-4:30 PM
    918-494-6339
    (for healthcare
    professionals only)

PENNSYLVANIA

PHILADELPHIA

Drug Information Center Temple University Hospital Dept. of Pharmacy

3401 N. Broad St.
Philadelphia, PA 19140
Mon.-Fri. 8 AM-4:30 PM
    215-707-4644

Drug Information Service Tenet Health System Hahnemann University Hospital Department of Pharmacy

MS 451
Broad and Vine Streets
Philadelphia, PA 19102
Mon.-Fri. 8 AM-4 PM
    215-762-DRUG (3784)
    (for healthcare
    professionals only)

Drug Information Service Dept. of Pharmacy Thomas Jefferson University Hospital

111 S. 11th St.
Philadelphia, PA 19107-5089
Mon.-Fri. 8 AM-5 PM
    215-955-8877

University of Pennsylvania Health System Drug Information Service Hospital of the University of Pennsylvania Department of Pharmacy

3400 Spruce St.
Philadelphia, PA 19104
Mon.-Fri. 8:30 AM-4 PM
    215-662-2903

DRUG INFORMATION CENTERS

PITTSBURGH

Pharmaceutical Information CenterMylan School of Pharmacy Duquesne University

431 Mellon Hall
Pittsburgh, PA 15282
Mon.-Fri. 8 AM-4 PM
412-396-4600

Drug Information Center University of Pittsburgh

302 Scaife Hall
200 Lothrop St.
Pittsburgh, PA 15213
Mon.-Fri. 8:30 AM-4:30 PM
412-647-3784
(for healthcare professionals only)

UPLAND

Drug Information Center Crozer-Chester Medical Center Dept. of Pharmacy

1 Medical Center Blvd.
Upland, PA 19013
Mon.-Fri. 8 AM-4:30 PM
610-447-2851
(for in-house healthcare professionals only)

PUERTO RICO
PONCE

Centro Informacion Medicamentos Escuela de Medicina de Ponce

P.O. Box 7004
Ponce, PR 00732-7004
Mon.-Fri. 8 AM-4:30 PM
787-840-2575

SAN JUAN

Centro de Informacion de Medicamentos-CIM Escuela de Farmacia-RCM

P.O. Box 365067
San Juan, PR 00936-5067
Mon.-Fri. 8 AM-5:30 PM
787-758-2525, ext. 1516

SOUTH CAROLINA
CHARLESTON

Drug Information Service Medical University of South Carolina

150 Ashley Ave.
Rutledge Tower Annex
Room 604
P.O. Box 250584
Charleston, SC 29425-0810
Mon.-Fri. 9 AM-5:30 PM
843-792-3896
800-922-5250

COLUMBIA

Drug Information Service University of South Carolina College of Pharmacy

Columbia, SC 29208
Mon.-Fri. 8 AM-5 PM
803-777-7804
www.pharm.sc.edu

SPARTANBURG

Drug Information Center Spartanburg Regional Healthcare System

101 E. Wood St.
Spartanburg, SC 29303
Mon.-Fri. 8 AM-4:30 PM
864-560-6910

TENNESSEE
KNOXVILLE

Drug Information Center University of Tennessee Medical Center at Knoxville

1924 Alcoa Highway
Knoxville, TN 37920-6999
Mon.-Fri. 8 AM-4:30 PM
865-544-9124

MEMPHIS

South East Regional Drug Information Center VA Medical Center

1030 Jefferson Ave.
Memphis, TN 38104
Mon.-Fri. 6:30 AM-4 PM
901-523-8990, ext. 6720

Drug Information Center University of Tennessee

875 Monroe Ave.
Suite 116
Memphis, TN 38163
Mon.-Fri. 8 AM-5 PM
901-448-5556

TEXAS
AMARILLO

Drug Information Center Texas Tech Health Sciences Center School of Pharmacy

1300 Coulter Rd.
Amarillo, TX 79106
Mon.-Fri. 8 AM-5 PM
806-356-4008

GALVESTON

Drug Information Center University of Texas Medical Branch

301 University Blvd.
Galveston, TX 77555-0701
Mon.-Fri. 8 AM-5 PM
409-772-2734

HOUSTON

Drug Information Center Ben Taub General Hospital Texas Southern University/HCHD

1504 Taub Loop
Houston, TX 77030
Mon.-Fri. 8:30 AM-5 PM
713-873-3710

LACKLAND A.F.B.

Drug Information Center Dept. of Pharmacy Wilford Hall Medical Center

2200 Bergquist Dr.
Suite 1
Lackland A.F.B., TX 78236
7 days/week, 24 hours
210-292-5414

LUBBOCK

Drug Information and Consultation Service Covenant Medical Center

3615 19th St.
Lubbock, TX 79410
Mon.-Fri. 8 AM-5 PM
806-725-0408

SAN ANTONIO

Drug Information Service University of Texas Health Science Center at San Antonio Department of Pharmacology

7703 Floyd Curl Drive
San Antonio, TX 78229-3900
Mon.-Fri. 8 AM-4 PM
210-567-4280

TEMPLE

Drug Information Center Scott and White Memorial Hospital

2401 S. 31st St.
Temple, TX 76508
Mon.-Fri. 8 AM-5 PM
254-724-4636

UTAH
SALT LAKE CITY

Drug Information Service University of Utah Hospital

421 Wakara Way
Suite 204
Salt Lake City, UT 84108
Mon.-Fri. 7 AM-5 PM
801-581-2073

DRUG INFORMATION CENTERS

VIRGINIA

HAMPTON

Drug Information Center
Hampton University School
of Pharmacy

Hampton Harbors Annex
Hampton, VA 23668
Mon.-Fri. 9 AM-4 PM
  757-728-6693

WEST VIRGINIA

MORGANTOWN

West Virginia Center for
Drug and Health Information
West Virginia University
Robert C. Byrd
Health Sciences Center

1124 HSN, P.O. Box 9520
Morgantown, WV 26506
Mon.-Fri. 8:30 AM-5 PM
  304-293-6640
  800-352-2501 **(WV only)**
www.hsc.wvu.edu/SOP

WYOMING

LARAMIE

Drug Information Center
University of Wyoming

P.O. Box 3375
Laramie, WY 82071
Mon.-Fri. 8:30 AM-4:30 PM
  307-766-6988

POISON ANTIDOTE CHART

WARNING: While every effort has been made to ensure the accuracy of this chart, it is not intended to serve as the sole source of information on antidotes. Guidelines may need to be adjusted based on factors such as anticipated usage in the hospital's local area, the nearest alternate sources of antidotes, and distance to tertiary care institutions. Contact your nearest regional poison control center (1-800-222-1222) for treatment information regarding any exposure, including indications for use of antidote therapy. Directions in this chart assume that all basic life support and decontamination measures have been initiated as needed.

ANTIDOTE	POISON/DRUG/TOXIN	SUGGESTED MINIMUM STOCK QUANTITY	COMMENTS
N-Acetylcysteine (Acetadote®, Mucomyst®)	Acetaminophen Carbon tetrachloride Other hepatotoxins	Oral product: 600 mL in 10 mL or 30 mL vials of 20% solution IV product: One carton of four 30 mL vials of 20% solution	Acetaminophen is the most common drug involved intentional and unintentional poisonings. 600 mL (120 g) of the oral product provides enough antidote to treat an adult for an entire 3-day course of therapy, or enough to treat three adults for 24 h. Several vials may be stocked in the ED to provide a loading dose and the remaining vials in the pharmacy for the q 4 h maintenance doses. The IV product dose of 120mL (24 g) will treat one adult patient for an entire 20-hour IV protocol.
Amyl nitrite, sodium nitrite, and sodium thiosulfate (Cyanide antidote kit)	Acetonitrile Acrylonitrile Bromates (thiosulfate only) Chlorates (thiosulfate only) Cyanide (e.g., HCN, KCN and NaCN) Cyanogen chloride Cyanogenic glycoside natural sources (e.g., apricot pits and peach pits) Hydrogen sulfide (nitrites only) Laetrile Mustard agents (thiosulfate only) Nitroprusside (thiosulfate only) Smoke inhalation (combustion of synthetic materials)	One to two kits	Stock one kit in the ED. Consider also stocking one kit in the pharmacy. Note: This kit has a short shelf life of 24 months.
Antivenin, Crotalidae Polyvalent (equine origin)	Pit viper envenomation (e.g., rattlesnakes, cottonmouths, and timber rattlers)	Ten vials	Stock in pharmacy. Advised in geographic areas with endemic populations of copperheads, water mocassins, or eastern massasauga ratlesnakes. In low-risk areas, know nearest alternate source of antivenin. Note: 20 to 40 vials or more may be needed for moderate to severe envenomations. The antivenin must be administered in a critical care setting since it is an equine-derived product. Refrigeration is unnecessary.

(Continued)

This chart is adapted from material furnished by the Illinois Poison Center, a program of the Metropolitan Chicago Healthcare Council (MCHC).

POISON ANTIDOTE CHART

ANTIDOTE	POISON/DRUG/TOXIN	SUGGESTED MINIMUM STOCK QUANTITY	COMMENTS
Antivenin, Crotalidae Polyvalent Immune Fab–Ovine (CroFab®)	Pit viper envenomation (e.g., rattlesnakes, cottonmouths, copperheads, and timber rattlers)	Four to six vials	Stock in pharmacy. This product is a possible alternate to equine product. May have lower risk of hypersensitivity reaction than equine product. Average dose in premarketing trials was 12 vials but more may be needed. Note: Store in refrigerator. See entry above for equine antivenin.
Antivenin, *Latrodectus mactans* (Black widow spider)	Black widow spider envenomation	Zero to one vial	Serious *Latrodectus* envenomations are rare. This product is only used for severe envenomations. Antivenin must be given in a critical care setting since it is an equine-derived product. Know the nearest source of antidote. Note: Product must be refrigerated at all times.
Atropine sulfate	Alpha^2 agonists (e.g., clonidine, guanabenz, and guanfacine) Alzheimer's drugs (e.g., donepezil, galantamine, rivastigmine, tacrine) Antimyesthenic agents (e.g., pyridostigmine) Bradyarrhythmia-producing agents (e.g., beta blockers, calcium channel blockers, and digitalis glycosides) Cholinergic agonists (e.g., bethanechol) Muscarine-containing mushrooms (e.g., Clitocybe and Inocybe) Nerve agents (e.g., sarin, soman, tabun, and VX) Organophosphate and carbamate insecticides	Total 100 mg to 150 mg Available in various formulations: 0.4 mg/mL (20 mL, 8 mg vials) 0.1 mg/mL (10 mL, 1 mg ampules) 0.1 mg/mL (10 mL, 1 mg ampules) Atropine sulfate military-style auto-injectors: 2mg 2 mg/0.7 mL, 1 mg/0.7 mL, 0.5 mg/0.7 mL, 0.25 mg/0.3 mL	The product should be immediately available in the ED. Some may also be stored in the pharmacy or other hospital sites, but should be easily mobilized if a severely poisoned patient needs treatment. Note: Product is necessary for adequate preparedness for a weapon of mass destruction (WMD) incident; the suggested amount may not be sufficient for mass-casualty events. Auto-injectors are available from Bound Tree Medical, Inc. Drug stocked in chempack container is intended only for use in mass-casualty events.
Calcium disodium EDTA (Versenate®)	Lead Zinc salts (e.g., zinc chloride)	One 5 mL amp (200 mg/mL)	Stock in pharmacy. One vial provides 1 day of therapy for a child. More may be needed in lead-endemic areas.
Calcium chloride and Calcium gluconate	Beta blockers Calcium channel blockers Fluoride salts (e.g., NaF) Hydrofluoric acid (HF) Hyperkalemia (not digoxin-induced) Hypermagnesemia	10% calcium chloride: fifteen 10 mL vials 10% calcium gluconate: five 10 mL vials	Stock in ED. More may be stocked in pharmacy. Many ampules of calcium chloride may be necessary in life-threatening calcium channel blocker or hydrofluoric acid poisoning.
Deferoxamine mesylate (Desferal®)	Iron	Twelve 500 mg vials	Stock in pharmacy. Note: Per package insert, the maximum daily dose is 6 g (12 vials). However, this dose may be exceeded in serious poisonigs.
Digoxin immune Fab (Digibind®, DigiFab®)	Cardiac glycoside-containing plants (e.g., foxglove and oleander) Digitoxin Digoxin	Ten vials	Stock in ED or pharmacy. This amount (ten vials) may be given to a digoxin-poisoned patient in whom the digoxin level is unknown. This amount would effectively neutralize a steady-state digoxin level of 14.2 ng/mL in a 70-kg patient. More may be necessary in severe intoxications. Know nearest source of additional supply.

(Continued)

POISON ANTIDOTE CHART

ANTIDOTE	POISON/DRUG/TOXIN	SUGGESTED MINIMUM STOCK QUANTITY	COMMENTS
Dimercaprol (BAL in oil)	Arsenic Copper Gold Lead Lewisite Mercury	Two 3 mL amps (100 mg/mL)	Stock in pharmacy. This amount provides two doses of 3 to 5 mg/kg/dose given q 4 h to treat one seriously poisoned adult or provides enough to treat a 15-kg child for 24 h.
Ethanol	Ethylene glycol Methanol	6 L of 5% alcohol in D5W 10% alcohol in D5W was discontinued in 2004; however, it can be prepared from 5% alcohol in D5W and dehydrated alcohol. Consult Poison Control Center.	Stock in pharmacy. This amount (6 L) provides enough to treat two adults with a loading dose followed by a maintenance infusion for 4 hours each. More alcohol or fomepizole will be needed during dialysis or prolonged treatment. 95% or 40% alcohol diluted in juice may be given po if IV alcohol is unavailable. Note: Ethanol is unnecessary if fomepizole is stocked.
Flumazenil (Romazicon®)	Benzodiazepines Zaleplon Zolpidem	Total 1 mg: two 5 mL vials (0.1 mg/mL)	Suggested minimum is for ED stocking. Due to risk of seizures, use with extreme caution, if at all, in poisoned patients. More may be stocked in the pharmacy for use in reversal of conscious sedation.
Folic acid and Folinic acid (Leucovorin)	Methanol Methotrexate, trimetrexate Pyrimethamine Trimethoprim	Folic acid: three 50 mg vials Folinic acid: one 50 mg vial	Stock in pharmacy. For methanol-poisoned patients with an acidosis, give 50mg folinic acid initially, then 50mg of folic acid q 4 h for six doses.
Fomepizole (Antizol®)	Ethylene glycol Methanol	Two 1.5 g vial Note: Available in a kit of four 1.5 g vials	Stock in pharmacy. Know where nearest alternate supply is located. One vial will provide at least one initial adult dose. Hospitals with critical care and hemodialysis capabilities should consider stocking one kit of four vials (enough to treat one patient for up to several days). Note: Product has a 2-year shelf life; however, the manufacturer offers a credit for unused, expired product.
Glucagon	Beta blockers Calcium channel blockers Hypoglycemia Hypoglycemic agents	Fifty 1 mg vials	Stock 20 mg in ED and remainder in pharmacy. The total amount (50 mg) provides approximately 5 to 10 hours of high-dose therapy in life-threatening beta blocker or calcium channel blocker poisoning. A protocol using high doses of insulin/dextrose also may be considered. Consult regional poison center for guidelines.
Hyperbaric oxygen (HBO)	Carbon monoxide Carbon tetrachloride Cyanide Hydrogen sulfide Methemoglobinemia	Post the location and phone number of nearest HBO chamber in the ED.	Consult regional poison center to determine if HBO treatment is indicated.

(Continued)

POISON ANTIDOTE CHART

ANTIDOTE	POISON/DRUG/TOXIN	SUGGESTED MINIMUM STOCK QUANTITY	COMMENTS
Methylene blue	Methemoglobin-inducing agents including: Aniline dyes Dapsone Dinitrophenol Local anesthetics (e.g., benzocaine) Metoclopramide Monomethylhydrazine-containing mushrooms (e.g., Gyromitra) Naphthalene Nitrates and nitrites Nitrobenzene Phenazopyridine	Three 10 mL amps (10 mg/mL)	Stock in pharmacy. This amount provides three doses of 1 to 2 mg/kg (0.1 to 0.2 mL/kg) for an adult patient.
Nalmefene (Revex®) and Naloxone (Narcan®)	ACE inhibitors Alpha$_2$ agonists (e.g., clonidine, guanabenz, and guanfacine) Coma of unknown cause Imidazoline decongestants (e.g., oxymetazoline and tetrahydrozoline) Loperamide Opioids (e.g., codeine, dextromethorphan, diphenoxylate, fentanyl, heroin, meperidine, morphine, and propoxyphene)	Nalmefene: none required Naloxone: total 40 mg, any combination of 0.4 mg 1 mg, and 2 mg ampules	Stock 20 mg naloxone in the the institution. Note: Nalmefene has a longer duration of action but it offers no therapeutic advantage over a naloxone infusion.
D-penicillamine (Cuprimine®)	Arsenic Copper Lead Mercury	None required as an antidote. Available in bottles of 100 capsules (125 mg or 250 mg/capsule)	D-penicillamine is no longer considered the drug of choice for heavy-metal poisonings. It may be stocked in the pharmacy for other indications such as Wilson's disease or rheumatoid arthritis.
Physostigmine salicylate (Antilirium®)	Anticholinergic alkaloid-containing plants (e.g., deadly nightshade and jimson weed) Antihistamines Atropine and other anticholinergic agents Intrathecal baclofen	Two 2 mL ampules (1 mg/mL)	Stock in ED or pharmacy. Usual adult dose is 1 to 2 mg slow IV push. Note: Duration of effect is 30 to 60 min.
Phytonadione (Vitamin K1) (AquaMEPHYTON®, Mephyton®)	Indandione derivatives Long-acting anticoagulant rodenticides (e.g., brodifacoum and bromadiolone) Warfarin	Two 0.5 mL ampules (2 mg/mL) and ten 1 mL ampules (10 mg/mL) 5 mg tablets available in packages of 10, 14, 20, 30, and 100	Stock in pharmacy.
Pralidoxime chloride (2-PAM) (Protopam®)	Antimyesthenic agents (e.g., pyridostigmine) Nerve agents (e.g., sarin, soman, tabun, and VX) Organophosphate insecticides Tacrine	Six 1 g vials Pralidoxime chloride military-style auto-injectors: 600 mg/2 mL	Stock in ED or pharmacy. Note: Serious intoxications may require 500 mg/h (12 g/day). Product is necessary for adequate preparedness for a weapon of mass destruction (WMD) incident; the suggested amount may not be sufficient for mass-casualty events. Auto-injectors are available from Bound Tree Medical, Inc. Drug stocked in chempack container is intended only for use in mass-casualty events.

(Continued)

POISON ANTIDOTE CHART

ANTIDOTE	POISON/DRUG/TOXIN	SUGGESTED MINIMUM STOCK QUANTITY	COMMENTS
Protamine sulfate	Enoxaparin Heparin	Variable, consider recommendation of hospital P&T Committee Available as 5 mL ampules (10 mg/mL) and 25 mL vials (250 mg/25 mL)	Stock in pharmacy.
Pyridoxine hydrochloride (Vitamin B6)	Acrylamide Ethylene glycol Hydrazine Isoniazid (INH) Monomethylhydrazine-containing mushrooms (e.g., Gyromitra)	Four 30 mL vials (100 mg/mL 3 g/vial) or one hundred 1 mL vials (100 mg/mL vials)	Stock in ED or pharmacy. Usual dose is 1 g pyridoxine HCl for each gram of INH ingested. If amount ingested is unknown, give 5 g of pyridoxine. Repeat dose if seizures are uncontrolled Know nearest source of additional supply. For ethylene glycol, a dose of 100 mg/day enhances the clearance of toxic metabolite.
Sodium bicarbonate	Chlorine gas Hyperkalemia Serum alkalinization: Agents producing a quinidine-like effect as noted by widened QRS complex on EKG (e.g., amantadine, carbamazepine, chloroquine, cocaine, diphenhydramine, flecainide, propafenone, propoxyphene, tricyclic antidepressants, quinidine, and related agents) Urine alkalinization: Weakly acidic agents (e.g., chlorophenoxy herbicides, chlorpropamide, phenobarbital, and salicylates)	Twenty 50 mEq vials	Stock 10 vials in the ED and 10 vials elsewhere in the hospital.
Succimer (Chemet®)	Arsenic Lead Lewisite Mercury	One bottle of 100 capsules (100 mg/capsule)	Stock in pharmacy. FDA-approved only for pediatric lead poisoning; however, it has shown efficacy for other heavy-metal poisonings.

POISON CONTROL CENTERS

The American Association of Poison Control Centers (AAPCC) uses a single, nationwide emergency number to automatically link callers with their regional poison center. This toll-free number, **800-222-1222**, also works for **teletype lines (TTY)** for the hearing-impaired and **telecommunication devices (TTD)** for individuals who are deaf. However, a few local poison centers and the ASPCA/Animal Poison Control Center are not part of this nationwide system and continue to use separate numbers.

Most of the centers listed below are certified by the AAPCC. Certified centers are marked by an asterisk after the name. Each has to meet certain criteria. It must, for example, serve a large geographic area; it must be open 24 hours a day and provide direct-dial or toll-free access; it must be supervised by a medical director; and it must have registered pharmacists or nurses available to answer questions from the public.

Within each state, centers are listed alphabetically by city. Some state poison centers also list their original emergency numbers (including TTY/TDD) that only work within that state. For these listings, callers may use either the state number or the nationwide 800 number.

ALABAMA

BIRMINGHAM

Regional Poison Control Center,
The Children's Hospital
of Alabama (*)

1600 7th Ave. South
Birmingham, AL 35233-1711
Business: 205-939-9201
Emergency: 800-222-1222
www.chsys.org

TUSCALOOSA

Alabama Poison Center (*)

2503 Phoenix Dr.
Tuscaloosa, AL 35405
Business: 205-345-0600
Emergency: 800-222-1222
800-462-0800 (AL)
www.alapoisoncenter.org

ALASKA

JUNEAU

Alaska Poison Control System

Section of Community
Health and EMS
410 Willoughby Ave., Room 103
Box 110616
Juneau, AK 99811-0616
Business: 907-465-3027
Emergency: 800-222-1222
www.chems.alaska.gov

(PORTLAND, OR)

Oregon Poison Center (*)
Oregon Health Sciences University

3181 SW Sam Jackson Park Rd.
CB550
Portland, OR 97239
Business: 503-494-8311
Emergency: 800-222-1222
www.oregonpoison.com

ARIZONA

PHOENIX

Banner Poison Control Center (*)
Banner Good Samaritan
Medical Center

901 E. Willetta St.
Room 2701
Phoenix, AZ 85006
Business: 602-495-4884
Emergency: 800-222-1222
www.bannerpoisoncontrol.com

TUCSON

Arizona Poison and Drug
Information Center (*)
Arizona Health Sciences Center

1501 N. Campbell Ave.
Room 1156
Tucson, AZ 85724
Business: 520-626-7899
Emergency: 800-222-1222

ARKANSAS

LITTLE ROCK

Arkansas Poison and
Drug Information Center
College of Pharmacy - UAMS

4301 West Markham St.
Mail Slot 522-2
Little Rock, AR 72205-7122
Business: 501-686-5540
Emergency: 800-222-1222
800-376-4766 (AR)
TDD/TTY: 800-641-3805

ASPCA/Animal Poison Control Center

1717 South Philo Rd.
Suite 36
Urbana, IL 61802
Business: 217-337-5030
Emergency: 888-426-4435
800-548-2423
www.napcc.aspca.org

CALIFORNIA

FRESNO/MADERA

California Poison Control System-
Fresno/Madera Div.(*)
Children's Hospital of Central
California

9300 Valley Children's Place MB 15
Madera, CA 93638-8762
Business: 559-622-2300
Emergency: 800-222-1222
800-876-4766 (CA)
TDD/TTY: 800-972-3323
www.calpoison.org

SACRAMENTO

California Poison Control System-
Sacramento Div.(*)
UC Davis Medical Center

Room HSF 1024
2315 Stockton Blvd.
Sacramento, CA 95817
Business: 916-227-1400
Emergency: 800-222-1222
800-876-4766 (CA)
TDD/TTY: 800-972-3323
www.calpoison.org

SAN DIEGO

California Poison Control
System-San Diego Div. (*)
UC San Diego Medical Center

200 West Arbor Dr.
San Diego, CA 92103-8925
Business: 858-715-6300
Emergency: 800-222-1222
800-876-4766 (CA)
TDD/TTY: 800-972-3323
www.calpoison.org

SAN FRANCISCO

California Poison Control
System-San Francisco Div.(*)
San Francisco General Hospital
University of California
San Francisco

Box 1369
San Francisco, CA 94143-1369
Business: 415-502-6000
Emergency: 800-222-1222
800-876-4766 (CA)
TDD/TTY: 800-972-3323
www.calpoison.org

Poison Control Centers

COLORADO
DENVER

Rocky Mountain Poison and Drug Center (*)

777 Bannock St.
Mail Code 0180
Denver, CO 80204-4507
Business: 303-739-1100
Emergency: 800-222-1222
TDD/TTY: 303-739-1127 (CO)
www.RMPDC.org

CONNECTICUT
FARMINGTON

Connecticut Regional Poison Control Center (*)
University of Connecticut Health Center

263 Farmington Ave.
Farmington, CT 06030-5365
Business: 860-679-4540
Emergency: 800-222-1222
TDD/TTY: 866-218-5372
http://poisoncontrol.uchc.edu

DELAWARE
(PHILADELPHIA, PA)

The Poison Control Center (*)
Children's Hospital of Philadelphia

34th St. & Civic Center Blvd.
Philadelphia, PA 19104-4303
Business: 215-590-2003
Emergency: 800-222-1222
800-722-7112 (DE)
TDD/TTY: 215-590-8789
www.poisoncontrol.chop.edu

DISTRICT OF COLUMBIA
WASHINGTON, DC

National Capital Poison Center (*)

3201 New Mexico Ave., NW
Suite 310
Washington, DC 20016
Business: 202-362-3867
Emergency: 800-222-1222
www.poison.org

FLORIDA
JACKSONVILLE

Florida Poison Information Center-Jacksonville (*)
SHANDS Hospital

655 West 8th St.
Jacksonville, FL 32209
Business: 904-244-4465
Emergency: 800-222-1222
http://fpicjax.org

MIAMI

Florida Poison Information Center-Miami (*) University of Miami–Department of Pediatrics

P.O. Box 016960 (R-131)
Miami, FL 33101
Business: 305-585-5250
Emergency: 800-222-1222
www.miami.edu/poison-center

TAMPA

Florida Poison Information Center-Tampa (*)
Tampa General Hospital

P.O. Box 1289
Tampa, FL 33601-1289
Business: 813-844-7044
Emergency: 800-222-1222
www.poisoncentertampa.org

GEORGIA
ATLANTA

Georgia Poison Center (*)
Hughes Spalding Children's Hospital, Grady Health System

80 Jesse Hill Jr. Dr., SE
P.O. Box 26066
Atlanta, GA 30303-3050
Business: 404-616-9237
Emergency: 800-222-1222
404-616-9000 (Atlanta)
TDD: 404-616-9287
www.georgiapoisoncenter.org

Hawaii
(DENVER, CO)

Rocky Mountain Poison and Drug Center (*)

777 Bannock St.
Mail Code 0180
Denver, CO 80204-4507
Business: 303-739-1100
Emergency: 800-222-1222
www.RMPDC.org

IDAHO
(DENVER, CO)

Rocky Mountain Poison and Drug Center (*)

777 Bannock St.
Mail Code 0180
Denver, CO 80204-4507
Business: 303-739-1100
Emergency: 800-222-1222
www.RMPDC.org

ILLINOIS
CHICAGO

Illinois Poison Center (*)

222 South Riverside Plaza
Suite 1900
Chicago, IL 60606
Business: 312-906-6136
Emergency: 800-222-1222
TDD/TTY: 312-906-6185
www.illinoispoisoncenter.org

INDIANA
INDIANAPOLIS

Indiana Poison Control Center (*)
Clarian Health Partners Methodist Hospital

I-65 at 21st St.
Indianapolis, IN 46206-1367
Business: 317-962-2335
Emergency: 800-222-1222
800-382-9097
317-962-2323
(Indianapolis)
TTY: 317-962-2336
www.clarian.org/poisoncontrol

IOWA
SIOUX CITY

Iowa Statewide Poison Control Center Iowa Health System and the University of Iowa Hospitals and Clinics

401 Douglas St., Suite 402
Sioux City, IA 51101
Business: 712-279-3710
Emergency: 800-222-1222
712-277-2222 (IA)
www.iowapoison.org

KANSAS
KANSAS CITY

Mid-America Poison Control Center
University of Kansas Medical Center

3901 Rainbow Blvd.
Room B-400
Kansas City, KS 66160-7231
Business 913-588-6638
Emergency: 800-222-1222
800-332-6633 (KS)
TDD: 913-588-6639
www.kumc.edu/poison

POISON CONTROL CENTERS

KENTUCKY
LOUISVILLE

Kentucky Regional Poison Center (*)

P.O. Box 35070
Louisville, KY 40232-5070
Business: 502-629-7264
Emergency: 800-222-1222
 502-589-8222
 (Louisville)
www.krpc.com

LOUISIANA
MONROE

Louisiana Drug and Poison Information Center (*)
University of Louisiana at Monroe

700 University Ave.
Monroe, LA 71209-6430
Business: 318-342-3648
Emergency: 800-222-1222
www.lapcc.org

MAINE
PORTLAND

Northern New England Poison Center

Maine Medical Center
22 Bramhall St.
Portland, ME 04102
Business: 207-662-7220
Emergency: 800-222-1222
 207-871-2879 (ME)
TDD/TTY: 877-299-4447 (ME)
 207-871-2879 (ME)
www.nnepc.org

MARYLAND
BALTIMORE

Maryland Poison Center (*)
University of Maryland at Baltimore School of Pharmacy

20 North Pine St., PH 772
Baltimore, MD 21201
Business: 410-706-7604
Emergency: 800-222-1222
TDD: 410-706-1858
www.mdpoison.com

(WASHINGTON, DC)

National Capital Poison Center (*)

3201 New Mexico Ave., NW
Suite 310
Washington, DC 20016
Business: 202-362-3867
Emergency: 800-222-1222
TDD/TTY: 202-362-8563 (MD)
www.poison.org

MASSACHUSETTS
BOSTON

Regional Center for Poison Control and Prevention (*)
(Serving Massachusetts and Rhode Island)

300 Longwood Ave.
Boston, MA 02115
Business: 617-355-6609
Emergency: 800-222-1222
TDD/TTY: 888-244-5313
www.maripoisoncenter.com

MICHIGAN
DETROIT

Regional Poison Control Center (*)
Children's Hospital of Michigan

4160 John R. Harper
 Professional Office Bldg.
Suite 616
Detroit, MI 48201
Business: 313-745-5335
Emergency: 800-222-1222
TDD/TTY: 800-356-3232
www.mitoxic.org/pcc

GRAND RAPIDS

DeVos Children's Hospital Regional Poison Center (*)

100 Michigan St., NE
Grand Rapids, MI 49503
Business: 616-391-3690
Emergency: 800-222-1222
http://poisoncenter.
 devoschildrens.org

MINNESOTA
MINNEAPOLIS

Minnesota Poison Control System (*)
Hennepin County Medical Center

701 Park Ave.
Mail Code RL
Minneapolis, MN 55415
Business: 612-873-3144
Emergency: 800-222-1222
www.mnpoison.org

MISSISSIPPI
JACKSON

Mississippi Regional Poison Control Center, University of Mississippi Medical Center

2500 North State St.
Jackson, MS 39216
Business: 601-984-1680
Emergency: 800-222-1222

MISSOURI
ST. LOUIS

Missouri Regional Poison Center (*) Cardinal Glennon Children's Hospital

7980 Clayton Rd.
Suite 200
St. Louis, MO 63117
Business: 314-772-5200
Emergency: 800-222-1222
TDD/TTY: 314-612-5705
www.cardinalglennon.com

MONTANA
(DENVER, CO)

Rocky Mountain Poison and Drug Center (*)

777 Bannock St.
Mail Code 0180
Denver, CO 80204-4507
Business: 303-739-1100
Emergency: 800-222-1222
TDD/TTY: 303-739-1127
www.RMPDC.org

NEBRASKA
OMAHA

The Poison Center (*)
Children's Hospital

8401 W. Dodge St., Suite 115
Omaha, NE 68114
Business: 402-955-5555
Emergency: 800-222-1222
www.nebraskapoison.com

NEVADA
(DENVER, CO)

Rocky Mountain Poison and Drug Center (*)

777 Bannock St.
Mail Code 0180
Denver, CO 80204-4507
Business: 303-739-1100
Emergency: 800-222-1222
www.RMPDC.org

(PORTLAND, OR)

Oregon Poison Center (*)
Oregon Health Sciences University

3181 SW Sam Jackson Park Rd.
Portland, OR 97201
Business: 503-494-8600
Emergency: 800-222-1222
www.oregonpoison.com

POISON CONTROL CENTERS

NEW HAMPSHIRE
(PORTLAND, ME)

Northern New England Poison Center

Maine Medical Center
22 Bramhall St.
Portland, ME 04102
Business: 207-662-7220
Emergency: 800-222-1222
www.nnepc.org

NEW JERSEY
NEWARK

New Jersey Poison Information and Education System (*) UMDNJ

65 Bergen St.
Newark, NJ 07101
Business: 973-972-9280
Emergency: 800-222-1222
TDD/TTY: 973-926-8008
www.njpies.org

NEW MEXICO
ALBUQUERQUE

New Mexico Poison and Drug Information Center (*)

MSC09-5080
1 University of New Mexico
Albuquerque, NM 87131-0001
Business: 505-272-4261
Emergency: 800-222-1222
http://HSC.UNM.edu/pharmacy/poison

NEW YORK
BUFFALO

Western New York Regional Poison Control Center (*) Children's Hospital of Buffalo

219 Bryant St.
Buffalo, NY 14222
Business: 716-878-7654
Emergency: 800-222-1222
www.fingerlakespoison.org

MINEOLA

Long Island Regional Poison and Drug Information Center (*) Winthrop University Hospital

259 First St.
Mineola, NY 11501
Business: 516-663-2650
Emergency: 800-222-1222
TDD: 516-747-3323 (Nassau)
516-924-8811 (Suffolk)
www.lirpdic.org

NEW YORK CITY

New York City Poison Control Center (*) NYC Dept. of Health

455 First Ave., Room 123
New York, NY 10016
Business: 212-447-8152
Emergency: 800-222-1222
(English) 212-340-4494
212-POISONS
(212-764-7667)

Emergency: 212-venenos
(Spanish) (212-836-3667)
TDD: 212-689-9014

ROCHESTER

Finger Lakes Regional Poison and Drug Information Center (*) University of Rochester Medical Center

601 Elmwood Ave.
Box 321
Rochester, NY 14642
Business: 585-273-4155
Emergency: 800-222-1222
TTY: 585-273-3854

SYRACUSE

Central New York Poison Center (*) SUNY Upstate Medical University

750 East Adams St.
Syracuse, NY 13210
Business: 315-464-7078
Emergency: 800-222-1222
www.cnypoison.org

NORTH CAROLINA
CHARLOTTE

Carolinas Poison Center (*) Carolinas Medical Center

P.O. Box 32861
Charlotte, NC 28232
Business: 704-512-3795
Emergency: 800-222-1222
TDD: 800-735-8262
TTY: 800-735-2962
www.ncpoisoncenter.org

NORTH DAKOTA
(MINNEAPOLIS, MN)

Minnesota Poison Control System (*) Hennepin County Medical Center

701 Park Ave.
Mail Code 820
Minneapolis, MN 55415
Business: 612-873-3144
Emergency: 800-222-1222
www.ndpoison.org

OHIO
CINCINNATI

Cincinnati Drug and Poison Information Center (*) Regional Poison Control System

3333 Burnet Ave.
Vernon Place, 3rd Floor
Cincinnati, OH 45229
Business: 513-636-5111
Emergency: 800-222-1222
TDD/TTY: 800-253-7955
www.cincinnatichildrens.org/dpic

CLEVELAND

Greater Cleveland Poison Control Center

11100 Euclid Ave.
MP 6007
Cleveland, OH 44106-6007
Business: 216-844-1573
Emergency: 800-222-1222
216-231-4455 (OH)

COLUMBUS

Central Ohio Poison Center (*)

700 Children's Dr.
Room L032
Columbus, OH 43205-2696
Business: 614-722-2635
Emergency: 800-222-1222
TTY: 614-228-2272
www.bepoisonsmart.com

OKLAHOMA
OKLAHOMA CITY

Oklahoma Poison Control Center (*) Children's Hospital at OU Medical Center

940 Northeast 13th St.
Room 3510
Oklahoma City, OK 73104
Business: 405-271-5062
Emergency: 800-222-1222
www.oklahomapoison.org

OREGON
PORTLAND

Oregon Poison Center (*) Oregon Health Sciences University

3181 S.W. Sam Jackson Park Rd.,
CB550
Portland, OR 97239
Business: 503-494-8968
Emergency: 800-222-1222
www.oregonpoison.com

POISON CONTROL CENTERS

PENNSYLVANIA
PHILADELPHIA

The Poison Control Center (*)
Children's Hospital of Philadelphia

34th Street & Civic Center Blvd.
Philadelphia, PA 19104-4399
Business: 215-590-2003
Emergency: 800-222-1222
 215-386-2100 (PA)
TDD/TTY: 215-590-8789
www.poisoncontrol.chop.edu

PITTSBURGH

Pittsburgh Poison Center (*)
Children's Hospital of Pittsburgh

3705 Fifth Ave.
Pittsburgh, PA 15213
Business: 412-390-3300
Emergency: 800-222-1222
 412-681-6669
www.chp.edu/clinical/03a_poison.php

PUERTO RICO
SANTURCE

San Jorge Children's Hospital Poison Center

268 San Jorge St.
Santurce, PR 00912
Business: 787-726-5660
Emergency: 800-222-1222
TTY: 787-641-1934
www.poisoncenter.net

RHODE ISLAND
(BOSTON, MA)

Regional Center for Poison Control and Prevention (*)
(Serving Massachusetts and Rhode Island)

300 Longwood Ave.
Boston, MA 02115
Business: 617-355-6609
Emergency: 800-222-1222
TDD/TTY: 888-244-5313
www.maripoisoncenter.com

SOUTH CAROLINA
COLUMBIA

Palmetto Poison Center (*)
College of Pharmacy
University of South Carolina

Columbia, SC 29208
Business: 803-777-7909
Drug Info: 803-777-7805
Emergency: 800-222-1222
 800-922-1117 (SC)
http://poison.sc.edu

SOUTH DAKOTA
(MINNEAPOLIS, MN)

Hennepin Regional Poison Center (*)
Hennepin County Medical Center

701 Park Ave.
Minneapolis, MN 55415
Business: 612-873-3144
Emergency: 800-222-1222
www.mnpoison.org

SIOUX FALLS

Provides education only—Does not manage exposure cases.

Sioux Valley Poison Control Center (*)

1305 W. 18th St.
Box 5039
Sioux Falls, SD 57117-5039
Business: 605-328-6670
www.sdpoison.org

TENNESSEE
NASHVILLE

Tennessee Poison Center (*)

1161 21st Ave. South
501 Oxford House
Nashville, TN 37232-4632
Business: 615-936-0760
Emergency: 800-222-1222
www.poisonlifeline.org

TEXAS
AMARILLO

Texas Panhandle Poison Center (*)
Northwest Texas Hospital

1501 S. Coulter Dr.
Amarillo, TX 79106
Business: 806-354-1630
Emergency: 800-222-1222
www.poisoncontrol.org

DALLAS

North Texas Poison Center (*)
Texas Poison Center Network
Parkland Health and Hospital System

5201 Harry Hines Blvd.
Dallas, TX 75235
Business: 214-589-0911
Emergency: 800-222-1222
www.poisoncontrol.org

EL PASO

West Texas Regional Poison Center (*)
Thomason Hospital

4815 Alameda Ave.
El Paso, TX 79905
Business 915-534-3800
Emergency: 800-222-1222
www.poisoncontrol.org

GALVESTON

Southeast Texas Poison Center (*)
The University of Texas Medical Branch

3.112 Trauma Bldg.
301 University Ave.
Galveston, TX 77555-1175
Business: 409-766-4403
Emergency: 800-222-1222
www.poisoncontrol.org

SAN ANTONIO

South Texas Poison Center (*)
The University of Texas Health Science Center–San Antonio

7703 Floyd Curl Dr., MC 7849
San Antonio, TX 78229-3900
Business: 210-567-5762
Emergency: 800-222-1222
www.poisoncontrol.org

TEMPLE

Central Texas Poison Center (*)
Scott & White Memorial Hospital

2401 South 31st St.
Temple, TX 76508
Business: 254-724-7401
Emergency: 800-222-1222
www.poisoncontrol.org

UTAH
SALT LAKE CITY

Utah Poison Control Center (*)

585 Komas Dr.
Suite 200
Salt Lake City, UT 84108
Business: 801-587-0600
Emergency: 800-222-1222
 801-587-0600 (UT)
http://uuhsc.utah.edu/poison

VERMONT
(PORTLAND, ME)

Northern New England Poison Center

Maine Medical Center
22 Bramhall St.
Portland, ME 04102
Business: 207-662-7220
Emergency: 800-222-1222
www.nnepc.org

A33

POISON CONTROL CENTERS

VIRGINIA
CHARLOTTESVILLE

Blue Ridge Poison Center (*)
University of Virginia Health System

P.O. Box 800774
Charlottesville, VA 22908-0774
Business: 434-924-0347
Emergency: 800-222-1222
www.healthsystem.virginia.edu.
  brpc

RICHMOND

Virginia Poison Center (*)
Virginia Commonwealth University

P.O. Box 980522
Richmond, VA 23298-0522
Business: 804-828-4780
Emergency: 800-222-1222
              804-828-9123
www.vcu.edu/mcved/vpc

WASHINGTON
SEATTLE

Washington Poison Center (*)

155 NE 100th St.
Suite 400
Seattle, WA 98125-8011
Business: 206-517-2350
Emergency: 800-222-1222
              206-526-2121 (WA)
TDD: 800-572-0638 (WA)
www.wapc.org

WEST VIRGINIA
CHARLESTON

West Virginia Poison Center (*)

3110 MacCorkle Ave. SE
Charleston, WV 25304
Business: 304-347-1212
Emergency: 800-222-1222
www.wvpoisoncenter.org

WISCONSIN
MILWAUKEE

Children's Hospital of Wisconsin
Statewide Poison Center

9000 W. Wisconsin Ave.
P.O. Box 1997, Mail Station 677A
Milwaukee, WI 53226
Business: 414-266-2952
Emergency: 800-222-1222
TDD/TTY: 414-266-2542
www.chw.org

Wyoming
(OMAHA, NE)

The Poison Center (*)
Children's Hospital

8401 W. Dodge St., Suite 115
Omaha, NE 68114
Business: 402-955-5555
Emergency: 800-222-1222
www.nebraskapoison.com

ACNE PRODUCTS

BRAND	INGREDIENT/STRENGTH	DOSE
BENZOYL PEROXIDE		
Clean & Clear Continuous Control Acne Cleanser	Benzoyl Peroxide 10%	**Adults & Peds:** Use bid.
Clean & Clear Persa-Gel 10, Maximum Strength	Benzoyl Peroxide 10%	**Adults & Peds:** Use qd-tid.
Clearasil Daily Acne Control cream	Benzoyl Peroxide 10%	**Adults & Peds:** Use qd-tid.
Clearasil Maximum Strength Acne Treatment vanishing cream	Benzoyl Peroxide 10%	**Adults & Peds:** Use qd-tid.
Clearasil Total Control Acne Crisis Clear Up	Benzoyl Peroxide 10%	**Adults & Peds:** Use qd-tid.
Clearasil Ultra Acne Treatment tinted cream	Benzoyl Peroxide 10%	**Adults & Peds:** Use tid.
Clearasil Ultra Acne Treatment vanishing cream	Benzoyl Peroxide 10%	**Adults & Peds:** Use tid.
Neutrogena Clear Pore Cleanser Mask	Benzoyl Peroxide 3.5%	**Adults & Peds:** Use biw-tiw.
Neutrogena On-the-Spot Acne Treatment vanishing cream	Benzoyl Peroxide 2.5%	**Adults & Peds:** Apply qd initially, then bid-tid.
Oxy 10 Balance Oil-Free Maximum Strength Acne Wash	Benzoyl Peroxide 10%	**Adults & Peds:** Use bid-tid.
Oxy Balance Acne Treatment for Sensitive Skin vanishing cream	Benzoyl Peroxide 5%	**Adults & Peds:** Use qd-tid.
Oxy Balance Maximum Acne Treatment tinted lotion	Benzoyl Peroxide 10%	**Adults & Peds:** Use qd-tid.
Oxy Spot Treatment	Benzoyl Peroxide 10%	**Adults & Peds:** Use qd-tid.
PanOxyl Aqua Gel Maximum Strength gel	Benzoyl Peroxide 10%	**Adults & Peds:** Apply qd initially, then bid-tid.
PanOxyl Bar 10% Maximum Strength	Benzoyl Peroxide 10%	**Adults & Peds:** Apply qd initially, then bid-tid.
PanOxyl Bar 5%	Benzoyl Peroxide 5%	**Adults & Peds:** Use qd initially, then bid-tid.
ZAPZYT Maximum Strength Acne Treatment gel	Benzoyl Peroxide 10%	**Adults & Peds:** Use qd-tid.
ZAPZYT Treatment Bar	Benzoyl Peroxide 10%	**Adults & Peds:** Use qd-tid.
SALICYLIC ACID		
Aveeno Clear Complexion Cleansing Bar	Salicylic Acid 0.5%	**Adults & Peds:** Use daily.
Aveeno Clear Complexion Foaming Cleanser	Salicylic Acid 0.5%	**Adults & Peds:** Use daily.
Aveeno Correcting Treatment, Clear Complexion	Salicylic Acid 1%	**Adults & Peds:** Use qd-tid.
Biore Blemish Fighting Cleansing Cloths	Salicylic Acid 0.5%	**Adults & Peds:** Use qd.
Biore Blemish Fighting Ice Cleanser	Salicylic Acid 2%	**Adults & Peds:** Use qd.
Bye Bye Blemish Acne Lemon Scrub	Salicylic Acid 1%	**Adults & Peds:** Use qd-tid.
Bye Bye Blemish Anti-Acne Moisturizer	Salicylic Acid 0.5%	**Adults & Peds:** Use qd-tid.
Bye Bye Blemish Anti-Acne Serum	Salicylic Acid 1%	**Adults & Peds:** Use qd-tid.
Bye Bye Blemish Drying Lotion	Salicylic Acid 2%	**Adults & Peds:** Use pm.

(Continued)

ACNE PRODUCTS

BRAND	INGREDIENT/STRENGTH	DOSE
SALICYLIC ACID *(Continued)*		
Bye Bye Blemish Purifying Acne Mask	Salicylic Acid 0.5%	**Adults & Peds:** Use qd.
Clean & Clear Advantage Acne Cleanser	Salicylic Acid 2%	**Adults & Peds:** Use qd.
Clean & Clear Advantage Acne Spot Treatment	Salicylic Acid 2%	**Adults & Peds:** Use qd.
Clean & Clear Advantage Daily Cleansing Pads	Salicylic Acid 2%	**Adults & Peds:** Use qd.
Clean & Clear Blackhead Clearing Astringent	Salicylic Acid 1%	**Adults & Peds:** Use qd.
Clean & Clear Blackhead Clearing Daily Cleansing Pads	Salicylic Acid 1%	**Adults & Peds:** Use qd.
Clean & Clear Blackhead Clearing Scrub	Salicylic Acid 2%	**Adults & Peds:** Use qd.
Clean & Clear Clear Advantage Daily Acne Clearing lotion	Salicylic Acid 1%	**Adults & Peds:** Use qd.
Clean & Clear Continuous Control Acne Wash, Oil Free	Salicylic Acid 2%	**Adults & Peds:** Use qd.
Clean & Clear Facial Cleansing Bar, Blackhead Clearing	Salicylic Acid 0.5%	**Adults & Peds:** Use qd.
Clean & Clear Oil-Free Dual Action Moisturizer lotion	Salicylic Acid 0.5%	**Adults & Peds:** Use qd-tid.
Clearasil 3 in 1 Acne Defense Cleanser	Salicylic Acid 2%	**Adults & Peds:** Use qd-tid.
Clearasil Acne Fighting Cleansing Wipes	Salicylic Acid 2%	**Adults & Peds:** Use qd.
Clearasil Acne Fighting Facial Moisturizer	Salicylic Acid 2%	**Adults & Peds:** Use qd-tid.
Clearasil Acne Fighting Foaming Cleanser	Salicylic Acid 2%	**Adults & Peds:** Use qd-tid.
Clearasil Blackhead Clearing Pads with Targeted Action	Salicylic Acid 2%	**Adults & Peds:** Use qd-tid.
Clearasil Blackhead Clearing Scrub	Salicylic Acid 2%	**Adults & Peds:** Use qd.
Clearasil Daily Acne Control Pore Cleansing Pads	Salicylic Acid 2%	**Adults & Peds:** Use qd.
Clearasil Daily Blackhead Control Astringent	Salicylic Acid 1%	**Adults & Peds:** Use qd.
Clearasil Daily Oil Control Cream Cleanser	Salicylic Acid 1%	**Adults & Peds:** Use qd.
Clearasil Icewash, Acne Gel Cleanser	Salicylic Acid 2%	**Adults & Peds:** Use qd.
Clearasil Maximum Strength Pore Cleansing Pads	Salicylic Acid 2%	**Adults & Peds:** Use qd-tid.
Clearasil Oil Control Acne Wash	Salicylic Acid 2%	**Adults & Peds:** Use qd.
Clearasil Overnight Acne Defense Gel	Salicylic Acid 2%	**Adults & Peds:** Use qd-tid.
Clearasil Total Control Daily Skin Perfecting Treatment	Salicylic Acid 0.5%	**Adults & Peds:** Use qd.
Clearasil Total Control Deep Pore Cream Cleanser	Salicylic Acid 2%	**Adults & Peds:** Use qd.
Clearasil Ultra Acne Clearing Scrub	Salicylic Acid 2%	**Adults & Peds:** Use qd.
Clearasil Ultra Deep Pore Cleansing Pads	Salicylic Acid 2%	**Adults & Peds:** Use qd-tid.
L'Oreal Pure Zone Pore Unclogging Scrub Cleanser	Salicylic Acid 1%	**Adults & Peds:** Use bid.
L'Oreal Pure Zone Skin Clearing Foaming Cleanser	Salicylic Acid 2%	**Adults & Peds:** Use bid.

(Continued)

ACNE PRODUCTS

BRAND	INGREDIENT/STRENGTH	DOSE
SALICYLIC ACID *(Continued)*		
Neutrogena Clear Pore Treatment - Night Time	Salicylic Acid 2%	**Adults & Peds:** Use qd.
Neutrogena Advanced Solutions Acne Mark Fading Peel with CelluZyme	Salicylic Acid 2%	**Adults & Peds:** Use qw-tiw.
Neutrogena Blackhead Eliminating Astringent	Salicylic Acid 0.5%	**Adults & Peds:** Use qd.
Neutrogena Blackhead Eliminating Daily Scrub	Salicylic Acid 2%	**Adults & Peds:** Use prn.
Neutrogena Blackhead Eliminating Treatment Mask	Salicylic Acid 0.5%	**Adults & Peds:** Use biw-tiw.
Neutrogena Body Clear Body Scrub	Salicylic Acid 2%	**Adults & Peds:** Use qd.
Neutrogena Body Clear Body Wash	Salicylic Acid 2%	**Adults & Peds:** Use qd.
Neutrogena Clear Pore Oil-Controlling Astringent	Salicylic Acid 2%	**Adults & Peds:** Use qd-tid.
Neutrogena Maximum Strength Oil Controlling Pads	Salicylic Acid 2%	**Adults & Peds:** Use qd-tid.
Neutrogena Multi-Vitamin Acne Treatment	Salicylic Acid 1.5%	**Adults & Peds:** Use prn.
Neutrogena Oil Free Acne Stress Control Power Clear scrub	Salicylic Acid 2%	**Adults & Peds:** Use qd.
Neutrogena Oil Free Acne Stress Control Power Foam wash	Salicylic Acid 2%	**Adults & Peds:** Use qd.
Neutrogena Acne Stress Control 3-in-1 Hydrating Acne Treatment	Salicylic Acid 2%	**Adults & Peds:** Use qd.
Neutrogena Oil Free Acne Wash Cleansing Cloths	Salicylic Acid 2%	**Adults & Peds:** Use qd.
Neutrogena Oil Free Acne Wash Cream Cleanser	Salicylic Acid 2%	**Adults & Peds:** Use qd.
Neutrogena Rapid Clear Acne Defense Lotion	Salicylic Acid 2%	**Adults & Peds:** Use qd-tid.
Neutrogena Rapid Clear Acne Eliminating Gel	Salicylic Acid 2%	**Adults & Peds:** Use qd-tid.
Neutrogena Skin Clearing Face Wash	Salicylic Acid 1.5%	**Adults & Peds:** Use bid.
Neutrogena Skin Clearing Moisturizer	Salicylic Acid 2%	**Adults & Peds:** Use prn.
Noxzema Continuous Clean Clarifying Toner	Salicylic Acid 2%	**Adults & Peds:** Use qd-tid.
Noxzema Continuous Clean Deep Foaming Cleanser	Salicylic Acid 2%	**Adults & Peds:** Use qd.
Noxzema Continuous Clean Microbead Cleanser	Salicylic Acid 2%	**Adults & Peds:** Use qd.
Noxzema Triple Clean Pads	Salicylic Acid 2%	**Adults & Peds:** Use qd-tid.
Olay Daily Facials Clarity Daily Scrub	Salicylic Acid 2%	**Adults & Peds:** Apply qd.
Olay Daily Facials Clarity, Purifying Toner	Salicylic Acid 2%	**Adults & Peds:** Apply qd-tid.
Olay Daily Facials Night Cleansing Cloths	Salicylic Acid 2%	**Adults & Peds:** Apply qd-tid.
Olay Daily Facials Self-Foaming Discs	Salicylic Acid 2%	**Adults & Peds:** Apply qd-tid.
Oxy Balance Daily Cleansing Pads, Sensitive Skin	Salicylic Acid 0.5%	**Adults & Peds:** Use qd-tid.
Oxy Balance Deep Pore Cleansing Pads, Gentle	Salicylic Acid 0.5%	**Adults & Peds:** Use qd-tid.

(Continued)

ACNE PRODUCTS

BRAND	INGREDIENT/STRENGTH	DOSE
SALICYLIC ACID *(Continued)*		
Oxy Deep Pore Acne Medicated Cleansing Pads, Maximum Strength	Salicylic Acid 2%	**Adults & Peds:** Use qd-tid.
Oxy Body Wash	Salicylic Acid 2%	**Adults & Peds:** Use qd.
Phisoderm Anti-Blemish Gel Facial Wash	Salicylic Acid 2%	**Adults & Peds:** Use qd.
St. Ives Medicated Apricot Scrub	Salicylic Acid 2%	**Adults & Peds:** Use qd.
Stridex Facewipes to Go with Acne Medication	Salicylic Acid 0.5%	**Adults & Peds:** Use qd-tid.
Stridex Triple Action Acne Pads Maximum Strength, Alcohol Free	Salicylic Acid 2%	**Adults & Peds:** Use qd-tid.
Stridex Triple Action Acne Pads with Salicylic Acid, Super Scrub	Salicylic Acid 0.5%	**Adults & Peds:** Use qd-tid.
Stridex Triple Action Medicated Acne Pads, Sensitive Skin	Salicylic Acid 0.5%	**Adults & Peds:** Use qd-tid.
ZAPZYT Acne Wash Treatment For Face & Body	Salicylic Acid 2%	**Adults & Peds:** Use bid.
ZAPZYT Acne Wash with Soothing Aloe & Chamomile	Salicylic Acid 2%	**Adults & Peds:** Use qd-tid.
ZAPZYT Pore Treatment Gel	Salicylic Acid 2%	**Adults & Peds:** Use qd-tid.

Antiseborrheal Products

BRAND	INGREDIENT/STRENGTH	DOSE
COAL TAR		
DHS Tar Dermatological Hair & Scalp Shampoo	Coal Tar 0.5%	**Adults & Peds:** Use biw.
DHS Tar Shampoo	Coal Tar 0.5%	**Adults & Peds:** Use at least biw.
Neutrogena T/Gel Shampoo Orignial Formula	Coal Tar 0.5%	**Adults & Peds:** Use at least biw.
Neutrogena T/Gel Stubborn Itch Shampoo	Coal Tar 0.5%	**Adults & Peds:** Use at least biw.
Polytar shampoo	Coal Tar 0.5%	**Adults & Peds:** Use at least biw.
Polytar soap	Coal Tar 0.5%	**Adults & Peds:** Apply to affected area prn.
Psoriasin Liquid dab-on	Coal Tar 0.66%	**Adults:** Apply to affected area qd-qid.
Ionil-T Shampoo	Coal Tar 1%	**Adults & Peds:** Use at least biw.
Neutrogena T/Gel Shampoo Extra Strength	Coal Tar 1%	**Adults & Peds:** Use at least biw.
Psoriasin gel	Coal Tar 1.25%	**Adults:** Apply to affected area qd-qid.
Ionil-T Plus Shampoo	Coal Tar 2%	**Adults & Peds:** Use at least biw.
MG217 Ointment	Coal Tar 2%	**Adults & Peds:** Apply to affected area qd-qid.
Denorex Therapeutic Protection 2-in-1 shampoo	Coal Tar 2.5%	**Adults & Peds:** Use at least biw.
Denorex Therapeutic Protection shampoo	Coal Tar 2.5%	**Adults & Peds:** Use at least biw.
MG217 Tar Shampoo	Coal Tar 3%	**Adults & Peds:** Use at least biw.
Ionil T Therapeutic Coal Tar Shampoo	Coal Tar 5%	**Adults & Peds:** Use biw.
CORTICOSTEROIDS		
Aveeno Anti-Itch Cream 1%	Hydrocortisone 1%	**Adults & Peds:** ≥2 yrs: Apply to affected area tid-qid.
Cortaid Advanced 12-Hour Anti-Itch Cream	Hydrocortisone 1%	**Adults & Peds:** ≥2 yrs: Apply to affected area tid-qid.
Cortaid Intensive Therapy Cooling Spray	Hydrocortisone 1%	**Adults & Peds:** ≥2 yrs: Apply to affected area tid-qid.
Cortaid Intensive Therapy Moisturizing Cream	Hydrocortisone 1%	**Adults & Peds:** ≥2 yrs: Apply to affected area tid-qid.
Cortaid Maximum Strength Cream	Hydrocortisone 1%	**Adults & Peds:** ≥2 yrs: Apply to affected area tid-qid.
Cortaid Maximum Strength Ointment	Hydrocortisone 1%	**Adults & Peds:** ≥2 yrs: Apply to affected area tid-qid.
Cortizone-10 Cream	Hydrocortisone 1%	**Adults & Peds:** ≥2 yrs: Apply to affected area tid-qid.
Cortizone-10 Maximum Strength Anti-Itch Ointment	Hydrocortisone 1%	**Adults & Peds:** ≥2 yrs: Apply to affected area tid-qid.
Cortizone-10 Ointment	Hydrocortisone 1%	**Adults & Peds:** ≥2 yrs: Apply to affected area tid-qid.
Cortizone-10 Plus Maximum Strength Cream	Hydrocortisone 1%	**Adults & Peds:** ≥2 yrs: Apply to affected area tid-qid.
Cortizone-10 Quick Shot Spray	Hydrocortisone 1%	**Adults & Peds:** ≥2 yrs: Apply to affected area tid-qid.

(Continued)

Antiseborrheal Products

BRAND	INGREDIENT/STRENGTH	DOSE
PYRITHIONE ZINC		
Denorex Dandruff Shampoo, Daily Protection	Pyrithione Zinc 2%	**Adults & Peds:** Use biw.
Garnier Fructis Fortifying Shampoo, Anti-Dandruff	Pyrithione Zinc 1%	**Adults & Peds:** Use biw.
Head & Shoulders Dandruff Conditioner, Dry Scalp Care	Pyrithione Zinc 0.5%	**Adults & Peds:** Use biw.
Head & Shoulders Dandruff Conditioner, Extra Fullness	Pyrithione Zinc 0.5%	**Adults & Peds:** Use biw.
Head & Shoulders Dandruff Shampoo Plus Conditioner, Smooth & Silky	Pyrithione Zinc 1%	**Adults & Peds:** Use biw.
Head & Shoulders Dandruff Shampoo, Citrus Breeze	Pyrithione Zinc 1%	**Adults & Peds:** Use biw.
Head & Shoulders Dandruff Shampoo, Classic Clean	Pyrithione Zinc 1%	**Adults & Peds:** Use biw.
Head & Shoulders Dandruff Shampoo, Dry Scalp Care	Pyrithione Zinc 1%	**Adults & Peds:** Use biw.
Head & Shoulders Dandruff Shampoo, Extra Volume	Pyrithione Zinc 1%	**Adults & Peds:** Use biw.
Head & Shoulders Dandruff Shampoo, Ocean Lift	Pyrithione Zinc 1%	**Adults & Peds:** Use biw.
Head & Shoulders Dandruff Shampoo, Refresh	Pyrithione Zinc 1%	**Adults & Peds:** Use biw.
Head & Shoulders Dandruff Shampoo, Restoring Shine	Pyrithione Zinc 1%	**Adults & Peds:** Use biw.
Head & Shoulders Dandruff Shampoo, Sensitive Care	Pyrithione Zinc 1%	**Adults & Peds:** Use biw.
Head & Shoulders Dandruff Shampoo, Smooth & Silky	Pyrithione Zinc 1%	**Adults & Peds:** Use biw.
L'Oreal VIVE for Men Shampoo, Thickening Anti-Dandruff	Pyrithione Zinc 1%	**Adults & Peds:** Use biw.
Neutrogena T-Gel Daily Control Dandruff Shampoo	Pyrithione Zinc 1%	**Adults & Peds:** Use biw.
Pantene Pro-V Shampoo + Conditioner, Anti-Dandruff	Pyrithione Zinc 1%	**Adults & Peds:** Use biw.
Pert Plus Shampoo Plus Conditioner, Dandruff Control	Pyrithione Zinc 1%	**Adults & Peds:** Use biw.
Selsun Blue Dandruff Conditioner	Pyrithione Zinc 0.75%	**Adults & Peds:** Use biw.
Suave for Men 2 in 1 Shampoo/Conditioner, Dandruff	Pyrithione Zinc 0.5%	**Adults & Peds:** Use biw.
SALICYLIC ACID		
Neutrogena T/Gel Conditioner	Salicylic Acid 2%	**Adults & Peds:** Use at least biw.
Psoriasin Therapeutic Body Wash With Aloe	Salicylic Acid 3%	**Adults & Peds:** Use biw.
Psoriasin Therapeutic Shampoo With Panthenol	Salicylic Acid 3%	**Adults & Peds:** Use biw.
Neutrogena T/Sal Shampoo, Scalp Build-up Control	Salicylic Acid 3%	**Adults & Peds:** Use biw.
Scalpicin Anti-Itch Liquid Scalp Treatment (Combe)	Salicylic Acid 3%	**Adults:** Apply to affected area qd-qid.
SALICYLIC ACID/SULFUR/COAL TAR		
Sebex-T Tar Shampoo	Salicylic acid/sulfur/coal tar 2%-2%-5%	**Adults & Peds:** Use qw to biw.
Sebutone	Salicylic acid/sulfur/coal tar 2%-2%-1.5%	**Adults & Peds:** Use qw to biw.

(Continued)

ANTISEBORRHEAL PRODUCTS

BRAND	INGREDIENT/STRENGTH	DOSE
SELENIUM SULFIDE		
Head & Shoulders Dandruff Shampoo, Intensive Treatment	Selenium Sulfide 1%	**Adults & Peds:** Use biw.
Selsun Blue Dandruff Shampoo, Medicated Treatment	Selenium Sulfide 1%	**Adults & Peds:** Use biw.
Selsun Blue Dandruff Shampoo Plus Conditioner	Selenium Sulfide 1%	**Adults & Peds:** Use biw.
	Selenium Sulfide 1%	**Adults & Peds:** Use biw.
Selsun Blue Dandruff Shampoo, Balanced Treatment	Selenium Sulfide 1%	**Adults & Peds:** Use biw.
	Selenium Sulfide 1%	**Adults & Peds:** Use biw.
Selsun Blue Dandruff Shampoo, Moisturizing Treatment	Selenium Sulfide 1%	**Adults & Peds:** Use biw.
SULFUR/SALICYLIC ACID		
Sebulex Medicated Dandruff Shampoo	Sulfur/Salicylic Acid 2%-2%	**Adults & Peds:** Use qd.

Contact Dermatitis Products

BRAND	INGREDIENT/STRENGTH	DOSE
ANTIHISTAMINE		
Benadryl Extra Strength Gel Pump	Diphenhydramine HCl 2%	**Adults & Peds ≥12 yrs:** Apply to affected area tid-qid.
ANTIHISTAMINE COMBINATION		
Benadryl Extra Strength Cream	Diphenhydramine HCl/Zinc Acetate 2%-0.1%	**Adults & Peds ≥12 yrs:** Apply to affected area tid-qid.
Benadryl Extra Strength Spray	Diphenhydramine HCl/Zinc Acetate 2%-0.1%	**Adults & Peds ≥12 yrs:** Apply to affected area tid-qid.
Benadryl Itch Relief Spray	Diphenhydramine HCl/Zinc Acetate 2%-0.1%	**Adults & Peds ≥2 yrs:** Apply to affected area tid-qid.
Benadryl Itch Relief Stick	Diphenhydramine HCl/Zinc Acetate 2%-0.1%	**Adults & Peds ≥2 yrs:** Apply to affected area tid-qid.
Benadryl Original Cream	Diphenhydramine HCl/Zinc Acetate 1%-0.1%	**Adults & Peds ≥2 yrs:** Apply to affected area tid-qid.
CalaGel Anti-Itch Gel	Diphenhydramine HCl/Zinc Acetate/Benzethonium Chloride 2%-0.215%-15%	**Adults & Peds ≥2 yrs:** Apply to affected area tid-qid.
Ivarest Anti-Itch Cream	Diphenhydramine HCl/Calamine 2%-14%	**Adults & Peds ≥2 yrs:** Apply to affected area tid-qid.
ASTRINGENT		
Domeboro Powder Packets	Aluminum Acetate/Aluminum Sulfate 938mg-1191mg	**Adults & Peds:** Dissolve 1-2 packets and apply to affected area for 15-30 min tid.
Ivy-Dry Super Lotion Extra Strength	Zinc Acetate/Benzyl Alcohol 2%-10%	**Adults & Peds: ≥ 6 yrs:** Apply to affected area qd-tid.
ASTRINGENT COMBINATION		
Aveeno Anti-Itch Cream	Calamine/Pramoxine HCl 3%-1%	**Adults & Peds ≥2 yrs:** Apply to affected area tid-qid.
Aveeno Anti-Itch Lotion	Calamine/Pramoxine HCl/Camphor 3%-1%-0.47%	**Adults & Peds ≥2 yrs:** Apply to affected area tid-qid.
Caladryl Clear Lotion	Zinc Acetate/Pramoxine HCl 0.1%-1%	**Adults & Peds ≥2 yrs:** Apply to affected area tid-qid.
Caladryl Lotion	Calamine/Pramoxine HCl 8%-1%	**Adults & Peds ≥2 yrs:** Apply to affected area tid-qid.
Calamine lotion (generic)	Calamine/Zinc Oxide 6.971%-6.971%	**Adults & Peds:** Apply to affected area prn.
CLEANSER		
Ivy-Dry Scrub	Polyethylene, sodium lauryl sulfoacetate, cetearyl alcohol, nonoxynol-9, camellia sinensis oil, phenoxyethanol, methylparaben, propylparaben, triethanolamine, carbomer, erythorbic acid, aloe barbadensis extract, tocopheryl acetate extract, tetrasodium EDTA	**Adults & Peds:** Wash affected area prn.
IvyStat! Gel/Exfoliant	Hydrocortisone 1% (gel); Cocamidopropyl-sultaine, PEG-4 laurate, cocamide DEA, polyethylene beads, sodium chloride, benzethonium chloride (cleanser)	**Adults & Peds:** Apply to affected area tid-qid.
CORTICOSTEROID		
Aveeno Anti-Itch Cream 1%	Hydrocortisone 1%	**Adults & Peds ≥2 yrs:** Apply to affected area tid-qid.
Cortaid Advanced 12-Hour Anti-Itch Cream	Hydrocortisone 1%	**Adults & Peds ≥2 yrs:** Apply to affected area tid-qid.
Cortaid Intensive Therapy Cooling Spray	Hydrocortisone 1%	**Adults & Peds ≥2 yrs:** Apply to affected area tid-qid.
Cortaid Intensive Therapy Moisturizing Cream	Hydrocortisone 1%	**Adults & Peds ≥2 yrs:** Apply to affected area tid-qid.
Cortaid Maximum Strength Cream	Hydrocortisone 1%	**Adults & Peds ≥2 yrs:** Apply to affected area tid-qid.

(Continued)

Contact Dermatitis Products

BRAND	INGREDIENT/STRENGTH	DOSE
Cortaid Maximum Strength Ointment	Hydrocortisone 1%	**Adults & Peds ≥2 yrs:** Apply to affected area tid-qid.
Cortizone-10 Cream	Hydrocortisone 1%	**Adults & Peds ≥2 yrs:** Apply to affected area tid-qid.
Cortizone-10 Maximum Strength Anti-Itch Ointment	Hydrocortisone 1%	**Adults & Peds ≥2 yrs:** Apply to affected area tid-qid.
Cortizone-10 Ointment	Hydrocortisone 1%	**Adults & Peds ≥2 yrs:** Apply to affected area tid-qid.
Cortizone-10 Plus Maximum Strength Cream	Hydrocortisone 1%	**Adults & Peds ≥2 yrs:** Apply to affected area tid-qid.
Cortizone-10 Quick Shot Spray	Hydrocortisone 1%	**Adults & Peds ≥2 yrs:** Apply to affected area tid-qid.
Dermarest Eczema Lotion	Hydrocortisone 1%	**Adults & Peds ≥2 yrs:** Apply to affected area tid-qid.
COUNTERIRRITANT		
Gold Bond First Aid Quick Spray	Menthol/Benzethonium Chloride 1%-0.13%	**Adults & Peds ≥2 yrs:** Apply to affected area tid-qid.
Gold Bond Medicated Maximum Strength Anti-Itch Cream	Menthol/Pramoxine HCl 1%-1%	**Adults & Peds ≥2 yrs:** Apply to affected area tid-qid.
Ivy Block Lotion	Bentoquatam 5%	**Adults & Peds ≥2 yrs:** Apply q4h for continued protection.
LOCAL ANESTHETIC		
Solarcaine Aloe Extra Burn Relief Gel	Lidocaine HCl 0.5%	**Adults & Peds ≥2 yrs:** Apply to affected area tid-qid.
Solarcaine Aloe Extra Spray	Lidocaine HCl 0.5%	**Adults & Peds ≥2 yrs:** Apply to affected area tid-qid.
Solarcaine First Aid Medicated Spray	Benzocaine/Triclosan 20%-0.13%	**Adults & Peds ≥2 yrs:** Apply to affected area qd-tid.
LOCAL ANESTHETIC COMBINATION		
Bactine First Aid Liquid	Lidocaine HCl/Benzalkonium Chloride 2.5%-0.13%	**Adults & Peds ≥2 yrs:** Apply to affected area qd-tid.
Bactine Pain Relieving Cleansing Spray	Lidocaine HCl/Benzalkonium Chloride 2.5%-0.13%	**Adults & Peds ≥2 yrs:** Apply to affected area qd-tid.
Lanacane Maximum Strength Cream	Benzocaine/Benzethonium Chloride 20%-0.2%	**Adults & Peds ≥2 yrs:** Apply to affected area qd-tid.
Lanacane Maximum Strength Spray	Benzocaine/Benzethonium Chloride/Ethanol 20%-0.2%-36%	**Adults & Peds ≥2 yrs:** Apply to affected area qd-tid.
Lanacane Original Formula Cream	Benzocaine/Benzethonium Chloride 6%-0.2%	**Adults & Peds ≥2 yrs:** Apply to affected area qd-tid.
SKIN PROTECTANT		
Aveeno Skin Relief Moisturizing Cream	Dimethicone 2.5%	**Adults & Peds:** Apply to affected area prn.
SKIN PROTECTANT COMBINATION		
Aveeno Itch Relief Lotion	Dimethicone/Menthol 2.5%-0.1%	**Adults & Peds ≥2 yrs:** Apply to affected area tid-qid.
Gold Bond Extra Strength Medicated Body Lotion	Dimethicone/Menthol 5%-0.5%	**Adults & Peds:** Apply to affected area prn.
Gold Bond Medicated Body Lotion	Dimethicone/Menthol 5%-0.15%	**Adults & Peds:** Apply to affected area prn.
Gold Bond Medicated Extra Strength Powder	Zinc Oxide/Menthol 5%-0.8%	**Adults & Peds ≥2 yrs:** Apply to affected area tid-qid.
Vaseline Intensive Care Lotion Advanced Healing	Dimethicone 1%-White Petrolatum	**Adults & Peds:** Apply to affected area prn.

Dandruff Products

BRAND	INGREDIENT/STRENGTH	DOSE
COAL TAR		
Denorex Dandruff Shampoo + Conditioner, Therapeutic	Coal Tar 2.5%	**Adults & Peds:** Use biw.
DHS Tar Dermatological Hair & Scalp Shampoo	Coal Tar 0.5%	**Adults & Peds:** Use biw.
Ionil T Therapeutic Coal Tar Shampoo	Coal Tar 2.5%	**Adults & Peds:** Use biw.
Neutrogena T-Gel Original Shampoo	Coal Tar 0.5%	**Adults & Peds:** Use biw.
Neutrogena T-Gel Shampoo, Extra Strength	Coal Tar 1%	**Adults & Peds:** Use biw.
Neutrogena T-Gel Shampoo, Stubborn Itch Control	Coal Tar 0.5%	**Adults & Peds:** Use biw.
KETOCONAZOLE		
Nizoral Anti-Dandruff Shampoo	Ketoconazole 1%	**Adults & Peds $\geq$12:** Use q3-4d prn.
PYRITHIONE ZINC		
Denorex Dandruff Shampoo, Daily Protection	Pyrithione Zinc 2%	**Adults & Peds:** Use biw.
Garnier Fructis Fortifying Shampoo, Anti-Dandruff	Pyrithione Zinc 1%	**Adults & Peds:** Use biw.
Head & Shoulders Dandruff Conditioner, Dry Scalp Care	Pyrithione Zinc 0.5%	**Adults & Peds:** Use biw.
Head & Shoulders Dandruff Conditioner, Extra Fullness	Pyrithione Zinc 0.5%	**Adults & Peds:** Use biw.
Head & Shoulders Dandruff Shampoo Plus Conditioner, Smooth & Silky	Pyrithione Zinc 1%	**Adults & Peds:** Use biw.
Head & Shoulders Dandruff Shampoo, Citrus Breeze	Pyrithione Zinc 1%	**Adults & Peds:** Use biw.
Head & Shoulders Dandruff Shampoo, Classic Clean	Pyrithione Zinc 1%	**Adults & Peds:** Use biw.
Head & Shoulders Dandruff Shampoo, Dry Scalp Care	Pyrithione Zinc 1%	**Adults & Peds:** Use biw.
Head & Shoulders Dandruff Shampoo, Extra Volume	Pyrithione Zinc 1%	**Adults & Peds:** Use biw.
Head & Shoulders Dandruff Shampoo, Ocean Lift	Pyrithione Zinc 1%	**Adults & Peds:** Use biw.
Head & Shoulders Dandruff Shampoo, Refresh	Pyrithione Zinc 1%	**Adults & Peds:** Use biw.
Head & Shoulders Dandruff Shampoo, Restoring Shine	Pyrithione Zinc 1%	**Adults & Peds:** Use biw.
Head & Shoulders Dandruff Shampoo, Sensitive Care	Pyrithione Zinc 1%	**Adults & Peds:** Use biw.
Head & Shoulders Dandruff Shampoo, Smooth & Silky	Pyrithione Zinc 1%	**Adults & Peds:** Use biw.
L'Oreal VIVE for Men Shampoo, Thickening Anti-Dandruff	Pyrithione Zinc 1%	**Adults & Peds:** Use biw.
Neutrogena T-Gel Daily Control Dandruff Shampoo	Pyrithione Zinc 1%	**Adults & Peds:** Use biw.
Pantene Pro-V Shampoo + Conditioner, Anti-Dandruff	Pyrithione Zinc 1%	**Adults & Peds:** Use biw.
Pert Plus Shampoo Plus Conditioner, Dandruff Control	Pyrithione Zinc 1%	**Adults & Peds:** Use biw.
Selsun Blue Dandruff Conditioner	Pyrithione Zinc 0.75%	**Adults & Peds:** Use biw.
Suave for Men 2 in 1 Shampoo/ Conditioner, Dandruff	Pyrithione Zinc 0.5%	**Adults & Peds:** Use biw.

(Continued)

DANDRUFF PRODUCTS

BRAND	INGREDIENT/STRENGTH	DOSE
SALICYLIC ACID		
Denorex Dandruff Shampoo, Extra Strength	Salicylic Acid 3%	**Adults & Peds:** Use biw.
Neutrogena T/Sal Shampoo, Scalp Build-up Control	Salicylic Acid 3%	**Adults & Peds:** Use biw.
Scalpicin Anti-Itch Liquid Scalp Treatment	Salicylic Acid 3%	**Adults & Peds:** Apply to affected area qd-qid.
SELENIUM SULFIDE		
Head & Shoulders Dandruff Shampoo, Intensive Treatment	Selenium Sulfide 1%	**Adults & Peds:** Use biw.
Selsun Blue Dandruff Shampoo, Medicated Treatment	Selenium Sulfide 1%	**Adults & Peds:** Use biw.
Selsun Blue Dandruff Shampoo Plus Conditioner	Selenium Sulfide 1%	**Adults & Peds:** Use biw.
Selsun Blue Dandruff Shampoo, Balanced Treatment	Selenium Sulfide 1%	**Adults & Peds:** Use biw.
Selsun Blue Dandruff Shampoo, Moisturizing Treatment	Selenium Sulfide 1%	**Adults & Peds:** Use biw.
SULFUR/SALICYLIC ACID		
Sebulex Medicated Dandruff Shampoo	Sulfur/Salicylic Acid 2%-2%	**Adults & Peds ≥12yrs:** Use qd.

Diaper Rash Products

BRAND	INGREDIENT/STRENGTH	DOSE
WHITE PETROLATUM		
Balmex Extra Protective Clear Ointment	White Petrolatum 51%	**Peds:** Apply prn.
Vaseline Baby, Baby Fresh Scent	White Petrolatum (strength n/a)	**Peds:** Apply prn.
Vaseline Petroleum Jelly	White Petrolatum (strength n/a)	**Peds:** Apply prn.
ZINC OXIDE		
Aveeno Baby Soothing Relief Diaper Rash Cream	Zinc Oxide 13%	**Peds:** Apply prn.
Balmex Diaper Rash Ointment with Aloe & Vitamin E	Zinc Oxide 11.3%	**Peds:** Apply prn.
Boudreaux's Butt Paste, Diaper Rash Ointment	Zinc Oxide 16%	**Peds:** Apply prn.
California Baby Diaper Rash Cream	Zinc Oxide 12%	**Peds:** Apply prn.
Canus Li'l Goat's Milk Ointment	Zinc Oxide 40%	**Peds:** Apply prn.
Desitin Diaper Rash Ointment, Creamy, Fresh Scent	Zinc Oxide 10%	**Peds:** Apply prn.
Desitin Diaper Rash Ointment, Hypoallergenic	Zinc Oxide 40%	**Peds:** Apply prn.
Huggies Diaper Rash Cream	Zinc Oxide 10%	**Peds:** Apply prn.
Johnson's Baby Diaper Rash Cream with Zinc Oxide	Zinc Oxide 13%	**Peds:** Apply prn.
Mustela Bebe Vitamin Barrier Cream	Zinc Oxide 10%	**Peds:** Apply prn.
Mustela Dermo-Pediatrics, Stelactiv Diaper Rash	Zinc Oxide 10%	**Peds:** Apply prn.
COMBINATION PRODUCTS		
A+D Original Ointment, Diaper Rash and All-Purpose Skincare Formula	Petrolatum/Lanolin 53.4%-15.5%	**Peds:** Apply prn.
A+D Zinc Oxide Diaper Rash Cream with Aloe	Dimethicone/Zinc Oxide 1%-10%	**Peds:** Apply prn.

Dry Skin Products

BRAND	INGREDIENTS	DOSE
AmLactin Moisturizing Cream	Lactic acid, ammonium hydroxide, light mineral oil, glyceryl stearate, PEG-100 stearate, glycerin, propylene glycol, magnesium aluminum silicate, laureth 4, polyoxyl 40 stearate, cetyl alcohol, methylcellulose, methyl and propylparabens	**Adults & Peds:** Apply to affected area bid.
AmLactin Moisturizing Lotion	Lactic acid, ammonium hydroxide, light mineral oil, glyceryl stearate, PEG-100 stearate, glycerin, propylene glycol, magnesium aluminum silicate, laureth 4, polyoxyl 40 stearate, cetyl alcohol, methylcellulose, methyl and propylparabens	**Adults & Peds:** Apply to affected area bid.
AmLactin XL Moisturizing Lotion Ultraplex Formulation	Ammonium lactate, potassium lactate, sodium lactate, emulsifyin wax, light mineral oil, white petrolatum, glycerin, propylene glycol, stearic acid, xanthum gum, methyl and propylparabens	**Adults & Peds:** Apply to affected area bid.
Aquaphor Baby Healing Ointment	Petrolatum, mineral oil, cerein, lanolin alcohol	**Adults & Peds:** Apply to affected area prn.
Aquaphor Original Ointment	Petrolatum, mineral oil, cerein, lanolin alcohol	**Adults & Peds:** Apply to affected area prn.
Aveeno Baby Essential Moisture Bath	Deionized water, cocamidopropyl betaine, decyl glucoside, PEG 80 sorbitan laurate, disodium lauroamphodiacetate, lauryl methyl gluceth 10 hydroxypropyl dimonium chloride, DI PPG 2 myreth-10 adipate, avena sativa kernel extract (oat), hydrolized oats, hydrolized milk protein, hydroxylated milk glycerides, hydrolized soy protein, PEG 25 soy sterol, coco glucoside, glycerol oleate, PEG 150 distearate, glycol distearate, acrylates/c10-30 alkyl acrylate crosspolymer, glycerin, tetrasodium EDTA, laureth-4, polyquaternium 10, PEG 14m, quaternium 15, sodium hydroxide, citric acid, fragrance	**Adults & Peds:** Apply to affected area prn.
Aveeno Baby Moisture Soothing Relief Cream	Glycerin, petrolatum, mineral oil, cetyl alcohol, dimethicone, avena sativa kernel flour, carbomer, sodium hydroxide, ceteareth-6, hydrolyzed milk protein, hydrolyzed oats, hydrolyzed soy protein, PEG-25 soya sterol, tetrasodium EDTA, methylparaben, citric acid, sodium citrate, benzalkonium chloride, benzaldehyde, butylene glycol, butylparaben, ethylparaben, ethyl alcohol, isobutylparaben, phenoxyethanol, propylparaben, stearyl alcohol	**Adults & Peds:** Apply to affected area prn.
Aveeno Bath Moisturizing Packets	Colloidal oatmeal 43%	**Adults & Peds:** Bathe in 1 packet for 15-20 min qd-bid.
Aveeno Daily Baby Lotion	Dimethicone 1.2%	**Peds:** Apply prn.
Aveeno Daily Moisturizer, Ultra-Calming SPF 15	Avobenzone/octinoxate/octisalate 3%-7.5%-2.%	**Adults:** Use qd.
Aveeno Daily Moisturizing Lotion	Dimethicone 1.25%	**Adults:** Use prn.
Aveeno Intense Relief Hand Cream	Glycerin, distearyldimonium chloride, petrolatum, isopropyl palmitate, cetyl alcohol, aluminum starch octenylsuccinate, dimethicone, avena sativa kernel flour, benzyl alcohol, sodium chloride	**Adults & Peds:** Apply to affected area prn.
Aveeno Moisturizing Bar for Dry Skin	Oat flour, cetearyl alcohol, stearic acid, sodium cocoyl isethionate, water, disodium lauryl sulfosuccinate, glycerin, hydrogenated vegetable oil, titanium dioxide, citric acid, sodium trideceth sulfate, hydrogenated castor oil	**Adults & Peds:** Wash face daily.
Aveeno Moisturizing Lotion, Skin Relief	Dimethicone 1.25%	**Adult & Peds:** ≥2 yrs: Use daily.

(Continued)

Dry Skin Products

BRAND	INGREDIENTS	DOSE
Aveeno Positively Radiant Moisturizing Lotion	Glycerin, emulsifying wax, ethylhexyl isononanoate, glycine soja (soybean) seed extract, propylene glycol isoceteth-3 acetate, dimethicone, polyacrylamide, cyclomethicone, stearic acid, phenoxyethanol, c13-14 isoparaffin, dimethicone copolyol, benzyl alcohol, titanium dioxide, fragrance, iodopropynyl butylcarbamate, glyceryl laurate, laureth-7, methylparaben, silica, mica, polymethyl-methacrylate, cetearyl alcohol, tetrasodium EDTA, butylparaben, ethylparaben, isobutylparaben, propylparaben, DMDM hydantoin, panthenyl ethyl ether, tocopheryl acetate, panthenol, BHT, citric acid	**Adults:** Apply daily.
Aveeno Positively Radiant Daily Moisturizer SPF 15	Avobenzone/octinoxate/octisalate arachidyl alcohol, arachidyl glucoside, behenyl alcohol, benzalkonium chloride, benzyl alcohol, BHT, bisphenylpropyl dimethicone, butylparaben, c12-15 alkyl benzoate, c13-14 isoparaffin, cetearyl alcohol, cetearyl glucoside, dimethicone, disodium EDTA, ethylene/acrylic acid copolymer, ethylparaben, fragrance, glycerin, glycine soja (soybean) seed extract, iodopropyl butylcarbamate, isobutylparaben, laureth-7, methylparaben, mica, panthenol, phenoxyethanol, polyacrylamide, polymethyl methacrylate, propylparaben, silica, steareth 2, steareth 21, titanium dioxide, water, sodium hydroxide, citric acid	**Adults:** Use daily.
Aveeno Positively Radiant Daily Cleansing Pads	Cocamidopropyl betaine, decyl glucoside, glycerin, disodium lauroamphodiacetate, PEG-16 soy sterol, polysorbate 20, PPG-2 hydroxyethyl cocamide, phenoxyethanol, tetrasodium EDTA, butylene glycol, sodium coco PG-dimonium chloride phosphate, sodium citrate, glycine soja (soybean) protein, citric acid, PEG-14m, methylparaben, butylparaben, ethylparaben, isobutylparaben, propylparaben, fragrance	**Adults:** Use daily.
Aveeno Positively Smooth Facial Moisturizer	C12-15 alkyl benzoate, cetearyl alcohol, bis-phenylpropyl dimethicone, glycine, soja seed extract, butylene glycol, arachidyl alcohol, glycine soja protein, dimethicone, glycerin, panthenol, polyacrylamide, phenoxyethanol, cetearyl glucoside, behenyl alcohol, benzyl alcohol, C13-14 isoparaffin, DMDM hydantoin, arachidyl glucoside, disodium EDTA, methylparaben, laureth 7, BHT, ethylparaben, butylparaben, propylparaben, isobutylparaben, fragrance, iodopropynyl butylcarbamate	**Adults:** Use prn.
Aveeno Positively Smooth Moisturizing Lotion	Glycerin, emulsifying wax, isononanoate, gylcine soja seed extract, propylene glycol isoceteth-3 acetate, dimethicone, cyclomethicone, polyacrylamide, stearic acid, panthenyl ethyl ether, tocopheryl acetate, panthenol, phenoxyethanol, C13-14 isoparaffin, dimethicone copolyol, benzyl alcohol, DMDM hydantoin, glyceryl laurate, laureth 7, methylparaben, cetearyl alcohol, tetrasodium EDTA, butylparaben, ethylparaben, BHT, propylparaben, isobutylparaben, fragrance, iodopropyl butylcarbamate	**Adults:** Use prn.
Aveeno Positively Smooth Moisturizing Pads	Cocamidopropyl betaine, decyl glucoside, glycerin, disodium lauroamphodiacetate, PEG-16 soy sterol, polysorbate 20, PPG-2 hydroxyethyl cocamide, phenoxyethanol, tetrasodium EDTA, butylene glycol, sodium coco PG-dimonium chloride phosphate, sodium citrate, glycine soja protein, citric acid, PEG-14M, methylparaben, butylparaben, ethylparaben, isobutylparaben, propylparaben, fragrance	**Adults:** Use daily.
Aveeno Radiant Skin Daily Moisturizer with SPF 15	Octinoxate (octyl methoxycinnamate)/avobenzone 3%/octisalate (octyl salicylate) 7.5%-3%-2%	**Adults:** Use prn.
Aveeno Skin Relief Body Wash, Fragrance Free	Glycerin, cocamidopropyl betaine, sodium laureth sulfate, decyl glucoside, oat flour, glycol stearate, sodium lauroampho-PG-acetate phosphate, guar hydroxypropyltrimonium chloride, hydroxypropyltrimonium hydrolyzed wheat protein, PEG 20 glycerides, hydroxypropyltrimonium hydrolyzed wheat starch, PEG 150 pentaerythrityl tetrastearate, PEG 120 methyl glucose trioleate, tetrasodium EDTA, PEG-6 caprylic/capric glyceride, quaternium 15, coriandum sativum extract, elettaria cardamomum seed extract, conmiphora myhrrha extract	**Adults:** Use prn.

(Continued)

DRY SKIN PRODUCTS

BRAND	INGREDIENTS	DOSE
Carmol-10 Lotion	Urea 10%	**Adults & Peds:** Apply to affected area qd-bid.
Carmol-20 Cream	Urea 20%	**Adults & Peds:** Apply to affected area qd-bid.
Cetaphil Daily Facial Moisturizer SPF 15	Avobenzone 3%, octocrylene 10%, diisopropyl adipate, cyclomethicone, glyceryl stearate, PEG-100 stearate, glycerin, polymethyl methacrylate, phenoxyethanol, benzyl alcohol, acrylates/C10-30 alkyl acrylate crosspolymer, tocopheryl acetate, carbomer 940, disodium EDTA, triethanolamine	**Adults & Peds:** Apply to affected area prn.
Cetaphil Moisturizing Cream	Glyceryl polymethacrylate, propylene glycol, petrolatum, dicaprylyl ether, PEG-5 glyceryl stearate, glycerin, dimethicone, dimethiconol, cetyl alcohol, sweet almond oil, acrylates/C10-30 alkylacrylate crosspolymer, tocopheryl acetate, phenoxyethanol, benzyl alcohol, disodium EDTA, sodium hydroxide, lactic acid	**Adults & Peds:** Apply to affected area prn.
Cetaphil Moisturizing Lotion	Glycerin, hydrogenated polyisobutene, cetearyl alcohol, ceteareth-20, macadamia nut oil, dimethicone, tocopheryl acetate, stearoxytrimethylsilane, stearyl alcohol, panthenol, farnesol, benzyl alcohol, phenoxyethanol, acrylates/C10-30 alkyl acrylate crosspolymer, sodium hydroxide, citric acid	**Adults & Peds:** Apply to affected area prn.
Cetaphil Therapeutic Hand Cream	Glycerin, cetearyl alcohol, oleth-2, PEG-2 stearate, butyrospermum parkii, ethylhexyl methoxycinnamate, dimethicone, stearyl alcohol, glyceryl stearate, PEG-100 stearate, methylparaben, tocopherol, arginine PCA, chlorhexidine digluconate	**Adults & Peds:** Apply to affected area prn.
Corn Huskers Lotion	Glycerin, SD alcohol 40, sodium calcium aginate, oleyl sarcosine, methylparaben, guar gum, triethanolamine, calcium sulfate, calcium chloride, fumaric acid, boric acid	**Adults & Peds:** Apply to affected area prn.
Eucerin Creme Original	Petrolatum, mineral oil, ceresin, lanolin alcohol, methylchloroisothiazolinone, methylisothiazolinone	**Adults & Peds:** Apply to affected area prn.
Eucerin Dry Skin Therapy Calming Crème	Glycerin, cetyl palmitate, mineral oil, caprylic/capric triglyceride, octyldodecanol, cetyl alcohol, glycerly stearate, colloidal oatmeal, dimethicone, PEG-40 stearate, phenoxyethanol, DMDM hydantoin	**Adults:** Apply to affected area prn.
Eucerin Dry Skin Therapy Plus Intensive Repair Lotion	Mineral oil, PEG-7 hydrogenated castor oil, isohexadecane, sodium lactate, urea, glycerin, isopropyl palmitate, panthenol, microcrystalline wax, magnesium sulfate, lanolin alcohol, bisabolol, methylchloroisothiazolinone, methylisothiazolinone	**Adults:** Apply to affected area prn.
Eucerin Gentle Hydrating Cleanser	Sodium laureth sulfate, cocamidopropyl betaine, disodium cocoamphodiacetate, glycol distearate, PEG-7 glyceryl cocoate, PEG-5 lanolate, cocamide MEA, laureth 10, citric acid, PEG-120 methyl glucose dioleate, lanolin alcohol, imidazolidinyl urea	**Adults:** Use on affected area qd.
Eucerin Hand Creme Extensive Repair	Glycerin, urea, glyceryl stearate, stearyl alcohol, dicaprylyl ether, sodium lactate, dimethicone, PEG-40 stearate, cyclopentasiloxane, cyclohexasiloxane, aluminum starch octenylsuccinate, lactic aid, xanthan gum, phenoxyethanol, methylparaben, propylparaben	**Adults & Peds:** Apply to affected area qd.
Eucerin Lotion Daily Replenishing	Sunflower seed oil, petrolatum, glycerin, glyceryl stearate SE, octyldodecanol, caprylic/capric triglyceride, stearic acid, dimethicone, cetearyl alcohol, lanolin alcohol, panthenol, tocopheryl acetate, cholesterol, carbomer, disodium EDTA, sodium hydroxide, phenoxyethanol, methylparaben, ethylparaben, propylparaben, butylparaben, BHT	**Adults & Peds:** Apply to affected area qd.
Eucerin Lotion Original	Mineral oil, isopropyl myristate, PEG-40 sorbitan peroleate, glyceryl lanolate, sorbitol, propylene glycol, cetyl palmitate, magnesium sulfate, aluminum stearate, lanolin alcohol, BHT, methylchloroisothiazolinone, methylisothiazolinone	**Adults & Peds:** Apply to affected area prn.
Eucerin Lotion Plus Intensive Repair	Mineral oil, PEG-7 hydrogenated castor oil, isohexadecane, sodium lactate, urea, glycerin, isopropyl palmitate, panthenol, microcrystalline wax, magnesium sulfate, lanolin alcohol, bisabolol, methylchloroisothiazolinone, methylisothiazolinone	**Adults & Peds:** Apply to affected area prn.

(Continued)

Dry Skin Products

BRAND	INGREDIENTS	DOSE
Eucerin Redness Relief Daily Perfecting Lotion	Octinoxate, octisalate, titanium dioxide, glycerin, dimethicone, olyglyceryl-3 methylglucose distearate, butyrospermum parkii, lauroyl lysine, squalane, alcohol Denat., sorbitan stearate, phenoxyethanol, butylene glycol, magnesium aluminum silicate, glycyrrhiza inflata root extract xanthan gum, methylparaben, propylparaben, ethylparaben, iodopropynyl butylcarbamate, trimethoxycaprylylsilane, chromium oxide greens, chromium hydroxide green, ultramarines	**Adults & Peds:** Apply to affected area prn.
Eucerin Redness Relief Soothing Cleanser	Glycerin, sodium laureth sulfate, carbomer, phenoxyethanol, PEG-40 hydrogenated castor oil, sodium methyl cocoyl taurate, PEG-7 glyceryl cocoate, decyl glucoside, glycyrrhiza inflata root extract, xanthan gum, sodium hydroxide, methylparaben, butylparaben, ethylparaben, isobutylparaben, propylparaben, benzophenone-4	**Adults & Peds:** Apply to affected area qam and qpm.
Eucerin Redness Relief Soothing Moisture Lotion	Octinoxate, octisalate, titanium dioxide, water, glycerin, dimethicone, polyglyceryl-3 methyl glucose distearate, butyrospermum parkii (shea butter), squalane, alcohol denat., dicaprylyl carbonate, sorbitan stearate, lauroyl lysine, glycyrrhiza inflata root extract, phenoxyethanol, 1,2-hexanediol, magnesium aluminum silicate, xanthan gum, trimethoxycaprylylsilane, methylparaben, propylparaben, ethylparaben	**Adults & Peds:** Apply to affected area qam and qpm.
Eucerin Redness Relief Soothing Night Creme	Glycerin, panthenol, caprylic/capric triglyceride, dicaprylyl carbonate, octyldodecanol, C12-15 alkyl benzoate, dimethicone, squalane, tapioca starch, cetearyl alcohol, glyceryl stearate citrate, myristyl myristate, butylene glycol, benzyl alcohol, glycyrrhiza inflata root extract, carbomer, phenoxyethanol, ammonium acryloyldimethyltaurate/VP copolymer, sodium hydroxide, methylparaben, propylparaben, iodopropynyl butylcarbamate	**Adults & Peds:** Apply to affected area qpm.
Gold Bond Ultimate Healing Skin Therapy Lotion	Glycerin, dimethicone, petrolatum, jojoba esters, cetyl alcohol, aloe barbadensis leaf juice, stearyl alcohol, distearyldimonium chloride, cetearyl alcohol, steareth-21, steareth-2, propylene glycol, chamomilla recutita flower extract, polysorbate 60, stearamidopropyl PG-dimonium chloride phosphate, methyl gluceth 20, tocopheryl acetate, magnesium ascorbyl phosphate, hydrolyzed collagen, hydrolyzed elastin, retinyl palmitate, hydrolyzed jojoba esters, glyceryl stearate, dipotassium EDTA, fragrance, triethanolamine, diazolidinyl urea, methylparaben, propylparaben	**Adults & Peds:** Apply to affected area prn.
Gold Bond Ultimate Healing Skin Therapy Powder	Corn starch, sodium bicarbonate, silica, fragrance, ascrobyl palmitate, aloe barbadensis leaf extract, lavandula angustifolia extract, chamomilla recutita flower extract, rosmarinus officinalis leaf extract, acacia farnesiana extract, tocopheryl acetate, retinyl palmitate, polyoxymethylene urea, isopropyl myristate, benzethonium chloride	**Adults & Peds:** Apply to affected area prn.
Keri Moisture Therapy Advance Extra Dry Skin Lotion	Glycerin, stearic acid, hydrogenated polyisobutene, petrolatum, cetyl alcohol, aloe barbadensis gel, tocopheryl acetate, cyclopentasiloxane, dimethicone copolyol, glyceryl stearate, PEG-100 stearate, dimethicone, carbomer, methylparaben, PEG-5 soya sterol, magnesium aluminum silicate, propylparaben, phenoxyethanol, disodium EDTA, diazolidinyl urea, sodium hydroxide	**Adults & Peds:** Apply to affected area prn.
Keri Moisture Therapy Lotion, Sensitive Skin	Glycerin, stearic acid, hydrogenated polyisobutene, petrolatum, cetyl alcohol, aloe barbadensis gel, tocopheryl acetate, cyclopentasiloxane, dimethicone copolyol, glyceryl stearate, PEG-100 Stearate, dimethicone, carborner, methylparaben, PEG-5 soya sterol, magnesium aluminum silicate, propylparaben, phenoxyethanol, disodium EDTA, diazolidinyl urea, sodium hydroxide	**Adults:** Apply to skin prn.
Keri Original Formula Lotion	Mineral oil, propylene glycol, PEG-40 stearate, glyceryl stearate/PEG-100 stearate, PEG-4 dilaurate, laureth-4, lanolin oil, methylparaben, carbomer, propylparaben, fragrance, triethanolamine, dioctyl sodium sulfosuccinate, quaternium-15	**Adults & Peds:** Apply to affected area prn.

(Continued)

Dry Skin Products

BRAND	INGREDIENTS	DOSE
Keri Shea Butter Moisture Therapy Lotion	Mineral oil, glycerin, butyrospermum parkii, PEG-40 stearate, glyceryl stearate, PEG-100 stearate, PEG-4 dilaurate, laureth 4, aloe barbadensis leaf juice, helianthus annuus seed oil, tocopheryl Acetate, carbomer, methylparaben, propylparaben, DMDM hydantoin, iodopropynyl butylcarbamate, sodium hydroxide, sodium EDTA	**Adults & Peds:** Apply to affected area prn.
Lac-Hydrin Five Lotion	Lactic acid, ammonium hydroxide, glycerin, petrolatum, squalane, stearth-2, POE-21-stearyl ether, propylene glycol dioctanoate, cetyl alcohol, dimethicone, methylchloroisothiazoline, methylisothiazolinone	**Adults & Peds:** Apply to affected area bid.
Lubriderm Advanced Therapy Lotion	Cetyl alcohol, glycerin, mineral oil, cyclomethicone, propylene glycol dicaprylate/dicaprate, PEG-40 stearate, isopropyl isostearate, emulsifying wax, lecithin, carbomer, diazolidinyl urea, titanium dioxide, sodium benzoate, BHT, PPG-3 myristyl ether citrate, disodium EDTA, retinyl palmitate, tocopheryl acetate, sodium pyruvate, fragrance, sodium hydroxide, xanthan gum, iodopropynyl butylcarbamate	**Adults & Peds:** Apply to affected area prn.
Lubriderm Daily Moisture Fragrance Free Lotion	Mineral oil, petrolatum, sorbitol solution, stearic acid, lanolin, lanolin alcohol, cetyl alcohol, glyceryl stearate/PEG-100 stearate, triethanolamine, dimethicone, propylene glycol, microcrystalline wax, PPG-3 myristyl ether citrate, disodium EDTA, methylparaben, ethylparaben, propylparaben, xanthan gum, butylparaben, methyldibromo glutaronitrile	**Adults & Peds:** Apply to affected area prn.
Lubriderm Daily Moisture Lotion	Mineral oil, petrolatum, sorbitol solution, stearic acid, lanolin, lanolin alcohol, cetyl alcohol, glyceryl stearate/PEG-100 stearate, triethanolamine, Dimethicone, Propylene Glycol, microcrystalline wax, PPG-3 myristyl ether citrate, disodium EDTA, methylparaben, ethylparaben, propylparaben, xanthan gum, butylparaben, methyldibromo glutaronitrile	**Adults & Peds:** Apply to affected area prn.
Lubriderm Sensitive Skin Lotion	Butylene glycol, mineral oil, petrolatum, glycerin, cetyl alcohol, propylene glycol dicaprylate/dicaprate, PEG-40 stearate, C11-13 isoparaffin, glyceryl stearate, PPG-3 myristyl ether citrate, emulsifying wax, dimethicone, DMDM hydantoin, methylparaben, carbomer 940, ethylparaben, propylparaben, titanium dioxide, disodium EDTA, sodium hydroxide, butylparaben, xanthan gum	**Adults & Peds:** Apply to affected area prn.
Lubriderm Daily UV Moisturizer Lotion, SPF 15	Octyl methoxycinnamate/octyl salicylate/oxybenzone 7.5%-4%-3%	**Adults & Peds: >6 mo:** Apply to skin prn.
Lubriderm Lotion, Skin Therapy, Fresh Scent	Mineral oil, petrolatum, sorbitol solution, stearic acid, lanolin, lanolin alcohol, cetyl alcohol, glyceryl stearate, PEG-100 stearate, triethanolamine, dimethicone, propylene glycol, tri (PPG-3 myristyl ether) citrate, disodium EDTA, methylparaben, ethylparaben, propylparaben, fragrance, xanthan gum, butylparaben, methyldibromo glutaronitrile	**Adults:** Apply to skin prn.
Lubriderm Skin Nourishing Moisturizing Lotion with Premium Oat Extract	Caprylic/capric triglycerides, glycerin, glyceryl stearate se, petrolatum, camellia oleifera seed oil, castor oil, cocoa butter, cetyl alcohol, wax, brassica alba seed extract, oat kernel extract, cassia angustifolia seed polysaccharide, glyceryl stearate, PEG 100 stearate, diazolidinyl urea, xanthan gum, disodium EDTA, fragrance, iodopropynyl butylcarbamate, soybean oil	**Adults:** Apply to skin prn.
Lubriderm Skin Nourishing Moisturizing Lotion with Shea and Cocoa Butters	Glycerin, cetyl alcohol, glyceryl stearate SE, petrolatum, emulsifying wax, caprylic/capric triglyceride, castor oil, octyldodecanol, shea butter, cocoa butter, dimethicone, tocopheryl acetate, diazolidinyl urea, xanthan gum, disodium EDTA, fragrance, iodopropynyl butylcarbamate	**Adults:** Apply to skin prn.
Lubriderm Skin Nourishing Moisturizing Lotion with Sea Kelp Extract	Glycerin, glyceryl, stearate SE, cetyl alcohol, emulsifying wax, petrolatum, caprylic/caprictriglyceride, castor oil, octyldodecanol, dimethicone, diazolidinyl urea, propylene glycol, xanthan gum, disodium EDTA, fragrance, giant kelp leaf extract, iodopropynyl butylcarbamate	**Adults:** Apply to skin prn.
Neutrogena Body Moisturizer Cream	Glycerin, emulsifying wax, octyl isononanoate, dimethicone, propylene glycol isoceteth-3 acetate, cyclomethicone, stearic acid, aloe extract, matricaria extract, tocopheryl acetate, dimethicone copolyol, acrylates/C10-30 alkyl acrylate crosspolymer, cetearyl alcohol, sodium cetearyl sulfate, sodium sulfate, hydrogenated lanolin, glyceryl laurate, tetrasodium EDTA, triethanolamine, BHT, geranium, dipropylene glycol, propylene glycol, methylparaben, ethylparaben, propylparaben, diazolidinyl urea, benzalkonium chloride	**Adults & Peds:** Apply to affected area prn.

(Continued)

Dry Skin Products

BRAND	INGREDIENTS	DOSE
Neutrogena Comforting Butter Body Cream	Glycerin, distearyldimonium chloride, petrolatum, isopropyl palmitate, cetyl alcohol, dimethicone, panthenol, butyrospermum parkii, cocoa (theobroma cacao) seed butter, mango (mangifera indica) seed butter, benzyl alcohol, BHT, sodium chloride, yellow 5, yellow 6, fragrance	**Adults & Peds:** Apply to affected area prn.
Neutrogena Comforting Butter Hand Cream	Glycerin, distearyldimonium chloride, petrolatum, isopropyl palmitate, cetyl alcohol, dimethicone, panthenol, butyrospermum parkii, cocoa (theobroma cacao) seed butter, mango (mangifera indica) seed butter, benzyl alcohol, phytantriol, BHT, sodium chloride, yellow 5, yellow 6, fragrance	**Adults & Peds:** Apply to affected area prn.
Neutrogena Fragrance-Free Body Moisturizer Cream	Glycerin, emulsifying wax, octyl isononanoate, dimethicone, propylene glycol isoceteth-3 acetate, cyclomethicone, stearic acid, aloe extract, matricaria extract, tocopheryl acetate, dimethicone copolyol, acrylates/C10-30 alkyl acrylate crosspolymer, cetearyl alcohol, sodium cetearyl sulfate, sodium sulfate, hydrogenated lanolin, glyceryl laurate, tetrasodium EDTA, triethanolamine, BHT, geranium, dipropylene glycol, propylene glycol, methylparaben, ethylparaben, propylparaben, diazolidinyl urea, benzalkonium chloride	**Adults & Peds:** Apply to affected area prn.
Neutrogena Moisture for Sensitive Skin	Glycerin, octyl palmitate, dimethicone, petrolatum, cyclomethicone, soy sterol, isopropyl isostearate, cetyl alcohol, PEG-10 soya sterol, glyceryl stearate, PEG-100 stearate, C12-15 alkyl benzoate, tetrasodium EDTA, sodium hydroxide, diazolidinyl urea, ethylparaben, methylparaben, propylparaben	**Adults & Peds:** Apply to affected area prn.
Neutrogena Norwegian Formula Body/Hand Cream	Glycerin, cetearyl alcohol, stearic acid, sodium cetearyl sulfate, methylparaben, propylparaben, dilauryl thiodipropionate, sodium sulfate	**Adults & Peds:** Apply to affected area qd.
Neutrogena Summer Glow Moisturizer	Avobenzone, octisalate, oxybenzone, glycerin, dimethicone, dihydroxy acetone, silica, diethylhexyl 2,6 naphthalate, c12-15 alkyl benzoate, potassium cetyl phosphate, hydroxypropyl starch phosphate, glyceryl stearate, PEG 100 stearate, hydrogenated palm glycerides, cetyl alcohol, BHT, magnesium aluminum silicate, chlorphenesin, tetrasodium EDTA, citric acid, sodium citrate, phenoxyethanol, methylparaben	**Adults & Peds:** Apply to affected area qd.
Nivea Body Age Defying Moisturizer	Glycerin, mineral oil, caprylic/capric triglycerides, cetyl alcohol, dimethicone, glyceryl stearate, cyclopentasiloxane, cyclohexasiloxane, PEG 40 stearate, creatine, 1-methylhydantoin-2-imide, ubiquinone, fragrance, carbomer, sodium hydroxide, phenoxyethanol, methylparaben, propylparaben	**Adults:** Apply to damp skin prn.
Nivea Body Creamy Conditioning Oil, Very Dry, Flaky Skin	Mineral oil, isopropyl myristate, PEG-40 sorbitan peroleate, glyceryl lanolate, sorbitol, propylene glycol, cetyl palmitate, magnesium sulfate, aluminum stearate, lanolin alcohol, fragrance, BHT, methylchloroisothiazolinone, methylisothiazolinone	**Adults:** Apply to damp skin prn.
Nivea Body Original Lotion, Dry Skin	Mineral oil, glycerin, isopropyl palmitate, glyceryl stearate SE, cetearyl alcohol, tocopheryl acetate, isopropyl myristate, simethicone, fragrance, carbomer, hydroxypropyl methylcellulose, sodium hydroxide, methylchloroisothiazolinone, methylisothiazolinone	**Adults:** Apply to damp skin prn.
Nivea Body Original Skin Oil, Extremely Dry, Chapped Skin	Mineral oil, triple purified water, lanolin, petrolatum, glyceryl lanolate, lanolin alcohol, fragrance, sodium borate, methylchloroisothiazolinone, methylisothiazolinone	**Adults:** Apply to affected area prn.
Nivea Body Sheer Moisture Lotion, Normal to Dry Skin	Mineral oil, caprylic/capric triglycerides, SD alcohol 40B, glycerin, glyceryl stearate citrate, cetearyl alcohol, dimethicone, tocopheryl acetate, panthenol, lanolin alcohol, fragrance, carbomer, sodium hydroxide, methylchloroisothiazolinone, methylisothiazolinone	**Adults:** Apply to damp skin prn.
Nivea Smooth Sensation Daily Lotion, Dry Skin	Glycerin, mineral oil, caprylic/capric triglycerides, cetyl alcohol, dimethicone, glyceryl stearate, cyclopentasiloxane, cyclohexasiloxane, PEG 40 stearate, ginkgo biloba leaf extract, tocopheryl acetate, butyrospermum parkii (shea butter), phenoxyethanol, fragrance, carbomer, sodium hydroxide, EDTA, methylparaben, propylparaben	**Adults:** Apply to damp skin prn.

(Continued)

Dry Skin Products

BRAND	INGREDIENTS	DOSE
Nivea Creme	Mineral oil, petrolatum, glycerin, isohexadecane, microcrystalline wax, lanolin alcohol, paraffin, panthenol, magnesium sulfate, decyl oleate, octyldodecanol, aluminum stearate, methylchloroisothiazolinone, methylisothiazolinone, citric acid, magnesium stearate	**Adults & Peds:** Apply to affected area prn.
Nivea Extra-Enriched Lotion	Mineral oil, isohexadecane, PEG-40 sorbitan peroleate, polyglyceryl-3 diisostearate, glycerin, petrolatum, isopropyl palmitate, cetyl palmitate, tocopheryl acetate (vitamin E), glyceryl lanolate, lanolin alcohol, magnesium sulfate, aluminum stearate, phenoxyethanol, methyldibromo glutaronitrile	**Adults & Peds:** Apply to damp skin after shower or bath.
Pacquin Hand & Body Cream	Glycerin, stearic acid, potassium stearate, sodium stearate, cetyl alcohol, fragrance, diisopropyl sebacate, carbomer 940, methylparaben, propylparaben	**Adults & Peds:** Apply to affected area qd.
Pacquin Plus Hand & Body Cream	Glycerin, stearic acid, potassium stearate, carbomer, cetyl alcohol, cetyl esters wax, diisopropyl sebacate, lanolin, myristyl lactate, sodium stearate, methyl- and propylparabens	**Adults & Peds:** Apply to affected area qd.
Vaseline Dual Action Petroleum Jelly Cream	Petrolatum, glycerin, potassium lactate, stearic acid, butylene glycol, glycol stearate, PEG-100 stearate, caprylic/capric triglyceride, lactic acid, dimethicone, helianthus annuus seed pil or glycine Soya (soybean) oil, glyceryl stearate, tocopheryl acetate, tocopheryl acetate, fragrance, cetyl alcohol, xanthan gum, glycine soja sterols, ethylhexyl methoxyethylcellulose, stearamide AMP, lecithin, methylparaben, DMDM hydantoin, disodium EDTA	**Adults & Peds:** Apply to affected area prn.
Vaseline Intensive Care Advanced Healing Fragrance Free	White petrolatum, glycerin, stearic acid, glycol stearate, helianthus annuus seed oil, glycine soja sterol, lecithin, tocopheryl acetate, retinyl palmitate, urea, collagen amino scids, sodium stearoyl lactate, mineral water, sodium PCA, potassium lactate, lactic acid, cetyl alcohol, glyceryl stearate, magnesium aluminum silicate, carbomer, stearamide AMP, ethylene brassylate, trolamine, corn oil, disodium EDTA, methylparaben, DMDM hydantoin, BHT, titanium dioxide	**Adults & Peds:** Apply to affected area prn.
Vaseline Intensive Care Cocoa Butter Deep Conditioning Lotion	Petrolatum, glycerin, stearic acid, isopropyl palmitate, glycol stearate, dimethicone, theobroma cacao seed butter (cocoa), butyrospermum parkii (shea butter), helianthus annuus seed oil or glycine soja oil (sunflower, soybean), glycine soja sterol (soybean), tocopheryl acetate (vitamin E acetate), retinyl palmitate (vitamin A palmitate), sodium stearoyl-2-lactylate, collagen amino acids, urea, glyceryl stearate, cetyl alcohol, magnesium aluminum silicate, carbomer, lecithin, mineral water, sodium pca, potassium lactate, lactic acid, fragrance, stearamide amp, triethanolamine, methylparaben, DMDM hydantoin, disodium EDTA, caramel, titanium dioxide	**Adults & Peds:** Apply to affected area prn.
Vaseline Intensive Care Firming & Radiance Age-Defying Lotion	Octinoxate 1.25%	**Adults & Peds:** Apply to affected area prn.
Vaseline Intensive Care Healthy Body Complexion Nourishing Body Lotion	Glycerin, dimethicone, potassium lactate, stearic acid, sodium hydroxypropyl starch phosphate, mineral oil, glycol stearate, lactic acid, glycine soja sterol, lecithin, petrolatum, tocopheryl acetate, retinyl palmitate, helianthus annuus seed acid, sodium PCA, sodium stearoyl lactate, urea, collagen amino acids, mineral water, glyceryl stearate, cetyl alcohol, magnesium aluminum silicate, fragrance, stearamide AMP, ethylhexyl methoxycinnamate, corn oil, methylparaben, DMDM hydantoin, disodium EDTA, xanthan gum, BHT	**Adults & Peds:** Apply to affected area prn.
Vaseline Intensive Care Healthy Hand & Nail Lotion	Potassium lactate, sodium hydroxypropyl starch phosphate, glycerin, stearic acid, mineral oil, dimethicone, lactic acid, glycol stearate, PEG 100 stearate, keratin, glycine soja sterol, lecithin, tocopheryl acetate, retinyl palmitate, healianthus annuus seed oil, sodium PCA, sodium stearoyl lactate, urea, collagen amino acids, ethylhexyl methoxycinnamate, petrolatum, mineral water, cetyl alcohol, stearamide AMP, cyclomethicone, magnesium aluminum silicate, glyceryl stearate, fragrance, xanthan gum, corn oil, BHT, disodium EDTA, methylparaben, DMDM hydantoin	**Adults & Peds:** Apply to affected area prn.

(Continued)

DRY SKIN PRODUCTS

BRAND	INGREDIENTS	DOSE
Vaseline Intensive Care Lotion Aloe and Naturals	Glycerin, stearic acid, aloe barbadensis leaf juice glycol stearate, helianthus annuus, seed oil, glycine soja sterols, lecithin, panthenol, tocopheryl acetate, retinyl palmitate, sucumis sativus extract, urea, collagen amino acids, sodium stearoyl lactate, mineral water, sodium PCA, potassium lactate, lactic acid, petrolatum, dimethicone, glyceryl stearate, cetyl alcohol, methyl palmitate, magnesium aluminum silicate, eucalyptus globulus oil, lavandula angustifolia oil, citrus aurantium dulcis oil, carbomer, stearamide AMP, triethanolamine, corn oil, butylene glycol, methylparaben, DMDM hydantoin, disodium EDTA, BHT, titanium dioxide	**Adults & Peds:** Apply to affected area prn.
Vaseline Intensive Care Lotion Total Moisture	Glycerin, stearic acid, glycol stearate, petrolatum, helianthus annuus seed oil, glycine soja sterols, lecithin, tocopheryl acetate, retinyl palmitate, urea, collagen amino acids, sodium stearoyl lactylate, mineral water, sodium PCA, potassium lactate, lactic acid, dimethicone, avena sativa kernel flour, keratin, glyceryl stearate, cetyl alcohol, magnesium aluminum silicate, fragrance, carbomer, stearamide AMP, triethanolamine, corn oil, methylparaben, DMDM hydantoin, iodopropynyl butylcarbamate, disodium EDTA, BHT, propylene glycol, titanium dioxide	**Adults & Peds:** Apply to affected area prn.
Vaseline Intensive Care Lotion Total Moisture	Glycerin, stearic acid, glycol stearate, petrolatum, helianthus annuus seed oil, glycine soja sterols, lecithin, tocopheryl acetate, retinyl palmitate, urea, collagen amino acids, sodium stearoyl lactylate, mineral water, sodium PCA, potassium lactate, lactic acid, dimethicone, avena sativa kernel flour, keratin, glyceryl stearate, cetyl alcohol, magnesium aluminum silicate, fragrance, carbomer, stearamide AMP, triethanolamine, corn oil, methylparaben, DMDM hydantoin, iodopropynyl butylcarbamate, disodium EDTA, BHT, propylene glycol, titanium dioxide	**Adults & Peds:** Apply to affected area prn.
Vaseline Intensive Care Nightly Renewal Light Body Lotion	Glycerin, isopropyl myristate, dimethicone, cyclopentasiloxane, stearic acid, tapioca starch, glycol stearate, helianthus annuus seed oil, glycine soja oil, glycine soja sterol (soybean), vitis vinefera seed extract, lavendula angustifolia extract, lecithin, tocopheryl acetate, retinyl palmitate, urea, collagen amino acids, sodium PCA, potassium lactate, lactic acid, cetyl alcohol, glyceryl stearate, magnesium aluminum silicate, carbomer, methyl methacrylate crosspolymer, fragrance	**Adults & Peds:** Apply to affected area prn.
Vaseline Intensive Rescue Moisture Locking Lotion	Glycerin, petrolatum, stearic acid, glycol stearate, dimethicone, isopropyl isostearate, tapioca starch, cetyl alcohol, glyceryl stearate, magnesium aluminum silicate, carbomer, ethylene brassylate, triethanolamine, disodium EDTA, phenoxyethanol, methylparaben, propylparaben, titanium dioxide	**Adults & Peds:** Apply to affected area prn.
Vaseline Jelly	White petrolatum	**Adults & Peds:** Apply to affected area prn.
Vaseline Petroleum Jelly Cream Deep Moisture	White petrolatum 10%	**Adults & Peds:** Apply to affected area prn.
Vaseline Soothing Moisture, Moisturizing Cream w/ Cocoa Butter	Petrolatum, caprylic/capric triglyceride, stearic acid, glycerin, sodium hydroxypropyl starch phosphate, glycol stearate, PEG-100 stearate, cocoa butter, cyclomethicone, glyceryl stearate, cetyl alcohol, tocopheryl acetate, acrylates/C10-30 alkyl acrylate crosspolymer, fragrance, stearamide AMP, potassium hydroxide, DMDM hydantoin, disodium EDTA, iodopropyl butylcarbamate, titanium dioxide	**Adults & Peds:** Apply to affected area prn.

Psoriasis Products

BRAND	INGREDIENT/ STRENGTH	DOSE
COAL TAR		
Denorex Psoriasis Overnight Treatment cream	Coal Tar (strength n/a)	**Adults & Peds:** Apply to affected area qhs prn.
Denorex Therapeutic Protection 2-in-1 shampoo	Coal Tar 2.5%	**Adults & Peds:** Use at least biw.
Denorex Therapeutic Protection shampoo	Coal Tar 2.5%	**Adults & Peds:** Use at least biw.
DHS tar Shampoo	Coal Tar 0.5%	**Adults & Peds:** Use at least biw.
Ionil-T Plus Shampoo	Coal Tar 2%	**Adults & Peds:** Use at least biw.
Ionil-T Shampoo	Coal Tar 1%	**Adults & Peds:** Use at least biw.
MG217 Ointment	Coal Tar 2%	**Adults & Peds:** Apply to affected area qd-qid.
MG217 tar Shampoo	Coal Tar 3%	**Adults & Peds:** Use at least biw.
Neutrogena T/Gel Shampoo Extra Strength	Coal Tar 1%	**Adults & Peds:** Use at least biw.
Neutrogena T/Gel Shampoo Orignial Formula	Coal Tar 0.5%	**Adults & Peds:** Use at least biw.
Neutrogena T/Gel Stubborn Itch Shampoo	Coal Tar 0.5%	**Adults & Peds:** Use at least biw.
Polytar shampoo	Coal Tar 0.5%	**Adults & Peds:** Use at least biw.
Polytar soap	Coal Tar 0.5%	**Adults & Peds:** Apply to affected area prn.
Psoriasin Multi-Symptom Psoriasis Relief Gel	Coal Tar 1.25%	**Adults & Peds:** Apply to affected area qd-qid.
Psoriasin Multi-Symptom Psoriasis Relief Ointment	Coal Tar 2%	**Adults & Peds:** Apply to affected area qd-qid.
CORTICOSTEROIDS		
Aveeno Anti-Itch Cream 1%	Hydrocortisone 1%	**Adults & Peds: >2 yrs:** Apply to affected area tid-qid.
Cortaid Advanced 12-Hour Anti-Itch Cream	Hydrocortisone 1%	**Adults & Peds: >2 yrs:** Apply to affected area tid-qid.
Cortaid Intensive Therapy Cooling Spray	Hydrocortisone 1%	**Adults & Peds: >2 yrs:** Apply to affected area tid-qid.
Cortaid Intensive Therapy Moisturizing Cream	Hydrocortisone 1%	**Adults & Peds: >2 yrs:** Apply to affected area tid-qid.
Cortaid Maximum Strength Cream	Hydrocortisone 1%	**Adults & Peds: >2 yrs:** Apply to affected area tid-qid.
Cortaid Maximum Strength Ointment	Hydrocortisone 1%	**Adults & Peds: >2 yrs:** Apply to affected area tid-qid.
Cortizone-10 Cream	Hydrocortisone 1%	**Adults & Peds: >2 yrs:** Apply to affected area tid-qid.
Cortizone-10 Maximum Strength Anti-Itch Ointment	Hydrocortisone 1%	**Adults & Peds: >2 yrs:** Apply to affected area tid-qid.
Cortizone-10 Ointment	Hydrocortisone 1%	**Adults & Peds: >2 yrs:** Apply to affected area tid-qid.
Cortizone-10 Plus Maximum Strength Cream	Hydrocortisone 1%	**Adults & Peds: >2 yrs:** Apply to affected area tid-qid.
Cortizone-10 Quick Shot Spray	Hydrocortisone 1%	**Adults & Peds: >2 yrs:** Apply to affected area tid-qid.
SALICYLIC ACID		
Denorex Psoriasis Daytime Treatment cream	Salicylic Acid 3%	**Adults & Peds:** Apply to affected area qd-qid.
Dermarest Psoriasis Medicated Foam Shampoo	Salicylic Acid 3%	**Adults & Peds:** Apply to affected are at least biw.
Dermarest Psoriasis Medicated Moisturizer	Salicylic Acid 2%	**Adults & Peds:** Apply to affected area qd-qid.

(Continued)

Psoriasis Products

BRAND NAME	INGREDIENT/STRENGTH	DOSE
SALICYLIC ACID *(Continued)*		
Dermarest Psoriasis Medicated Scalp Treatment	Salicylic Acid 3%	**Adults & Peds:** Apply to affected area qd-qid.
Dermarest Psoriasis Medicated Scalp Treatment mousse	Salicylic Acid 3%	**Adults & Peds:** Apply to affected area qd-qid.
Dermarest Psoriasis Medicated Shampoo/Conditioner	Salicylic Acid 3%	**Adults & Peds:** Apply to affected area at least biw.
Dermarest Psoriasis Skin Treatment	Salicylic Acid 3%	**Adults & Peds:** Apply to affected area qd-qid.
Neutrogena T/Gel Conditioner	Salicylic Acid 2%	**Adults & Peds:** Use at least biw.
Psoriasin Therapeutic Body Wash With Aloe	Salicylic Acid 3%	**Adults & Peds:** Use biw.
Psoriasin Therapeutic Shampoo With Panthenol	Salicylic Acid 3%	**Adults & Peds:** Use biw.

Wound Care Products

BRAND	INGREDIENT/STRENGTH	DOSE
NEOMYCIN/POLYMYXIN B/BACITRACIN COMBINATIONS		
Bacitracin ointment	Bacitracin 500 U	**Adults & Peds:** Apply to affected area qd-tid.
Bactine Pain Relieving Protective Antibiotic	Neomycin/polymyxin B/bacitracin/pramoxine 3.5mg-10,000 U- 500 U- 1%	**Adults & Peds:** Apply to affected area qd-tid.
Neosporin ointment	Neomycin/polymyxin B/bacitracin 3.5mg-5,000 U-400 U	**Adults & Peds:** Apply to affected area qd-tid.
Neosporin Plus Pain Relief cream	Neomycin/polymyxin B/pramoxine 3.5mg-10,000 U-10mg	**Adults & Peds:** Apply to affected area qd-tid.
Neosporin Plus Pain Relief ointment	Neomycin/polymyxin B/bacitracin/pramoxine 3.5mg-10,000 U-500 U-10mg	**Adults & Peds:** Apply to affected area qd-tid.
Neosporin To Go ointment	Neomycin/polymyxin B/bacitracin 3.5mg-5,000 U-400 U	**Adults & Peds:** Apply to affected area qd-tid.
Polysporin ointment	Polymyxin B/bacitracin 10,000 U-500 U	**Adults & Peds:** Apply to affected area qd-tid.
BENZALKONIUM CHLORIDE COMBINATIONS		
Bactine First Aid Liquid	Lidocaine HCl/benzalkonium chloride 2.5%-0.13%	**Adults & Peds:** ≥2 yrs: Apply to affected area qd-tid.
Bactine Pain Relieving Cleansing Spray	Lidocaine HCl/benzalkonium chloride 2.5%-0.13%	**Adults & Peds:** ≥2 yrs: Apply to affected area qd-tid.
Bactine Pain Relieving Cleansing Wipes	Benzalkonium chloride/pramoxine HCl 0.13%-1.0%	**Adults & Peds:** ≥2 yrs: Use 1 wipe qd-tid.
Band-Aid Antiseptic Foam, One-Step Cleansing and Infection Protection	Benzalkonim chloride 0.13%	**Adults & Peds:** ≥3 yrs: Use tid.
BENZETHONIUM CHLORIDE COMBINATIONS		
Gold Bond First Aid Quick Spray	Menthol/benzethonium chloride 1%-0.13%	**Adults & Peds:** ≥2 yrs: Apply to affected area tid-qid.
Lanacane Maximum Strength Cream	Benzocaine/benzethonium chloride 20%-0.1%	**Adults & Peds:** ≥2 yrs: Apply to affected area tid-qid.
CHLORHEXIDINE GLUCONATE		
Hibiclens	Chlorhexidine gluconate 4%	**Adults & Peds:** Apply sparingly to affected area prn.
IODINE		
Betadine Skin Cleanser	Povidone-iodine 7.5%	**Adults & Peds:** Apply to affected area for 3 minutes and rinse. Repeat bid-tid.
Betadine solution	Povidone-iodine 10%	**Adults & Peds:** Apply to affected area qd-tid.
Betadine spray	Povidone-iodine 10%	**Adults & Peds:** Apply to affected area qd-tid.
Betadine Surgical Scrub	Povidone-iodine 7.5%	**Adults & Peds:** Apply to affected area for 5 minutes.
Betadine swab	Povidone-iodine 10%	**Adults & Peds:** Apply to affected area qd-tid.
MISCELLANEOUS		
Aquaphor Healing Ointment	Petrolatum, mineral oil, ceresin, lanolin, alcohol, panthenol, glycerin, bisabolol	**Adults & Peds:** Apply to affected area prn.
Curad Spray Bandage	Ethyl acetate, pentane, methylacrylate, menthol, carbon dioxide	**Adults & Peds:** Apply to affected area prn.
Proxacol Hydrogen Peroxide	Hydrogen peroxide 3%	**Adults:** Apply to affected area qd-tid.
Wound Wash Sterile Saline spray	Sterile sodium chloride solution 0.9%	**Adults & Peds:** Apply to affected area prn.

Antacid and Heartburn Products

BRAND	INGREDIENT/STRENGTH	DOSE
ANTACID		
Alka-Mints chewable tablets	Calcium Carbonate 850mg	**Adults & Peds: ≥12 yrs:** 1-2 tabs q2h. **Max:** 9 tabs q24h.
Alka-Seltzer Gold tablets	Citric Acid/Potassium Bicarbonate/Sodium Bicarbonate 1000mg-344mg-1050mg	**Adults: ≥60 yrs:** 2 tabs q4h prn. **Max:** 6 tabs q24h. **Adults & Peds: ≥12 yrs:** 2 tabs q4h prn. **Max:** 8 tabs q24h. **Peds:** ≤12 yrs: 1 tab q4h prn. **Max:** 4 tabs q24h.
Alka-Seltzer Heartburn Relief tablets	Citric Acid/Sodium Bicarbonate 1000mg-1940mg	**Adults: ≥60 yrs:** 2 tabs q4h prn. **Max:** 4 tabs q24h. **Adults & Peds: ≥12 yrs:** 2 tabs q4h prn. **Max:** 8 tabs q24h.
Alka-Seltzer tablets, Extra-Strength	Aspirin/Sodium Bicarbonate/Citric Acid 500mg-1985mg-1000mg	**Adults: ≥60 yrs:** 2 tabs q6h prn. **Max:** 3 tabs q24h. **Adults & Peds: ≥12 yrs:** 2 tabs q6h prn. **Max:** 7 tabs q24h.
Brioschi powder	Sodium Bicarbonate/Tartaric Acid 2.69g-2.43g/dose	**Adults & Peds: ≥12 yrs:** 1 capful (6g) dissolved in 4-6 oz water q1h. **Max:** 6 doses q24h.
Dulcolax Milk of Magnesia liquid	Magnesium Hydroxide 400mg/5mL	**Adults & Peds: ≥12 yrs:** 1-3 tsp (5-15mL) qd-qid.
Gaviscon Extra Strength liquid	Aluminum Hydroxide/Magnesium Carbonate 254mg-237.5mg/5mL	**Adults:** 2-4 tsp (10-20mL) qid.
Gaviscon Extra Strength tablets	Aluminum Hydroxide/Magnesium Carbonate 160mg-105mg	**Adults:** 2-4 tabs qid.
Gaviscon Original chewable tablets	Aluminum Hydroxide/Magnesium Trisilicate 80mg-20mg	**Adults:** 2-4 tabs qid.
Gaviscon Regular Strength liquid	Aluminum Hydroxide/Magnesium Carbonate 95mg-358mg/5mL	**Adults:** 2-4 tsp (10-20mL) qid.
Gaviscon Acid Breakthrough, chewable tablets	Calcium Carbonate 500mg	**Adults:** 2 tabs prn.
Maalox Quick Dissolve Regular Strength chewable tablets	Calcium Carbonate 600mg	**Adults:** 1-2 tabs prn. **Max:** 12 tabs q24h.
Mylanta, Children's	Calcium Carbonate 400 mg	**Peds: 6-11 yrs (48-95 lbs):** Take 2 tab prn. **Peds: 2-5 yrs (24-47 lbs):** Take 1 tab prn
Mylanta gelcaps	Calcium Carbonate/Magnesium Hydroxide 550mg-125mg	**Adults:** 2-4 caps prn. **Max:** 12 caps q24h.
Mylanta Supreme Antacid liquid	Calcium Carbonate/Magnesium Hydroxide 400mg-135mg/5mL	**Adults:** 2-4 tsp (10-20mL) qid. **Max:** 18 tsp (90mL) q24h.
Mylanta Ultra chewable tablets	Calcium Carbonate/Magnesium Hydroxide 700mg-300mg	**Adults:** 2-4 tabs qid. **Max:** 10 tabs q24h.
Pepto-Bismol Children's Chewable Tablets	Calcium Carbonate 400 mg	**Peds: 2-5 yrs (24-47 lbs):** Take 1 tab q24h. **Peds: 6-11 yrs (48-95 lbs):** Take 2 tab q24h.
Phillips Milk of Magnesia liquid	Magnesium Hydroxide 400mg/5mL	**Adults & Peds: ≥12 yrs:** 30-60mL qd. **Peds: 6-11 yrs:** 15-30mL qd. **2-5 yrs:** 5-15mL qd.
Rolaids Extra Strength Softchews	Calcium Carbonate 1177mg	**Adults:** 2-3 chews q1h prn. **Max:** 6 chews q24h.
Rolaids Extra Strength tablets	Calcium Carbonate/Magnesium Hydroxide 675mg-135mg	**Adults:** 2-4 tabs q1h prn. **Max:** 10 tabs q24h.
Rolaids tablets	Calcium Carbonate/Magnesium Hydroxide 550mg-110mg	**Adults:** 2-4 tabs q1h prn. **Max:** 12 tabs q24h.
Titralac chewable tablets	Calcium Carbonate 420mg	**Adults:** 2 tabs q2-3h prn. **Max:** 19 tabs q24h.

(Continued)

ANTACID AND HEARTBURN PRODUCTS

BRAND	INGREDIENT/STRENGTH	DOSE
ANTACID *(Continued)*		
Tums chewable tablets	Calcium Carbonate 500mg	**Adults:** 2-4 tabs q1h prn. **Max:** 15 tabs q24h.
Tums E-X chewable tablets	Calcium Carbonate 750mg	**Adults:** 2-4 tabs prn. **Max:** 10 tabs q24h.
Tums Lasting Effects chewable tablets	Calcium Carbonate 500mg	**Adults:** 2 tabs prn. **Max:** 15 tabs q24h.
Tums Smooth Dissolve tablets	Calcium Carbonate 750mg	**Adults:** 2-4 tabs prn. **Max:** 10 tabs q24h.
Tums Ultra Maximum Strength chewable tablets	Calcium Carbonate 1000mg	**Adults:** 2-3 tabs prn. **Max:** 7 tabs q24h.
ANTACID/ANTIFLATULENT		
Gas-X with Maalox capsules	Calcium Carbonate/Simethicone 250mg-62.5mg	**Adults:** 2-4 caps prn. **Max:** 8 caps q24h.
Gas-X Extra Strength with Maalox capsules	Calcium Carbonate/Simethicone 500mg-125mg	**Adults:** 1-2 caps prn. **Max:** 4 caps q24h.
Gelusil chewable tablets	Aluminum Hydroxide/Magnesium Hydroxide/Simethicone 200mg-200mg-20mg	**Adults:** 2-4 tabs qid.
Maalox Max liquid	Aluminum Hydroxide/Magnesium Hydroxide/Simethicone 400mg-400mg-40mg/5mL	**Adults & Peds:** ≥12 yrs: 2-4 tsp (10-20mL) qid. **Max:** 12 tsp (60mL) q24h.
Maalox Max Quick Dissolve Maximum Strength tablets	Calcium Carbonate/Simethicone 1000mg-60mg	**Adults:** 1-2 tabs prn. **Max:** 8 tabs q24h.
Maalox Regular Strength liquid	Aluminum Hydroxide/Magnesium Hydroxide/Simethicone 200mg-200mg-20mg/5mL	**Adults & Peds:** ≥12 yrs: 2-4 tsp (10-20mL) qid. **Max:** 16 tsp (80mL) q24h.
Mylanta Maximum Strength liquid	Aluminum Hydroxide/Magnesium Hydroxide/Simethicone 400mg-400mg-40mg/5mL	**Adults & Peds:** ≥12 yrs: 2-4 tsp (10-20mL) qid. **Max:** 12 tsp (60mL) q24h.
Mylanta Regular Strength liquid	Aluminum Hydroxide/Magnesium Hydroxide/Simethicone 200mg-200mg-20mg/5mL	**Adults & Peds:** ≥12 yrs: 2-4 tsp (10-20mL) qid. **Max:** 12 tsp (60mL) q24h.
Rolaids Multi-Sympton chewable tablets	Calcium Carbonate/Magnesium Hydroxide/Simethicone 675mg-135mg-60mg	**Adults:** 2 tabs qid prn. **Max:** 8 tabs q24h.
Titralac Plus chewable tablets	Calcium Carbonate/Simethicone 420mg-21mg	**Adults:** 2 tabs q2-3h prn. **Max:** 19 tabs q24h.
BISMUTH SUBSALICYLATE		
Maalox Total Stomach Relief Maximum Strength liquid	Bismuth Subsalicylate 525mg/15mL	**Adults & Peds:** ≥12 yrs: 2 tbl (30mL) q1/2-1h. **Max:** 8 tbl (120mL) q24h.
Pepto Bismol chewable tablets	Bismuth Subsalicylate 262mg	**Adults & Peds:** ≥12 yrs: 2 tabs q1/2-1h. **Max:** 8 doses q24h.
Pepto Bismol caplets	Bismuth Subsalicylate 262mg	**Adults & Peds:** ≥12 yrs: 2 tabs q1/2-1h. **Max:** 8 doses q24h.
Pepto Bismol liquid	Bismuth Subsalicylate 262mg/15mL	**Adults & Peds:** ≥12 yrs: 2 tbl (30mL) q1/2-1h. **Max:** 8 doses (240mL) q24h.
Pepto Bismol Maximum Strengtth liquid	Bismuth Subsalicylate 525mg/15mL	**Adults & Peds:** ≥12 yrs: 2 tbl (30mL) q1h. **Peds: 9-12 yrs:** 1 tbl (15mL) q1h. **6-9 yrs:** 2 tsp (10mL) q1h. **3-6 yrs:** 1 tsp (5mL) q1h. **Max:** of 8 doses (240mL) q24h.
H₂-RECEPTOR ANTAGONIST		
Pepcid AC chewable tablets	Famotidine 10mg	**Adults & Peds:** ≥12 yrs: 1 tab qd. **Max:** 2 tabs q24h.

(Continued)

Antacid and Heartburn Products

BRAND	INGREDIENT/STRENGTH	DOSE
H_2-RECEPTOR ANTAGONIST *(Continued)*		
Pepcid AC gelcaps	Famotidine 10mg	**Adults & Peds: ≥12 yrs:** 1 tab qd. **Max:** 2 tabs q24h.
Pepcid AC Maximum Strength tablets	Famotidine 20mg	**Adults & Peds: ≥12 yrs:** 1 tab qd. **Max:** 2 tabs q24h.
Pepcid AC tablets	Famotidine 10mg	**Adults & Peds: ≥12 yrs:** 1 tab qd. **Max:** 2 tabs q24h.
Tagamet HB tablets	Cimetidine 200mg	**Adults & Peds: ≥12 yrs:** 1 tab qd. **Max:** 2 tabs q24h.
Zantac 150 tablets	Ranitidine 150mg	**Adults & Peds: ≥12 yrs:** 1 tab qd. **Max:** 2 tabs q24h.
Zantac 75 tablets	Ranitidine 75mg	**Adults & Peds: ≥12 yrs:** 1 tab qd. **Max:** 2 tabs q24h.
H_2-RECEPTOR ANTAGONIST/ANTACID		
Pepcid Complete chewable tablets	Famotidine/Calcium Carbonate/ Magnesium Hydroxide 10mg-800mg-165mg	**Adults & Peds: ≥12 yrs:** 1 tab qd. **Max:** 2 tabs q24h.
PROTON PUMP INHIBITOR		
Prilosec OTC tablets	Omeprazole 20mg	**Adults:** 1 tab qd x 14 days. May repeat 14 day course q 4 months.

Antidiarrheal Products

BRAND	INGREDIENT/STRENGTH	DOSE
ABSORBENT AGENTS		
Equalactin chewable tablets	Calcium Polycarbophil 625mg	**Adults:** ≥**12 yrs:** 2 tabs q30min prn. **Max:** 6 doses q24h. **Peds: 6-12 yrs:** 1 tab q30min. **Max:** 6 doses q24h. **3-6 yrs:** 1 tab q30min. **Max:** 3 doses q24h.
Fibercon caplets	Calcium Polycarbophil 625mg	**Adults:** ≥**12 yrs:** 2 tabs q30min prn. **Max:** 6 doses q24h. **Peds: 6-12 yrs:** 1 tab q30min. **Max:** 6 doses q24h. **3-6 yrs:** 1 tab q30min. **Max:** 3 doses q24h.
Fiber-Lax tablets	Calcium Polycarbophil 625mg	**Adults:** ≥**12 yrs:** 2 tabs q30min prn. **Max:** 6 doses q24h. **Peds: 6-12 yrs:** 1 tab q30min. **Max:** 6 doses q24h. **3-6 yrs:** 1 tab q30min. **Max:** 3 doses q24h.
Kapectolin	Kaolin/Pectin 90g-2g/30mL	**Adults:** 60-120mL after each loose bowel movement. **Peds:** ≥**12 yrs:** 45-60mL after each loose bowel movement. **6-12 yrs:** 30-60mL after each loose bowel movement. **3-6 yrs:** 15-30mL after each loose bowel movement.
Konsyl Fiber tablets	Calcium Polycarbophil 625mg	**Adults:** ≥**12 yrs:** 2 tabs q30min prn. **Max:** 6 doses q24h. **Peds: 6-12 yrs:** 1 tab q30min. **Max:** 6 doses q24h. **3-6 yrs:** 1 tab q30min. **Max:** 3 doses q24h.
Phillip's Fibercaps	Calcium Polycarbophil 625mg	**Adults:** ≥**12 yrs:** 2 tabs q30min prn. **Max:** 6 doses q24h. **Peds: 6-12 yrs:** 1 tab q30min. **Max:** 6 doses q24h. **3-6 yrs:** 1 tab q30min. **Max:** 3 doses q24h.
ANTIPERISTALTIC AGENTS		
Imodium A-D caplet	Loperamide HCl 2mg	**Adults:** ≥**12 yrs:** 2 caplets after first loose stool; 1 caplet after each subsequent loose stool. **Max:** 4 caplets q24h. **Peds: 9-11 yrs (60-95lbs):** 1 caplet after first loose stool; ½ caplet after each subsequent loose stool. **Max:** 3 caplets q24h. **6-8 yrs (48-59 lbs):** 1 caplet after first loose stool; ½ caplet after each subsequent loose stool. **Max:** 2 caplets q24h.
Imodium A-D E-Z Chews	Loperamide HCl 2mg	**Adults:** ≥**12 yrs:** 2 caplets after first loose stool; 1 caplet after each subsequent loose stool. **Max:** 4 caplets q24h. **Peds: 9-11 yrs (60-95 lbs):** 1 caplet after first loose stool; ½ caplet after each subsequent loose stool. **Max:** 3 caplets q24h. **6-8 yrs (48-59 lbs):** 1 caplet after first loose stool; 1/2 caplet after each subsequent loose stool. **Max:** 2 caplets q24h.
Imodium A-D liquid	Loperamide HCl 1mg/7.5mL	**Adults:** ≥**12 yrs:** 30mL (6 tsp) after first loose stool; 15mL (3 tsp) after each subsequent loose stool. **Max:** 60mL (12 tsp) q24h. **Peds: 9-11 yrs (60-95 lbs):** 15mL (3 tsp) after first loose stool; 7.5mL (1½ tsp) after each subsequent loose stool. **Max:** 45mL (9 tsp) q24h. **6-8 yrs (48-59 lbs):** 15 mL (3 tsp) after first loose stool; 7.5mL (1½ tsp) after each subsequent loose stool. **Max:** 30mL (6 tsp) q24h.

(Continued)

ANTIDIARRHEAL PRODUCTS

BRAND	INGREDIENT/STRENGTH	DOSE
ANTIPERISTALTIC/ANTIFLATULENT AGENTS		
Imodium Advanced caplet	Loperamide HCl/Simethicone 2mg-125mg	**Adults: ≥12 yrs:** 2 caplets after first loose stool; 1 caplet after each subsequent loose stool. **Max:** 4 caplets q24h. **Peds: 9-11 yrs (60-95 lbs):** 1 caplet after first loose stool; 1/2 caplet after each subsequent loose stool. **Max:** 3 caplets q24h. **6-8 yrs (48-59 lbs):** 1 caplet after first loose stool; ½ caplet after each subsequent loose stool. **Max:** 2 caplets q24h.
Imodium Advanced chewable tablet	Loperamide HCl/Simethicone 2mg-125mg	**Adults: ≥12 yrs:** 2 caplets after first loose stool; 1 caplet after each subsequent loose stool. **Max:** 4 caplets q24h. **Peds: 9-11 yrs (60-95 lbs):** 1 caplet after first loose stool; ½ caplet after each subsequent loose stool. **Max:** 3 caplets q24h. **6-8 yrs (48-59lbs):** 1 caplet after first loose stool; ½ caplet after each subsequent loose stool. **Max:** 2 caplets q24h.
BISMUTH SUBSALICYLATE		
Kaopectate caplet	Bismuth Subsalicylate 262mg	**Adults & Peds: ≥12 yrs:** 2 caplets q½-1h. **Max:** 8 doses q24h.
Kaopectate Extra Strength liquid	Bismuth Subsalicylate 525mg/15mL	**Adults: ≥12 yrs:** 2 tbl (30mL). **Peds: 9-12 yrs:** 1 tbl (15mL) q1h prn. **6-9 yrs:** 2 tsp (10mL) q1h prn. **3-6 yrs:** 1 tsp (5mL) q1h prn. **Max:** 8 doses q24h.
Kaopectate liquid	Bismuth Subsalicylate 262mg/15mL	**Adults: ≥12 yrs:** 2 tbl (30mL). **Peds: 9-12 yrs:** 1 tbl (15mL) q1h prn. **6-9 yrs:** 2 tsp (10mL) q1h prn. **3-6 yrs:** 1 tsp (5mL) q1h prn. **Max:** 8 doses q24h.
Pepto Bismol chewable tablets	Bismuth Subsalicylate 262mg	**Adults & Peds: ≥12 yrs:** 2 tabs q½-1h. **Max:** 8 doses q24h.
Pepto Bismol caplets	Bismuth Subsalicylate 262mg	**Adults & Peds: ≥12 yrs:** 2 tabs q½-1h. **Max:** 8 doses q24h.
Pepto Bismol liquid	Bismuth Subsalicylate 262mg/15mL	**Adults & Peds: ≥12 yrs:** 2 tbl (30mL) q½-1h. **Max:** 8 doses q24h.
Pepto Bismol Maximum Strength	Bismuth Subsalicylate 525mg/15mL	**Adults: ≥12 yrs:** 2 tbl (30mL). **Peds: 9-12 yrs:** 1 tbl (15mL) q1h prn. **6-9 yrs:** 2 tsp (10mL) q1h prn. **3-6 yrs:** 1 tsp (5mL) q1h prn. **Max:** 8 doses q24h.

Antiflatulant Products

BRAND	INGREDIENT/STRENGTH	DOSE
ALPHA-GALACTOSIDASE		
Beano Food Enzyme Dietary Supplement drops	Alpha-Galactosidase Enzyme 150 GalU	**Adults:** Add 5 drops before meals.
Beano Food Enzyme Dietary Supplement tablets	Alpha-Galactosidase Enzyme 150 GalU	**Adults:** Take 3 tabs before meals.
ANTACID/ANTIFLATULENCE		
Gas-X with Maalox capsules	Calcium Carbonate/Simethicone 250mg-62.5mg	**Adults:** 2-4 caps prn. **Max:** 8 caps q24h.
Gas-X Extra Strength with Maalox capsules	Calcium Carbonate/Simethicone 500mg-125mg	**Adults:** 1-2 caps prn. **Max:** 4 caps q24h.
Gelusil chewable tablets	Aluminum Hydroxide/Magnesium Hydroxide/Simethicone 200mg-200mg-20mg	**Adults:** 2-4 tabs qid.
Maalox Max liquid	Aluminum Hydroxide/Magnesium Hydroxide/Simethicone 400mg-400mg-40mg/5mL	**Adults & Peds: ≥12 yrs:** 2-4 tsp (10-20mL) qid. **Max:** 12 tsp (60mL) q24h.
Maalox Max Quick Dissolve Maximum Strength tablets	Calcium Carbonate/Simethicone 1000mg-60mg	**Adults:** 1-2 tabs prn. **Max:** 8 tabs q24h.
Maalox Regular Strength liquid	Aluminum Hydroxide/Magnesium Hydroxide/Simethicone 200mg-200mg-20mg/5mL	**Adults & Peds: ≥12 yrs:** 2-4 tsp (10-20mL) qid. **Max:** 16 tsp (80mL) q24h.
Mylanta Maximum Strength liquid	Aluminum Hydroxide/Magnesium Hydroxide/Simethicone 400mg-400mg-40mg/5mL	**Adults & Peds: ≥12 yrs:** 2-4 tsp (10-20mL) qid. **Max:** 12 tsp (60mL) q24h.
Mylanta Regular Strength liquid	Aluminum Hydroxide/Magnesium Hydroxide/Simethicone 200mg-200mg-20mg/5mL	**Adults & Peds: ≥12 yrs:** 2-4 tsp (10-20mL) qid. **Max:** 24 tsp (120mL) q24h.
Rolaids Antacid & Antigas Soft Chews	Calcium Carbonate/Simethicone 1177mg-80mg	**Adults:** 2-3 chews hourly prn.
Titralac Plus chewable tablets	Calcium Carbonate/Simethicone 420mg-21mg	**Adults:** 2 tabs q2-3h prn. **Max:** 19 tabs q24h.
SIMETHICONE		
GasAid Maximum Strength Anti-Gas softgels	Simethicone 125mg	**Adults:** Take 1-2 caps prn and qhs. **Max:** 4 caps q24h.
Gas-X Infant Drops	Simethicone 20mg/0.3mL	**Peds: ≥2 yrs (≥24 lbs):** 0.6mL prn. **Peds: <2 yrs (<24 lbs):** 0.3mL prn. **Max:** 6 doses q24h.
Gas-X Thin Strips	Simethicone 62.5mg	**Adults:** Allow 2-4 strips to dissolve prn. **Max:** 8 strips q24h.
Gas-X Antigas Chewable tablets	Simethicone 80mg	**Adults:** Take 1-2 caps prn and qhs. **Max:** 6 caps q24h.
Gas-X Extra Strength Antigas softgels	Simethicone 125mg	**Adults:** Take 1-2 caps prn and qhs. **Max:** 4 caps q24h.
Gas-X Maximum Strength Antigas softgels	Simethicone 166mg	**Adults:** Take 1-2 caps prn and qhs. **Max:** 3 caps q24h.
Little Tummys Gas Relief drops	Simethicone 20mg/0.3mL	**Peds: ≥2 yrs (≥24 lbs):** 0.6mL prn. **Peds: <2 yrs (<24 lbs):** 0.3mL prn. **Max:** 12 doses q24h.
Mylanta Gas Maximum Strength Chewable tablets	Simethicone 125mg	**Adults:** Chew 1-2 tab prn and qhs.
Mylanta Gas Regular Strength Chewable tablets	Simethicone 80mg	**Adults:** Chew 1-2 tab prn and qhs.
Mylicon Infant's Gas Relief drops	Simethicone 20mg/0.3mL	**Peds: ≥2 yrs (≥24 lbs):** 0.6mL prn. **Peds: <2 yrs (<24 lbs):** 0.3mL prn. **Max:** 12 doses q24h.

LAXATIVE PRODUCTS

BRAND	INGREDIENT/STRENGTH	DOSE
BULK-FORMING		
Citrucel caplets	Methylcellulose 500mg	**Adults:** ≥**12 yrs:** 2-4 tabs qd. **Max:** 12 tabs q24h. **Peds: 6-12 yrs:** 1 tabs qd. **Max:** 6 tabs q24h.
Citrucel powder	Methylcellulose 2g/tbl	**Adults:** ≥**12 yrs:** 1 tbl (11.5g) qd tid. **Peds: 6-12 yrs:** 1/2 tbl (5.75g) qd.
Equalactin chewable tablet	Calcium Polycarbophil 625mg	**Adults & Peds:** ≥**12 yrs:** 2 tabs qd. **Max:** 8 tabs qd.
Fibercon caplets	Calcium Polycarbophil 625mg	**Adults & Peds:** ≥**12 yrs:** 2 tabs qd. **Max:** 8 tabs qd.
Fiber-Lax tablets	Calcium Polycarbophil 625mg	**Adults & Peds:** ≥**12 yrs:** 2 tabs qd. **Max:** 8 tabs qd.
Konsyl Easy Mix powder	Psyllium 6g/tsp	**Adults:** ≥**12 yrs:** 1 tsp qd-tid. **Peds: 6-12 yrs:** 1/2 tsp qd-tid.
Konsyl Fiber tablets	Calcium Polycarbophil 625mg	**Adults & Peds:** ≥**12 yrs:** 2 tabs qd. **Max:** 8 tabs qd.
Konsyl Orange powder	Psyllium 3.4g	**Adults:** ≥**12 yrs:** 1 tsp qd-tid. **Peds: 6-12 yrs:** 1/2 tsp qd-tid.
Konsyl Original powder	Psyllium 6g/tsp	**Adults:** ≥**12 yrs:** 1 tsp qd-tid. **Peds: 6-12 yrs:** 1/2 tsp qd-tid.
Konsyl-D powder	Psyllium 3.4g/tsp	**Adults:** ≥**12 yrs:** 1 tsp qd-tid. **Peds: 6-12 yrs:** 1/2 tsp qd-tid.
Metamucil capsules	Psyllium 0.52g	**Adults & Peds:** ≥**12 yrs:** 5 caps qd-tid.
Metamucil Original Texture powder	Psyllium 3.4g/tbs	**Adults:** ≥**12 yrs:** 1 tbs qd-tid. **Peds: 6-12 yrs:** 1/2 tsp qd-tid.
Metamucil Smooth Texture powder	Psyllium 3.4g/tbs	**Adults:** ≥**12 yrs:** 1 tbs qd-tid. **Peds: 6-12 yrs:** 1/2 tsp qd-tid.
Metamucil wafers	Psyllium 3.4 g/dose	**Adults:** ≥**12 yrs:** 2 wafers qd-tid. **Peds: 6-12 yrs:** 1 wafer qd-tid.
HYPEROSMOTICS		
Fleet Children's Babylax suppositories	Glycerin 2.3g	**Peds: 2-5 yrs:** 1 supp. qd.
Fleet Glycerin suppositories	Glycerin 2g	**Adults & Peds:** ≥**6 yrs:** 1 supp qd.
Fleet Liquid Glycerin suppositories	Glycerin 5.6g	**Adults & Peds:** ≥**6 yrs:** 1 supp qd.
Fleet Mineral Oil Enema	Mineral Oil 133mL	**Adults:** ≥**12 yrs:** 1 bottle (133mL). **Peds: 2-12 yrs:** 1/2 bottle (66.5mL)
HYPEROSMOTIC COMBINATION		
Fleet Pain Relief Pre-Moistened Anorectal Pads	Glycerin/Pramoxine HCl 12%-1%	**Adults & Peds:** ≥**12 yrs:** Apply to affected area five times daily.
SALINES		
Ex-Lax Milk of Magnesia liquid	Magnesium Hydroxide 400mg/5mL	**Adults & Peds:** ≥**12 yrs:** Take 2-4 tbs hs. **Peds: 6-11 yrs:** 1-2 tbs hs. **2-5 yrs:** 1-3 tbs hs.
Fleet Children's Enema	Monobasic Sodium Phosphate/Dibasic Sodium Phosphate 9.5g-3.5g/66mL	**Peds: 5-11 yrs:** 1 bottle (66mL). **2-5 yrs:** 1/2 bottle (33mL).
Fleet Enema	Monobasic Sodium Phosphate/Dibasic Sodium Phosphate 19g-7g/133mL	**Adults & Peds:** ≥**12 yrs:** 1 bottle (133mL).
Fleet Phospho-Soda	Monobasic Sodium Phosphate/Dibasic Sodium Phosphate 2.4g-0.9g/5mL	**Adults:** ≥**12 yrs:** 4-9 tsp qd. **Peds: 10-11 yrs:** 2-4 tsp qd. **5-9 yrs:** 1-2 tsp qd.
Magnesium Citrate solution	Magnesium Citrate 1.75gm/30mL	**Adults:** ≥**12 yrs:** 300mL. **Peds: 6-12 yrs:** 90-210mL. **2-6 yrs:** 60-90mL.

(Continued)

LAXATIVE PRODUCTS

BRAND	INGREDIENT/STRENGTH	DOSE
SALINES *(Continued)*		
Phillips Antacid/Laxative chewable tablets	Magnesium Hydroxide 311mg	**Adults:** ≥ 12 yrs: 6-8 tabs qd. **Peds: 6-11 yrs:** 3-4 tabs qd. **2-5 yrs:** 1-2 tabs qd.
Phillips Soft Chews, Laxative	Magnesium/Sodium 500mg-10 mg	**Adults & Peds:** ≥12 yrs: Take 2-4 tab qd. **Max:** 4 tab q24h.
Phillips Cramp-free Laxative caplets	Magnesium 500 mg	**Adults & Peds:** ≥12 yrs: Take 2-4 tab qd. **Max:** 4 tab q24h.
Phillips Milk of Magnesia Concentrated liquid	Magnesium Hydroxide 800mg/5mL	**Adults:** ≥12 yrs: 15-30mL qd. **Peds: 6-11 yrs:** 7.5-15mL qd. **2-5 yrs:** 2.5-7.5mL qd.
Phillips Milk of Magnesia liquid	Magnesium Hydroxide 400mg/5mL	**Adults:** ≥12 yrs: 30-60mL qd. **Peds: 6-11 yrs:** 15-30mL qd. **2-5 yrs:** 5-15mL qd.
SALINE COMBINATION		
Phillips M-O liquid	Magnesium Hydroxide/Mineral Oil 300mg-1.25mL/5mL	**Adults:** ≥12 yrs: 30-60mL qd. **Peds: 6-11 yrs:** 5-15mL qd.
STIMULANTS		
Alophen Enteric Coated Stimulant Laxative pills	Bisacodyl 5mg	**Adults:** ≥12 yrs: Take 1-3 tab qd. **Peds: 6-12 yrs:** Take 1 tab qd.
Carter's Laxative, Sodium Free pills	Bisacodyl 5mg	**Adults:** ≥12 yrs: Take 1-3 tab (usually 2 tab) qd. **Peds: 6-12 yrs:** Take 1 tab qd.
Castor Oil	Castor Oil	**Adults:** ≥12 yrs: 15-60mL. **Peds: 2-12 yrs:** 5-15mL.
Correctol Stimulant Laxative Tablets For Women	Bisacodyl 5mg	**Adults:** ≥12 yrs: Take 1-3 tab qd. **Peds: 6-12 yrs:** Take 1 tab qd.
Doxidan capsules	Bisacodyl 5mg	**Adults:** ≥12 yrs: 1-3 caps (usually 2) qd. **Peds: 6-12 yrs:** 1 cap qd.
Dulcolax Overnight Relief Laxative tablets	Bisacodyl 5mg	**Adults:** ≥12 yrs: 1-3 tabs (usually 2) qd. **Peds:** 6-12 yo: 1 tab qd.
Dulcolax suppository	Bisacodyl 10mg	**Adults:** ≥12 yrs: 1 supp qd. **Peds: 6-12 yrs:** 1/2 supp qd.
Dulcolax tablets	Bisacodyl 5mg	**Adults:** ≥12 yrs: 1-3 tabs (usually 2) qd. **Peds: 6-12 yrs:** 1 tab qd.
Ex-Lax Maximum Strength tablets	Sennosides 25mg	**Adults:** ≥12 yrs: 2 tabs qd-bid. **Peds: 6-12 yrs:** 1 tab qd-bid.
Ex-Lax tablets	Sennosides 15mg	**Adults:** ≥12 yrs: 2 tabs qd-bid. **Peds: 6-12 yrs:** 1 tab qd-bid.
Ex-Lax Ultra Stimulant Laxative tablets	Bisacodyl 5mg	**Adults:** ≥12 yrs: 1-3 tabs qd. **Peds: 6-12 yrs:** 1 tab qd.
Fleet Bisacodyl suppositories	Bisacodyl 10mg	**Adults:** ≥12 yrs: 1 supp. qd. **Peds: 6-12 yrs:** 1/2 supp. qd.
Fleet Stimulant Laxative tablets	Bisacodyl 5mg	**Adults:** ≥12 yrs: 1-3 tabs (usually 2) qd. **Peds: 6-12 yrs:** 1 tab qd.
Nature's Remedy caplets	Aloe/Cascara Sagrada 100mg-150mg	**Adults:** ≥12 yrs: 2 tabs qd-bid. **Max:** 4 tabs bid. **Peds: 6-12 yrs:** 1 tab qd-bid. **Max:** 2 tab bid. **2-6 yrs:** 1/2 tab qd-bid. **Max:** 1 tab bid.
Perdiem Overnight Relief tablets	Sennosides 15mg	**Adults:** ≥12 yrs: 2 tabs qd-bid. **Peds: 6-12 yrs:** 1 tab qd-bid.
Senokot tablets	Sennosides 8.6mg	**Adults:** ≥12 yrs: 2 tabs qd. **Max:** 4 tabs bid. **Peds: 6-12 yrs:** 1 tab qd. **Max:** 2 tabs bid. **2-6 yrs:** 1/2 tab qd. **Max:** 1 tab bid.
STIMULANT COMBINATIONS		
Perdiem powder	Senna/Psyllium 0.74g-3.25g/6g	**Adults:** ≥12 yrs: 1-2 tsp qd-bid. **Peds:** 6-12 yo: 1 tsp qd-bid.

(Continued)

LAXATIVE PRODUCTS

BRAND	INGREDIENT/STRENGTH	DOSE
STIMULANT COMBINATIONS *(Continued)*		
Peri-Colace tablets	Sennosides/Docusate 8.6mg-50mg	**Adults: ≥12 yrs:** 2-4 tabs qd. **Peds: 6-12 yrs:** 1-2 tabs qd. **2-6 yrs:** 1 tab qd.
SennaPrompt capsules	Sennosides/Psyllium 500mg/9mg	**Adults & Peds: ≥12 yrs:** 5 caps qd-bid.
Senokot S tablets	Sennosides/Docusate 8.6mg-50mg	**Adults: ≥12 yrs:** 2 tabs qd. **Max:** 4 tabs bid. **Peds: 6-12 yrs:** 1 tab qd. **Max:** 2 tabs bid. **2-6 yrs:** 1/2 tab qd. **Max:** 1 tab bid.
SURFACTANTS (STOOL SOFTENERS)		
Colace capsules	Docusate Sodium 100mg	**Adults: ≥12 yrs:** 1-3 caps qd. **Peds: 2-12 yrs:** 1 cap qd.
Colace capsules	Docusate Sodium 50mg	**Adults: ≥12 yrs:** 1-6 caps qd. **Peds: 2-12 yrs:** 1-3 caps qd.
Colace Glycerin suppositories	Glycerin 2.1g; 1.2g	**Adults: ≥6 yrs:** 2.1g supp qd. **Peds: 2-6 yrs:** 1.2g supp qd.
Colace liquid	Docusate Sodium 10mg/mL	**Adults: ≥12 yrs:** 5-15mL qd-bid. **Peds: 2-12 yrs:** 5-15mL qd.
Colace syrup	Docusate Sodium 60mg/15mL	**Adults: ≥12 yrs:** 15-90mL qd. **Peds: 2-12 yrs:** 5-37.5mL qd.
Correctol Stool Softener Laxative soft-gels	Docusate Sodium 100mg	**Adults: ≥12 yrs:** Take 1-3 cap qd. **Peds: 6-12 yrs:** Take 1 cap qd
Docusol Constipation Relief, mini enemas	Docusate Sodium 283mg	**Adults: ≥12 yrs:** Take 1-3 units qd. **Peds: 6-12 yrs:** Take 1 unit qd
Dulcolax Stool Softener capsules	Docusate Sodium 100mg	**Adults: ≥12 yrs:** 1-3 caps qd. **Peds: 2-12 yrs:** 1 cap qd.
Ex-Lax Stool Softener tablets	Docusate Sodium 100mg	**Adults: ≥12 yrs:** 1-3 caps qd. **Peds: 2-12 yrs:** 1 cap qd.
Fleet Sof-Lax tablets	Docusate Sodium 100mg	**Adults: ≥12 yrs:** 1-3 caps qd. **Peds: 2-12 yrs:** 1 cap qd.
Kaopectate Liqui-Gels	Docusate Calcium 240mg	**Adults & Peds: ≥12 yrs:** 1 cap qd until normal bowel movement.
Phillips Stool Softener capsules	Docusate Sodium 100mg	**Adults: ≥12 yrs:** 1-3 caps qd. **Peds: 2-12 yrs:** 1 cap qd.

ALLERGIC RHINITIS PRODUCTS

BRAND	INGREDIENT/STRENGTH	DOSE
ANTIHISTAMINE		
Alavert 24-Hour Allergy tablets	Loratadine 10mg	**Adults & Peds:** ≥**6 yrs:** 1 tab qd. **Max:** 1 tab q24h.
Benadryl Allergy capsules	Diphenhydramine HCl 25mg	**Adults:** ≥**12 yrs:** 1-2 caps q4-6h. **Peds:** 6-12 yrs: 1 cap q4-6h. **Max:** 6 doses q24h.
Benadryl Allergy chewable tablets	Diphenhydramine HCl 12.5mg	**Adults:** ≥**12 yrs:** 2-4 tabs q4-6h. **Peds:** 6-12 yrs: 1-2 tabs q4-6h. **Max:** 6 doses q24h.
Benadryl Allergy liquid	Diphenhydramine HCl 12.5mg/5mL	**Adults:** ≥**12 yrs:** 2-4 tsp (10-20mL) q4-6h. **Peds: 6-12 yrs:** 1-2 tsp (5-10mL) q4-6h. **Max:** 6 doses q24h.
Benadryl Allergy Ultratab	Diphenhydramine HCl 25mg	**Adults:** ≥**12 yrs:** 1-2 tabs q4-6h. **Peds:** 6-12 yrs: 1 tab q4-6h. **Max:** 6 doses q24h.
Benadryl Children's Allergy fastmelt tablets	Diphenhydramine Citrate HCl 19mg	**Adults:** ≥**12 yrs:** 2-4 tabs q4-6h. **Peds:** 6-12 tant **Max:** 6 doses q24h.
Chlor-Trimeton 4-Hour Allergy tablets	Chlorpheniramine Maleate 4mg	**Adults:** ≥**12 yrs:** 1 tab q4-6h. **Max:** 6 tabs q24h. **Peds: 6-12 yrs:** 1/2 tab q4-6h. **Max:** 3 tabs q24h.
Claritin 24 Hour Allergy tablets	Loratadine 10mg	**Adults & Peds:** ≥**6 yrs:** 1 tab qd. **Max:** 1 tab q24h.
Claritin Children's syrup	Loratadine 5mg/5mL	**Adults:** ≥**6 yrs:** 2 tsp qd. **Max:** 2 tsp q24h. **Peds: 2-6 yrs:** 1 tsp qd. **Max:** 1 tsp q24h.
Claritin RediTabs	Loratadine 10mg	**Adults & Peds:** ≥**6 yrs:** 1 tab qd. **Max:** 1 tab q24h.
Dimetapp ND Children's Allergy liquid	Loratadine 5mg/5mL	**Adults:** ≥**6 yrs:** 2 tsp qd. **Max:** 2 tsp q24h. **Peds: 2-6 yrs:** 1 tsp qd. **Max:** 1 tsp q24h.
Dimetapp ND Children's Allergy tablets	Loratadine 10mg	**Adults & Peds:** ≥**6 yrs:** 1 tab qd. **Max:** 1 tab q24h.
Tavist Allergy tablets	Clemastine Fumarate 1.34mg	**Adults & Peds:** ≥**12 yrs:** 1 tab q12h. **Max:** 2 tabs q24h.
Tavist ND 24-Hour Allergy tablets	Loratadine 10mg	**Adults & Peds:** ≥**6 yrs:** 1 tab qd. **Max:** 1 tab q24h.
Triaminic Allerchews	Loratadine 10mg	**Adults & Peds:** ≥**6 yrs:** 1 tab qd. **Max:** 1 tab q24h.
ANTIHISTAMINE COMBINATIONS		
Advil Allergy Sinus caplets	Chlorpheniramine Maleate/ Ibuprofen/Pseudoephedrine HCl 2mg-200mg-30mg	**Adults & Peds:** ≥**12 yrs:** 1 tab q4-6h. **Max:** 6 tabs q24h.
Alavert D-12 Hour Allergy tablets	Loratadine/Pseudoephedrine Sulfate 5mg-120mg	**Adults & Peds:** ≥**12 yrs:** 1 tab q12h. **Max:** 2 tabs q24h.
Benadryl Allergy & Sinus Headache caplets	Diphenhydramine HCl/ Acetaminophen/Phenylephrine HCl/ 12.5mg-325mg-5mg	**Adults & Peds:** ≥**12 yrs:** 2 caps q4h. **Max:** 12 caps q24h.
Benadryl Severe Allergy & Sinus Headache caplets	Diphenhydramine HCl/ Acetaminophen/Phenylephrine HCl 25mg-325mg-5mg	**Adults & Peds:** ≥**12 yrs:** 2 tabs q4h. **Max:** 12 tabs q24h.
Benadryl-D Allergy & Sinus Liquid	Diphenhydramine HCl/ Pseudoephedrine HCl 12.5mg-30mg/5mL	**Adults & Peds:** ≥**12 yrs:** 2 tsp q4-6h. **Peds: 6-12 yrs:** 1 tsp q4-6h. **Max:** 4 doses q24h.
Benadryl-D Allergy & Sinus tablets	Diphenhydramine HCl/ Phenylephrine HCl 25mg-10mg	**Adults & Peds:** ≥**12 yrs:** 1 tab q4h. **Max:** 6 tabs q24h.

(Continued)

ALLERGIC RHINITIS PRODUCTS

BRAND	INGREDIENT/STRENGTH	DOSE
ANTIHISTAMINE COMBINATIONS *(Continued)*		
Claritin-D 12 Hour Allergy & Congestion tablets	Loratadine/Pseudoephedrine Sulfate 5mg-120mg	**Adults & Peds:** ≥12 yrs: 1 tab q12h. **Max:** 2 tabs q24h.
Claritin-D 24 Hour Allergy & Congestion tablets	Loratadine/Pseudoephedrine Sulfate 10mg-240mg	**Adults & Peds:** ≥12 yrs: 1 tab q12h. **Max:** 1 tabs q24h.
Drixoral Allergy Sinus sustained-action tablets	Dexbrompheniramine Maleate/Acetaminophen/ Pseudoephedrine HCl 3mg-500mg-60mg	**Adults & Peds:** ≥12 yrs: 2 tabs q12h. **Max:** 4 tabs q24h.
Sinutab Sinus caplets	Acetaminophen/Phenylephrine HCl 325mg-5mg	**Adults & Peds:** ≥12 yrs: 2 tabs q4h. **Max:** 12 tabs q24h.
Sudafed PE Sinus & Allergy tablets	Chlorpheniramine Maleate/Phenylephrine HCl 4mg-10mg	**Adults:** ≥12 yrs: 1 tab q4h. **Peds:** 6-12 yrs: 1/2 tab q4h. **Max:** 6 doses q24h.
Tylenol Allergy Complete Multi-Symptom Cool Burst caplets	Chlorpheniramine Maleate/ Acetaminophen/Phenylephrine HCl 2mg-325mg-5mg	**Adults & Peds:** ≥12 yrs: 2 tabs q4h. **Max:** 12 tabs q24h.
Tylenol Allergy Complete Nighttime Cool Burst caplets	Diphenhydramine HCl/ Acetaminophen/Phenylephrine HCl 25mg-325mg-5mg	**Adults & Peds:** ≥12 yrs: 2 tabs q4h. **Max:** 12 tabs q24h.
Tylenol Allergy Complete caplets	Chlorpheniramine Maleate/ Acetaminophen/Pseudoephedrine HCl 2mg-500mg-30mg	**Adults & Peds:** ≥12 yrs: 2 tabs q4-6h. **Max:** 8 tabs q24h.
Tylenol Allergy Complete Night Time caplets	Diphenhydramine HCl/ Acetaminophen/Pseudoephedrine HCl 25mg-500mg-30mg	**Adults & Peds:** ≥12 yrs: 2 tabs q4-6h. **Max:** 8 tabs q24h.
Tylenol Severe Allergy caplets	Diphenhydramine HCl/ Acetaminophen 12.5mg-500mg	**Adults & Peds:** ≥12 yrs: 2 tabs q4-6h. **Max:** 8 tabs q24h.
TOPICAL NASAL DECONGESTANTS		
4-Way Fast Acting Nasal Decongestant Spray	Phenylephrine HCl 1%	**Adults & Peds:** ≥12 yrs: Instill 2-3 sprays per nostril q4h.
4-Way Nasal Decongestant Spray, 12 Hour	Phenylephrine HCl 1%	**Adults & Peds:** ≥12 yrs: Instill 2-3 sprays per nostril q4h.
4-Way No Drip Nasal Decongestant Spray	Phenylephrine HCl 1%	**Adults & Peds:** ≥12 yrs: Instill 2-3 sprays per nostril q4h.
Afrin Extra Moisturizing Nasal Spray	Oxymetazoline HCl 0.05%	**Adults & Peds:** ≥6 yrs: Instill 2-3 sprays per nostril q10-12h.
Afrin No Drip Nasal Spray	Oxymetazoline HCl 0.05%	**Adults & Peds:** ≥6 yrs: Instill 2-3 sprays per nostril q10-12h.
Afrin No Drip Sinus Nasal Spray	Oxymetazoline HCl 0.05%	**Adults & Peds:** ≥6 yrs: Instill 2-3 sprays per nostril q10-12h.
Afrin Original Nasal Spray	Oxymetazoline HCl 0.05%	**Adults & Peds:** ≥6 yrs: Instill 2-3 sprays per nostril q10-12h.
Afrin Original Pumpmist Nasal Spray	Oxymetazoline HCl 0.05%	**Adults & Peds:** ≥6 yrs: Instill 2-3 sprays per nostril q10-12h.
Afrin Severe Congestion Nasal Spray	Oxymetazoline HCl 0.05%	**Adults & Peds:** ≥6 yrs: Instill 2-3 sprays per nostril q10-12h.
Afrin Sinus Nasal Spray	Oxymetazoline HCl 0.05%	**Adults & Peds:** ≥6 yrs: Instill 2-3 sprays per nostril q10-12h.
Benzedrex Inhaler	Propylhexedrine 250mg	**Adults & Peds:** ≥6 yrs: Inhale 2 sprays per nostril q2h
Neo-Synephrine 12 Hour Extra Moisturizing Nasal Spray	Oxymetazoline HCl 0.05%	**Adults & Peds:** ≥6 yrs: Instill 2-3 sprays per nostril q10-12h.
Neo-Synephrine 12 Hour Nasal Decongestant Spray	Oxymetazoline HCl 0.05%	**Adults & Peds:** ≥6 yrs: Instill 2-3 sprays per nostril q10-12h.
Neo-Synephrine Extra Strength Nasal Decongestant Drops	Phenylephrine HCl 1%	**Adults & Peds:** ≥12 yrs: Instill 2-3 drops per nostril q4h.

(Continued)

ALLERGIC RHINITIS PRODUCTS

BRAND	INGREDIENT/STRENGTH	DOSE
TOPICAL NASAL DECONGESTANTS *(Continued)*		
Neo-Synephrine Extra Strength Nasal Spray	Phenylephrine HCl 1%	**Adults & Peds:** ≥6 yrs: Instill 2-3 sprays per nostril q4h.
Neo-Synephrine Mild Formula Nasal Spray	Phenylephrine HCl 0.25%	**Adults & Peds:** ≥6 yrs: Instill 2-3 sprays per nostril q4h.
Neo-Synephrine Regular Strength Nasal Decongestant Spray	Phenylephrine HCl 0.5%	**Adults & Peds:** ≥12 yrs: Instill 2-3 sprays per nostril q4h.
Nostrilla 12 Hour Nasal Decongestant	Oxymetazoline HCl 0.05%	**Adults & Peds:** ≥6 yrs: Instill 2-3 sprays per nostril q10-12h.
Vicks Sinex 12 Hour Ultra Fine Mist For Sinus Relief	Oxymetazoline HCl 0.05%	**Adults & Peds:** ≥12 yrs: Instill 2-3 sprays per nostril q10-12h.
Vicks Sinex Long Acting Nasal Spray For Sinus Relief	Oxymetazoline HCl 0.05%	**Adults & Peds:** ≥12 yrs: Instill 2-3 sprays per nostril q10-12h.
Vicks Sinex Nasal Spray For Sinus Relief	Phenylephrine HCl 0.5%	**Adults & Peds:** ≥12 yrs: Instill 2-3 sprays per nostril q4h.
TOPICAL NASAL MOISTURIZERS		
4-Way Saline Moisturizing Mist	Water, Boric Acid, Glycerin, Sodium Chloride, Sodium Borate, Eucalyptol, Menthol, Polysorbate 80, Benzalkonium Chloride	**Adults & Peds:** ≥2 yrs: Instill 2-3 sprays per nostril prn.
Ayr Baby's Saline Nose Spray, Drops	Sodium Chloride 0.65%	**Peds:** Instill 2 to 6 drops in each nostril.
Ayr Saline Nasal Gel	Aloe Vera Gel, Carbomer, Diazolidinyl Urea, Dimethicone Copolyol, FD&C Blue 1, Geranium Oil, Glycerin, Glyceryl Polymethacrylate, Methyl Gluceth 10, Methylparaben, Poloxamer 184, Propylene Glycol, Propylparaben, Sodium Chloride, Tocopherol Acetate, Triethanolamine, Xanthan Gum, Water	**Adults & Peds:** ≥12 yrs: Apply to nostril prn.
Ayr Saline Nasal Gel, No-Drip Sinus Spray	Water, Sodium Carbomethyl Starch, Propylene Glycol, Glycerin, Aloe Barbadensis Leaf Juice (Aloe Vera Gel), Sodium Chloride, Cetyl Pyridinium Chloride, Citric Acid, Disodium EDTA, Glycine Soja (Soybean Oil), Tocopheryl Acetate, Benzyl Alcohol, Benzalkonium Chloride, Geranium Maculatum Oil	**Adults & Peds:** ≥12 yrs: Use prn as directed.
Ayr Saline Nasal Mist	Sodium Chloride 0.65%	**Adults & Peds:** ≥12 yrs: Instill 2 sprays per nostril prn.
ENTSOL Mist, Buffered Hypertonic Nasal Irrigation Mist	Purified Water, Sodium Chloride, Sodium Phosphate Dibasic Edetate Disodium, Potassium Phosphate Monobasic, Benzalkonium Chloride	**Adults & Peds:** ≥12 yrs: Instill 1-2 sprays per nostril prn.
ENTSOL Single Use, Pre-Filled Nasal Wash Squeeze Bottle	Purified Water, Sodium Chloride, Sodium Phosphate Dibasic, Potassium Phosphate Monobasic	**Adults & Peds:** ≥12 yrs: Use as directed.
ENTSOL Spray, Buffered Hypertonic Saline Nasal Spray	Purified Water, Sodium Chloride Phosphate Dibasic, Potassium Phosphate Monobasic	**Adults & Peds:** ≥12 yrs: Instill 1 spray per nostril bid, 6 times daily
Little Noses Saline Spray/Drops, Non-Medicated	Sodium Chloride 0.65%	**Peds:** 2-6 drops per nostril as directed.
Ocean Premium Saline Nasal Spray	Sodium Chloride 0.65%, Phenylcarbinol, Benzalkonium Chloride	**Adults & Peds:** ≥6 yrs: Instill 2 sprays per nostril prn.
Simply Saline Sterile Saline Nasal Mist	Sodium Chloride 0.9%	**Adults & Peds:** ≥12 yrs: Use prn as directed.

(Continued)

Allergic Rhinitis Products

BRAND	INGREDIENT/STRENGTH	DOSE
TOPICAL NASAL MOISTURIZERS *(Continued)*		
SinoFresh Moisturizing Nasal & Sinus Spray	Cetylpyridinium Chloride 0.05%	**Adults & Peds: ≥12 yrs:** Instill 1-3 sprays per nostril qd.
Zicam Nasal Moisturizer	Purified Water, High Purity Sodium Chloride, Aloe Vera	**Adults & Peds: ≥12 yrs:** Use as directed.
MISCELLANEOUS		
NasalCrom Allergy Prevention Nasal Spray	Cromolyn Sodium 5.2mg	**Adults & Peds: ≥6 yrs:** Instill 1 spray per nostril q4-6h.
NasalCrom Nasal Allergy Symptom Controller, Nasal Spray	Cromolyn Sodium 5.2mg	**Adults & Peds: ≥2 yrs:** Instill 1 spray per nostril q4-6h.
Similasan Hay Fever Relief, Non-Drowsy Formula, Nasal Spray	Cardiospermum HPUS 6X, Galphimia Glauca HPUS 6X, Luffa Operculata HPUS 6X, Sabadilla HPUS 6x	**Adults & Peds: ≥12 yrs:** Use as directed.
Zicam Allergy Relief, Homeopathic Nasal Solution, Pump	Luffa Operculata 4x, 12x, 30x, Galphimia Glauca 12x, 30x, Histaminum Hydrochloricum 12x, 30x, 200x, Sulphur 12x, 30x, 200x	**Adults & Peds: ≥6 yrs:** Instill 2-3 sprays per nostril q4h.

Is it a Cold, the Flu, or an Allergy?

	COLD	FLU	AIRBORNE ALLERGY
SYMPTOMS			
Chest discomfort	Mild to moderate	Common; can become severe	Sometimes
Cough	Common (hacking cough)	Sometimes	Sometimes
Duration	3-14 days	Days to weeks	Weeks (eg, 6 weeks for ragweed or grass pollen seasons)
Extreme exhaustion	Never	Early and prominent	Never
Fatigue, weakness	Sometimes	Can last up to 2-3 weeks	Sometimes
Fever	Rare	Characteristic, high (100-102 °F); lasts 3-4 days	Never
General aches, pains	Slight	Usual; often severe	Never
Headache	Rare	Prominent	Sometimes
Itchy eyes	Rare or never	Rare or never	Common
Runny nose	Common		Common
Sneezing	Usual	Sometimes	Usual
Sore throat	Common	Sometimes	Sometimes
Stuffy nose	Common	Sometimes	Common
TREATMENT			
	Antihistamines	Amantadine	Antihistamines
	Decongestants	Rimantadine	Nasal steroids
	Nonsteroidal antiflammatories	Oseltamivir	Decongestants
	Temporary symptom relief	Zanamavir	
PREVENTION			
	Wash your hands often; avoid close contact with anyone with a cold	Annual vaccination Amantadine Rimantadine Oseltamivir	Avoid allergens such as pollen, house flies, dust mites, mold pet dander, cockroaches
COMPLICATIONS			
	Sinus infection	Bronchitis	Sinus infections
	Middle ear infection	Pneumonia	Asthma
	Asthma	Can be life-threatening	

Adapted from the National Institute of Allergy and Infectious Diseases, September 2005.

Cough-Cold-Flu Products

BRAND NAME	ANALGESIC	ANTIHISTAMINE	DECONGESTANT	COUGH SUPPRESSANT	EXPECTORANT	DOSE
ANTIHISTAMINE + DECONGESTANT						
Actifed Cold & Allergy tablets		Chlorpheniramine Maleate 4mg	Phenylephrine HCl 10mg			**Adults:** ≥12 yrs: 1 tabs q4-6h. **Max:** 4 tabs q24h. **Peds: 6-12 yrs:** 1/2 tab q4-6h. **Max:** 2 tabs q24h.
Benadryl Children's Allergy & Cold Fastmelt tablets		Diphenhydramine HCl 19mg	Pseudoephedrine HCl 30mg			**Adults:** ≥12 yrs: 2 tabs q4h. **Max:** 8 tabs q24h. **Peds: 6-12 yrs:** 1 tab q4h. **Max:** 4 tabs q24h.
Benadryl-D Allergy/Sinus Tablets		Diphenhydramine HCl 25mg	Phenylephrine HCl 10mg			**Adults & Peds:** ≥12 yrs: 1 tab q4h. **Max:** 6 tab q24h.
Children's Benadryl-D Allergy & Sinus Liquid		Diphenhydramine HCl 12.5mg/5mL	Pseudoephedrine HCl 30mg/5mL			**Adults:** ≥12 yrs: 2 tsp (10mL) q4-6h. **Peds: 6-12 yrs:** 1 tsp (5mL) q4-6h. **Max:** 4 doses q24h.
Children's Benadryl Allergy & Cold Fastmelt Tablets		Diphenhydramine HCl 19mg	Pseudoephedrine HCl 30mg			**Adult & Peds** ≥12 yrs: 2 tabs q4h. **Max:** 8 tabs q24h. **Peds: 6-12 yrs:** 1 tab q4h. **Max:** 6 doses q24h.
Dimetapp Children's Cold & Allergy elixir		Brompheniramine Maleate 1mg/5mL	Phenylephrine HCl 2.5mg/5mL			**Adults:** ≥12 yrs: 4 tsp (20mL) q4h. **Peds: 6-12 yrs:** 2 tsp (10mL) q4h. **Max:** 6 doses q24h.
Triaminic Cold & Allergy liquid		Chlorpheniramine Maleate 1mg/5mL	Phenylephrine HCl 2.5mg/5mL			**Adults:** ≥12 yrs: 1 tsp (5mL) q4h. **Max:** 6 doses q24h. **Peds: 6-12 yrs:** 2 tsp (10mL).
Triaminic Nighttime Cough & Cold liquid		Diphenhydramine HCl 6.25mg/5mL	Phenylephrine HCl 2.5mg/5mL			**Adults:** ≥12 yrs: 1 tsp (5mL) q4h. **Max:** 6 doses q24h. **Peds: 6-12 yrs:** 2 tsp (10mL).
ANTIHISTAMINE + DECONGESTANT + ANALGESIC						
Actifed Cold & Sinus caplets	Acetaminophen 500mg	Chlorpheniramine Maleate 2mg	Pseudoephedrine HCl 30mg			**Adults & Peds:** ≥12 yrs: 2 tabs q6h. **Max:** 8 tabs q24h.
Advil Multi-Symptom Cold caplets	Ibuprofen 200mg	Chlorpheniramine Maleate 2mg	Pseudoephedrine HCl 30mg			**Adults & Peds:** ≥12 yrs: 1 tab q4-6h. **Max:** 6 tabs q24h.
Alka-Seltzer Plus Cold effervescent tablets	Acetaminophen 250mg	Chlorpheniramine Maleate 2mg	Phenylephrine HCl 5mg			**Adults & Peds:** ≥12 yrs: 2 tabs q4h. **Max:** 8 tabs q24h.

COUGH-COLD-FLU PRODUCTS

BRAND NAME	ANALGESIC	ANTIHISTAMINE	DECONGESTANT	COUGH SUPPRESSANT	EXPECTORANT	DOSE
Benadryl Allergy & Cold caplets	Acetaminophen 500mg	Diphenhydramine HCl 12.5mg	Phenylephrine HCl 5mg			**Adults & Peds: ≥12 yrs:** 2 cap q4h. **Max:** 12 q24h. **Peds: 6-12 yrs:** 1 cap q4h. **Max:** 5 tabs q24h.
Benadryl Allergy & Sinus Headache caplets	Acetaminophen 325mg	Diphenhydramine HCl 12.5mg	Phenylephrine HCl 5mg			**Adults & Peds: ≥12 yrs:** 2 tab q4h. **Max:** 12 tab q24h. **Peds: 6-12 yrs:** 1 cap q4h. **Max:** 5 tabs q24h.
Benadryl Severe Allergy & Sinus Headache caplets	Acetaminophen 325mg	Diphenhydramine HCl 25mg	Phenylephrine HCl 5mg			**Adults & Peds: ≥12 yrs:** 2 caps q4h. **Max:** 12 caps q24h.
Comtrex Acute Head Cold caplets	Acetaminophen 500mg	Brompheniramine Maleate 2mg	Pseudoephedrine HCl 30mg			**Adults & Peds: ≥12 yrs:** 2 tabs q6h. **Max:** 8 tabs q24h.
Comtrex Flu Therapy Nightime liquid	Acetaminophen 1000mg/30mL	Chlorpheniramine Maleate 4mg/30mL	Pseudoephedrine HCl 60mg/30mL			**Adults & Peds: ≥12 yrs:** 2 tbl (30mL) q6h. **Max:** 8 tbl (240mL) q24h.
Comtrex Flu Therapy Day & Night tablets	Acetaminophen 500mg	Chlorpheniramine Maleate 2mg	Pseudoephedrine HCl 30mg			**Adults & Peds: ≥12 yrs:** 2 tabs q6h. **Max:** 4 daytime tabs q24h.
Comtrex Nighttime Acute Head Cold liquid	Acetaminophen 1000mg/30mL	Brompheniramine Maleate 4mg/30mL	Pseudoephedrine HCl 60mg/30mL			**Adults & Peds: ≥12 yrs:** 2 tbl (30mL) q6h. **Max:** 8 tbl (240mL) q24h.
Contac Cold & Flu Maximum Strength caplets	Acetaminophen 500mg	Chlorpheniramine Maleate 2mg	Phenylephrine HCl 5mg			**Adults & Peds: ≥12 yrs:** 2 caps q4-6h **Max:** 8 caps q24h.
Dristan Cold Multi-Symptom tablets	Acetaminophen 325mg	Chlorpheniramine Maleate 2mg	Phenylephrine HCl 5mg			**Adults & Peds: ≥12 yrs:** 2 tabs q4h. **Max:** 12 caps q24h.
Robitussin Cold & Congestion tablets	Acetaminophen 325mg	Chlorpheniramine Maleate 2mg	Phenylephrine HCl 5mg			**Adults & Peds: ≥12 yrs:** 2 tabs q4h. **Max:** 12 caps q24h.
Sudafed Sinus PE Nighttime Cold caplets	Acetaminophen 325mg	Diphenhydramine HCl 25mg	Phenylephrine HCl 5mg			**Adults & Peds: ≥12 yrs:** 2 tabs q4h. **Max:** 12 tabs q24h.
Sudafed PE Severe Cold caplets	Acetaminophen 325mg	Diphenhydramine HCl 12.5mg	Phenylephrine HCl 5mg			**Adults & Peds: ≥12 yrs:** 2 tabs q4h. **Max:** 12 tabs q24h. **Peds: 6-12 yrs:** 1 tab q4h. **Max:** 5 tabs q24h.
Theraflu Cold & Sore Throat Hot Liquid	Acetaminophen 325mg/packet	Pheniramine Maleate 20mg/packet	Phenylephrine HCl 10mg/packet			**Adults & Peds: ≥12 yrs:** 1 packet q4h. **Max:** 6 packets q24h.
Theraflu Nighttime Severe Cold Hot Liquid	Acetaminophen 650mg/packet	Pheniramine Maleate 20mg/packet	Phenylephrine HCl 10mg/packet			**Adults & Peds: ≥12 yrs:** 1 packet q4h. **Max:** 6 packets q24h.

(Continued)

COUGH-COLD-FLU PRODUCTS

BRAND NAME	ANALGESIC	ANTIHISTAMINE	DECONGESTANT	COUGH SUPPRESSANT	EXPECTORANT	DOSE
ANTIHISTAMINE + DECONGESTANT + ANALGESIC *(Continued)*						
Theraflu Flu & Sore Throat Liquid	Acetaminophen 650mg/packet	Pheniramine Maleate 20mg/packet	Phenylephrine HCl 10mg/packet			**Adults & Peds: ≥12 yrs:** 1 packet q4h. **Max:** 6 packets q24h.
Tylenol Children's Plus Cold liquid	Acetaminophen 160mg/5mL	Chlorpheniramine Maleate 1mg/5mL	Phenylephrine HCl 2.5mg/5mL			**Peds: 6-11 yrs (48-95 lbs):** 2 tsp (10mL) q4h. **Max:** 5 doses q24h.
Tylenol Children's Plus Cold & Allergy liquid	Acetaminophen 160mg/5mL	Diphenhydramine HCl 12.5mg/5mL	Phenylephrine HCl 2.5mg/5mL			**Peds: 6-11 yrs (48-95 lbs):** 2 tsp (10mL) q4-6h. **Max:** 4 doses q24h.
Tylenol Children's Plus Cold Nighttime suspension	Acetaminophen 160mg/5mL	Chlorpheniramine Maleate 1mg/5mL	Pseudoephedrine HCl 15mg/5mL			**Peds: 6-12 yrs (48-95 lbs):** 2 tsp (10mL) q4-6h. **Max:** 8 tsp (40mL) q24h.
Tylenol Flu Nighttime gelcaps	Acetaminophen 500mg	Diphenhydramine HCl 25mg	Pseudoephedrine HCl 30mg			**Adults & Peds: ≥12 yrs:** 2 caps q6h. **Max:** 8 caps q24h.
Tylenol Sinus Congestion & Pain Nighttime caplets	Acetaminophen 325mg	Chlorpheniramine Maleate 2mg	Phenylephrine HCl 5mg			**Adults & Peds: ≥12 yrs:** 2 caps q4h. **Max:** 12 caps q24h.
Tylenol Sinus Nighttime caplets	Acetaminophen 500mg	Doxylamine Succinate 6.25mg	Pseudoephedrine HCl 30mg			**Adults & Peds: ≥12 yrs:** 2 tabs q4-6h. **Max:** 8 tabs q24h.
COUGH SUPPRESSANT						
Delsym 12 Hour Cough Relief liquid				Dextromethorphan Polistirex 30mg/5mL		**Adults: ≥12 yrs:** 2 tsp (10mL) q12h. **Peds: 6-12 yrs:** 1 tsp (5mL) q12h. 2-6 yrs: 1/2 tsp (2.5mL) q12h. **Max:** 4 doses q24h.
PediaCare Long-Acting Cough liquid				Dextromethorphan HBr 7.5mg/5mL		**Peds: 6-12 yrs:** 2 tsp q6-8h. 2-6 yrs: 1 tsp q6-8h. **Max:** 4 doses q24h.
Robitussin Cough Long-Acting liquid				Dextromethorphan HBr 15mg/5mL		**Adults & Peds: ≥12 yrs:** 2 tsp (10mL) q6-8h. **Max:** 8 tsp (40mL) q24h.
Robitussin CoughGels liqui-gels				Dextromethorphan HBr 15mg		**Adults & Peds: ≥12 yrs:** 2 caps q6-8h. **Max:** 8 caps q24h.
Robitussin Pediatric Cough liquid				Dextromethorphan HBr 7.5mg/5mL		**Adults: ≥12 yrs (≥96 lbs):** 4 tsp (20mL) q6-8h. **Peds: 6-12 yrs (48-95 lbs):** 2 tsp (10mL) q6-8h. 2-6yrs: 1 tsp (5mL) q6-8h. **Max:** 4 doses q24h.

COUGH-COLD-FLU PRODUCTS

BRAND NAME	ANALGESIC	ANTIHISTAMINE	DECONGESTANT	COUGH SUPPRESSANT	EXPECTORANT	DOSE
Simply Cough liquid				Dextromethorphan HBr 5mg/5mL		**Peds: 6-12 yrs (48-95 lbs):** 2 tsp (10mL) q4h. **2-6 yrs (24-47 lbs):** 1 tsp (5mL) q4h. **Max:** 4 doses q24h.
Theraflu Long Acting Cough thin strips				Dextromethorphan 11mg/strip		**Adults & Peds: ≥12 yrs:** 2 strips q6-8h. **Max:** 8 strips q24h.
Triaminic Long Acting Cough thin strips				Dextromethorphan 5.5mg/strip		**Peds: 6-12 yrs:** 2 strips q6-8h. **Max:** 8 strips q24h.
Vicks DayQuil Cough liquid				Dextromethorphan HBr 15mg/15mL		**Adults & Peds: ≥12 yrs:** 2 tbl (30mL) q6-8h. **Peds: 6-12 yrs:** 1 tbl (15mL) q6-8h. **Max:** 4 doses q24h.
Vicks 44 liquid				Dextromethorphan HBr 30mg/15mL		**Adults & Peds: ≥12 yrs:** 1 tbl (15mL) q6-8h. **Peds: 6-12 yrs:** 1.5 tsp (7.5mL) q6-8h. **Max:** 4 doses q24h.
Vicks BabyRub				Eucalyptus, petrolatum, fragrance, aloe extract, eucalyptus oil, lavender oil, rosemary oil		**Peds: ≥3 mth:** Apply q8h.
Vicks Cough Drops Cherry Flavor				Menthol 1.7mg		**Adults & Peds: ≥5 yrs:** 3 drops q1-2h.
Vicks Cough Drops Original Flavor				Menthol 3.3mg		**Adults & Peds: ≥5 yrs:** 2 drops q1-2h.
Vicks VapoRub				Camphor 5.2% Menthol 2.8%, Eucalyptus 1.2%		**Adults & Peds: ≥2 yrs:** Apply q8h.
Vicks VapoRub cream				Camphor 4.8% Menthol 2.6%, Eucalyptus 1.2%		**Adults & Peds: ≥2 yrs:** Apply q8h.
Vicks VapoSteam				Camphor 6.2%		**Adults & Peds: ≥2 yrs:** 1 tbl/quart q8h.
COUGH SUPPRESSANT + ANTIHISTAMINE						
Coricidin HBP Cough & Cold tablets		Chlorpheniramine Maleate 4mg		Dextromethorphan HBr 30mg		**Adults & Peds: ≥12 yrs:** 1 tabs q6h. **Max:** 4 tabs q24h.
Dimetapp Long-Acting Cold Plus Cough elixir		Chlorpheniramine Maleate 1mg/5mL		Dextromethorphan HBr 7.5mg/5mL		**Peds: ≥12 yrs:** 4 tsp (20mL) q6h. **6-12 yrs:** 2 tsp (10 mL) q6h. **Max:** 4 doses q24h.

(Continued)

COUGH-COLD-FLU PRODUCTS

BRAND NAME	ANALGESIC	ANTIHISTAMINE	DECONGESTANT	COUGH SUPPRESSANT	EXPECTORANT	DOSE
COUGH SUPPRESSANT + ANTIHISTAMINE (Continued)						
Robitussin Cough & Cold Long-Acting liquid		Chlorpheniramine Maleate 2mg/5mL		Dextromethorphan HBr 15mg/5mL		**Adults:** ≥**12 yrs:** 2 tsp (10mL) q6h. **Max:** 4 doses q24h.
Triaminic Softchews Cough & Runny Nose		Chlorpheniramine Maleate 1mg		Dextromethorphan HBr 5mg		**Adults & Peds:** ≥**12 yrs:** 1 tabs q4-6h. **Max:** 6 tabs q24h.
Vicks Children's NyQuil liquid		Chlorpheniramine Maleate 2mg/15mL		Dextromethorphan HBr 15mg/15mL		**Adults:** ≥**12 yrs:** 2 tbl (30mL) q6h. **Peds: 6-11 yrs:** 1 tbl (15mL) q6h. **Max:** 4 doses q24h.
Vicks NyQuil Cough liquid		Doxylamine Succinate 6.25mg/15mL		Dextromethorphan HBr 15mg/15mL		**Adults & Peds:** ≥**12 yrs:** 2 tbl (30mL) q6h. **Max:** 8 tbl (120mL) q24h.
COUGH SUPPRESSANT + ANTIHISTAMINE + ANALGESIC						
Alka-Seltzer Plus Flu effervescent tablets	Aspirin 500mg	Chlorpheniramine Maleate 2mg		Dextromethorphan HBr 15mg		**Adults & Peds:** ≥**12 yrs:** 2 tabs q6h. **Max:** 8 tabs q24h.
Alka-Seltzer Plus Nighttime Liquid Gels	Acetaminophen 325mg	Doxylamine Succinate 6.25mg		Dextromethorphan HBr 15mg		**Adults & Peds:** ≥**12 yrs:** 2 tabs q6h. **Max:** 12 tabs q24h.
Coricidin HBP Maximum Strength Flu tablets	Acetaminophen 500mg	Chlorpheniramine Maleate 2mg		Dextromethorphan HBr 15mg		**Adults & Peds:** ≥**12 yrs:** 2 tabs q6h. **Max:** 8 tabs q24h.
Triaminic Flu Cough & Fever liquid	Acetaminophen 160mg/5mL	Chlorpheniramine Maleate 1mg/5mL		Dextromethorphan HBr 7.5mg/5mL		**Adults & Peds:** ≥**12 yrs:** 1 tsp (5mL) q6h. **Max:** 4 doses (20mL) q24h.
Tylenol Nighttime Cough & Sore Throat Cool Burst liquid	Acetaminophen 1000mg/30mL	Doxylamine 12.5mg/30mL		Dextromethorphan HBr 30mg/30mL		**Adults & Peds:** ≥**12 yrs:** 2 tbl (30mL) q6h. **Max:** 8 tbl (120mL) q24h.
Vicks 44M liquid	Acetaminophen 162.5mg/5mL	Chlorpheniramine Maleate 1mg/5mL		Dextromethorphan HBr 7.5mg/5mL		**Adults & Peds:** ≥**12 yrs:** 4 tsp (20mL) q6h. **Max:** 16 tsp (80mL) q24h.
Vicks NyQuil liquicaps	Acetaminophen 325mg	Doxylamine Succinate 6.25mg		Dextromethorphan HBr 15mg		**Adults & Peds:** ≥**12 yrs:** 2 caps q6h. **Max:** 8 caps q24h.
Vicks NyQuil liquid	Acetaminophen 500mg/15mL	Doxylamine Succinate 6.25mg/15mL		Dextromethorphan HBr 15mg/15mL		**Adults & Peds:** ≥**12 yrs:** 2 tbl (30mL) q6h. **Max:** 8 tbl (120mL) q24h.
COUGH SUPPRESSANT + ANTIHISTAMINES + ANALGESIC + DECONGESTANT						
Alka-Seltzer Plus Cough & Cold Liquid Gels	Acetaminophen 325mg	Chlorpheniramine Maleate 2mg	Phenylephrine HCl 5mg	Dextromethorphan HBr 10mg		**Adults & Peds:** ≥**12 yrs:** 2 tabs q4h. **Max:** 12 tabs q24h.
Alka-Seltzer Plus Nighttime effervescent tablets	Acetaminophen 250mg	Doxlamine Succinate 6.25mg	Phenylephrine HCl 5mg	Dextromethorphan HBr 10mg		**Adults & Peds:** ≥**12 yrs:** 2 tabs q4h. **Max:** 8 tabs q24h.

COUGH-COLD-FLU PRODUCTS

BRAND NAME	ANALGESIC	ANTIHISTAMINE	DECONGESTANT	COUGH SUPPRESSANT	EXPECTORANT	DOSE
Alka-Seltzer Plus Cough & Cold effervescent tablets	Acetaminophen 250mg	Chlorpheniramine Maleate 2mg	Phenylephrine HCl 5mg	Dextromethorphan HBr 10mg		**Adults & Peds: ≥12 yrs:** 2 tabs q4h. **Max:** 8 tabs q24h.
Alka-Seltzer Plus Cough & Cold liquid	Acetaminophen 162.5mg/5mL	Chlorpheniramine Maleate 1mg/5mL	Phenylephrine HCl 2.5mg/5mLmg	Dextromethorphan HBr 5mg/5mL		**Adults & Peds: ≥12 yrs:** 4 tsp q4h. **Max:** 24 tsp q24h.
Comtrex Cold & Cough Nighttime caplets	Acetaminophen 500mg	Chlorpheniramine Maleate 2mg	Pseudoephedrine HCl 30mg	Dextromethorphan HBr 15mg		**Adults & Peds: ≥12 yrs:** 2 tabs q6h. **Max:** 8 tabs q24h.
Comtrex Nighttime Cold & Cough liquid	Acetaminophen 1000mg/30mL	Chlorpheniramine Maleate 4mg/30mL	Pseudoephedrine HCl 60mg/30mL	Dextromethorphan HBr 30mg/30mL		**Adults & Peds: ≥12 yrs:** 2 tbl (30mL) q6h. **Max:** 8 tbl (240mL) q24h.
Dimetapp Children's Nighttime Flu liquid	Acetaminophen 160mg/5mL	Chlorpheniramine Maleate 1mg/5mL	Phenylephrine HCl 2.5mg/5mL	Dextromethorphan HBr 5mg/5mL		**Adults: ≥12 yrs:** 4 tsp (20mL) q4h. **Peds: 6-12 yrs:** 2 tsp (10mL) q4h. **Max:** 5 doses q24h.
Robitussin Cold Cough & Flu liquid	Acetaminophen 160mg/5mL	Chlorpheniramine Maleate 1mg/5mL	Phenylephrine HCl 2.5mg/5mL	Dextromethorphan HBr 5mg/5mL		**Adults: ≥12 yrs:** 4 tsp (20mL) q4h. **Peds: 6-12 yrs:** 2 tsp (10mL) q4h. **Max:** 5 doses q24h.
Tylenol Children's Plus Flu liquid	Acetaminophen 160mg/5mL	Chlorpheniramine Maleate 1mg/5mL	Phenylephrine HCl 2.5mg/5mL	Dextromethorphan HBr 7.5mg/5mL		**Peds: 6-11 yrs (48-95 lbs);** 2 tsp (10mL) q6-8h. **Max:** 4 doses q24h.
Tylenol Cold & Flu Severe Nighttime Cool Burst liquid	Acetaminophen 1000mg/30mL	Doxylamine 12.5mg/30mL	Pseudoephedrine HCl 60mg/30mL	Dextromethorphan HBr 30mg/30mL		**Adults & Peds: ≥12 yrs:** 2 tbl (30mL) q6h. **Max:** 8 tbl (120mL) q24h.
Tylenol Cold Head Congestion Nighttime caplets	Acetaminophen 325mg	Chlorpheniramine Maleate 2mg	Phenylephrine HCl 5mg	Dextromethorphan HBr 10mg		**Adults & Peds: ≥12 yrs:** 2 caps q4h. **Max:** 12 caps q24h.
Tylenol Cold Multi-Symptom Nighttime caplets	Acetaminophen 325mg	Chlorpheniramine Maleate 2mg	Phenylephrine HCl 5mg	Dextromethorphan HBr 10mg		**Adults & Peds: ≥12 yrs:** 2 caps q4h. **Max:** 12 caps q24h.
Tylenol Cold Multi-Symptom Nighttime liquid	Acetaminophen 325mg/15mL	Doxylamine 6.25mg/30mL	Phenylephrine HCl 5mg/15mL	Dextromethorphan HBr 10mg/15mL		**Adults & Peds: ≥12 yrs:** 2 tbl (30mL) q4h. **Max:** 12 tbl (180mL) q24h.
Tylenol Cold Nighttime Cool Burst caplets	Acetaminophen 325mg	Chlorpheniramine Maleate 2mg	Pseudoephedrine HCl 30mg	Dextromethorphan HBr 15mg		**Adults & Peds: ≥12 yrs:** 2 tabs q6h. **Max:** 8 tabs q24h.
COUGH SUPPRESSANT + ANTIHISTAMINE + DECONGESTANT						
Dimetapp DM Children's Cold & Cough elixir		Brompheniramine Maleate 1mg/5mL	Phenylephrine HCl 2.5mg/5mL	Dextromethorphan HBr 5mg/5mL		**Adults: ≥12 yrs:** 4 tsp (20mL) q4h. **Peds: 6-12 yrs:** 2 tsp (10mL) q4h. **Max:** 6 doses q24h.
Robitussin Allergy & Cough liquid		Chlorpheniramine Maleate 2mg/5mL	Phenylephrine HCl 5mg/5mL	Dextromethorphan HBr 10mg/5mL		**Adults: ≥12 yrs:** 2 tsp (10mL) q4h. **Peds: 6-12 yrs:** 1 tsp (5mL) q4h. **Max:** 6 doses q24h.

(Continued)

COUGH-COLD-FLU PRODUCTS

BRAND NAME	ANALGESIC	ANTIHISTAMINE	DECONGESTANT	COUGH SUPPRESSANT	EXPECTORANT	DOSE
COUGH SUPPRESSANT + ANTIHISTAMINE + DECONGESTANT (Continued)						
Robitussin Pediatric Cough & Cold Nighttime liquid		Chlorpheniramine Maleate 1mg/5mL	Phenylephrine HCl 2.5mg/5mL	Dextromethorphan HBr 5mg/5mL		**Adults & Peds: ≥12 yrs** (≥ 96 lbs): 4 tsp (20mL) q4h. **Peds: 6-12 yrs (48-95 lbs):** 2 tsp (10mL) q4h.
Robitussin Cough & Cold Nighttime liquid		Chlorpheniramine Maleate 1mg/5mL	Phenylephrine HCl 2.5mg/5mL	Dextromethorphan HBr 5mg/5mL		**Adults: ≥12 yrs:** 4 tsp (20mL) q4h. **Peds: 6-12 yrs:** 2 tsp (10mL) q4h. **Max:** 6 doses q24h.
Theraflu Cold & Cough Hot Liquid		Pheniramine Maleate 20mg/packet	Phenylephrine HCl 10mg/packet	Dextromethorphan HBr 20mg/packet		**Adults & Peds: ≥12 yrs:** 1 packet q4h. **Max:** 6 packets q24h.
COUGH SUPPRESSANT + DECONGESTANT						
PediaCare Children's Multi-Symptom Cold Liquid			Phenylephrine HCl 2.5mg/5mL	Dextromethorphan HBr 5mg/5mL		**Peds: 6-12 yrs:** 2 tsp (10mL) q4h. 2-6 yrs: 1 tsp (5mL) q4h. **Max:** 6 doses q24h.
PediaCare Decongestant & Cough Infants' drops			Phenylephrine HCl 1.25mg/0.8mL	Dextromethorphan HBr 2.5mg/0.8mL		**Peds: 2-3 yrs:** 1.6mL q4h. **Max:** 6 doses q24h.
Vicks 44D Cough & Congestion Relief liquid			Phenylephrine HCl 10mg/15mL	Dextromethorphan HBr 30mg/15mL		**Adults: ≥12 yrs:** 1 tbl (15mL) q4h. **Peds: 6-12 yrs:** 1.5 tsp (7.5mL) q4h. **Max:** 6 doses q24h.
COUGH SUPPRESSANT + DECONGESTANT + ANALGESIC						
Alka-Seltzer Plus Day Cold liquid gels	Acetaminophen 325mg		Phenylephrine HCl 5mg	Dextromethorphan HBr 10mg		**Adults & Peds: ≥12 yrs:** 2 tabs q4h. **Max:** 12 tabs q24h.
Alka-Seltzer Plus Day & Night liquid gels	Acetaminophen 325mg		Phenylephrine HCl 5mg	Dextromethorphan HBr 10mg		**Adults & Peds: ≥12 yrs:** 2 tabs q4h. **Max:** 12 tabs q24h.
Alka-Seltzer Plus Day & Night effervescent tablets	Acetaminophen 250mg		Phenylephrine HCl 5mg	Dextromethorphan HBr 10mg		**Adults & Peds: ≥12 yrs:** 2 tabs q4h. **Max:** 8 tabs q24h.
Alka-Seltzer Plus Day Cold Liquid	Acetaminophen 162.5mg/5mL		Phenylephrine HCl 2.5mg/5mL	Dextromethorphan HBr 5mg/5mL		**Adults & Peds: ≥12 yrs:** 4 tsps q4h. **Max:** 6 doses q24h.
Sudafed PE Cold & Cough caplets	Acetaminophen 325mg		Phenylephrine HCl 5mg	Dextromethorphan HBr 10mg		**Adults & Peds: ≥12 yrs:** 2 caps q4h. **Max:** 12 tabs q24h.
Theraflu Daytime Severe Cold caplets	Acetaminophen 325mg		Phenylephrine HCl 5mg	Dextromethorphan HBr 5mg		**Adults & Peds: ≥12 yrs:** 2 tabs q6h. **Max:** 8 tabs q24h.

COUGH-COLD-FLU PRODUCTS

BRAND NAME	ANALGESIC	ANTIHISTAMINE	DECONGESTANT	COUGH SUPPRESSANT	EXPECTORANT	DOSE
Tylenol Cold & Flu Severe Daytime Cool Burst liquid	Acetaminophen 1000mg/30mL		Pseudoephedrine HCl 60mg/30mL	Dextromethorphan HBr 30mg/30mL		**Adults & Peds: ≥12 yrs:** 2 tbl (30mL) q6h. **Max:** 8 tbl (120mL) q24h.
Tylenol Cold Daytime Cool Burst caplets	Acetaminophen 325mg		Pseudoephedrine HCl 30mg	Dextromethorphan HBr 15mg		**Adults & Peds: ≥12 yrs:** 2 tabs q6h. **Max:** 8 tabs q24h.
Tylenol Cold Head Congestion Daytime capsules	Acetaminophen 325mg		Phenylephrine HCl 5mg	Dextromethorphan HBr 10mg		**Adults & Peds: ≥12 yrs:** 2 caps q4h. **Max:** 12 caps q24h.
Tylenol Cold Head Congestion Day/Night pack	Acetaminophen 325mg		Phenylephrine HCl 5mg	Dextromethorphan HBr 10mg		**Adults & Peds: ≥12 yrs:** 2 caps q4h. **Max:** 12 caps q24h.
Tylenol Cold Multi-Symptom Daytime capsules	Acetaminophen 325mg		Phenylephrine HCl 5mg	Dextromethorphan HBr 10mg		**Adults & Peds: ≥12 yrs:** 2 caps q4h. **Max:** 12 caps q24h.
Tylenol Cold Multi-Symptom Day/Night pack	Acetaminophen 325mg		Phenylephrine HCl 5mg	Dextromethorphan HBr 10mg		**Adults & Peds: ≥12 yrs:** 2 caps q4h. **Max:** 12 caps q24h.
Tylenol Plus Cold & Cough Infants' drops	Acetaminophen 80mg/0.8mL		Phenylephrine HCl 1.25mg/0.8mL	Dextromethorphan HBr 2.5mg/0.8mL		**Peds: 2-3 yrs (24-35 lbs):** 1.6mL q4h. **Max:** 5 doses q24h.
Tylenol Flu Daytime gelcaps	Acetaminophen 500mg		Pseudoephedrine HCl 30mg	Dextromethorphan HBr 15mg		**Adults & Peds: ≥12 yrs:** 2 caps q6h. **Max:** 8 caps q24h.
Vicks DayQuil liquicaps	Acetaminophen 325mg		Phenylephrine HCl 5mg	Dextromethorphan HBr 10mg		**Adults & Peds: ≥12 yrs:** 2 caps q4. **Max:** 6 caps q24h.
Vicks DayQuil liquid	Acetaminophen 325mg/15mL		Phenylephrine HCl 5mg/15mL	Dextromethorphan HBr 10mg/15mL		**Adults & Peds: ≥12 yrs:** 2 tbl (30mL) q4h. **Max:** 12 tbl (120mL) q24h.
COUGH SUPPRESSANT + DECONGESTANT + EXPECTORANT						
Robitussin CF liquid			Phenylephrine HCl 5mg/5mL	Dextromethorphan HBr 10mg/5mL	Guaifenesin 100mg/5mL	**Adults: ≥12 yrs:** 2 tsp (10mL) q4h. **Peds: 6-12 yrs:** 1 tsp (5mL) q4h. **2-6 yrs:** 1/2 tsp (2.5mL) q4h. **Max:** 6 doses q24h.
COUGH SUPPRESSANT + DECONGESTANT + EXPECTORANT + ANALGESIC						
Comtrex Chest Cold capsules	Acetaminophen 250mg		Pseudoephedrine HCl 30mg	Dextromethorphan HBr 10mg	Guaifenesin 100mg	**Adults & Peds: ≥12 yrs:** 2 caps q4h. **Max:** 12 caps q24h.
Tylenol Cold Multi-Symptom Severe liquid	Acetaminophen 325mg/15mL		Phenylephrine HCl 5mg/15ml	Dextromethorphan HBr 10mg/15mL	Guaifenesin 200mg/15mL	**Adults & Peds: ≥12 yrs:** 2 tbs q4h. **Max:** 12 tbs q24h.
Tylenol Cold Multi-Symptom Severe caplets	Acetaminophen 325mg		Phenylephrine HCl 5mg	Dextromethorphan HBr 10mg	Guaifenesin 200mg	**Adults & Peds: ≥12 yrs:** 2 tabs q4h. **Max:** 12 tabs q24h.

(Continued)

COUGH-COLD-FLU PRODUCTS

BRAND NAME	ANALGESIC	ANTIHISTAMINE	DECONGESTANT	COUGH SUPPRESSANT	EXPECTORANT	DOSE
COUGH SUPPRESSANT + DECONGESTANT + EXPECTORANT + ANALGESIC *(Continued)*						
Tylenol Severe Head Congestion caplets	Acetaminophen 325mg		Phenylephrine HCl 5mg	Dextromethorphan HBr 10mg	Guaifenesin 200mg	**Adults & Peds: ≥12 yrs:** 2 tabs q4h. **Max:** 12 tabs q24h.
COUGH SUPPRESSANT & EXPECTORANT						
Coricidin HBP Chest Congestion & Cough softgels				Dextromethorphan HBr 10mg	Guaifenesin 200mg	**Adults & Peds: ≥12 yrs:** 1-2 caps q4h. **Max:** 12 caps q24h.
Mucinex DM extended-release tablets				Dextromethorphan HBr 30mg	Guaifenesin 600mg	**Adults & Peds: ≥12 yrs:** 1-2 tabs q12h. **Max:** 4 tabs q24h.
Robitussin Cough & Congestion liquid				Dextromethorphan HBr 10mg/5mL	Guaifenesin 200mg/5mL	**Adults:** ≥12 yrs: 2 tsp (10mL) q4h. **Peds: 6-12 yrs:** 1 tsp (5mL) q4h. **2-6 yrs:** 1/2 tsp (2.5mL) q4h. **Max:** 6 doses q24h.
Robitussin DM Infant Drops				Dextromethorphan HBr 5mg/2.5mL	Guaifenesin 100mg/2.5mL	**Peds 2-6 yrs (24-47lbs):** 2.5mL q4h. **Max:** 6 doses q24h.
Robitussin DM liquid				Dextromethorphan HBr 10mg/5mL	Guaifenesin 100mg/5mL	**Adults: ≥12 yrs:** 2 tsp (10mL) q4h. **Peds: 6-12 yrs:** 1 tsp (5mL) q4h. **2-6 yrs:** 1/2 tsp (2.5mL) q4h. **Max:** 6 doses q24h.
Robitussin Sugar Free Cough liquid				Dextromethorphan HBr 10mg/5mL	Guaifenesin 100mg/5mL	**Adults: ≥12 yrs:** 2 tsp (10mL) q4h. **Peds: 6-12 yrs:** 1 tsp (5mL) q4h. **2-6 yrs:** 1/2 tsp (2.5mL) q4h. **Max:** 6 doses q24h.
Vicks 44E liquid				Dextromethorphan HBr 20mg/15mL	Guaifenesin 200mg/15mL	**Adults: ≥12 yrs:** 1 tbl (15mL) q4h. **Peds: 6-12 yrs:** 1.5 tsp (7.5mL) q4h. **Max:** 6 doses q24h.
Vicks 44E Pediatric liquid				Dextromethorphan HBr 10mg/15mL	Guaifenesin 100mg/15mL	**Adults: ≥12 yrs:** 2 tbl (30mL) q4h. **Peds: 6-12 yrs:** 1 tbl (15mL) q4h. **2-5 yrs:** 0.5 tbl (7.5mL) q4h. **Max:** 6 doses q24h.
DECONGESTANT						
Contac-D Cold Decongestant tablets			Phenylephrine HCl 10mg			**Adults & Peds: ≥12 yrs:** 1 tabs q4h. **Max:** 6 tabs q24h.

COUGH-COLD-FLU PRODUCTS

BRAND NAME	ANALGESIC	ANTIHISTAMINE	DECONGESTANT	COUGH SUPPRESSANT	EXPECTORANT	DOSE
Dimetapp Children's Cold & Allergy Chewable tablets			Phenylephrine HCl 1.25mg			**Peds: 6-12 yrs:** 2 tabs q4h. **Max:** 6 tabs q24h.
Dimetapp Toddler's Drops Decongestant			Phenylephrine HCl 1.25mg/0.8mL			**Peds: 2-6 yrs:** 1.6mL q4h. **Max:** 6 doses q24h.
PediaCare Decongestant Infants' drops			Phenylephrine HCl 1.25mg/0.8mL			**Peds: 2-3 yrs:** 1.6mL q4h. **Max:** 6 doses q24h.
PediaCare Children's Decongestant liquid			Phenylephrine HCl 2.5mg/5mL			**Peds: 6-12 yrs:** 2 tsp (10mL) q4h. **2-6 yrs:** 1 tsp (5mL) q4h. **Max:** 6 doses q24h.
Sudafed 12 Hour tablets			Pseudoephedrine HCl 120mg			**Adults & Peds: ≥12 yrs:** 1 tab q12h. **Max:** 2 tabs q24h.
Sudafed 24 Hour tablets			Pseudoephedrine HCl 240mg			**Adults & Peds: ≥12 yrs:** 1 tab q24h. **Max:** 1 tab q24h.
Sudafed Children's liquid			Pseudoephedrine HCl 15mg/5mL			**Adults: ≥12 yrs:** 4 tsp (20mL) q4-6h. **Peds: 6-12 yrs:** 2 tsp (10mL) q4-6h. **2-6 yrs:** 1 tsp (5mL) q4-6h. **Max:** 4 doses q24h.
Sudafed PE tablets			Phenylephrine HCl 10mg			**Adults & Peds: ≥12 yrs:** 1 tab q4h. **Max:** 6 tabs q24h.
Sudafed PE Quick Dissolve Strips			Phenylephrine HCl 10mg			**Adults & Peds: ≥12 yrs:** 1 film q4h. **Max:** 6 films q24h.
Sudafed tablets			Pseudoephedrine HCl 30mg			**Adults: ≥12 yrs:** 2 tabs q4-6h. **Peds: 6-12 yrs:** 1 tab q4-6h. **Max:** 4 doses q24h.
Vicks Sinex 12-hour nasal spray			Oxymetazoline HCl 0.05%			**Adults & Peds: ≥6 yrs:** 2-3 sprays q10-12h. **Max:** 2 doses q24h.
Vicks Sinex Nasal Spray			Phenylephrine HCl 0.5%			**Adults & Peds: ≥12 yrs:** 2-3 sprays q4h. **Max:** 18 sprays q24h.
Vicks Sinex UltraFine Mist			Phenylephrine HCl 0.5%			**Adults & Peds: ≥12 yrs:** 2-3 sprays q4h. **Max:** 18 sprays q24h.
Vicks Sinex 12 Hour UltraFine Mist			Oxymetazoline HCl 0.05%			**Adults & Peds: ≥6 yrs:** 2-3 sprays q10-12h. **Max:** 2 doses q24h.

(Continued)

COUGH-COLD-FLU PRODUCTS

BRAND NAME	ANALGESIC	ANTIHISTAMINE	DECONGESTANT	COUGH SUPPRESSANT	EXPECTORANT	DOSE
DECONGESTANT *(Continued)*						
Vicks Vapor Inhaler			Levmetamfetamine 50mg			**Adults: ≥12 yrs:** 2 inhalations q2h. **Max:** 24 inhalations q24h. **Peds: 6-12 yrs:** 1 inhalation q2h. **Max:** 12 inhalations q24h.
DECONGESTANT + ANALGESIC						
Advil Children's Cold liquid	Ibuprofen 100mg		Pseudoephedrine HCl 15mg			**Peds: 6-11 yrs (48-95 lbs):** 2 tsp (10mL) q6h. **2-5 yrs (24-47 lbs):** 1 tsp (5mL) q6h. **Max:** 4 doses q24h
Advil Cold & Sinus caplets/liqui-gels	Ibuprofen 200mg		Pseudoephedrine HCl 30mg			**Adults & Peds: ≥12 yrs:** 1-2 caps q4-6h. **Max:** 6 caps q24h.
Alka-Seltzer Plus Cold & Sinus tablets	Acetaminophen 250mg		Phenylephrine HCl 5mg			**Adults & Peds: ≥12 yrs:** 2 tabs q4h. **Max:** 8 tab q24h.
Alka-Seltzer Plus Cold & Sinus Effervescent tablets	Acetaminophen 250mg		Phenylephrine HCl 5mg			**Adults & Peds: ≥12 yrs:** 2 tabs q4h. **Max:** 8 tab q24h.
Contac Cold & Flu Day & Night caplets	Acetaminophen 500mg		Phenylephrine HCl 5mg			**Adults & Peds: ≥12 yrs:** 2 caps q4-6h. **Max:** 8 tab q24h.
Contac Cold & Flu Maximum Strength caplets	Acetaminophen 500mg		Phenylephrine HCl 5mg			**Adults & Peds: ≥12 yrs:** 2 caps q4-6h. **Max:** 8 tab q24h.
Motrin Children's Cold suspension	Ibuprofen 100mg/5mL		Pseudoephedrine HCl 15mg/5mL			**Peds: 6-12 yrs (48-95 lbs):** 2 tsp (10mL) q6h. **2-6 yrs (24-47 lbs):** 1 tsp (5mL) q6h. **Max:** 4 doses q24h.
Sinutab Sinus tablets	Acetaminophen 500mg		Phenylephrine HCl 5mg			**Adults & Peds: ≥12 yrs:** 2 tabs q6h. **Max:** 8 tabs q24h.
Sudafed PE Sinus Headache caplets	Acetaminophen 325mg		Phenylephrine HCl 5mg			**Adults & Peds: ≥12 yrs:** 2 caps q4h. **Max:** 12 caps q24h.
Theraflu Daytime Severe Cold Hot liquid	Acetaminophen 650mg		Phenylephrine HCl 10mg			**Adults & Peds: ≥12 yrs:** 1 packet q4h. **Max:** 6 packets q24h.
Tylenol Sinus Congestion & Pain Daytime gelcaps	Acetaminophen 325mg		Phenylephrine HCl 5mg			**Adults & Peds: ≥12 yrs:** 2 caps q4h. **Max:** 12 caps q24h.
Tylenol Sinus Congestion & Pain Day/Night pack	Acetaminophen 325mg		Phenylephrine HCl 5mg			**Adults & Peds: ≥12 yrs:** 2 caps q4h. **Max:** 12 caps q24h.

COUGH-COLD-FLU PRODUCTS

BRAND NAME	ANALGESIC	ANTIHISTAMINE	DECONGESTANT	COUGH SUPPRESSANT	EXPECTORANT	DOSE
Vicks DayQuil Sinus liquicaps	Acetaminophen 325mg		Phenylephrine HCl 5mg			**Adults & Peds: ≥12 yrs:** 2 caps q4h. **Max:** 6 caps q24h.
DECONGESTANT + EXPECTORANT						
Robitussin PE Head & Chest liquid			Phenylephrine HCl 5mg/5mL		Guaifenesin 100mg/5mL	**Adults: ≥12 yrs:** 2 tsp (10mL) q4h. **Peds: 6-12 yrs:** 1 tsp (5mL) q4h. **Max:** 6 doses q24h.
Sinutab Non-Drying liquid caps			Pseudoephedrine HCl 30mg		Guaifenesin 200mg	**Adults & Peds: ≥12 yrs:** 2 cap q4h. **Max:** 12 q24h
Sudafed Non-Drying Sinus liquid caps			Phenylephrine HCl 5mg		Guaifenesin 200mg	**Adults & Peds: ≥12 yrs:** 2 caps q4h. **Max:** 8 caps q24h.
Triaminic Chest & Nasal liquid			Phenylephrine HCl 2.5mg/5mL		Guaifenesin 50mg/5mL	**Adults & Peds: ≥12 yrs:** 1 tsp q 4h. **Max:** 6 doses q24h. **Peds: 6-12 yrs:** 2 tsp (10mL). **2-6 yrs:** 1 tsp (5mL).
DECONGESTANT + EXPECTORANT + ANALGESIC						
Tylenol Sinus Congestion & Severe pain caplets	Acetaminophen 325 mg		Phenylephrine HCl 5mg		Guaifenesin 200mg	**Adults & Peds: ≥12 yrs:** 2 caps q4h. **Max:** 12 caps q24h.
EXPECTORANT						
Mucinex extended-release tablets					Guaifenesin 600mg	**Adults & Peds: ≥12 yrs:** 1-2 tabs q12h. **Max:** 4 tabs q24h.
Robitussin liquid					Guaifenesin 100mg/5mL	**Adults: ≥12 yrs:** 2-4 tsp (10-20mL) q4h. **Peds: 6-12 yrs:** 1-2 tsp (5-10mL) q4h. **2-6 yrs:** 1/2-1 tsp (2.5-5mL) q4h. **Max:** 6 doses q24h.

NASAL DECONGESTANT/MOISTURIZING PRODUCTS

BRAND	INGREDIENT/STRENGTH	DOSE
PSEUDOEPHEDRINE		
Dimetapp Decongestant Toddler's drops	Phenylephrine HCl 1.25mg/0.8mL	**Peds: 2-6 yrs:** 1.6mL q4h. **Max:** 6 doses/day.
Sudafed 12 Hour tablets	Pseudoephedrine HCl 120mg	**Adults & Peds: ≥12 yrs:** 1 tab q12h. **Max:** 2 tabs/day.
Sudafed 24 Hour tablets	Pseudoephedrine HCl 240mg	**Adults & Peds: ≥12 yrs:** 1 tab q24h. **Max:** 1 tab/day.
Sudafed Children's Nasal Decongestant chewable tablets	Pseudoephedrine HCl 15mg	**Peds: 6-12 yrs:** 2 tabs q4-6h. **Max:** 4 doses/day.
Sudafed Children's Nasal Decongestant liquid	Pseudoephedrine HCl 15mg	**Adults: ≥12 yrs:** 4 tsp q4-6h. **Peds: 6-12 yrs:** 2 tsp q4-6h. **2-6 yrs:** 1 tsp q4-6h. **Max:** 4 doses/day.
Sudafed Nasal Decongestant tablets	Pseudoephedrine HCl 30mg	**Adults: ≥12 yrs:** 2 tabs q4-6h. **Peds: 6-12 yrs:** 1 tab q4-6h. **Max:** 4 doses/day.
TOPICAL NASAL DECONGESTANTS		
4-Way Fast Acting Nasal Decongestant spray	Phenylephrine HCl 1%	**Adults & Peds: ≥12 yrs:** Instill 2-3 sprays per nostril q4h.
4-Way Nasal Decongestant spray, 12 Hour	Phenylephrine HCl 1%	**Adults & Peds: ≥12 yrs:** Instill 2-3 sprays per nostril q4h.
4-Way No Drip Nasal Decongestant spray	Phenylephrine HCl 1%	**Adults & Peds: ≥12 yrs:** Instill 2-3 sprays per nostril q4h.
Afrin Extra Moisturizing Nasal spray	Oxymetazoline HCl 0.05%	**Adults & Peds: ≥6 yrs:** Instill 2-3 sprays per nostril q10-12h.
Afrin No Drip Nasal Spray	Oxymetazoline HCl 0.05%	**Adults & Peds: ≥6 yrs:** Instill 2-3 sprays per nostril q10-12h.
Afrin No Drip Sinus Nasal spray	Oxymetazoline HCl 0.05%	**Adults & Peds: ≥6 yrs:** Instill 2-3 sprays per nostril q10-12h.
Afrin Original Nasal spray	Oxymetazoline HCl 0.05%	**Adults & Peds: ≥6 yrs:** Instill 2-3 sprays per nostril q10-12h.
Afrin Original Pumpmist Nasal spray	Oxymetazoline HCl 0.05%	**Adults & Peds: ≥6 yrs:** Instill 2-3 sprays per nostril q10-12h.
Afrin Severe Congestion Nasal spray	Oxymetazoline HCl 0.05%	**Adults & Peds: ≥6 yrs:** Instill 2-3 sprays per nostril q10-12h.
Afrin Sinus Nasal spray	Oxymetazoline HCl 0.05%	**Adults & Peds: ≥6 yrs:** Instill 2-3 sprays per nostril q10-12h.
Benzedrex Inhaler	Propylhexedrine 250 mg	**Adults & Peds: ≥6 yrs:** Inhale 2 sprays per nostril q2h.
Neo-Synephrine 12 Hour Extra Moisturizing Nasal spray	Oxymetazoline HCl 0.05%	**Adults & Peds: ≥6 yrs:** Instill 2-3 sprays per nostril q10-12h.
Neo-Synephrine 12 Hour Nasal Decongestant spray	Oxymetazoline HCl 0.05%	**Adults & Peds: ≥6 yrs:** Instill 2-3 sprays per nostril q10-12h.
Neo-Synephrine Extra Strength Nasal Decongestant Drops	Phenylephrine HCl 1%	**Adults & Peds: ≥12 yrs:** Instill 2-3 drops per nostril q4h.
Neo-Synephrine Extra Strength Nasal spray	Phenylephrine HCl 1%	**Adults & Peds: ≥6 yrs:** Instill 2-3 sprays per nostril q4h.
Neo-Synephrine Mild Formula Nasal spray	Phenylephrine HCl 0.25%	**Adults & Peds: ≥6 yrs:** Instill 2-3 sprays per nostril q4h.
Neo-Synephrine Regular Strength Nasal Decongestant spray	Phenylephrine HCl 0.5%	**Adults & Peds: ≥12 yrs:** Instill 2-3 sprays per nostril q4h.
Nostrilla 12 Hour Nasal Decongestant	Oxymetazoline HCl 0.05%	**Adults & Peds: ≥6 yrs:** Instill 2-3 sprays per nostril q10-12h.
Vicks Sinex 12 Hour Ultra Fine Mist For Sinus Relief	Oxymetazoline HCl 0.05%	**Adults & Peds: ≥12 yrs:** Instill 2-3 sprays per nostril q10-12h.
Vicks Sinex Long Acting Nasal Spray For Sinus Relief	Oxymetazoline HCl 0.05%	**Adults & Peds: ≥12 yrs:** Instill 2-3 sprays per nostril q10-12h.
Vicks Sinex Nasal Spray For Sinus Relief	Phenylephrine HCl 0.5%	**Adults & Peds: ≥12 yrs:** Instill 2-3 sprays per nostril q4h.

(Continued)

NASAL DECONGESTANT/MOISTURIZING PRODUCTS

BRAND	INGREDIENT/STRENGTH	DOSE
TOPICAL NASAL MOISTURIZERS		
4-Way Saline Moisturizing Mist	Water, Boric Acid, Glycerin, Sodium Chloride, Sodium Borate, Eucalyptol, Menthol, Polysorbate 80, Benzalkonium Chloride	**Adults & Peds: ≥2 yrs:** Instill 2-3 sprays per nostril prn.
Ayr Baby's Saline Nose Spray, Drops	Sodium Chloride 0.65%	**Peds:** Instill 2 to 6 drops in each nostril.
Ayr Saline Nasal Gel	Aloe Vera Gel, Carbomer, Diazolidinyl Urea, Dimethicone Copolyol, FD&C Blue 1, Geranium Oil, Glycerin, Glyceryl Polymethacrylate, Methyl Gluceth 10, Methylparaben, Poloxamer 184, Propylene Glycol, Propylparaben, Sodium Chloride, Tocopherol Acetate, Triethanolamine, Xanthan Gum, Water	**Adults & Peds: ≥12 yrs:** Apply to nostril prn.
Ayr Saline Nasal Gel, No-Drip Sinus Spray	Water, Sodium Carbomethyl Starch, Propylene Glycol, Glycerin, Aloe Barbadensis Leaf Juice (Aloe Vera Gel), Sodium Chloride, Cetyl Pyridinium Chloride, Citric Acid, Disodium EDTA, Glycine Soja (Soybean Oil), Tocopheryl Acetate, Benzyl Alcohol, Benzalkonium Chloride, Geranium Maculatum Oil	**Adults & Peds: ≥12 yrs:** Use prn as directed.
Ayr Saline Nasal Mist	Sodium Chloride 0.65%	**Adults & Peds: ≥12 yrs:** Instill 2 sprays per nostril prn.
ENTSOL Mist, Buffered Hypertonic Nasal Irrigation Mist	Purified Water, Sodium Chloride, Sodium Phosphate Dibasic Edetate Disodium, Potassium Phosphate Monobasic, Benzalkonium Chloride	**Adults & Peds: ≥12 yrs:** Instill 1-2 sprays per nostril prn.
ENTSOL Single Use, Pre-Filled Nasal Wash Squeeze Bottle	Purified Water, Sodium Chloride, Sodium Phosphate Dibasic, Potassium Phosphate Monobasic	**Adults & Peds: ≥12 yrs:** Use as directed.
ENTSOL Spray, Buffered Hypertonic Saline Nasal Spray	Purified Water, Sodium Chloride Phosphate Dibasic, Potassium Phosphate Monobasic	**Adults & Peds: ≥12 yrs:** Instill 1 spray per nostril bid, 6 times daily
Little Noses Saline Spray/Drops, Non-Medicated	Sodium Chloride 0.65%	**Peds:** 2-6 drops per nostril as directed.
Ocean Premium Saline Nasal Spray	Sodium Chloride 0.65%, Phenylcarbinol, Benzalkonium Chloride	**Adults & Peds: ≥6 yrs:** Instill 2 sprays per nostril prn.
Simply Saline Sterile Saline Nasal Mist	Sodium Chloride 0.9%	**Adults & Peds: ≥12 yrs:** Use prn as directed.
SinoFresh Moisturizing Nasal & Sinus spray	Cetylpyridinium Chloride 0.05%	**Adults & Peds: ≥12 yrs:** Instill 1-3 sprays per nostril qd.
Zicam Nasal Moisturizer	Purified Water, High Purity Sodium Chloride, Aloe Vera	**Adults & Peds: ≥12 yrs:** Use as directed.

Analgesic Products

BRAND	INGREDIENT/STRENGTH	DOSE
ACETAMINOPHEN		
Anacin Aspirin Free tablets	Acetaminophen 500mg	**Adults & Peds: ≥12 yrs:** 2 tabs q6h. **Max:** 8 tabs q24h.
Feverall Childrens' suppositories	Acetaminophen 120mg	**Peds: 3-6 yrs:** 1-2 supp. q4-6h. max 6 supp. q24h.
Feverall Infants' suppositories	Acetaminophen 80mg	**Peds: 3-11 months:** 1 supp. q6h. **12-36 months:** 1 supp. q4h. **Max:** 6 supp. q24h.
Feverall Jr. Strength suppositories	Acetaminophen 325mg	**Peds: 6-12 yrs:** 1 supp. q4-6h. **Max:** 6 supp. q24h.
Tylenol 8 Hour caplets	Acetaminophen 650mg	**Adults & Peds: ≥12 yrs:** 2 tabs q8h prn. **Max:** 6 tabs q24h.
Tylenol 8 Hour geltabs	Acetaminophen 650mg	**Adults & Peds: ≥12 yrs:** 2 tabs q8h prn. **Max:** 6 tabs q24h.
Tylenol Arthritis caplets	Acetaminophen 650mg	**Adults:** 2 tabs q8h prn. **Max:** 6 tabs q24h.
Tylenol Arthritis geltabs	Acetaminophen 650mg	**Adults:** 2 tabs q8h prn. **Max:** 6 tabs q24h.
Tylenol Children's Meltaways tablets	Acetaminophen 80mg	**Peds: 2-3 yrs (24-35 lbs):** 2 tabs **4-5 yrs (36-47 lbs):** 3 tabs. **6-8 yrs (48-59 lbs):** 4 tabs. **9-10 yrs (60-71 lbs):** 5 tabs. **11 yrs (72-95 lbs):** 6 tabs. May repeat q4h. **Max:** 5 doses q24h.
Tylenol Children's suspension	Acetaminophen 160mg/5mL	**Peds: 2-3 yrs (24-35 lbs):** 1 tsp (5mL). **4-5 yrs (36-47 lbs):** 1.5 tsp (7.5mL). **6-8 yrs (48-59 lbs):** 2 tsp (10mL). **9-10 yrs (60-71 lbs):** 2.5 tsp (12.5mL). **11 yrs (72-95 lbs):** 3 tsp (15mL). May repeat q4h. **Max:** 5 doses q24h.
Tylenol Extra Strength caplets	Acetaminophen 500mg	**Adults & Peds: ≥12 yrs:** 2 tabs q4-6h prn. **Max:** 8 tabs q24h.
Tylenol Extra Strength Cool caplets	Acetaminophen 500mg	**Adults & Peds: ≥12 yrs:** 2 tabs q4-6h prn. **Max:** 8 tabs q24h.
Tylenol Extra Strength gelcaps	Acetaminophen 500mg	**Adults & Peds: ≥ 12 yrs:** 2 caps q4-6h prn. **Max:** 8 caps q24h.
Tylenol Rapid Blast liquid	Acetaminophen 500mg/15mL	**Adults & Peds: ≥12 yrs:** 2 tbl (30mL) q4-6h prn. **Max:** 8 tbl (120mL) q24h.
Tylenol Extra Strength EZ tablets	Acetaminophen 500mg	**Adults & Peds: ≥12 yrs:** 2 tabs q4-6h prn. **Max:** 8 tabs q24h.
Tylenol Extra Strength Go tablets	Acetaminophen 500mg	**Adults & Peds: ≥12 yrs:** 2 tabs q4-6h prn. **Max:** 8 tabs q24h.
Tylenol Infants' suspension	Acetaminophen 80mg/0.8mL	**Peds: 2-3 yrs (24-35 lbs):** 1.6 mL q4h prn. **Max:** 5 doses (8mL) q24h.
Tylenol Junior Meltaways tablets	Acetaminophen 160mg	**Peds: 6-8 yrs (48-59 lbs):** 2 tabs. **9-10 yrs (60-71 lbs):** 2.5 tabs. **11 yrs (72-95 lbs):** 3 tabs. **12 yrs (≥96 lbs):** 4 tabs. May repeat q4h. **Max:** 5 doses q24h.
Tylenol Regular Strength tablets	Acetaminophen 325mg	**Adults & Peds: ≥12 yrs:** 2 tabs q4-6h prn. **Max:** 12 tabs q24h. **Peds: 6-11 yrs:** 1 tab q4-6h. **Max:** 5 tabs q24h.
ACETAMINOPHEN COMBINATIONS		
Anacin Advanced Headache tablets	Acetaminophen/Aspirin/Caffeine 250mg-65mg	**Adults & Peds: ≥12 yrs:** 2 tabs q6h. Max: 8 tabs q24h.

(Continued)

ANALGESIC PRODUCTS

BRAND	INGREDIENT/STRENGTH	DOSE
ACETAMINOPHEN COMBINATIONS *(Continued)*		
Excedrin Back & Body caplets	Acetaminophen/Aspirin Buffered 250mg-250mg	**Adults & Peds:** ≥**12 yrs:** 2 tabs q6h. **Max:** 8 tabs q24h.
Excedrin Extra Strength caplets	Acetaminophen/Aspirin/Caffeine 250mg-250mg-65mg	**Adults & Peds:** ≥**12 yrs:** 2 tabs q6h. **Max:** 8 tabs q24h.
Excedrin Extra Strength geltabs	Acetaminophen/Aspirin/Caffeine 250mg-250mg-65mg	**Adults & Peds:** ≥**12 yrs:** 2 tabs q6h. **Max:** 8 tabs q24h.
Excedrin Extra Strength tablets	Acetaminophen/Aspirin/Caffeine 250mg-250mg-65mg	**Adults & Peds:** ≥**12 yrs:** 2 tabs q6h. **Max:** 8 tabs q24h.
Excedrin Migraine caplets	Acetaminophen/Aspirin/Caffeine 250mg-250mg-65mg	**Adults:** 2 tabs prn. **Max:** 2 tabs q24h.
Excedrin Migraine geltabs	Acetaminophen/Aspirin/Caffeine 250mg-250mg-65mg	**Adults:** 2 tabs prn. **Max:** 2 tabs q24h.
Excedrin Migraine tablets	Acetaminophen/Aspirin/Caffeine 250mg-250mg-65mg	**Adults:** 2 tabs prn. **Max:** 2 tabs q24h.
Excedrin Quicktabs tablets	Acetaminophen/Caffeine 500mg-65mg	**Adults & Peds:** ≥**12 yrs:** 2 tabs q6h. **Max:** 8 tabs q24h.
Excedrin Sinus Headache caplets	Acetaminophen/Phenylephrine HCl 325mg-5mg	**Adults & Peds:** ≥**12 yrs:** 2 tabs q4h. **Max:** 12 tabs q24h.
Excedrin Sinus Headache tablets	Acetaminophen/Phenylephrine HCl 325mg-5mg	**Adults & Peds:** ≥**12 yrs:** 2 tabs q4h. **Max:** 12 tabs q24h.
Excedrin Tension Headache caplets	Acetaminophen/Caffeine 500mg-65mg	**Adults & Peds:** ≥**12 yrs:** 2 tabs q6h. **Max:** 8 tabs q24h.
Excedrin Tension Headache geltabs	Acetaminophen/Caffeine 500mg-65mg	**Adults & Peds:** ≥**12 yrs:** 2 tabs q6h. **Max:** 8 tabs q24h.
Excedrin Tension Headache tablets	Acetaminophen/Caffeine 500mg-65mg	**Adults & Peds:** ≥**12 yrs:** 2 tabs q6h. **Max:** 8 tabs q24h.
Goody's Extra Strength Headache Powders	Acetaminophen/Aspirin/Caffeine 260mg-520mg-32.5mg	**Adults & Peds:** ≥**12 yrs:** 1 powder q4-6h. **Max:** 4 powders q24h.
Midol Menstrual Headache caplets	Acetaminophen/Caffeine 500mg-65g	**Adults & Peds:** ≥**12 yrs:** 2 tabs q6h. **Max:** 8 tabs q24h.
Midol Menstrual Complete caplets	Acetaminophen/Caffeine/Pyrilamine Maleate 500mg-60mg-15mg	**Adults & Peds:** ≥**12 yrs:** 2 tabs q6h. **Max:** 8 tabs q24h.
Midol Menstrual Complete caplets	Acetaminophen/Caffeine/Pyrilamine Maleate 500mg-60mg-15mg	**Adults & Peds:** ≥**12 yrs:** 2 tabs q6h. **Max:** 8 tabs q24h.
Midol PMS caplets	Acetaminophen/Pamabrom/Pyrilamine 500mg-25mg-15mg	**Adults & Peds:** ≥**12 yrs:** 2 tabs q6h. **Max:** 8 tabs q24h.
Midol Teen caplets	Acetaminophen/Pamabrom 500mg-25mg	**Adults & Peds:** ≥**12 yrs:** 2 tabs q6h. **Max:** 8 tabs q24h.
Pamprin Multi-Symptom caplets	Acetaminophen/Pamabrom/Pyrilamine 500mg-25mg-15mg	**Adults & Peds:** ≥**12 yrs:** 2 tabs q4-6h. **Max:** 8 tabs q24h.
Premsyn PMS caplets	Acetaminophen/Pamabrom/Pyrilamine 500mg-25mg-15mg	**Adults & Peds:** ≥**12 yrs:** 2 tabs q4-6h. **Max:** 8 tabs q24h.
Tylenol Women's caplets	Acetaminophen/Pamabrom 500mg-25mg	**Adults & Peds:** ≥**12 yrs:** 2 tabs q4-6h. **Max:** 8 tabs q24h.
Vanquish caplets	Acetaminophen/Aspirin/Caffeine 194mg-227mg-33mg	**Adults & Peds:** ≥**12 yrs:** 2 tabs q6h. **Max:** 8 tabs q24h.
ACETAMINOPHEN/SLEEP AIDS		
Excedrin PM caplets	Acetaminophen/Diphenhydramine 500mg-38mg	**Adults & Peds:** ≥**12 yrs:** 2 tabs qhs.
Excedrin PM geltabs	Acetaminophen/Diphenhydramine citrate 500mg-38 mg	**Adults & Peds:** ≥**12 yrs:** 2 tabs qhs.
Excedrin PM tablets	Acetaminophen/Diphenhydramine citrate 500mg-38 mg	**Adults & Peds:** ≥**12 yrs:** 2 tabs qhs.
Goody's PM Powder	Acetaminophen/Diphenhydramine 1000mg-76mg/dose	**Adults & Peds:** ≥**12 yrs:** 1 packet (2 powders) qhs.
Tylenol PM caplets	Acetaminophen/Diphenhydramine 500mg-25mg	**Adults & Peds:** ≥**12 yrs:** 2 tabs qhs.
Tylenol PM gelcaps	Acetaminophen/Diphenhydramine 500mg-25mg	**Adults & Peds:** ≥**12 yrs:** 2 caps qhs.

(Continued)

ANALGESIC PRODUCTS

BRAND	INGREDIENT/STRENGTH	DOSE
ACETAMINOPHEN/SLEEP AIDS *(Continued)*		
Tylenol PM geltabs	Acetaminophen/Diphenhydramine 500mg-25mg	**Adults & Peds: ≥12 yrs:** 2 tabs qhs.
Tylenol PM liquid	Acetaminophen/Diphenhydramine 1000g-50mg/30 mL	**Adults & Peds: ≥12 yrs:** 2 tbl (30mL) qhs. **Max:** 8 tbl (120mL) q24h.
NSAIDs		
Advil caplets	Ibuprofen 200mg	**Adults & Peds: ≥12 yrs:** 1-2 tabs q4-6h. **Max:** 6 tabs q24h.
Advil Children's Chewables tablets	Ibuprofen 50mg	**Peds: 2-3 yr (24-35 lb):** 2 tabs q6-8h. **4-5 yr (36-47 lb):** 3 tabs q6-8h. **6-8 yr (45-89 lb):** 4 tabs q6-8h. **9-10 yr (60-71 lb):** 5 tabs q6-8h. **11 yr (72-95 lb):** 6 tabs q6-8h. **Max:** 4 doses q24h.
Advil Children's suspension	Ibuprofen 100mg/5mL	**Peds: 2-3 yrs (24-35 lbs):** 1 tsp (5mL). **4-5 yrs (36-47 lbs):** 1.5 tsp (7.5mL). **6-8 yrs (48-59 lbs):** 2 tsp (10mL). **9-10 yrs (60-71 lbs):** 2.5 tsp (12.5mL). **11 yrs (72-95 lbs):** 3 tsp (15mL). May repeat q6-8h. **Max:** 4 doses q24h.
Advil gelcaps	Ibuprofen 200mg	**Adults & Peds: ≥12 yrs:** 1-2 caps q4-6h. **Max:** 6 caps q24h.
Advil Infants' Drops	Ibuprofen 50mg/1.25mL	**Peds: 6-11 months (12-17 lbs):** 1.25mL. **12-23 months (18-23 lbs):** 1.875mL. May repeat q6-8h. **Max:** 4 doses q24h.
Advil Junior Strength tablets	Ibuprofen 100mg	**Peds: 6-10 yrs (48-71 lbs):** 2 tabs. **11 yrs (72-95 lbs):** 3 tabs. May repeat q6-8h. **Max:** 4 doses q24h.
Advil Junior Strength Chewable tablets	Ibuprofen 100mg	**Peds: 6-10 yrs (48-71 lbs):** 2 tabs. **11 yrs (72-95 lbs):** 3 tabs. May repeat q6-8h. **Max:** 4 doses q24h.
Advil liqui-gels	Ibuprofen 200mg	**Adults & Peds: ≥12 yrs:** 1-2 caps q4-6h. **Max:** 6 caps q24h.
Advil Migraine capsules	Ibuprofen 200mg	**Adults:** 2 caps prn. **Max:** 2 caps q24h.
Advil tablets	Ibuprofen 200mg	**Adults & Peds: ≥12 yrs:** 1-2 tabs q4-6h. **Max:** 6 tabs q24h.
Aleve caplets	Naproxen Sodium 220mg	**Adults: ≥65 yrs:** 1 tab q12h. **Max:** 2 tabs q24h. **Adults & Peds: ≥12 yrs:** 1 tab q8-12h. **Max:** 3 tabs q24h.
Aleve gelcaps	Naproxen Sodium 220mg	**Adults: ≥65 yrs:** 1 cap q12h. **Max:** 2 caps q24h. **Adults & Peds: ≥12 yrs:** 1 cap q8-12h. **Max:** 3 caps q24h.
Aleve tablets	Naproxen Sodium 220mg	**Adults: ≥65 yrs:** 1 tab q12h. **Max:** 2 tabs q24h. **Adults & Peds: ≥12 yrs:** 1 tab q8-12h. **Max:** 3 tabs q24h.
Midol Cramps and Body Aches tablets	Ibuprofen 200mg	**Adults & Peds: ≥12 yrs:** 1-2 tabs q4-6h. **Max:** 6 tabs q24h.
Midol Extended Relief caplets	Naproxen Sodium 220mg	**Adults & Peds: ≥12 yrs:** 1 tabs q8-12h. **Max:** 3 tabs q24h.
Motrin Children's suspension	Ibuprofen 100mg/5mL	**Peds: 2-3 yrs (24-35 lbs):** 1 tsp (5mL). **4-5 yrs (36-47 lbs):** 1.5 tsp (7.5mL). **6-8 yrs (48-59 lbs):** 2 tsp (10mL). **9-10 yrs (60-71 lbs):** 2.5 tsp (12.5mL). **11 yrs (72-95 lbs):** 3 tsp (15mL). May repeat q6-8h. **Max:** 4 doses q24h.

(Continued)

ANALGESIC PRODUCTS

BRAND	INGREDIENT/STRENGTH	DOSE
NSAIDs *(Continued)*		
Motrin IB caplets	Ibuprofen 200mg	**Adults & Peds: ≥12 yrs:** 1-2 tabs q4-6h. **Max:** 6 tabs q24h.
Motrin IB gelcaps	Ibuprofen 200mg	**Adults & Peds: ≥12 yrs:** 1-2 tabs q4-6h. **Max:** 6 tabs q24h.
Motrin IB tablets	Ibuprofen 200mg	**Adults & Peds: ≥12 yrs:** 1-2 tabs q4-6h. **Max:** 6 tabs q24h.
Motrin Infants' Drops	Ibuprofen 50mg/1.25mL	**Peds: 6-11 months (12-17 lbs):** 1.25mL. **12-23 months (18-23 lbs):** 1.875mL. May repeat q6-8h. **Max:** 4 doses q24h.
Motrin Junior Strength chewable tablets	Ibuprofen 100mg	**Peds: 6-8 yrs (48-59 lbs):** 2 tabs. **9-10 yrs (60-71 lbs):** 2.5 tabs. **11 yrs (72-95 lbs):** 3 tabs. May repeat q6-8h. **Max:** 4 doses q24h.
Nuprin caplets	Ibuprofen 200mg	**Adults & Peds: ≥12 yrs:** 1-2 tabs q4-6h. **Max:** 6 tabs q24h.
Nuprin tablets	Ibuprofen 200mg	**Adults & Peds: ≥12 yrs:** 1-2 tabs q4-6h. **Max:** 6 tabs q24h.
SALICYLATES		
Anacin 81 tablets	Aspirin 81mg	**Adults & Peds: ≥12 yrs:** 4-8 tabs q4h. **Max:** 48 tabs q24h.
Aspergum chewable tablets	Aspirin 227mg	**Adults & Peds: ≥12 yrs:** 2 tabs q4h. **Max:** 16 tabs q24h.
Bayer Aspirin Extra Strength caplets	Aspirin 500mg	**Adults & Peds: ≥12 yrs:** 1-2 tabs q4-6h. **Max:** 8 tabs q24h.
Bayer Aspirin safety coated caplets	Aspirin 325mg	**Adults & Peds: ≥12 yrs:** 1-2 tabs q4h or 3 tabs q6h. **Max:** 12 tabs q24h.
Bayer Children's Aspirin chewable tablets	Aspirin 81mg	**Adults & Peds: ≥12 yrs:** 4-8 tabs q4h. **Max:** 48 tabs q24h.
Bayer Low Dose Aspirin tablets	Aspirin 81mg	**Adults & Peds: ≥12 yrs:** 4-8 tabs q4h. **Max:** 48 tabs q24h.
Bayer Sugar Free Low Dose Aspirin tablets	Aspirin 81mg	**Adults & Peds: ≥12 yrs:** 4-8 tabs q4h. **Max:** 48 tabs q24h.
Bayer Genuine Aspirin tablets	Aspirin 325mg	**Adults & Peds: ≥12 yrs:** 1-2 tabs q4h or 3 tabs q6h. **Max:** 12 tabs q24h.
Bayer Extra-Strength Plus caplets	Aspirin 500mg	**Adults & Peds: ≥12 yrs:** 2 tabs q6h. **Max:** 8 tabs q24h.
Doan's Regular Strength caplets	Magnesium Salicylate Tetrahydrate 377mg	**Adults & Peds: ≥12 yrs:** 2 tabs q4h. **Max:** 12 tabs q24h.
Ecotrin Adult Low Strength tablets	Aspirin 81mg	**Adults:** 4-8 tabs q4h. **Max:** 48 tabs q24h.
Ecotrin Enteric Low Strength tablets	Aspirin 81mg	**Adults:** 4-8 tabs q4h. **Max:** 48 tabs q24h.
Ecotrin Enteric Regular Strength tablets	Aspirin 325mg	**Adults & Peds: ≥12 yrs:** 1-2 tabs q4h. **Max:** 12 tabs q24h.
Ecotrin Maximum Strength tablets	Aspirin 500mg	**Adults & Peds: ≥12 yrs:** 2 tabs q6h. **Max:** 8 tabs q24h.
Ecotrin Regular Strength tablets	Aspirin 325mg	**Adults & Peds: ≥12 yrs:** 1-2 tabs q4h. **Max:** 12 tabs q24h.
Halfprin 162mg tablets	Aspirin 162mg	**Adults & Peds: ≥12 yrs:** 2-4 tabs q4h. **Max:** 24 tabs q24h.
Halfprin 81mg tablets	Aspirin 81mg	**Adults & Peds: ≥12 yrs:** 4-8 tabs q4h. **Max:** 48 tabs q24h.
St. Joseph Adult Low Strength chewable tablets	Aspirin 81mg	**Adults & Peds: ≥12 yrs:** 4-8 tabs q4h. **Max:** 48 tabs q24h.
St. Joseph Adult Low Strength tablets	Aspirin 81mg	**Adults & Peds: ≥12 yrs:** 4-8 tabs q4h. **Max:** 48 tabs q24h.

(Continued)

ANALGESIC PRODUCTS

BRAND	INGREDIENT/STRENGTH	DOSE
SALICYLATES, BUFFERED		
Ascriptin Maximum Strength tablets	Aspirin Buffered with Maalox/Calcium Carbonate 500mg	**Adults & Peds:** ≥12 yrs: 2 tabs q4h. **Max:** 8 tabs q24h.
Ascriptin Regular Strength tablets	Aspirin Buffered with Maalox/Calcium Carbonate 325mg	**Adults & Peds:** ≥12 yrs: 2 tabs q4h. **Max:** 12 tabs q24h.
Bayer Extra Strength Plus caplets	Aspirin Buffered with Calcium Carbonate 500mg	**Adults & Peds:** ≥12 yrs: 1-2 tabs q4-6h. **Max:** 8 tabs q24h.
Bufferin Extra Strength tablets	Aspirin Buffered with Calcium Carbonate/Magnesium Oxide/Magnesium Carbonate 500mg	**Adults & Peds:** ≥12 yrs: 2 tabs q6h. **Max:** 8 tabs q24h.
Bufferin tablets	Aspirin Buffered with Calcium Carbonate/Magnesium Oxide/Magnesium Carbonate 325mg	**Adults & Peds:** ≥12 yrs: 2 tabs q4h. **Max:** 12 tabs q24h.
SALICYLATE COMBINATIONS		
Alka-Seltzer effervescent tablets	Aspirin/Citric Acid/Sodium Bicarbonate 325mg-1000mg-1916mg	**Adults & Peds:** ≥12 yrs: 2 tabs q4h. **Max:** 8 tabs q24h.
Alka-Seltzer Extra Strength effervescent tablets	Aspirin/Citric Acid/Sodium Bicarbonate 500mg-1000mg-1985mg	**Adults & Peds:** ≥12 yrs: 2 tabs q6h. **Max:** 7 tabs q24h.
Alka-Seltzer Morning Relief effervescent tablets	Aspirin/Caffeine 500mg-65mg	**Adults & Peds:** ≥12 yrs: 2 tabs q6h. **Max:** 8 tabs q24h.
Anacin Pain Reliever caplets	Aspirin/Caffeine 400mg-32mg	**Adults & Peds:** ≥12 yrs: 2 tabs q6h. **Max:** 8 tabs q24h.
Anacin Extra Strength tablets	Aspirin/Caffeine 500mg-32mg	**Adults & Peds:** ≥12 yrs: 2 tabs q6h. **Max:** 8 tabs q24h.
Anacin tablets	Aspirin/Caffeine 400mg-32mg	**Adults & Peds:** ≥12 yrs: 2 tabs q6h. **Max:** 8 tabs q24h.
Bayer Back & Body Pain caplets	Aspirin/Caffeine 500mg-32.5mg	**Adults & Peds:** ≥12 yrs: 2 tabs q6h. **Max:** 8 tabs q24h.
BC Arthritis Strength powders	Aspirin/Caffeine/Salicylamide 742mg-38mg-222mg	**Adults & Peds:** ≥12 yrs: 1 powder q3-4h. **Max:** 4 powders q24h.
BC Original powders	Aspirin/Caffeine/Salicylamide 650mg-33.3mg-195mg	**Adults & Peds:** ≥12 yrs: 1 powder q3-4h.
SALICYLATE/SLEEP AID		
Alka-Seltzer PM Pain Reliever & Sleep Aid, effervescent tablets	Aspirin/Diphenhydramine Citrate 325mg-38 mg	**Adults & Peds:** ≥12 yrs: 2 tabs qpm.
Bayer PM Relief caplets	Aspirin/Diphenhydramine 500mg-38.3mg	**Adults & Peds:** ≥12 yrs: 2 tabs qhs.
Doan's Extra Strength PM caplets	Magnesium Salicylate Tetrahydrate/Diphenhydramine 580mg-25mg	**Adults & Peds:** ≥12 yrs: 2 tabs 2 tabs qhs.

ANTIPYRETIC PRODUCTS

ACETAMINOPHEN

BRAND	INGREDIENT/STRENGTH	DOSE
Anacin Aspirin Free tablets	Acetaminophen 500mg	**Adults & Peds: ≥12 yrs:** 2 tabs q6h. **Max:** 8 tabs q24h.
Feverall Childrens' suppositories	Acetaminophen 120mg	**Peds: 3-6 yrs:** 1-2 supp. q4-6h. **Max:** 6 supp q24h.
Feverall Infants' suppositories	Acetaminophen 80mg	**Peds: 3-11 months:** 1 supp q6h. **12-36 months:** 1 supp q4h. **Max:** 6 supp q24h.
Feverall Jr. Strength suppositories	Acetaminophen 325mg	**Peds: 6-12 yrs:** 1 supp q4-6h. **Max:** 6 supp q24h.
Tylenol 8 Hour caplets	Acetaminophen 650mg	**Adults & Peds: ≥12 yrs:** 2 tabs q8h prn. **Max:** 6 tabs q24h.
Tylenol 8 Hour geltabs	Acetaminophen 650mg	**Adults & Peds: ≥12 yrs:** 2 tabs q8h prn. **Max:** 6 tabs q24h.
Tylenol Arthritis caplets	Acetaminophen 650mg	**Adults:** 2 tabs q8h prn. **Max:** 6 tabs q24h.
Tylenol Arthritis geltabs	Acetaminophen 650mg	**Adults:** 2 tabs q8h prn. **Max:** 6 tabs q24h.
Tylenol Children's Meltaways tablets	Acetaminophen 80mg	**Peds: 2-3 yrs (24-35 lbs):** 2 tabs. **4-5 yrs (36-47 lbs):** 3 tabs. **6-8 yrs (48-59 lbs):** 4 tabs. **9-10 yrs (60-71 lbs):** 5 tabs. **11 yrs (72-95 lbs):** 6 tabs. May repeat q4h. **Max:** 5 doses q24h.
Tylenol Children's suspension	Acetaminophen 160mg/5mL	**Peds: 2-3 yrs (24-35 lbs):** 1 tsp (5mL). **4-5 yrs (36-47 lbs):** 1.5 tsp (7.5mL). **6-8 yrs (48-59 lbs):** 2 tsp (10mL). **9-10 yrs (60-71 lbs):** 2.5 tsp (12.5mL). **11 yrs (72-95 lbs):** 3 tsp (15mL). May repeat q4h. **Max:** 5 doses q24h.
Tylenol Extra Strength caplets	Acetaminophen 500mg	**Adults & Peds: ≥12 yrs:** 2 tabs q4-6h prn. **Max:** 8 tabs q24h.
Tylenol Extra Strength Cool caplets	Acetaminophen 500mg	**Adults & Peds: ≥12 yrs:** 2 tabs q4-6h prn. **Max:** 8 tabs q24h.
Tylenol Extra Strength gelcaps	Acetaminophen 500mg	**Adults & Peds: ≥ 12 yrs:** 2 caps q4-6h prn. **Max:** 8 caps q24h.
Tylenol Extra Strength Geltabs	Acetaminophen 500mg	**Adults & Peds: ≥12 yrs:** 2 tabs q4-6h prn. **Max:** 8 tabs q24h.
Tylenol Extra Strength liquid	Acetaminophen 1000mg/30mL	**Adults & Peds: ≥12 yrs:** 2 tbl (30mL) q4-6h prn. **Max:** 8 tbl (120mL) q24h.
Tylenol Extra Strength tablets	Acetaminophen 500mg	**Adults & Peds: ≥12 yrs:** 2 tabs q4-6h prn. **Max:** 8 tabs q24h.
Tylenol Infants' suspension	Acetaminophen 80mg/0.8mL	**Peds: 2-3 yrs (24-35 lbs):** 1.6 mL q4h prn. **Max:** 5 doses (8mL) q24h.
Tylenol Junior Meltaways tablets	Acetaminophen 160mg	**Peds: 6-8 yrs (48-59 lbs):** 2 tabs. **9-10 yrs (60-71 lbs):** 2.5 tabs. **11 yrs (72-95 lbs):** 3 tabs. **12 yrs (≥96 lbs):** 4 tabs. May repeat q4h. **Max:** 5 doses q24h.
Tylenol Regular Strength tablets	Acetaminophen 325mg	**Adults & Peds: ≥12 yrs:** 2 tabs q4-6h prn. **Max:** 12 tabs q24h. **Peds: 6-11 yrs:** 1 tab q4-6h. **Max:** 5 tabs q24h.

(Continued)

ANTIPYRETIC PRODUCTS

BRAND	INGREDIENT/STRENGTH	DOSE
NONSTEROIDAL ANTI-INFLAMMATORY DRUGS (NSAIDs)		
Advil Children's Chewables tablets	Ibuprofen 50mg	**Peds: 2-3 yr (24-35 lb):** 2 tabs q6-8h. **4-5 yr (36-47 lb):** 3 tabs q6-8h. **6-8 yr (45-89 lb):** 4 tabs q6-8h. **9-10 yr (60-71 lb):** 5 tabs q6-8h. **11 yr (72-95 lb):** 6 tabs q6-8h. **Max:** 4 doses q24h
Advil Children's suspension	Ibuprofen 100mg/5mL	**Peds: 2-3 yrs (24-35 lbs):** 1 tsp (5mL). **4-5 yrs (36-47 lbs):** 1.5 tsp (7.5mL). **6-8 yrs (48-59 lbs):** 2 tsp (10mL). **9-10 yrs (60-71 lbs):** 2.5 tsp (12.5mL). **11 yrs (72-95 lbs):** 3 tsp (15mL). May repeat q6-8h. **Max:** 4 doses q24h.
Advil gelcaps	Ibuprofen 200mg	**Adults & Peds: ≥12 yrs:** 1-2 caps q4-6h. **Max:** 6 caps q24h.
Advil Infants' drops	Ibuprofen 50mg/1.25mL	**Peds: 6-11 months (12-17 lbs):** 1.25mL. **12-23 months (18-23 lbs):** 1.875mL. May repeat q6-8h. **Max:** 4 doses q24h.
Advil Junior Strength tablets	Ibuprofen 100mg	**Peds: 6-10 yrs (48-71 lbs):** 2 tabs. **11 yrs (72-95 lbs):** 3 tabs. May repeat q6-8h. **Max:** 4 doses q24h.
Advil liqui-gels	Ibuprofen 200mg	**Adults & Peds: ≥12 yrs:** 1-2 caps q4-6h. **Max:** 6 caps q24h.
Advil tablets	Ibuprofen 200mg	**Adults & Peds: ≥12 yrs:** 1-2 tabs q4-6h. **Max:** 6 tabs q24h.
Aleve caplets	Naproxen Sodium 220mg	**Adults: ≥65 yrs:** 1 tab q12h. **Max:** 2 tabs q24h. **Adults & Peds: ≥12 yrs:** 1 tab q8-12h. **Max:** 3 tabs q24h.
Aleve gelcaps	Naproxen Sodium 220mg	**Adults: ≥65 yrs:** 1 cap q12h. **Max:** 2 caps q24h. **Adults & Peds: ≥12 yrs:** 1 cap q8-12h. **Max:** 3 caps q24h.
Aleve tablets	Naproxen Sodium 220mg	**Adults: ≥65 yrs:** 1 tab q12h. **Max:** 2 tabs q24h. **Adults & Peds: ≥12 yrs:** 1 tab q8-12h. **Max:** 3 tabs q24h.
Motrin Children's suspension	Ibuprofen 100mg/5mL	**Peds: 2-3 yrs (24-35 lbs):** 1 tsp (5mL). **4-5 yrs (36-47 lbs):** 1.5 tsp (7.5mL). **6-8 yrs (48-59 lbs):** 2 tsp (10mL). **9-10 yrs (60-71 lbs):** 2.5 tsp (12.5mL). **11 yrs (72-95 lbs):** 3 tsp (15mL). May repeat q6-8h. **Max:** 4 doses q24h.
Motrin IB caplets	Ibuprofen 200mg	**Adults & Peds: ≥12 yrs:** 1-2 tabs q4-6h. **Max:** 6 tabs q24h.
Motrin IB tablets	Ibuprofen 200mg	**Adults & Peds: ≥12 yrs:** 1-2 tabs q4-6h. **Max:** 6 tabs q24h.
Motrin Infants' drops	Ibuprofen 50mg/1.25mL	**Peds: 6-11 months (12-17 lbs):** 1.25mL. **12-23 months (18-23 lbs):** 1.875mL. May repeat q6-8h. **Max:** 4 doses q24h.
Motrin Junior Strength chewable tablets	Ibuprofen 100mg	**Peds: 6-8 yrs (48-59 lbs):** 2 tabs. **9-10 yrs (60-71 lbs):** 2.5 tabs. **11 yrs (72-95 lbs):** 3 tabs. May repeat q6-8h. **Max:** 4 doses q24h.
Nuprin caplets	Ibuprofen 200mg	**Adults & Peds: ≥12 yrs:** 1-2 tabs q4-6h. **Max:** 6 tabs q24h.
Nuprin tablets	Ibuprofen 200mg	**Adults & Peds: ≥12 yrs:** 1-2 tabs q4-6h. **Max:** 6 tabs q24h.

(Continued)

ANTIPYRETIC PRODUCTS

BRAND	INGREDIENT/STRENGTH	DOSE
SALICYLATES		
Anacin 81 tablets	Aspirin 81mg	**Adults & Peds:** ≥**12 yrs:** 4-8 tabs q4h. **Max:** 48 tabs q24h.
Aspergum chewable tablets	Aspirin 227mg	**Adults & Peds:** ≥**12 yrs:** 2 tabs q4h. **Max:** 16 tabs q24h.
Bayer Aspirin Extra Strength caplets	Aspirin 500mg	**Adults & Peds:** ≥**12 yrs:** 1-2 tabs q4-6h. **Max:** 8 tabs q24h.
Genuine Bayer Aspirin coated caplets	Aspirin 325mg	**Adults & Peds:** ≥**12 yrs:** 1-2 tabs q4h or 3 tabs q6h. **Max:** 12 tabs q24h.
Bayer Aspirin safety coated caplets	Aspirin 325mg	**Adults & Peds:** ≥**12 yrs:** 1-2 tabs q4h or 3 tabs q6h. **Max:** 12 tabs q24h.
Bayer Children's Aspirin chewable tablets	Aspirin 81mg	**Adults & Peds:** ≥**12 yrs:** 4-8 tabs q4h. **Max:** 48 tabs q24h.
Bayer Low Dose Aspirin tablets	Aspirin 81mg	**Adults & Peds:** ≥**12 yrs:** 4-8 tabs q4h. **Max:** 48 tabs q24h.
Ecotrin Adult Low Strength tablets	Aspirin 81mg	**Adults:** 4-8 tabs q4h. **Max:** 48 tabs q24h.
Ecotrin Enteric Low Strength tablets	Aspirin 81mg	**Adults:** 4-8 tabs q4h. **Max:** 48 tabs q24h.
Ecotrin Enteric Regular Strength tablets	Aspirin 325mg	**Adults & Peds:** ≥**12 yrs:** 1-2 tabs q4h. **Max:** 12 tabs q24h.
Ecotrin Maximum Strength tablets	Aspirin 500mg	**Adults & Peds:** ≥**12 yrs:** 2 tabs q6h. **Max:** 8 tabs q24h.
Ecotrin Regular Strength tablets	Aspirin 325mg	**Adults & Peds:** ≥**12 yrs:** 1-2 tabs q4h. **Max:** 12 tabs q24h.
Halfprin 162mg tablets	Aspirin 162mg	**Adults & Peds:** ≥**12 yrs:** 2-4 tabs q4h. **Max:** 24 tabs q24h.
Halfprin 81mg tablets	Aspirin 81mg	**Adults & Peds:** ≥**12 yrs:** 4-8 tabs q4h. **Max:** 48 tabs q24h.
St. Joseph Adult Low Strength chewable tablets	Aspirin 81mg	**Adults & Peds:** ≥**12 yrs:** 4-8 tabs q4h. **Max:** 48 tabs q24h.
St. Joseph Adult Low Strength tablets	Aspirin 81mg	**Adults & Peds:** ≥**12 yrs:** 4-8 tabs q4h. **Max:** 48 tabs q24h.
SALICYLATES, BUFFERED		
Bayer Extra Strength Plus caplets	Aspirin Buffered with Calcium Carbonate 500mg	**Adults & Peds:** ≥**12 yrs:** 1-2 tabs q4-6h. **Max:** 8 tabs q24h.
Bufferin Extra Strength tablets	Aspirin Buffered with Calcium Carbonate/ Magnesium Oxide/Magnesium Carbonate 500mg	**Adults & Peds:** ≥**12 yrs:** 2 tabs q6h. **Max:** 8 tabs q24h.
Bufferin tablets	Aspirin Buffered with Calcium Carbonate/ Magnesium Oxide/Magnesium Carbonate 325mg	**Adults & Peds:** ≥**12 yrs:** 2 tabs q4h. **Max:** 12 tabs q24h.

ACNE MANAGEMENT: TOPICAL THERAPIES

DRUG (BRAND)	HOW SUPPLIED	DOSAGE	SIDE EFFECTS
ANTIBACTERIAL/KERATOLYTIC AGENTS & COMBINATIONS			
Benzoyl peroxide (Benzac AC, Benzagel, Triaz)	Benzac AC: (Gel) 5%, 10% [60g], (Wash) 10% [60g]; Benzagel: (Gel) 5%, 10% [42.5g], (Wash) 10% [60g]; Triaz: (Gel) 3%, 6%, 9% [42.5g], (Cleanser) 3%, 6%, 9% [170.3g, 240.2g], (Pads) 3%, 6%, 9% [30g]	(Benzac) Apply qd-bid. (Benzagel) Apply wash qd-bid; apply gel qd initially or qhs for light skin. (Triaz) Apply gel/wash qd-bid.	Erythema, peeling, contact dermatitis, dryness
Benzoyl peroxide/ Sulfur (Sulfoxyl Lotion Regular/Strong)	Lot: (Regular): 10%-2% [59mL]; (Strong): 10%-5% [59mL]	Apply initially once daily for the first week then twice daily, as tolerated.	Erythema, peeling, contact, dermatitis, dryness, irritation, itching, redness
Clindamycin/ Benzoyl peroxide (Benzaclin, Duac)	Benzaclin: (Gel) 1%-5% [25g, 50g]; Duac: (Gel) 1%-5% [45g]	(Benzaclin) Apply qd. (Duac) Apply once in the evening.	Dry skin, erythema, peeling, and burning
Benzoyl peroxide/ Erythromycin (Benzamycin)	Gel: 5%-3% [46.6g, 60s]	Apply bid.	Dryness, urticaria, skin irritation, skin discoloration, oiliness
Benzoyl peroxide (Brevoxyl, Zoderm)	Brevoxyl: (Gel) 4%, 8% [42.5g, 90g], (Lot, Cleanser) 4%, 8% [297g], (Lot, Creamy Wash) 4%, 8% [170g]; Zoderm: (Cleanser) 4.5%, 6.5%, 8.5% [400mL], (Cre/Gel) 4.5%, 6.5%, 8.5% [125mL]	(Brevoxyl) Apply gel qd-bid; apply lotion qd for first week then bid as tolerated. (Zoderm) Apply qd-bid.	Erythema, peeling, contact dermatitis, dryness
ANTIBIOTICS & COMBINATIONS			
Clindamycin (Cleocin T, Clindagel, Clindets, Evoclin Foam)	Cleocin T: (Gel) 1% [30g, 60g], (Lot) 1% [60mL], (Sol) 1% [30mL, 60mL], (Swab, Pledgets) 1% [60s]; Clindagel: 1% [40, 75mL]; Clindets: (Swab) 1% [69]; Evoclin: (Foam) 1% [50g, 100g]	(Cleocin T) Apply bid. (Clindagel) Apply qd. (Clindets) Apply bid. (Evoclin Foam) Apply qd.	Local irritation, stains clothing
Clindamycin/ Tretinoin (Ziana)	Gel: 1.2%-0.025% [2g, 30g, 60g]	Apply qd at bedtime.	Nasopharyngitis, erythema, scaling, itching, burning
Dapsone (Aczone)	Gel: 5% [30g]	Apply bid.	Erythema, dryness, oiliness/peeling, nasopharyngitis, headache
Erythromycin (A/T/S, Emgel, Erycette, Erygel)	A/T/S: (Gel) 2% [30g], (Sol) 2% [60mL]; Emgel: (Gel) 2% [27g, 50g]; Erycette: (Swab) 2% [60g]; Erycette: (Swab) 2% [60g]; Erygel: 2% [30g, 60g]	(A/T/S) Apply gel qd-bid; apply solution bid. (Emgel) Apply bid. (Erycette) Apply bid. (Erygel) Apply qd-bid.	Local irritation, stains clothing
Gentamicin (Garamycin Topical)	Cre, Oint: 0.1% [15g]	Apply tid-qid.	Irritation (erythema and pruritus)
Sulfacetamide (Klaron)	Lot: 10% [118mL]	Apply bid.	Itching, redness, irritation
Sulfacetamide/ Sulfur (Plexion TS, Sulfacet-R, Zetacet)	Plexion TS: (Lot) 10%-5% [30g]; Sulfacet-R/Zetacet: (Lot) 10%-5% [25g]	Apply qd-tid.	Itching, redness, irritation
Sulfacetamide/ Sulfur (Plexion SCT, Rosac)	Plexion SCT: (Cre) 10%-5% [120g]; Rosac: (Cre) 10%-5% [45g]	Apply qd-tid.	Local irritation
Sulfacetamide/ Sulfur (Clenia, Plexion, Rosula)	Clenia: (Cleanser) 10%-5% [170g, 340g], Cre, 10%-5% [28g]; Plexion: (Cleanser) 10%-5% [170.3g, 340.2g]; Rosula: (Cleanser) 10%-5% [355mL], Gel 10%-5% [45mL]	Apply cream qd initially then titrate to bid-tid prn. (Plexion) Apply qd-bid. (Rosula) Apply cleanser qd-bid; apply gel qd-tid.	Local irritation

(Continued)

ACNE MANAGEMENT: TOPICAL THERAPIES

DRUG (BRAND)	HOW SUPPLIED	DOSAGE	SIDE EFFECTS
ANTIBIOTICS & COMBINATIONS *(Continued)*			
Sulfacetamide/ Urea (Rosula NS Dicarboxylic Acids)	(Swab) 10%-10% [30s]	Apply qd-bid.	Local hypersensitivity, instances of Stevens-Johnson syndrome
Azelaic acid (Azelex, Finevin)	(Cre) 20% [30g, 50g]	Apply bid.	Dryness, scaling, erythema, burning, irritation, pruritus; rarely, hypopigmentation
Azelaic acid (Finacea, Retinoids)	(Gel) 15% [30g]	Apply bid.	Burning, stinging, tingling, pruritus, scaling, dry skin
Adapalene (Differin)	(Cre, Gel) 0.1% [45g]; (Pledglets) 0.1% [60s]; (Sol) 0.1% [30mL]	Apply hs.	Erythema, scaling, dryness, pruritus, burning, sunburn, acne flares
Tazarotene (Tazorac)	(Cre) 0.05%, 0.1% [30g, 60g]; (Gel) 0.05%, 0.1% [30g, 100g]	Apply hs.	Pruritus, burning/stinging, erythema, irritation, skin pain, desquamation, dry skin, rash
Tretinoin (Avita, Retin-A)	(Cre) 0.025%, 0.05%, 0.1% [20g, 45g]; (Gel) 0.01%, 0.025% [15g, 45g]; (Sol) 0.05% [28mL]	Apply hs.	Local skin reactions (red, edematous, blistered, crusted), photosensitivity, temporary skin pigmentation changes
Tretinoin microsphere (Retin-A-Micro)	(Gel) 0.04%, 0.1% [20g, 45g]	Apply hs.	

Source:
FDA-Approved Product Labeling.

ACNE MANAGEMENT: SYSTEMIC THERAPIES

DRUG (BRAND)	HOW SUPPLIED	DOSAGE	SIDE EFFECTS
ANTIBIOTICS			
Doxycycline hyclate (Doryx, Vibramycin)	Cap: 75mg, 100mg	100mg q12h on 1st day, followed by 100mg qd.	Anorexia, nausea, vomiting, diarrhea, dysphagia, enterocolitis, rash, exfoliative dermatitis, renal toxicity, hypersensitivity reactions, blood dyscrasias
Doxycycline monohydrate (Minodox)	Cap: 50mg, 100mg	100mg q12h or 50mg q6h for 1 day, then 100mg/day.	GI effects, photosensitivity, rash, monohydrate, blood dyscrasias, hypersensitivity reactions
Minocycline hydrochloride (Dynacin, Minocin)	Cap: 50mg, 75mg, 100mg; Tab: 50mg, 75mg, 100mg	200mg initially, then 100mg q12h; alternative is 100-200mg initially, then 50mg qid.	Anorexia, nausea, vomiting, diarrhea, dysphagia, enterocolitis, pancreatitis, increased LFTs, hepatitis, liver failure, renal toxicity, rash, exfoliative, dermatitis, Stevens-Johnson syndrome, skin and mucous, membrane, pigmentation, blood, dyscrasias, headache, tooth discoloration
Minocycline hydrochloride (Solodyn)	Tab, Extended-Release: 45mg, 90mg, 135mg.	1mg/kg qd for 12 weeks.	Headache, fatigue, dizziness, pruritus, malaise, mood alteration
Tetracycline hydrochloride (Sumycin)	Sus: 125mg/5mL; Tab: 250mg, 500mg	Mild-Moderate: 250mg qid or 500mg bid. Severe: 500mg qid. Severe Acne: Initial: 1g/day in divided doses. Maint: After improvement, 125-500mg/day	GI effects, photosensitivity, increased BUN, hypersensitivity reactions, blood dyscrasias, dizziness, headache
RETINOID			
Isotretinoin (Accutane)	Cap: 10mg, 20mg, 40mg	0.5-1mg/kg/day given bid for 15-20 weeks.	Cheilitis, dry skin and mucous membranes, conjunctivitis, blood dyscrasias, epistaxis, decreased HDL, elevated cholesterol and TG, elevated blood sugar, arthralgias, back pain, hearing/vision impairment, rash, photosensitivity reactions, psychiatric disorders
VITAMIN/MINERAL			
Nicotinamide/ Folic acid/Zinc (Nicomide)	Tab: (Nicotinamide-Folic acid-Zinc) 750mg-500mcg-25mg	1 tab qd-bid.	Nausea, vomiting, transient LFT elevations, allergic sensitization

Source:
FDA-Approved Product Labeling.

Antibiotic Sensitivity – Aminoglycosides*

ORGANISMS	Amikacin	Gentamicin	Streptomycin	Tobramycin
ANAEROBES				
Actinomyces				
Bacillus anthracis				
Bacteroides fragilis				
Clostridium difficile				
Clostridium species				
GRAM-NEGATIVE AEROBES				
Acinetobacter baumannii	++	+		++
Aeromonas hydrophila	++	++		++
Bartonella henselae		++		
Bordetella species				
Burkholderia cepacia				
Campylobacter jejuni		+		
Citrobacter species	++	+++		+++
Coxiella burnetti				
Enterobacter species	+++	+++		+++
Escherichia coli	+	++		++

+++ = excellent activity (1st line recommendation). ++ = good activity (2nd line recommendation). + = moderate activity (acceptable in vitro data suggesting some isolates may be sensitive).
Blank = no or insufficient activity, or unknown.
†† 2nd line against *S. typhi*. † Penicillin sensitive; MIC ≤1.0 mcg/mL. §§ Penicillin resistant; MIC ≥2.0 mcg/mL.
*These are generalizations. There are major differences among countries, areas, and hospitals depending on antibiotic usage patterns.

ANTIBIOTIC SENSITIVITY – AMINOGLYCOSIDES

ORGANISMS	Amikacin	Gentamicin	Streptomycin	Tobramycin
GRAM-NEGATIVE AEROBES *(Continued)*				
Francisella tularensis		+++	+++	+
Haemophilus influenzae	+	+		+
Klebsiella species	++	++		++
Legionella species				
Moraxella catarrhalis	+	+		+
Morganella morganii	++	++		++
Neisseria gonorrhoeae				
Neisseria meningitidis				
Pasturella multocida				
Proteus mirabilis	++	+++		++
Proteus vulgaris	++	+++		++
Providencia stuartii	++	++		++
Pseudomonas aeruginosa	+++	+++		+++
Rickettsia species				
Salmonella species				
Serratia species	++	++		++
Shigella species	+	+		+
Stenotrophomonas maltophilia				

+++ = excellent activity (1st line recommendation).   ++ = good activity (2nd line recommendation).   + = moderate activity (acceptable in vitro data suggesting some isolates may be sensitive).
Blank = no or insufficient activity, or unknown.   † Penicillin sensitive; MIC ≤1.0 mcg/mL.   §§ Penicillin resistant; MIC ≥2.0 mcg/mL.
†† 2nd line against *S. typhi*.
*These are generalizations. There are major differences among countries, areas, and hospitals depending on antibiotic usage patterns.

ANTIBIOTIC SENSITIVITY – AMINOGLYCOSIDES

AMINOGLYCOSIDES (CONTINUED)

ORGANISMS	Amikacin	Gentamicin	Streptomycin	Tobramycin
GRAM-NEGATIVE AEROBES *(Continued)*				
Vibrio vulnificus				
Yersinia enterocolitica	++	++		++
Yersinia pestis		++	+++	+
GRAM-POSITIVE AEROBES				
Enterococcus faecalis		++	++	
Enterococcus faecium		+	+	
Enterococcus faecium (VRE)		+	+	
Listeria monocytogenes	+	+		+
Nocardia	++			
Staphylococcus aureus (MSSA)				
Staphylococcus aureus (MRSA)				
Staphylococcus epidermidis		+		
Staphylococcus epidermidis (MRSE)		+		
Streptococcus pneumoniae†				
Streptococcus pneumoniae§§				

+++ = excellent activity (1st line recommendation). ++ = good activity (2nd line recommendation). + = moderate activity (acceptable in vitro data suggesting some isolates may be sensitive).
Blank = no or insufficient activity, or unknown.
†† 2nd line against *S. typhi*. † Penicillin sensitive; MIC ≤1.0 mcg/mL. §§ Penicillin resistant; MIC ≥2.0 mcg/mL.
*These are generalizations. There are major differences among countries, areas, and hospitals depending on antibiotic usage patterns.

ANTIBIOTIC SENSITIVITY - AMINOGLYCOSIDES

ORGANISMS	Amikacin	Gentamicin	Streptomycin	Tobramycin
GRAM-POSITIVE AEROBES (Continued)				
Streptococcus (Group A,B,C,F,G)				
Streptococcus species		+		
MISCELLANEOUS				
Chlamydia pneumoniae				
Chlamydia trachomatis				
Ehrlichia/Anaplasma species				
MYCOBACTERIA				
Mycobacterium avium (MAI) (non-HIV)	++		+	
Mycoplasma pneumoniae				
SPIROCHETES				
Leptospira interrogans				
Treponema pallidum (syphilis)				

+++ = excellent activity (1st line recommendation). ++ = good activity (2nd line recommendation). + = moderate activity (acceptable in vitro data suggesting some isolates may be sensitive).
Blank = no or insufficient activity, or unknown.
†† 2nd line against *S. typhi*. † Penicillin sensitive; MIC ≤1.0 mcg/mL. §§ Penicillin resistant; MIC ≥2.0 mcg/mL.
*These are generalizations. There are major differences among countries, areas, and hospitals depending on antibiotic usage patterns.

ANTIBIOTIC SENSITIVITY – CARBAPENEMS/MONOBACTAMS*

ORGANISMS	Aztreonam	Ertapenem	Imipenem/Cilastatin	Meropenem
ANAEROBES				
Actinomyces			++	++
Bacillus anthracis				
Bacteroides fragilis		+++	+++	+++
Clostridium difficile				
Clostridium species		++	++	++
GRAM-NEGATIVE AEROBES				
Acinetobacter baumannii	+		+++	+++
Aeromonas hydrophila	++	+	++	++
Bartonella henselae				
Bordetella species		+	+	+
Burkholderia cepacia		+	+	++
Campylobacter jejuni		+	+	+
Citrobacter species	++	+++	+++	+++
Coxiella burnetti				
Enterobacter species	++	++	+++	+++
Escherichia coli	++	++	++	++

+++ = excellent activity (1st line recommendation). ++ = good activity (2nd line recommendation). + = moderate activity (acceptable in vitro data suggesting some isolates may be sensitive).
Blank = no or insufficient activity, or unknown.
†† 2nd line against *S. typhi*. † Penicillin sensitive: MIC ≤1.0 mcg/mL. §§ Penicillin resistant; MIC ≥2.0 mcg/mL
*These are generalizations. There are major differences among countries, areas, and hospitals depending on antibiotic usage patterns.

ANTIBIOTIC SENSITIVITY - CARBAPENEMS/MONOBACTAMS

ORGANISMS	Aztreonam	Ertapenem	Imipenem/Cilastatin	Meropenem
GRAM-NEGATIVE AEROBES *(Continued)*				
Francisella tularensis				
Haemophilus influenzae	++	++	++	++
Klebsiella species	++	++	++	++
Legionella species				
Moraxella catarrhalis	++	++	++	++
Morganella morganii	++	++	++	++
Neisseria gonorrhoeae	+		+	+
Neisseria meningitidis	++		++	++
Pasturella multocida			++	++
Proteus mirabilis	++	++	++	++
Proteus vulgaris	++	++	++	++
Providencia stuartii	++	++	++	++
Pseudomonas aeruginosa	+++		+++	+++
Rickettsia species				
Salmonella species	++	++	++	++
Serratia species	++	++	++	++
Shigella species	++	++	++	++
Stenotrophomonas maltophilia				

+++ = excellent activity (1st line recommendation).   ++ = good activity (2nd line recommendation).   + = moderate activity (acceptable in vitro data suggesting some isolates may be sensitive).
Blank = no or insufficient activity, or unknown.
†† 2nd line against *S. typhi*.   † Penicillin sensitive; MIC ≤1.0 mcg/mL.   §§ Penicillin resistant; MIC ≥2.0 mcg/mL.
* These are generalizations. There are major differences among countries, areas, and hospitals depending on antibiotic usage patterns.

ANTIBIOTIC SENSITIVITY - CARBAPENEMS/MONOBACTAMS

CARBAPENEMS/MONOBACTAMS (CONTINUED)

ORGANISMS	Aztreonam	Ertapenem	Imipenem/Cilastatin	Meropenem
GRAM-NEGATIVE AEROBES *(Continued)*				
Vibrio vulnificus				
Yersinia enterocolitica	++			
Yersinia pestis				
GRAM-POSITIVE AEROBES				
Enterococcus faecalis		+	++	+
Enterococcus faecium			+	
Enterococcus faecium (VRE)				
Listeria monocytogenes			+	+
Nocardia			++	
Staphylococcus aureus (MSSA)		++	++	++
Staphylococcus aureus (MRSA)				
Staphylococcus epidermidis		++	++	++
Staphylococcus epidermidis (MRSE)				
Streptococcus pneumoniae†		++	++	++
Streptococcus pneumoniae§§		++	++	++

+++ = excellent activity (1st line recommendation).   ++ = good activity (2nd line recommendation).   + = moderate activity (acceptable in vitro data suggesting some isolates may be sensitive).
Blank = no or insufficient activity, or unknown.
†† 2nd line against *S. typhi*.   † Penicillin sensitive; MIC ≤1.0 mcg/mL.   §§ Penicillin resistant; MIC ≥2.0 mcg/mL.
*These are generalizations. There are major differences among countries, areas, and hospitals depending on antibiotic usage patterns.

Antibiotic Sensitivity – Carbapenems/Monobactams

ORGANISMS	Aztreonam	Ertapenem	Imipenem/Cilastatin	Meropenem
GRAM-POSITIVE AEROBES *(Continued)*				
Streptococcus (Group A,B,C,F,G)		++	++	++
Streptococcus species		++	++	++
MISCELLANEOUS				
Chlamydia pneumoniae				
Chlamydia trachomatis				
Ehrlichia/Anaplasma species				
MYCOBACTERIA				
Mycobacterium avium (MAI) (non-HIV)				
Mycoplasma pneumoniae				
SPIROCHETES				
Leptospira interrogans				
Treponema pallidum (syphilis)				

+++ = excellent activity (1st line recommendation). ++ = good activity (2nd line recommendation). + = moderate activity (acceptable in vitro data suggesting some isolates may be sensitive).
Blank = no or insufficient activity, or unknown.
†† 2nd line against *S. typhi*.   † Penicillin sensitive; MIC ≤1.0 mcg/mL.   §§ Penicillin resistant; MIC ≥2.0 mcg/mL.
*These are generalizations. There are major differences among countries, areas, and hospitals depending on antibiotic usage patterns.

Antibiotic Sensitivity – Cephalosporins*

Organisms	Cefaclor	Cefadroxil	Cefazolin	Cefdinir	Cefepime	Cefixime	Cefotaxime	Cefoxitin	Cefpodoxime Proxetil	Cefprozil	Ceftazidime	Ceftibuten	Ceftizoxime	Ceftriaxone	Cefuroxime Axetil	Cephalexin
ANAEROBES																
Actinomyces							+						+	++		
Bacillus anthracis																
Bacteroides fragilis								++					+			
Clostridium difficile																
Clostridium species	+		+		+		+	++		+	+		+	+	+	
GRAM-NEGATIVE AEROBES																
Acinetobacter baumannii					++		+				++		+	+		
Aeromonas hydrophila					++	++	++	+			++		++	++	+	
Bartonella henselae																
Bordetella species																
Burkholderia cepacia					+		+				++		+			
Campylobacter jejuni					+		+							+		
Citrobacter species					+++	++	++				++		++	++		
Coxiella burnetti																
Enterobacter species					+++		+				++		++	++	++	
Escherichia coli	++	+++	+++	++	++	++	+++	++	++	+++	++	++	++	+++	++	+++

+++ = excellent activity (1st line recommendation). ++ = good activity (2nd line recommendation). + = moderate activity (acceptable in vitro data suggesting some isolates may be sensitive).
Blank = no or insufficient activity, or unknown.
†† 2nd line against *S. typhi*. † Penicillin sensitive; MIC ≤1.0 mcg/mL. §§ Penicillin resistant; MIC ≥2.0 mcg/mL.
*These are generalizations. There are major differences among countries, areas, and hospitals depending on antibiotic usage patterns.

ANTIBIOTIC SENSITIVITY – CEPHALOSPORINS

ORGANISMS	Cefaclor	Cefadroxil	Cefazolin	Cefdinir	Cefepime	Cefixime	Cefotaxime	Cefoxitin	Cefpodoxime Proxetil	Cefprozil	Ceftazidime	Ceftibuten	Ceftizoxime	Ceftriaxone	Cefuroxime Axetil	Cephalexin
GRAM-NEGATIVE AEROBES *(Continued)*																
Francisella tularensis																
Haemophilus influenzae	++			+++	++	++	+++	++	+++	++	++	++	+++	+++	++	
Klebsiella species	+	++	++	++	++	++	+++	++	++	++	++	++	+++	+++	++	++
Legionella species																
Moraxella catarrhalis	+++	+	+	+++	++	++	+++	+	+++	+++	+	+++	+++	+++	+++	+
Morganella morganii					++		+++	+		+	++	++	+++	+++	+	
Neisseria gonorrhoeae	+				++	+++	++	++	++	+	+	++	++	++	++	
Neisseria meningitidis					++	+	++	+			+	++	++	++	++	
Pasturella multocida			+		++	++	++		++		++	++	++	++	++	+
Proteus mirabilis	++	++	++	+++	++	++	+++	++	+++	+++	++	+++	+++	+++	+++	++
Proteus vulgaris					++	++	+++	+	+		++	+	+++	+++	++	
Providencia stuartii					+++		+++	+	+		+++	+	+++	+++	+	
Pseudomonas aeruginosa					+++						+++					
Rickettsia species																
Salmonella species							+++††							+++		
Serratia species				+	+++	+	+++	+	+		++		+++	+++		

+++ = excellent activity (1st line recommendation). ++ = good activity (2nd line recommendation). + = moderate activity (acceptable in vitro data suggesting some isolates may be sensitive).
Blank = no or insufficient activity, or unknown.
†† 2nd line against *S. typhi*. † Penicillin sensitive; MIC ≤1.0 mcg/mL. §§ Penicillin resistant; MIC ≥2.0 mcg/mL.
*These are generalizations. There are major differences among countries, areas, and hospitals depending on antibiotic usage patterns.

ANTIBIOTIC SENSITIVITY – CEPHALOSPORINS

CEPHALOSPORINS (CONTINUED)

ORGANISMS	Cefaclor	Cefadroxil	Cefazolin	Cefdinir	Cefepime	Cefixime	Cefotaxime	Cefoxitin	Cefpodoxime Proxetil	Cefprozil	Ceftazidime	Ceftibuten	Ceftizoxime	Ceftriaxone	Cefuroxime Axetil	Cephalexin
GRAM-NEGATIVE AEROBES *(Continued)*																
Shigella species				+	++		++	+	++	+	++	+	++	++	++	
Stenotrophomonas maltophilia											+					
Vibrio vulnificus							++				+++					
Yersinia enterocolitica				++	++	++	++	+	++		++	++	++	++	+	
Yersinia pestis							+							+		
GRAM-POSITIVE AEROBES																
Enterococcus faecalis																
Enterococcus faecium																
Enterococcus faecium (VRE)																
Listeria monocytogenes																
Nocardia							++							++		
Staphylococcus aureus (MSSA)	+	+++	+++	++	++		++	+	++	+	+	+	++	++	++	++
Staphylococcus aureus (MRSA)																

+++ = excellent activity (1st line recommendation). ++ = good activity (2nd line recommendation). + = moderate activity (acceptable in vitro data suggesting some isolates may be sensitive).
Blank = no or insufficient activity, or unknown.
†† 2nd line against *S. typhi*. † Penicillin sensitive; MIC ≤1.0 mcg/mL. §§ Penicillin resistant; MIC ≥2.0 mcg/mL.
*These are generalizations. There are major differences among countries, areas, and hospitals depending on antibiotic usage patterns.

ANTIBIOTIC SENSITIVITY - CEPHALOSPORINS

ORGANISMS	Cefaclor	Cefadroxil	Cefazolin	Cefdinir	Cefepime	Cefixime	Cefotaxime	Cefoxitin	Cefpodoxime Proxetil	Cefprozil	Ceftazidime	Ceftibuten	Ceftizoxime	Ceftriaxone	Cefuroxime Axetil	Cephalexin
GRAM-POSITIVE AEROBES (Continued)																
Staphylococcus epidermidis	+	++	++		+		+	+	+	++			+	+	++	++
Staphylococcus epidermidis (MRSE)																
Streptococcus pneumoniae†	++	++	++	++	++	++	++	+	++	++	+	+	++	++	++	++
Streptococcus pneumoniae§§					+		+++		+				++	+++		
Streptococcus (Group A,B,C,F,G)	++	++	++	++	++	++	++	+	++	++	+	+	++	++	++	++
Streptococcus species	++	++	++	++	++	++	++	+	++	++	+	+	+	++	++	++
MISCELLANEOUS																
Chlamydia pneumoniae																
Chlamydia trachomatis																
Ehrlichia/Anaplasma species																
MYCOBACTERIA																
Mycobacterium avium (MAI) (non-HIV)																

+++ = excellent activity (1st line recommendation). ++ = good activity (2nd line recommendation). + = moderate activity (acceptable in vitro data suggesting some isolates may be sensitive).
Blank = no or insufficient activity, or unknown. † Penicillin sensitive; MIC ≤1.0 mcg/mL. §§ Penicillin resistant; MIC ≥2.0 mcg/mL.
†† 2nd line against *S. typhi*.
* These are generalizations. There are major differences among countries, areas, and hospitals depending on antibiotic usage patterns.

ANTIBIOTIC SENSITIVITY – CEPHALOSPORINS

CEPHALOSPORINS (CONTINUED)

ORGANISMS	Cefaclor	Cefadroxil	Cefazolin	Cefdinir	Cefepime	Cefixime	Cefotaxime	Cefoxitin	Cefpodoxime Proxetil	Cefprozil	Ceftazidime	Ceftibuten	Ceftizoxime	Ceftriaxone	Cefuroxime axetil	Cephalexin
MYCOBACTERIA *(Continued)*																
Mycoplasma pneumoniae																
SPIROCHETES																
Leptospira interrogans							++							++		
Treponema pallidum (syphilis)													+	++		

+++ = excellent activity (1st line recommendation). ++ = good activity (2nd line recommendation). + = moderate activity (acceptable in vitro data suggesting some isolates may be sensitive).
Blank = no or insufficient activity, or unknown.
†† 2nd line against *S. typhi*.   † Penicillin sensitive; MIC ≤1.0 mcg/mL.   §§ Penicillin resistant; MIC ≥2.0 mcg/mL.
*These are generalizations. There are major differences among countries, areas, and hospitals depending on antibiotic usage patterns.

Antibiotic Sensitivity – Fluoroquinolones*

ORGANISMS	Ciprofloxacin	Gemifloxacin	Levofloxacin	Moxifloxacin	Norfloxacin	Ofloxacin
ANAEROBES						
Actinomyces				+		
Bacillus anthracis	+++		++	++		++
Bacteroides fragilis				+		
Clostridium difficile						
Clostridium species				+		
GRAM-NEGATIVE AEROBES						
Acinetobacter baumannii	++		++	+		+
Aeromonas hydrophila	+++		+++	+++	+	+++
Bartonella henselae	+					
Bordetella species	+		+	+		
Burkholderia cepacia	++		+	+		
Campylobacter jejuni	+++		++	+++	++	++
Citrobacter species	++		++	+	+	+
Coxiella burnetti	++		++			++
Enterobacter species	++		++	++	++	++
Escherichia coli	++		++	++	+++	++

+++ = excellent activity (1st line recommendation). ++ = good activity (2nd line recommendation). + = moderate activity (acceptable in vitro data suggesting some isolates may be sensitive).
Blank = no or insufficient activity, or unknown.
† Penicillin sensitive; MIC ≤1.0 mcg/mL. §§ Penicillin resistant; MIC ≥2.0 mcg/mL.
†† 2nd line against S. typhi.
*These are generalizations. There are major differences among countries, areas, and hospitals depending on antibiotic usage patterns.

ANTIBIOTIC SENSITIVITY – FLUOROQUINOLONES

FLUOROQUINOLONES (CONTINUED)

ORGANISMS	Ciprofloxacin	Gemifloxacin	Levofloxacin	Moxifloxacin	Norfloxacin	Ofloxacin
GRAM-NEGATIVE AEROBES *(Continued)*						
Francisella tularensis	++					
Haemophilus influenzae	++	++	++	++		++
Klebsiella species	++	+	++	++	++	++
Legionella species	+++	++	+++	+++		+++
Moraxella catarrhalis	++	++	++	++		++
Morganella morganii	++		++	+		+
Neisseria gonorrhoeae	+++		+++	++	++	+++
Neisseria meningitidis	++		++	++	+	++
Pasturella multocida	++		+			+
Proteus mirabilis	++		++	++	+++	++
Proteus vulgaris	++		++	++	+++	++
Providencia stuartii	++		++	+	++	+
Pseudomonas aeruginosa	+++		+++	++	++	++
Rickettsia species	++		++	+		++
Salmonella species	+++	++††	+++	+++	+++	+++
Serratia species	+++		+++	++	++	++
Shigella species	+++		+++	+++	+++	+++
Stenotrophomonas maltophilia	+		+	++	+	+

+++ = excellent activity (1st line recommendation).   ++ = good activity (2nd line recommendation).   + = moderate activity (acceptable in vitro data suggesting some isolates may be sensitive).
Blank = no or insufficient activity, or unknown.
† Penicillin sensitive; MIC ≤1.0 mcg/mL.   §§ Penicillin resistant; MIC ≥2.0 mcg/mL.
†† 2nd line against *S. typhi*.
*These are generalizations. There are major differences among countries, areas, and hospitals depending on antibiotic usage patterns.

ANTIBIOTIC SENSITIVITY - FLUOROQUINOLONES

ORGANISMS	Ciprofloxacin	Gemifloxacin	Levofloxacin	Moxifloxacin	Norfloxacin	Ofloxacin
GRAM-NEGATIVE AEROBES *(Continued)*						
Vibrio vulnificus	+		+	+		
Yersinia enterocolitica	++		++	++	++	++
Yersinia pestis	+		+			
GRAM-POSITIVE AEROBES						
Enterococcus faecalis	+		++	++	+	+
Enterococcus faecium	+		+	+		+
Enterococcus faecium (VRE)						
Listeria monocytogenes						
Nocardia						
Staphylococcus aureus (MSSA)	+	++	++	++	+	+
Staphylococcus aureus (MRSA)			+	+		
Staphylococcus epidermidis	+		+	+	+	+
Staphylococcus epidermidis (MRSE)	+		+	+		+
Streptococcus pneumoniae†	+	++	++	++		+
Streptococcus pneumoniae§§	+	+++	+++	+++		+

+++ = excellent activity (1st line recommendation). ++ = good activity (2nd line recommendation). + = moderate activity (acceptable in vitro data suggesting some isolates may be sensitive).
Blank = no or insufficient activity, or unknown.
†† 2nd line against *S. typhi*. † Penicillin sensitive; MIC ≤1.0 mcg/mL. §§ Penicillin resistant; MIC ≥2.0 mcg/mL.
*These are generalizations. There are major differences among countries, areas, and hospitals depending on antibiotic usage patterns.

ANTIBIOTIC SENSITIVITY – FLUOROQUINOLONES

FLUOROQUINOLONES (CONTINUED)

ORGANISMS	Ciprofloxacin	Gemifloxacin	Levofloxacin	Moxifloxacin	Norfloxacin	Ofloxacin
GRAM-POSITIVE AEROBES *(Continued)*						
Streptococcus (Group A,B,C,F,G)	+	+	+	+		+
Streptococcus species	+	++	++	++	+	+
MISCELLANEOUS						
Chlamydia pneumoniae	++	++	++	++		++
Chlamydia trachomatis			++	++		++
Ehrlichia/Anaplasma species	+		+			+
MYCOBACTERIA						
Mycobacterium avium (MAI) (non-HIV)	++		++	++		++
Mycoplasma pneumoniae	++	++	++	++		++
SPIROCHETES						
Leptospira interrogans						
Treponema pallidum (syphilis)						

+++ = excellent activity (1st line recommendation). ++ = good activity (2nd line recommendation). + = moderate activity (acceptable in vitro data suggesting some isolates may be sensitive). Blank = no or insufficient activity, or unknown.
† Penicillin sensitive; MIC ≤1.0 mcg/mL.   §§ Penicillin resistant; MIC ≥2.0 mcg/mL.
†† 2nd line against *S. typhi*.
*These are generalizations. There are major differences among countries, areas, and hospitals depending on antibiotic usage patterns.

ANTIBIOTIC SENSITIVITY – MACROLIDES & CLINDAMYCIN*

ORGANISMS	Azithromycin	Clarithromycin	Clindamycin	Erythromycin	Telithromycin
ANAEROBES					
Actinomyces	++	++	++	++	
Bacillus anthracis		+	++	+	
Bacteroides fragilis			++		
Clostridium difficile			++		
Clostridium species			++		
GRAM-NEGATIVE AEROBES					
Acinetobacter baumannii					
Aeromonas hydrophila					
Bartonella henselae	+++	+++		+++	
Bordetella species	+++	+++		+++	++
Burkholderia cepacia					
Campylobacter jejuni	+++	+++	++	+++	
Citrobacter species					
Coxiella burnetti				+	
Enterobacter species					
Escherichia coli					

+++ = excellent activity (1st line recommendation).   ++ = good activity (2nd line recommendation).   + = moderate activity (acceptable in vitro data suggesting some isolates may be sensitive).
Blank = no or insufficient activity, or unknown.
†† 2nd line against *S. typhi*.   † Penicillin sensitive; MIC ≤1.0 mcg/mL.   §§ Penicillin resistant; MIC ≥2.0 mcg/mL.
*These are generalizations. There are major differences among countries, areas, and hospitals depending on antibiotic usage patterns.

ANTIBIOTIC SENSITIVITY – MACROLIDES & CLINDAMYCIN

MACROLIDES & CLINDAMYCIN (CONTINUED)

ORGANISMS	Azithromycin	Clarithromycin	Clindamycin	Erythromycin	Telithromycin
GRAM-NEGATIVE AEROBES *(Continued)*					
Francisella tularensis					
Haemophilus influenzae	++	++		+	++
Klebsiella species					
Legionella species	+++	+++		++	++
Moraxella catarrhalis	+++	+++		++	++
Morganella morganii					
Neisseria gonorrhoeae	++			+	
Neisseria meningitidis					
Pasturella multocida	+				
Proteus mirabilis					
Proteus vulgaris					
Providencia stuartii					
Pseudomonas aeruginosa					
Rickettsia species				+	+
Salmonella species	++				
Serratia species					
Shigella species	+				
Stenotrophomonas maltophilia					

+++ = excellent activity (1st line recommendation). ++ = good activity (2nd line recommendation). + = moderate activity (acceptable in vitro data suggesting some isolates may be sensitive). Blank = no or insufficient activity, or unknown. † Penicillin sensitive; MIC ≤1.0 mcg/mL. §§ Penicillin resistant; MIC ≥2.0 mcg/mL.
†† 2nd line against *S. typhi*.
*These are generalizations. There are major differences among countries, areas, and hospitals depending on antibiotic usage patterns.

ANTIBIOTIC SENSITIVITY - MACROLIDES & CLINDAMYCIN

ORGANISMS	Azithromycin	Clarithromycin	Clindamycin	Erythromycin	Telithromycin
GRAM-NEGATIVE AEROBES *(Continued)*					
Vibrio vulnificus					
Yersinia enterocolitica					
Yersinia pestis					
GRAM-POSITIVE AEROBES					
Enterococcus faecalis					
Enterococcus faecium					
Enterococcus faecium (VRE)					
Listeria monocytogenes				++	
Nocardia	++	++		+	++
Staphylococcus aureus (MSSA)			++		
Staphylococcus aureus (MRSA)	+	+	++	+	
Staphylococcus epidermidis	+	+	++	+	
Staphylococcus epidermidis (MRSE)	++	++	++	++	++
Streptococcus pneumoniae†			++		+++
Streptococcus pneumoniae§§	++	++	++	++	++

+++ = excellent activity (1st line recommendation).   ++ = good activity (2nd line recommendation).   + = moderate activity (acceptable in vitro data suggesting some isolates may be sensitive).
Blank = no or insufficient activity, or unknown.
†† 2nd line against *S. typhi*.   † Penicillin sensitive: MIC ≤1.0 mcg/mL.   §§ Penicillin resistant: MIC ≥2.0 mcg/mL.
*These are generalizations. There are major differences among countries, areas, and hospitals depending on antibiotic usage patterns.

ANTIBIOTIC SENSITIVITY – MACROLIDES & CLINDAMYCIN

MACROLIDES & CLINDAMYCIN (CONTINUED)

ORGANISMS	Azithromycin	Clarithromycin	Clindamycin	Erythromycin	Telithromycin
GRAM-POSITIVE AEROBES *(Continued)*					
Streptococcus (Group A,B,C,F,G)	++	++	++	++	
Streptococcus species					
MISCELLANEOUS					
Chlamydia pneumoniae	+++	+++		+++	++
Chlamydia trachomatis	+++	++	++	++	
Ehrlichia/Anaplasma species	++	+++			
MYCOBACTERIA					
Mycobacterium avium (MAI) (non-HIV)	+++	+++		+++	++
Mycoplasma pneumoniae				++	
SPIROCHETES					
Leptospira interrogans	+			+	
Treponema pallidum (syphilis)					

+++ = excellent activity (1st line recommendation). ++ = good activity (2nd line recommendation). + = moderate activity (acceptable in vitro data suggesting some isolates may be sensitive).
Blank = no or insufficient activity, or unknown.
†† 2nd line against *S. typhi*.   † Penicillin sensitive; MIC ≤1.0 mcg/mL.   §§ Penicillin resistant; MIC ≥2.0 mcg/mL.
*These are generalizations. There are major differences among countries, areas, and hospitals depending on antibiotic usage patterns.

ANTIBIOTIC SENSITIVITY – PENICILLINS*

ORGANISMS	Amoxicillin	Amoxicillin + Clavulanate	Ampicillin	Ampicillin + Sulbactam	Dicloxacillin	Nafcillin/ Oxacillin	Penicillin	Piperacillin	Piperacillin + Tazobactam	Ticarcillin + Clavulanic Acid
ANAEROBES										
Actinomyces	+++	++	+++	++			+++			++
Bacillus anthracis	++	+	++	+			++			+
Bacteroides fragilis		+++		+++				+	+++	+++
Clostridium difficile										
Clostridium species	++	++	++	++			+++	++	++	++
GRAM-NEGATIVE AEROBES										
Acinetobacter baumannii				++				+	++	++
Aeromonas hydrophila								+	+	+
Bartonella henselae										
Bordetella species										
Burkholderia cepacia									+	+
Campylobacter jejuni	++	+								+
Citrobacter species								++	++	++
Coxiella burnetti										
Enterobacter species								++	++	++
Escherichia coli	+++	++	+++	++				++	++	++

+++ = excellent activity (1st line recommendation). ++ = good activity (2nd line recommendation). + = moderate activity (acceptable in vitro data suggesting some isolates may be sensitive).
Blank = no or insufficient activity, or unknown.
†† 2nd line against *S. typhi*. † Penicillin sensitive; MIC ≤1.0 mcg/mL. §§ Penicillin resistant; MIC ≥2.0 mcg/mL.
*These are generalizations. There are major differences among countries, areas, and hospitals depending on antibiotic usage patterns.

ANTIBIOTIC SENSITIVITY - PENICILLINS

PENICILLINS (CONTINUED)

ORGANISMS	Amoxicillin	Amoxicillin + Clavulanate	Ampicillin	Ampicillin + Sulbactam	Dicloxacillin	Nafcillin/ Oxacillin	Penicillin	Piperacillin	Piperacillin + Tazobactam	Ticarcillin + Clavulanic Acid
GRAM-NEGATIVE AEROBES *(Continued)*										
Francisella tularensis										
Haemophilus influenzae	+	+++	+	++					++	++
Klebsiella species		++		++				++	++	++
Legionella species										
Moraxella catarrhalis		+++		++					++	++
Morganella morganii								++	++	++
Neisseria gonorrhoeae		++	++	++						++
Neisseria meningitidis	+	++	++				+++	++		
Pasturella multocida	++	+++	++	++			+++	++	++	++
Proteus mirabilis	+++	++	+++	++				++	++	++
Proteus vulgaris								++	++	++
Providencia stuartii								++	++	++
Pseudomonas aeruginosa								+++	+++	
Rickettsia species										
Salmonella species	+	++	+	++				++	++	++
Serratia species								++	++	++
Shigella species	++	++	++	+				+	+	+

+++ = excellent activity (1st line recommendation). ++ = good activity (2nd line recommendation). + = moderate activity (acceptable in vitro data suggesting some isolates may be sensitive).
Blank = no or insufficient activity, or unknown.
†† 2nd line against *S. typhi*. † Penicillin sensitive; MIC ≤1.0 mcg/mL. §§ Penicillin resistant; MIC ≥2.0 mcg/mL.
*These are generalizations. There are major differences among countries, areas, and hospitals depending on antibiotic usage patterns.

ANTIBIOTIC SENSITIVITY - PENICILLINS

ORGANISMS	Amoxicillin	Amoxicillin + Clavulanate	Ampicillin	Ampicillin + Sulbactam	Dicloxacillin	Nafcillin/ Oxacillin	Penicillin	Piperacillin	Piperacillin + Tazobactam	Ticarcillin + Clavulanic Acid
GRAM-NEGATIVE AEROBES *(Continued)*										
Stenotrophomonas maltophilia										
Vibrio vulnificus				++				+	+	++
Yersinia enterocolitica		+		++					++	
Yersinia pestis	+		+					++	++	++
GRAM-POSITIVE AEROBES										
Enterococcus faecalis	+++	++	+++	++			+++	++	++	
Enterococcus faecium	+	+	+	+			+	+	+	
Enterococcus faecium (VRE)										
Listeria monocytogenes	+++	++	+++	++			++	++	++	
Nocardia	+	++	+	++						
Staphylococcus aureus (MSSA)		++		++	+++	+++			++	++
Staphylococcus aureus (MRSA)										
Staphylococcus epidermidis		++		++	+++	+++			++	++
Staphylococcus epidermidis (MRSE)										
Streptococcus pneumoniae†	+++	++	++	++	+	+	+++	++	++	++
Streptococcus pneumoniae§§	++	++	++	++			++	+	+	+

+++ = excellent activity (1st line recommendation). ++ = good activity (2nd line recommendation). + = moderate activity (acceptable in vitro data suggesting some isolates may be sensitive).
Blank = no or insufficient activity, or unknown.   † Penicillin sensitive; MIC ≤1.0 mcg/mL.   §§ Penicillin resistant; MIC ≥2.0 mcg/mL.
†† 2nd line against *S. typhi*.
*These are generalizations. There are major differences among countries, areas, and hospitals depending on antibiotic usage patterns.

ANTIBIOTIC SENSITIVITY – PENICILLINS

PENICILLINS (CONTINUED)

ORGANISMS	Amoxicillin	Amoxicillin + Clavulanate	Ampicillin	Ampicillin + Sulbactam	Dicloxacillin	Nafcillin/ Oxacillin	Penicillin	Piperacillin	Piperacillin + Tazobactam	Ticarcillin + Clavulanic Acid
GRAM-POSITIVE AEROBES *(Continued)*										
Streptococcus (Group A,B,C,F,G)	+++	+	+++	+	+	+	+++	+	+	+
Streptococcus species	+++	+	++	+	+	+	+++	++	+	+
MISCELLANEOUS										
Chlamydia pneumoniae										
Chlamydia trachomatis										
Ehrlichia/Anaplasma species										
MYCOBACTERIA										
Mycobacterium avium (MAI) (non-HIV)										
Mycoplasma pneumoniae										
SPIROCHETES										
Leptospira interrogans	++		+++				+++			
Treponema pallidum (syphilis)	++		++				+++			

+++ = excellent activity (1st line recommendation). ++ = good activity (2nd line recommendation). + = moderate activity (acceptable in vitro data suggesting some isolates may be sensitive). Blank = no or insufficient activity, or unknown. † Penicillin sensitive; MIC ≤1.0 mcg/mL. §§ Penicillin resistant; MIC ≥2.0 mcg/mL.
†† 2nd line against *S. typhi*.
*These are generalizations. There are major differences among countries, areas, and hospitals depending on antibiotic usage patterns.

Antibiotic Sensitivity – Sulfonamides and Tetracyclines

Antibiotic Sensitivity – Sulfonamides*

ORGANISMS	Trimethoprim + Sulfamethoxazole
ANAEROBES	
Actinomyces	
Bacillus anthracis	
Bacteroides fragilis	
Clostridium difficile	
Clostridium species	
GRAM-NEGATIVE AEROBES	
Acinetobacter baumannii	+
Aeromonas hydrophila	++
Bartonella henselae	
Bordetella species	++
Burkholderia cepacia	+++
Campylobacter jejuni	
Citrobacter species	++
Coxiella burnetti	
Enterobacter species	++

Antibiotic Sensitivity – Tetracyclines*

ORGANISMS	Doxycycline	Minocycline	Tetracycline
ANAEROBES			
Actinomyces	++	++	++
Bacillus anthracis	++		++
Bacteroides fragilis	+		+
Clostridium difficile			
Clostridium species	+		+
GRAM-NEGATIVE AEROBES			
Acinetobacter baumannii	++	++	++
Aeromonas hydrophila	++	++	++
Bartonella henselae	+++	++	++
Bordetella species	+	++	+
Burkholderia cepacia		++	
Campylobacter jejuni	++	++	++
Citrobacter species			
Coxiella burnetti	+++	+++	+++
Enterobacter species			

+++ = excellent activity (1st line recommendation).   ++ = good activity (2nd line recommendation).   + = moderate activity (acceptable in vitro data suggesting some isolates may be sensitive).
Blank = no or insufficient activity, or unknown.
† Penicillin sensitive: MIC ≤1.0 mcg/mL.   §§ Penicillin resistant; MIC ≥2.0 mcg/mL.
†† 2nd line against S. typhi.
*These are generalizations. There are major differences among countries, areas, and hospitals depending on antibiotic usage patterns.

ANTIBIOTIC SENSITIVITY – SULFONAMIDES AND TETRACYCLINES

SULFONAMIDES (CONTINUED)

ORGANISMS	Trimethoprim + Sulfamethoxazole
GRAM-NEGATIVE AEROBES *(Continued)*	
Escherichia coli	+++
Francisella tularensis	
Haemophilus influenzae	+++
Klebsiella species	+++**
Legionella species	++
Moraxella catarrhalis	+++
Morganella morganii	
Neisseria gonorrhoeae	
Neisseria meningitidis	
Pasturella multocida	++
Proteus mirabilis	++
Proteus vulgaris	++
Providencia stuartii	++
Pseudomonas aeruginosa	
Rickettsia species	
Salmonella species	++
Serratia species	+

TETRACYCLINES (CONTINUED)

ORGANISMS	Doxycycline	Minocycline	Tetracycline
GRAM-NEGATIVE AEROBES *(Continued)*			
Escherichia coli	+	+	+
Francisella tularensis	++	++	++
Haemophilus influenzae	++	++	++
Klebsiella species	+	+	
Legionella species	++	++	++
Moraxella catarrhalis	++	++	++
Morganella morganii	++	++	++
Neisseria gonorrhoeae	+	+	+
Neisseria meningitidis	+	+	+
Pasturella multocida	++		++
Proteus mirabilis	+	+	+
Proteus vulgaris	+	+	+
Providencia stuartii			
Pseudomonas aeruginosa			
Rickettsia species	+++	+++	+++
Salmonella species	+	+	+
Serratia species			

+++ = excellent activity (1st line recommendation). ++ = good activity (2nd line recommendation). + = moderate activity (acceptable in vitro data suggesting some isolates may be sensitive).
Blank = no or insufficient activity, or unknown.
†† 2nd line against *S. typhi.* † Penicillin sensitive; MIC ≤1.0 mcg/mL. §§ Penicillin resistant; MIC ≥2.0 mcg/mL.
*These are generalizations. There are major differences among countries, areas, and hospitals depending on antibiotic usage patterns.

Antibiotic Sensitivity – Sulfonamides and Tetracyclines

ORGANISMS	Trimethoprim + Sulfamethoxazole	Doxycycline	Minocycline	Tetracycline
GRAM-NEGATIVE AEROBES (Continued)				
Shigella species	++	+	+	+
Stenotrophomonas maltophilia	+++		+	
Vibrio vulnificus		+++	+++	+++
Yersinia enterocolitica	+++	+		
Yersinia pestis	+	++	++	++
GRAM-POSITIVE AEROBES				
Enterococcus faecalis		+	+	+
Enterococcus faecium				
Enterococcus faecium (VRE)		+	+	+
Listeria monocytogenes	++	+	+	+
Nocardia	+++	++	++	+
Staphylococcus aureus (MSSA)	++	++	++	+
Staphylococcus aureus (MRSA)	++	++	++	+
Staphylococcus epidermidis	++	++	++	+
Staphylococcus epidermidis (MRSE)	++	++	++	++
Streptococcus pneumoniae†	++	++	++	++

+++ = excellent activity (1st line recommendation).   ++ = good activity (2nd line recommendation).   + = moderate activity (acceptable in vitro data suggesting some isolates may be sensitive).
Blank = no or insufficient activity, or unknown.   † Penicillin sensitive; MIC ≤1.0 mcg/mL.   §§ Penicillin resistant; MIC ≥2.0 mcg/mL.
†† 2nd line against S. typhi.
*These are generalizations. There are major differences among countries, areas, and hospitals depending on antibiotic usage patterns.

ANTIBIOTIC SENSITIVITY – SULFONAMIDES AND TETRACYCLINES

SULFONAMIDES (CONTINUED)

ORGANISMS	Trimethoprim + Sulfamethoxazole
GRAM-POSITIVE AEROBES (Continued)	
Streptococcus pneumoniae§§	
Streptococcus (Group A,B,C,F,G)	++
Streptococcus species	++
MISCELLANEOUS	
Chlamydia pneumoniae	
Chlamydia trachomatis	+
Ehrlichia/Anaplasma species	
MYCOBACTERIA	
Mycobacterium avium (MAI) (non-HIV)	
Mycoplasma pneumoniae	
SPIROCHETES	
Leptospira interrogans	
Treponema pallidum (syphilis)	

+++ = excellent activity (1st line recommendation). ++ = good activity (2nd line recommendation). + = moderate activity (acceptable in vitro data suggesting some isolates may be sensitive).
Blank = no or insufficient activity, or unknown.
†† 2nd line against S. typhi.   † Penicillin sensitive; MIC ≤1.0 mcg/mL.   §§ Penicillin resistant; MIC ≥2.0 mcg/mL.
*These are generalizations. There are major differences among countries, areas, and hospitals depending on antibiotic usage patterns.

TETRACYCLINES (CONTINUED)

ORGANISMS	Doxycycline	Minocycline	Tetracycline
GRAM-POSITIVE AEROBES (Continued)			
Streptococcus pneumoniae§§	+	+	+
Streptococcus (Group A,B,C,F,G)	+	+	+
Streptococcus species	+	+	+
MISCELLANEOUS			
Chlamydia pneumoniae	+++	+++	+++
Chlamydia trachomatis	+++	+++	+++
Ehrlichia/Anaplasma species	+++	+++	+++
MYCOBACTERIA			
Mycobacterium avium (MAI) (non-HIV)			
Mycoplasma pneumoniae	++	++	++
SPIROCHETES			
Leptospira interrogans	++	++	++
Treponema pallidum (syphilis)	++	++	++

ANTIBIOTIC SENSITIVITY – MISCELLANEOUS*

ORGANISMS	Chloramphenicol	Colistin	Daptomycin	Fosfomycin	Linezolid	Metronidazole	Nitrofurantoin	Quinupristin + Dalfopristin	Rifampin	Vancomycin
ANAEROBES										
Actinomyces										
Bacillus anthracis	++							+		+
Bacteroides fragilis	++					+++		+	++	++
Clostridium difficile					+	+++			+	++
Clostridium species	++				+	++		+	+	+
GRAM-NEGATIVE AEROBES										
Aeromonas hydrophila	+									
Bartonella henselae	+								++	
Bordetella species	+								+	
Burkholderia cepacia	++								+	
Campylobacter jejuni	++									
Citrobacter species	+	+		+			++			
Coxiella burnetii	+								++	
Enterobacter species		+		+						
Escherichia coli	+	+		++			++		+	
Francisella tularensis	++									

+++ = excellent activity (1st line recommendation). ++ = good activity (2nd line recommendation). + = moderate activity (acceptable in vitro data suggesting some isolates may be sensitive).
Blank = no or insufficient activity, or unknown.
†† 2nd line against *S. typhi*. † Penicillin sensitive; MIC ≤1.0 mcg/mL. §§ Penicillin resistant; MIC ≥2.0 mcg/mL.
*These are generalizations. There are major differences among countries, areas, and hospitals depending on antibiotic usage patterns.

ANTIBIOTIC SENSITIVITY - MISCELLANEOUS

MISCELLANEOUS (CONTINUED)

ORGANISMS	Chloramphenicol	Colistin	Daptomycin	Fosfomycin	Linezolid	Metronidazole	Nitrofurantoin	Quinupristin + Dalfopristin	Rifampin	Vancomycin
GRAM-NEGATIVE AEROBES *(Continued)*										
Haemophilus influenzae	++							+	+	
Klebsiella species	+	+		+						
Legionella species								+	++	
Moraxella catarrhalis	++							+	+	
Morganella morganii				+			+			
Neisseria gonorrhoeae				+				+	++	
Neisseria meningitidis	++							+	++	
Pasturella multocida									+	
Proteus mirabilis				++			++		+	
Proteus vulgaris				+			+		+	
Providencia stuartii	+			+			++			
Pseudomonas aeruginosa		++								
Rickettsia species	++								+	
Salmonella species	++	+								
Serratia species	+			+			+		+	
Shigella species	++	+								
Stenotrophomonas maltophilia	+									

+++ = excellent activity (1st line recommendation). ++ = good activity (2nd line recommendation). + = moderate activity (acceptable in vitro data suggesting some isolates may be sensitive).
Blank = no or insufficient activity, or unknown.
†† 2nd line against *S. typhi*. † Penicillin sensitive; MIC ≤1.0 mcg/mL. §§ Penicillin resistant; MIC ≥2.0 mcg/mL.
*These are generalizations. There are major differences among countries, areas, and hospitals depending on antibiotic usage patterns.

ANTIBIOTIC SENSITIVITY - MISCELLANEOUS

ORGANISMS	Chloramphenicol	Colistin	Daptomycin	Fosfomycin	Linezolid	Metronidazole	Nitrofurantoin	Quinupristin + Dalfopristin	Rifampin	Vancomycin
GRAM-NEGATIVE AEROBES *(Continued)*										
Vibrio vulnificus										
Yersinia enterocolitica	++									
Yersinia pestis	++									
GRAM-POSITIVE AEROBES										
Enterococcus faecalis	+			++	++		++			++
Enterococcus faecium	++		++	++	+++		++	++	+	+++
Enterococcus faecium (VRE)	++		++	+	+++		++	+++	+	
Listeria monocytogenes	++				+			+	++	+
Nocardia					+					
Staphylococcus aureus (MSSA)	+		++		++		++	++	++	++
Staphylococcus aureus (MRSA)	+		++		++		+	++	++	+++
Staphylococcus epidermidis	+		++		++		++	++	++	+++
Staphylococcus epidermidis (MRSE)	+		++		++		+	++		+++
Streptococcus pneumoniae†	+		++		++			++	++	++
Streptococcus pneumoniae§§	+		++		++			++	++	+++

+++ = excellent activity (1st line recommendation). ++ = good activity (2nd line recommendation). + = moderate activity (acceptable in vitro data suggesting some isolates may be sensitive).
Blank = no or insufficient activity, or unknown.
†† 2nd line against *S. typhi*. † Penicillin sensitive; MIC ≤1.0 mcg/mL. §§ Penicillin resistant; MIC ≥2.0 mcg/mL.
*These are generalizations. There are major differences among countries, areas, and hospitals depending on antibiotic usage patterns.

ANTIBIOTIC SENSITIVITY - MISCELLANEOUS

MISCELLANEOUS (CONTINUED)

ORGANISMS	Chloramphenicol	Colistin	Daptomycin	Fosfomycin	Linezolid	Metronidazole	Nitrofurantoin	Quinupristin + Dalfopristin	Rifampin	Vancomycin
GRAM-POSITIVE AEROBES *(Continued)*										
Streptococcus (Group A,B,C,F,G)	+		+					++	+	++
Streptococcus species	++		+		++			+	+	++
MISCELLANEOUS										
Chlamydia pneumoniae								+	+	
Chlamydia trachomatis							+		+	
Ehrlichia/Anaplasma species	++								++	
MYCOBACTERIA										
Mycobacterium avium (MAI) (non-HIV)					+				++	
Mycoplasma pneumoniae								+		
SPIROCHETES										
Leptospira interrogans										
Treponema pallidum (syphilis)	++									

+++ = excellent activity (1st line recommendation). ++ = good activity (2nd line recommendation). + = moderate activity (acceptable in vitro data suggesting some isolates may be sensitive).
Blank = no or insufficient activity, or unknown. † 2nd line against *S. typhi*. ‡ Penicillin sensitive; MIC ≤1.0 mcg/mL. §§ Penicillin resistant; MIC ≥2.0 mcg/mL.
*These are generalizations. There are major differences among countries, areas, and hospitals depending on antibiotic usage patterns.

Oral Antibiotics

DRUG	BRAND	FORMULATIONS (mg or mg/5mL)*
CEPHALOSPORINS		
Cefaclor	Ceclor	Cap: 250, 500 Sus: 125, 187, 250, 375
	Ceclor CD	Tab, ER: 375, 500
Cefadroxil	Duricef	Cap: 500 Sus: 125, 250, 500 Tab: 1g
Cefdinir	Omnicef	Cap: 300 Sus: 125, 250
Cefditoren	Spectracef	Tab: 200
Cefixime	Suprax	Sus: 100, 200
Cefpodoxime	Vantin	Sus: 50, 100 Tab: 100, 200
Cefprozil	Cefzil	Sus: 125, 250 Tab: 250, 500
Ceftibuten	Cedax	Cap: 400 Sus: 90
Cefuroxime	Ceftin	Sus: 125, 250 Tab: 125, 250, 500
Cephalexin	Keflex	Cap: 250, 333, 500, 750
FLUOROQUINOLONES		
Ciprofloxacin**	Cipro	Sus: 250, 500 Tab: 100, 250, 500, 750
	Cipro XR	Tab, ER: 500, 1000
	ProQuin XR	Tab, ER: 500
Levofloxacin**	Levaquin	Sol: 125 Tab: 250, 500, 750
Moxifloxacin	Avelox	Tab: 400
Norfloxacin	Noroxin	Tab: 400
Ofloxacin	Floxin	Tab: 200, 300, 400
MACROLIDES		
Azithromycin**	Zithromax	Sus: 100, 200, 1g/pkt Tab: 250, 500, 600
	Zmax	Sus, ER: 2g
Clarithromycin	Biaxin	Sus: 125, 250 Tab: 250, 500
	Biaxin XL	Tab, ER: 500, 1000
Dirithromycin		Tab: 250
Erythromycin ethylsuccinate	E.E.S.	Granules: 200 Sus: 200, 400 Tab: 400
	EryPed	Drops: 100mg/2.5mL Granules: 200, 400 Sus: 200, 400
	Eryc	Cap, DR: 250
	Ery-Tab	Tab, DR: 250, 333, 500
	PCE	Tab: 333, 500
PENICILLINS		
Amoxicillin	Amoxil	Cap: 250, 500 Chew, Tab: 200, 400 Drops: 50mg/mL Sus: 125, 200, 250, 400 Tab: 500, 875
Ampicillin	Principen	Cap: 250, 500 Sus: 125, 250
Penicillin V	Veetids	Sus: 125, 250 Tab: 250, 500

(Continued)

ORAL ANTIBIOTICS

DRUG	BRAND	FORMULATIONS (mg or mg/5mL)*
TETRACYCLINES		
Doxycycline	Doryx	Cap: 75, 100
	Monodox	Cap: 50, 100
	Vibramycin	Cap: 50, 100 Syr: 50 Sus: 25
	Vibra-Tabs	Tab: 100
Minocycline**	Minocin	Cap: 50, 100
	Dynacin	Cap: 75, 100
Tetracycline	Sumycin	Cap: 250, 500 Sus: 125 Tab: 250, 500
OTHER		
Loracarbef	Lorabid	Cap: 200, 400 Sus: 100, 200
Clindamycin**	Cleocin	Cap: 75, 150, 300 Sus: 75
Fosfomycin	Monurol	Powder: 3g/packet
Linezolid**	Zyvox	Sus: 100 Tab: 600
Metronidazole	Flagyl	Cap: 375 Tab: 250, 500
	Flagyl ER	Tab, ER: 750
Nitrofurantoin	Macrobid	Cap: 100
	Macrodantin	Cap: 25, 50, 100
Telithromycin	Ketek	Tab: 300, 400
Trimethoprim	Primsol	Sol: 50
Vancomycin**	Vancocin	Cap: 125, 250
COMBINATIONS		
Erythromycin ethylsuccinate/ Sulfisoxazole	Pediazole	Sus: 200/600
Amoxicillin/Clavulanate	Augmentin	Chew, Tab: 125/31.25, 250/62.5, 200/28.5, 400/57 Sus: 125/31.2, 200/28.5, 400/57, 250/62.5 Tab: 250/125, 500/125, 875/125
	Augmentin ES	Sus: 600/42.9
	Augmentin XR	Tab, ER: 1000/62.5
Sulfamethoxazole/ Trimethoprim	Bactrim, Septra**	Tab: 400/80 Sus: (Septra) 200/40
	Bactrim DS, Septra DS	Tab, DS: 800/160

* Unless otherwise indicated.   **Injection formulation available.

ANTIBIOTICS: NEONATAL RECOMMENDED CONCENTRATIONS FOR ADMINISTRATION

GENERIC NAME	ROUTE	UNITS	CONCENTRATION AVAILABLE	DEFAULT	HIGH	LOW
Acyclovir	IV	mg/mL	50*	7	7	5
Amikacin	IV	mg/mL	50*	10	10	5
Amikacin	IM	mg/mL	50	50	50	10
Amphotericin B	IV	mg/mL	5*	0.1	0.1	0.05
Amphotericin B Lipid Complex	IV	mg/mL	5*	2	2	0.5
Amphotericin B Liposome	IV	mg/mL	4*	2	5	1
Ampicillin	IV	mg/mL	125 or 250*	50	100	20
Ampicillin	IM	mg/mL	250	250	250	125
Azithromycin	IV	mg/mL	100*	2	2	2
Aztreonam	IV	mg/mL	50	50	66	20
Aztreonam	IM	mg/mL	125 or 250	167	333	83
Caspofungin	IV	mg/mL	5.2*	0.2	0.5	0.2
Cefepime	IV	mg/mL	100	100	160	100
Cefepime	IM	mg/mL	280	280	280	160
Cefazolin	IV	mg/mL	225*	100	125	20
Cefazolin	IM	mg/mL	225	330	330	100
Cefotaxime	IV	mg/mL	50 or 100	50	100	25
Cefotaxime	IM	mg/mL	230 or 300	300	330	100
Cefoxitin	IV	mg/mL	100*	40	100	20
Cefoxitin	IM	mg/mL	400*	200	400	100
Ceftazidime	IV	mg/mL	200	100	200	50
Ceftazidime	IM	mg/mL	200	200	100	50
Ceftriaxone	IV	mg/mL	40 or 100*	40	40	20
Ceftriaxone	IM	mg/mL	250	250	250	100
Chloramphenicol	IV	mg/mL	100*	10	100	5
Clindamycin	IV	mg/mL	150*	10	18	6
Erythromycin Lactobionate	IV	mg/mL	50*	5	5	1
Fluconazole	IV	mg/mL	2	2	2	2
Ganciclovir	IV	mg/mL	50*	5	10	5
Gentamicin	IV	mg/mL	10	10	10	2
Gentamicin	IM	mg/mL	40	10	40	10
Imipenem - Cilastatin	IV	mg/mL	2.5 or 5	5	5	2.5
Linezolid	IV	mg/mL	2	2	2	2
Meropenem	IV	mg/mL	50	50	50	25
Metronidazole	IV	mg/mL	5	5	5	5
Nafcillin	IV	mg/mL	250*	40	40	20
Netilmicin	IM	mg/mL	100*	5	100	2.5
Oxacillin	IV	mg/mL	100*	25	100	25
Penicillin G	IV	U/mL	500,000	100,000	500,000	50,000
Piperacillin	IV	mg/mL	400*	100	200	50
Piperacillin	IM	mg/mL	400	300	400	100
Piperacillin - Tazobactam	IV	mg/mL	200	100	200	50
Rifampin	IV	mg/mL	60*	3	6	3
Ticarcillin -Clavulanate	IV	mg/mL	200	50	100	10
Tobramycin	IV	mg/mL	10	10	10	2
Tobramycin	IM	mg/mL	40	40	40	10
Vancomycin	IV	mg/mL	50*	5	5	2.5
Zidovudine (ZDV, AZT)	IV	mg/mL	10*	4	4	2

* See Special Consideration/Preparation section in the NeoFax drug profile for dilution details.
Adapted from *NeoFax 2007*.

SYSTEMIC ANTIBIOTICS

BRAND NAME (Generic)	DOSAGE FORM/ STRENGTH	INDICATIONS	ADULT DOSE	PEDIATRIC DOSE
AMINOGLYCOSIDES				
Amikin (amikacin sulfate)	Inj: 50mg/mL, 250mg/mL	Short-term treatment of serious infections caused by gram-negative bacteria such as septicemia, and respiratory tract, bone/joint, CNS (including meningitis), skin and soft tissue, and intra-abdominal infections; burns and postoperative infections; complicated and recurrent urinary tract infections (UTI); and staphylococcal disease.	(IM/IV)15mg/kg/day given q8h or q12h. Max: 15mg/kg/day. Heavier Weight Patients: Max: 1.5g/day. Recurrent Uncomplicated UTI: 250mg bid. Duration: 7-10 days. Stop therapy if no response after 3-5 days. Reduce dose if suspect renal dysfunction. Discontinue if azotemia increases or if a progressive decrease in urinary output occurs.	15mg/kg/day given bid-tid. Newborns: LD: 10mg/kg. MD: 7.5mg/kg q12h. Duration: 7-10 days.
Amikin Pediatric (amikacin sulfate)	Inj: 50mg/mL	Short-term treatment of serious infections caused by gram-negative bacteria such as septicemia, and respiratory tract, bone/joint, CNS (including meningitis), skin and soft tissue, and intra-abdominal infections; burns and postoperative infections; complicated and recurrent urinary tract infections (UTI); and staphylococcal disease.		15mg/kg/day given bid-tid. Newborns: LD: 10mg/kg. MD: 7.5mg/kg q12h. Duration: 7-10 days.
Gentamicin sulfate	Inj: 10mg/mL, 40mg/mL	Treatment of bacterial neonatal sepsis, bacterial septicemia, and serious bacterial infections of the CNS (meningitis), urinary tract, respiratory tract, gastrointestinal tract (including peritonitis), skin, bone and soft tissue (including burns) caused by susceptible strains of microorganisms.	(IM/IV) Serious Infections: 3mg/kg/day given q8h. Life-Threatening Infections: 5mg/kg/day tid-qid; reduce to 3mg/kg/day as soon as clinically indicated. Treat for 7-10 days; may need longer course in difficult and complicated infections. Renal Impairment: Reduced dose given q8h or usual dose given at prolonged intervals based on either CrCl or serum creatinine. Dialysis: 1-1.7mg/kg, depending on severity of infection, at end of each dialysis period. Obese Patients: Calculate dose based on estimated lean body mass.	6-7.5mg/kg/day (2-2.5mg/kg given q8h). Infants and Neonates: 7.5mg/kg/day (2.5mg/kg given q8h). Premature and Full-Term Neonates 1 week: 5mg/kg/day (2.5mg/kg given q12h). Treat for 7-10 days; may need longer course in difficult and complicated infections. Renal Impairment: Reduced dose given q8h or usual dose given at prolonged intervals based on either CrCl or serum creatinine. Dialysis: 2mg/kg at end of each dialysis period. Obese Patients: Calculate dose based on estimated lean body mass.

SYSTEMIC ANTIBIOTICS

BRAND NAME (Generic)	DOSAGE FORM/ STRENGTH	INDICATIONS	ADULT DOSE	PEDIATRIC DOSE
Nebcin (tobramycin sulfate)	Inj: 10mg/mL, 40mg/mL, 1.2g	Treatment of serious lower respiratory tract, CNS (eg, meningitis), intra-abdominal, bone, skin and skin structure, and complicated/recurrent urinary tract infections; and septicemia.	(IM/IV) Serious Infections: 3mg/kg/day given q8h. Life-Threatening Infections: Up to 5mg/kg/day given tid-qid. Reduce to 3mg/kg/day as soon as clinically indicated. Max: 5mg/kg/day unless serum levels monitored. Treat for 7-10 days; may need longer course in difficult and complicated infections. Severe Cystic Fibrosis: Initial: 10mg/kg/day given qid. Measure levels to determine subsequent doses. Renal Impairment: LD: 1mg/kg followed by reduced doses given q8h or normal doses given at prolonged intervals based on either CrCl or serum creatinine. Do not use either method during dialysis. Obese Patients: Calculate dose based on estimated lean body weight plus 40% of the excess as the basic weight on which to figure mg/kg. ADD-Vantage vials are not for IM use.	>1 week: (IM/IV) 6-7.5mg/kg/day given tid-qid (eg, 2-2.5mg/kg q8h or 1.5-1.89mg/kg q6h). 1 week: Up to 2mg/kg q12h. Treat for 7-10 days; may need longer course in difficult and complicated infections. Severe Cystic Fibrosis: Initial: 10mg/kg/day given qid. Measure levels to determine subsequent doses. Renal Impairment: LD: 1mg/kg, followed by reduced doses given q8h or normal doses given at prolonged intervals based on either method during dialysis. Obese Patients: Calculate dose based on estimated lean body weight plus 40% of the excess as the basic weight on which to figure mg/kg. ADD-Vantage vials are not for IM use.
Streptomycin sulfate	Inj: 1g	Treatment of moderate to severe infections such as mycobacterium tuberculosis (TB) and non-TB infections (eg, plague, tularemia, chancroid, granuloma inguinale, *H.influenzae* and *K.pneumoniae* infections, UTI, gram-negative bacillary bacteremia, endocardial infections).	IM only. TB: 15mg/kg/day (Max: 1g), or 25-30mg/kg twice weekly (Max: 1.5g), or 25-30mg/kg three times weekly (Max: 1.5g). Do not exceed a total dose of 120g over the course of therapy unless no other therapeutic options exist. Elderly (>60 yrs): Reduce dose. Treat for minimum of 1 year if possible. Tularemia: 1-2g/day in divided doses for 7-14 days until afebrile for 5-7 days. Plague: 1g bid for minimum of 10 days. Streptococcal Endocarditis: With PCN, 1g bid for week 1, then 500mg bid for week 2. Enterococcal Endocarditis: With PCN, 1g bid for 2 weeks, then 500mg bid for 4 weeks. Renal Impairment: Reduce dose. Moderate/Severe Infections: 1-2g/day in divided doses q6-12h. Max: 2g/day.	IM only. TB: 20-40mg/kg/day (Max: 1g), or 25-30 mg/kg twice weekly (Max: 1.5g), or 25-30mg/kg three times weekly (Max: 1.5g). Do not exceed a total dose of 120g over the course of therapy unless no other therapeutic options exist. Treat for minimum of 1 year if possible. Moderate/Severe Infections: 20-40mg/kg/day (8-20mg/lb/day) in dividedddoses q6-12h.

(Continued)

SYSTEMIC ANTIBIOTICS

BRAND NAME (Generic)	DOSAGE FORM/ STRENGTH	INDICATIONS	ADULT DOSE	PEDIATRIC DOSE
AMINOGLYCOSIDES *(Continued)*				
TOBI (tobramycin)	Sol: 60mg/mL (300mg/ampule)	Management of cystic fibrosis patients with *P. aeruginosa*.	Inhale via nebulizer 300mg q12h for 28 days, then stop for 28 days. Resume therapy for next 28-day on/28-day off cycle.	≥6 yrs: Inhale via nebulizer 300mg q12h for 28 days, then stop for 28 days. Resume therapy for next 28-day on/28-day off cycle.
Trobicin (spectinomycin HCl)	Inj: 2g	Treatment of acute gonorrheal urethritis and proctitis in men and acute gonorrheal cervicitis in women due to *Neisseria gonorrhoeae*. Treatment of men and women recently exposed to gonorrhea.	Administer 2g (5mL) IM into upper outer quandrant of gluteal muscle. Use 4g (10mL) for treatment in geographic areas with prevalent antibiotic resistance. Divide dose between 2 gluteal sites.	
CARBAPENEMS				
Invanz (ertapenem sodium)	Inj: 1g	Treatment of complicated intra-abdominal infections; skin and skin structure infections (SSSI), including diabetic foot infections without osteomyelitis; community acquired pneumonia (CAP); complicated urinary tract infections (UTI) including pyelonephritis; acute pelvic infections including postpartum endomyometritis, septic abortion, and post surgical gynecologic infections; prophylaxis of surgical site infection following elective colorectal surgery.	Treatment: 1g IM/IV qd. Duration: Intra-Abdominal Infections: 5-14 days. SSSI: 7-14 days. CAP/UTI: 10-14 days. Pelvic Infection: 3-10 days. May administer IV for up to 14 days and IM for up to 7 days. CrCl ≤30mL/min/1.73m²: 500mg IM/IV qd. Hemodialysis: Give 150mg IM/IV after dialysis only if 500mg dose was given within 6 hrs prior to dialysis. Prophylaxis: 1g IV as single dose given 1 hr prior to surgical incision.	≥13 yrs: 1g IM/IV qd. 3 mo-12 yrs: 15mg/kg IM/IV bid (not to exceed 1g/day). Treatment Duration: Intra-Abdominal Infections: 5-14 days. SSSI: 7-14 days. CAP/UTI: 10-14 days. Pelvic Infections: 3-10 days. May administer IV for up to 14 days and IM for up to 7 days. CrCl ≤30mL/min/1.73 m²: 500mg IM/IV qd.
CEPHALOSPORINS, FIRST GENERATION				
Duricef (cefadroxil monohydrate)	Cap: 500mg; Sus: 250mg/5mL [50mL, 100mL], 500mg/5mL [50mL, 75mL, 100mL]; Tab: 1g	Skin and skin structure infections (SSSI) and urinary tract infections (UTI), pharyngitis, and tonsillitis.	Uncomplicated Lower UTI: 1-2g/day given qd or bid. Other UTI: 1gm bid. SSSI: 1g qd or 500mg bid. Group A β-hemolytic Strep Pharyngitis/Tonsillitis: 1g qd or 500mg bid for 10 days. CrCl ≤50mL/min: Initial: 1g. Maint: CrCl 25-50mL/min: 500mg q12h; CrCl 10-25mL/min: 500mg q24h; CrCl 0-10mL/min: 500mg q36h	UTI/SSSI: 15mg/kg q12h. Pharyngitis/Tonsillitis/Impetigo: 30mg/kg qd or 15mg/kg q12h. Treat β-hemolytic strep infections for at least 10 days.
Keflex (cephalexin)	Cap: 250mg, 333mg, 500mg, 750mg; Sus: 125mg/5mL, 250mg/5mL [100mL, 200mL]	Treatment of otitis media and skin and skin structure infections (SSSI); bone, genitourinary tract, and respiratory tract infections.	Usual: 25-50mg/kg/day in divided doses. Streptococcal Pharyngitis/SSSI/Uncomplicated Cystitis (>15 yrs): 500mg q12h. Treat cystitis for 7-14 days. Max: 4g/day.	Usual: 25-50mg/kg/day in divided doses. Streptococcal Pharyngitis (>1 yr)/SSSI: May divide dose and give q12h. Otitis Media: 75-100mg/kg/day in divided doses. Administer for ≥10 days in, β-hemolytic streptococcal infections.

SYSTEMIC ANTIBIOTICS

BRAND NAME (Generic)	DOSAGE FORM/ STRENGTH	INDICATIONS	ADULT DOSE	PEDIATRIC DOSE
CEPHALOSPORINS, SECOND GENERATION				
Cefaclor	Cap: 250mg, 500mg; Sus: 125mg/5mL [75mL, 150mL], 187mg/5mL [50mL, 100mL], 250mg/5mL [75mL, 150mL], 375mg/5mL [50mL, 100mL]	Treatment of otitis media, pharyngitis, tonsillitis, lower respiratory tract, urinary tract, and skin and skin structure infections caused by susceptible strains of microorganisms.	Usual: 250mg q8h. Severe Infections/Pneumonia: 500mg q8h. Treat ß-hemolytic strep for 10 days.	≥1 mo: Usual: 20mg/kg/day given q8h. Otitis Media/Serious Infections: 40mg/kg/day. Max: 1g/day. May administer q12h for otitis media and pharyngitis. Treat ß-hemolytic strep for 10 days.
Cefaclor ER	Tab, Extended-Release: 375mg, 500mg	Acute bacterial exacerbation of chronic bronchitis (ABECB), secondary bacterial infections of acute bronchitis, pharyngitis, tonsillitis, and uncomplicated skin and skin structure infections (SSSI) caused by susceptible strains of microorganisms.	ABECB/Acute Bronchitis: 500mg q12h for 7 days. Pharyngitis/Tonsillitis: 375mg q12h for 10 days. SSSI: 375mg q12h for 7-10 days. Take with meals. Do not crush, cut or chew tab.	≥16 yrs: ABECB/Acute Bronchitis: 500mg q12h for 7 days. Pharyngitis/Tonsillitis: 375mg q12h for 10 days. SSSI: 375mg q12h for 7-10 days. Take with meals. Do not crush, cut or chew tab.
Cefoxitin (cefoxitin sodium)	Inj: 1g, 1g/50mL, 2g, 2g/50mL, 10g	Treatment of lower respiratory tract, urinary tract, intra-abdominal, gynecological, skin and skin structure, and bone and joint infections, and septicemia. For surgical prophylaxis.	Usual: 1-2g IV q6-8h. Moderate-Severe: 1g IV q6h or 2g IV q6-8h. Gas Gangrene/Other Infections Requiring Higher Dose: 2g IV q4h or 3g IV q6h. Renal Insufficiency: LD: 1-2g IV. Maint: CrCl 30-50mL/min: 1-2g IV q8-12h. CrCl 10-29mL/min: 1-2g IV q12-24h. CrCl 5-9mL/min: 0.5-1g IV q12-24h. CrCl <5mL/min: 0.5-1g IV q24-48h. Hemodialysis: LD: 1-2g IV after dialysis. Maint: See renal insufficiency doses above. Prophylaxis: Uncontaminated GI Surgery/Hysterectomy: 2g IV 0.5-1 hr prior to surgery, then 2g IV q6h after first dose up to 24 hrs. C-Section: 2g IV single dose after umbilical cord is clamped, or 2g IV after umbilical cord is clamped followed by 2g IV 4 and 8 hrs after initial dose.	≥3 mo: 80-160mg/kg/day divided into 4-6 equal doses. Max: 12g/day. Prophylaxis: Uncontaminated GI Surgery/Hysterectomy: 30-40mg/kg IV 0.5-1 hr prior to surgery, then 30-40mg/kg IV q6h after first dose up to 24 hrs.

(Continued)

SYSTEMIC ANTIBIOTICS

CEPHALOSPORINS, SECOND GENERATION *(Continued)*

BRAND NAME (Generic)	DOSAGE FORM/ STRENGTH	INDICATIONS	ADULT DOSE	PEDIATRIC DOSE
Ceftin (cefuroxime axetil)	Sus: 125mg/5mL [100mL], 250mg/5mL [50mL, 100mL]; Tab: 125mg, 250mg, 500mg	(Sus/Tab) Pharyngitis/tonsillitis, acute otitis media, and impetigo. (Tab) Uncomplicated skin and skin structure (SSSI), and urinary tract infection (UTI), gonorrhea, early lyme disease, acute bacterial maxillary sinusitis, acute bacterial exacerbations of chronic bronchitis (ABECB) and secondary bacterial infections of acute bronchitis.	(Tab) Pharyngitis/Tonsillitis/Sinusitis: 250mg bid for 10 days. ABECB/SSSI: 250-500mg bid for 10 days. Acute Bronchitis: 250-500mg bid for 5-10 days. UTI: 125-250mg bid for 7-10 days. Gonorrhea: 1000mg single dose. Lyme Disease: 500mg bid for 20 days.	≥13 yrs: (Tab) Pharyngitis/Tonsillitis/Sinusitis: 250mg bid for 10 days. ABECB/SSSI: 250-500mg bid for 10 days. Acute Bronchitis: 250-500mg bid for 5-10 days. UTI: 125-250mg bid for 7-10 days. Gonorrhea: 1000mg single dose. Lyme Disease: 500mg bid for 20 days. 3 mo-12 yrs: (Sus) Pharyngitis/Tonsillitis: 10mg/kg bid for 10 days. Max: 500mg/day. Otitis Media/Sinusitis/Impetigo: 15mg/kg bid for 10 days. Max: 1000mg/day. (Tab-If can swallow whole) Pharyngitis/Tonsillitis: 125mg bid for 10 days. Otitis Media/Sinusitis: 250mg bid for 10 days.
Cefzil (cefprozil)	Sus: 125mg/5mL, 250mg/5mL [50mL, 75mL, 100mL]; Tab: 250mg, 500mg	Mild to moderate pharyngitis/tonsillitis, otitis media, acute sinusitis, secondary bacterial infection of acute bronchitis, acute bacterial exacerbation of chronic bronchitis (ABECB), and uncomplicated skin and skin structure infections (SSSI).	≥13 yrs: Pharyngitis/Tonsillitis: 500mg q24h for 10 days. Acute Sinusitis: 250-500mg q12h for 10 days. ABECB/Acute Bronchitis: 500mg q12h for 10 days. SSSI: 250-500mg q12h or 500mg q24h. CrCl <30mL/min: 50% of standard dose.	2-12 yrs: Pharyngitis/Tonsillitis: 7.5mg/kg q12h for 10 days. SSSI: 20mg/kg q24h for 10 days. 6 mos-12 yrs: Otitis Media: 15mg/kg q12h for 10 days. Acute Sinusitis: 7.5-15mg/kg q12h for 10 days. Do not exceed adult dose. CrCl <30mL/min: 50% of standard dose.
Mefoxin (cefoxitin sodium)	Inj: 1g, 1g/50mL, 2g, 2g/50mL, 10g	Treatment of lower respiratory tract, urinary tract, intra-abdominal, gynecological, skin and skin structure, and bone and joint infections, and septicemia. For surgical prophylaxis.	Usual: 1-2g IV q6-8h. Uncomplicated Infections: 1g IV q6-8h. Moderate-Severe: 1g IV q4h or 2g IV q6-8h. Gas Gangrene/Other Infections Requiring Higher Dose: 2g IV q4h or 3g IV q6h. Renal Insufficiency: LD: 1-2g IV. Maint: CrCl 30-50mL/min: 1-2g IV q8-12h. CrCl 10-29mL/min: 1-2g IV q12-24h. CrCl 5-9mL/min: 0.5-1g IV q12-24h. CrCl <5mL/min: 0.5-1g IV q24-48h. Hemodialysis: LD: 1-2g IV after dialysis. Maint: See renal insufficiency doses above. Prophylaxis: Uncontaminated GI Surgery/Hysterectomy: 2g IV 0.5-1 hr prior to surgery, then 2g IV q6h after first dose up to 24 hrs. C-Section: 2g IV single dose after umbilical cord is clamped, or 2g IV after umbilical cord is clamped followed by 2g IV 4 and 8 hrs after initial dose.	≥3 mos: 80-160mg/kg/day divided into 4-6 equal doses. Max: 12g/day. Prophylaxis: Uncontaminated GI Surgery/Hysterectomy: 30-40mg/kg IV 0.5-1 hr prior to surgery, then 30- 40mg/kg IV q6h after first dose up to 24 hrs.

SYSTEMIC ANTIBIOTICS

BRAND NAME (Generic)	DOSAGE FORM/ STRENGTH	INDICATIONS	ADULT DOSE	PEDIATRIC DOSE
CEPHALOSPORINS, THIRD GENERATION				
Cedax (ceftibuten)	Cap: 400mg; Sus: 90mg/5mL [30mL, 60mL, 90mL, 120mL]	Acute bacterial exacerbations of chronic bronchitis (ABECB), acute bacterial otitis media, pharyngitis and tonsillitis.	ABECB/Otitis Media/Pharyngitis/Tonsillitis: 400mg qd for 10 days. Max: 400mg/day. CrCl 30-49mL/min: 4.5mg/kg or 200mg qd. CrCl 5-29mL/min: 2.25mg/kg or 100mg qd. Take 2 hrs before or at least 1 hr after a meal.	≥6 mo: Pharyngitis/Tonsillitis/Otitis Media: 9mg/kg qd for 10 days. Max: 400mg. ABECB/Otitis Media/ Pharyngitis/Tonsillitis: ≥12 yrs: 400mg qd for 10 days Max: 400mg/day. CrCl 30-49mL/min: 4.5mg/kg or 200mg qd. CrCl 5-29mL/min: 2.25mg/kg or 100mg qd. Take 2 hrs before or at least 1 hr after a meal.
Cefizox (ceftizoxime)	Inj: 1g, 2g, 10g	Treatment of lower respiratory tract, skin and skin structure, intra-abdominal, bone and joint, and urinary tract infections (UTI), gonorrhea, pelvic inflammatory disease (PID), meningitis, and septicemia.	Uncomplicated UTI: 500mg q12h IM/IV. Other Sites: 1g q8-12h IM/IV. Severe/Refractory Infections: 1-2g IM/IV q8-12h. PID: 2g IV q8h. Life Threatening Infections: 3-4g IV q8h. Uncomplicated Gonorrhea: 1g IM as single dose. Renal Impairment: LD: 500mg-1g IM/IV. Less Severe Infection: Maint: CrCl 50-79mL/min: 500 mg q8h. CrCl 5-49mL/min: 250-500mg q12h. CrCl 0-4mL/min (Dialysis): 500mg q48h or 250mg q24h. Life Threatening Infection: Maint: CrCl 50-79mL/min: 0.75-1.5g q8h. CrCl 5-49mL/min: 0.5-1g q12h. CrCl 0-4mL/min (Dialysis): 0.5-1g q48h or 0.5g q24h.	≥6 mos: 50mg/kg IM/IV q6-8h, up to 200mg/kg/day. Max: 6g/day for serious infections.

(Continued)

SYSTEMIC ANTIBIOTICS

BRAND NAME (Generic)	DOSAGE FORM/ STRENGTH	INDICATIONS	ADULT DOSE	PEDIATRIC DOSE
CEPHALOSPORINS, THIRD GENERATION *(Continued)*				
Ceptaz (ceftazidime)	Inj: 10g	Treatment of lower respiratory tract (eg, pneumonia), skin and skin structure (SSSI), bone and joint, gynecologic, CNS (eg, meningitis), intra-abdominal, and urinary tract infections (UTI), and septicemia. For use in sepsis.	Usual: 1g IM/IV q8-12h. Uncomplicated UTI: 250mg IM/IV q12h. Complicated UTI: 500mg IM/IV q8-12h. Bone and Joint Infection: 2g IV q12h. Uncomplicated Pneumonia/SSSI: 500mg-1g IM/IV q8h. Gynecological/Intra-Abdominal/Meningitis/Severe Life-Threatening Infection: 2g IV q8h. Lung Infection caused by Pseudomonas spp. in Cystic Fibrosis (normal renal function): 30-50mg/kg IV q8h. Max: 6g/day. CrCl 31-50mL/min: 1g q12h. CrCl 16-30mL/min: 1g q24h. CrCl 6-15mL/min: 500mg q48h. For severe infections (6g/day), increase renal impairment dose by 50% or increase dosing interval. Apply reduced dosage recommendations after initial 1g LD is given. Hemodialysis: Give 1g before then 1g after each hemodialysis. Intra-Peritoneal Dialysis/Continuous Ambulatory Peritoneal Dialysis: Give 1g followed by 500mg q24h.	≥12 yrs: Usual: 1g IM/IV q8-12h. Uncomplicated UTI: 250mg IM/IV q12h. Complicated UTI: 500mg IM/IV q8-12h. Bone and Joint Infection: 2g IV q12h. Uncomplicated Pneumonia/SSSI: 500mg-1g IM/IV q8h. Gynecological/Intra-Abdominal/Meningitis/Severe Life-Threatening Infection: 2g IV q8h. Lung Infection caused by Pseudomonas spp. in Cystic Fibrosis (normal renal function): 30-50mg/kg IV q8h. Max: 6g/day. CrCl 31-50mL/min: 1g q12h. CrCl 16-30mL/min: 1g q24h. CrCl 6-15mL/min: 500mg q48h. CrCl <5mL/min: 500mg q24h. For severe infections (6g/day), increase renal impairment dose by 50% or increase dosing interval. Apply reduced dosage recommendations after initial 1g LD is given. Hemodialysis: Give 1g before then 1g after each hemodialysis. Intra-Peritoneal Dialysis/Continuous Ambulatory Peritoneal Dialysis: Give 1g followed by 500mg q24h.
Claforan (cefotaxime sodium)	Inj: 500mg, 1g, 2g, 10g	Treatment of lower respiratory tract, genitourinary, gynecologic, intra-abdominal, skin and skin structure, bone and joint, and CNS infections (eg, meningitis), bacteremia, and septicemia. For surgical prophylaxis.	Gonococcal Urethritis/Cervicitis (Males/Females): 500mg single dose IM. Rectal Gonorrhea: 0.5g (females) or 1g (males) single dose IM. Uncomplicated Infections: 1g IM/IV q12h. Moderate-Severe Infections: 1-2g IM/IV q8h. Septicemia: 2g IV q6-8h. Life-Threatening Infections: 2g IV q4h. Max: 12g/day. Surgical Prophylaxis: 1g IM/IV 30-90 min before surgery. Cesarean Section: 1g IV when umbilical cord is clamped, then 1g IV at 6 and 12 hrs after 1st dose. CrCl <20mL/min/1.73 m²: Give 1/2 of usual dose.	>50kg: Use adult dose. Max: 12g/day. 1mo-12 yrs and ≤50kg: 50-180mg/kg/day IM/IV divided in 4-6 doses. 1-4 weeks: 50mg/kg IV q8h. 0-1 week: 50mg/kg IV q12h. CrCl <20mL/min/1.73 m²: Give 1/2 of usual dose.

SYSTEMIC ANTIBIOTICS

BRAND NAME (Generic)	DOSAGE FORM/ STRENGTH	INDICATIONS	ADULT DOSE	PEDIATRIC DOSE
Fortaz (ceftazidime)	Inj: 500mg, 1g, 1g/50mL, 2g, 2g/50mL, 6g	Treatment of lower respiratory tract (eg, pneumonia), skin and skin structure (SSSI), bone and joint, gynecologic, CNS (eg, meningitis), intra-abdominal, and urinary tract infections (UTI), and septicemia. For use in sepsis.	Usual: 1g IM/IV q8-12h. Uncomplicated UTI: 250mg IM/IV q12h. Complicated UTI: 500mg IM/IV q8-12h. Bone and Joint Infection: 2g IV q12h. Uncomplicated Pneumonia/SSSI: 500mg-1g IM/IV q8h. Gynecological/Intra-Abdominal/Meningitis/Severe Life-Threatening Infection: 2g IV q8h. Lung Infection Caused by Pseudomonas spp. in Cystic Fibrosis (Normal Renal Function): 30-50mg/kg IV q8h. Max: 6g/day. CrCl 31-50mL/min: 1g q12h. CrCl 16-30mL/min: 1g q24h. CrCl 6-15mL/min: 500mg q24h. CrCl <5mL/min: 500mg q48h. For severe renal impairment dose (6g/day), increase dosing interval. Apply reduced dosage recommendations after initial 1g LD is given Hemodialysis: Give 1g before then 1g after each hemodialysis. Intra-Peritoneal Dialysis/Continuous Ambulatory Peritoneal Dialysis: Give 1g followed by 500mg q24h, or add to fluid at 250mg/2L.	1 mo-12 yrs: 30-50mg/kg IV q8h. Max: 6g/day. Neonates (0-4 weeks): 30mg/kg IV q12h. Higher doses for cystic fibrosis or meningitis. CrCl 31-50 mL/min: 1g q12h. CrCl 16-30mL/min: 1g q24h. CrCl 6-15mL/min: 500mg q24h. CrCl <5mL/min: 500mg q48h. For severe infections (6g/day), increase renal impairment dose by 50% or increase dosing interval. Apply reduced dosage recommendations after initial 1g LD is given. Hemodialysis: Give 1g before then 1g after each hemodialysis. Intra-Peritoneal Dialysis/Continuous Ambulatory Peritoneal Dialysis: Give 1g followed by 500mg q24h, or add to fluid at 250mg/2L.
Omnicef (cefdinir)	Cap: 300mg; Sus: 125mg/5mL, 250mg/5mL [60mL, 100mL]	Community acquired pneumonia (CAP), acute exacerbations of chronic bronchitis (AECB), acute maxillary sinusitis, pharyngitis/tonsillitis, uncomplicated skin and structure infections (SSSI), and acute bacterial otitis media.	(Cap) SSSI/CAP: 300mg q12h for 10 days. AECB/Pharyngitis/Tonsillitis: 300mg q12h for 5-10 days or 600mg q24h for 10 days. Sinusitis: 300mg q12h or 600mg q24h for 10 days. CrCl <30mL/min: 300mg qd.	(Sus) 6 mo-12 yrs: Otitis Media/Pharyngitis/Tonsillitis: 7mg/kg q12h for 5-10 days or 14mg/kg q24h for 10 days. Sinusitis: 7mg/kg q12h or 14mg/kg q24h for 10 days. SSSI: 7mg/kg q12h for 10 days. (Cap) ≥13 yrs: CAP/SSSI: 300mg q12h for 10 days. AECB/Pharyngitis/Tonsillitis: 300mg q12h for 5-10 days or 600mg q24h for 10 days. Sinusitis: 300mg q12h or 600mg q24h for 10 days. CrCl <30mL/min/1.73m²: 7mg/kg qd. Max: 300mg qd.
Rocephin (ceftriaxone sodium)	Inj: 250mg, 500mg, 1g, 2g, 10g	Treatment of lower respiratory tract infections, skin and skin structure infections, bone and joint infections, intra-abdominal infections, acute otitis media, uncomplicated gonorrhea, pelvic inflammatory disease, UTI, septicemia, and meningitis. For surgical prophylaxis.	Usual: 1-2g/day IV/IM given qd-bid. Max: 4g/day. Gonorrhea: 250mg IM single dose. Surgical Prophylaxis: 1g IV 1/2-2 hrs before surgery.	Skin Infections: 50-75mg/kg/day IV/IM given qd-bid. Max: 2g/day. Otitis Media: 50mg/kg (up to 1g) IM single dose. Serious Infections: 50-75mg/kg/day IM/IV given q12h. Max: 2g/day. Meningitis: Initial: 100mg/kg (up to 4g), then 100mg/kg/day given qd-bid for 7-14 days. Max: 4g/day.

(Continued)

SYSTEMIC ANTIBIOTICS

BRAND NAME (Generic)	DOSAGE FORM/ STRENGTH	INDICATIONS	ADULT DOSE	PEDIATRIC DOSE
CEPHALOSPORINS, THIRD GENERATION *(Continued)*				
Spectracef (cefditoren pivoxil)	Tab: 200mg	Treatment of acute bacterial exacerbations of chronic bronchitis (ABECB), pharyngitis/tonsillitis, community acquired pneumonia (CAP), and uncomplicated skin and skin-structure infections (SSSI).	ABECB: 400mg bid for 10 days. Pharyngitis/Tonsillitis/SSSI: 200mg bid for 10 days. CAP: 400mg bid for 14 days. CrCl 30-49mL/min: 200mg bid. CrCl<30mL/min: 200mg qd. Take with meals.	≥12 yrs: ABECB: 400mg bid for 10 days. Pharyngitis/Tonsillitis/SSSI: 200mg bid for 10 days. CAP: 400mg bid for 14 days. CrCl 30-49mL/min: 200mg bid. CrCl<30mL/min: 200mg qd. Take with meals.
Suprax (cefixime)	Sus: 100mg/5mL [50mL, 75mL, 100mL]	Otitis media, pharyngitis, tonsillitis, acute bronchitis, acute exacerbation of chronic bronchitis, uncomplicated UTIs, and cervical/urethral gonorrhea caused by susceptible strains.	Usual: 400mg qd. Gonorrhea: 400mg single dose. CrCl 21-60mL/min/Hemodialysis: Give 75% of standard dose. CrCl <20mL/min/CAPD: Give 50% of standard dose.	>12 yrs or >50kg: (Tab/Sus) Usual: 400mg qd. ≥6 mos: (Sus) 8mg/kg qd or 4mg/kg bid. Treat for at least 10 days with *S. pyogenes*. CrCl 21-60mL/min/Hemodialysis: Give 75% of standard dose. CrCl <20mL/min/CAPD: Give 50% of standard dose.
Tazicef (ceftazidime)	Inj: 1g, 2g, 6g	Treatment of lower respiratory tract (eg, pneumonia), skin and skin structure (SSSI), bone and joint, gynecologic, CNS (eg, meningitis), intra-abdominal, and urinary tract infections (UTI), and septicemia. For use in sepsis.	Usual: 1g IM/IV q8-12h. Uncomplicated UTI: 250mg IM/IV q12h. Complicated UTI: 500mg IM/IV q8-12h. Bone and Joint Infection: 2g IV q12h. Uncomplicated Pneumonia/SSSI: 500mg-1g IM/IV q8h. Gynecological/Intra-Abdominal/Meningitis/Severe Life-Threatening Infection: 2g IV q8h. Lung Infection caused by Pseudomonas in Cystic Fibrosis (normal renal function): 30-50mg/kg IV q8h. Max: 6g/day. Renal Impairment: CrCl 31-50mL/min: 1g q12h. CrCl 16-30mL/min: 1g q24h. CrCl 6-15mL/min: 500mg q24h. CrCl <5mL/min: 500mg q48h. For severe infections (6g/day), increase renal impairment dose by 50% or increase dosing interval. Apply reduced dosage recommendations after initial 1g LD is given. Hemodialysis: Give 1g before and 1g after each hemodialysis. Intra-Peritoneal Dialysis/Continuous Ambulatory Peritoneal Dialysis: Give 1g followed by 500mg q24h, or add to fluid at 250mg/2L.	Neonates (0-4 weeks): 30mg/kg IV q12h. 1 mo-12 yrs: 30-50mg/kg IV q8h. Max: 6g/day. Higher doses for patients with cystic fibrosis or when treating meningitis. Renal Impairment: CrCl 31-50mL/min: 1g q12h. CrCl 16-30mL/min: 1g q24h. CrCl 6-15mL/min: 500mg q24h. CrCl <5mL/min: 500mg q48h. For severe infections (6g/day), increase renal impairment dose by 50% or increase dosing interval. Apply reduced dosage recommendations after initial 1g LD is given. Hemodialysis: Give 1g before and 1g after each hemodialysis. Intra-Peritoneal Dialysis/Continuous Ambulatory Peritoneal Dialysis: Give 1g followed by 500mg q24h, or add fluid at 250mg/2L.

SYSTEMIC ANTIBIOTICS

BRAND NAME (Generic)	DOSAGE FORM/ STRENGTH	INDICATIONS	ADULT DOSE	PEDIATRIC DOSE
Tazidime (ceftazidime)	Inj: 1g, 2g, 6g	Treatment of lower respiratory tract (eg, pneumonia), skin and skin structure (SSSI), bone and joint, gynecologic, CNS (eg, meningitis), intra-abdominal, and urinary tract infections (UTI), and septicemia. For use in sepsis.	Usual: 1g IM/IV Q8-12h. Uncomplicated UTI: 250mg IM/IV q12h. Complicated UTI: 500mg IM/IV q8-12h. Bone and Joint Infection: 2g IV q12h. Uncomplicated Pneumonia/Skin and Skin Structure Infection: 500mg-1g IM/IV q8h. Gynecological/Intra-Abdominal/Meningitis/Severe Life-Threatening Infection: 2g IV q8h. Lung Infection caused by Pseudomonas spp. in Cystic Fibrosis (normal renal function): 30-50mg/kg IV q8h. Max: 6g/day. Renal impairment: CrCl 31-50mL/min: 1g q12h. CrCl 16-30mL/min: 1g q24h. CrCl 6-15mL/min: 500mg q24h. CrCl <5mL/min: 500mg q48h. For severe infections (6g/day), increase renal impairment dose by 50% or increase dosing interval. Apply reduced dosage recommendations after initial 1g LD is given. Hemodialysis: Give 1g before then 1g after each hemodialysis. Intra-Peritoneal Dialysis/Continuous Ambulatory Peritoneal Dialysis: Give 1g followed by 500mg q24h, or add to fluid at 250mg/2L.	Neonates (0-4 weeks): 30mg/kg IV q12h. 1 mo-12 yrs: 30-50mg/kg IV q8h. Max: 6g/day. Higher doses for cystic fibrosis and meningitis. Renal Impairment: CrCl 31-50mL/min: 1g q12h. CrCl 16-30mL/min: 1g q24h. CrCl 6-15mL/min: 500mg q24h. CrCl <5mL/min: 500mg q48h. For severe infections (6g/day), increase renal impairment dose by 50% or increase dosing interval. Apply reduced dosage recommendations after initial 1g LD is given. Hemodialysis: Give 1g before then 1g after each hemodialysis. Intra-Peritoneal Dialysis/Continuous Ambulatory Peritoneal Dialysis: Give 1g followed by 500mg q24h, or add to fluid at 250mg/2L.
Vantin (cefpodoxime proxetil)	Sus: 50mg/5mL [50mL, 100mL], 100mg/5mL [50mL, 75mL, 100mL]; Tab: 100mg, 200mg	Acute otitis media, pharyngitis/tonsillitis, community acquired pneumonia (CAP), acute bacterial exacerbation of chronic bronchitis (ABECB), acute uncomplicated urethral and cervical gonorrhea, acute uncomplicated ano-rectal infections in women, uncomplicated skin and skin structure infections (SSSI), acute maxillary sinusitis, uncomplicated urinary tract infections (UTI).	Take tabs with food. Pharyngitis/Tonsillitis: 100mg q12h for 5-10 days. CAP: 200mg q12h for 14 days. ABECB: 200mg q12h for 10 days. Uncomplicated Gonorrhea (Men and Women)/Rectal Gonococcal Infections (women): 200mg single dose. SSSI: 400mg q12h for 7-14 days. Sinusitis: 200mg q12h for 10 days. UTI: 100mg q12h for 7 days. CrCl<30mL/min: Increase interval to q24h. Hemodialysis: Dose 3 times weekly after dialysis.	≥12 yrs: Take tabs with food. Pharyngitis/Tonsillitis: 100mg q12h for 5-10 days. CAP: 200mg q12h for 14 days. ABECB: 200mg q12h for 10 days. Uncomplicated Gonorrhea (men and women)/Rectal Gonococcal Infections (women): 200mg single dose. SSSI: 400mg q12h for 7-14 days. Sinusitis: 200mg q12h for 10 days. UTI: 100mg q12h for 7 days. 2 mos-11 yrs: Otitis Media: 5mg/kg q12h for 5 days. Max: 200mg/dose. Pharyngitis/Tonsillitis: 5mg/kg q12h for 5-10 days. Max: 100mg/dose. Sinusitis: 5mg/kg q12h for 10 days. Max: 200mg/dose. CrCl<30mL/min: Increase interval to q24h. Hemodialysis: Dose 3 times weekly after dialysis.

(Continued)

SYSTEMIC ANTIBIOTICS

BRAND NAME (Generic)	DOSAGE FORM/ STRENGTH	INDICATIONS	ADULT DOSE	PEDIATRIC DOSE
CEPHALOSPORIN, FOURTH GENERATION				
Maxipime (cefepime HCl)	Inj: 500mg, 1g, 2g	Treatment of uncomplicated/complicated urinary tract (UTI), uncomplicated skin and skin structure (SSSI), and complicated intra-abdominal infections, and pneumonia. Emperic therapy for febrile neutropenia.	Moderate-Severe Pneumonia: 1-2g IV q12h for 10 days. Febrile Neutropenia Emperic Therapy: 2g IV q8h for 7 days or until neutropenia resolved. Mild-Moderate UTI: 0.5-1g IM/IV q12h for 7-10 days. Severe UTI/Moderate-Severe SSSI: 2g IV q12h for 10 days. Complicated Intra-Abdominal Infections: 2g IV q12h for 7-10 days. CrCl<60mL/min: Initial: Same dose as normal renal function. Maint: Refer to prescribing information for dose-adjustment.	2 months-16 yrs: ≤40kg: UTI/SSSI/Pneumonia: 50mg/kg IV q12h. Febrile Neutropenia: 50mg/kg IV q8h. Max: Do not exceed adult dose. CrCl ≤60mL/min: Initial: Same dose as normal renal function. Maint: Refer to prescribing information for dose adjustment.
FLUOROQUINOLONES				
Avelox (moxifloxacin HCl)	Inj: 400mg/250mL; Tab: 400mg [ABC pack, 5 tabs]	Acute bacterial sinusitis, acute bacterial exacerbation of chronic bronchitis (ABECB), uncomplicated skin and skin structure infections (SSSI), complicated skin and skin structure infections (cSSSI), complicated intra-abdominal infections (cIAI), and community acquired pneumonia (CAP), including multi-drug resistant *S.pneumoniae*.	≥18 yrs: Sinusitis: 400mg PO/IV q24h for 10 days. ABECB: 400mg PO/IV q24h for 5 days. SSSI: 400mg PO/IV q24h for 7 days. cSSSI: 400mg PO/IV q24h for 7-21 days. cIAI: 400mg IV q24h for 5-14 days. CAP: 400mg PO/IV q24h for 7-14 days.	

SYSTEMIC ANTIBIOTICS

BRAND NAME (Generic)	DOSAGE FORM/ STRENGTH	INDICATIONS	ADULT DOSE	PEDIATRIC DOSE
Cipro (ciprofloxacin HCl)	Sus: 250mg/5mL, 500mg/5mL [100mL]; Tab: 250mg, 500mg, 750mg	Treatment of lower respiratory tract (LRTI), complicated intra-abdominal, skin and skin structure (SSSI), bone and joint, and urinary tract infections (UTI), acute exacerbations of chronic bronchitis, acute sinusitis, acute uncomplicated cystitis in females, chronic bacterial prostatitis, infectious diarrhea, typhoid fever, post-exposure inhalational anthrax, uncomplicated cervical and urethral gonorrhea, complicated UTI and pyelonephritis in pediatrics.	≥18 yrs: Acute Sinusitis/Typhoid Fever: 500mg q12h for 10 days. LRTI/SSSI: Mild-Moderate: 500mg q12h for 7-14 days. Severe/Complicated: 750mg q12h for 7-14 days. Cystitis/Acute Uncomplicated UTI: 250mg q12h for 3 days. Mild-Moderate UTI: 250mg q12h for 7-14 days. Severe/Complicated UTI: 500mg q12h for 7-14 days. Chronic Bacterial Prostatitis: 500mg q12h for 28 days. Intra-Abdominal: 500mg q12h (w/ metronidazole) for 7-14 days. Bone and Joint: Mild-Moderate: 500mg q12h for ≥4-6 weeks. Severe/Complicated: 750mg q12h for ≥4-6 weeks. Infectious Diarrhea: 500mg q12h for 5-7 days. Uncomplicated Urethral/Cervical Gonococcal: 250mg single dose. Inhalational Anthrax: 500mg q12h for 60 days. CrCl 30-50mL/min: 250-500mg q12h. CrCl 5-29mL/min: 250-500mg q18h. Hemodialysis/Peritoneal Dialysis: 250-500mg q24h (after dialysis). Administer at least 2 hrs before or 6 hrs after magnesium or aluminum containing antacids, sucralfate, Videx (didanosine) chewable/buffered tablets or pediatric powder, or other products containing calcium, iron or zinc.	<18 yrs: Inhalational Anthrax: 15mg/kg q12h for 60 days. Max: 500mg/dose. 1-17 yrs: Complicated UTI/Pyelonephritis: 10-20mg/kg q12h for 10-21 days. Max: 750mg/dose.

(Continued)

SYSTEMIC ANTIBIOTICS

BRAND NAME (Generic)	DOSAGE FORM/ STRENGTH	INDICATIONS	ADULT DOSE	PEDIATRIC DOSE
FLUOROQUINOLONES *(Continued)*				
Cipro IV (ciprofloxacin)	Inj: 10mg/mL, 200mg/100mL, 400mg/200mL	Treatment of skin and skin structure (SSSI), bone and joint, complicated intra-abdominal infections, lower respiratory (LRTI), and urinary tract infections (UTI), nosocomial pneumonia, acute sinusitis, chronic bacterial prostatitis, post-exposure inhalational anthrax, empirical therapy for febrile neutropenia, complicated UTI and pyelonephritis in pediatrics	≥18 yrs: IV: UTI: Mild-Moderate: 200mg q12h for 7-14 days. Complicated/Severe: 400mg q12h for 7-14 days. LRTI/SSSI: Mild-Moderate: 400mg q12h for 7-14 days. Complicated/Severe: 400mg q8h for 7-14 days. Bone and Joint: Mild-Moderate: 400mg q12h for ≥4-6 weeks. Complicated/Severe: 400mg q8h for ≥4-6 weeks. Nosocomial Pneumonia: 400mg q8h for 10-14 days. Complicated Intra-Abdominal: 400mg q12h (w/metronidazole) for 7-14 days. Acute Sinusitis: 400mg q12h for 10 days. Chronic Bacterial Prostatitis: 400mg q12h for 28 days. Febrile Neutropenia: 400mg q8h (w/piperacillin 50mg/kg q4h) for 7-14 days. Max: 24g/day. Inhalational Anthrax: 400mg q12h for 60 days. Administer over 60 min. CrCl 5-29mL/min: 200-400mg q18-24h.	<18 yrs: Inhalational Anthrax: 10mg/kg q12h for 60 days. Max: 400mg/dose, 800mg/day. 1-17 yrs: Complicated UTI/Pyleonephritis: 6-10mg/kg q8h for 10-21 days. Max: 400mg/dose.
Cipro XR (ciprofloxacin)	Tab, Extended-Release: 500mg, 1000mg	Uncomplicated (acute cystitis) and complicated urinary tract infections (UTI), and acute uncomplicated pyelonephritis due to *E.coli*.	≥18 yrs: Uncomplicated UTI: 500mg qd for 3 days. Complicated UTI: 1000mg qd for 7-14 days. CrCl <30mL/min: 500 mg qd. Acute Uncomplicated Pyelonephritis: 1000mg qd for 7-14 days. CrCl <30mL/min: 500mg qd. Take with fluids. Administer at least 2 hrs before or 6 hrs after magnesium or aluminum containing antacids, sucralfate, Videx (didanosine) chewable/buffered tablets or pediatric powder, metal cations (eg, iron), multivitamins with zinc. Avoid concomitant administration with dairy products alone, or with calcium-fortified products. Space concomitant calcium intake (>800mg) by at least 2 hrs. Do not split, crush, or chew. Swallow tab whole. Dialysis: Give after procedure is completed.	

SYSTEMIC ANTIBIOTICS

BRAND NAME (Generic)	DOSAGE FORM/ STRENGTH	INDICATIONS	ADULT DOSE	PEDIATRIC DOSE
Factive (gemifloxacin mesylate)	Tab: 320mg	Treatment of community-acquired pneumonia (CAP), including multi-drug resistant *Streptococcus pneumoniae* (MDRSP), and acute bacterial exacerbation of chronic bronchitis (ABECB).	≥18 yrs: ABECB: 320mg qd for 5 days. CAP: 320mg qd for 5 days *S.pneumoniae, H.influenzae, M. pneumoniae,* or *C.pneumoniae* or 7 days (MDRSP, K.pneumoniae,* or *M.catarrhalis).* Renal Impairment: CrCl ≤40mL/min or Dialysis: 160mg qd. Take with fluids.	
Floxin (ofloxacin)	Tab: 200mg, 300mg, 400mg	Treatment of acute urinary tract (UTI) and uncomplicated skin and skin structure infection (SSSI), acute bacterial exacerbation of chronic bronchitis (ABECB), community acquired pneumonia (CAP), acute uncomplicated urethral and cervical gonorrhea, nongonococcal urethritis and cervicitis, mixed infections of the urethra and cervix, acute pelvic inflammatory disease (PID), uncomplicated cystitis, prostatitis.	≥18 yrs: ABECB/CAP/SSSI: 400mg q12h for 10 days. Cervicitis/Urethritis: 300mg q12h for 7 days. Gonorrhea: 400mg single dose. PID: 400mg q12h for 10-14 days. Uncomplicated Cystitis: 200mg q12h for 3 days *(E.coli* or *K.pneumoniae)* or 7 days (other pathogens). Complicated UTI: 200mg q12h for 10 days. Prostatitis: *(E.coli)* 300mg q12h for 6 weeks. CrCl 20-50mL/min: Dose q24h. CrCl <20mL/min: After regular initial dose, give 50% of normal dose q24h. Severe Hepatic Impairment: Max. 400mg/day.	
Floxin IV (ofloxacin)	Inj: 4mg/mL, 40mg/mL	Treatment of acute bacterial exacerbation of chronic bronchitis, community-acquired pneumonia, uncomplicated skin and skin structure infections, acute uncomplicated urethral and cervical gonorrhea, nongonococcal urethritis and cervicitis, urethral and cervical infections, acute pelvic inflammatory disease (PID), uncomplicated cystitis, urinary tract infections (UTI), prostatitis.	Lower Respiratory Tract Infection/Skin Structure Infections: 400mg q12h for 10 days. Cervicitis/Urethritis: 300mg q12h for 7 days. Gonorrhea: 400mg single dose. PID: 400mg q12h for 10-14 days. Uncomplicated Cystitis: 200mg q12h for 3 days. Other Uncomplicated UTIs: 200mg q12h for 7 days. Complicated UTI: 200mg q12h for 10 days. Prostatitis: 300mg q12h for 6 weeks. Renal Impairment: CrCl 20-50mL/min: increase dosing interval to 24 hrs. CrCl<20mL/min: give normal initial dose then 50% of normal dose and increase dosing interval to 24 hrs. Severe Hepatic Impairment: Max. 400mg qdy. Switch to oral form when appropriate. Max. 10 days IV.	

(Continued)

SYSTEMIC ANTIBIOTICS

FLUOROQUINOLONES (Continued)

BRAND NAME (Generic)	DOSAGE FORM/ STRENGTH	INDICATIONS	ADULT DOSE	PEDIATRIC DOSE
Levaquin (levofloxacin)	Inj: 5mg/mL, 25mg/mL; Sol: 25mg/mL; Tab: 250mg, 500mg, 750mg [Leva-pak, 5]	Uncomplicated and complicated skin and skin structure (SSSI), and urinary tract infections (UTI), acute bacterial sinusitis, acute bacterial exacerbation of chronic bronchitis (ABECB), community acquired pneumonia (CAP), including multi-drug resistant *Streptococcus pneumoniae*, nosocomial pneumonia, chronic bacterial prostatitis (CBP), and acute pyelonephritis caused by susceptible strains of microorganisms. Prevention of inhalational anthrax following exposure to *Bacillus anthracis*.	≥18 yrs: IV/PO: ABECB: 500mg qd for 7 days. CAP: 500mg qd for 7-14 days or 750mg qd for 5 days.Sinusitis: 500mg qd for 10-14 days or 750mg qd for 5 days. CBP: 500mg qd for 28 days. Uncomplicated SSSI: 500mg qd for 7-10 days. Complicated SSSI/Nosocomial Pneumonia: 750mg qd for 7-14 days. Inhalational Anthrax: 500mg qd for 60 days.Complicated SSSI/Nosocomial Pneumonia/CAP/Sinusitis: CrCl 20-49mL/min: 750mg, then 750mgq48h. CrCl 10-19mL/min/ Hemodialysis/CAPD: 750mg, then 500mg q48h. ABECB/CAP/Sinusitis/Uncomplicated SSSI/CBP/ Inhalational Anthrax:CrCl 20-49mL/min: 500mg, then 250mg q24h. CrCl 10-19mL/min/Hemodialysis/ CAPD: 500mg,then 250mg q48h. Complicated UTI/ Acute Pyelonephritis: 250mg qd for 10 days. CrCl 10-19mL/min: 250mg, then 250mg q48h. Uncomplicated UTI: 250mg qd for 3 days. Take oral solution 1 hr before or 2 hrs after eating.	
Maxaquin (lomefloxacin HCl)	Tab: 400mg	Treatment of acute bacterial exacerbation of chronic bronchitis (ABECB) and uncomplicated/complicated urinary tract infections (UTI). Preoperatively for the prevention of infections from transrectal prostate biopsy (TRPB) and in transurethral surgical procedures (TUSP).	≥18 yrs: ABECB: 400mg qd for 10 days. Uncomplicated Cystitis: 400mg qd for 3 days *E.coli* or 10 days *K.pneumoniae*, *P.mirabilis*, or *S.saprophyticus*. Complicated UTI: 400mg qd for 14 days. Hemodialysis/CrCl>10 to <40mL/min: LD: 400mg. Maint: 200mg qd. Preoperative Prevention: TRPB: 400mg single dose 1-6 hrs before procedure. TUSP: 400mg single dose 2-6 hrs before procedure.	
Proquin XR (ciprofloxacin HCl)	Tab, Extended-Release: 500mg	Treatment of uncomplicated urinary tract infections (acute cystitis) caused by *E.coli* and *K.pneumoniae*.	500mg qd with pm meal for 3 days. Administer at least 4 hrs before or 2 hrs after magnesium or aluminum containing antacids, sucralfate, Videx (didanosine) chewable/buffered tablets of pediatric powder, metal cations (eg, iron), multivitamins with zinc. Do not split, crush, or chew. Swallow tab whole.	

SYSTEMIC ANTIBIOTICS

BRAND NAME (Generic)	DOSAGE FORM/ STRENGTH	INDICATIONS	ADULT DOSE	PEDIATRIC DOSE
MACROLIDES				
Biaxin (clarithromycin)	Sus: 125mg/5mL, 250mg/5mL [50mL, 100mL]; Tab: 250mg, 500mg	Adults: Pharyngitis/tonsillitis, acute maxillary sinusitis, acute bacterial exacerbation of chronic bronchitis (ABECB), community acquired pneumonia (CAP), uncomplicated skin and skin structure infections (SSSI), disseminated mycobacterial infections, combination therapy for *H.pylori* infection with duodenal ulcers. MAC prophylaxis in advanced HIV. Pediatrics: Pharyngitis/tonsillitis, CAP, acute maxillary sinusitis, acute otitis media, uncomplicated SSSI, disseminated mycobacterial infections. MAC prophylaxis in advanced HIV.	Pharyngitis/Tonsillitis: 250mg q12h for 10 days. Sinusitis: 500mg q12h for 14 days. ABECB: 250-500mg q12h for 7-14 days. SSSI/CAP: 250mg q12h for 7-14 days. MAC Prophylaxis/Treatment: 500mg bid. *H.pylori:* Triple Therapy: 500mg + amoxicillin 1g + omeprazole 20mg, all q12h for 10 days; or 500mg + amoxicillin 1g + lansoprazole 30mg, all q12h for 10-14 days. Give additional omeprazole 20mg qd for 18 days with active ulcer. Dual Therapy: 500mg q8h + omeprazole 40mg qd for 14 days (give additional omeprazole 20mg qd for 14 days with active ulcer); or 500mg q8h or q12h + ranitidine bismuth citrate 400mg q12h for 14 days (give additional ranitidine bismuth citrate 400mg bid for 14 days with active ulcer). Avoid Biaxin and ranitidine bismuth citrate combination with CrCl<25mL/min.	≥6 mo: Usual: 7.5mg/kg q12h for 10 days. MAC Prophylaxis/Treatment: ≥20 mo: 7.5mg/kg bid, up to 500mg bid. CrCl <30mL/min: Give 50% dose or double interval.
Biaxin XL (clarithromycin)	Tab, Extended-Release: 500mg [PAC 14 tabs]	Treatment of acute maxillary sinusitis, community acquired pneumonia (CAP), and acute bacterial exacerbation of chronic bronchitis (ABECB).	Sinusitis: 1000mg qd for 14 days. ABECB/CAP: 1000mg qd for 7 days. CrCl <30mL/min: Give 50% dose or double interval. Take with food.	
E.E.S. (erythromycin ethylsuccinate)	Sus: 200mg/5mL, 400mg/5mL (100mL, 480mL]; Tab: 400mg	Mild to moderate upper and lower respiratory tract and skin and skin structure infections, listeriosis, pertussis, diphtheria, erythrasma, intestinal amebiasis, acute pelvic inflammatory disease (PID) *N.gonorrhea*, primary syphilis in PCN allergy, Legionnaires' disease, chlamydial infections (eg, newborn conjunctivitis urethral, endocervical, or rectal, etc), and nongonococcal urethritis. Prophylaxis of endocarditis or rheumatic fever.	Usual: 1600mg/day given q6h, q8h or q12h. Max: 4g/day. Treat strep infections for 10 days. Streptococcal Infection Prophylaxis with Rheumatic Heart Disease: 400mg bid. Urethritis *C.trachomatis* or *U. urealyticum*: 800mg tid for 7 days. Primary Syphilis: 48-64g in divided doses over 10-15 days. Intestinal Amebiasis: 400mg qid for 10-14 days. Pertussis: 40-50mg/kg/day in divided doses for 5-14 days. Legionnaires' Disease: 1.6-4g/day in divided doses.	Usual: 30-50mg/kg/day in divided doses q6h, q8h or q12h. Double dose for more severe infections. Treat strep infections for 10 days. Intestinal Amebiasis: 30-50mg/kg/day in divided doses for 10-14 days. Pertussis: 40-50mg/kg/day in divided doses for 5-14 days.

(Continued)

SYSTEMIC ANTIBIOTICS

MACROLIDES (Continued)

BRAND NAME (Generic)	DOSAGE FORM/ STRENGTH	INDICATIONS	ADULT DOSE	PEDIATRIC DOSE
ERYC (erythromycin)	Cap, Delayed-Release: 250mg	Mild to moderate upper and lower respiratory tract and skin and soft tissue infections, pertussis, diphtheria, erythrasma, intestinal amebiasis, acute pelvic inflammatory disease (PID) (*N. gonorrhea*), *Listeria monocytogenes* infections, primary syphilis in PCN allergy, Legionnaires' disease, chlamydial infections (eg, newborn conjunctivitis, urethral, endocervical, or rectal, etc), and nongonococcal urethritis. Prophylaxis of endocarditis or rheumatic fever in PCN allergy.	Usual: 250mg q6h or 500mg q12h. Max: 4g/day. Treat strep infections for 10 days. Chlamydial Urogenital Infection During Pregnancy: 500mg qid for at least 7 days or 250mg qid for 14 days. Urethral/Endocervical/Rectal Chlamydial Infections: 500mg qid for 7 days. Primary Syphilis: 30-40g in divided doses for 10-15 days. Acute PID: 500mg (erythromycin lactobionate) IV q6h for 3 days, then 250mg PO q6h for 7 days. Streptococcal Infection Long-Term Prophylaxis of Rheumatic Fever: 250mg bid. Intestinal Amebiasis: 250mg qid for 10-14 days. Pertussis: 40-50mg/kg/day in divided doses for 5-14 days. Legionnaires' Disease: 1-4g/day in divided doses. Bacterial Endocarditis Prophylaxis: 1g 1 hr before procedure, then 500mg 6 hrs later.	Usual: 30-50mg/kg/day in divided doses without food. Max: 4g/day. Severe Infections: Double dose up to 4g/day. Treat strep infections for 10 days. Intestinal Amebiasis: 30-50mg/kg/day in divided doses for 10-14 days. Bacterial Endocarditis Prophylaxis: 20mg/kg 1 hr before procedure, then 10mg/kg 6 hrs later.
EryPed (erythromycin ethylsuccinate)	Sus: 100mg/2.5mL [50mL], 200mg/5mL, 400mg/5mL [5mL, 100mL, 200mL]; Tab, Chewable: 200mg	Treatment of mild to moderate upper and lower respiratory tract and skin and skin structure infections, listeriosis, pertussis, diphtheria, erythrasma, intestinal amebiasis, acute pelvic inflammatory disease (PID) *N.gonorrhea*, primary syphilis in PCN allergy, Legionnaires' disease, chlamydial infections (eg, newborn conjunctivitis, urethral, endocervical, or rectal, etc), and nongonococcal urethritis. Prophylaxis of endocarditis or rheumatic fever.	Usual: 1600mg/day given q6h, q8h or q12h. Max: 4g/day. Treat strep infections for 10 days. Streptococcal Infection Prophylaxis with Rheumatic Heart Disease: 400mg bid. Urethritis *C.trachomatis* or *U. urealyticum*: 800mg tid for 7 days. Primary Syphilis:48-64g in divided doses over 10-15 days. Intestinal Amebiasis: 400mg qid for 10-14 days. Pertussis:40-50mg/kg/day in divided doses for 5-14 days. Legionnaires' Disease: 1.6-4g/day in divided doses.	Usual: 30-50mg/kg/day in divided doses q6h, q8h or q12h. Double dose for more severe infections. Treat strep infections for 10 days. Intestinal Amebiasis: 30-50mg/kg/day in divided doses for 10-14 days. Pertussis: 40-50mg/kg/day in divided doses for 5-14 days.

SYSTEMIC ANTIBIOTICS

BRAND NAME (Generic)	DOSAGE FORM/ STRENGTH	INDICATIONS	ADULT DOSE	PEDIATRIC DOSE
Ery-Tab (erythromycin)	Tab, Delayed-Release: 250mg, 333mg, 500mg	Mild to moderate upper and lower respiratory tract and skin and skin structure infections, listeriosis, pertussis, diphtheria, erythrasma, intestinal amebiasis, acute pelvic inflammatory disease (PID) (*N.gonorrhea*), primary syphilis in PCN allergy, Legionnaires' disease, chlamydial infections (eg, newborn conjunctivitis urethral, endocervical, rectal, etc), and nongonococcal urethritis. Prophylaxis of rheumatic fever.	Usual: 250mg qid, 333mg q8h or 500mg q12h without food. Max: 4g/day. Do not take bid when dose is ≥1g/day. Chlamydial Urogenital Infection During Pregnancy: 500mg qid or 666mg q8h for 7 days, or 500mg q 12h, 333mg q8h or 250mg qid for 14 days. Urethral/Endocervical/Rectal Chlamydial Infections and Nongonococcal Urethritis: 500mg qid or 666mg q8h for at least 7 days. Primary Syphilis: 30-40g in divided doses for 10-15 days. Acute PID: 500mg (erythromycin lactobionate) IV q6h for 3 days, then 500mg PO q12h or 333mg q8h for 7 days. Streptococcal Infection Long-Term Prophylaxis of Rheumatic Fever: 250mg bid. Intestinal Amebiasis: 500mg q12h, 333mg q8h or 250mg q6h for 10-14 days. Pertussis: 40-50mg/kg/day in divided doses for 5-14 days. Legionnaires' Disease: 1-4g/day in divided doses.	Usual: 30-50mg/kg/day in divided doses without food. Severe Infections: Double dose up to 4g/day. Treat strep infections for 10 days. Chlamydial Conjunctivitis of Newborns and Chlamydial Pneumonia in Infancy: 12.5mg/kg qid for 2 weeks and 3 weeks, respectively. Intestinal Amebiasis: 30-50mg/kg/day in divided doses for 10-14 days. Long-Term Prophylaxis of Rheumatic Fever: 250mg bid. Intestinal Amebiasis: 30-50mg/kg/day in divided doses for 10-14 days. Pertussis: 40-50mg/kg/day in divided doses. Legionnaire's Disease: 1-4g/day in divided doses.
Erythrocin (erythromycin stearate)	Tab: 250mg, 500mg	Mild to moderate upper and lower respiratory tract, and skin and skin structure infections, listeriosis, pertussis, diphtheria, erythrasma, intestinal amebiasis, acute pelvic inflammatory disease (PID) (gonorrhea), primary syphilis in PCN allergy, Legionnaires' disease, chlamydial infections (eg, newborn conjunctivitis urethral, endocervical, or rectal, etc), and nongonococcal urethritis. Prophylaxis of rheumatic fever.	Usual: 250mg q6h or 500mg q12h without food. Max: 4g/day. Treat strep infections for 10 days. Streptococcal Infection Prophylaxis of Rheumatic Fever: 250mg bid. Chlamydial Urogenital Infection During Pregnancy: 500mg qid for 7 days or 250mg qid for 14 days. Urethral/Endocervical/Rectal Chlamydial Infections and Nongonococcal Urethritis: 500mg qid for at least 7 days. Primary Syphilis: 30-40g in divided doses over 10-15 days. Acute PID: 500mg (erythromycin lactobionate) IV q6h for 3 days, then 500mg PO q12h for 7 days. Intestinal Amebiasis: 250mg qid for 10-14 days. Pertussis: 40-50mg/kg/day in divided doses for 5-14 days. Legionnaires' Disease: 1-4g/day in divided doses.	Usual: 30-50mg/kg/day in divided doses without food. Severe Infections: Double dose up to 4g/day. Treat strep infections for 10 days. Streptococcal Infection Prophylaxis of Rheumatic Fever: 250mg bid. Chlamydial Conjunctivitis of Newborns/Chlamydial Pneumonia in Infancy: 12.5mg/kg qid for 2 weeks and 3 weeks, respectively. Intestinal Amebiasis: 30-50mg/kg/day in divided doses for 10-14 days. Pertussis: 40-50mg/kg/day in divided doses for 5-14 days.

(Continued)

SYSTEMIC ANTIBIOTICS

MACROLIDES (Continued)

BRAND NAME (Generic)	DOSAGE FORM/ STRENGTH	INDICATIONS	ADULT DOSE	PEDIATRIC DOSE
Erythromycin	Cap, Delayed-Release: 250mg	Mild to moderate upper and lower respiratory tract and skin and skin structure infections, listeriosis, pertussis, diphtheria, erythrasma, intestinal amebiasis, primary syphilis in PCN allergy, Legionnaires' disease, chlamydial infections (eg, newborn conjunctivitis urethral, endocervical, rectal, etc), and nongonococcal urethritis. Prophylaxis of endocarditis or rheumatic fever.	Usual: 250mg q6h or 500mg q12h without food. Max: 4g/day. Treat strep infections for 10 days. Streptococcal Infection Prophylaxis of Rheumatic Fever: 250mg bid. Chlamydial Urogenital Infection During Pregnancy: 500mg qid for 7 days or 250mg qid for 14 days. Urethral/Endocervical/Rectal Chlamydial Infections: 500mg qid for at least 7 days. Primary Syphilis: 30-40g in divided doses over 10-15 days. Intestinal Amebiasis: 250mg q6h for 10-14 days. Pertussis: 40-50mg/kg/day in divided doses for 5-14 days. Legionnaires' Disease: 1-4g/day in divided doses. Bacterial Endocarditis Prophylaxis: 1g 1 hr before procedure, then 500mg 6 hrs later.	Usual: 30-50mg/kg/day in divided doses without food. Severe Infections: Double dose up to 4g/day. Treat strep infections for 10 days. Streptococcal Infection Prophylaxis of Rheumatic Fever: 250mg bid. Intestinal Amebiasis: 30-50mg/kg/day in divided doses for 10-14 days. Pertussis: 40-50mg/kg/day in divided doses for 5-14 days. Bacterial Endocarditis Prophylaxis: 20mg/kg 1 hr before procedure, then 10mg/kg 6 hrs later.
Erythromycin Base	Tab: 250mg	Mild to moderate upper and lower respiratory tract and skin and skin structure infections, listeriosis, pertussis, diphtheria, erythrasma, intestinal amebiasis, acute pelvic inflammatory disease (PID) (*N.gonorrhea*), primary syphilis in PCN allergy, Legionnaires' disease, chlamydial infections (eg, newborn conjunctivitis urethral, endocervical, rectal, etc), and nongonococcal urethritis. Prophylaxis of rheumatic fever.	Usual: 250mg q6h or 500mg q12h without food. Max: 4g/day. Treat strep infections for 10 days. Streptococcal Infection Prophylaxis of Rheumatic Fever: 250mg bid. Chlamydial Urogenital Infection During Pregnancy: 500mg qid for 7 days or 250mg qid for 14 days. Urethral/Endocervical/Rectal Chlamydial Infections and Nongonococcal Urethritis: 500mg qid for at least 7 days. Primary Syphilis: 30-40g in divided doses over 10-15 days. Acute PID: 500mg (erythromycin lactobionate) IV q6h for 3 days, then 500mg PO q12h for 7 days. Pertussis: 250mg qid for 10-14 days. Intestinal Amebiasis: 40-50mg/kg/day in divided doses for 5-14 days. Legionnaires' Disease: 1-4g/day in divided doses.	Usual: 30-50mg/kg/day in divided doses without food. Severe Infections: Double dose up to 4g/day. Treat strep infections for 10 days. Streptococcal Infection Prophylaxis of Rheumatic Fever: 250mg bid. Chlamydial Conjunctivitis of Newborns and Chlamydial Pneumonia in Infancy: 12.5mg/kg qid for 2 weeks and 3 weeks, respectively. Intestinal Amebiasis: 30-50mg/kg/day in divided doses for 10-14 days. Pertussis: 40-50mg/kg/day in divided doses for 5-14 days.
Pediazole (sulfisoxazole acetyl-erythromycin ethysuccinate)	Sus: (Erythromycin Ethylsuccinate-Sulfisoxazole Acetyl) 200mg-600mg/5mL [100 mL, 150mL, 200mL]	Acute otitis media caused by *H.influenzae*.		>2 mos: Dose based on 50mg/kg/day erythromycin or 150mg/kg/day sulfisoxazole given tid-qid for 10 days. Max: 6g/day sulfisoxazole.

SYSTEMIC ANTIBIOTICS

BRAND NAME (Generic)	DOSAGE FORM/ STRENGTH	INDICATIONS	ADULT DOSE	PEDIATRIC DOSE
PCE (erythromycin)	Tab, Extended-Release: 333mg, 500mg	Mild to moderate upper and lower respiratory tract and skin and skin structure infections, listeriosis, pertussis, diphtheria, erythrasma, intestinal amebiasis, acute pelvic inflammatory disease (PID) (*N gonorrhea*), primary syphilis in PCN allergy, Legionnaires' disease, chlamydial infections (eg, newborn conjunctivitis urethral, endocervical, or rectal, etc), and nongonococcal urethritis. Prophylaxis of rheumatic fever.	Usual: 333mg q8h or 500mg q12h without food. Max: 4g/day. Do not take bid when dose is ≥1g/day. Treat strep infections for 10 days. Chlamydial Urogenital Infection During Pregnancy: 500mg qid or 666mg q8h for 7 days, or 500mg q12h, 333mg q8h or 250mg qid for 14 days. Urethral/Endocervical/ Rectal Chlamydial Infections and Nongonococcal Urethritis: 500mg qid or 666mg q8h for at least 7 days. Primary Syphilis: 30-40g in divided doses for 10-15 days. Acute PID: 500mg (erythromycin lactobionate) IV q6h for 3 days, then 500mg PO q12h or 333mg q8h for 7 days. Streptococcal Infection Long-Term Prophylaxis of Rheumatic Fever: 250mg bid. Intestinal Amebiasis: 500mg q12h, or 333mg q8h or 250mg q6h for 10-14 days. Pertussis: 40-50mg/kg/day in divided doses for 5-14 days. Legionnaires' Disease: 1-4g/day in divided doses.	Usual: 30-50mg/kg/day in divided doses without food. Max: 4g/day. Severe Infections: Double dose up to 4g/day. Treat strep infections for 10 days. Chlamydial Conjunctivitis of Newborns and Chlamydial Pneumonia in Infancy: 12.5mg/kg qid for 2 weeks and 3 weeks, respectively. Intestinal Amebiasis: 30-50mg/kg/day in divided doses for 10-14 days. Long-Term Prophylaxis of Rheumatic Fever: 250mg bid. Pertussis: 40-50mg/kg/day in divided doses for 5-14 days. Legionnaires' Disease: 1-4g/day in divided doses.
Zithromax (azithromycin)	Inj: 500mg; Sus: 100mg/5mL [15mL], 200mg/5mL [15mL, 22.5mL, 30mL], 1g/pkt [3 10⁵]; Tab: 250mg [Z-Pak, 6 tabs], 500mg [Tri-Pak, 3 tabs], 600mg	(PO) Treatment of acute bacterial exacerbations of COPD, acute bacterial sinusitis (ABS), community acquired pneumonia (CAP), pharyngitis/tonsillitis, uncomplicated skin and skin structure, urethritis/ cervicitis, genital ulcer disease (men), acute otitis media, prevention of disseminated *Mycobacterium avium* complex (MAC) disease in advanced HIV infection. (IV) Treatment of CAP and pelvic inflammatory disease (PID).	(PO) COPD/CAP/Pharyngitis/Tonsillitis (second line therapy)/SSSIs: ≥16 yrs: 500mg on day 1, then 250 mg qd on days 2-5. COPD: 500mg qd for 3 days. ABS: 500mg qd for 3 days. Genital Ulcer Disease and Non-Gonococcal Urethritis/Cervicitis: 1g single dose. Urethritis/Cervicitis due to gonorrhea: 2g single dose. MAC Prophylaxis: 1200mg once weekly. MAC Treatment: 600mg qd with ethambutol 15mg/kg/day. (IV) ≥16 yrs: CAP: 500mg qd for at least 2 days, then 500mg PO to complete 7-10 day course. PID: 500mg qd for 1-2 days, then 250mg PO to complete 7-day course.	(Sus) Otitis Media: ≥6 mo: 30mg/kg single dose; 10mg/kg for 3 days; or 10mg/kg qd on day 1, then 5mg/kg qd on days 2-5. ABS: ≥6 mo: 10mg/kg qd for 3 days. CAP: ≥6 mo: 10mg/kg qd on day 1, then 5mg/kg qd on days 2-5. (Sus, Tab) Pharyngitis/Tonsillitis: ≥2 yrs: 12mg/kg qd for 5 days. 1g suspension is not for pediatric use.
Zmax (azithromycin)	Sus, Extended-Release: 2g	Treatment of mild to moderate acute bacterial sinusitis due to *Haemophilus influenzae*, *Moraxella catarrhalis*, or *Streptococcus pneumoniae*. Treatment of community-acquired pneumonia due to *Chlamydophila pneumoniae*, *Haemophilus influenzae*, *Mycoplasma pneumoniae*, or *Streptococcus pneumoniae* in patients appropriate for oral therapy.	2g single dose. Take on an empty stomach (1 hr before or 2 hrs after a meal).	

(Continued)

SYSTEMIC ANTIBIOTICS

BRAND NAME (Generic)	DOSAGE FORM/ STRENGTH	INDICATIONS	ADULT DOSE	PEDIATRIC DOSE
PENICILLINS				
Amoxil (amoxicillin)	Cap: 250mg, 500mg; Sus: 50mg/mL [15mL, 30mL], 125mg/5mL [80mL, 100mL, 150mL], 200mg/5mL [5mL, 50mL, 75mL, 100mL], 250mg/5mL [80mL, 100mL, 150mL], 400mg/5mL [5mL, 50mL, 75mL, 100mL]; Tab: 500mg, 875mg; Tab, Chewable: 200mg, 400mg	Infections of the ear, nose, throat, genitourinary tract, skin and skin structure, lower respiratory tract due to susceptible (beta lactamase negative) organisms; gonorrhea (acute uncomplicated). *H.pylori* eradication to reduce the risk of duodenal ulcer recurrence.	Ear/Nose/Throat/SSSI/GU: (Mild/Moderate): 500mg q12h or 250mg q8h. (Severe): 875mg q12h or 500mg q8h. LRTI: 875mg q12h or 500mg q8h. Gonorrhea: 3g as single dose. *H.pylori*: (Dual Therapy) 1g + 30mg lansoprazole, both tid for 14 days. (Triple Therapy) 1g + 30mg lansoprazole + 500mg clarithromycin, all q12h X 14 days. CrCl 10-30mL/min: 250-500mg q12h. <10mL/min: 250-500mg q24h. Hemodialysis: 250-500mg or 250mg q24h, additional dose during and at the end.	Neonates: ≤12 weeks: Max: 30mg/kg/day divided q12h. >3 mo: Ear/Nose/Throat/SSSI/GU: (Mild/Moderate): 25mg/kg/day given q12h or 20mg/kg/day given q8h. (Severe): 45mg/kg/day given q12h or 40 mg/kg/day given q8h. LRTI: 45mg/kg/day given q12h or 40mg/kg/day given q8h. Gonorrhea: (Prepubertal) 50mg/kg with 25mg/kg probenecid as single dose. (Not for <2 yrs). >40kg: Dose as adult.
Ampicillin (ampicillin sodium)	Inj: 125mg, 250mg, 500mg, 1g, 2g, 10g	Treatment of respiratory tract, urinary tract, and GI infections, bacterial meningitis, septicemia, endocarditis.	IM/IV: Respiratory Tract: ≥40kg: 250-500mg q8h. <40kg: 25-50mg/kg/day given q6-8h. GU/GI Caused by *N.gonorrhea* (Females): ≥40kg: 500mg q6h. <40kg: 50mg/kg/day given q6-8h. Urethritis Caused by *N.gonorrhea* (Males): 500mg q8-12h for 2 doses; may retreat if needed. Bacterial Meningitis: 150-200mg/kg/day given q3-4h. Septicemia: 150-200mg/kg/day IV for 3 days, continue with IM q3-4h. Treat for minimum of 10 days and 48-72 hrs after being asymptomatic.	Bacterial Meningitis: 150-200mg/kg/day given q3-4h. Septicemia: 150-200mg/kg/day IV given q3-4h for 3 days, continue with IM q3-4h. Treat for minimum of 10 days and 48-72 hrs after being asymptomatic.

SYSTEMIC ANTIBIOTICS

BRAND NAME (Generic)	DOSAGE FORM/ STRENGTH	INDICATIONS	ADULT DOSE	PEDIATRIC DOSE
Augmentin (amoxicillin-clavulanate potassium)	(Amoxicillin-Clavulanate) Sus: 125-31.25mg/5mL [75mL, 100mL], 200-28.5mg/5mL [50mL, 75mL, 100mL], 250-62.5mg/5mL [75mL, 100mL], 400-57mg/5mL [50mL, 75mL, 100mL]; Tab: 250-125mg, 500-125mg, 875-125mg; Tab, Chewable: 200-28.5mg, 250-62.5mg, 400-57mg	Treatment of lower respiratory tract (LRTI), skin and skin structure (SSSI), and urinary tract infections (UTI), otitis media (OM), sinusitis.	(Dose based on amoxicillin) 500mg q12h or 250mg q8h. Severe Infections/RTI: 875mg q12h or 500mg q8h. May use 125mg/5mL or 250mg/5mL sus in place of 500mg tab and 200mg/5mL sus or 400mg/5mL sus, in place of 875mg tab. CrCl <30mL/min: Do not give 875mg tab. CrCl 10-30mL/min: 250-500mg q12h. CrCl <10mL/min: 250-500mg q24h. Hemodialysis: 250-500mg q24h, give additional dose during and at the end of dialysis.	(Dose based on amoxicillin) ≥40kg: Use adult dose. ≥12 weeks: Sinusitis/OM/LRTI/Severe Infections: (Sus/Tab, Chewable) 45mg/kg/day given q12h or 40mg/kg/day given q8h. Less Severe Infections: 25mg/kg/day given q12h or 20mg/kg/day given q8h. <12 weeks:15mg/kg q12h (use 125mg/5mL sus).
Augmentin ES-600 (amoxicillin-clavulanate potassium)	Sus: (Amoxicillin-Clavulanate) 600mg-42.9mg/5mL [50mL, 75mL, 100mL, 150mL]	Treatment of recurrent or persistent acute otitis media.		(Dose based on amoxicillin) 3 mo-12 yrs: <40kg: 45mg/kg q12h for 10 days.
Augmentin XR (amoxicillin-clavulanate potassium)	Tab, Extended-Release: (Amoxicillin-Clavulanate) 1000 mg-62.5mg	Treatment of community acquired pneumonia (CAP) or acute bacterial sinusitis due to confirmed or suspected β-lactamase producing pathogens.	Sinusitis: 2 tabs q12h for 10 days. CAP: 2 tabs q12h for 7-10 days. Take at the start of a meal.	≥16 yrs: Sinusitis: 2 tabs q12h for 10 days. CAP: 2 tabs q12h for 7-10 days. Take at the start of a meal.
Bicillin C-R (penicillin G benzathine-penicillin G procaine)	Inj: (Penicillin G Benzathine-Penicillin G Procaine) 300,000-300,000 U/mL	Treatment of moderately severe to severe upper-respiratory tract (URT) and skin and soft-tissue infections (SSTI), scarlet fever and erysipelas due to streptococci. Treatment of moderately severe pneumonia and otitis media due to pneumococci.	Group A Strep: URTI/SSTI/Scarlet Fever/Erysipelas: 2.4 MU IM. Treat at a single session using multiple IM sites, or use an alternative schedule and give 1/2 of the total dose on Day 1 and 1/2 on Day 3. Pneumococcal Infections (Except Meningitis): 1.2 MU IM, repeat every 2-3 days until temperature is normal for 48 hrs. Administer IM into upper, outer quadrant of buttock.	Group A Strep: URTI/SSTI/Scarlet Fever/Erysipelas: >60 lbs: 2.4 MU IM. 30-60 lbs: 900,000 U-1.2 MU IM. <30 lbs: 600,000 U IM. Treat at a single session using multiple IM sites, or use an alternative schedule and give 1/2 of the total dose on Day 1 and 1/2 on Day 3. Pneumococcal Infections (Except Meningitis): 600,000 U IM, repeat every 2-3 days until temperature is normal for 48 hrs. Administer IM into upper, outer quadrant of buttock. Use the midlateral aspect of thigh in neonates, infants, and small children.

(Continued)

SYSTEMIC ANTIBIOTICS

PENICILLINS (Continued)

BRAND NAME (Generic)	DOSAGE FORM/ STRENGTH	INDICATIONS	ADULT DOSE	PEDIATRIC DOSE
Bicillin C-R 900/300 (penicillin G benzathine-penicillin G procaine)	Inj: (Penicillin G Benzathine-Penicillin G Procaine) 900,000-300,000 U/2mL	Treatment of moderately severe to severe upper-respiratory tract (URT) and skin and soft-tissue infections (SSTI), scarlet fever and erysipelas due to streptococci. Treatment of moderately severe pneumonia and otitis media due to pneumococci.		Group A Strep: URTI/SSTI/Scarlet Fever/Erysipelas: 1.2 MU IM single dose. Pneumococcal Infections (Except Meningitis): 1.2 MU IM every 2-3 days until temperature is normal for 48 hrs. Administer IM into upper, outer quadrant of buttock. Use midlateral aspect of thigh in neonates, infants, and small children.
Bicillin L-A (penicillin G benzathine)	Inj: 600,000 U/mL	Treatment of mild to moderate upper respiratory tract infections (URTI) due to streptococci and venereal infections (eg, syphilis, yaws, bejel, pinta). Prophylaxis to prevent recurrence of rheumatic fever or chorea.	Group A Strep: URTI: 1.2 MU IM single dose. Primary/Secondary/Latent Syphilis: 2.4 MU IM single dose. Late Syphilis (Tertiary/Neurosyphilis): 2.4 MU IM every 7 days for 3 doses. Yaws/Bejel/Pinta: 1.2 MU IM single dose. Rheumatic Fever/Glomerulonephritis Prophylaxis: 1.2 MU IM once a mo or 600,000 U IM every 2 weeks. Administer IM into upper, outer quadrant of buttock.	Group A Strep: URTI: Older Pediatrics: 900,000 U IM single dose. <60lbs: 300,000-600,000 U IM single dose. Congenital Syphilis: 2-12 yrs: Adjust dose based on adult schedule. <2 yrs: 50,000 U/Kg IM single dose. Rheumatic Fever/Glomerulonephritis Prophylaxis: 1.2 MU IM once a mo or 600,000 U every 2 weeks. Administer IM into upper, outer quadrant of buttock. Use the midlateral aspect of thigh in neonates, infants, and small children.
Dicloxacillin (dicloxacillin sodium)	Cap: 250mg, 500mg; Sus: 62.5mg/5mL [100mL]	Infections caused by penicillinase-producing staphylococci.	Mild-Moderate Infection: 125mg q6h. Severe Infection: 250mg q6h for at least 14 days.	<40kg: Mild-Moderate Infection: 12.5mg/kg/day in divided doses q6h. Severe Infection: 25mg/kg/day in divided doses q6h for at least 14 days.
Geocillin (carbenicillin disodium)	Tab: 382mg	Treatment of acute and chronic infections of the upper and lower urinary tract (UTI) and asymptomatic bacteriuria.	UTI: E.coli, Proteus, and Enterobacter: 1-2 tabs qid. Pseudomonas, Enterococcus: 2 tabs qid. Prostatitis: E.coli, Proteus, Enterococcus and Enterobacter: 2 tabs qid. CrCl 10-20mL/min: Adjust dose.	
Penicillin VK, Veetids (penicillin V potassium)	Sus: 125mg/5mL, 250mg/5mL [100mL, 200mL]; Tab: 250mg, 500mg	Mild to moderately severe bacterial infections including conditions of the respiratory tract, oropharynx, skin and soft tissue. Prevention of recurrence following rheumatic fever and/or chorea.	Usual: Streptococcal Infections (Scarlet Fever, Erysipelas, Upper Respiratory Tract): 125-250mg q6-8h for 10 days. Pneumococcal Infections (Otitis Media, Respiratory Tract): 250-500mg q6h until afebrile for at least 2 days. Staphylococcus Infections (Skin/Soft Tissue): 250-500mg q6-8h. Fusospirochetosis Infections (Oropharynx): 250-500mg q6-8h. Rheumatic Fever/Chorea Prevention: 250-500mg bid.	≥12 yrs: Usual: Streptococcal Infections (Scarlet Fever, Erysipelas, Upper Respiratory Tract): 125-250mg q6-8h for 10 days. Pneumococcal Infections (Otitis media, Respiratory Tract): 250-500mg q6h until afebrile for at least 2 days. Staphylococcus Infections (Skin/Soft Tissue): 250-500mg q6-8h. Fusospirochetosis Infections (Oropharynx): 250-500mg q6-8h. Rheumatic Fever/Chorea Prevention: 125-250mg bid.

SYSTEMIC ANTIBIOTICS

BRAND NAME (Generic)	DOSAGE FORM/ STRENGTH	INDICATIONS	ADULT DOSE	PEDIATRIC DOSE
Pfizerpen (penicillin G potassium)	Inj: 1 MU, 5 MU, 20 MU	For therapy of severe infections when rapid and high blood levels of penicillin required. Management of streptococcal, pneumococcal, staphylococcal, clostridial, fusospirochetal, listeria, and gram negative bacillary, and pasteurella infections. For anthrax, actinomycosis, diphtheria, erysipeloid, meningitis, endocarditis, bacteremia, rat-bite fever, syphilis, and gonorrheal endocarditis and arthritis. With combined oral therapy, prophylaxis against endocarditis in patients with congenital heart disease, rheumatic, or other acquired valvular heart disease undergoing dental procedures or surgical procedures of upper respiratory tract.	Anthrax/Gonorrheal Endocarditis/Severe Infections (Streptococci, Pneumococci, Staphylococci): Minimum of 5 MU/day. Syphilis: Administer in hospital. Determine dose and duration based on age and weight. Meningococcic Meningitis: 1-2 MU IM q2h or 20-30 MU/day continuous IV. Actinomycosis: 1-6 MU/day for cervicofacial cases; 10-20 MU/day for thoracic and abdominal disease. Clostridial Infections: 20 MU/day (adjunct to antitoxin). Fusospirochetal Severe Infections: 5-10 MU/day for oropharynx, lower respiratory tract, and genital area infection. Rat-bite Fever: 12-15 MU/day for 3-4 weeks. Listeria Endocarditis: 15-20 MU/day for 4 weeks. Pasteurella Bacteremia/Meningitis: 4-6 MU/day for 2 weeks. Erysipeloid Endocarditis: 2-20 MU/day for 4-6 weeks. Gram Negative Bacillary Bacteremia: 20-80 MU/day. Diphtheria (carrier state): 0.3-0.4 MU/day in divided doses for 10-12 days. Endocarditis Prophylaxis: 1 MU IM mixed with 0.6 MU procaine penicillin G 0.5-1 hr before procedure. Renal/Cardiac/Vascular Dysfunction: Consider dose reduction. For streptococcal infection, treat for minimum 10 days.	Listeria Infections: Neonates: 0.5-1 MU/day. Congenital Syphilis: Administer in hospital. Determine dose and duration based on age and weight. Endocarditis Prophylaxis: 30,000 U/kg IM mixed with 0.6 MU procaine penicillin G 0.5-1 hr before procedure. For streptococcal infection, treat for minimum 10 days.
Permapen (penicillin G benzathine)	Inj: 600,000 U/mL	Treatment of microorganisms susceptible to low and very prolonged serum levels in upper respiratory tract infections (streptococci group A—without bacteremia), syphilis, yaws, bejel, and pinta. Prophylaxis for rheumatic fever and/or chorea. Follow-up prophylactic therapy for rheumatic heart disease and acute glomerulonephritis.	Streptococcal Infection: 1.2 MU IM single dose. Primary/Secondary/Latent Syphilis: 1 MU IM single dose. Late (Tertiary/Neurosyphilis) Syphilis: 3 MU IM every 7 days for total of 6-9 MU. Yaws/Bejel/Pinta: 1.2 MU IM single dose. Rheumatic Fever/Glomerulonephritis Prophylaxis: 1.2 MU IM once moly or 600,000 U IM twice moly. Use upper outer quadrant of buttock. Rotate injection site.	≤12 yrs: Adjust dose according to age and weight and severity of infection. Streptococcal Infection: 900,000 U IM single dose in older children. Congenital Syphilis: <2 yrs: 50,000 U/kg IM single dose. 2-12 yrs: Adjust dose based on adult schedule. Use midlateral aspect of thigh in infants and small children. May divide dose between 2 buttocks in peds <2 yrs. Rotate injection site.

(Continued)

SYSTEMIC ANTIBIOTICS

BRAND NAME (Generic)	DOSAGE FORM/ STRENGTH	INDICATIONS	ADULT DOSE	PEDIATRIC DOSE
PENICILLINS *(Continued)*				
Piperacillin	Inj: 2g, 3g, 4g	Treatment of serious intra-abdominal, urinary tract, gynecologic, lower respiratory tract, skin and skin structure, bone and joint, and gonococcal infections, septicemia, and perioperative surgical prophylaxis.	Usual: 3-4g IM/IV q4-6h. Max: 24g/day; IM: 2g/site. Serious Infections: 200-300mg/kg/day IV divided q4-6h. Complicated UTI: 125-200mg/kg/day IV divided q6-8h. Uncomplicated UTI/Community Acquired Pneumonia: 100-125mg/kg/day IM/IV divided q6-12h. Uncomplicated Gonorrhea: 2g IM single dose with 1g PO probenecid 1/2 hr before injection. Surgical Prophylaxis: 2g IV 20-30 min just prior to anesthesia (See labeling for follow-up dosing). C-Section: 2g IV after cord is clamped, then 2g IV at 4 hrs and 8 hrs after 1st dose. Renal Impairment: Uncomplicated/Complicated UTI: CrCl<20mL/min: 3g q12h. Complicated UTI: CrCl 20-40mL/min: 3g q8h. Serious Infection: CrCl 20-40mL/min: 4g q8h. CrCl <20mL/min: 4g q12h. Hemodialysis: Give 1g additional dose after each dialysis. Max: 2g q8h. Usual treatment is for 3-10 days; treat gynecologic infections for 3-10 days; treat *S.pyogenes* infections for at least 10 days.	≥12 yrs: Usual: 3-4g IM/IV q4-6h. Max: 24g/day; IM: 2g/site. Serious Infections: 200-300mg/kg/day IV divided q4-6h. Complicated UTI: 125-200mg/kg/day IV divided q6-8h. Uncomplicated UTI/Community Acquired Pneumonia: 100-125mg/kg/day IM/IV divided q6-12h. Uncomplicated Gonorrhea: 2g IM single dose with 1g PO probenecid 1/2 hr before injection. Surgical Prophylaxis: 2g IV 20-30 minute just prior to anesthesia (See labeling for follow-up dosing). C-section: 2g IV after cord is clamped, then 2g IV at 4 hrs and 8 hrs after 1st dose. Renal Impairment: Uncomplicated/Complicated UTI: CrCl <20mL/min: 3g q12h. Complicated UTI: CrCl 20-40mL/min: 3g q8h. Serious Infection: CrCl 20-40mL/min: 4g q8h. CrCl <20mL/min: 4g q12h. Hemodialysis: Give 1g additional dose after each dialysis. Max: 2g q8h. Usual treatment is for 7-10 days; treat gynecologic infections for 3-10 days; treat *S.pyogenes* nfections for at least 10 days.
Timentin (ticarcillin-clavulanate potassium)	Inj: (Ticarcillin-Clavulanate) 3g-100mg, 3g-100mg/100mL, 30g-1g	Treatment of lower respiratory tract, bone and joint, skin and skin structure, urinary tract (UTI), gynecologic, and intra-abdominal infections, and septicemia.	≥60kg: UTI/Systemic Infection: 3g-100mg (3.1g vial) IV q4-6h. Gynecologic Infections: Moderate: 200mg/kg/day ticarcillin IV given q6h. Severe: 300mg/kg/day ticarcillin IV given q4h. <60kg: Usual: 200-300mg/kg/day ticarcillin IV given q4-6h. UTI: 3g-200mg (3.2g vial) q8h. Renal Impairment (based on ticarcillin): CrCl 60-30mL/min: 2g IV q4h. CrCl 30-10mL/min: 2g IV q8h. CrCl<10mL/min: 2g IV q12h (2g IV q24h with hepatic dysfunction). Peritoneal Dialysis: 3.1g IV q12h. Hemodialysis: 2g IV q12h, and 3.1g after each dialysis. Apply reduced dosage after initial 3.1g LD is given.	≥3 mo: >60kg: Mild to Moderate: 3g-100mg (3.1g vial) IV q6h. Severe: 3g-100mg (3.1g vial) IV q4h. <60kg: Mild to Moderate: 50mg/kg ticarcillin IV q6h. Severe: 50mg/kg ticarcillin IV q4h. Renal Impairment (based on ticarcillin): CrCl 60-30mL/min: 2g IV q4h. CrCl 30-10mL/min: 2g IV q8h. CrCl<10mL/min: 2g IV q12h (2g IV q24h with hepatic dysfunction). Peritoneal Dialysis: 3.1g IV q12h. Hemodialysis: 2g IV q12h, and 3.1g after each dialysis. Apply reduced dosage after initial 3.1g LD is given.

SYSTEMIC ANTIBIOTICS

BRAND NAME (Generic)	DOSAGE FORM/ STRENGTH	INDICATIONS	ADULT DOSE	PEDIATRIC DOSE
Unasyn (ampicillin sodium/ sulbactam sodium)	Inj: (Ampicillin-Sulbactam) 1g-0.5g, 2g-1g, 10g-5g	Treatment of skin and skin structure (SSSI), intra-abdominal, and gynecological infections caused by susceptible microorganisms.	1.5-3g (ampicillin + sulbactam) IM/IV q6h. Max: 4g/day sulbactam. Renal Impairment: CrCl ≥30mL/min: 1.5-3g q6-8h. CrCl 15-29mL/min: 1.5-3g q12h. CrCl 5-14mL/min: 1.5-3g q24h.	≥1 yr: SSSI: 1.5-3g (ampicillin + sulbactam) IM/IV q6h. Max: 4g/day sulbactam.
Veetids (penicillin V potassium)	Sus: 125mg/5mL, 250mg/5mL [100mL, 200mL]; Tab: 250mg, 500mg	Mild to moderately severe bacterial infections including conditions of the respiratory tract, oropharynx, skin and soft tissue. Prevention of recurrence following rheumatic fever and/or chorea.	Streptococcal Infections (Scarlet Fever, Erysipelas, Upper Respiratory Tract): 125-250mg q6-8h for 10 days. Pneumococcal Infections (Otitis media. Respiratory Tract): 250-500mg q6h until afebrile for at least 2 days. Staphylococcus Infections (Skin/Soft Tissue): 250-500mg q6-8h. Fusospirochetosis Infections (Oropharynx): 250-500mg q6-8h. Rheumatic Fever/Chorea Prevention: 125-250mg bid.	Streptococcal Infections (Scarlet fever, Erysipelas, Upper Respiratory Tract): 125-250mg q6-8h for 10 days. Pneumococcal Infections (Otitis media. Respiratory Tract): 250-500mg q6h until afebrile for at least 2 days. Staphylococcus Infections (Skin/Soft Tissue): 250-500mg q6-8h. Fusospirochetosis Infections (Oropharynx): 250-500mg q6-8h. Rheumatic Fever/Chorea Prevention: 125-250mg bid.
Zosyn (piperacillin sodium-tazobactam)	Inj: (Piperacillin-Tazobactam) 40mg-5mg/mL, 60mg-7.5mg/mL, 2g-0.25g, 3g-0.375g, 4g-0.5g, 4g-0.5g/100mL, 36g-4.5g	Treatment of appendicitis, peritonitis, uncomplicated/complicated skin and skin structure infections, postpartum endometritis, pelvic inflammatory disease, moderate severity of community acquired pneumonia, and moderate to severe nosocomial pneumonia.	Usual: 3.375g q6h for 7-10 days. Nosocomial Pneumonia: 4.5g q6h for 7-14 days plus aminoglycoside. CrCl 20-40mL/min: 2.25g q6h. CrCl <20mL/min: 2.25g q8h. Hemodialysis: Max: 2.25g q12h. Give 1 additional 0.75g dose after each dialysis period.	

STREPTOMYCES DERIVATIVES

BRAND NAME (Generic)	DOSAGE FORM/ STRENGTH	INDICATIONS	ADULT DOSE	PEDIATRIC DOSE
Sumycin (tetracycline HCl)	Sus: 125mg/5mL; Tab: 250mg, 500mg	Treatment of respiratory tract, urinary tract, and skin and skin structure infections, lymphogranuloma, psittacosis, trachoma, uncomplicated urethral/endocervical/rectal infection caused by *Chlamydia*, nongonococcal urethritis, chancroid, plague, cholera, brucellosis, and others. When PCN is contraindicated, treatment of uncomplicated gonorrhea, syphilis, listeriosis, anthrax, *Clostridium* species, and others. Adjunct therapy for amebicides and severe acne.	Mild-Moderate: 250mg qid or 500mg bid. Severe: 500mg qid. Continue for 24-48 hrs after symptoms subside (minimum 10 days with Group A β-hemolytic streptococci). Severe Acne: Initial: 1g/day in divided doses. Maint: After improvement, 125-500mg/day. Brucellosis: 500mg qid for 3 weeks plus streptomycin 1g IM bid for 1 week, then qd for 1 week. Syphilis: 30-40g equally divided over 10-15 days. Gonorrhea: 500mg q6h for 7 days. Chlamydia: 500mg qid for at least 7 days. Renal Dysfunction: Reduce dose or extend dose interval.	Usual: 25-50mg/kg divided bid-qid. Continue for 24-48 hrs after symptoms subside (minimum 10 days with Group A β-hemolytic streptococci). Severe Acne: Initial: 1g/day in divided doses. Maint: After improvement, 125-500mg/day. Renal Dysfunction: Reduce dose or extend dose interval.

(Continued)

SYSTEMIC ANTIBIOTICS

BRAND NAME (Generic)	DOSAGE FORM/ STRENGTH	INDICATIONS	ADULT DOSE	PEDIATRIC DOSE
STREPTOMYCES DERIVATIVES *(Continued)*				
Lincocin (lincomycin HCl)	Inj: 300mg/mL	Treatment of serious infections due to streptococci, pneumococci, and staphylococci. Reserve for PCN allergy or if PCN is inappropriate.	IM: Serious Infection: 600mg q24h. More Severe Infection: 600mg q12h or more often. IV: Dose depends on severity. Serious Infection: 600mg-1g q8-12h. More Severe Infection: Increase dose. Infuse over ≥1 hr. Life-Threatening Situation: Up to 8g/day has been given. Max: 8g/day. Severe Renal Dysfunction: 25-30% of normal dose.	>1 mo: IM: Serious Infection: 10mg/kg q24h. More Severe Infection: 10mg/kg q12h or more often. IV: 10-20mg/kg/day, depending on severity infused in divided doses as described for adults. Severe Renal Dysfunction: 25-30% of normal dose.
TETRACYCLINE DERIVATIVES				
Declomycin (demeclocycline HCl)	Tab: 150mg, 300mg	Treatment of infections due to *rickettsiae*, *Mycoplasma pneumoniae*, *B.recurrentis*, agents of psittacosis, ornithosis, lymphogranuloma venereum or granuloma inguinale. Treatment of gram-negative infections (eg, respiratory, urinary tract), gram-positive infections (eg, respiratory tract, skin and soft tissue), trachoma, inclusion conjunctivitis. When PCN is contraindicated, treatment of gonorrhea, syphilis, listeriosis, anthrax, *Clostridium* species, and others. Adjunct therapy for amebicides.	Usual: 150mg qid or 300mg q12h bid. Gonorrhea: Initial: 600mg, then 300mg q12h for 4 days. Gonorrhea: 600mg followed by 300mg q12h for 4 days to a total of 3g. Renal/Hepatic Impairment: Reduce dose and/or extend dose intervals. Continue therapy for at least 24-48 hrs after symptoms subside. Treat strep infections for at least 10 days. Take at least 1 hr before or 2 hrs after meals with plenty of fluids.	>8 yrs: Usual: 3-6mg/lb/day given bid-qid. Gonorrhea: 600mg followed by 300mg q12h for 4 days to a total of 3g. Renal/Hepatic Impairment: Reduce dose and/or extend dose intervals. Continue therapy for at least 24-48 hrs after symptoms subside. Treat strep infections for at least 10 days. Take at least 1 hr before or 2 hrs after meals with plenty of fluids.
Doryx (doxycycline hyclate)	Cap: 75mg, 100mg	Treatment of susceptible infections including respiratory, urinary, skin and skin structure, lymphogranuloma, psittacosis, trachoma, uncomplicated urethral/endocervical/rectal, nongonococcal urethritis, rickettsiae, chancroid, plague, cholera, brucellosis, anthrax. When penicillin is contraindicated, treatment of syphilis, listeriosis, *Clostridium* species, and others. Adjunct therapy for amebiasis and severe acne.	Usual: 100mg q12h on 1st day, followed by 100mg qd. Severe Infections/Chronic UTI: 100mg q12h. Uncomplicated Gonococcal Infections (Men, except anorectal infections): 100mg bid for 7 days, or 300mg followed in 1 hr by another 300mg dose. Acute Epididymo-Orchitis: 100mg bid for at least 10 days. Primary/Secondary Syphilis: 300mg/day in divided doses for at least 10 days. Nongonococcal Urethritis, Uncomplicated Urethral/Endocervical/Rectal Infection: 100mg bid for at least 7 days. Inhalational Anthrax (post-exposure): 100mg bid for 60 days. Treat Strep infections for 10 days.	>8 yrs: >100 lbs: 100mg q12h on 1st day, followed by 100mg qd. Severe Infections/Chronic UTI: 100mg q12h. ≤100 lbs: 2mg/lb given bid on Day 1, followed by 1mg/lb given qd-bid thereafter. Severe Infections: Up to 2mg/lb. Inhalational Anthrax (post-exposure): <100 lbs: 1mg/lb bid for 60 days. >100 lbs: 100mg bid for 60 days.

SYSTEMIC ANTIBIOTICS

BRAND NAME (Generic)	DOSAGE FORM/ STRENGTH	INDICATIONS	ADULT DOSE	PEDIATRIC DOSE
Dynacin (minocycline HCl)	Cap: 50mg, 75mg, 100mg; Tab: 50mg, 75mg, 100mg	Treatment of inclusion conjunctivitis, nongonococcal urethritis, and other infections (eg, respiratory tract, endocervical, rectal, urinary tract, skin and skin structure) caused by susceptible strains of microorganisms. Alternative treatment in certain other infections (eg, urethritis, gonococcal, syphilis, anthrax). Adjunctive therapy in acute intestinal amebiasis and severe acne. Treatment of *Mycobacterium marinum* and asymptomatic carriers of *Neisseria meningitidis*.	Usual: 200mg initially, then 100mg q12h; alternative is 100-200mg initially, then 50mg qid. Uncomplicated Gonococcal Infection (Men, Other Than Urethritis and Anorectal Infections): 200mg initially, then 100mg q12h for minimum 4 days. Uncomplicated Gonococcal Urethritis (Men): 100mg q12h for 5 days. Syphilis: Administer usual dose for 10-15 days. Meningococcal Carrier State: 100mg q12h for 5 days. *Mycobacterium marinum*: 100mg q12h for 6-8 weeks. Uncomplicated urethral, endocervical, or rectal infection: 100mg q12h for at least 7 days. Renal Dysfunction: Reduce dose and/or extend dose intervals.	>8 yrs: 4mg/kg initially followed by 2mg/kg q12h. Take with plenty of fluids.
Minocin (minocycline HCl)	Cap: 50mg, 100mg; Inj: 100mg; Sus: 50mg/5mL [60mL]	Treatment of inclusion conjunctivitis, nongonococcal urethritis, and other infections (eg, respiratory tract, endocervical, rectal, urinary tract, skin and skin structure) caused by susceptible strains of microorganisms. Alternative treatment in certain other infections (eg, urethritis, gonococcal, syphilis, anthrax). Adjunctive therapy in acute intestinal amebiasis and severe acne. Treatment of *Mycobacterium marinum* and asymptomatic carriers of *Neisseria meningitidis*.	Usual: 200mg initially, then 100mg q12h; alternative is 100-200mg initially, then 50mg qid. Uncomplicated Gonococcal Infection (Men, other than urethritis and anorectal infections): 200mg initially, then 100mg q12h for minimum 4 days. Uncomplicated Gonococcal Urethritis (Men): 100mg q12h for 5 days. Syphilis: Administer usual dose for 10-15 days. Meningococcal Carrier State: 100mg q12h for 5 days. *Mycobacterium marinum*: 100mg q12h for 6-8 weeks. Uncomplicated Urethral, Endocervical, or Rectal Infection Caused by *Chlamydia trachomatis* or *Ureaplasma urealyticum*: 100mg q12h for at least 7 days. Gonorrhea in Patients Sensitive to PCN: 200mg initially, then 100mg q12h for at least 4 days, with post-therapy cultures within 2-3 days. Take with plenty of fluids. Renal Dysfunction: Max: 200mg/24hrs.	>8 yrs: 4mg/kg initially followed by 2mg/kg q12h. Take with plenty of fluids. Renal Dysfunction: Max: 200mg/24 hrs.

(Continued)

SYSTEMIC ANTIBIOTICS

(Generic)	BRAND NAME STRENGTH	DOSAGE FORM/ INDICATIONS	DOSE	ADULT DOSE	PEDIATRIC
TETRACYCLINE DERIVATIVES *(Continued)*					
Monodox (doxycycline monohydrate)	Cap: 50mg, 100mg	Treatment of respiratory tract, urinary tract, skin and skin structure, uncomplicated urethral/endocervical/rectal infection caused by *C.trachomatis*, nongonococcal urethritis caused by *C.trachomatis* and *U.urealyticum*, lymphogranuloma, psittacosis, trachoma, chancroid, plague, cholera, brucellosis. Treatment of uncomplicated gonorrhea, syphilis, listeriosis, anthrax, *Clostridium* species when PCN is contraindicated. Adjunct therapy for amebicides and severe acne.	Usual: 100mg q12h or 50mg q6h for 1 day, then 100 mg/day. Severe Infection: 100mg q12h. Uncomplicated Gonococcal Infections (except anorectal infections in men): 100mg bid for 7 days or 300mg stat, then repeat in 1 hr. Acute Epididymo-Orchitis caused by *N.gonorrhea* or *C.trachomatis*: 100mg bid for at least 10 days. Primary/Secondary Syphilis: 300mg/day in divided dose for at least 10 days. Uncomplicated Urethral/Endocervical/Rectal Infection caused by *C.trachomatis*: 100mg bid for at least 7 days. Nongonococcal Urethritis caused by *C.trachomatis* and *U.urealyticum*: 100mg bid for at least 7 days. Take with full glass of water. Take with food if GI upset occurs.		>8 yrs: ≤100 lbs: 2mg/lb divided in 2 doses for 1 day, then 1mg/lb daily in single or 2 divided doses. Severe Infection: May use up to 2mg/lb/day. >100 lbs: 100mg q12h or 50mg q6h for 1 day, then 100mg/day. Severe Infection: 100mg q12h. Take with a full glass of water. Take with food if GI upset occurs.
Oracea (doxycycline)	Cap: 40mg	Treatment of only inflammatory lesions (papules and pustules) of rosacea.	40mg qd in am. Take on empty stomach.		
Periostat (doxycycline hyclate)	Tab: 20mg	Adjunct to scaling and root planing to promote attachment level gain and reduces pocket depth in patients with adult periodontitis.	Following scaling and root planing, 20mg bid, 1 hour prior to morning and evening meals for up to 9 mos. Maintain adequate fluid intake with caps to reduce risk of esophageal irritation and ulceration.		
Solodyn (minocycline HCl)	Tab, Extended-Release: 45mg, 90mg, 135mg.	Treatment of inflammatory lesions of non-nodular moderate to severe acne vulgaris in patients ≥12 yrs.	1mg/kg qd for 12 weeks. Reduce dose with renal impairment.	≥12 yrs: 1mg/kg qd for 12 weeks. Reduce dose with renal impairment.	
Vibra-tabs (doxycycline hyclate)	Tab: 100mg	Treatment of susceptible infections including respiratory, urinary, skin and skin structure, lymphogranuloma, psittacosis, trachoma, uncomplicated urethral/endocervical/rectal, nongonococcal urethritis, rickettsiae, chancroid, plague, cholera, brucellosis, anthrax. When penicillin is contraindicated, treatment of uncomplicated gonorrhea, syphilis, listeriosis, *Clostridium species*, and others. Adjunct therapy for amebiasis and severe acne. Prophylaxis of malaria.	Usual: 100mg q12h on day 1, then 100mg qd or 50mg q12h. Severe Infection: 100mg q12h. Treat for 10 days with strep infection. Uncomplicated Gonococcal Infection (Except Anorectal in Men): 100mg bid for 7 days or 300mg followed by 300mg in 1 hr. Uncomplicated Urethral/Endocervical/Rectal Infection and Nongonococcal Urethritis: 100mg bid for 7 days. Syphilis: 100mg bid for 2 weeks. Syphilis for >1 yr: 100mg bid for 4 weeks. Acute Epididymo-orchitis: 100mg bid for at least 10 days. Inhalation Anthrax (Post-Exposure): 100mg bid for 60 days. Malaria Prophylaxis: 100mg qd. Begin 1-2 days before travel and continue for 4 weeks after leaving malarious area.		

SYSTEMIC ANTIBIOTICS

BRAND NAME (Generic)	DOSAGE FORM/ STRENGTH	INDICATIONS	ADULT DOSE	PEDIATRIC DOSE
Vibramycin (doxycycline)	Cap: (Doxycycline Hyclate) 50mg, 100mg; Syrup: (Doxycycline Calcium) 50mg/5mL; Sus: (Doxycycline Monohydrate) 25mg/5mL [60mL]	Treatment of susceptible infections including respiratory, urinary, skin and skin structure, lymphogranuloma, psittacosis, trachoma, uncomplicated urethral/endocervical/rectal, nongonococcal urethritis, rickettsiae, chancroid, plague, cholera, brucellosis, anthrax. When penicillin is contraindicated, treatment of uncomplicated gonorrhea, syphilis, listeriosis, *Clostridium species*, and others. Adjunct therapy for amebiasis and severe acne. Prophylaxis of malaria.	Usual: 100mg q12h on day 1, then 100mg qd or 50mg q12h. Severe Infection: 100mg q12h. Treat for 10 days with strep infection. Uncomplicated Gonococcal Infection (Except Anorectal in Men): 100mg bid for 7 days or 300mg followed by 300mg in 1 hr. Uncomplicated Urethral/Endocervical/Rectal Infection and Nongonococcal Urethritis: 100mg bid for 7 days. Syphilis: 100mg bid for 2 weeks. Acute Epididymo-orchitis: 100mg bid for at least 10 days. Inhalation Anthrax (Post-Exposure): 100mg bid for 60 days. Malaria Prophylaxis: 100mg qd. Begin 1-2 days before travel and continue for 4 weeks after leaving malarious area.	>8 yrs: ≤100 lbs: 1mg/lb bid on day 1, then 1mg/lb qd or 0.5mg/lb bid. Severe Infections: Maint: 2mg/lb. >100 lbs: Usual: 100mg q12h on day 1, then 100mg qd or 50mg q12h. Severe Infection: 100mg q12h. Treat for 10 days with strep infection. Inhalation Anthrax (Post-Exposure): <100 lbs: 1mg/lb bid for 60 days. ≥100 lbs: 100mg bid for 60 days. Malaria Prophylaxis: 2mg/kg qd. Max: 100mg/day. Begin 1-2 days before travel and continue for 4 weeks after leaving malarious area.
Vibramycin IV (doxycycline hyclate)	Inj: 100mg, 200mg	Treatment of *rickettsiae, Mycoplasma pneumoniae, psittacosis,* ornithosis, lymphogranuloma venereum, granuloma inguinale, relapsing fever, chancroid, *Pasteurella pestis, Pasteurella tularensis, Bartonella bacilliformis, Bacteroides species, Vibrio comma, Vibrio fetus, Brucella species, E.coli, Enterobacter aerogenes, Shigella species, Mirna species, Herellea species, Haemophilus influenzae, Klebsiella species, Streptococcus species, Diplococcus pneumoniae, Staphylococcus aureus,* anthrax, and trachoma. When PCN is contraindicated; treatment of *Neisseria gonorrheae, N.meningitidis,* syphilis, yaws, *Listeria monocytogenes, Clostridium species, Fusobacterium fusiforme* and *Actinomyces species.* Adjunct therapy for amebiasis.	Usual: 200mg IV divided qd-bid on Day 1 then 100-200mg/day IV depending on severity, with 200mg administered in 1 or 2 infusions. Primary/Secondary Syphilis: 300mg/day IV for at least 10 days. Inhalational Anthrax (Post-Exposure): Institute oral therapy as soon as possible and continue therapy for a total of 60 days.	>8 yrs: >100 lbs: Usual: 200mg IV divided qd-bid on Day 1 then 100-200mg/day IV depending on severity, with 200mg administered in 1 or 2 infusions. ≤100 lbs: 2mg/lb IV divided qd-bid on Day 1 then 1-2mg/lb/day IV divided qd-bid depending on severity. Inhalational Anthrax (Post-Exposure): <100 lbs: 1mg/lb IV bid. Institute oral therapy as soon as possible and continue therapy for a total of 60 days.

(Continued)

SYSTEMIC ANTIBIOTICS

MISCELLANEOUS

BRAND NAME (Generic)	DOSAGE FORM/ STRENGTH	INDICATIONS	ADULT DOSE	PEDIATRIC DOSE
Bactrim (trimethoprim-sulfamethoxazole)	(Sulfamethoxazole [SMX]-Trimethoprim [TMP]) Tab: 400mg-80mg; Tab, DS: 800mg-160mg	Treatment of urinary tract infection (UTI), acute otitis media, acute exacerbation of chronic bronchitis (AECB), travelers' diarrhea, Shigellosis, and pneumocystitis carinii pneumonia (PCP).	UTI: 800mg SMX-160mg TMP q12h for 10-14 days. Shigellosis: 800mg SMX-160mg TMP q12h for 5 days. AECB: 800mg SMX-160mg TMP q12h for 14 days. PCP Treatment: 15-20mg/kg TMP and 75-100 mg/kg SMX per 24 hrs given q6h for 14-21 days. PCP Prophylaxis: 800mg SMX-160mg TMP qd. Traveler's Diarrhea: 800mg SMX-160mg TMP q12h for 5 days. CrCl: 15-30mL/min: 50% usual dose. CrCl: <15mL/min: Not recommended.	≥2 mo: UTI/Otitis Media: 4mg/kg TMP and 20mg/kg SMX q12h for 10 days. Shigellosis: 8mg/kg TMP and 40mg/kg SMX per 24 hrs given q12h for 5 days. PCP Treatment: 15-20mg/kg TMP and 75-100mg/kg SMX per 24 hrs given q6h for 14-21 days. PCP Prophylaxis: 150mg/m2/day TMP with 750mg/m2/day SMX given bid, on 3 consecutive days/week. Max: 320mg TMP/1600mg SMX/day. CrCl: 15-30mL/min: 50% usual dose. CrCl: <15mL/min: Not recommended.
Cleocin (clindamycin)	Cap: (HCl) 75mg, 150mg, 300mg; Inj: (Phosphate) 150mg/mL, 300mg/50mL, 600mg/50mL, 900mg/50mL; Sus: (HCl) 75mg/5mL [100g]	Serious infections caused by anaerobes, streptococci, pneumococci and staphylococci.	Serious Infection: 150-300mg PO q6h or 600-1200 mg/day IM/IV given bid-qid. More Severe Infection: 300-450mg PO q6h or 1200-2700mg/day IM/IV given bid-qid. Life-threatening infections: Up to 4800mg/day IV. Max: 600mg per IM injection. Take oral form with full glass of water. Treat B-hemolytic strep for at least 10 days.	Birth-16 yrs: Serious Infection: 8-16mg/kg/day PO. More Severe Infection: 16-20mg/kg/day PO. 1 mo-16 yrs: 20-40mg/kg/day IM/IV given tid-qid; use higher dose for more severe infection. <1 mo: 15-20mg/kg/day IM/IV given tid-qid. Take oral form with full glass of water. Treat B-hemolytic strep for at least 10 days.
Coly-Mycin M (colistimethate sodium)	Inj: 150mg	Treatment of acute or chronic infections due to certain gram-negative bacilli (eg, Pseudomonas aeruginosa, Enterobacter aerogenes, E.coli, Klebsiella pneumoniae).	Usual: 2.5-5mg/kg/day IV/IM in 2-4 divided doses. Max: 5mg/kg/day. SCr 1.3-1.5mg/dL: 2.5-3.8mg/kg/day IV/IM in 2 divided doses. SCr 1.6-2.5mg/dL: 2.5mg/kg/day IV/IM in 1-2 divided doses. SCr 2.6-4mg/dL: 1.5mg/kg/day IV/IM q36h. Obesity: Base dose on IBW.	Usual: 2.5-5mg/kg/day IV/IM in 2-4 divided doses. Max: 5mg/kg/day. SCr 1.3-1.5mg/dL: 2.5-3.8mg/kg/day IV/IM in 2 divided doses. SCr 1.6-2.5mg/dL: 2.5mg/kg/day IV/IM in 1-2 divided doses. SCr 2.6-4mg/dL: 1.5mg/kg/day IV/IM q36h. Obesity: Base dose on IBW.
Cubicin (daptomycin)	Inj: 500mg	Susceptible complicated skin and skin structure infections (cSSSI). Staphylococcus aureus blood stream infections (bacteremia).	≥18 yrs: Administer as IV infusion over 30 minutes. cSSSI: 4mg/kg once every 24 hrs for 7-14 days. S.aureus Bacteremia: 6mg/kg once every 24 hrs for minimum 2-6 weeks. Renal impairment: CrCl <30 mL/min, Hemodialysis or CAPD: (cSSSI) 4mg/kg or (S.aureus bacteremia) 6mg/kg once every 48 hrs.	
Flagyl IV (metronidazole HCl)	Inj: 500mg, 500mg (RTU)	Treatment of anaerobic intra-abdominal, skin and skin structure, gynecologic, bone and joint, CNS, lower respiratory tract infections, endocarditis, and septicemia.	LD: 15mg/kg IV. Maint: 6 hrs later, 7.5mg/kg IV q6h for 7-10 days or more. Max: 4g/24 hrs.	

SYSTEMIC ANTIBIOTICS

BRAND NAME (Generic)	DOSAGE FORM/ STRENGTH	INDICATIONS	ADULT DOSE	PEDIATRIC DOSE
Hiprex (methenamine hippurate)	Tab: 1g	Prophylaxis or suppression of recurrent urinary tract infections when long-term therapy is necessary. For use only after infection is eradicated by other appropriate antimicrobials.	1g bid.	>12 yrs: 1g bid. 6 to 12 yrs: 0.5g-1g bid.
Ketek (telithromycin)	Tab: 300mg [20^S], 400mg [60^S], Ketek Pak, 100^S]	Treatment of mild to moderate community-acquired pneumonia (CAP).	800mg qd for 7-10 days. Severe Renal Impairment (CrCl <30mL/min): 600mg qd. Hemodialysis: Give after dialysis session on dialysis days. Severe Renal Impairment (CrCl <30mL/min) with Hepatic Impairment: 400mg qd.	
Macrobid (nitrofurantoin monohydrate)	Cap: 100mg	Treatment of acute uncomplicated urinary tract infections (acute cystitis).	100mg every 12 hrs for 7 days. Take with food.	>12 yrs: 100mg every 12 hrs for 7 days. Take with food.
Macrodantin (nitrofurantoin macrocrystals)	Cap: 25mg, 50mg, 100mg	Treatment of urinary tract infection.	50-100mg qid for at least 7 days. Take with food. Long-term Suppressive Use: 50-100mg at bedtime.	≥1 mo: 5-7mg/kg/day given qid for at least 7 days. Take with food. Long-term Suppressive Use: 1mg/kg/day given qd-bid.
Monurol (fosfomycin tromethamine)	Pow: 3g/sachet	Uncomplicated urinary tract infection (acute cystitis) in women.	≥18 yrs: 1 single-dose sachet. Mix with 3-4oz of water before ingesting.	
Primsol (trimethoprim HCl)	Sol: 50mg/5mL	Treatment of acute otitis media in pediatrics and urinary tract infection (UTI) in adults.	UTI: Usual: 100mg q12h or 200mg q24h for 10 days. CrCl: 15-30mL/min: Give 50% of usual dose.	Otitis Media: ≥6 mos: 5mg/kg q12h for 10 days. CrCl: 15-30mL/min: Give 50% of usual dose.
Rifadin (rifampin)	Cap: 150mg, 300mg; Inj: 600mg	Treatment of all forms of tuberculosis (TB). Treatment of asymptomatic carriers of *Neisseria meningitidis* to eliminate meningococci from the nasopharynx.	TB: 10mg/kg PO/IV qd. Max: 600mg/day. Meningococcal Carriers: 600mg bid for 2 days. Take 1 hr before or 2 hrs after a meal with a full glass of water. TB: 10-20mg/kg PO/IV qd. Max: 600mg/day.	Meningococcal Carriers: ≥1 mo: 10mg/kg q12h for 2 days. Max: 600mg/dose. <1 mo: 5mg/kg q12h for 2 days. Take 1 hr before or 2 hrs after a meal with a full glass of water.
Rifamate (isoniazid-rifampin)	Cap: (Isoniazid-Rifampin) 150mg-300mg	For pulmonary tuberculosis (TB). Not for initial therapy or prevention of TB.	2 caps. Take 1 hr before or 2 hrs after meals. Give with pyridoxine in the malnourished, those predisposed to neuropathy (eg, alcoholics, diabetics), and adolescents.	

(Continued)

SYSTEMIC ANTIBIOTICS

BRAND NAME (Generic)	DOSAGE FORM/ STRENGTH	INDICATIONS	ADULT DOSE	PEDIATRIC DOSE
MISCELLANEOUS *(Continued)*				
Rifater (isoniazid-rifampin-pyrazinamide)	Tab: (Isoniazid-Pyrazinamide-Rifampin) 50mg-300mg-120mg	For initial phase of pulmonary tuberculosis treatment	≥44kg: 4 tabs single dose qd. 45-54kg: 5 tabs qd single dose. ≥55kg: 6 tabs single dose. Give pyridoxine in malnourished, if predisposed to neuropathy (eg, alcoholics, diabetics), and adolescents. Take 1 hr before or 2 hrs after meals with full glass of water. Treatment usually lasts 2 months.	≥15 yrs: ≤44kg: 4 tabs single dose qd. 45-54kg: 5 tabs qd single dose. ≥55kg: 6 tabs qd single dose. Give pyridoxine in malnourished, if predisposed to neuropathy (eg, alcoholics, diabetics), and adolescents. Take 1 hr before or 2 hrs after meals with full glass of water. Treatment usually lasts 2 months.
Septra (sulfamethoxazole-trimethoprim)	(Sulfamethoxazole [SMX]-Trimethoprim [TMP]) Inj: 80mg-16mg/mL; Sus: 200mg-40mg/5mL [100mL, 473mL]; Tab: 400mg-80mg; Tab: DS: 800mg-160mg	(Inj, Sus, Tab) Treatment of urinary tract infection (UTI), pneumocystis carinii pneumonia (PCP) and enteritis caused by *Shigella*. (Sus, Tab). Treatment of acute exacerbation of chronic bronchitis (AECB), travelers' diarrhea, and acute otitis media.	(Sus, Tab) UTI: 800mg-160mg PO q12h for 10-14 days. Shigellosis/Traveler's Diarrhea: 800mg-160mg PO q12h for 5 days. AECB: 800mg-160mg PO q12h for 14 days. PCP Treatment: 15-20mg/kg TMP and 75-100mg/kg SMX per 24 hrs given PO q6h for 14-21 days PCP Prophylaxis: 800mg-160mg PO qd. (Inj) Severe UTI: 8-10mg/kg TMP IV given in divided doses q6, 8 or 12h for up to 14 days. PCP Treatment: 15-20mg/kg TMP IV given in divided doses q6-8h for up to 14 days. Shigellosis: 8-10mg/kg TMP IV given in divided doses q6, 8 or 12h for 5 days. (Inj, Sus, Tab) Renal Impairment: CrCl 15-30 mL/min: 50% usual dose. CrCl <15mL/min: Not recommended.	(Sus, Tab) ≥2 mo: UTI/Otitis Media: 4mg/kg TMP and 20mg/kg SMX q12h for 10 days. Shigellosis/Traveler's Diarrhea: 4mg/kg TMP and 20mg/kg SMX q12h for 5 days. PCP Treatment: 15-20mg/kg TMP and 75-100mg/kg SMX/24 hrs given q6h for 14-21 days. PCP Prophylaxis: 150mg/m2/day TMP and 750mg/m2/day SMX PO given bid, on 3 consecutive days per week. Max: 320mg TMP and 1600mg SMX per day. (Inj) Severe UTI: 8-10mg/kg TMP IV given in divided doses q6, 8 or 12h for up to 14 days. PCP Treatment: 15-20mg/kg TMP IV given in divided doses q6-8h for up to 14 days. Shigellosis: 8-10mg/kg TMP IV given in divided doses q6, 8 or 12h for 5 days. (Inj, Sus, Tab) Renal Impairment: CrCl 15-30mL/min: 50% usual dose. CrCl <15mL/min: Not recommended.
Synercid (dalfopristin-quinupristin)	Inj: (Dalfopristin-Quinupristin) 350mg-150mg per 500mg vial	Treatment of serious or life-threatening *Enterococcus faecium* (VREF) bacteremia and complicated skin and skin structure infections (SSSI) caused by *Staphylococcus aureus* (methicillin susceptible) or *Streptococcus pyogenes*.	VREF: 7.5mg/kg IV q8h. Duration depends on site and severity of infection. Complicated SSSI: 7.5mg/kg IV q12h for at least 7 days. Hepatic Cirrhosis (Child Pugh A or B): May need dose reduction.	≥16 yrs: VREF: 7.5mg/kg IV q8h. Duration depends on site and severity of infection. Complicated SSSI: 7.5mg/kg IV q12h for at least 7 days. Hepatic Cirrhosis (Child Pugh A or B): May need dose reduction.

SYSTEMIC ANTIBIOTICS

BRAND NAME (Generic)	DOSAGE FORM/ STRENGTH	INDICATIONS	ADULT DOSE	PEDIATRIC DOSE
Vancocin (vancomycin HCl)	Inj: 500mg/100mL, 1g/200mL	Treatment of severe infections caused by susceptible strains of methicillin-resistant staphylococci. Indicated for penicillin-allergic patients, those who cannot receive or have failed to respond to other drugs, and for vancomycin-susceptible organisms that are resistant to other antimicrobials.	Usual: 500mg IV q6h or 1g IV q12h. Mild to Moderate Renal Impairment: Initial: 15mg/kg/day. Maint: 1.9mg/kg/d. Administer 10mg/min or over at least 60 min, whichever is longer. Renal Dysfunction: Initial: 15mg/kg. Dose is about 15x the GFR in mL/min (refer to table in labeling). Elderly: Require greater dose reduction. Functionally Anephric: Initial: 15mg/kg, then 1.9mg/kg/24hrs. Marked Renal Dysfunction: 250-1000mg every several days. Anuria: 1000mg every 7-10 days.	Usual: 10mg/kg IV q6h. Infants/Neonates: Initial: 15mg/kg, then 10mg/kg q12h for neonates in the 1st week of life and q8h thereafter until 1 mo of age. Administer over at least 60 min. Renal Dysfunction: Initial: 15mg/kg. Dose is about 15x the GFR in mL/min (refer to table in labeling). Premature Infants: Require greater dose reduction.
Vancocin Oral (vancomycin HCl)	Cap: 125mg, 250mg	Staphylococcal enterocolitis and antibiotic-associated pseudomembranous colitis caused by *C. difficile*.	500mg-2g/day given tid-qid for 7-10 days.	40mg/kg/day given tid-qid for 7-10 days. Max: 2g/day.
Zyvox (linezolid)	Inj: 2mg/mL [100mL, 200mL, 300mL]; Sus: 100mg/5mL; Tab: 400mg, 600mg	Vancomycin resistant *Enterococcus faecium* (VRE) infections, nosocomial pneumonia caused by *Staphylococcus aureus* (methicillin-susceptible and-resistant strains) or *Streptococcus pneumoniae* (including multi-drug resistant strains [MDRSP]), complicated skin and skin structure infections (SSSI) including diabetic foot infections without concomitant osteomyelitis caused by *Staphylococcus aureus* (methicillin-susceptible and -resistant strains), *Streptococcus pyogenes*, or *Streptococcus agalactiae*, uncomplicated SSSI caused by *Staphylococcus aureus* (methicillin-susceptible only) or *Streptococcus pyogenes*, community-acquired pneumonia (CAP) caused by *Streptococcus pneumoniae* (MDRSP), including concurrent bacteremia, or *Staphylococcus aureus* (methicillin-susceptible strains only).	Complicated SSSI/CAP/Nosocomial Pneumonia: 600mg IV/PO q12h for 10-14 days. VRE: 600mg IV/PO q12h for 14-28 days. Uncomplicated SSSI: 400mg PO q12h for 10-14 days.	Complicated SSSI/CAP/Nosocomial Pneumonia: Treat for 10-14 days. ≥12 yrs: 600mg IV/PO q12h. Birth-11 yrs: 10mg/kg IV/PO q8h. VRE: Treat for 14-28 days: ≥12 yrs: 600mg IV/PO q12h. Birth-11 yrs: 10mg/kg IV/PO q8h. Uncomplicated SSSI: Treat for 10-14 days: ≥12 yrs: 600mg PO q12h. 5-11 yrs: 10mg/kg PO q12h. <5 yrs: 10mg/kg PO q8h. Neonates <7 days should be initiated with dosing regimen of 10mg/kg q12h; may increase to 10mg/kg q8h if suboptimal response. All neonatal patients should receive 10mg/kg q8h by 7 days of life.

Asthma Management

DRUG (BRAND)	DOSAGE FORM	ADULT DOSE	CHILD DOSE*
SYSTEMIC CORTICOSTEROIDS			
Methylprednisolone	Tab: 2, 4, 8, 16, 32mg	7.5-60mg qd in a single dose or qod prn for control. Short course "burst": 40-60 mg/day as single dose or 2 divided doses for 3-10 days.	0.25-2mg/kg qd in a single dose or qod prn for control. Short course "burst": 1-2mg/kg/day. Max: 60mg/day for 3-10 days.
Prednisolone	Tab: 5mg; Liq: 5mg/5mL, 15mg/5mL		
Prednisone	Tab: 1, 2.5, 5, 10, 20, 50mg Liq: 5mg/mL, 5mg/5mL		
CROMOLYN & NEDOCROMIL			
Cromolyn (Intal)	MDI: 800mcg/puff	2 puffs qid	1-2 puffs tid-qid
	Neb Sol: 20mg/ampule	1 ampule tid-qid	1 ampule tid-qid
Nedocromil (Tilade)	MDI: 1.75mg/puff	2-4 puffs bid-qid	1-2 puffs bid-qid
LONG-ACTING BETA$_2$-AGONISTS			
Salmeterol (Serevent)	MDI: 21mcg/puff	2 puffs q 12 hours	1-2 puffs q 12 hours
	DPI: 50mcg/blister	1 blister q 12 hours	1 blister q 12 hours
Formoterol (Foradil)	DPI: 12mcg	1 cap q 12 hours	1 cap q 12 hours
COMBINATION AGENTS			
Fluticasone/ Salmeterol (Advair)	DPI: 100, 250, 500mcg/50mcg	1 puff bid	(100mcg/50mcg) 1 puff bid
METHYLXANTHINE			
Theophylline	Liquid, Capsules, Sustained-Release Tabs	Initial: 10mg/kg/day up to 300mg max. Usual Max: 800mg/day.	Initial: 10mg/kg/day. Usual Max: <1 yr: 0.2 x age in weeks + 5 = mg/kg/day. 1 yr: 16mg/kg/day.
LEUKOTRIENE MODIFIERS			
Montelukast (Singulair)	Tab: 10mg; Chewable: 4mg, 5mg	10mg qhs	2-5 yrs: 4mg qhs. 6-14 yrs: 5mg qhs. 15 yrs: 10mg qhs.
Zafirlukast (Accolate)	Tab: 10mg, 20mg	20mg bid	≥12 yrs: 20mg bid. 5-11 yrs: 10mg bid.
Zileuton (Zyflo)	Tab: 600mg	600mg qid	≥12 yr: 600mg qid

ESTIMATED COMPARATIVE DAILY DOSAGES FOR INHALED CORTICOSTEROIDS						
	LOW DAILY DOSE		MEDIUM DAILY DOSE		HIGH DAILY DOSE	
DRUG	ADULT	CHILD*	ADULT	CHILD*	ADULT	CHILD*
Beclomethasone HFA 40, 80mcg/puff (QVAR)	80-240mcg	80-160mcg	240-480mcg	160-320mcg	>480mcg	>320mcg
Budesonide DPI 200mcg/inhalation (Pulmicort Turbuhaler)	200-600mcg	200-400mcg	600-1200mcg	400-800mcg	>1200mcg	>800mcg
Budesonide Neb Sol: 0.25, 0.5mg/2mL (Pulmicort Respules)	N/A	0.5mg	N/A	1.0mg	N/A	2.0mg
Flunisolide 250mcg/puff (Aerobid)	500-1000mcg	500-750mcg	1000-2000mcg	1000-1250mcg	>2000mcg	>1250mcg
Fluticasone MDI 44, 110, or 220mcg/puff (Flovent)	88-264mcg	88-176mcg	264-660mcg	176-440mcg	>660mcg	>440mcg
Triamcinolone acetonide 100mcg/puff (Azmacort)	400-1000mcg	400-800mcg	1000-2000mcg	800-1200mcg	>2000mcg	>1200mcg

*Children ≤12 yrs unless otherwise noted. MDI: metered-dose inhaler; DPI: dry powder inhaler.
Adopted from: The NAEPP Expert Panel Report: Guidelines for the Diagnosis and Management of Asthma– Update on Selected Topics 2002. http://www.nhlbi.nih.gov/guidelines/asthma/asthsumm.htm

ASTHMA TREATMENT PLAN

CLASSIFICATION	LUNG FUNCTION	STEPWISE APPROACH TO THERAPY IN PATIENTS OVER 5 YEARS OF AGE
Mild intermittent • Symptoms ≤2 times a week • Asymptomatic and normal PEF between exacerbations • Brief exacerbations (from a few hours to a few days); intensity may vary • Nighttime symptoms ≤twice/month	• FEV_1 or PEF ≥80% predicted • PEF variability <20%	**Step 1** • **No daily medication required.** • **Short-acting inhaled ß₂-agonists as needed (2-4 puffs prn).** • Severe exacerbations may occur, separated by long periods of normal lung function and no symptoms; a course of systemic corticosteroids is recommended.
Mild persistent • Symptoms >2 times a week but <1 time a day • Exacerbations may affect activity • Nighttime symptoms >twice/month	• FEV_1 or PEF ≥80% predicted • PEF variability 20% to 30%	**Step 2** • **Low-dose inhaled corticosteroids.** • **Short-acting inhaled ß₂-agonists as needed (2-4 puffs prn).** ALTERNATIVE TREATMENT: • Cromolyn, leukotriene modifier, nedocromil OR • Sustained-release theophylline to serum concentration of 5 to 15mcg/mL.
Moderate persistent • Daily symptoms • Daily use of inhaled short-acting ß₂-agonist • Exacerbations affect activity • Exacerbations ≥2 times a week; may last days • Nighttime symptoms >once/week	• FEV_1 or PEF >60% to <80% predicted • PEF variability >30%	**Step 3** • **Low- to medium-dose inhaled corticosteroids** AND • **Long-acting inhaled ß₂-agonists.** • **Short-acting inhaled ß₂-agonists as needed (2-4 puffs prn).** ALTERNATIVE TREATMENT: • Increase inhaled corticosteroids within medium-dose range OR • Low- to medium-dose inhaled corticosteroids and either leukotriene modifier or theophylline. IF NEEDED: • Increase inhaled corticosteroids within medium-dose range, and add long-acting inhaled ß₂-agonists. ALTERNATIVE TREATMENT: Increase inhaled corticosteroids in medium-dose range, and add either leukotriene modifier or theophylline.
Severe persistent • Continual symptoms • Limited physical activity • Frequent exacerbations • Nighttime symptoms are frequent	• FEV_1 or PEF ≤60% predicted • PEF variability >30%	**Step 4** • **High-dose inhaled corticosteroids** AND • **Long-acting inhaled ß₂-agonists.** • **Short-acting inhaled ß₂-agonists as needed (2-4 puffs prn).** AND, IF NEEDED: • Long-term corticosteroid tablets or syrup (2mg/kg/day; Usual Max: 60mg/day). Make repeat attempts to reduce systemic corticosteroids and maintain control with high-dose inhaled corticosteroids.

Note: Preferred treatments are in bold.
Key Points:

- Stepwise approach presents general guidelines. Review treatment every 1 to 6 months; a gradual stepwise reduction in treatment may be possible. If control is not maintained, consider step up.
- The presence of one of the features of severity is sufficient to place a patient in that category. An individual should be assigned to the most severe grade in which any feature occurs (PEF is % of personal best; FEV is % predicted).
- Intensity of treatment will depend on severity of exacerbation; up to 3 treatments at 20-minute intervals or a single nebulizer treatment as needed. Course of systemic corticosteroids may be needed.
- Use of short-acting beta₂-agonists on a daily basis, or increasing use, indicates the need to initiate or increase long-term control therapy.
- Airflow obstruction is indicated by reduced FEV_1 and FEV_1/FVC values relative to reference or predicted values.
- Abnormalities of lung function are categorized as restrictive and obstructive defects. A reduced ratio of FEV_1/FVC (eg, <65%) indicates obstruction to the flow of air from the lungs, whereas a reduced FVC with a normal FEV_1/FVC ratio suggests a restrictive pattern.

Abbreviations: FEV_1: Forced expiratory volume in one second. FVC: Forced vital capacity.
*Adapted from the *1997 Guidelines for the Diagnosis and Management of Asthma* and the *Update on Selected Topics 2002.* Executive Summary of the NAEPP Expert Panel Report II.

HIV/AIDS PHARMACOTHERAPY

DRUG	BRAND	HOW SUPPLIED	USUAL DOSE	FOOD EFFECT
NUCLEOSIDE REVERSE TRANSCRIPTASE INHIBITORS (NRTIs)				
Abacavir (ABC)	Ziagen	Sol: 20mg/mL [240mL]; Tab: 300mg	*Adults:* >16 yrs: or 600mg qd. *Pediatrics:* 3 months-16 yrs: 8mg/kg bid. Max: 300mg bid.	Take without regard to meals.
Didanosine (ddI)	Videx Powder for Oral Sol; Videx EC	Powder for Sol: 2g, 4g; Cap, Delayed Release: (Videx EC) 125mg, 200mg, 250mg, 400mg	*Adults:* ≥60kg: (Cap) 400mg qd; (Sol) 200mg bid or 400mg qd. <60kg: (Cap) 250mg qd. (Sol) 125mg bid or 250mg qd. *Pediatrics:* 2 weeks-8 months: (Sol) 100mg/m² bid. >8 months: 120mg/m² bid.	Take on empty stomach at least 30 minutes before or 2 hrs after meals. Swallow caps whole.
Emtricitabine (FTC)	Emtriva	Cap: 200mg; Sol: 10mg/mL	*Adults:* ≥18 yrs: Cap: 200mg qd. Sol: 240mg (24mL) qd. *Pediatrics:* 0-3 mos: 3mg/kg qd. 3 mos-17 yrs: Cap: >33kg: 200mg qd. Sol: 6mg/kg qd. Max: 240mg (24mL).	Take without regard to meals.
Lamivudine	Epivir	Sol: 10mg/mL [240mL]; Tab: 150mg, 300mg	*Adults:* 150mg bid or 300mg qd. *Pediatrics:* 3 months-16 yrs: 4mg/kg bid. Max: 150mg bid.	Take without regard to meals.
Stavudine (d4T)	Zerit	Cap: 15mg, 20mg, 30mg, 40mg; Sol: 1mg/mL [200mL]	*Adults:* ≥60kg: 40mg q12h. <60kg: 30mg q12h. *Pediatrics:* ≥60kg: 40mg q12h. 30-59 kg: 30mg q12h. ≥14 days and <30kg: 1mg/kg q12h. Birth-13 days: 0.5mg/kg q12h.	Take without regard to meals
Tenofovir Disoproxil Fumarate (TDF)	Viread	Tab: 300mg	*Adults:* 300mg once daily.	Take without regard to meals.
Zalcitabine (ddC)	Hivid	Tab: 0.375mg, 0.75mg	*Adults:* 0.75mg q8h. *Pediatrics:* >13 yrs: 0.75mg q8h.	Take without regard to meals.
Zidovudine (AZT, ZDV)	Retrovir	Cap: 100mg; Inj: 10mg/mL; Sol: 10mg/mL; Tab: 300mg	*Adults:* (Cap, Tab) 600mg/day in divided doses. (Inj) 1mg/kg IV over 1 hr 5-6 times/day. *Pediatrics:* 6 weeks-12 yrs: 160mg/m² PO q8h. Max: 200mg PO q8h.	Take without regard to meals.
NON NUCLEOSIDE REVERSE TRANSCRIPTATSE INHIBITORS (NNRTIs)				
Delavirdine (DLV)	Rescriptor	Tab: 100mg, 200mg	*Adults:* Usual: 400mg tid. *Pediatrics:* ≥16yrs: Usual: 400mg tid.	Take without regard to meals.
Efavirenz (EFV)	Sustiva	Cap: 50mg, 100mg, 200mg; Tab: 600mg	*Adults:* Initial: 600mg qd at bedtime. *Pediatrics:* ≥3 yrs: 10 to <15kg: 200mg qd. 15 to <20kg: 250mg qd. 20 to <25kg: 300mg qd. 25 to <32.5kg: 350mg qd. 32.5 to <40kg: 400mg qd. ≥40kg: 600mg qd at bedtime.	Take on an empty stomach.

(Continued)

HIV/AIDS PHARMACOTHERAPY

DRUG	BRAND	HOW SUPPLIED	USUAL DOSE	FOOD EFFECT
NON NUCLEOSIDE REVERSE TRANSCRIPTATSE INHIBITORS (NNRTIs) *(Continued)*				
Nevirapine (NVP)	Viramune	Sus: 50mg/5mL [240mL]; Tab: 200mg* *scored	*Adults:* 200mg qd for 14 days (lead-in period), then 200mg bid. *Pediatrics:* 2 months-8 yrs: 4mg/kg qd for 14 days, then 7mg/kg bid. Max: 400mg/day. 8 yrs: 4mg/kg qd for 14 days, then 4mg/kg bid. Max: 400mg/day.	Take without regard to meals.
PROTEASE INHIBITORS (PIs)				
Amprenavir (APV)	Agenerase	Cap: 50mg; Sol: 15mg/mL [240mL]	*Adults:* (Cap) 1200mg bid. (Sol): 1400mg bid. *Pediatrics:* (Cap) 13-16 yrs: 1200mg bid. 13-16 yrs and <50kg or 4-12yrs: 20mg/kg bid or 15mg/kg tid. Max: 2400mg/day. (Sol) >16 yrs or 13-16 yrs and ≥50kg: 1400mg bid. 4-12 yrs or 13-16 yrs and <50kg: 22.5mg/kg bid or 17mg/kg tid. Max: 2800mg/day.	Take without regard to meals but avoid high fat foods.
Atazanavir (ATV)	Reyataz	Cap: 100mg, 150mg, 200mg, 300mg	*Adults:* Therapy-naive: 400mg qd. Therapy Experienced: (ATV 300mg + RTV 100mg)qd.	Take with food; avoid taking with antacids.
Darunavir (DRV)	Prezista	Tab: 300mg	*Adults:* (DRV 600mg + RTV 100mg) bid.	Take with food.
Fosamprenavir (fAPV)	Lexiva	Tab: 700mg	*Adults:* Therapy-naive: 1400mg bid OR 1400mg qd + RTV 200mg qd OR 700mg bid + RTV 100mg bid. PI-Experienced: 700mg bid + RTV 100mg bid.	Take without regard to meals.
Indinavir (IDV)	Crixivan	Cap: 100mg, 200mg, 333mg, 400mg	*Adults:* 800mg q8h OR (IDV 800mg + RTV 100 or 200mg) q12h.	Take 1 hr before or 2 hr after meals; may take with skim milk or low-fat meal. RTV-boosted, take with or without food.
Nelfinavir (NFV)	Viracept	Sus: (powder) 50mg/g [144g] Tab: 250mg, 625mg	*Adults:* 1250mg bid or 750mg tid. *Pediatrics:* 2-13 yrs: 45-55mg/kg bid; 25-35mg/kg tid. Max: 2500mg/day	Take with meal.
Ritonavir (RTV)	Norvir	Cap: 100mg Sol: 80mg/mL [240mL]	*Adults:* Initial: 300mg bid. Titrate: Increase every 2-3 days by 100mg bid. Maint: 600mg bid. *Pediatrics:* >1 month: Initial: 250mg/m^2 po bid. Titrate: Increase by 50mg/m^2 every 2-3 days. Maint: 350-400mg/m^2 po bid or highest tolerated dose. Max: 600mg bid.	Take with food, may improve tolerability.

(Continued)

HIV/AIDS Pharmacotherapy

DRUG	BRAND	HOW SUPPLIED	USUAL DOSE	FOOD EFFECT
PROTEASE INHIBITORS (PIs) *(Continued)*				
Saquinavir (SQV)	Invirase*	Hard Gel Cap: 200mg Tab: 500mg	*Adults/Pediatrics:* >16 yrs: 1000mg bid with RTV 100mg bid OR 1000mg bid with LPV/RTV 400/100mg bid (no additional RTV).	Take within 2 hrs after a meal when taken with RTV.
	Fortovase*	Soft Gelatin Cap: 200mg	*Adults/Pediatrics:* >16 yrs: 1200mg tid OR 1000mg bid with RTV 100mg bid.	Take with a meal or up to 2 hrs after a meal.
Tipranavir (TPV)	Aptivus	Cap: 250mg	*Adults:* (500mg + RTV 200mg) bid.	Take with food.
FUSION INHIBITORS				
Enfuvirtide (T20)	Fuzeon	Inj: 90mg/1ml (60s)	*Adults:* 90mg SQ bid. *Pediatrics:* 6-16 yrs: 2mg/kg SQ bid. Max: 90mg bid. 11-15.5kg: 27mg bid. 15.6-20.0kg: 36mg bid. 20.1-24.5kg: 45mg bid. 24.6-29.0kg: 54mg bid. 29.1-33.5kg: 63mg bid. 33.6-38.0kg: 72mg bid. 38.1-42.5kg: 81mg bid. ≥42.6kg: 90mg bid.	
COMBINATIONS				
EFV/FTC/TDF	Atripla	Tab: (Efavirenz-Emtricitabine-Tenofovir DF) 600mg-200mg-300mg	*Adults:* ≥18 yrs: 1 tab qd.	Take on empty stomach.
3TC/ZDV	Combivir	Tab: (Lamivudine-Zidovudine) 150mg-300mg	*Adults:* 1 tab bid. *Pediatrics:* ≥12 yrs: 1 tab bid. Do not give if CrCl ≤50mL/min.	Take without regard to meals.
ABC/3TC	Epzicom	Tab: (Abacavir Sulfate-Lamivudine) 600mg-300mg	*Adults:* ≥18 yrs: CrCl >50mL min: 1 tab qd.	Take without regard to meals.
LPV/RTV	Kaletra	Tab: (Lopinavir-Ritonavir) 200mg-50mg; Sol: (Lopinavir-Ritonavir) 80mg-20mg/mL [160mL]	*Adults:* Therapy-Naive: 400/100mg (2 tabs or 5mL) bid or 800/200mg qd (4 tabs or 10mL). Therapy Experienced: 400/100mg bid (2 tabs or 5mL).	Take without regard to meals. Sol: Take with meal.
ABC/ZDV/3TC	Trizivir	Tab: (Abacavir-Lamivudine-Zidovudine) 300mg-150mg-300mg	*Adults:* >40kg and CrCl >50mL/min: 1 tab bid.	Take without regard to meals.
FTC/TDF	Truvada	Tab: (Emtricitabine-Tenofovir Disoproxil Fumarate) 200mg-300mg	*Adults:* ≥18 years: CrCl ≥50mL/min: 1 tab qd. CrCl 30-49mL/min: 1 tab q48h.	Take without regard to meals.

*Invirase and Fortovase are not bioequivalent and cannot be used interchangeably.

Sources: FDA Approved Labeling; Guidelines for the Use of Antiretroviral Agents in HIV-1-Infected Adults and Adolescents - October 10, 2006.

Insulin Formulations

TYPE OF INSULIN	BRAND	ONSET* (hrs)	PEAK* (hrs)	DURATION* (hrs)	COMMON PITFALLS**
Rapid-acting Insulin Glulisine Human Insulin Inhalation Powder Insulin Lispro Insulin Aspart	Apidra Exubera Humalog Novolog	– 10-20 min <0.25 <0.25	0.5 to 1.7 0.5 to 1.5 0.5 to 1.5 0.5 to 1	1 to 3 6 3 to 5 3 to 5	See individual comments. See individual comments. Hypoglycemia occurs if lag time is too long or the patient exercises within 1 hr of dose; with high-fat meals, the dose should be adjusted downward.
Short-acting Regular Insulin	Humulin R† Novolin R	0.5 to 1 0.5 to 1	2 to 4 2 to 5	4 to 12 8	Lag time is not used appropriately; the insulin should be given 20 to 30 minutes before the patient eats.
Intermediate-acting NPH (Isophane)	Humulin N Novolin R	1 to 3	6 to 12	18 to 24	In many patients, breakfast injection does not last the evening until the evening meal; administration with the evening meal does not meet insulin needs on awakening.
Long-acting Insulin glargine Insulin detemir	Lantus Levemir	1 –	Flat 6 to 8	24 24	Administer once daily at the same time every day. See individual comments.
Combinations Isophane insulin suspension (70%)/regular insulin (30%)	Humulin 70/30 Novolin 70/30	0.5 to 1	4 to 6	24	See individual comments.
Isophane insulin suspension (50%)/regular insulin (50%)	Humulin 50/50	0.5 to 1	3 to 5	24	See individual comments.
Insulin lispro protamine (75%)/insulin lispro (25%)	Humalog Mix 75/25	≤0.25	0.5 to 4	24	See individual comments.
Insulin aspart protamine (70%)/ insulin aspart (30%)	Novolog Mix 70/30	≤0.25	1 to 4	24	See individual comments.

*Approximate parameters following SC injection of an average patient dose; insulin concentration: 100U/mL. (Not applicable for inhalation insulin.)

**Source: Hirsch, IB. Type 1 Diabetes Mellitus and the Use of Flexible Insulin Regimens. *Am Fam Physician.* November 1999;60(8):2343-2352, 2355-2356.

†Also available 500 U/mL for insulin resistant patients (rapid onset; up to 24 hour duration).

ORAL CONTRACEPTIVES

DRUG	ESTROGEN	PROGESTIN	STRENGTH (ESTROGEN/PROGESTIN)
MONOPHASIC			
Alesse, Levlite	Ethinyl Estradiol	Levonorgestrel	20mcg/0.1mg
Brevicon, Modicon	Ethinyl Estradiol	Norethindrone	35mcg/0.5mg
Demulen 1/35	Ethinyl Estradiol	Ethynodiol Diacetate	35mcg/1mg
Demulen 1/50	Ethinyl Estradiol	Ethynodiol Diacetate	50mcg/1mg
Desogen, Ortho-Cept	Ethinyl Estradiol	Desogestrel	30mcg/0.15mg
Levlen, Nordette-28	Ethinyl Estradiol	Levonorgestrel	30mcg/0.15mg
Loestrin 21 1/20, Loestrin Fe 1/20	Ethinyl Estradiol	Norethindrone Acetate	20mcg/1mg
Loestrin 21 1.5/30, Loestrin Fe 1.5/30	Ethinyl Estradiol	Norethindrone Acetate	30mcg/1.5mg
Lo/Ovral	Ethinyl Estradiol	Norgestrel	30mcg/0.3mg
Lybrel	Ethinyl Estradiol	Levonorgestrel	20mcg/90mcg
Norinyl 1/35, Ortho-Novum 1/35	Ethinyl Estradiol	Norethindrone	35mcg/1mg
Norinyl 1/50, Ortho-Novum 1/50	Mestranol	Norethindrone	50mcg/1mg
Ortho-Cyclen	Ethinyl Estradiol	Norgestimate	35mcg/0.25mg
Ovcon 35	Ethinyl Estradiol	Norethindrone	35mcg/0.4mg
Ovcon 50	Ethinyl Estradiol	Norethindrone	50mcg/1mg
Seasonale	Ethinyl Estradiol	Levonorgestrel	30mcg/0.15mg
Seasonique	Ethinyl Estradiol	Levonorgestrel	0.01mg, 0.15mg/0.03mg
Yasmin	Ethinyl Estradiol	Drospirenone	30mcg/3mg
YAZ	Ethinyl Estradiol	Drospirenone	0.02mg/3mg
BIPHASIC			
Ortho-Novum 10/11	Ethinyl Estradiol	Norethindrone	**Phase 1:** 35mcg/0.5mg **Phase 2:** 35mcg/1mg
Mircette	Ethinyl Estradiol	Desogestrel	**Phase 1:** 20mcg/0.15mg **Phase 2:** 10mcg/NONE
TRIPHASIC			
Cyclessa	Ethinyl Estradiol	Desogestrel	**Phase 1:** 25mcg/0.1mg **Phase 2:** 25mcg/0.125mg **Phase 3:** 25mcg/0.15mg
Estrostep Fe	Ethinyl Estradiol	Norethindrone Acetate	**Phase 1:** 20mcg/1mg **Phase 2:** 30mcg/1mg **Phase 3:** 35mcg/1mg
Ortho-Novum 7/7/7	Ethinyl Estradiol	Norethindrone	**Phase 1:** 35mcg/0.5mg **Phase 2:** 35mcg/0.75mg **Phase 3:** 35mcg/1mg
Ortho Tri-Cyclen	Ethinyl Estradiol	Norgestimate	**Phase 1:** 35mcg/0.18mg **Phase 2:** 35mcg/0.215mg **Phase 3:** 35mcg/0.25mg
Ortho Tri-Cyclen Lo	Ethinyl Estradiol	Norgestimate	**Phase 1:** 25mcg/0.18mg **Phase 2:** 25mcg/0.215mg **Phase 3:** 25mcg/0.25mg
Tri-Levlen, Triphasil, Trivora 28	Ethinyl Estradiol	Levonorgestrel	**Phase 1:** 30mcg/0.05mg **Phase 2:** 40mcg/0.075mg **Phase 3:** 30mcg/0.125mg

(Continued)

Oral Contraceptives

DRUG	ESTROGEN	PROGESTIN	STRENGTH (ESTROGEN/PROGESTIN)
TRIPHASIC *(Continued)*			
Tri-Norinyl	Ethinyl Estradiol	Norethindrone	**Phase 1:** 35mcg/0.5mg **Phase 2:** 35mcg/1mg **Phase 3:** 35mcg/0.5mg
PROGESTIN ONLY			
Nor-Q.D., Ortho-Micronor		Norethindrone	0.35mg

Topical Corticosteroids

STEROID	DOSAGE FORM(S)	STRENGTH (%)	POTENCY	FREQUENCY
Alclometasone Dipropionate (Aclovate)	Cre, Oint	0.05	Low	bid/tid
Augmented Betamethasone Dipropionate	Oint	0.05	Very High	qd/bid
(Diprolene, Diprolene AF)	Cre, Lot	0.05	High	qd/bid
Betamethasone Dipropionate	Cre, Lot, Oint	0.05	High	qd/bid
Betamethasone Valerate (Beta-Val)	Cre, Lot	0.1	Medium	qd/tid
(Luxiq)	Foam, Lot	0.12, 0.1	Medium	bid
Clobetasol Propionate (Clobex, Cormax, Olux, Temovate, Temovate-E)	Cre, Foam (Olux), Gel, Lotion (Clobex), Oint, Shampoo (Clobex), Sol	0.05	Very High	bid qd (shampoo)
Clocortolone Pivalate (Cloderm)	Cre	0.1	Low	tid
Desonide (DesOwen, Verdeso)	Cre, Foam, Lot, Oint	0.05	Low	bid/tid
Desoximetasone	Cre	0.05	Medium	bid
(Topicort, Topicort LP)	Cre, Oint	0.25	High	bid
	Gel	0.05	High	bid
Diflorasone Diacetate	Cre, Oint (Maxiflor)	0.05	High	qd/tid
(Maxiflor, Psorcon)	Oint (Psorcon)	0.05	Very High	qd/qid
Fluocinolone Acetonide	Cre, Oint	0.025	Medium	bid/qid
(Capex, Derma-Smoothe/FS, Synalar)	Sol	0.01	Medium	bid/qid
	Oil (Derma-Smoothe/FS)	0.01	Medium	qd/tid
	Shampoo (Capex)	0.01	Medium	qd
Fluocinonide	Cre, Gel, Oint, Sol	0.05	High	bid/qid
(Lidex, Lidex-E, Vanos)	Cre	0.1	Very High	qd/bid
Flurandrenolide	Cre, Oint	0.025	Medium	bid/tid
(Cordran, Cordran SP)	Cre, Lot, Oint	0.05	Medium	bid/tid
	Tape	4mcg/cm^2	Medium	qd/bid
Fluticasone Propionate	Cre, Lot	0.05	Medium	qd/bid
(Cutivate)	Oint	0.005	Medium	bid
Halcinonide (Halog, Halog-E)	Cre, Oint, Sol	0.1	High	qd/tid
Halobetasol Propionate (Ultravate)	Cre, Oint	0.05	Very High	qd/bid
Hydrocortisone	Cre, Lot, Oint	0.5	Low	tid/qid
(Ala-Cort, Ala-Scalp, Anusol HC, Cetacort, Hi-Cort, Hytone, Nutracort, Stie-Cort, Synacort, Texacort)	Cre, Lot, Oint, Sol	1	Low	tid/qid
	Lot	2	Low	tid/qid
	Cre, Lot, Oint, Sol	2.5	Low	tid/qid
Hydrocortisone Butyrate (Locoid, Locoid Lipo Cream)	Cre, Lot, Oint, Sol	0.1	Medium	bid/tid
Hydrocortisone Probutate (Pandel)	Cre	0.1	Medium	qd/bid
Hydrocortisone Valerate (Westcort)	Cre, Oint	0.2	Medium	bid/tid
Mometasone Furoate (Elocon)	Cre, Lot, Oint	0.1	Medium	qd
Prednicarbate (Dermatop)	Cre, Oint	0.1	Medium	bid
Triamcinolone Acetonide	Cre, Lot, Oint	0.025	Medium	bid/qid
(Kenalog, Triderm)	Cre, Lot, Oint	0.1	Medium	bid/tid
	Cre, Oint	0.5	High	bid/tid
	Spray	0.147	Medium	tid/qid

IMMUNIZATION SCHEDULE FOR PERSONS 0-6 YEARS

RECOMMENDED IMMUNIZATION SCHEDULE FOR PERSONS AGED 0-6 YEARS

Vaccine ▼ Age ▶	Birth	1 month	2 months	4 months	6 months	12 months	15 months	18 months	19–23 months	2–3 years	4–6 years
Hepatitis B[1]	HepB	HepB	see footnote 1		HepB					HepB Series	
Rotavirus[2]			Rota	Rota	Rota						
Diphtheria, Tetanus, Pertussis[3]			DTaP	DTaP	DTaP		DTaP				DTaP
Haemophilus influenzae type b[4]			Hib	Hib	Hib[4]	Hib			Hib		
Pneumococcal[5]			PCV	PCV	PCV	PCV				PCV / PPV	
Inactivated Poliovirus			IPV	IPV		IPV					IPV
Influenza[6]						Influenza (Yearly)					
Measles, Mumps, Rubella[7]						MMR					MMR
Varicella[8]						Varicella					Varicella
Hepatitis A[9]						HepA (2 doses)				HepA Series	
Meningococcal[10]											MPSV4

Range of recommended ages   Catch-up immunization   Certain high-risk groups

This schedule indicates the recommended ages for routine administration of currently licensed childhood vaccines, as of December 1, 2006, for children aged 0–6 years. Additional information is available at **http://www.cdc.gov/nip/recs/child-schedule.htm**. Any dose not administered at the recommended age should be administered at any subsequent visit, when indicated and feasible. Additional vaccines may be licensed and recommended during the year. Licensed combination vaccines may be used whenever any components of the combination are indicated and other components of the vaccine are not contraindicated and if approved by the Food and Drug Administration for that dose of the series. Providers should consult the respective Advisory Committee on Immunization Practices statement for detailed recommendations. Clinically significant adverse events that follow immunization should be reported to the Vaccine Adverse Event Reporting System (VAERS). Guidance about how to obtain and complete a VAERS form is available at **http://www.vaers.hhs.gov** or by telephone, **800-822-7967**.

1. **Hepatitis B vaccine (HepB).** *(Minimum age: birth)*
   At birth:
   - Administer monovalent HepB to all newborns before hospital discharge.
   - If mother is hepatitis surface antigen (HBsAg)-positive, administer HepB and 0.5 mL of hepatitis B immune globulin (HBIG) within 12 hours of birth.
   - If mother's HBsAg status is unknown, administer HepB within 12 hours of birth. Determine the HBsAg status as soon as possible and if HBsAg-positive, administer HBIG (no later than age 1 week).
   - If mother is HBsAg-negative, the birth dose can only be delayed with physician's order and mother's negative HBsAg laboratory report documented in the infant's medical record.

   After the birth dose:
   - The HepB series should be completed with either monovalent HepB or a combination vaccine containing HepB. The second dose should be administered at age 1–2 months. The final dose should be administered at age ≥24 weeks. Infants born to HBsAg-positive mothers should be tested for HBsAg and antibody to HBsAg after completion of ≥3 doses of a licensed HepB series, at age 9–18 months (generally at the next well-child visit).

   4-month dose:
   - It is permissible to administer 4 doses of HepB when combination vaccines are administered after the birth dose. If monovalent HepB is used for doses after the birth dose, a dose at age 4 months is not needed.

2. **Rotavirus vaccine (Rota).** *(Minimum age: 6 weeks)*
   - Administer the first dose at age 6–12 weeks. Do not start the series later than age 12 weeks.
   - Administer the final dose in the series by age 32 weeks. Do not administer a dose later than age 32 weeks.
   - Data on safety and efficacy outside of these age ranges are insufficient.

3. **Diphtheria and tetanus toxoids and acellular pertussis vaccine (DTaP).** *(Minimum age: 6 weeks)*
   - The fourth dose of DTaP may be administered as early as age 12 months, provided 6 months have elapsed since the third dose.
   - Administer the final dose in the series at age 4–6 years.

4. **Haemophilus influenzae type b conjugate vaccine (Hib).** *(Minimum age: 6 weeks)*
   - If PRP-OMP (PedvaxHIB® or ComVax® [Merck]) is administered at ages 2 and 4 months, a dose at age 6 months is not required.
   - TriHiBit® (DTaP/Hib) combination products should not be used for primary immunization but can be used as boosters following any Hib vaccine in children aged ≥12 months.

(Continued)

A191

Immunization Schedule for Persons 0-6 Years

5. **Pneumococcal vaccine.** *(Minimum age: 6 weeks for pneumococcal conjugate vaccine [PCV]; 2 years for pneumococcal polysaccharide vaccine [PPV])*
   - Administer PCV at ages 24–59 months in certain high-risk groups. Administer PPV to children aged ≥2 years in certain high-risk groups. See *MMWR* 2000;49(No. RR-9):1–35.

6. **Influenza vaccine.** *(Minimum age: 6 months for trivalent inactivated influenza vaccine [TIV]; 5 years for live, attenuated influenza vaccine [LAIV])*
   - All children aged 6–59 months and close contacts of all children aged 0–59 months are recommended to receive influenza vaccine.
   - Influenza vaccine is recommended annually for children aged ≥59 months with certain risk factors, health-care workers, and other persons (including household members) in close contact with persons in groups at high risk. See *MMWR* 2006;55(No. RR-10):1–41.
   - For healthy persons aged 5–49 years, LAIV may be used as an alternative to TIV.
   - Children receiving TIV should receive 0.25 mL if aged 6–35 months or 0.5 mL if aged ≥3 years.
   - Children aged <9 years who are receiving influenza vaccine for the first time should receive 2 doses (separated by ≥4 weeks for TIV and ≥6 weeks for LAIV).

7. **Measles, mumps, and rubella vaccine (MMR).** *(Minimum age: 12 months)*
   - Administer the second dose of MMR at age 4–6 years. MMR may be administered before age 4–6 years, provided ≥4 weeks have elapsed since the first dose and both doses are administered at age ≥12 months.

8. **Varicella vaccine.** *(Minimum age: 12 months)*
   - Administer the second dose of varicella vaccine at age 4–6 years. Varicella vaccine may be administered before age 4–6 years, provided that ≥3 months have elapsed since the first dose and both doses are administered at age ≥12 months. If second dose was administered ≥28 days following the first dose, the second dose does not need to be repeated.

9. **Hepatitis A vaccine (HepA).** *(Minimum age: 12 months)*
   - HepA is recommended for all children aged 1 year (i.e., aged 12–23 months). The 2 doses in the series should be administered at least 6 months apart.
   - Children not fully vaccinated by age 2 years can be vaccinated at subsequent visits.
   - HepA is recommended for certain other groups of children, including in areas where vaccination programs target older children. See *MMWR* 2006;55(No. RR-7):1–23.

10. **Meningococcal polysaccharide vaccine (MPSV4).** *(Minimum age: 2 years)*
    - Administer MPSV4 to children aged 2–10 years with terminal complement deficiencies or anatomic or functional asplenia and certain other high-risk groups. See MMWR 2005;54(No. RR-7):1–21.

The Recommended Immunization Schedules for Persons Aged 0–18 Years are approved by the Advisory Committee on Immunization Practices **(http://www.cdc.gov/nip/acip)**, the American Academy of Pediatrics **(http://www.aap.org)**, and the American Academy of Family Physicians **(http://www.aafp.org)**.

Recommended Immunization Schedule for Persons Aged 7-18 Years

This schedule indicates the recommended ages for routine administration of currently licensed childhood vaccines, as of December 1, 2006, for children aged 7-18 years. Additional information is available at http://www.cdc.gov/nip/recs/child-schedule.htm. Any dose not administered at the recommended age should be administered at any subsequent visit, when indicated and feasible. Additional vaccines may be licensed and recommended during the year. Licensed combination vaccines may be used whenever any components of the combination are indicated and other components of the vaccine are not contraindicated and if approved by the Food and Drug Administration for that dose of the series. Providers should consult the respective Advisory Committee on Immunization Practices statement for detailed recommendations. Clinically significant adverse events that follow immunization should be reported to the Vaccine Adverse Event Reporting System (VAERS). Guidance about how to obtain and complete a VAERS form is available at http://www.vaers.hhs.gov or by telephone, 800-822-7967.

1. **Tetanus and diphtheria toxoids and acellular pertussis vaccine (Tdap).** *(Minimum age: 10 years for BOOSTRIX® and 11 years for ADACEL™)*

   - Administer at age 11–12 years for those who have completed the recommended childhood DTP/DTaP vaccination series and have not received a tetanus and diphtheria toxoids vaccine (Td) booster dose.
   - Adolescents aged 13–18 years who missed the 11–12 year Td/Tdap booster dose should also receive a single dose of Tdap if they have completed the recommended childhood DTP/DTaP vaccination series.

2. **Human papillomavirus vaccine (HPV).** *(Minimum age: 9 years)*

   - Administer the first dose of the HPV vaccine series to females at age 11–12 years.
   - Administer the second dose 2 months after the first dose and the third dose 6 months after the first dose.
   - Administer the HPV vaccine series to females at age 13–18 years if not previously vaccinated.

3. **Meningococcal vaccine.** *(Minimum age: 11 years for meningococcal conjugate vaccine [MCV4]; 2 years for meningococcal polysaccharide vaccine [MPSV4])*

   - Administer MCV4 at age 11–12 years and to previously unvaccinated adolescents at high school entry (at approximately age 15 years).
   - Administer MCV4 to previously unvaccinated college freshmen living in dormitories; MPSV4 is an acceptable alternative.
   - Vaccination against invasive meningococcal disease is recommended for children and adolescents aged ≥2 years with terminal complement deficiencies or anatomic or functional asplenia and certain other high-risk groups. See MMWR 2005;54(No. RR-7):1–21. Use MPSV4 for children aged 2–10 years and MCV4 or MPSV4 for older children.

4. **Pneumococcal polysaccharide vaccine (PPV).** *(Minimum age: 2 years)*

   - Administer for certain high-risk groups. See MMWR 1997;46(No. RR-8):1–24, and MMWR 2000;49(No. RR-9):1–35.

5. **Influenza vaccine.** *(Minimum age: 6 months for trivalent inactivated influenza vaccine [TIV]; 5 years for live, attenuated influenza vaccine [LAIV])*

   - Influenza vaccine is recommended annually for persons with certain risk factors, health-care workers, and other persons (including household members) in close contact with persons in groups at high risk. See MMWR 2006;55 (No. RR-10):1–41.
   - For healthy persons aged 5–49 years, LAIV may be used as an alternative to TIV.
   - Children aged <9 years who are receiving influenza vaccine for the first time should receive 2 doses (separated by >4 weeks for TIV and >6 weeks for LAIV).

(Continued)

Immunization Schedule for Persons 7-18 Years

6. **Hepatitis A vaccine (HepA).** *(Minimum age: 12 months)*
   - The 2 doses in the series should be administered at least 6 months apart.
   - HepA is recommended for certain other groups of children, including in areas where vaccination programs target older children. See *MMWR* 2006;55 (No. RR-7):1–23.

7. **Hepatitis B vaccine (HepB).** *(Minimum age: birth)*
   - Administer the 3-dose series to those who were not previously vaccinated.
   - A 2-dose series of Recombivax HB® is licensed for children aged 11–15 years.

8. **Inactivated poliovirus vaccine (IPV).** *(Minimum age: 6 weeks)*
   - For children who received an all-IPV or all-oral poliovirus (OPV) series, a fourth dose is not necessary if the third dose was administered at age ≥4 years.
   - If both OPV and IPV were administered as part of a series, a total of 4 doses should be administered, regardless of the child's current age.

9. **Measles, mumps, and rubella vaccine (MMR).** *(Minimum age: 12 months)*
   - If not previously vaccinated, administer 2 doses of MMR during any visit, with >4 weeks between the doses.

10. **Varicella vaccine.** *(Minimum age: 12 months)*
    - Administer 2 doses of varicella vaccine to persons without evidence of immunity.
    - Administer 2 doses of varicella vaccine to persons aged <13 years at least 3 months apart. Do not repeat the second dose, if administered ≥28 days after the first dose.
    - Administer 2 doses of varicella vaccine to persons aged ≥13 years at least 4 weeks apart.

The Recommended Immunization Schedules for Persons Aged 0–18 Years are approved by the Advisory Committee on Immunization Practices (**http://www.cdc.gov/nip/acip**), the American Academy of Pediatrics (**http://www.aap.org**), and the American Academy of Family Physicians (**http://www.aafp.org**).

Catch-up Immunization Schedule for Persons Aged 4 Months–18 Years Who Start Late or Who Are More Than 1 Month Behind

Vaccine	Minimum Age for Dose 1	Dose 1 to Dose 2	Dose 2 to Dose 3	Dose 3 to Dose 4	Dose 4 to Dose 5
CATCH-UP SCHEDULE FOR PERSONS AGED 4 MONTHS–6 YEARS					
Hepatitis B[1]	Birth	4 weeks	8 weeks (and 16 weeks after first dose)		
Rotavirus[2]	6 wks	4 weeks	4 weeks		
Diphtheria, Tetanus, Pertussis[3]	6 wks	4 weeks	4 weeks	6 months	6 months[a]
Haemophilus influenzae type b[4]	6 wks	4 weeks if first dose administered at age <12 months; 8 weeks (as final dose) if first dose administered at age 12-14 months; No further doses needed if first dose administered at age ≥15 months	4 weeks if current age <12 months; 8 weeks (as final dose)[a] if current age ≥12 months and second dose administered at age <15 months; No further doses needed if previous dose administered at age ≥15 months	8 weeks (as final dose) This dose only necessary for children aged 12 months–5 years who received 3 doses before age 12 months	
Pneumococcal[5]	6 wks	4 weeks if first dose administered at age <12 months and current age <24 months; 8 weeks (as final dose) if first dose administered at age ≥12 months or current age 24–59 months; No further doses needed for healthy children if first dose administered at age ≥24 months	4 weeks if current age <12 months; 8 weeks (as final dose) if current age ≥12 months; No further doses needed for healthy children if previous dose administered at age ≥24 months	8 weeks (as final dose) This dose only necessary for children aged 12 months–5 years who received 3 doses before age 12 months	
Inactivated Poliovirus[6]	6 wks	4 weeks	4 weeks	4 weeks[a]	
Measles, Mumps, Rubella[7]	12 mos	4 weeks			
Varicella[8]	12 mos	3 months			
Hepatitis A[9]	12 mos	6 months			
CATCH-UP SCHEDULE FOR PERSONS AGED 7–18 YEARS					
Tetanus, Diphtheria/Tetanus, Diphtheria, Pertussis[10]	7 yrs[10]	4 weeks	8 weeks if first dose administered at age <12 months; 6 months if first dose administered at age ≥12 months	6 months if first dose administered at age <12 months	
Human Papillomavirus[11]	9 yrs	4 weeks	12 weeks		
Hepatitis A[9]	12 mos	6 months			
Hepatitis B[1]	Birth	4 weeks	8 weeks (and 16 weeks after first dose)		
Inactivated Poliovirus[6]	6 wks	4 weeks	4 weeks	4 weeks[a]	
Measles, Mumps, Rubella[7]	12 mos	4 weeks			
Varicella[8]	12 mos	4 weeks if first dose administered at age ≥13 years; 3 months if first dose administered at age <13 years			

The table above provides catch-up schedules and minimum intervals between doses for children whose vaccinations have been delayed. A vaccine series does not need to be restarted, regardless of the time that has elapsed between doses. Use the section appropriate for the child's age.

1. **Hepatitis B vaccine (HepB).** *(Minimum age: birth)*
   - Administer the 3-dose series to those who were not previously vaccinated.
   - A 2-dose series of Recombivax HB® is licensed for children aged 11–15 years.

2. **Rotavirus vaccine (Rota).** *(Minimum age: 6 weeks)*
   - Do not start the series later than age 12 weeks.
   - Administer the final dose in the series by age 32 weeks. Do not administer a dose later than age 32 weeks.
   - Data on safety and efficacy outside of these age ranges are insufficient.

3. **Diphtheria and tetanus toxoids and acellular pertussis vaccine (DTaP).** *(Minimum age: 6 weeks)*
   - The fifth dose is not necessary if the fourth dose was administered at age ≥4 years.
   - DTaP is not indicated for persons aged ≥7 years.

4. **Haemophilus influenzae type b conjugate vaccine (Hib).** *(Minimum age: 6 weeks)*
   - Vaccine is not generally recommended for children aged ≥5 years.
   - If current age <12 months and the first 2 doses were PRP-OMP (PedvaxHIB® or ComVax® [Merck]), the third (and final) dose should be administered at age 12–15 months and at least 8 weeks after the second dose.
   - If first dose was administered at age 7–11 months, administer 2 doses separated by 4 weeks plus a booster at age 12–15 months.

5. **Pneumococcal conjugate vaccine (PCV).** *(Minimum age: 6 weeks)*
   - Vaccine is not generally recommended for children aged ≥5 years.

6. **Inactivated poliovirus vaccine (IPV).** *(Minimum age: 6 weeks)*
   - For children who received an all-IPV or all-oral poliovirus (OPV) series, a fourth dose is not necessary if third dose was administered at age ≥4 years.
   - If both OPV and IPV were administered as part of a series, a total of 4 doses should be administered, regardless of the child's current age.

(Continued)

Catch-up Immunization Schedule for Persons 4 Months–18 Years

7. **Measles, mumps, and rubella vaccine (MMR).** *(Minimum age: 12 months)*

   - The second dose of MMR is recommended routinely at age 4–6 years but may be administered earlier if desired.
   - If not previously vaccinated, administer 2 doses of MMR during any visit with ≥4 weeks between the doses.

8. **Varicella vaccine.** *(Minimum age: 12 months)*

   - The second dose of varicella vaccine is recommended routinely at age 4–6 years but may be administered earlier if desired.
   - Do not repeat the second dose in persons aged <13 years if administered ≥28 days after the first dose.

9. **Hepatitis A vaccine (HepA).** *(Minimum age: 12 months)*

   - HepA is recommended for certain groups of children, including in areas where vaccination programs target older children. See *MMWR* 2006;55(No. RR-7):1–23.

10. **Tetanus and diphtheria toxoids vaccine (Td) and tetanus and diphtheria toxoids and acellular pertussis vaccine (Tdap).** *(Minimum ages: 7 years for Td, 10 years for BOOSTRIX®, and 11 years for ADACEL™)*

    - Tdap should be substituted for a single dose of Td in the primary catch-up series or as a booster if age appropriate; use Td for other doses.
    - A 5-year interval from the last Td dose is encouraged when Tdap is used as a booster dose. A booster (fourth) dose is needed if any of the previous doses were administered at age <12 months. Refer to ACIP recommendations for further information. See *MMWR* 2006;55(No. RR-3).

11. **Human papillomavirus vaccine (HPV).** *(Minimum age: 9 years)*

    - Administer the HPV vaccine series to females at age 13–18 years if not previously vaccinated.

Information about reporting reactions after immunization is available online at http://www.vaers.hhs.gov or by telephone via the 24-hour national toll-free information line 800-822-7967. Suspected cases of vaccine-preventable diseases should be reported to the state or local health department. Additional information, including precautions and contraindications for immunization, is available from the National Center for Immunization and Respiratory Diseases at **http://www.cdc.gov/nip/default.htm** or telephone, **800-CDC-INFO (800-232-4636).**

ADULT IMMUNIZATION SCHEDULE BY VACCINE AND AGE GROUP

RECOMMENDED ADULT IMMUNIZATION SCHEDULE, BY VACCINE AND AGE GROUP

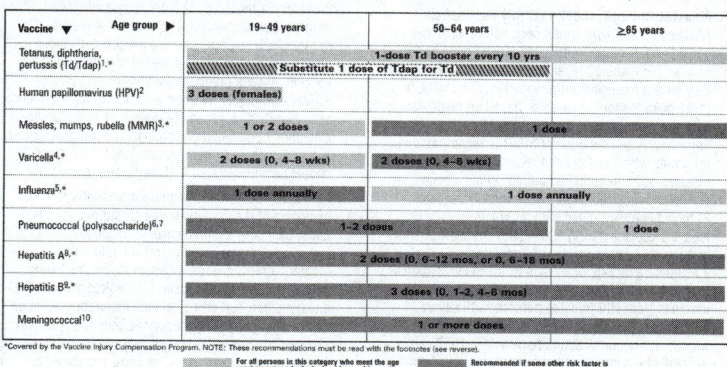

*Covered by the Vaccine Injury Compensation Program. NOTE: These recommendations must be read with the footnotes (see reverse).

For all persons in this category who meet the age requirements and who lack evidence of immunity (e.g., lack documentation of vaccination or have no evidence of prior infection)

Recommended if some other risk factor is present (e.g., on the basis of medical, occupational, lifestyle, or other indications)

This schedule indicates the recommended age groups and medical indications for routine administration of currently licensed vaccines for persons aged ≥19 years, as of October 1, 2006. Licensed combination vaccines may be used whenever any components of the combination are indicated and when the vaccine's other components are not contraindicated. For detailed recommendations on all vaccines, including those used primarily for travelers or that are issued during the year, consult the manufacturers' package inserts and the complete statements from the Advisory Committee on Immunization Practices (www.cdc.gov/nip/publications/acip-list.htm).

Report all clinically significant postvaccination reactions to the Vaccine Adverse Event Reporting System (VAERS). Reporting forms and instructions on filing a VAERS report are available at www.vaers.hhs.gov or by telephone, 800-822-7967.

Information on how to file a Vaccine Injury Compensation Program claim is available at www.hrsa.gov/vaccinecompensation or by telephone, 800-338-2382. To file a claim for vaccine injury, contact the U.S. Court of Federal Claims, 717 Madison Place, N.W., Washington, D.C. 20005; telephone, 202-357-6400.

Additional information about the vaccines in this schedule and contraindications for vaccination is also available at www.cdc.gov/nip or from the CDC-INFO Contact Center at 800-CDC-INFO (800-232-4636) in English and Spanish, 24 hours a day, 7 days a week.

1. **Tetanus, diphtheria, and acellular pertussis (Td/Tdap) vaccination.** Adults with uncertain histories of a complete primary vaccination series with diphtheria and tetanus toxoid–containing vaccines should begin or complete a primary vaccination series. A primary series for adults is 3 doses; administer the first 2 doses at least 4 weeks apart and the third dose 6–12 months after the second. Administer a booster dose to adults who have completed a primary series and if the last vaccination was received ≥10 years previously. Tdap or tetanus and diphtheria (Td) vaccine may be used; Tdap should replace a single dose of Td for adults aged <65 years who have not previously received a dose of Tdap (either in the primary series, as a booster, or for wound management). Only one of two Tdap products (Adacel® [sanofi pasteur]) is licensed for use in adults. If the person is pregnant and received the last Td vaccination ≥10 years previously, administer Td during the second or third trimester; if the person received the last Td vaccination in <10 years, administer Tdap during the immediate postpartum period. A one-time administration of 1 dose of Tdap with an interval as short as 2 years from a previous Td vaccination is recommended for postpartum women, close contacts of infants aged <12 months, and all healthcare workers with direct patient contact. In certain situations, Td can be deferred during pregnancy and Tdap substituted in the immediate postpartum period, or Tdap can be given instead of Td to a pregnant woman after an informed discussion with the woman (see www.cdc.gov/nip/publications/acip-list.htm). Consult the ACIP statement for recommendations for administering Td as prophylaxis in wound management (www.cdc.gov/mmwr/preview/mmwrhtml/00041645.htm).

2. **Human papillomavirus (HPV) vaccination.** HPV vaccination is recommended for all women aged ≤26 years who have not completed the vaccine series. Ideally, vaccine should be administered before potential exposure to HPV through sexual activity; however, women who are sexually active should still be vaccinated. Sexually active women who have not been infected with any of the HPV vaccine types receive the full benefit of the vaccination. Vaccination is less beneficial for women who have already been infected with one or more of the four HPV vaccine types. A complete series consists of 3 doses. The second dose should be administered 2 months after the first dose; the third dose should be administered 6 months after the first dose. Vaccination is not

(Continued)

ADULT IMMUNIZATION SCHEDULE BY VACCINE AND AGE GROUP

recommended during pregnancy. If a woman is found to be pregnant after initiating the vaccination series, the remainder of the 3-dose regimen should be delayed until after completion of the pregnancy.

3. **Measles, mumps, rubella (MMR) vaccination.**
Measles component: adults born before 1957 can be considered immune to measles. Adults born during or after 1957 should receive ≥1 dose of MMR unless they have a medical contraindication, documentation of ≥1 dose, history of measles based on healthcare provider diagnosis, or laboratory evidence of immunity. A second dose of MMR is recommended for adults who 1) have been recently exposed to measles or in an outbreak setting; 2) have been previously vaccinated with killed measles vaccine; 3) have been vaccinated with an unknown type of measles vaccine during 1963–1967; 4) are students in postsecondary educational institutions; 5) work in a healthcare facility; or 6) plan to travel internationally. Withhold MMR or other measles-containing vaccines from HIV-infected persons with severe immunosuppression.

Mumps component: adults born before 1957 can generally be considered immune to mumps. Adults born during or after 1957 should receive 1 dose of MMR unless they have a medical contraindication, history of mumps based on healthcare provider diagnosis, or laboratory evidence of immunity. A second dose of MMR is recommended for adults who 1) are in an age group that is affected during a mumps outbreak; 2) are students in postsecondary educational institutions; 3) work in a healthcare facility; or 4) plan to travel internationally. For unvaccinated healthcare workers born before 1957 who do not have other evidence of mumps immunity, consider giving 1 dose on a routine basis and strongly consider giving a second dose during an outbreak.

Rubella component: administer 1 dose of MMR vaccine to women whose rubella vaccination history is unreliable or who lack laboratory evidence of immunity. For women of childbearing age, regardless of birth year, routinely determine rubella immunity and counsel women regarding congenital rubella syndrome. Do not vaccinate women who are pregnant or who might become pregnant within 4 weeks of receiving vaccine. Women who do not have evidence of immunity should receive MMR vaccine upon completion or termination of pregnancy and before discharge from the healthcare facility.

4. **Varicella vaccination.** All adults without evidence of immunity to varicella should receive 2 doses of varicella vaccine. Special consideration should be given to those who 1) have close contact with persons at high risk for severe disease (e.g., healthcare workers and family members of immunocompromised persons) or 2) are at high risk for exposure or transmission (e.g., teachers of young children; child care employees; residents and staff members of institutional settings, including correctional institutions; college students; military personnel; adolescents and adults living in households with children; nonpregnant women of childbearing age; and international travelers). Evidence of immunity to varicella in adults includes any of the following: 1) documentation of 2 doses of varicella vaccine at least 4 weeks apart; 2) U.S.-born before 1980 (although for healthcare workers and pregnant women, birth before 1980 should not be considered evidence of immunity); 3) history of varicella based on diagnosis or verification of varicella by a healthcare provider (for a patient reporting a history of or presenting with an atypical case, a mild case, or both, healthcare providers should seek either an epidemiologic link with a typical varicella case or evidence of laboratory confirmation, if it was performed at the time of acute disease); 4) history of herpes zoster based on healthcare provider diagnosis; or 5) laboratory evidence of immunity or laboratory confirmation of disease. Do not vaccinate women who are pregnant or might become pregnant within 4 weeks of receiving the vaccine. Assess pregnant women for evidence of varicella immunity. Women who do not have evidence of immunity should receive dose 1 of varicella vaccine upon completion or termination of pregnancy and before discharge from the healthcare facility. Dose 2 should be administered 4–8 weeks after dose 1.

5. **Influenza vaccination.** Medical indications: chronic disorders of the cardiovascular or pulmonary systems, including asthma; chronic metabolic diseases, including diabetes mellitus, renal dysfunction, hemoglobinopathies, or immunosuppression (including immunosuppression caused by medications or HIV); any condition that compromises respiratory function or the handling of respiratory secretions or that can increase the risk of aspiration (e.g., cognitive dysfunction, spinal cord injury, or seizure disorder or other neuromuscular disorder); and pregnancy during the influenza season. No data exist on the risk for severe or complicated influenza disease among persons with asplenia; however, influenza is a risk factor for secondary bacterial infections that can cause severe disease among persons with asplenia. Occupational indications: healthcare workers and employees of long-term–care and assisted living facilities. Other indications: residents of nursing homes and other long-term–care and assisted living facilities; persons likely to transmit influenza to persons at high risk (e.g., in-home household contacts and care-givers of children aged 0–59 months, or persons of all ages with high-risk conditions); and anyone who would like to be vaccinated. Healthy, nonpregnant persons aged 5–49 years without high-risk medical conditions who are not contacts of severely immunocompromised persons in special care units can receive either intranasally administered influenza vaccine (FluMist®) or inactivated vaccine. Other persons should receive the inactivated vaccine.

6. **Pneumococcal polysaccharide vaccination.** Medical indications: chronic disorders of the pulmonary system (excluding asthma); cardiovascular diseases; diabetes mellitus; chronic liver diseases, including liver disease as a result of alcohol abuse (e.g., cirrhosis); chronic renal failure or nephrotic syndrome; functional or anatomic asplenia (e.g., sickle cell disease or splenectomy [if elective splenectomy is planned, vaccinate at least 2 weeks before surgery]); immunosuppressive conditions (e.g., congenital immunodeficiency, HIV infection [vaccinate as close to diagnosis as possible when CD4 cell counts are highest], leukemia, lymphoma, multiple myeloma, Hodgkin disease, generalized malignancy, or organ or bone marrow transplantation); chemotherapy with alkylating agents, antimetabolites, or high-dose, long-term corticosteroids; and cochlear implants. Other indications: Alaska Natives and certain American Indian populations and residents of nursing homes or other long-term–care facilities.

7. **Revaccination with pneumococcal polysaccharide vaccine.** One-time revaccination after 5 years for persons with chronic renal failure or nephrotic syndrome; functional or anatomic asplenia (e.g., sickle cell disease or splenectomy); immunosuppressive conditions (e.g., congenital immunodeficiency, HIV

Adult Immunization Schedule by Vaccine and Age Group

infection, leukemia, lymphoma, multiple myeloma, Hodgkin disease, generalized malignancy, or organ or bone marrow transplantation); or chemotherapy with alkylating agents, antimetabolites, or high-dose, long-term corticosteroids. For persons aged ≥65 years, one-time revaccination if they were vaccinated ≥5 years previously and were aged <65 years at the time of primary vaccination.

8. **Hepatitis A vaccination.** *Medical indications:* persons with chronic liver disease and persons who receive clotting factor concentrates. *Behavioral indications:* men who have sex with men and persons who use illegal drugs. *Occupational indications:* persons working with hepatitis A virus (HAV)–infected primates or with HAV in a research laboratory setting. *Other indications:* persons traveling to or working in countries that have high or intermediate endemicity of hepatitis A (a list of countries is available at *www.cdc.gov/travel/diseases.htm*) and any person who would like to obtain immunity. Current vaccines should be administered in a 2-dose schedule at either 0 and 6–12 months, or 0 and 6–18 months. If the combined hepatitis A and hepatitis B vaccine is used, administer 3 doses at 0, 1, and 6 months.

9. **Hepatitis B vaccination.** *Medical indications:* persons with end-stage renal disease, including patients receiving hemodialysis; persons seeking evaluation or treatment for a sexually transmitted disease (STD); persons with HIV infection; persons with chronic liver disease; and persons who receive clotting factor concentrates. *Occupational indications:* healthcare workers and public-safety workers who are exposed to blood or other potentially infectious body fluids. *Behavioral indications:* sexually active persons who are not in a long-term, mutually monogamous relationship (i.e., persons with >1 sex partner during the previous 6 months); current or recent injection-drug users; and men who have sex with men. *Other indications:* household contacts and sex partners of persons with chronic hepatitis B virus (HBV) infection; clients and staff members of institutions for persons with developmental disabilities; all clients of STD clinics; international travelers to countries with high or intermediate prevalence of chronic HBV infection (a list of countries is available at *www.cdc.gov/travel/diseases.htm*); and any adult seeking protection from HBV infection. Settings where hepatitis B vaccination is recommended for all adults: STD treatment facilities; HIV testing and treatment facilities; facilities providing drug-abuse treatment and prevention services; healthcare settings providing services for injection-drug users or menwho have sex with men; correctional facilities; end-stage renal disease programs and facilities for chronic hemodialysis patients; and institutions and nonresidential daycare facilities for persons with developmental disabilities. Special formulation indications: for adultpatients receiving hemodialysis and other immunocompromised adults, 1 dose of 40 Ìg/mL (Recombivax HB®) or 2 doses of 20 Ìg/mL (Engerix-B®).

10. **Meningococcal vaccination.** *Medical indications:* adults with anatomic or functional asplenia, or terminal complement component deficiencies. *Other indications:* first-year college students living in dormitories; microbiologists who are routinely exposed to isolates of *Neisseria meningitidis*; military recruits; and persons who travel to or live in countries in which meningococcal disease is hyperendemic or epidemic (e.g., the "meningitis belt" of sub-Saharan Africa during the dry season [December–June]), particularly if their contact with local populations will be prolonged. Vaccination is required by the government of Saudi Arabia for all travelers to Mecca during the annual Hajj. Meningococcal conjugate vaccine is preferred for adults with any of the preceding indications who are aged ≤55 years, although meningococcal polysaccharide vaccine (MPSV4) is an acceptable alternative. Revaccination after 5 years might be indicated for adults previously vaccinated with MPSV4 who remain at high risk for infection (e.g., persons residing in areas in which disease is epidemic).

11. **Selected conditions for which *Haemophilus influenzae* type b (Hib) vaccine may be used.** Hib conjugate vaccines are licensed for children aged 6 weeks–71 months. No efficacy data are available on which to base a recommendation concerning use of Hib vaccine for older children and adults with the chronic conditions associated with an increased risk for Hib disease. However, studies suggest good immunogenicity in patients who have sickle cell disease, leukemia, or HIV infection or whohave had splenectomies; administering vaccine to these patients is not contraindicated.

Recommended Adult Immunization Schedule, by Vaccine and Medical and Other Indications

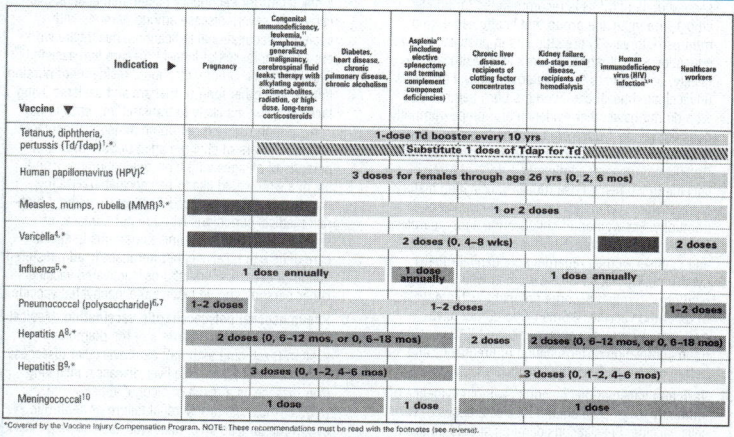

1. **Tetanus, diphtheria, and acellular pertussis (Td/Tdap) vaccination.** Adults with uncertain histories of a complete primary vaccination series with diphtheria and tetanus toxoid–containing vaccines should begin or complete a primary vaccination series. A primary series for adults is 3 doses; administer the first 2 doses at least 4 weeks apart and the third dose 6–12 months after the second. Administer a booster dose to adults who have completed a primary series and if the last vaccination was received ≥10 years previously. Tdap or tetanus and diphtheria (Td) vaccine may be used; Tdap should replace a single dose of Td for adults aged <65 years who have not previously received a dose of Tdap (either in the primary series, as a booster, or for wound management). Only one of two Tdap products (Adacel® [sanofi pasteur]) is licensed for use in adults. If the person is pregnant and received the last Td vaccination ≥10 years previously, administer Td during the second or third trimester; if the person received the last Td vaccination in <10 years, administer Tdap during the immediate postpartum period. A one-time administration of 1 dose of Tdap with an interval as short as 2 years from a previous Td vaccination is recommended for postpartum women, close contacts of infants aged <12 months, and all healthcare workers with direct patient contact. In certain situations, Td can be deferred during pregnancy and Tdap substituted in the immediate postpartum period, or Tdap can be given instead of Td to a pregnant woman after an informed discussion with the woman (see www.cdc.gov/nip/publications/acip-list.htm). Consult the ACIP statement for recommendations for administering Td as prophylaxis in wound management (www.cdc.gov/mmwr/preview/mmwrhtml/00041645.htm).

2. **Human papillomavirus (HPV) vaccination.** HPV vaccination is recommended for all women aged ≤26 years who have not completed the vaccine series. Ideally, vaccine should be administered before potential exposure to HPV through sexual activity; however, women who are sexually active should still be vaccinated. Sexually active women who have not been infected with any of the HPV vaccine types receive the full benefit of the vaccination. Vaccination is less beneficial for women who have already been infected with one or more of the four HPV vaccine types. A complete series consists of 3 doses. The second dose should be administered 2 months after the first dose; the third dose should be administered 6 months after the first dose. Vaccination is not recommended during pregnancy. If a woman is found to be pregnant after initiating the vaccination series, the remainder of the 3-dose regimen should be delayed until after completion of the pregnancy.

3. **Measles, mumps, rubella (MMR) vaccination.** *Measles component:* adults born before 1957 can be considered immune to measles. Adults born during or after 1957 should receive ≥1 dose of MMR unless they have a medical contraindication, documentation of ≥1 dose, history of measles based on healthcare provider diagnosis, or laboratory evidence of immunity. A second dose of MMR is recommended for adults who 1) have been recently exposed to measles or in an outbreak setting; 2) have been previously vaccinated with killed measles vaccine; 3) have been vaccinated with an unknown type of measles vaccine during 1963–1967; 4) are students in postsecondary educational institutions; 5) work in a healthcare facility; or 6) plan to travel internationally. Withhold MMR or other measles-containing vaccines from HIV-infected persons with severe immunosuppression.

(Continued)

Adult Immunization Schedule by Vaccine and Medical and Other Indications

Mumps component: adults born before 1957 can generally be considered immune to mumps. Adults born during or after 1957 should receive 1 dose of MMR unless they have a medical contraindication, history of mumps based on healthcare provider diagnosis, or laboratory evidence of immunity. A second dose of MMR is recommended for adults who 1) are in an age group that is affected during a mumps outbreak; 2) are students in postsecondary educational institutions; 3) work in a healthcare facility; or 4) plan to travel internationally. For unvaccinated healthcare workers born before 1957 who do not have other evidence of mumps immunity, consider giving 1 dose on a routine basis and strongly consider giving a second dose during an outbreak. *Rubella component:* administer 1 dose of MMR vaccine to women whose rubella vaccination history is unreliable or who lack laboratory evidence of immunity. For women of childbearing age, regardless of birth year, routinely determine rubella immunity and counsel women regarding congenital rubella syndrome. Do not vaccinate women who are pregnant or who might become pregnant within 4 weeks of receiving vaccine. Women who do not have evidence of immunity should receive MMR vaccine upon completion or termination of pregnancy and before discharge from the healthcare facility.

4. **Varicella vaccination.** All adults without evidence of immunity to varicella should receive 2 doses of varicella vaccine. Special consideration should be given to those who 1) have close contact with persons at high risk for severe disease (e.g., healthcare workers and family contacts of immunocompromised persons) or 2) are at high risk for exposure or transmission (e.g., teachers of young children; child care employees; residents and staff members of institutional settings, including correctional institutions; college students; military personnel; adolescents and adults living in households with children; nonpregnant women of childbearing age; and international travelers). Evidence of immunity to varicella in adults includes any of the following: 1) documentation of 2 doses of varicella vaccine at least 4 weeks apart; 2) U.S.-born before 1980 (although for healthcare workers and pregnant women, birth before 1980 should not be considered evidence of immunity); 3) history of varicella based on diagnosis or verification of varicella by a healthcare provider (for a patient reporting a history of or presenting with an atypical case, a mild case, or both, healthcare providers should seek either an epidemiologic link with a typical varicella case or evidence of laboratory confirmation, if it was performed at the time of acute disease); 4) history of herpes zoster based on healthcare provider diagnosis; or 5) laboratory evidence of immunity or laboratory confirmation of disease. Do not vaccinate women who are pregnant or might become pregnant within 4 weeks of receiving the vaccine. Assess pregnant women for evidence of varicella immunity. Women who do not have evidence of immunity should receive dose 1 of varicella vaccine upon completion or termination of pregnancy and before discharge from the healthcare facility. Dose 2 should be administered 4–8 weeks after dose 1.

5. **Influenza vaccination.** *Medical indications:* chronic disorders of the cardiovascular or pulmonary systems, including asthma; chronic metabolic diseases, including diabetes mellitus, renal dysfunction, hemoglobinopathies, or immunosuppression (including immunosuppression caused by medications or HIV); any condition that compromises respiratory function or the handling of respiratory secretions or that can increase the risk of aspiration (e.g., cognitive dysfunction, spinal cord injury, or seizure disorder or other neuromuscular disorder); and pregnancy during the influenza season. No data exist on the risk for severe or complicated influenza disease among persons with asplenia; however, influenza is a risk factor for secondary bacterial infections that can cause severe disease among persons with asplenia. *Occupational indications:* healthcare workers and employees of long-term–care and assisted living facilities. *Other indications:* residents of nursing homes and other long-term–care and assisted living facilities; persons likely to transmit influenza to persons at high risk (e.g., in-home household contacts and care-givers of children aged 0–59 months, or persons of all ages with high-risk conditions); and anyone who would like to be vaccinated. Healthy, nonpregnant persons aged 5–49 years without high-risk medical conditions who are not contacts of severely immunocompromised persons in special care units can receive either intranasally administered influenza vaccine (FluMist®) or inactivated vaccine. Other persons should receive the inactivated vaccine.

6. **Pneumococcal polysaccharide vaccination.** *Medical indications:* chronic disorders of the pulmonary system (excluding asthma); cardiovascular diseases; diabetes mellitus; chronic liver diseases, including liver disease as a result of alcohol abuse (e.g., cirrhosis); chronic renal failure or nephrotic syndrome; functional or anatomic asplenia (e.g., sickle cell disease or splenectomy [if elective splenectomy is planned, vaccinate at least 2 weeks before surgery]); immunosuppressive conditions (e.g., congenital immunodeficiency, HIV infection [vaccinate as close to diagnosis as possible when CD4 cell counts are highest], leukemia, lymphoma, multiple myeloma, Hodgkin disease, generalized malignancy, or organ or bone marrow transplantation); chemotherapy with alkylating agents, antimetabolites, or high-dose, long-term corticosteroids; and cochlear implants. *Other indications:* Alaska Natives and certain American Indian populations and residents of nursing homes or other long-term–care facilities.

7. **Revaccination with pneumococcal polysaccharide vaccine.** One-time revaccination after 5 years for persons with chronic renal failure or nephrotic syndrome; functional or anatomic asplenia (e.g., sickle cell disease or splenectomy); immunosuppressive conditions (e.g., congenital immunodeficiency, HIV infection, leukemia, lymphoma, multiple myeloma, Hodgkin disease, generalized malignancy, or organ or bone marrow transplantation); or chemotherapy with alkylating agents, antimetabolites, or high-dose, long-term corticosteroids. For persons aged ≥65 years, one-time revaccination if they were vaccinated ≥5 years previously and were aged <65 years at the time of primary vaccination.

8. **Hepatitis A vaccination.** *Medical indications:* persons with chronic liver disease and persons who receive clotting factor concentrates. *Behavioral indications:* men who have sex with men and persons who use illegal drugs. *Occupational indications:* persons working with hepatitis A virus (HAV)–infected primates or with HAV in a research laboratory setting. *Other indications:* persons traveling to or working in countries that have high or intermediate endemicity of hepatitis A (a list of countries is available at *www.cdc.gov/travel/diseases.htm*) and any person who would wish to obtain immunity. Current vaccines should be administered in a 2-dose schedule at either 0 and

Adult Immunization Schedule by Vaccine and Medical and other Indications

6–12 months, or 0 and 6–18 months. If the combined hepatitis A and hepatitis B vaccine is used, administer 3 doses at 0, 1, and 6 months.

9. **Hepatitis B vaccination.** *Medical indications:* persons with end-stage renal disease, including patients receiving hemodialysis; persons seeking evaluation or treatment for a sexually transmitted disease (STD); persons with HIV infection; persons with chronic liver disease; and persons who receive clotting factor concentrates. Occupational indications: healthcare workers and public-safety workers who are exposed to blood or other potentially infectious body fluids. Behavioral indications: sexually active persons who are not in a long-term, mutually monogamous relationship (i.e., persons with >1 sex partner during the previous 6 months); current or recent injection-drug users; and men who have sex with men. *Other indications:* household contacts and sex partners of persons with chronic hepatitis B virus (HBV) infection; clients and staff members of institutions for persons with developmental disabilities; all clients of STD clinics; international travelers to countries with high or intermediate prevalence of chronic HBV infection (a list of countries is available at *www.cdc.gov/travel/diseases.htm*); and any adult seeking protection from HBV infection. Settings where hepatitis B vaccination is recommended for all adults: STD treatment facilities; HIV testing and treatment facilities; facilities providing drug-abuse treatment and prevention services; healthcare settings providing services for injection-drug users or menwho have sex with men; correctional facilities; end-stage renal disease programs and facilities for chronic hemodialysis patients; and institutions and nonresidential daycare facilities for persons with developmental disabilities. Special formulation indications: for adultpatients receiving hemodialysis and other immunocompromised adults, 1 dose of 40 Ìg/mL (Recombivax HB®) or 2 doses of 20 Ìg/mL (Engerix-B®).

10. **Meningococcal vaccination.** *Medical indications:* adults with anatomic or functional asplenia, or terminal complement component deficiencies. Other indications: first-year college students living in dormitories; microbiologists who are routinely exposed to isolates of *Neisseria meningitidis*; military recruits; and persons who travel to or live in countries in which meningococcal disease is hyperendemic or epidemic (e.g., the "meningitis belt" of sub-Saharan Africa during the dry season [December–June]), particularly if their contact with local populations will be prolonged. Vaccination is required by the government of Saudi Arabia for all travelers to Mecca during the annual Hajj. Meningococcal conjugate vaccine is preferred for adults with any of the preceding indications who are aged ≤55 years, although meningococcal polysaccharide vaccine (MPSV4) is an acceptable alternative. Revaccination after 5 years might be indicated for adults previously vaccinated with MPSV4 who remain at high risk for infection (e.g., persons residing in areas in which disease is epidemic).

11. **Selected conditions for which *Haemophilus influenzae* type b (Hib) vaccine may be used.** Hib conjugate vaccines are licensed for children aged 6 weeks–71 months. No efficacy data are available on which to base a recommendation concerning use of Hib vaccine for older children and adults with the chronic conditions associated with an increased risk for Hib disease. However, studies suggest good immunogenicity in patients who have sickle cell disease, leukemia, or HIV infection or whohave had splenectomies; administering vaccine to these patients is not contraindicated.

Drugs Excreted in Breast Milk

The following list is not comprehensive; generic forms and alternate brands of some products may be available. When recommending drugs to pregnant or nursing patients, always check product labeling for specific precautions.

Accolate
Accuretic
Aciphex
Actiq
Activella
Actonel with Calcium
ActoPlus Met
Actos
Adalat
Adderall
Advicor
Aggrenox
Aldactazide
Aldactone
Aldomet
Aldoril
Alesse
Allegra-D
Alfenta
Aloprim
Altace
Ambien
Anaprox
Ancef
Androderm
Antara
Apresoline
Aralen
Arthrotec
Asacol
Ativan
Augmentin
Avalide
Avandia
Avelox
Axid
Axocet
Azactam
Azasan
Azathioprine
Azulfidine
Bactrim
Baraclude
Benadryl
Bentyl
Betapace
Bextra
Bexxar
Bicillin
Blocadren
Boniva
Brethine
Brevicon
Brontex
Byetta
Caduet
Cafergot
Calan
Campral
Capoten
Capozide
Captopril
Carbatrol

Cardizem
Cataflam
Catapres
Ceclor
Cefizox
Cefobid
Cefotan
Ceftin
Celebrex
Celexa
Ceptaz
Cerebyx
Ceredase
Cipro
Ciprodex
Claforan
Clarinex
Claritin
Claritin-D
Cleocin
Climara
Clozaril
Codeine
CombiPatch
Combipres
Combivir
Combunox
Compazine
Cordarone
Corgard
Cortisporin
Corzide
Cosopt
Coumadin
Covera-HS
Cozaar
Crestor
Crinone
Cyclessa
Cymbalta
Cystospaz
Cytomel
Cytotec
Cytoxan
Dapsone
Daraprim
Darvon
Darvon-N
Decadron
Deconsal II
Demerol
Demulen
Depacon
Depakene
Depakote
DepoDur
Depo-Provera
Desogen
Desoxyn
Desyrel
Dexedrine
DextroStat
D.H.E. 45

Diabinese
Diastat
Diflucan
Digitek
Dilacor
Dilantin
Dilaudid
Diovan
Diprivan
Diuril
Dolobid
Dolophine
Doral
Doryx
Droxia
Duraclon
Duragesic
Duramorph
Duratuss
Duricef
Dyazide
Dyrenium
E.E.S.
EC-Naprosyn
Ecotrin
Effexor
Elestat
EMLA
Enduron
Epzicom
Equetro
ERYC
EryPed
Ery-Tab
Erythrocin
Erythromycin
Esgic-plus
Eskalith
Estrogel
Estrostep
Ethmozine
Evista
FazaClo
Felbatol
Feldene
femhrt
Fiorinal
Florinef
Floxin
Foradil
Fortamet
Fortaz
Fosamax Plus D
Furosemide
Gabitril
Galzin
Garamycin
Glucophage
Glyset
Guaifed
Halcion
Haldol

Helidac
Hydrocet
Hydrocortone
HydroDIURIL
Iberet-Folic
Ifex
Imitrex
Imuran
Inderal
Inderide
Indocin
INFeD
Inspra
Invanz
Inversine
Isoptin
Kadian
Keflex
Keppra
Kerlone
Ketek
Klonopin
Kronofed-A
Kutrase
Lamictal
Lamisil
Lamprene
Lanoxicaps
Lanoxin
Lariam
Lescol
Levbid
Levitra
Levlen
Levlite
Levora
Levothroid
Levoxyl
Levsin
Levsinex
Lexapro
Lexiva
Lexxel
Lindane
Lioresal
Lipitor
Lithium
Lithobid
Lo/Ovral
Loestrin
Lomotil
Loniten
Lopressor
Lortab
Lotensin
Lotrel
Luminal
Luvox
Lyrica
Macrobid
Macrodantin
Marinol
Maxipime

Drugs Excreted in Breast Milk

- Maxzide
- Mefoxin
- Menostar
- Methergine
- Methotrexate
- MetroCream/Gel/Lotion
- Mexitil
- Micronor
- Microzide
- Midamor
- Migranal
- Miltown
- Minizide
- Minocin
- Mirapex
- Mircette
- M-M-R II
- Mobic
- Modicon
- Moduretic
- Monodox
- Monopril
- Morphine
- MS Contin
- MSIR
- Myambutol
- Mycamine
- Mysoline
- Namenda
- Naprelan
- Naprosyn
- Nascobal
- Necon
- NegGram
- Nembutal
- Neoral
- Niaspan
- Nicotrol
- Niravam
- Nizoral
- Norco
- Nor-QD
- Nordette
- Norinyl
- Noritate
- Normodyne
- Norpace
- Norplant
- Novantrone
- Nubain
- Nucofed
- Nydrazid
- Oramorph
- Oretic
- Ortho-Cept
- Ortho-Cyclen
- Ortho-Novum
- Ortho Tri-Cyclen
- Orudis
- Ovcon
- Oxistat
- OxyContin
- OxyFast
- OxyIR
- Pacerone
- Pamelor
- Pancrease
- Paxil
- PCE
- Pediapred
- Pediazole
- Pediotic
- Pentasa
- Pepcid
- Periostat
- Persantine
- Pfizerpen
- Phenergan
- Phenobarbital
- Phrenilin
- Pipracil
- Plan B
- Ponstel
- Pravachol
- Premphase
- Prempro
- Prevacid
- Prevacid NapraPAC
- PREVPAC
- Prinzide
- Procanbid
- Prograf
- Proloprim
- Prometrium
- Pronestyl
- Propofol
- Prosed/DS
- Protonix
- Provera
- Prozac
- Pseudoephedrine
- Pulmicort
- Pyrazinamide
- Quinidex
- Quinine
- Raptiva
- Reglan
- Relpax
- Renese
- Requip
- Reserpine
- Restoril
- Retrovir
- Rifadin
- Rifamate
- Rifater
- Rimactane
- Risperdal
- Rocaltrol
- Rocephin
- Roferon A
- Roxanol
- Rozerem
- Sanctura
- Sandimmune
- Sarafem
- Seconal
- Sectral
- Semprex-D
- Septra
- Seroquel
- Sinequan
- Slo-bid
- Soma
- Sonata
- Spiriva
- Sporanox
- Stadol
- Streptomycin
- Stromectol
- Symbyax
- Symmetrel
- Synthroid
- Tagamet
- Tambocor
- Tapazole
- Tarka
- Tavist
- Tazicef
- Tazidime
- Tegretol
- Tenoretic
- Tenormin
- Tenuate
- Tequin
- Testoderm
- Thalitone
- Theo-24
- Theo-Dur
- Thorazine
- Tiazac
- Timolide
- Timoptic
- Tindamax
- Tobi
- Tofranil
- Tolectin
- Toprol-XL
- Toradol
- Trandate
- Tranxene
- Trental
- Tricor
- Triglide
- Trilafon
- Trileptal
- Tri-Levlen
- Trilisate
- Tri-Norinyl
- Triostat
- Triphasil
- Trivora
- Trizivir
- Trovan
- Truvada
- Tygacil
- Tylenol
- Tylenol with Codeine
- Ultane
- Ultram
- Unasyn
- Uniphyl
- Uniretic
- Unithroid
- Urimax
- Valium
- Valtrex
- Vanceril
- Vancocin
- Vantin
- Vascor
- Vaseretic
- Vasotec
- Ventavis
- Verelan
- Vermox
- Versed
- Vibramycin
- Vibra-Tabs
- Vicodin
- Vigamox
- Viramune
- Voltaren
- Vytorin
- Wellbutrin
- Xanax
- Xolair
- Zantac
- Zarontin
- Zaroxolyn
- Zegerid
- Zemplar
- Zestoretic
- Zetia
- Ziac
- Zinacef
- Zithromax
- Zocor
- Zomig
- Zonalon
- Zonegran
- Zosyn
- Zovia
- Zovirax
- Zyban
- Zydone
- Zyloprim
- Zyprexa
- Zyrtec

USE-IN-PREGNANCY RATINGS

The U.S. Food and Drug Administration's Use-in-Pregnancy rating system weighs the degree to which available information has ruled out risk to the fetus against the drug's potential benefit to the patient. Below is a listing of drugs (by generic name) for which ratings are available.

X

Contraindicated in pregnancy

Studies in animals or humans, or investigational or postmarketing reports, have demonstrated fetal risk which clearly outweighs any possible benefit to the patient.

Acetohydroxamic Acid
Acitretin
Amlodipine Besylate/
    Atorvastatin Calcium
Amprenavir
Anisindione
Atorvastatin Calcium
Bexarotene
Bicalutamide
Bosentan
Cetrorelix Acetate
Choriogonadotropin Alfa
Chorionic Gonadotropin
Clomiphene Citrate
Desogestrel/Ethinyl Estradiol
Diclofenac Sodium/Misoprostol
Dihydroergotamine Mesylate
Dutasteride
Estazolam
Estradiol
Estradiol Acetate
Estradiol Cypionate/
    Medroxyprogesterone Acetate
Estradiol Valerate
Estradiol/Levonorgestrel
Estradiol/Norethindrone Acetate
Estrogens, Conjugated
Estrogens, Conjugated, Synthetic A
Estrogens, Conjugated/
    Medroxyprogesterone Acetate
Estrogens, Esterified
Estrogens, Esterified/
    Methyltestosterone
Estropipate
Ethinyl Estradiol/Drospirenone
Ethinyl Estradiol/
    Ethynodiol Diacetate
Ethinyl Estradiol/Etonogestrel
Ethinyl Estradiol/Ferrous Fumarate/
    Norethindrone Acetate
Ethinyl Estradiol/Levonorgestrel
Ethinyl Estradiol/Norelgestromin
Ethinyl Estradiol/Norethindrone
Ethinyl Estradiol/Norethindrone
    Acetate
Ethinyl Estradiol/Norgestimate
Ethinyl Estradiol/Norgestrel
Ezetimibe/Simvastatin
Finasteride
Fluorouracil
Fluoxymesterone
Flurazepam Hydrochloride
Fluvastatin Sodium
Follitropin Alfa
Follitropin Beta
Ganirelix Acetate
Goserelin Acetate
Histrelin Acetate
Hydromorphone Hydrochloride
Interferon Alfa-2B,
    Recombinant/Ribavirin
Iodine I 131 Tositumomab/
    Tositumomab
Isotretinoin
Leflunomide
Leuprolide Acetate
Levonorgestrel
Lovastatin
Lovastatin/Niacin
Medroxyprogesterone Acetate
Megestrol Acetate
Menotropins
Mequinol/Tretinoin
Mestranol/Norethindrone
Methotrexate Sodium
Methyltestosterone
Miglustat
Misoprostol
Nafarelin Acetate
Norethindrone
Norethindrone Acetate
Norgestrel
Oxandrolone
Oxymetholone
Plicamycin
Pravastatin Sodium
Pravastatin Sodium/Aspirin Buffered
Raloxifene Hydrochloride
Ribavirin
Rosuvastatin Calcium
Simvastatin
Tazarotene
Testosterone
Testosterone Enanthate
Thalidomide
Tositumomab
Triptorelin Pamoate
Urofollitropin
Warfarin Sodium

D

Positive evidence of risk

Investigational or postmarketing data show risk to the fetus. Nevertheless, potential benefits may outweigh the potential risk.

Alitretinoin
Alprazolam
Altretamine
Amiodarone Hydrochloride
Amlodipine Besylate/
    Benazepril Hydrochloride
Anastrozole
Arsenic Trioxide
Aspirin Buffered/Pravastatin Sodium
Aspirin/Dipyridamole
Atenolol
Azathioprine
Azathioprine Sodium
Benazepril Hydrochloride*
Benazepril Hydrochloride/
    Hydrochlorothiazide*
Bortezomib
Busulfan
Candesartan Cilexetil*
Candesartan Cilexetil/
    Hydrochlorothiazide*
Capecitabine
Captopril*
Carbamazepine
Carboplatin
Carmustine (Bcnu)
Chlorambucil
Cladribine
Clofarabine
Clonazepam
Cytarabine Liposome
Dactinomycin
Daunorubicin Citrate Liposome
Daunorubicin Hydrochloride
Demeclocycline Hydrochloride
Diazepam
Divalproex Sodium
Docetaxel
Doxorubicin Hydrochloride
Doxorubicin Hydrochloride Liposome
Doxycycline Calcium
Doxycycline Hyclate
Doxycycline Monohydrate
Efavirenz
Enalapril Maleate*
Enalapril Maleate/Hydrochlorothiazide*
Epirubicin Hydrochloride
Eprosartan Mesylate

* Category C or D depending on the trimester the drug is given.

USE-IN-PREGNANCY RATINGS

Erlotinib
Exemestane
Felodipine/Enalapril Maleate
Floxuridine
Fludarabine Phosphate
Flutamide
Fosinopril Sodium*
Fosinopril Sodium/
  Hydrochlorothiazide*
Fosphenytoin Sodium
Fulvestrant
Gefitinib
Gemcitabine Hydrochloride
Gemtuzumab Ozogamicin
Goserelin Acetate
Ibritumomab Tiuxetan
Idarubicin Hydrochloride
Ifosfamide
Imatinib Mesylate
Irbesartan*
Irbesartan/Hydrochlorothiazide*
Irinotecan Hydrochloride
Letrozole
Lisinopril*
Lisinopril/Hydrochlorothiazide*
Lithium Carbonate
Losartan Potassium*
Losartan Potassium/
  Hydrochlorothiazide*
Mechlorethamine Hydrochloride
Melphalan
Melphalan Hydrochloride
Mephobarbital
Mercaptopurine
Methimazole
Midazolam Hydrochloride
Minocycline Hydrochloride
Mitoxantrone Hydrochloride
Moexipril Hydrochloride*
Moexipril Hydrochloride/
  Hydrochlorothiazide*
Nelarabine
Neomycin Sulfate/
  Polymyxin B Sulfate
Nicotine
Olmesartan Medoxomil
Oxaliplatin
Pamidronate Disodium
Pemetrexed
Penicillamine
Pentobarbital Sodium
Pentostatin
Perindopril Erbumine*
Phenytoin
Procarbazine Hydrochloride
Quinapril Hydrochloride*
Quinapril Hydrochloride/
  Hydrochlorothiazide*
Ramipril*
Sorafenib
Streptomycin Sulfate
Sunitinib
Tamoxifen Citrate
Telmisartan

Telmisartan/Hydrochlorothiazide
Temozolomide
Thioguanine
Tigecycline
Tobramycin
Topotecan Hydrochloride
Toremifene Citrate
Trandolapril*
Trandolapril/Verapamil
  Hydrochloride*
Tretinoin
Valproate Sodium
Valproic Acid
Valsartan*
Valsartan/Hydrochlorothiazide*
Vinorelbine Tartrate
Voriconazole
Zoledronic Acid

Risk cannot be ruled out

Human studies are lacking, and animal studies are either positive for risk or are lacking as well. However, potential benefits may outweigh the potential risk.

Abacavir Sulfate
Abacavir Sulfate/Lamivudine
Abacavir Sulfate/
  Lamivudine/Zidovudine
Abciximab
Acamprosate Calcium
Acetaminophen
Acetaminophen/
  Butalbital/Caffeine
Acetaminophen/Caffeine/
  Chlorpheniramine Maleate/
  Hydrocodone Bitartrate/
  Phenylephrine Hydrochloride
Acetazolamide
Acetazolamide Sodium
Acyclovir
Adapalene
Adefovir Dipivoxil
Adenosine
Alatrofloxacin Mesylate
Albendazole
Albumin (Human)
Albuterol
Albuterol Sulfate
Albuterol Sulfate/Ipratropium
  Bromide
Alclometasone Dipropionate
Aldesleukin
Alemtuzumab
Alendronate Sodium
Alendronate Sodium/Cholecalciferol
Allopurinol Sodium
Almotriptan Malate

Alpha1-Proteinase Inhibitor (Human)
Alprostadil
Alteplase
Amantadine Hydrochloride
Amifostine
Aminocaproic Acid
Aminohippurate Sodium
Aminolevulinic Acid Hydrochloride
Aminosalicylic Acid
Amlodipine Besylate
Amlodipine Besylate/Benazepril
  Hydrochloride
Amoxicillin/Clarithromycin/
  Lansoprazole
Amphetamine Aspartate/
  Amphetamine Sulfate/
  Dextroamphetamine Saccharate/
  Dextroamphetamine Sulfate
Amprenavir
Anagrelide Hydrochloride
Anthralin
Antihemophilic Factor (Human)
Antihemophilic Factor (Recombinant)
Anti-Inhibitor Coagulant Complex
Anti-Thymocyte Globulin
Apomorphine Hydrochloride
Aripiprazole
Arnica Montana/Herbals, Multiple/
  Sulfur
Asparaginase
Atomoxetine Hydrochloride
Atovaquone
Atovaquone/Proguanil Hydrochloride
Atropine Sulfate/Benzoic Acid/
  HyoscyamineSulfate/
  Methenamine/Methylene Blue/
  Phenyl Salicylate
Atropine Sulfate/Hyoscyamine
  Sulfate/Scopolamine
  Hydrobromide
Azelastine Hydrochloride
Bacitracin Zinc/Neomycin Sulfate/
  Polymyxin B Sulfate
Baclofen
Bcg, Live (Intravesical)
Becaplermin
Beclomethasone Dipropionate
Beclomethasone Dipropionate
  Monohydrate
Benazepril Hydrochloride*
Benazepril Hydrochloride/
  Hydrochlorothiazide*
Bendroflumethiazide
Benzocaine
Benzonatate
Benzoyl Peroxide
Benzoyl Peroxide/Clindamycin
Benzoyl Peroxide/Erythromycin
Betamethasone Dipropionate
Betamethasone Dipropionate/
  Clotrimazole
Betamethasone Valerate
Betaxolol Hydrochloride
Bethanechol Chloride

USE-IN-PREGNANCY RATINGS

Bevacizumab
Bimatoprost
Bisacodyl/Polyethylene Glycol/
　Potassium Chloride/
　Sodium Bicarbonate/
　Sodium Chloride
Bisoprolol Fumarate
Bisoprolol Fumarate/
　Hydrochlorothiazide
Bitolterol Mesylate
Black Widow Spider Antivenin
　(Equine)
Botulinum Toxin Type A
Botulinum Toxin Type B
Brinzolamide
Brompheniramine Maleate/
　Dextromethorphan Hydrobromide/
　Phenylephrine Hydrochloride
Budesonide
Bupivacaine Hydrochloride
Bupivacaine Hydrochloride/
　Epinephrine Bitartrate
Buprenorphine Hydrochloride
Buprenorphine Hydrochloride/
　Naloxone Hydrochloride
Butabarbital/Hyoscyamine
　Hydrobromide/Phenazopyridine
　Hydrochloride
Butalbital/Acetaminophen
Butenafine Hydrochloride
Butoconazole Nitrate
Butorphanol Tartrate
Caffeine Citrate
Calcipotriene
Calcitonin-Salmon
Calcitriol
Calcium Acetate
Candesartan Cilexetil*
Candesartan Cilexetil/
　Hydrochlorothiazide*
Capreomycin Sulfate
Captopril*
Carbetapentane Tannate/
　Chlorpheniramine Tannate
Carbetapentane
　Tannate/Chlorpheniramine
　Tannate/Ephedrine
　Tannate/Phenylephrine Tannate
Carbidopa/Entacapone/Levodopa
Carbidopa/Levodopa
Carbinoxamine Maleate/
　Dextromethorphan Hydrobromide/
　Pseudoephedrine Hydrochloride
Carteolol Hydrochloride
Carvedilol
Caspofungin Acetate
Celecoxib
Cetirizine Hydrochloride
Cetuximab
Cevimeline Hydrochloride
Chloramphenicol
Chloroprocaine Hydrochloride
Chlorothiazide
Chlorothiazide Sodium

Chlorpheniramine Maleate/
　Methscopolamine Nitrate/
　Phenylephrine Hydrochloride
Chlorpheniramine Maleate/
　Pseudoephedrine Hydrochloride
Chlorpheniramine Polistirex/
　Hydrocodone Polistirex
Chlorpheniramine Tannate/
　Phenylephrine Tannate
Chlorpropamide
Chlorthalidone/Clonidine Hydrochloride
Choline Magnesium Trisalicylate
Cidofovir
Cilostazol
Cinacalcet Hydrochloride
Ciprofloxacin Hydrochloride
Ciprofloxacin Hydrochloride/
　Hydrocortisone
Ciprofloxacin/Dexamethasone
Citalopram Hydrobromide
Clarithromycin
Clobetasol Propionate
Clonidine
Clonidine Hydrochloride
Codeine Phosphate/Acetaminophen
Colistimethate Sodium
Colistin Sulfate/Hydrocortisone
　Acetate/Neomycin Sulfate/
　Thonzonium Bromide
Corticorelin Ovine Triflutate
Cycloserine
Cyclosporine
Cytomegalovirus Immune Globulin
Dacarbazine
Daclizumab
Dantrolene Sodium
Dapsone
Darbepoetin Alfa
Darifenacin
Deferoxamine Mesylate
Delavirdine Mesylate
Denileukin Diftitox
Desloratadine
Desloratadine/Pseudoephedrine
　Sulfate
Desoximetasone
Dexamethasone
Dexamethasone Sodium Phosphate
Dexmethylphenidate Hydrochloride
Dexrazoxane
Dextroamphetamine Sulfate
Diazoxide
Dichlorphenamide
Diclofenac Potassium
Diclofenac Sodium
Diflorasone Diacetate
Diflunisal
Digoxin
Digoxin Immune Fab (Ovine)
Diltiazem Hydrochloride
Dimethyl Sulfoxide
Dinoprostone
Diphtheria & Tetanus Toxoids and
　Acellular Pertussis Vaccine Adsorbed

Diphtheria & Tetanus Toxoids and
　Acellular Pertussis Vaccine
　Adsorbed/Hepatitis B Vaccine,
　Recombinant/Poliovirus Vaccine
　Inactivated
Dirithromycin
Dofetilide
Donepezil Hydrochloride
Dorzolamide Hydrochloride
Dorzolamide Hydrochloride/
　Timolol Maleate
Doxazosin Mesylate
Dronabinol
Drotrecogin Alfa (Activated)
Duloxetine Hydrochloride
Echothiophate Iodide
Econazole Nitrate
Efalizumab
Eflornithine Hydrochloride
Eletriptan Hydrobromide
Enalapril Maleate*
Enalapril Maleate/Felodipine*
Enalapril Maleate/Hydrochlorothiazide*
Entacapone
Entecavir
Epinastine Hydrochloride
Epinephrine
Epoetin Alfa
Eprosartan Mesylate
Erythromycin Ethylsuccinate/
　Sulfisoxazole Acetyl
Escitalopram Oxalate
Esmolol Hydrochloride
Eszopiclone
Ethionamide
Ethotoin
Etidronate Disodium
Exenatide
Ezetimibe
Factor IX Complex
Felodipine
Fenofibrate
Fentanyl
Fentanyl Citrate
Ferrous Fumarate/Folic Acid/
　Intrinsic Factor Concentrate/
　Liver Preparations/
　Vitamin B12/Vitamin C/
　Vitamins with Iron
Fexofenadine Hydrochloride
Fexofenadine Hydrochloride/
　Pseudoephedrine Hydrochloride
Filgrastim
Flecainide Acetate
Fluconazole
Flucytosine
Fludrocortisone Acetate
Flumazenil
Flunisolide
Fluocinolone Acetonide
Fluocinolone Acetonide/
　Hydroquinone/Tretinoin
Fluocinonide
Fluorometholone

*Category C or D depending on the trimester the drug is given.

A209

Use-in-Pregnancy Ratings

Fluorometholone/Sulfacetamide Sodium
Fluoxetine Hydrochloride
Fluoxetine Hydrochloride/Olanzapine
Flurandrenolide
Flurbiprofen Sodium
Fluticasone Propionate
Fluticasone Propionate Hfa
Fluticasone Propionate/Salmeterol Xinafoate
Fomivirsen Sodium
Formoterol Fumarate
Fosamprenavir Calcium
Foscarnet Sodium*
Fosinopril Sodium*
Fosinopril Sodium/Hydrochlorothiazide*
Frovatriptan Succinate
Furosemide
Gabapentin
Gallium Nitrate
Ganciclovir
Ganciclovir Sodium
Gatifloxacin
Gemfibrozil
Gemifloxacin Mesylate
Gentamicin Sulfate
Gentamicin Sulfate/Prednisolone Acetate
Glimepiride
Glipizide
Glipizide/Metformin Hydrochloride
Globulin, Immune (Human)
Globulin, Immune (Human)/Rho (D) Immune Globulin (Human)
Glyburide
Gramicidin/Neomycin Sulfate/Polymyxin B Sulfate
Guaifenesin/Hydrocodone Bitartrate
Haemophilus B Conjugate Vaccine
Haemophilus B Conjugate Vaccine/Hepatitis B Vaccine, Recombinant
Halobetasol Propionate
Haloperidol Decanoate
Hemin
Heparin Sodium
Hepatitis A Vaccine, Inactivated
Hepatitis A Vaccine, Inactivated/Hepatitis B Vaccine, Recombinant
Hepatitis B Immune Globulin (Human)
Hepatitis B Vaccine, Recombinant
Homatropine Methylbromide/Hydrocodone Bitartrate
Homeopathic Formulations
Hydralazine Hydrochloride/Isosorbide Dinitrate
Hydrochlorothiazide
Hydrocodone Bitartrate
Hydrocodone Bitartrate/Acetaminophen
Hydrocodone Bitartrate/Ibuprofen
Hydrocortisone
Hydrocortisone Acetate
Hydrocortisone Acetate/Neomycin Sulfate/Polymyxin B Sulfate
Hydrocortisone Acetate/Pramoxine Hydrochloride
Hydrocortisone Butyrate
Hydrocortisone Probutate
Hydrocortisone/Neomycin Sulfate/Polymyxin B Sulfate
Hydromorphone Hydrochloride
Hydroquinone
Hyoscyamine Sulfate
Ibandronate Sodium
Ibutilide Fumarate
Iloprost
Imiglucerase
Imipenem/Cilastatin
Imiquimod
Immune Globulin Intravenous (Human)
Indinavir Sulfate
Indocyanine Green
Influenza Virus Vaccine
Insulin Aspart
Insulin Aspart Protamine,Human/Insulin Aspart, Human
Insulin Glargine
Insulin Glulisine
Interferon Alfa-2A, Recombinant
Interferon Alfa-2B, Recombinant
Interferon Alfacon-1
Interferon Alfa-N3 (Human Leukocyte Derived)
Interferon Beta-1A
Interferon Beta-1B
Interferon Gamma-1B
Iodoquinol/Hydrocortisone
Irbesartan*
Irbesartan/Hydrochlorothiazide*
Iron Dextran
Isoniazid/Pyrazinamide/Rifampin
Isosorbide Mononitrate
Isradipine
Itraconazole
Ivermectin
Ketoconazole
Ketorolac Tromethamine
Ketotifen Fumarate
Labetalol Hydrochloride
Lamivudine
Lamivudine/Zidovudine
Lamotrigine
Lanthanum Carbonate
Latanoprost
Levalbuterol Hydrochloride
Levalbuterol Tartrate
Levamisole Hydrochloride
Levetiracetam
Levobunolol Hydrochloride
Levofloxacin
Linezolid
Lisinopril*
Lisinopril/Hydrochlorothiazide*
Lopinavir/Ritonavir
Losartan Potassium*
Losartan Potassium/Hydrochlorothiazide*
Loteprednol Etabonate
Mafenide Acetate
Magnesium Salicylate Tetrahydrate
Measles Virus Vaccine, Live
Measles, Mumps & Rubella Virus Vaccine, Live
Mebendazole
Mecamylamine Hydrochloride
Mecasermin [Rdna Origin]
Medrysone
Mefenamic Acid
Mefloquine Hydrochloride
Meloxicam
Meningoccal Polysaccharide Diphtheria Toxoid Conjugate Vaccine
Meningococcal Polysaccharide Vaccine
Meperidine Hydrochloride
Mepivacaine Hydrochloride
Metaproterenol Sulfate
Metaraminol Bitartrate
Metformin Hydrochloride/Pioglitazone Hydrochloride
Metformin Hydrochloride/Rosiglitazone Maleate
Methamphetamine Hydrochloride
Methazolamide
Methenamine Mandelate/Sodium Acid Phosphate
Methocarbamol
Methoxsalen
Methscopolamine Nitrate/Pseudoephedrine Hydrochloride
Methyldopa/Chlorothiazide
Methyldopa/Hydrochlorothiazide
Methylphenidate Hydrochloride
Metipranolol
Metoprolol Succinate
Metoprolol Tartrate
Metoprolol Tartrate/Hydrochlorothiazide
Metyrosine
Mexiletine Hydrochloride
Micafungin Sodium
Midodrine Hydrochloride
Mivacurium Chloride
Modafinil
Moexipril Hydrochloride*
Moexipril Hydrochloride/Hydrochlorothiazide*
Mometasone Furoate
Mometasone Furoate Monohydrate
Morphine Sulfate
Morphine Sulfate, Liposomal
Moxifloxacin Hydrochloride
Mumps Virus Vaccine, Live
Muromonab-Cd3
Mycophenolate Mofetil
Mycophenolate Mofetil Hydrochloride
Mycophenolic Acid
Nabumetone
Nadolol

Use-in-Pregnancy Ratings

Nadolol/Bendroflumethiazide
Naloxone Hydrochloride/
 Pentazocine Hydrochloride
Naltrexone Hydrochloride
Naphazoline Hydrochloride
Naproxen
Naproxen Sodium
Naratriptan Hydrochloride
Natamycin
Nateglinide
Nefazodone Hydrochloride
Neomycin Sulfate/
 Dexamethasone Sodium
 Phosphate
Neomycin Sulfate/Polymyxin B
 Sulfate/Prednisolone Acetate
Nesiritide
Nevirapine
Niacin
Nicardipine Hydrochloride
Nifedipine
Nilutamide
Nimodipine
Nisoldipine
Nitroglycerin
Norfloxacin
Ofloxacin
Olanzapine
Olmesartan Medoxomil/
 Hydrochlorothiazide
Olopatadine Hydrochloride
Olsalazine Sodium
Omega-3-Acid Ethyl Esters
Omeprazole
Oprelvekin
Orphenadrine Citrate
Oseltamivir Phosphate
Oxcarbazepine
Oxycodone Hydrochloride/
 Acetaminophen
Oxycodone Hydrochloride/Ibuprofen
Oxymorphone Hydrochloride
Palifermin
Palivizumab
Pancrelipase
Paricalcitol
Paroxetine Hydrochloride
Paroxetine Mesylate
Peg-3350/Potassium Chloride/
 Sodium Bicarbonate/
 Sodium Chloride
Pegademase Bovine
Pegaspargase
Pegfilgrastim
Peginterferon Alfa-2A
Peginterferon Alfa-2B
Pemirolast Potassium
Pentazocine Hydrochloride/
 Acetaminophen
Pentoxifylline
Perindopril Erbumine*
Phenoxybenzamine Hydrochloride
Phentermine Hydrochloride
Pilocarpine Hydrochloride

Pimecrolimus
Pimozide
Pioglitazone Hydrochloride
Pirbuterol Acetate
Piroxicam
Plasma Fractions, Human/
 Rabies Immune Globulin (Human)
Plasma Protein Fraction (Human)
Pneumococcal Vaccine, Diphtheria
 Conjugate
Pneumococcal Vaccine, Polyvalent
Podofilox
Polyethylene Glycol
Polyethylene Glycol/Potassium
 Chloride/Sodium Bicarbonate/
 Sodium Chloride
Polyethylene Glycol/Potassium
 Chloride/Sodium
 Bicarbonate/Sodium
 Chloride/Sodium Sulfate
Polymyxin B Sulfate/
 Trimethoprim Sulfate
Polythiazide/Prazosin Hydrochloride
Porfimer Sodium
Potassium Acid Phosphate
Potassium Chloride
Potassium Citrate
Potassium Phosphate/
 Sodium Phosphate
Pralidoxime Chloride
Pramipexole Dihydrochloride
Pramlintide Acetate
Pramoxine Hydrochloride/
 Hydrocortisone Acetate
Prazosin Hydrochloride
Prednisolone Acetate
Prednisolone Acetate/
 Sulfacetamide Sodium
Prednisolone Sodium Phosphate
Pregabalin
Procainamide Hydrochloride
Promethazine Hydrochloride
Propafenone Hydrochloride
Proparacaine Hydrochloride
Propranolol Hydrochloride
Pseudoephedrine Hydrochloride
Pyrimethamine
Quetiapine Fumarate
Quinapril Hydrochloride*
Quinidine Sulfate
Rabies Vaccine
Ramelteon
Ramipril*
Rasburicase
Remifentanil Hydrochloride
Repaglinide
Reteplase
Rho (D) Immune Globulin (Human)
Rifampin
Rifapentine
Rifaximin
Riluzole
Rimantadine Hydrochloride
Risedronate Sodium

Risedronate Sodium/Calcium
 Carbonate
Risperidone
Rituximab
Rizatriptan Benzoate
Rocuronium Bromide
Rofecoxib
Ropinirole Hydrochloride
Rosiglitazone Maleate
Rubella Virus Vaccine, Live
Salmeterol Xinafoate
Sargramostim
Scopolamine
Selegiline Hydrochloride
Sertaconazole Nitrate
Sertraline Hydrochloride
Sevelamer Hydrochloride
Sibutramine Hydrochloride Monohydrate
Sirolimus
Sodium Benzoate/
 Sodium Phenylacelate
Sodium Phenylbutyrate
Sodium Sulfacetamide/Sulfur
Solifenacin Succinate
Somatropin
Somatropin (rDNA origin)
Stavudine
Streptokinase
Succimer
Sulfacetamide Sodium
Sulfamethoxazole/Trimethoprim
Sulfanilamide
Sumatriptan
Sumatriptan Succinate
Tacrine Hydrochloride
Tacrolimus
Telithromycin
Telmisartan*
Telmisartan/Hydrochlorothiazide*
Tenecteplase
Terazosin Hydrochloride
Teriparatide
Tetanus & Diphtheria Toxoids
 Adsorbed
Tetanus Immune Globulin (Human)
Theophylline
Theophylline Anhydrous
Thiabendazole
Thrombin
Thyrotropin Alfa
Tiagabine Hydrochloride
Tiludronate Disodium
Timolol Hemihydrate
Timolol Maleate
Timolol Maleate/Hydrochlorothiazide
Tinidazole
Tiotropium Bromide
Tipranavir
Tizanidine Hydrochloride
Tobramycin/Dexamethasone
Tobramycin/Loteprednol Etabonate
Tolcapone
Tolterodine Tartrate
Topiramate

* Category C or D depending on the trimester the drug is given.

USE-IN-PREGNANCY RATINGS

Tramadol Hydrochloride
Tramadol Hydrochloride/
  Acetaminophen
Trandolapril*
Trandolapril/Verapamil Hydrochloride*
Travoprost
Tretinoin
Triamcinolone Acetonide
Triamterene
Triamterene/Hydrochlorothiazide
Trientine Hydrochloride
Triethanolamine Polypeptide Oleate-
  Condensate
Trifluridine
Trimethoprim Hydrochloride
Trimipramine Maleate
Tropicamide/Hydroxyamphetamine
  Hydrobromide
Trospium Chloride
Trovafloxacin Mesylate
Tuberculin Purified Protein Derivative,
  Diluted
Typhoid Vaccine Live Oral Ty21A
Unoprostone Isopropyl
Urea
Valdecoxib
Valganciclovir Hydrochloride
Valsartan*
Valsartan/Hydrochlorothiazide*
Varicella Virus Vaccine, Live
Venlafaxine Hydrochloride
Verapamil Hydrochloride
Verteporfin
Vitamin K1
Yellow Fever Vaccine
Zalcitabine
Zaleplon
Zanamivir
Zidovudine
Zileuton
Ziprasidone Mesylate
Zolmitriptan
Zonisamide

No evidence of risk in humans

*Either animal findings show risk
while human findings do not, or, if no
adequate human studies have been
done, animal findings are negative.*

Acarbose
Acrivastine
Acyclovir
Acyclovir Sodium
Adalimumab
Agalsidase Beta
Alefacept
Alfuzosin Hydrochloride
Alosetron Hydrochloride
Amiloride Hydrochloride
Amiloride Hydrochloride/
  Hydrochlorothiazide
Amoxicillin
Amoxicillin/Clavulanate Potassium
Amphotericin B
Amphotericin B Lipid Complex
Amphotericin B, Liposomal
Amphotericin B/Cholesteryl Sulfate
  Complex
Ampicillin Sodium/Sulbactam Sodium
Anakinra
Antithrombin III
Aprepitant
Aprotinin
Argatroban
Arginine Hydrochloride
Atazanavir Sulfate
Azelaic Acid
Azithromycin
Azithromycin Dihydrate
Aztreonam
Balsalazide Disodium
Basiliximab
Bivalirudin
Brimonidine Tartrate
Budesonide
Bupropion Hydrochloride
Cabergoline
Carbenicillin Indanyl Sodium
Cefaclor
Cefazolin Sodium
Cefdinir
Cefditoren Pivoxil
Cefepime Hydrochloride
Cefixime
Cefoperazone Sodium
Cefotaxime Sodium
Cefotetan Disodium
Cefoxitin Sodium
Cefpodoxime Proxetil
Cefprozil
Ceftazidime Sodium
Ceftibuten Dihydrate
Ceftizoxime Sodium
Ceftriaxone Sodium
Cefuroxime
Cefuroxime Axetil
Cephalexin
Cetirizine Hydrochloride
Ciclopirox
Ciclopirox Olamine
Cimetidine
Cimetidine Hydrochloride
Cisatracurium Besylate
Clindamycin Hydrochloride/
  Clindamycin Phosphate
Clindamycin Palmitate Hydrochloride
Clindamycin Phosphate
Clopidogrel Bisulfate
Clotrimazole
Clozapine
Colesevelam Hydrochloride
Cromolyn Sodium
Cyclobenzaprine Hydrochloride
Cyproheptadine Hydrochloride
Dalfopristin/Quinupristin
Dalteparin Sodium
Dapiprazole Hydrochloride
Daptomycin
Desflurane
Desmopressin Acetate
Dicyclomine Hydrochloride
Didanosine
Diphenhydramine Hydrochloride
Dipivefrin Hydrochloride
Dipyridamole
Dolasetron Mesylate
Dornase Alfa
Doxapram Hydrochloride
Doxepin Hydrochloride
Doxercalciferol
Edetate Calcium Disodium
Emtricitabine
Emtricitabine/Tenofovir Disoproxil
  Fumarate
Enfuvirtide
Enoxaparin Sodium
Eplerenone
Epoprostenol Sodium
Ertapenem
Erythromycin
Erythromycin Ethylsuccinate
Erythromycin Stearate
Esomeprazole Magnesium
Esomeprazole Sodium
Etanercept
Ethacrynate Sodium
Ethacrynic Acid
Famciclovir
Famotidine
Fenoldopam Mesylate
Fondaparinux Sodium
Galantamine Hydrobromide
Glatiramer Acetate
Glucagon
Glyburide/Metformin Hydrochloride
Granisetron Hydrochloride
Hydrochlorothiazide
Ibuprofen
Indapamide
Infliximab
Insulin Lispro Protamine, Human/
  Insulin Lispro, Human
Insulin Lispro, Human
Ipratropium Bromide
Iron Sucrose
Isosorbide Mononitrate
Lactulose
Lansoprazole
Lansoprazole/Naproxen
Laronidase
Lepirudin
Levocarnitine
Lidocaine
Lidocaine Hydrochloride
Lidocaine/Prilocaine
Lindane
Loperamide Hydrochloride

USE-IN-PREGNANCY RATINGS

Loracarbef
Loratadine
Malathion
Meclizine Hydrochloride
Memantine Hydrochloride
Meropenem
Mesalamine
Metformin Hydrochloride
Methohexital Sodium
Methyldopa
Metolazone
Metronidazole
Miglitol
Montelukast Sodium
Mupirocin
Mupirocin Calcium
Naftifine Hydrochloride
Nalbuphine Hydrochloride
Nalmefene Hydrochloride
Naloxone Hydrochloride
Naproxen Sodium
Nedocromil Sodium
Nelfinavir Mesylate
Nitazoxanide
Nitrofurantoin Macrocrystals
Nitrofurantoin Macrocrystals/
 Nitrofurantoin Monohydrate
Nizatidine
Octreotide Acetate
Omalizumab
Ondansetron
Ondansetron Hydrochloride
Orlistat
Oxiconazole Nitrate
Oxybutynin
Oxybutynin Chloride
Oxycodone Hydrochloride

Palonosetron Hydrochloride
Pancrelipase
Pantoprazole Sodium
Pegvisomant
Pemoline
Penciclovir
Penicillin G Benzathine
Penicillin G Benzathine/
 Penicillin G Procaine
Penicillin G Potassium
Pentosan Polysulfate Sodium
Pergolide Mesylate
Permethrin
Piperacillin Sodium
Piperacillin Sodium/
 Tazobactam Sodium
Praziquantel
Progesterone
Propofol
Pseudoephedrine Hydrochloride
Pseudoephedrine Sulfate
Psyllium Preparations
Rabeprazole Sodium
Ranitidine Hydrochloride
Rifabutin
Ritonavir
Rivastigmine Tartrate
Ropivacaine Hydrochloride
Saquinavir
Saquinavir Mesylate
Sevoflurane
Sildenafil Citrate
Silver Sulfadiazine
Sodium Ferric Gluconate
Somatropin
Sotalol Hydrochloride

Sucralfate
Sulfasalazine
Tadalafil
Tamsulosin Hydrochloride
Tegaserod Maleate
Tenofovir Disoproxil Fumarate
Terbinafine Hydrochloride
Ticarcillin Disodium/
 Clavulanate Potassium
Ticlopidine Hydrochloride
Tirofiban Hydrochloride
Torsemide
Trastuzumab
Treprostinil Sodium
Urokinase
Ursodiol
Valacyclovir Hydrochloride
Vancomycin Hydrochloride
Vardenafil Hydrochloride
Zafirlukast
Zolpidem Tartrate

Controlled studies show no risk

Adequate, well-controlled studies in pregnant women have failed to demonstrate risk to the fetus.

Levothyroxine Sodium
Liothyronine Sodium
Liotrix
Nystatin

---

* Category C or D depending on the trimester the drug is given.

VITAMIN COMPARISON TABLE

For easy comparison, the grid below lists the contents of an assortment of widely available vitamin/mineral supplements. It includes entries for all vitamins and minerals—except sodium—assigned a Recommended Dietary Allowance (Daily Value) by the U.S. Food and Drug Administration.

The grid is divided into two parts: the first covers general multivitamin/mineral supplements for adults; the second focuses on supplements sold especially for children.

Many of the brands in the grid include other ingredients that have nutritional importance but lack an official Recommended Dietary Allowance from the government. The presence of additional ingredients is noted in the last column of the grid.

Ingredient	Measure
Vitamin A (retinol, beta-carotene)	International Units
Vitamin B1 (thiamin)	Milligrams
Vitamin B2 (riboflavin)	Milligrams
Vitamin B3 (niacin)	Milligrams
Vitamin B5 (pantothenic acid)	Milligrams
Vitamin B6 (pyridoxine)	Milligrams
Vitamin B9 (folic acid)	Micrograms

Ingredient	Measure
Vitamin B12 (cobalamin)	Micrograms
Vitamin C (ascorbic acid)	Milligrams
Vitamin D	International Units
Vitamin E	International Units
Biotin	Micrograms
Calcium	Milligrams
Copper	Milligrams

Ingredient	Measure
Iodine	Micrograms
Iron	Milligrams
Magnesium	Milligrams
Phosphorus	Milligrams
Potassium	Milligrams
Zinc	Milligrams

The amounts listed are drawn from the manufacturer's package labeling, primarily as published in the *Physicians' Desk Reference®* and *PDR® for Nonprescription Drugs, Dietary Supplements and Herbs*. For easy comparison, the figures have been converted as necessary from the unit of measure used by the manufacturer to the measurement most frequently employed in the industry. **Amounts listed are those found in a single tablet, capsule, packet, or dose.** Check package labeling for the total daily dose recommended by the manufacturer.

To conserve space, units of measure are not shown in the grid. They are as follows:

BRAND	A	B-1	B-2	B-3	B-5	B-6	B-9	B-12	C	D	E	BIOTIN	CALCIUM	COPPER	IODINE	IRON	MAGNESIUM	PHOSPHORUS	POTASSIUM	ZINC	OTHER
ADULTS																					
ACES (Carlson)	5,000	—	—	—	—	—	—	—	500	—	200	—	—	—	—	—	—	—	—	—	Y
Active Calcium	—	—	—	—	—	—	—	—	—	100	—	—	200	—	—	—	100	—	—	—	Y
Anti-Aging Daily Premium Pak	11,250	9	9	15	9	9	300	6	575	400	130	375	202	0.75	75	7.5	80	—	—	7.5	Y

VITAMIN COMPARISON TABLE

BRAND	A	B-1	B-2	B-3	B-5	B-6	B-9	B-12	C	D	E	BIOTIN	CALCIUM	COPPER	IODINE	IRON	MAGNESIUM	PHOSPHORUS	POTASSIUM	ZINC	OTHER
Caltrate 600 Plus	—	—	—	—	—	—	—	—	—	400	—	—	600	1	—	—	50	—	—	7.5	Y
Centrum	3,500	1.5	1.7	20	10	2	400	6	60	400	30	30	162	2	150	18	100	109	80	15	Y
Centrum Performance	3,500	4.5	5.1	40	10	6	400	18	120	400	60	40	100	2	150	18	40	48	80	15	Y
Centrum Silver	3,500	1.5	1.7	20	10	3	400	25	60	400	45	30	200	2	150	—	100	48	80	15	Y
Chelated Mineral Tablets	—	—	—	—	—	—	—	—	—	—	—	—	67.5	0.5	56.25	—	75	—	—	5	Y
Chromagen	—	—	—	—	—	—	—	10	150	—	—	—	—	—	—	70	—	—	—	—	—
Chromagen FA	—	—	—	—	—	—	1,000	10	150	—	—	—	—	—	—	70	—	—	—	—	—
Chromagen Forte	—	—	—	—	—	—	1,000	10	60	—	—	—	—	—	—	151	—	—	—	—	—
Citracal Prenatal Rx	2,700	3	3.4	20	—	20	1,000	—	120	400	30	—	125	2	150	27	—	—	—	25	—
Dextrim Results, Ephedrine Free	—	—	—	—	5	2	—	—	10	—	5	—	90	—	—	—	6.7	70	—	2.5	Y
Duet by Stuartnatal	3,000	1.8	4	20	—	25	1,000	12	120	400	30	—	200	2	—	29	25	—	—	25	—
Duet Chewable by Stuartnatal	3,000	1.8	4	20	—	25	1,000	12	120	400	30	—	100	2	—	29	25	—	—	25	—
Eldertonic	—	0.5	0.6	7	3	0.7	—	2	—	—	—	—	—	—	—	—	0.7	—	—	5	Y
Estroven	—	2	2	20	—	10	400	6	—	—	30	—	150	—	—	—	—	—	—	—	Y
Folgard Rx 2.2	—	—	—	—	—	25	2,200	1,000	—	—	—	—	—	—	—	—	—	—	—	—	—
Hep-Forte	1,200	1	1	10	2	0.5	60	1	10	—	10	3.3	—	—	—	—	—	—	—	2	Y
Mega Antioxidant	5,000	9	9	13.3	30	9	333	20	433	150	150	100	—	—	—	—	—	—	—	—	Y

A215

Vitamin Comparison Table

BRAND	A	B-1	B-2	B-3	B-5	B-6	B-9	B-12	C	D	E	BIOTIN	CALCIUM	COPPER	IODINE	IRON	MAGNESIUM	PHOSPHORUS	POTASSIUM	ZINC	OTHER
Mega-B	—	100	100	100	100	100	100	100	—	—	—	100	—	—	—	—	—	—	—	—	Y
Megadose	25,000*	80	80	80	80	80	400	80	250	1,000*	100	80	50	0.5	150	10	7	—	10	25	Y
NataChew	1,000	2	3	20	—	10	1	12	120	400	11	—	—	—	—	29	—	—	—	—	—
Nephrocaps	—	1.5	1.7	20	5	10	1,000	6	100	—	—	150	—	—	—	—	—	—	—	—	—
Nicomide Tablets	—	—	—	750	—	—	500	—	—	—	—	—	—	—	—	—	—	—	—	25	—
Niferex-150 Forte	—	—	—	—	—	—	1,000	25	60	—	—	—	—	—	—	150	—	—	—	—	—
Nu-Iron V	4,000	3	3	10	—	2	1	3	50	400	—	—	312	—	—	60	—	—	—	—	—
Obegyn Prenatal	5,000	1.7	2	20	10	10	1	12	120	400	60	300	455	2	150	18	150	—	—	25	—
One-A-Day Active	5,000	4.5	5.1	40	10	6	400	18	120	400	60	40	110	2	150	9	40	48	200	15	Y
One-A-Day Men's Health	3,500	1.2	1.7	16	5	3	400	18	90	400	45	30	210	2	—	—	120	—	100	15	Y
One-A-Day Women's	2,500	1.5	1.7	10	5	2	400	6	60	400	30	—	450	—	—	18	50	—	—	15	—
PreCare Chewable	—	—	—	—	—	2	1,000	—	50	6mcg	3.5	—	250	2	—	40	50	—	—	15	—
PreCare Conceive	—	3	3.4	20	—	50	1,000	12	60	—	30	—	200	2	—	30	100	—	—	15	—
PreCare Prenatal	—	3	3.4	20	—	50	1,000	12	50	6mcg	3.5	—	250	2	—	40	50	—	—	15	—
PremesisRx Tablets	—	—	—	—	—	75	1,000	12	—	—	—	—	200	—	—	—	—	—	—	—	—
Prenate GT.	2,700	3	3.4	20	6	20	1,000	12	120	400	10	30	200	2	—	90	30	—	—	15	—
PrimaCare AM Capsules	—	—	—	—	—	—	—	—	—	170	30	—	150	—	—	—	—	—	—	—	—
PrimaCare PM Tablets	—	3	3.4	20	7	50	1,000	12	100	230	—	35	250	1.3	—	30	—	—	—	11	Y
Right Choice AM	833	8.3	5	16.6	16.6	8.3	266.6	66.6	200	—	66.6	100	—	—	—	—	—	—	—	—	Y

*USP units.

VITAMIN COMPARISON TABLE

BRAND	A	B-1	B-2	B-3	B-5	B-6	B-9	B-12	C	D	E	BIOTIN	CALCIUM	COPPER	IODINE	IRON	MAGNESIUM	PHOSPHORUS	POTASSIUM	ZINC	OTHER
Right Choice PM	—	—	—	—	—	—	—	—	—	133.3	—	—	166.6	0.66	50	—	83.3	—	33	5	Y
StrongStart Caplets	1,000	3	3.4	20	7	75	1,000	12	50	400	30	35	225	—	—	40	30	—	—	15	Y
Strovite Advance	3,000	20	5	25	15	25	1,000	50	300	400	100	100	—	1.5	—	—	50	—	—	25	Y
Vicon Forte	8,000	10	5	25	10	2	1,000	10	150	—	50	—	—	—	—	—	70	—	—	80	Y

CHILDREN

BRAND	A	B-1	B-2	B-3	B-5	B-6	B-9	B-12	C	D	E	BIOTIN	CALCIUM	COPPER	IODINE	IRON	MAGNESIUM	PHOSPHORUS	POTASSIUM	ZINC	OTHER
Centrum, Kids	3,500	1.5	1.7	20	10	2	400	6	60	400	30	45	108	2	150	18	40	50	—	15	Y
Flintstones	3,000	1.5	1.7	15	10	2	400	6	60	400	30	40	100	2	150	18	20	100	—	12	—
My First Flintstones	1,998	1.05	1.2	10	—	1.05	300	4.5	60	400	15	—	—	—	—	—	—	—	—	—	—
One-A-Day Kids Bugs Bunny and Friends	3,000	1.5	1.7	15	10	2	400	6	60	400	30	40	100	2	150	18	20	100	—	12	—
One-A-Day Kids Scooby-Doo	3,000	1.5	1.7	15	10	2	400	6	60	400	30	40	100	2	150	18	20	100	—	12	—
One-A-Day Kids Scooby-Doo Plus Calcium	2,500	1.05	1.2	13.5	—	1.05	300	4.5	60	400	15	—	250	—	—	—	—	—	—	—	—

Boys Head Circumference-for-age and Weight-for-length
Birth to 36 months (5th–95th percentile)

Girls Length-for-age and Weight-for-age
Birth to 36 months (5th-95th percentile)

Girls Head Circumference-for-Age and Weight-for-Length
Birth to 36 Months (5th-95th Percentile)

Boys Stature-for-age and Weight-for-age Children 2 to 20 years (5th-95th percentile)

Boys BMI-for-age
Children 2 to 20 years (5th-95th percentile)

Girls Stature-for-age and Weight-for-age Children 2 to 20 years (5th-95th percentile)

Girls BMI-for-age
Children 2 to 20 years (5th-95th percentile)

Boys Weight-for-stature
(5th-95th percentile)

A235

Girls Weight-for-stature
(5th-95th Percentile)

Boys Length-for-age and Weight-for-age
Birth to 36 months (3rd-97th percentile)

A239

Boys Head Circumference-for-age and Weight-for-length
Birth to 36 months (3rd-97th percentile)

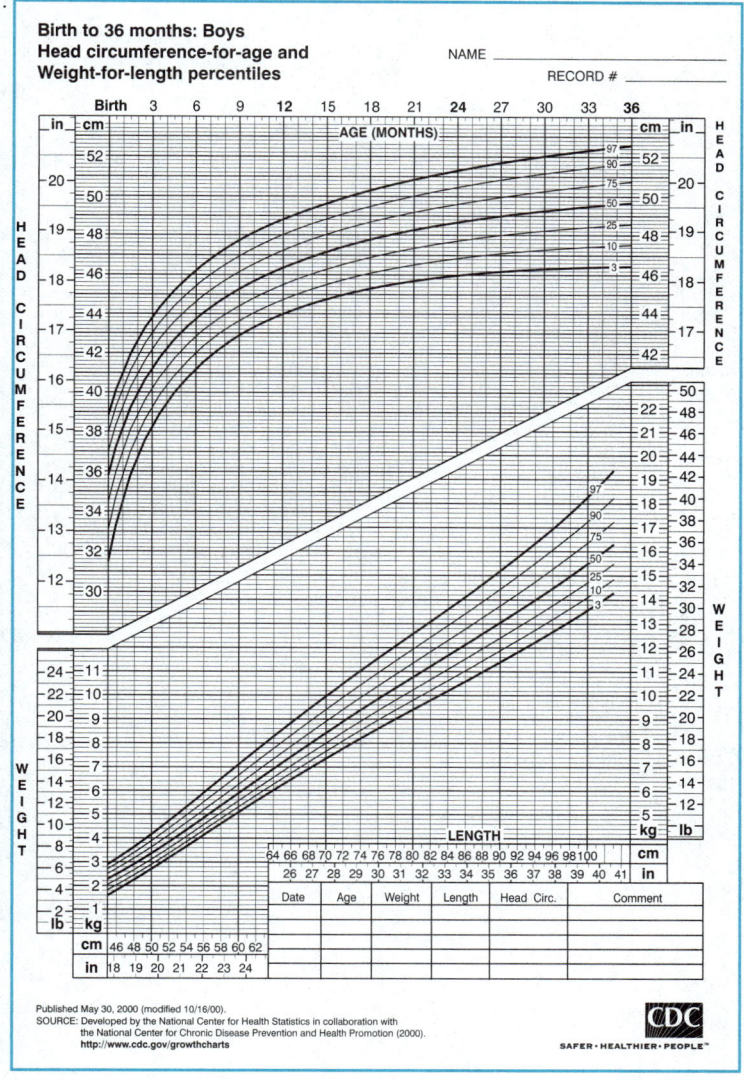

Girls Length-for-age and Weight-for-age
Birth to 36 months (3rd-97th percentile)

Girls Head Circumference-for-Age and Weight-for-Length
Birth to 36 months (3rd–97th percentile)

Boys BMI-for-age
Children 2 to 20 years (3rd-97th percentile)

Girls Stature-for-age and Weight-for-age
Children 2 to 20 years (3rd-97th percentile)

Boys Weight-for-stature (3rd-97th Percentile)

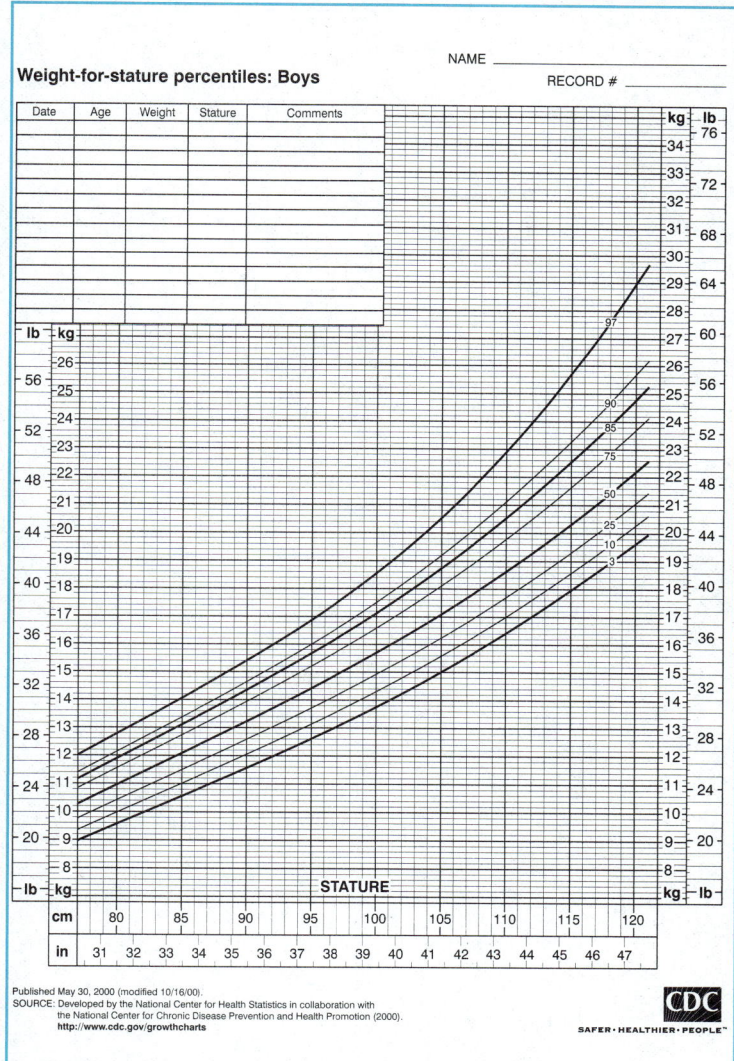

Girls Weight-for-stature
(3rd-97th percentile)

Weight-for-stature percentiles: Girls

Indices

Brand/Generic Index

Organized alphabetically, this index includes the brand and generic names of each product described in the PDR and NeoFax drug sections (*NeoFax page numbers are shown in italics*). Brand-name drug entries are capitalized; generic names are not. If more than one brand name is associated with a generic, each brand can be found under the generic entry.

A

Abacavir Sulfate
   Trizivir 367
   Ziagen 412
ABELCET 1
ABREVA 1
ACCOLATE 1
ACCUNEB 2
ACCUTANE 2
Acetaminophen
   Acetaminophen *421*
   Esgic 135
   Esgic-Plus 135
   Feverall 139
   Fioricet 140
   Lortab 201
   Phrenilin 271
   Phrenilin Forte 271
   Tylenol 371
   Tylenol 8 Hour 371
   Tylenol Arthritis Pain 371
   Tylenol Children's 371
   Tylenol Extra Strength 371
   Tylenol Infant's 371
   Tylenol Junior 371
   Tylenol Regular
     Strength 371
   Tylenol with Codeine 372
Acetic Acid
   Acetasol HC 398
   VoSol HC 398
Acetylcysteine
   Mucomyst 226
ACLOVATE 3
Acrivastine
   Semprex-D 317
ACTHIB 3
ACTICIN 4
ACTIQ 4
ACULAR 5
Acyclovir
   Acyclovir *421*
   Zovirax 416
   Zovirax Cream 416
ADACEL 5
Adapalene
   Differin 108
ADDERALL 6
ADDERALL XR 6
ADENOCARD 7
Adenosine
   Adenosine *422*
   Adenocard 7
ADIPEX-P 8
ADRIAMYCIN 8
ADVAIR 9
ADVAIR HFA 10

AEROBID 11
AGENERASE 11
AGRYLIN 12
AK-FLUOR 13
ALACOL DM 13
ALAMAST 14
Albendazole
   Albenza 14
ALBENZA 14
ALBUTEROL 14, *423*
Albuterol Sulfate
   AccuNeb 2
   Albuterol 14
   ProAir HFA 283
   Proventil 14
   Proventil HFA 292
   Ventolin HFA 384
   VoSpire ER 398
Alclometasone
   Dipropionate
   Aclovate 3
ALCORTIN 15
ALDARA 15
ALEVE 16
Alglucosidase Alfa
   Myozyme 230
ALINIA 16
ALL CLEAR 17
ALL CLEAR AR 17
ALLEGRA 17
ALLEGRA-D 18
ALLERX 18
Allopurinol
   Zyloprim 417
Allopurinol Sodium
   Aloprim 19
ALOCRIL 19
ALOMIDE 19
ALOPRIM 19
ALPHAGAN P 20
Alprostadil
   Alprostadil *424*
   Prostin VR Pediatric 291
ALTABAX 20
Alteplase
   Cathflo Activase 55
Aluminum Hydroxide
   Mylanta Maximum
     Strength Liquid 229
   Mylanta Regular
     Strength Liquid 229
Amantadine HCl
   Symmetrel 336
AMBISOME 20
Amcinonide
   Cyclocort 84
AMIDATE 21

Amikacin Sulfate
   Amikacin *425*
   Amikin 21
   Amikin Pediatric 21
AMIKIN 21
AMINOPHYLLINE *427*
Aminosalicylic Acid
   Paser 261
AMINODARONE *428*
Amlodipine Besylate
   Caduet 53
   Norvasc 243
Ammonium Lactate
   Lac-Hydrin 186
Amoxicillin
   Amoxil 22
   Augmentin 33
   Augmentin ES-600 33
   Augmentin XR 34
   DisperMox 112
AMOXIL 22
Amphetamine Salt Combo
   Adderall 6
   Adderall XR 6
AMPHOTEC 23
Amphotericin B
   Amphotericin B *429*
   AmBisome 20
Amphotericin B Cholesteryl
   Sulfate
   Amphotec 23
Amphotericin B (Lipid
   Complex)
   Amphotericin B (Lipid
     Complex) *430*
   Abelcet 1
AMPHOTERICIN B
   (LIPOSOME) *431*
AMPICILLIN 23
Ampicillin
   Ampicillin 23, *432*
AMPICILLIN INJECTION 23
   Ampicillin Injection 23
   Unasyn 374
Amprenavir
   Agenerase 11
Amyl Nitrite
   Cyanide Antidote
     Package 83
Amylase
   Cotazym 81
   Pancrease 259
   Pancrease MT 259
   Viokase 392
   Zymase 418
ANAFRANIL 24

I-1

Brand/Generic Index

Anagrelide HCl
  Agrylin 12
ANALPRAM-HC 25
ANCEF 25
ANDRODERM 25
ANECTINE 26
Antazoline Phosphate
  Vasocon-A 382
Antihemophilic Factor
  Kogenate FS 185
ANTIVERT 27
ANUSOL-HC CREAM 27
ANZEMET 27
ARALEN 28
ARMOUR THYROID 28
ARRANON 29
Arsenic Trioxide
  Trisenox 367
Articaine HCl
  Septocaine 320
ASMANEX 29
Aspirin
  Bayer Aspirin 41
  Bayer Aspirin Children's 41
  Bayer Aspirin Extra
    Strength 42
  Bayer Aspirin Regimen ... 41
  Bayer Aspirin Regimen
    with Calcium 41
  Bayer Extra Strength 41
  Ecotrin 120
  Equagesic 130
  Genuine Bayer Aspirin 41
  Soma Cmpd/Codeine ... 325
  Soma Compound 326
  Synalgos-DC 337
ASTELIN 30
ATGAM 30
ATIVAN 31
Atomoxetine HCl
  Strattera 326
Atorvastatin Calcium
  Caduet 53
  Lipitor 196
Atovaquone
  Malarone 205
  Malarone Pediatric 205
  Mepron 211
Atracurium Besylate
  Tracrium 362
ATROPINE SULFATE 31, 432
Atropine Sulfate
  Atropine Sulfate 31, 432
  Donnatal 114
  Donnatal Extentabs 114
  Lomotil 200
  Lonox 200
  Prosed DS 290
  Prosed EC 290
  Urised 377
ATROVENT 32
ATROVENT NASAL 32
AUGMENTIN 33
AUGMENTIN ES-600 33
AUGMENTIN XR 34
AVAPRO 34
AXID 35

AZACTAM 35
AZASITE 36
Azelaic Acid
  Azelex 36
  Finevin 140
Azelastine HCl
  Astelin 30
  Optivar 254
AZELEX 36
Azithromycin
  Azasite 36
  Azithromycin 433
  Zithromax 412
  Zithromax 412
AZMACORT 36
Aztreonam
  Azactam 35
  Aztreonam 434
AZULFIDINE 37
AZULFIDINE EN 37

B

Bacitracin
  Bacitracin Injection 38
  Neosporin + Pain Relief
    Maximum Strength 236
BACITRACIN INJECTION 38
Bacitracin Zinc
  Neosporin Ointment 236
BACLOFEN 38
Baclofen
  Baclofen 38
  Kemstro 38
BACTRIM 39
BACTROBAN 39
BALAMINE DM 40
Balsalazide Disodium
  Colazal 74
BARACLUDE 40
Basiliximab
  Simulect 321
BAYER ASPIRIN 41
BAYER ASPIRIN EXTRA
  STRENGTH 42
Becaplermin
  Regranex 299
Beclomethasone
dipropionate
  Beconase 42
  Beconase AQ 42
  Qvar 297
BECONASE AQ 42
BENADRYL ALLERGY 42
Benazepril HCl
  Lotensin 201
BENZACLIN 43
BENZAGEL 43
BENZAMYCIN 43
Benzoic Acid
  Prosed DS 290
  Prosed EC 290
  Urised 377
Benzonatate
  Tessalon 348
Benzoyl Peroxide
  BenzaClin 43

Benzagel 43
Benzagel Wash 43
Benzamycin 43
Brevoxyl 52
Duac 116
Benzphetamine HCl
  Didrex 107
Betamethasone
  Celestone 60
Betamethasone Acetate
  Celestone Soluspan 60
Betamethasone
(Augmented)
Dipropionate
  Diprolene 111
  Diprolene AF 111
BETAMETHASONE
  DIPROPIONATE 44
Betamethasone Sodium
Phosphate
  Celestone Soluspan 60
BETAPACE 44
BETAPACE AF 45
BIAXIN 46
BICILLIN C-R 46
BICILLIN C-R 900/300 47
BICILLIN L-A 47
BILTRICIDE 48
Bisacodyl
  Dulcolax 116
  Fleet Bisacodyl 141
Bismuth Subsalicylate
  Pepto-Bismol 266
  Pepto-Bismol Maximum
    Strength 266
BLEPH-10 48
BLEPHAMIDE 49
BONTRIL SLOW-RELEASE 49
BOOSTRIX 50
Bosentan
  Tracleer 361
Botanical/Mineral
Substances
  Traumeel 363
  Traumeel Topical 363
BOTOX 50
Botulinum Toxin Type A
  Botox 50
BREVITAL 51
BREVOXYL 52
Brimonidine Tartrate
  Alphagan P 20
BROMFED 52
Bromocriptine Mesylate
  Parlodel 260
Brompheniramine Maleate
  Alacol DM 13
  Bromfed 52
  Bromfed-PD 52
  Bromfenex 52
  Bromfenex-PD 52
  Carbofed DM 313
  Cardec DM 313
  Lodrane 24 199
  Rondec Syrup 312
  Rondec-DM Syrup 313

Brand/Generic Index

Budesonide
  Pulmicort 294
  Pulmicort Flexhaler 294
  Pulmicort Respules 294
  Rhinocort Aqua 303
Budesonide Fumarate
Dihydrate
  Symbicort 335
BUMETANIDE *435*
Bupivacaine HCl
  Marcaine 205
  Marcaine with
    Epinephrine 206
  Sensorcaine 318
  Sensorcaine with
    Epinephrine 319
  Sensorcaine-MPF 318
  Sensorcaine-MPF
    w/Epinephrine 319
BUPRENEX 52
Buprenorphine
  Suboxone 329
  Subutex 329
Buprenorphine HCl
  Buprenex 52
Busulfan
  Myleran 230
Butalbital
  Esgic 135
  Esgic-Plus 135
  Fioricet 140
  Phrenilin 271
  Phrenilin Forte 271
Butenafine HCl
  Lotrimin Ultra 202
  Mentax 210
Butoconazole Nitrate
  Mycelex-3 227

C

CADUET 53
CAFCIT 54
Caffeine
  Esgic 135
  Esgic-Plus 135
  Fioricet 140
  Synalgos-DC 337
Caffeine Citrate
  Caffeine Citrate *436*
  Cafcit 54
Calcitriol
  Rocaltrol 308
Calcium Carbonate
  Calcium carbonate *437*
  Calcium glubionate *438*
  Calcium gluconate *438*
  Calcium - Oral *439*
  Children's Mylanta 63
  Pepcid Complete 266
Calfactant
  Infasurf *489*
CAPTOPRIL *439*
Carbamazepine
  Carbatrol 54
  Tegretol 345
  Tegretol-XR 345
CARBATROL 54

Carbetapentane Tannate
  Rynatuss 315
  Rynatuss Pediatric 315
  Tussi-12 370
Carbinoxamine Maleate
  Balamine DM 40
  Palgic 258
  Rondec 311
  Rondec Oral Drops 311
  Rondec-DM Drops 312
  Rondec-TR 311
Carisoprodol
  Soma 325
  Soma Cmpd/Codeine ... 325
  Soma Compound 326
Castor Oil
  Granulex 158
CASPOFUNGIN *440*
CATHFLO ACTIVASE 55
CEDAX 55
CEENU 55
CEFACLOR
  Cefaclor 56
  Cefaclor ER 56
CEFACLOR ER 56
Cefadroxil Monohydrate
  Duricef 118
Cefazolin
  Ancef 25
Cefdinir
  Omnicef 252
Cefditoren Pivoxil
  Spectracef 326
Cefepime HCl
  Cefepime *442*
  Maxipime 208
Cefixime
  Suprax 334
CEFIZOX 57
Cefotaxime Sodium
  Cefotaxime *443*
  Claforan 69
CEFOXITIN 57
Cefoxitin Sodium
  Cefoxitin 57, *444*
  Mefoxin 57
Cefpodoxime Proxetil
  Vantin 381
Cefprozil
  Cefzil 58
Ceftazidime
  Ceftazidime *445*
  Ceptaz 61
  Fortaz 149
  Tazicef 343
  Tazidime 344
Ceftibuten
  Cedax 55
CEFTIN 58
Ceftizoxime
  Cefizox 57
Ceftriaxone Sodium
  Ceftriaxone *446*
  Rocephin 309
Cefuroxime Axetil
  Ceftin 58
CEFZIL 58

CELEBREX 59
Celecoxib
  Celebrex 59
CELESTONE 60
CELESTONE SOLUSPAN ... 60
CELONTIN 61
Cephalexin
  Keflex 182
  Panixine 260
CEPTAZ 61
CEREZYME 62
CERUBIDINE 62
Cetirizine HCl
  Zyrtec 418
  Zyrtec-D 419
CHERACOL W/CODEINE .. 63
CHILDREN'S MYLANTA ... 63
CHLORAL HYDRATE ... 64, *447*
CHLORAMPHENICOL *447*
Chlordiazepoxide HCl
  Librium 194
Chloroprocaine HCl
  Nesacaine 237
  Nesacaine-MPF 237
Chloroquine
  Aralen 28
Chlorothiazide
  Chlorothiazide *448*
  Diuril 113
Chloroxylenol
  Cortane-B 78
  Zoto HC 78
Chlorpheniramine Maleate
  AlleRx 18
  Chlor-Trimeton 65
  Dallergy 87
  Dallergy Jr 87
  Deconamine 93
  Deconamine SR 93
  De-Congestine TR 93
  Hista-Vent DA 163
  Kronofed-A 93
  Tussend 369
Chlorpheniramine Polistirex
  Tussionex Pennkinetic 370
Chlorpheniramine Tannate
  Rynatan Pediatric 314
  Rynatuss 315
  Rynatuss Pediatric 315
  Tussi-12 370
CHLORPROMAZINE 64
CHLOR-TRIMETON 65
Cholestyramine
  Questran 295
  Questran Light 295
Choline Magnesium
Trisalicylate
  Trilisate 366
Chorionic Gonadotropin
  Novarel 244
  Pregnyl 278
  Profasi 286
Ciclesonide
  Omnaris 251
Ciclopirox
  Loprox 200
  Loprox TS 200

I-3

Brand/Generic Index

Cilastatin
  Primaxin I.M. 282
  Primaxin I.V. 282
CILOXAN 65
CIMETIDINE 66
Cimetidine
  Cimetidine 66, *449*
  Tagamet 66
CIPRO HC 66
CIPRO IV 67
CIPRO ORAL 67
CIPRODEX 68
Ciprofloxacin
  Cipro IV 67
  Ciprodex 68
Ciprofloxacin HCl
  Ciloxan 65
  Cipro HC 66
  Cipro Oral 67
Cisatracurium Besylate
  Nimbex 239
CLAFORAN 69
CLARINEX 69
CLARINEX-D 24 HOUR 69
CLARIPEL 70
Clarithromycin
  Biaxin 46
CLARITIN OTC 70
CLARITIN-D OTC 70
Clavulanate Potassium
  Augmentin 33
  Augmentin ES-600 33
  Augmentin XR 34
  Timentin 354
Clemastine Fumarate
  Tavist Allergy 342
CLENIA 71
CLEOCIN 71
CLEOCIN T 72
CLEOCIN VAGINAL 72
CLINDAGEL 72
Clindamycin
  BenzaClin 43
  Clindamycin *450*
  Duac 116
Clindamycin HCl
  Cleocin 71
Clindamycin Phosphate
  Cleocin T 72
  Cleocin Vaginal 72
  Cleocin Vaginal Ovules ... 72
  Clindagel 72
  Clindamax Vaginal 72
  Evoclin 137
  Ziana 412
Clobetasol Propionate
  Clobevate 73
  Cormax 78
  Cormax Scalp 78
  Embeline E 124
  Olux 251
  Olux-E 251
  Temovate 346
  Temovate Scalp 346
  Temovate-E 346
CLOBEVATE 73

Clocortolone Pivalate
  Cloderm 73
CLODERM 73
Clofarabine
  Clolar 73
CLOLAR 73
Clomipramine HCl
  Anafranil 24
Clonazepam
  Klonopin 184
  Klonopin Wafers 184
Clorazepate Dipotassium
  Tranxene T-Tab 362
  Tranxene-SD 362
  Tranxene-SD Half
    Strength 362
Clotrimazole
  Gyne-Lotrimin 160
  Gyne-Lotrimin 3 160
  Gyne-Lotrimin 3
    Combination Pack 160
  Gyne-Lotrimin
    Combination Pack 160
  Lotrimin 202
  Lotrimin AF 202
  Mycelex Troche 227
  Mycelex-7 228
Codeine Phosphate
  Cheracol w/Codeine 63
  Cheratussin AC 63
  Guaituss AC 63
  Guaituss DAC 160
  Halotussin AC 63
  Mytussin AC 63
  Mytussin DAC 248
  Nucofed 247
  Nucofed Pediatric
    Expectorant 248
  Promethazine
    VC/Codeine 288
  Promethazine
    w/Codeine 289
  Soma Cmpd/Codeine ... 325
  Tylenol with Codeine 372
COLACE 74
COLAZAL 74
Colfosceril palmitate
  Exosurf 468
Colistimethate Sodium
  Coly-Mycin M 75
Colistin sulfate
  Cortisporin-TC Otic 79
COLY-MYCIN M 75
COMBIVIR 75
COMPAZINE 76
CONCERTA 76
CORDRAN 77
CORMAX 78
CORTANE-B 78
CORTEF 78
CORTISPORIN OTIC 79
CORTISPORIN-TC OTIC 79
CORTROSYN 80
COSMEGEN 80
COSOPT 81
Cosyntropin
  Cortrosyn 80

COTAZYM 81
CROFAB 82
Cromolyn Sodium
  Intal 177
  Opticrom 254
Crotalidae Polyvalent
Immune Fab (Ovine)
  Crofab 82
CUPRIMINE 82
CUROSURF *451*
CUTIVATE 83
CYANIDE ANTIDOTE
  PACKAGE 83
Cyclobenzaprine HCl
  Flexeril 141
CYCLOCORT 84
CYCLOPENTOLATE
  (OPHTHALMIC) *451*
Cyclophosphamide
  Cytoxan 86
  Neosar 235
Cyclosporine
  Restasis 302
  Sandimmune 316
CYPROHEPTADINE 84
Cytarabine
  Cytosar-U 85
CYTOMEL 85
CYTOSAR-U 85
CYTOXAN 86

D

Daclizumab
  Zenapax 411
Dactinomycin
  Cosmegen 80
Dalfopristin
  Synercid 339
DALLERGY 87
DALLERGY JR 87
DALMANE 87
DANTRIUM 88
DANTRIUM IV 88
Dantrolene Sodium
  Dantrium 88
  Dantrium IV 88
DAPSONE 89
DAPTACEL 89
DARAPRIM 90
Daunorubicin HCl
  Cerubidine 62
DAYPRO 90
DAYTRANA 91
DDAVP 92
DECLOMYCIN 92
DECONAMINE 93
Deferasirox
  Exjade 137
Deferoxamine Mesylate
  Desferal 101
DELATESTRYL 94
Delavirdine Mesylate
  Rescriptor 301
Demeclocycline HCl
  Declomycin 92
DEMEROL INJECTION 94

Brand/Generic Index

DEMEROL ORAL 95
DEMSER 95
DEPACON 96
DEPAKENE 97
DEPAKOTE 97
DEPAKOTE ER 98
DEPO-MEDROL 99
DEPO-TESTOSTERONE 100
DERMA-SMOOTHE/FS 101
DERMATOP 101
DESFERAL 101
Desflurane
   Suprane 333
Desloratadine
   Clarinex 69
   Clarinex RediTabs 69
   Clarinex Syrup 69
   Clarinex-D 24 Hour 69
DESMOPRESSIN
   ACETATE 102
Desmopressin Acetate
   DDAVP 92
   DDAVP Nasal Spray 92
   DDAVP Rhinal Tube 92
   Desmopressin Acetate ... 102
DESONATE 103
Desonide
   Desonate 103
   Verdeso 385
Desoximetasone
   Topicort 361
   Topicort LP 361
DESOXYN 103
DEXAMETHASONE 103
Dexamethasone
   Ciprodex 68
   Decadron 103
   Dexamethasone 103, *452*
   TobraDex 357
DEXEDRINE 104
Dexmethylphenidate HCl
   Focalin 147
   Focalin XR 147
Dextran 70
   Visine Advanced
     Relief 395
Dextroamphetamine
Sulfate
   Dexedrine 104
   Dexedrine Spansules ... 104
   DextroStat 105
Dextromethorphan HBr
   Alacol DM 13
   Balamine DM 40
   Carbofed DM 313
   Cardec DM 313
   Promethazine DM 288
   Rondec DM Drops 312
   Rondec-DM Syrup 313
Dextromethorphan
Hydrobromide
   Duratuss DM 118
   Gani-Tuss-DM NR 370
   Mucinex DM 225
   Tussi-Organidin DM NR ... 370
   Tussi-Organidin DM S
     NR 370

DEXTROSTAT 105
DIASTAT 106
Diazepam
   Diastat 106
   Diazepam Injection 106
   Valium 379
DIAZEPAM INJECTION 106
DIAZOXIDE *453*
DICLOXACILLIN 107
Dicloxacillin Sodium
   Dicloxacillin 107
Didanosine
   Videx 389
   Videx EC 389
DIDREX 107
Diethylpropion HCl
   Tenuate 347
   Tenuate Dospan 347
DIFFERIN 108
DIFLUCAN 108
Diflunisal
   Dolobid 113
DIGIBIND 109
Digoxin
   Digitek 188
   Digoxin *454*
   Lanoxicaps 188
   Lanoxin 188
Digoxin Immune Fab
(Ovine)
   Digibind 109
Dihydrocodeine Bitartrate
   Synalgos-DC 337
DILANTIN 109
Diphenhydramine HCl
   Benadryl Allergy 42
   Diphenhydramine HCl
     Injection 110
DIPHENHYDRAMINE
   HCL INJECTION 110
Diphenoxylate HCl
   Lomotil 200
   Lonox 200
Diphtheria Toxoid
   Boostrix 50
   Daptacel 89
   Infanrix 176
   Pediarix 263
   Tetanus & Diphtheria
     Toxoids Adsorbed 349
   Tripedia 366
Diphtheria Toxoid,
Reduced
   Adacel 5
DIPRIVAN 111
DIPROLENE 111
Disopyramide Phosphate
   Norpace 242
   Norpace CR 242
DISPERMOX 112
DITROPAN XL 112
DIURIL 113
Divalproex Sodium
   Depakote 97
   Depakote ER 98
DOBUTAMINE *455*

Docetaxel
   Taxotere 342
Docosanol
   Abreva 1
Docusate Sodium
   Colace 74
   Peri-Colace 266
Dolasetron Mesylate
   Anzemet 27
DOLOBID 113
DONNATAL 114
DOPAMINE *457*
DORYX 115
Dorzolamide HCl
   Cosopt 81
   Trusopt 368
Doxorubicin HCl
   Adriamycin 8
Doxycycline Hyclate
   Doryx 115
   Vibramycin 387
   Vibramycin IV 388
   Vibra-Tabs 387
Doxycycline Monohydrate
   Monodox 223
Doxylamine Succinate
   Unisom 375
Droperidol
   Inapsine 173
Drospirenone
   YAZ 407
DRYVAX 115
DT VACCINE *459*
DTaP VACCINE *459*
DTaP-HepB-IPV
COMBINATION
VACCINE *460*
DUAC 116
DULCOLAX 116
DURAGESIC 117
DURATUSS 117
DURATUSS DM 118
DURATUSS G 118
DURICEF 118
DYNACIN 119

E

Echothiophate Iodide
   Phospholine Iodide 271
ECOTRIN 120
EDECRIN 121
E.E.S. 119
Efavirenz
   Sustiva 335
Eflornithine HCl
   Vaniqa 381
ELDOPAQUE FORTE 121
ELESTAT 122
ELIDEL 122
ELIMITE 122
ELITEK 123
ELMIRON 123
ELOCON 124
EMADINE 124
EMBELINE E 124

I-5

Brand/Generic Index

Emedastine Difumarate
  Emadine 124
EMLA 125, *461*
Emtricitabine
  Emtriva 125
EMTRIVA 125
Enalapril Maleate
  Enalapril Maleate *462*
  Vasotec 383
ENALAPRILAT *462*
ENBREL 126
Enfuvirtide
  Fuzeon 151
ENOXAPARIN *463*
Entecavir
  Baraclude 40
ENTEX HC 126
ENTEX LA 127
ENTEX PSE 127
Ephedrine Tannate
  Rynatuss 315
  Rynatuss Pediatric 315
EPIFOAM 128
Epinastine HCl
  Elestat 122
Epinephrine
  Epinephrine *464*
  EpiPen 128
  EpiPen Jr. 128
  Marcaine with
    Epinephrine 206
  Sensorcaine with
    Epinephrine 319
  Sensorcaine-MPF
    w/Epinephrine 319
  Septocaine 320
  Twinject 371
  Xylocaine with
    Epinephrine 405
  Xylocaine-MPF with
    Epinephrine 405
EPIPEN 128
EPIQUIN MICRO 128
EPIVIR 129
EPIVIR-HBV 129
Epoetin Alfa
  Epoetin Alfa *465*
  Epogen 130
  Procrit 284
EPOGEN 130
EQUAGESIC 130
ERTACZO 131
Ertapenem Sodium
  Invanz 178
ERYC 131
ERYPED 132
ERY-TAB 132
ERYTHROCIN 133
ERYTHROMYCIN 134
Erythromycin
  Benzamycin 43
  ERYC 131
  Ery-Tab 132
  Erythromycin 134, *466*
  Erythromycin Base 134
  Erythromycin
    Ophthalmic 135

  PCE 262
ERYTHROMYCIN BASE 134
Erythromycin
  Ethylsuccinate
  E.E.S. 119
  EryPed 132
  Pediazole 264
ERYTHROMYCIN
  OPHTHALMIC 135
Erythromycin Stearate
  Erythrocin 133
ESGIC 135
ESGIC-PLUS 135
ESKALITH 136
ESMOLOL *467*
Esomeprazole Magnesium
  Nexium 239
ESTROSTEP FE 136
Etanercept
  Enbrel 126
Ethacrynic Acid
  Edecrin 121
Ethambutol HCl
  Myambutol 227
Ethinyl Estradiol
  Estrostep Fe 136
  Ortho Tri-Cyclen 256
  Tri-Previfem 256
  Tri-Sprintec 256
  YAZ 407
Ethionamide
  Trecator 364
Ethosuximide
  Zarontin 409
Etodolac
  Lodine XL 199
Etomidate
  Amidate 21
EVOCLIN 137
EXJADE 137
EXOSURF *468*

F

Famotidine
  Famotidine *469*
  Pepcid 265
  Pepcid AC 266
  Pepcid Complete 266
  Pepcid RPD 265
Felbamate
  Felbatol 138
FELBATOL 138
Fentanyl
  Duragesic 117
  Fentanyl *469*
Fentanyl Citrate
  Actiq 4
  Sublimaze 329
FEOSOL 139
FERO-GRAD-500 139
FERRLECIT 139
Ferrous Sulfate
  Feosol 139
  Fero-Grad-500 139
  Ferrous Sulfate *470*
FEVERALL 139

Fexofenadine HCl
  Allegra 17
  Allegra-D 18
FINEVIN 140
FIORICET 140
FLAGYL 140
Flavoxate HCl
  Urispas 378
Flecainide Acetate
  Flecainide *471*
  Tambocor 341
FLEET BISACODYL 141
FLEET GLYCERIN
  LAXATIVES 141
FLEXERIL 141
FLONASE 142
FLOVENT HFA 142
FLOXIN OTIC 143
Fluconazole
  Fluconazole *472*
  Diflucan 108
FLUCYTOSINE *473*
FLUMADINE 143
Flumazenil
  Flumazenil *473*
  Romazicon 311
FLUMIST 144
Flunisolide
  Aerobid 11
  Aerobid-M (with
    menthol) 11
  Flunisolide Nasal Spray ... 144
  Nasarel 233
FLUNISOLIDE NASAL
  SPRAY 144
Fluocinolone Acetonide
  Derma-Smoothe/FS 101
  Synalar 337
Fluocinonide
  Lidex 194
  Lidex-E 194
  Vanos 381
Fluorescein Sodium
  AK-Fluor 13
Fluorometholone
  FML 146
  FML Forte 146
Fluoxetine HCl
  Prozac 293
Fluoxymesterone
  Halotestin 161
Flurandrenolide
  Cordran 77
  Cordran SP 77
Flurazepam HCl
  Dalmane 87
Fluticasone Furoate
  Veramyst 385
Fluticasone Propionate
  Advair 9
  Advair HFA 10
  Cutivate 83
  Flonase 142
  Flovent HFA 142
Fluvastatin Sodium
  Lescol 190
  Lescol XL 190

BRAND/GENERIC INDEX

FLUVIRIN 145
FLUVOXAMINE
  MALEATE 145
FLUZONE 146
FML 146
FOCALIN 147
FOCALIN XR 147
FOLIC ACID 148
Folic Acid
  Irofol 180
FORADIL 149
Formoterol
  Symbicort 335
Formoterol Fumarate
  Foradil 149
FORTAZ 149
FORTOVASE 150
FOSPHENYTOIN *474*
FURADANTIN 150
FUROSEMIDE 151
Furosemide
  Furosemide 151, *475*
  Lasix 151
FUZEON 151

G

Gabapentin
  Neurontin 238
GABITRIL 152
GAMMAR-P 152
Ganciclovir
  Ganciclovir *476*
  Vitrasert 397
GANTRISIN PEDIATRIC 153
GARDASIL 153
Gatifloxacin
  Zymar 418
GENOTROPIN 154
GENTAMICIN
  OPHTHALMIC 154
Gentamicin Sulfate
  Gentamicin
    Ophthalmic 154
Gentamicin Sulfate
  Injection 155, *477*
  Gentamicin Topical 155
GENTAMICIN SULFATE
  INJECTION 155, *477*
GENTAMICIN TOPICAL 155
GLEEVEC 156
GLUCAGON 156, *478*
GLUCOPHAGE XR 157
Glycerin
  Fleet Glycerin
    Laxatives 141
  Visine for Contacts 395
  Visine Tears 396
Glycopyrrolate
  Robinul 307
  Robinul Forte 307
  Robinul Injection 308
Granisetron HCl
  Kytril 185
GRANULEX 158
GRIFULVIN V 158

Griseofulvin
  Grifulvin V 158
  Gris-PEG 158
GRIS-PEG 158
GUAIFED-PD 159
Guaifenesin
  Ami-Tex PSE 127
  Cheracol w/Codeine 63
  Cheratussin AC 63
  Codiclear DH 159
  Duratuss 117
  Duratuss DM 118
  Duratuss G 118
  Entex HC 126
  Entex LA 127
  Entex PSE 127
  Gani-Tuss-DM NR 370
  Guaifed-PD 159
  Guaifenesin ER 118
  Guaifenex G 118
  Guaifenex PSE 120 127
  Guaituss AC 63
  Guiatuss DAC 160
  Halotussin AC 63
  Humibid 166
  Hycotuss 167
  Liquibid-D 118
  Mucinex 225
  Mucinex D 225
  Mucinex DM 225
  Muco-Fen 1200 118
  Mytussin AC 63
  Mytussin DAC 248
  Nucofed Pediatric
    Expectorant 248
  Tussend Expectorant 369
  Tussi-Organidin DM NR ... 370
  Tussi-Organidin DM S
    NR 370
  Vicodin Tuss 159
  Vi-Q-Tuss 167
GUAIFENESIN-HYDROCODONE
  BITARTRATE 159
GUIATUSS DAC 160
GYNE-LOTRIMIN 160

H

Haemophilus B Conjugate
  ActHIB 3, *479*
Halcinonide
  Halog 160
  Halog-E 160
Halobetasol Propionate
  Ultravate 374
HALOG 160
HALOPERIDOL 161
Haloperidol
  Haldol 161
  Haldol Decanoate 161
HALOTESTIN 161
HAVRIX 162
HEPARIN SODIUM 162, *480*
Hepatitis A Vaccine
  (Inactivated)
  Havrix 162

Hepatitis A Vaccine
  (inactivated)
  Vaqta 382
HEPATITIS B IMMUNE
  GLOBULIN (HUMAN) *481*
Hepatitis B (Recombinant)
  Hepatitis B Vaccine
    (Recombinant) *482*
  Pediarix 263
  Recombivax HB 299
  Recombivax HB Adult 299
  Recombivax HB
    Dialysis 299
  Recombivax HB
    Pediatric/Adolescent ... 299
Hexachlorophene
  pHisoHex 271
Hib CONJUGATE HEPATITIS
  B COMBINATION
  VACCINE *482*
HIPREX 163
HISTA-VENT DA 163
Histrelin Acetate
  Supprelin LA 333
HISTUSSIN D 164
HIVID 164
HUMALOG 165
Human Papillomavirus
  Recombinant Vaccine,
  Quadrivalent
  Gardasil 153
HUMATROPE 165
HUMIBID 166
HUMULIN 166
HUMULIN 70/30 167
HYALURONIDASE *483*
HYCOTUSS 167
HYDRALAZINE 168, *483*
HYDROCHLOROTHIAZIDE
  .... 168, *484*
Hydrocodone Bitartrate
  Codiclear DH 159
  Entex HC 126
  Histussin D 164
  Hycotuss 167
  Lortab 201
  Reprexain 389
  Tussend 369
  Tussend Expectorant 369
  Vicodin Tuss 159
  Vicoprofen 389
  Vi-Q-Tuss 167
Hydrocodone Polistirex
  Tussionex Pennkinetic 370
Hydrocortisone
  Acetasol HC 398
  Alcortin 15
  Anusol-HC Cream 27
  Cipro HC 66
  Cortane-B 78
  Cortef 78
  Cortisporin Otic 79
  Hydrocortisone *485*
  Hytone 170
  Pediotic 264
  Proctocort Cream 285
  Proctocream HC 27

I-7

Brand/Generic Index

Proctosol HC 27
Proctozone-HC 27
VoSoL HC 398
Vytone 399
Zoto HC 78
HYDROCORTISONE
ACETATE 168
Hydrocortisone Acetate
  Analpram-HC 25
  Cortisporin-TC Otic 79
  Epifoam 128
  Novacort 244
  Pramosone 276
  ProctoFoam-HC 285
Hydrocortisone Butyrate
  Locoid 198
Hydrocortisone Sodium
Succinate
  Solu-Cortef 323
Hydrocortisone Valerate
  Westcort 400
Hydroquinone
  Claripel 70
  Eldopaque Forte 121
  Eldoquin Forte 121
  Epiquin Micro 128
  Lustra 203
  Lustra-AF 203
  Solaquin Forte 323
Hydroxychloroquine Sulfate
  Plaquenil 273
Hydroxypropyl
Methylcellulose
  All Clear AR 17
  Visine for Contacts 395
  Visine Tears 396
HYDROXYZINE HCL 169
Hydroxyzine HCl
  Atarax 169
HYDROXYZINE
PAMOATE 170
Hydroxyzine Pamoate
  Vistaril 170
Hyoscyamine Sulfate
  Donnatal 114
  Donnatal Extentabs 114
  IB-Stat 171
  Levbid 190
  Levsin 190
  Levsinex 190
  NuLev 248
  Prosed DS 290
  Prosed EC 290
  Urimax 377
  Urised 377
  Urogesic Blue 378
HYTONE 170
HYTONE 1% 170
  Hydrocortisone 170

I

IB-STAT 171
Ibuprofen
  Ibuprofen Lysine 486
  Motrin 223
  Motrin, Children's 224
  Motrin IB 224

Motrin, Infants 224
Motrin, Junior 224
Reprexain 389
Vicoprofen 389
IC-GREEN 171
Imatinib Mesylate
  Gleevec 156
Imiglucerase
  Cerezyme 62
Imipenem
  Imipenem/Cilastatin 487
  Primaxin I.M. 282
  Primaxin I.V. 282
Imipramine HCl
  Tofranil 358
Imipramine Pamoate
  Tofranil-PM 359
Imiquimod
  Aldara 15
Immune Globulin
  Gammar-P 152
IMODIUM A-D 172
IMOGAM RABIES-HT 172
IMOVAX RABIES
VACCINE 172
INAPSINE 173
INDERAL 174
INDOCIN I.V. 174
Indocyanine Green
  IC-Green 171
INDOMETHACIN 175, 487
Indomethacin
  Indocin 175
  Indomethacin 175, 487
Indomethacin Sodium
trihydrate
  Indocin I.V. 174
INFANRIX 176
INFASURF 489
INFED 176
Infliximab
  Remicade 300
Influenza Virus Vaccine
  Fluvirin 145
  Fluzone 146
Influenza Virus Vaccine Live
  FluMist 144
INFUVITE PEDIATRIC 489
INSULIN 490
Insulin Aspart
  Novolog 246
Insulin Detemir, rDNA Origin
  Levemir 191
Insulin Glargine, Human
  Lantus 188
Insulin, Human Isophane
  Humulin 166
  Humulin N 166
  Humulin R 166
  Novolin 245
  Novolin N 245
  Novolin R 245
Insulin, Human (Isophane/
Regular)
  Humulin 50/50 167
  Humulin 70/30 167
  Novolin 70/30 245

Insulin Human, rDNA Origin
  Humulin 166
  Humulin 50/50 167
  Humulin 70/30 167
  Humulin N 166
  Humulin R 166
  Novolin 245
  Novolin 70/30 245
  Novolin N 245
  Novolin R 245
Insulin, Human Regular
  Humulin 166
  Humulin N 166
  Humulin R 166
  Novolin 245
  Novolin N 245
  Novolin R 245
Insulin Lispro
  Humalog 165
INTAL 177
Interferon Alfa-2a,
Recombinant
  Roferon-A 310
Interferon Alfa-2b
  Intron A 177
INTRAVENOUS IMMUNE
GLOBULIN (HUMAN) 491
INTRON A 177
INVANZ 178
INVIRASE 178
Iodoquinol
  Alcortin 15
  Vytone 399
IONAMIN 179
Ipratropium Bromide
  Atrovent 32
  Atrovent HFA 32
  Atrovent Nasal 32
  Ipratropium 492
IQUIX 179
Irbesartan
  Avapro 34
IROFOL 180
Iron
  Niferex 239
Iron Carbonyl
  Feosol 139
Iron Dextran
  INFeD 176
  Iron Dextran 493
ISONIAZID 180
Isoniazid
  Nydrazid 180
  Rifater 304
ISOPROTERENOL 494
Isotretinoin
  Accutane 2
  Amnesteem 2
  Claravis 2
  Sotret 2
Ivermectin
  Stromectol 328

K

KALETRA 180
KAYEXALATE 181

I-8 PDR® Concise Drug Guide

Brand/Generic Index

KEFLEX 182
KEPPRA 182
KETAMINE 183
Ketamine HCl
  Ketamine 183
Ketoconazole
  Nizoral 241
  Nizoral A-D 241
KETOROLAC 183
Ketorolac Tromethamine
  Acular 5
  Ketorolac 183
  Toradol 183
Ketotifen Fumarate
  Zaditor 408
KLARON 184
KLONOPIN 184
KOGENATE FS 185
KYTRIL 185

L

LAC-HYDRIN 186
LAMICTAL 186
LAMISIL AT 187
Lamivudine
  Combivir 75
  Epivir 129
  Epivir-HBV 129
  Lamivudine *495*
  Trizivir 367
Lamotrigine
  Lamictal 186
  Lamictal CD 186
LANOXIN 188
Lansoprazole
  Lansoprazole *495*
  Prevacid 279
  Prevacid IV 279
  Prevacid Solutab 279
LANTUS 188
LARIAM 189
LESCOL XL 190
Leuprolide Acetate
  Lupron Depot-Ped 203
  Lupron Pediatric 203
Levalbuterol HCl
  Xopenex 403
Levalbuterol Tartrate
  Xopenex HFA 403
LEVBID 190
LEVEMIR 191
Levetiracetam
  Keppra 182
Levocabastine HCl
  Livostin 198
Levocetirizine
Dihydrochloride
  Xyzal 406
Levofloxacin
  Iquix 179
  Quixin 297
LEVOTHROID 192
Levothyroxine Sodium
  Levothroid 192
  Levothyroxin (T_4) *496*
  Levoxyl 193

Synthroid 339
Tirosint 355
Unithroid 376
LEVOXYL 193
LIBRIUM 194
LIDEX 194
Lidocaine
  EMLA 125
  EMLA Anesthetic Disc 125
  Lidocaine -
Antiarrhythmic,
Anticonvulsant *497, 498*
  Lidocaine Ointment 194
  Synera 338
Lidocaine HCl
  Xylocaine Injection 403
  Xylocaine Jelly 404
  Xylocaine Viscous 404
  Xylocaine with
Epinephrine 405
  Xylocaine-MPF 403
  Xylocaine-MPF with
Epinephrine 405
LIDOCAINE OINTMENT 194
LINCOCIN 195
Lincomycin HCl
  Lincocin 195
LINDANE 195
Linezolid
  Linezolid *498*
  Zyvox 419
Liothyronine Sodium
  Cytomel 85
Liotrix
  Thyrolar 353
Lipase
  Cotazym 81
  Pancrease 259
  Pancrease MT 259
  Viokase 392
  Zymase 418
LIPITOR 196
Lisdexamfetamine
Dimesylate
  Vyvanse 399
LITHIUM CARBONATE 197
Lithium Carbonate
  Eskalith 136
  Eskalith CR 136
  Lithobid 197
LITHOBID 197
LIVOSTIN 198
LOCOID 198
LODINE XL 199
Lodoxamide Tromethamine
  Alomide 19
LODRANE 24 199
LOMOTIL 200
Lomustine
  CeeNU 56
Loperamide HCl
  Imodium A-D 172
Lopinavir
  Kaletra 180
LOPROX 200
Loratadine
  Claritin OTC 70

Claritin Reditab OTC 70
Claritin-D OTC 70
Lorazepam
  Ativan 31
  Lorazepam *500*
LORTAB 201
LOTENSIN 201
LOTRIMIN 202
LOTRIMIN AF 202
LOTRIMIN AF SPRAY &
  POWDER 202
LOTRIMIN ULTRA 202
Lovastatin
  Mevacor 218
LUPRON PEDIATRIC 203
LURIDE 203
LUSTRA 203
Lymphocyte Immune
Globulin, Anti-thymocyte
Globulin (Equine)
  Atgam 30

M

MACROBID 204
MACRODANTIN 204
Mafenide Acetate
  Sulfamylon 332
Magnesium Hydroxide
  Mylanta Maximum
Strength Liquid 229
  Mylanta Regular
Strength Liquid 229
  Pepcid Complete 266
MALARONE 205
Malathion
  Ovide 257
MARCAINE 205
MARCAINE WITH
  EPINEPHRINE 206
MATULANE 207
MAXAIR 207
MAXIPIME 208
Measles Vaccine Live
  ProQuad 290
MEBARAL 208
MEBENDAZOLE 209
Meclizine HCl
  Antivert 27
MECLOFENAMATE 209
Meclofenamate Sodium
  Meclofenamate 209
MEDROL 209
Mefenamic Acid
  Ponstel 275
Mefloquine HCl
  Lariam 189
Meloxicam
  Mobic 221
MENACTRA 210
Meningococcal
Polysaccharide Diptheria
Toxoid Conjugate
Vaccine
  Menactra 210
MENTAX 210

I-9

Brand/Generic Index

Meperidine HCl
  Demerol Injection 94
  Demerol Oral 95
Mephobarbital
  Mebaral 208
Meprobamate
  Equagesic 130
  Miltown 218
MEPRON 211
Mercaptopurine
  Purinethol 294
MERIDIA 211
Meropenem
  Meropenem *500*
  Merrem 212
MERREM 212
MERUVAX II 212
METADATE CD 213
METADATE ER 213
METAPROTERENOL 214
Metaproterenol Sulfate
  Alupent 214
  Metaproterenol 214
Metaxalone
  Skelaxin 322
Metformin HCl
  Glucophage 157
  Glucophage XR 157
  Riomet 157
METHADONE *501*
Methamphetamine HCl
  Desoxyn 103
Methenamine
  Prosed DS 290
  Prosed EC 290
  Urimax 377
  Urised 377
  Urogesic Blue 378
Methenamine Hippurate
  Hiprex 163
Methimazole
  Tapazole 342
Methocarbamol
  Robaxin 307
  Robaxin Injection 307
  Robaxin-750 307
Methohexital Sodium
  Brevital 51
METHOTREXATE
  SODIUM 214
Methotrexate Sodium
  Rheumatrex 214
Methoxsalen
  Oxsoralen 258
Methscopolamine Nitrate
  AlleRx 18
  Dallergy 87
  Hista-Vent DA 163
Methsuximide
  Celontin 61
METHYLDOPA 215
METHYLDOPATE HCL 216
Methylene Blue
  Prosed DS 290
  Prosed EC 290
  Urimax 377
  Urised 377

Urogesic Blue 378
METHYLIN 216
Methylphenidate
  Daytrana 91
Methylphenidate HCl
  Concerta 76
  Metadate CD 213
  Metadate ER 213
  Methylin 216
  Methylin ER 216
  Ritalin 306
  Ritalin LA 306
  Ritalin SR 306
Methylprednisolone
  Medrol 209
  Medrol Dose Pack 209
Methylprednisolone
  Acetate
  Depo-Medrol 99
Methylprednisolone Sodium
  Succinate
  Solu-Medrol 324
Methyltestosterone
  Testred 348
METOCLOPRAMIDE 217
Metoclopramide HCl
  Metoclopramide 217, *502*
  Reglan 217
  Reglan Injection 217
Metronidazole
  Flagyl 140
  Metronidazole *502*
Metyrosine
  Demser 95
MEVACOR 218
Miconazole Nitrate
  Lotrimin AF Spray &
    Powder 202
  Monistat 222
  Monistat 1
    Combination Pack 222
  Monistat 3 222
  Monistat 7 222
Midazolam HCl
  Midazolam *503*
  Versed Injection 385
  Versed Syrup 386
MILRINONE *505*
MILTOWN 218
Mineral Oil
  Tucks Ointment 368
MINOCIN 219
Minocycline HCl
  Dynacin 119
  Minocin 219
  Solodyn 323
MINOXIDIL 220
MINTEZOL 220
MIRALAX 221
MIVACURIM *506*
MOBAN 221
MOBIC 221
Modafinil
  Provigil 292
Molindone HCl
  Moban 221

Mometasone Furoate
  Asmanex 29
  Elocon 124
Mometasone Furoate
  Monohydrate
  Nasonex 234
MONISTAT 222
MONISTAT 1
  COMBINATION PACK ..222
MONODOX 223
Montelukast Sodium
  Singulair 322
MORPHINE *506*
MOTRIN 223
MOTRIN, CHILDREN'S 224
MOTRIN IB 224
Moxifloxacin HCl
  Vigamox 390
MUCINEX 225
MUCINEX D 225
MUCINEX DM 225
MUCOMYST 226
Multiple Vitamin
  Poly-Vi-Flor 275
Mumps Vaccine Live
  ProQuad 290
Mumps Virus Vaccine Live
  Mumpsvax 226
MUMPSVAX 226
Mupirocin
  Bactroban 39
  Mupirocin *507*
MYAMBUTOL 227
MYCELEX TROCHE 227
MYCELEX-3 227
MYCELEX-7 228
MYCOLOG-II 228
Mycophenolic Acid
  Myfortic 229
MYCOSTATIN TOPICAL ...228
MYFORTIC 229
MYLANTA MAXIMUM
  STRENGTH LIQUID 229
MYLERAN 230
MYOZYME 230
MYSOLINE 231

N

Nafarelin Acetate
  Synarel 338
NAFCILLIN *508*
Nalidixic Acid
  NegGram 234
NALOXONE 231
Naloxone
  Suboxone 329
  Subutex 329
Naloxone HCl
  Naloxone 231, *509*
  Narcan 231
  Talwin NX 340
Naphazoline HCl
  All Clear 17
  All Clear AR 17
  Naphcon-A 232
  Opcon-A 253

Brand/Generic Index

Vasocon-A ... 382
Visine-A ... 396
NAPHCON-A ... 232
NAPROSYN ... 232
Naproxen
  EC-Naprosyn ... 232
  Naprosyn ... 232
Naproxen Sodium
  Aleve ... 16
NASACORT AQ ... 233
NASAREL ... 233
NASONEX ... 234
NAVANE ... 234
Nedocromil Sodium
  Alocril ... 19
  Tilade ... 353
NEGGRAM ... 234
Nelarabine
  Arranon ... 29
Nelfinavir Mesylate
  Viracept ... 392
NEMBUTAL SODIUM ... 235
Neomycin
  Cortisporin Otic ... 79
  Neosporin + Pain Relief
    Maximum Strength ... 236
  Neosporin Ointment ... 236
Neomycin Sulfate
  Cortisporin-TC Otic ... 79
  Pediotic ... 264
NEOSAR ... 235
NEOSPORIN + PAIN
RELIEF MAXIMUM
STRENGTH ... 236
NEOSPORIN OINTMENT ... 236
NEOSTIGMINE ... 509
NEO-SYNEPHRINE
OPHTHALMIC ... 237
NESACAINE ... 237
NETILMICIN ... 510
NEURONTIN ... 238
Nevirapine
  Nevirapine ... 511
  Viramune ... 393
NEXIUM ... 239
NICARDIPINE ... 512
NIFEREX ... 239
NIMBEX ... 239
Nitazoxanide
  Alinia ... 16
Nitisinone
  Orfadin ... 256
NITRIC OXIDE ... 513
Nitrofurantoin
  Furadantin ... 150
Nitrofurantoin
Macrocrystals
  Macrodantin ... 204
Nitrofurantoin
Monohydrate
  Macrobid ... 204
NIX ... 240
Nizatidine
  Axid ... 35
  Axid Oral Solution ... 35
  Nizatidine ... 514
NIZORAL ... 241

NIZORAL A-D ... 241
NORDITROPIN ... 241
Norethindrone Acetate
  Estrostep Fe ... 136
Norgestimate
  Ortho Tri-Cyclen ... 256
  Tri-Previfem ... 256
  Tri-Sprintec ... 256
NORPACE ... 242
NORVASC ... 243
NORVIR ... 243
NOVACORT ... 244
NOVAREL ... 244
NOVOLIN ... 245
NOVOLIN 70/30 ... 245
NOVOLOG ... 246
NOXAFIL ... 246
NUCOFED ... 247
NUCOFED PEDIATRIC
EXPECTORANT ... 248
NULEV ... 248
NULYTELY ... 249
NUTROPIN ... 249
Nystatin
  Mycolog-II ... 228
  Mycostatin Topical ... 228
  Nystatin ... 514
  Nystop ... 250
NYSTOP ... 250

O

OCTREOTIDE ... 515
OCUFLOX ... 250
Ofloxacin
  Floxin Otic ... 143
  Floxin Otic Singles ... 143
  Ocuflox ... 250
Olopatadine HCl
  Patanol ... 261
OLUX ... 251
OLUX-E ... 251
Omalizumab
  Xolair ... 402
Omeprazole
  Omeprazole ... 515
  Prilosec ... 281
OMNARIS ... 251
OMNICEF ... 252
OMNITROPE ... 252
ONCASPAR ... 253
Ondansetron
  Zofran ... 414
1-DAY ... 1
OPCON-A ... 253
OPTICROM ... 254
OPTIVAR ... 254
ORAP ... 254
ORAPRED ... 255
ORFADIN ... 256
Orlistat
  Xenical ... 401
ORTHO TRI-CYCLEN ... 256
Oseltamivir Phosphate
  Tamiflu ... 341
OVIDE ... 257
OXACILLIN ... 516

OXANDRIN ... 257
Oxandrolone
  Oxandrin ... 257
Oxaprozin
  Daypro ... 90
Oxcarbazepine
  Trileptal ... 365
Oxiconazole Nitrate
  Oxistat ... 258
OXISTAT ... 258
OXSORALEN ... 258
Oxybutynin Chloride
  Ditropan ... 112
  Ditropan XL ... 112
Oxymetazoline HCl
  Visine L.R. ... 395

P

PALGIC ... 258
Palivizumab
  Palivizumab ... 517
  Synagis ... 337
PANCREASE ... 259
PANCURONIUM ... 259
Pancuronium Bromide
  Pancuronium ... 259, 518
PANIXINE ... 260
PAPAVERINE ... 519
Paricalcitol
  Zemplar IV ... 410
PARLODEL ... 260
PASER ... 261
PATANOL ... 261
PCE ... 262
PEDIAPRED ... 262
PEDIARIX ... 263
PEDIAZOLE ... 264
PEDIOTIC ... 264
Pegaspargase
  Oncaspar ... 253
Pemirolast Potassium
  Alamast ... 14
Penicillamine
  Cuprimine ... 82
  Depen ... 82
Penicillin G Benzathine
  Bicillin C-R ... 46
  Bicillin C-R 900/300 ... 47
  Bicillin L-A ... 47
  Permapen ... 267
Penicillin G Potassium
  Penicillin G ... 519
  Pfizerpen ... 268
Penicillin G Procaine
  Bicillin C-R ... 46
  Bicillin C-R 900/300 ... 47
Penicillin V Potassium
  Penicillin VK ... 265
  Veetids ... 265
PENICILLIN VK ... 265
Pentazocine HCl
  Talwin NX ... 340
Pentobarbital Sodium
  Nembutal Sodium ... 235
  Pentobarbital ... 520

Brand/Generic Index

Pentosan Sodium
  Elmiron 123
PEPCID 265
PEPCID AC 266
PEPCID COMPLETE ... 266
PEPTO-BISMOL 266
PERI-COLACE 266
PERMAPEN 267
Permethrin
  Acticin 4
  Elimite 122
  Nix 240
PERPHENAZINE 267
Pertussis Vaccine, Acellular
  Boostrix 50
  Infanrix 176
  Pediarix 263
  Tripedia 366
Pertussis Vaccine Acellular, Adsorbed
  Adacel 5
  Daptacel 89
Peruvian Balsam
  Granulex 158
PFIZERPEN 268
Phendimetrazine tartrate
  Bontril PDM 49
  Bontril Slow-Release ... 49
PHENERGAN INJECTION 269
Pheniramine Maleate
  Naphcon-A 232
  Opcon-A 253
  Visine-A 396
PHENOBARBITAL 269
Phenobarbital
  Donnatal 114
  Donnatal Extentabs ... 114
  Phenobarbital 269, 520
Phentermine
  Ionamin 179
Phentermine HCl
  Adipex-P 8
PHENTOLAMINE 522
Phenyl Salicylate
  Prosed DS 290
  Prosed EC 290
  Urimax 377
  Urised 377
  Urogesic Blue 378
Phenylephrine HCl
  Alacol DM 13
  Dallergy 87
  Dallergy Jr 87
  Entex HC 126
  Entex LA 127
  Guaifed-PD 159
  Hista-Vent DA 163
  Neo-Synephrine Ophthalmic 237
  Phenylephrine (Ophthalmic) 522
  Promethazine VC ... 288
Promethazine VC/Codeine 288
Phenylephrine Tannate
  Rynatan Pediatric ... 314

Rynatuss 315
Rynatuss Pediatric ... 315
PHENYTEK 270
Phenytoin
  Dilantin 109
  Phenytoin 523
Phenytoin Sodium
  Phenytek 270
PHISOHEX 271
PHOSPHOLINE IODIDE ... 271
PHRENILIN FORTE 271
PHYTONADIONE 272
Pimecrolimus
  Elidel 122
Pimozide
  Orap 254
PIPERACILLIN 272
Piperacillin Sodium
  Piperacillin 272, 524
PIPERACILLIN-TAZOBACTAM 524
Pirbuterol Acetate
  Maxair 207
  Maxair Autohaler ... 207
PLAQUENIL 273
PNEUMOCOCCAL 7-VALENT CONJUGATE VACCINE 525
PLEXION 274
Pneumococcal Vaccine
  Pneumovax 23 274
PNEUMOVAX 23 274
Poliovirus Vaccine, Inactivated
  Pediarix 263
Poliovirus Vaccine Enhanced-Inactivated 526
Polyethylene Glycol 300
  All Clear 17
Polyethylene Glycol 3350
  MiraLax 221
  NuLYTELY 249
  Trilyte 249
Polyethylene Glycol 400
  Visine Advanced Relief 395
  Visine Tears 396
Polymyxin B
  Neosporin + Pain Relief Maximum Strength ... 236
Polymyxin B Sulfate
  Cortisporin Otic ... 79
  Neosporin Ointment ... 236
  Pediotic 264
  Polytrim 275
Polysaccharide Iron Complex
  Irofol 180
POLYTRIM 275
POLY-VI-FLOR 275
POLY-VI-SOL MVI DROPS 527
PONSTEL 275
Posaconazole
  Noxafil 246

Poractant Alfa
  Curosurf 451
POTABA 276
Potassium Chloride
  NuLYTELY 249
  Potassium Chloride ... 527
  Trilyte 249
Potassium p-aminobenzoate
  Potaba 276
Povidone
  Visine Advanced Relief 395
PRAMOSONE 276
Pramoxine HCl
  Analpram-HC 25
  Cortane-B 78
  Epifoam 128
  Neosporin + Pain Relief Maximum Strength ... 236
  Novacort 244
  Pramosone 276
  ProctoFoam-HC ... 285
  Tucks Ointment ... 368
  Zoto HC 78
PRAVACHOL 277
Pravastatin Sodium
  Pravachol 277
Praziquantel
  Biltricide 48
Prednicarbate
  Dermatop 101
Prednisolone
  Prelone 278
Prednisolone Acetate
  Blephamide 49
Prednisolone Acetate
  Blephamide S.O.P. ... 49
Prednisolone Sodium Phosphate
  Orapred 255
  Pediapred 262
PREDNISONE 277
Prednisone
  Deltasone 277
PREGNYL 278
PRELONE 278
PREVACID 279
PREVIDENT 280
PRIFTIN 280
Prilocaine
  EMLA 125
  EMLA Anesthetic Disc ... 125
PRILOSEC 281
PRIMAXIN I.M. 282
PRIMAXIN I.V. 282
Primidone
  Mysoline 231
PRIMSOL 283
PROAIR HFA 283
PROBENECID 283
PROCAINAMIDE 528
Procarbazine HCl
  Matulane 207
Prochlorperazine
  Compazine 76
  Compro 76

Brand/Generic Index

PROCRIT 284
PROCTOCORT CREAM ... 285
PROCTOFOAM-HC 285
PROFASI 286
PROGRAF 286
Proguanil HCl
  Malarone 205
  Malarone Pediatric 205
PROMETHAZINE 287
PROMETHAZINE DM 288
Promethazine HCl
  Phenergan 287
  Phenergan Injection 269
  Promethazine 287
  Promethazine DM 288
  Promethazine VC 288
  Promethazine
    VC/Codeine 288
  Promethazine
    w/Codeine 289
  Promethegan 287
PROMETHAZINE VC 288
PROMETHAZINE
  VC/CODEINE 288
PROMETHAZINE
  W/CODEINE 289
Propofol
  Diprivan 111
Propranolol HCl
  Inderal 174
  Propanolol *529*
PROPYLTHIOURACIL 289
PROQUAD 290
PROSED EC 290
PROSTIN VR PEDIATRIC ... 291
PROTAMINE *529*
Protease
  Cotazym 81
  Pancrease 259
  Pancrease MT 259
  Viokase 392
  Zymase 418
PROTOPIC 291
Protriptyline HCl
  Vivactil 397
PROVENTIL HFA 292
PROVIGIL 292
PROZAC 293
Pseudoephedrine HCl
  Allegra-D 18
  AlleRx 18
  Ami-Tex PSE 127
  Balamine DM 40
  Bromfed 52
  Bromfed-PD 52
  Bromfenex 52
  Bromfenex-PD 52
  Carbofed DM 313
  Cardec DM 313
  Deconamine 93
  Deconamine SR 93
  De-Congestine TR 93
  Duratuss 117
  Entex PSE 127
  Guaifenex PSE 120 127
  Guaituss DAC 160
  Histussin D 164
  Kronofed-A 93
  Mucinex D 225
  Mytussin DAC 248
  Nucofed 247
  Nucofed Pediatric
    Expectorant 248
  Rondec 311
  Rondec Oral Drops 311
  Rondec Syrup 312
  Rondec-DM Drops 312
  Rondec-DM Syrup 313
  Rondec-TR 311
  Semprex-D 317
  Sudafed 330
  Tussend 369
  Tussend Expectorant 369
  Zyrtec-D 419
Pseudoephedrine Sulfate
  Clarinex-D 24 Hour 69
  Claritin-D OTC 70
PULMICORT 294
PURINETHOL 294
PYRAZINAMIDE 295
Pyrazinamide
  Rifater 304
PYRIDOXINE *530*
Pyrimethamine
  Daraprim 90

Q

QUESTRAN 295
QUINIDINE GLUCONATE
  INJECTION 296
Quinupristin
  Quinupristin/
    Dalfopristin *530*
  Synercid 339
QUIXIN 297
QVAR 297

R

Rabies Immune Globulin
  Imogam Rabies-HT 172
Rabies Vaccine
  Imovax Rabies
    Vaccine 172
Ranitidine HCl
  Ranitidine *531*
  Zantac 408
  Zantac 150 409
  Zantac 75 409
  Zantac OTC 409
RAPAMUNE 297
Rasburicase
  Elitek 123
REBETOL 298
RECOMBIVAX HB 299
REGRANEX 299
RELENZA 300
REMICADE 300
Remifentanil HCl
  Ultiva 373
RESCRIPTOR 301
RESTASIS 302
Retapamulin
  Altabax 20
RETIN-A 302
RETROVIR 303
RHINOCORT AQUA 303
Rho (D) Immune Globulin
  WinRho SDF 400
Ribavirin
  Rebetol 298
  Rifampin *532*
  Virazole 394
RIFADIN 304
Rifampin
  Rifadin 304
  Rifater 304
Rifapentine
  Priftin 280
RIFATER 304
Rifaximin
  Xifaxan 402
Rimantadine HCl
  Flumadine 143
RISPERDAL 305
Risperidone
  Risperdal 305
  Risperdal M-Tab 305
RITALIN 306
Ritonavir
  Kaletra 180
  Norvir 243
ROBAXIN 307
ROBINUL 307
ROBINUL INJECTION 308
ROCALTROL 308
ROCEPHIN 309
Rocuronium Bromide
  Zemuron 410
ROFERON-A 310
ROMAZICON 311
RONDEC 311
RONDEC SYRUP 312
RONDEC-DM DROPS 312
RONDEC-DM SYRUP 313
ROSAC 313
ROSULA 313
ROSULA NS 314
ROTATEQ 314
Rotavirus Vaccine, Live
  RotaTeq 314
  Rotavirus Vaccine *533*
RSV IMMUNE
  GLOBULIN *534*
Rubella Vaccine Live
  Meruvax II 212
  ProQuad 290
RYNATAN PEDIATRIC 314
RYNATUSS 315

S

SAIZEN 315
Salmeterol Xinafoate
  Advair 9
  Advair HFA 10
  Serevent 321
SANDIMMUNE 316
Saquinavir
  Fortovase 150

I-13

Brand/Generic Index

Saquinavir Mesylate
  Invirase 178
Scopolamine Hydrobromide
  Donnatal 114
  Donnatal Extentabs 114
Secobarbital Sodium
  Seconal Sodium 317
SECONAL SODIUM 317
SEMPREX-D 317
Senna
  Peri-Colace 266
  Senokot 318
SENOKOT 318
SENSORCAINE 318
SENSORCAINE WITH EPINEPHRINE 319
SEPTOCAINE 320
SEPTRA 320
SEREVENT 321
Sertaconazole Nitrate
  Ertaczo 131
Sertraline HCl
  Zoloft 415
Sevoflurane
  Ultane 373
Sibutramine HCl Monohydrate
  Meridia 211
SILDENAFIL 534
Simethicone
  Mylanta Maximum Strength Liquid 229
  Mylanta Regular Strength Liquid 229
SIMULECT 321
Simvastatin
  Zocor 413
SINGULAIR 322
Sirolimus
  Rapamune 297
SKELAXIN 322
Smallpox Vaccine, Dried
  Dryvax 115
Sodium Bicarbonate
  NuLYTELY 249
  Sodium Bicarbonate 535
  Trilyte 249
Sodium Biphosphate
  Urimax 377
  Urogesic Blue 378
Sodium Chloride
  NuLYTELY 249
  Trilyte 249
Sodium Ferric Gluconate Complex
  Ferrlecit 139
Sodium Fluoride
  Luride 203
  Poly-Vi-Flor 275
  PreviDent 280
  PreviDent 5000 Plus 280
Sodium Nitrite
  Cyanide Antidote Package 83
SODIUM NITROPRUSSIDE .. 536

Sodium Oxybate
  Xyrem 406
Sodium Polystyrene Sulfonate
  Kayexalate 181
Sodium Thiosulfate
  Cyanide Antidote Package 83
SOLAQUIN FORTE 323
SOLODYN 323
SOLU-CORTEF 323
SOLU-MEDROL 324
SOMA 325
SOMA CMPD/CODEINE 325
SOMA COMPOUND 326
Somatropin
  Genotropin 154
  Genotropin MiniQuick 154
  Humatrope 165
  Norditropin 241
  Norditropin Nordiflex 241
  Nutropin 249
  Nutropin AQ 249
  Omnitrope 252
  Saizen 315
  Tev-Tropin 349
Sotalol HCl
  Betapace 44
  Betapace AF 45
  Sotalol 537
SPECTRACEF 326
SPIRONOLACTONE 537
Starch
  Tucks Suppositories 368
Stavudine
  Zerit 411
STRATTERA 326
STREPTOMYCIN 327
Streptomycin Sulfate
  Streptomycin 327
STROMECTOL 328
SUBLIMAZE 329
SUBOXONE 329
Succinylcholine Chloride
  Anectine 26
SUCROSE 538
SUDAFED 330
SUFENTA 331
Sufentanil Citrate
  Sufenta 331
Sulbactam Sodium
  Unasyn 374
Sulfacetamide Sodium
  AK-Sulf 48
  Bleph-10 48
  Blephamide 49
  Blephamide S.O.P. 49
  Clenia 71
  Klaron 184
  Plexion 274
  Plexion SCT 274
  Plexion TS 274
  Rosac 313
  Rosula 313
  Rosula NS 314
  Sulfacet-R 331

  Zetacet 411
SULFACET-R 331
Sulfamethoxazole
  Bactrim 39
  Bactrim DS 39
  Septra 320
  Septra DS 320
  Sulfatrim Pediatric 320
SULFAMYLON 332
Sulfasalazine
  Azulfidine 37
  Azulfidine EN 37
Sulfisoxazole
  Gantrisin Pediatric 153
Sulfisoxazole Acetyl
  Pediazole 264
Sulfur
  Clenia 71
  Plexion 274
  Plexion SCT 274
  Plexion TS 274
  Rosac 313
  Rosula 313
  Sulfacet-R 331
  Zetacet 411
SUMYCIN 332
SUPPRELIN LA 333
SUPRANE 333
SUPRAX 334
SURFACTANT (NATURAL, ANIMAL-DERIVED) 538
SURVANTA 539
SURMONTIL 334
SUSTIVA 335
SYMBICORT 335
SYMMETREL 336
SYNAGIS 337
SYNALAR 337
SYNALGOS-DC 337
SYNAREL 338
SYNERA 338
SYNERCID 339
SYNTHROID 339

T

Tacrolimus
  Prograf 286
  Protopic 291
TALWIN NX 340
TAMBOCOR 341
TAMIFLU 341
TAPAZOLE 342
TAVIST ALLERGY 342
TAXOTERE 342
Tazarotene
  Tazorac 345
TAZICEF 343
TAZIDIME 344
TAZORAC 345
TEGRETOL 345
Telbivudine
  Tyzeka 372
TEMOVATE 346
Teniposide
  Vumon 398
TENUATE 347

Brand/Generic Index

Terbinafine HCl
  Lamisil AT 187
TERBUTALINE 347
Terbutaline Sulfate
  Terbutaline 347
TESSALON 348
Testosterone
  Androderm 25
Testosterone Cypionate
  Depo-Testosterone 100
Testosterone Enanthate
  Delatestryl 94
TESTRED 348
TETANUS & DIPHTHERIA
  TOXOIDS ADSORBED 349
Tetanus Toxoid
  Adacel 5
  Boostrix 50
  Daptacel 89
  Infanrix 176
  Pediarix 263
Tetanus & Diphtheria
  Toxoids Adsorbed 349
Tetanus Toxoid
  Adsorbed 349
  Tripedia 366
TETANUS TOXOID
  ADSORBED 349
Tetracaine
  Synera 338
Tetracycline HCl
  Sumycin 332
Tetrahydrozoline HCl
  Visine A.C. 394
  Visine Advanced
    Relief 395
  Visine Original 396
TEV-TROPIN 349
Thalidomide
  Thalomid 350
THALOMID 350
THAM ACETATE *540*
THEO-24 351
THEOLAIR 351
Theophylline
  Theo-24 351
  Theolair 351
  Uniphyl 375
Thiabendazole
  Mintezol 220
THIOGUANINE 352
THIORIDAZINE 352
Thioridazine HCl
  Thioridazine 352
Thiothixene
  Navane 234
Thonzonium Bromide
  Cortisporin-TC Otic 79
Thyroid
  Armour Thyroid 28
THYROLAR 353
Tiagabine HCl
  Gabitril 152
Ticarcillin Disodium
  Ticarcillin/Clavulanate ... *541*
  Timentin 354
TILADE 353

TIMENTIN 354
Timolol Maleate
  Cosopt 81
TINDAMAX 354
Tinidazole
  Tindamax 354
Tioconazole
  1-Day 1
TIROSINT 355
TOBI 356
TOBRADEX 357
Tobramycin
  TOBI 356
  TobraDex 357
  Tobramycin *541*
TOBRAMYCIN SULFATE 357
TOFRANIL 358
TOFRANIL-PM 359
TOLMETIN 359
Tolmetin Sodium
  Tolectin 359
  Tolmetin 359
TOPAMAX 360
TOPICORT 361
Topiramate
  Topamax 360
TRACLEER 361
TRACRIUM 362
TRANXENE-SD 362
TRAUMEEL 363
TRAUMEEL TOPICAL 363
TRECATOR 364
Tretinoin
  Retin-A 302
  Retin-A Micro 302
  Vesanoid 387
  Vesanoid 387
  Ziana 412
Triamcinolone Acetonide
  Azmacort 36
  Mycolog-II 228
  Nasacort AQ 233
  Nasacort HFA 233
TRIFLUOPERAZINE HCL 364
Trifluridine
  Viroptic 394
TRILEPTAL 365
TRILISATE 366
Trimethoprim
  Bactrim 39
  Bactrim DS 39
  Septra 320
  Septra DS 320
  Sulfatrim Pediatric 320
Trimethoprim HCl
  Primsol 283
Trimethoprim Sulfate
  Polytrim 275
Trimipramine Maleate
  Surmontil 334
TRIPEDIA 366
TRISENOX 367
TRI-VI-SOL MVI DROPS *543*
TRIZIVIR 367
TROPICAMIDE
  (OPHTHALMIC) *543*
TRUSOPT 368

Trypsin
  Granulex 158
TUCKS OINTMENT 368
TUCKS SUPPOSITORIES 368
TUSSEND 369
TUSSEND
  EXPECTORANT 369
TUSSI-12 370
TUSSIONEX
  PENNKINETIC 370
TUSSI-ORGANIDIN DM
  NR 370
TWINJECT 371
TYLENOL 371
TYLENOL WITH
  CODEINE 372
TYZEKA 372

U

ULTANE 373
ULTIVA 373
ULTRAVATE 374
UNASYN 374
UNIPHYL 375
UNISOM 375
UNITHROID 376
Urea
  Rosula NS 314
URIMAX 377
URISED 377
URISPAS 378
UROGESIC BLUE 378
Ursodiol *544*

V

Valacyclovir HCl
  Valtrex 379
VALIUM 379
Valproate Sodium
  Depacon 96
Valproic acid
  Depakene 97
VALTREX 379
VANCOCIN 380
VANCOCIN ORAL 380
Vancomycin HCl
  Vancocin 380
  Vancocin Oral 380
  Vancomycin *544*
VANIQA 381
VANOS 381
VANTIN 381
VAQTA 382
Varicella Virus Vaccine Live
  ProQuad 290
VASOCON-A 382
VASOTEC 383
VECURONIUM 383
Vecuronium Bromide
  Vecuronium 383, *546*
VENTOLIN HFA 384
VERAMYST 385
VERDESO 385
VERSED INJECTION 385
VERSED SYRUP 386

Brand/Generic Index

VESANOID 387
VIBRAMYCIN 387
VIBRAMYCIN IV 388
VICOPROFEN 389
Vidarabine
  Vira-A 392
VI-DAYLIN ADC DROPS ... *547*
VI-DAYLIN
  MULTIVITAMIN
  PRODUCTS *547*
VI-DAYLIN MVI DROPS *548*
VIDEX 389
VIGAMOX 390
VINBLASTINE 390
Vinblastine Sulfate
  Vinblastine 390
VINCRISTINE SULFATE 391
VIOKASE 392
VIRA-A 392
VIRACEPT 392
VIRAMUNE 393
VIRAZOLE 394
VIROPTIC 394
VISINE A.C. 394
VISINE ADVANCED
  RELIEF 395
VISINE FOR CONTACTS ... 395
VISINE L.R. 395
VISINE ORIGINAL 396
VISINE TEARS 396
VISINE-A 396
VI-SOL MULTIVITAMIN
  PRODUCTS *548*
VITAMIN A *549*
Vitamin C
  Fero-Grad-500 139
VITAMIN E *549*
VITAMIN K$_1$ *550*
VITRASERT 397
VIVACTIL 397
VOSOL HC 398
VOSPIRE ER 398
VUMON 398
VYTONE 399
VYVANSE 399

W

WESTCORT 400
WINRHO SDF 400

X

XENICAL 401
XIFAXAN 402
XOLAIR 402
XOPENEX 403
XOPENEX HFA 403
XYLOCAINE INJECTION ... 403
XYLOCAINE JELLY 404
XYLOCAINE VISCOUS 404
XYLOCAINE WITH
  EPINEPHRINE 405
XYREM 406
XYZAL 406

Y

YAZ 407
Yellow Fever Vaccine
  YF-Vax 407
YF-VAX 407

Z

ZADITOR 408
Zafirlukast
  Accolate 1
Zalcitabine
  Hivid 164
Zanamivir
  Relenza 300
ZANTAC 408
ZANTAC OTC 409
ZARONTIN 409
ZEMPLAR IV 410
ZEMURON 410
ZENAPAX 411
ZERIT 411
ZETACET 411
ZIAGEN 412
ZIANA 412
Zidovudine
  Combivir 75
  Retrovir 303
  Trizivir 367
  Zidovudine (ZDV, AZT) *551*
Zileuton
  Zyflo 417
  Zyflo CR 417
Zinc Oxide
  Tucks Ointment 368
Zinc Sulfate
  Visine A.C. 394
ZITHROMAX 412
ZOCOR 413
ZOFRAN 414
ZOLOFT 415
ZONEGRAN 416
Zonisamide
  Zonegran 416
ZOVIRAX 416
ZOVIRAX CREAM 416
ZYFLO CR 417
ZYLOPRIM 417
ZYMAR 418
ZYMASE 418
ZYRTEC 418
ZYRTEC-D 419
ZYVOX 419

Therapeutic Class Index

Organized alphabetically, this index includes the therapeutic class for each drug described in the PDR concise drug section. Therapeutic class headings are based on information provided in the drug monographs. The drug entries listed under each bold therapeutic class are organized alphabetically by brand name or monograph title (shown in capitalized letters), followed by the generic name in parentheses. (Note: Does not include NeoFax drug monographs.)

A

ACE INHIBITOR
LOTENSIN (benazepril HCl) 201
VASOTEC (enalapril maleate) 383

ACETAMIDE LOCAL ANESTHETIC
EMLA ANESTHETIC DISC (prilocaine) 125
LIDOCAINE OINTMENT (lidocaine) 194
SYNERA (tetracaine) 338
XYLOCAINE JELLY (lidocaine HCl) 404
XYLOCAINE VISCOUS (lidocaine HCl) 404

ACETAMINOPHEN ANTIDOTE/MUCOLYTIC
MUCOMYST (acetylcysteine) 226

ACID-STABLE PENICILLIN
VEETIDS (penicillin V potassium) 265

ACTINOMYCIN ANTIBIOTIC
COSMEGEN (dactinomycin) 80

ADAMANTANE CLASS ANTIVIRAL
FLUMADINE (rimantadine HCl) 143

ALKYLAMINE ANTIHISTAMINE
LODRANE 24 (brompheniramine maleate) 199

ALKYLATING AGENT
MYLERAN (busulfan) 230

ALLYLAMINE ANTIFUNGAL
LAMISIL AT (terbinafine HCl) 187

AMINOGLYCOSIDE
AMIKIN PEDIATRIC (amikacin sulfate) 21
GENTAMICIN OPHTHALMIC (gentamicin sulfate) 154
GENTAMICIN SULFATE INJECTION (gentamicin sulfate) 155
GENTAMICIN TOPICAL (gentamicin sulfate) 155
STREPTOMYCIN (streptomycin sulfate) 327
TOBI (tobramycin) 356
TOBRAMYCIN SULFATE (tobramycin sulfate) 357

AMINOGLYCOSIDE/CORTICOSTEROID
TOBRADEX (dexamethasone) 357

AMINOPENICILLIN/BETA LACTAMASE INHIBITOR
AUGMENTIN (clavulanate potassium) 33
AUGMENTIN ES-600 (clavulanate potassium) 33
AUGMENTIN XR (clavulanate potassium) 34

AMINOQUINOLONE
ARALEN (chloroquine) 28

ANABOLIC STEROID
OXANDRIN (oxandrolone) 257

ANALGESIC
FEVERALL (acetaminophen) 139
TYLENOL REGULAR STRENGTH (acetaminophen) 371

ANALGESIC, URINARY
ELMIRON (pentosan sodium) 123

ANDROGEN
ANDRODERM (testosterone) 25
DELATESTRYL (testosterone enanthate) 94
DEPO-TESTOSTERONE (testosterone cypionate) 100
HALOTESTIN (fluoxymesterone) 161
TESTRED (methyltestosterone) 348

ANESTHETIC
SEPTOCAINE (articaine HCl) 320

ANESTHETIC AGENT
TUCKS OINTMENT (pramoxine HCl) 368
TUCKS SUPPOSITORIES (starch) 368

ANGIOTENSIN II RECEPTOR ANTAGONIST
AVAPRO (irbesartan) 34

ANORECTIC SYMPATHOMIMETIC AMINE
ADIPEX-P (phentermine HCl) 8
BONTRIL PDM (phendimetrazine tartrate) 49
DIDREX (benzphetamine HCl) 107
IONAMIN (phentermine) 179

ANTACID
CHILDREN'S MYLANTA (calcium carbonate) 63

ANTACID/ANTIGAS
MYLANTA REGULAR STRENGTH LIQUID (magnesium hydroxide) 229

ANTHRACYCLINE
ADRIAMYCIN (doxorubicin HCl) 8
CERUBIDINE (daunorubicin HCl) 62

ANTIBACTERIAL COMBINATION
NEOSPORIN OINTMENT (polymyxin B sulfate) 236

ANTIBACTERIAL/ANALGESIC
NEOSPORIN + PAIN RELIEF MAXIMUM STRENGTH (pramoxine HCl) 236

ANTIBACTERIAL/CORTICOSTEROID COMBINATION
ACETASOL HC (hydrocortisone) 398
CIPRO HC (ciprofloxacin HCl) 66
CIPRODEX (dexamethasone) 68
CORTISPORIN OTIC (polymyxin B sulfate) 79
CORTISPORIN-TC OTIC (hydrocortisone acetate) 79
PEDIOTIC (polymyxin B sulfate) 264

ANTIBACTERIAL/KERATOLYTIC
BENZACLIN (benzoyl peroxide) 43
BENZAGEL WASH (benzoyl peroxide) 43
BENZAMYCIN (benzoyl peroxide) 43
BREVOXYL (benzoyl peroxide) 52
DUAC (benzoyl peroxide) 116

ANTIBIOTIC
BACITRACIN INJECTION (bacitracin) 38

I-17

Therapeutic Class Index

ANTICHOLINERGIC
ATROPINE SULFATE 31
IB-STAT (hyoscyamine sulfate) 171
LEVSINEX (hyoscyamine sulfate) 190
NULEV (hyoscyamine sulfate) 248
ROBINUL FORTE (glycopyrrolate) 307
ROBINUL INJECTION (glycopyrrolate) 308

ANTICHOLINERGIC AGENT
ATROVENT NASAL (ipratropium
   bromide) 32
DITROPAN (oxybutynin chloride) 112

ANTICHOLINERGIC BRONCHODILATOR
ATROVENT HFA (ipratropium bromide) 32

**ANTICHOLINERGIC/ANTIBACTERIAL/
ANTISEPTIC/ANALGESIC/ACIDIFIER**
URIMAX (hyoscyamine sulfate) 377
UROGESIC BLUE (hyoscyamine
   sulfate) 378

**ANTICHOLINERGIC/ANTISEPTIC/
ANTIBACTERIAL/ANALGESIC**
URISED (hyoscyamine sulfate) 377

ANTICHOLINERGIC/BARBITURATE
DONNATAL EXTENTABS (scopolamine
   hydrobromide) 114

ANTIDOTE
CYANIDE ANTIDOTE PACKAGE (sodium
   thiosulfate) 83

ANTIDOTE, DIGOXIN TOXICITY
DIGIBIND (digoxin immune fab
   (ovine)) 109

ANTIHEMOPHILIC FACTOR (Recombinant)
KOGENATE FS (antihemophilic factor) 185

ANTIHISTAMINE
ANTIVERT (meclizine HCl) 27
ASTELIN (azelastine HCl) 30
BENADRYL ALLERGY (diphenhydramine
   HCl) 42
CHLOR-TRIMETON (chlorpheniramine
   maleate) 65
DIPHENHYDRAMINE HCL INJECTION
   (diphenhydramine HCl) 110
TAVIST ALLERGY (clemastine
   fumarate) 342
UNISOM (doxylamine succinate) 375

**ANTIHISTAMINE/ANTICHOLINERGIC/
SYMPATHOMIMETIC**
DALLERGY (chlorpheniramine
   maleate) 87

**ANTIHISTAMINE/ANTICHOLINERGIC/
DECONGESTANT**
ALLERX (chlorpheniramine maleate) 18

**ANTIHISTAMINE/ANTICHOLINERGIC/
SYMPATHOMIMETIC**
HISTA-VENT DA (chlorpheniramine
   maleate) 163

**ANTIHISTAMINE/ANTITUSSIVE/
SYMPATHOMIMETIC**
ALACOL DM (brompheniramine
   maleate) 13

**ANTIHISTAMINE/COUGH SUPPRESSANT/
DECONGESTANT**
BALAMINE DM (carbinoxamine
   maleate) 40

ANTIHISTAMINE/DECONGESTANT
BROMFENEX-PD (brompheniramine
   maleate) 52
DECONAMINE SR (chlorpheniramine
   maleate) 93
RONDEC ORAL DROPS
   (carbinoxamine maleate) 311
RONDEC SYRUP (brompheniramine
   maleate) 312
SEMPREX-D (pseudoephedrine HCl) 317
VASOCON-A (antazoline phosphate) 382
ZYRTEC-D (pseudoephedrine HCl) 419

**ANTIHISTAMINE/DECONGESTANT/
ANTITUSSIVE**
CARBOFED DM (brompheniramine
   maleate) 313
RONDEC-DM DROPS (carbinoxamine
   maleate) 312

ANTIHISTAMINE/SYMPATHOMIMETIC
RYNATAN PEDIATRIC
   (chlorpheniramine tannate) 314

ANTIHISTAMINE/SYMPATHOMIMETIC AMINE
DALLERGY JR (chlorpheniramine
   maleate) 87

ANTI-INFLAMMATORY AGENT
COLAZAL (balsalazide disodium) 74

ANTIMANIC AGENT
LITHOBID (lithium carbonate) 197

ANTIMANIC AGENTS
ESKALITH CR (lithium carbonate) 136
LITHIUM CARBONATE 197

ANTIMETABOLITE
CLOLAR (clofarabine) 73
CYTOSAR-U (cytarabine) 85

ANTIMICROBIAL
PEPTO-BISMOL MAXIMUM STRENGTH
   (bismuth subsalicylate) 266

**ANTIMICROBIAL/CORTICOSTEROID/TOPICAL
ANESTHETIC**
ZOTO HC (pramoxine HCl) 78

ANTIMICROTUBULE AGENT
TAXOTERE (docetaxel) 342

ANTI-PERISTALSIS AGENT
IMODIUM A-D (loperamide HCl) 172

ANTIPROTOZOAL AGENT
ALINIA (nitazoxanide) 16
TINDAMAX (tinidazole) 354

ANTITUSSIVE/ANTIHISTAMINE
TUSSI-12 (chlorpheniramine tannate) 370

**ANTITUSSIVE/ANTIHISTAMINE/
BRONCHODILATOR/ SYMPATHOMIMETIC
COMBINATION**
RYNATUSS PEDIATRIC
   (chlorpheniramine tannate) 315

ANTITUSSIVE/DECONGESTANT
NUCOFED (pseudoephedrine HCl) 247

ANTITUSSIVE/EXPECTORANT
TUSSI-ORGANIDIN DM S NR
   (dextromethorphan hydrobromide) 370

ANTITUSSIVE/EXPECTORANT/DECONGESTANT
MYTUSSIN DAC (pseudoephedrine
   HCl) 248

ANTIVIRAL
ABREVA (docosanol) 1

ARYLOXYACETIC ACID DERIVATIVE
EDECRIN (ethacrynic acid) 121

THERAPEUTIC CLASS INDEX

AVERMECTINS DERIVATIVE
STROMECTOL (ivermectin) 328

AZOLE ANTIFUNGAL
ERTACZO (sertaconazole nitrate) 131
GYNE-LOTRIMIN 3 COMBINATION
  PACK (clotrimazole) 160
LOTRIMIN (clotrimazole) 202
LOTRIMIN AF (clotrimazole) 202
LOTRIMIN AF SPRAY & POWDER
  (miconazole nitrate) 202
MONISTAT 1 COMBINATION PACK
  (miconazole nitrate) 222
MONISTAT 7 (miconazole nitrate) 222
MYCELEX-3 (butoconazole nitrate) 227
MYCELEX-7 (clotrimazole) 228
NIZORAL (ketoconazole) 241
NIZORAL A-D (ketoconazole) 241
1-DAY (tioconazole) 1
OXISTAT (oxiconazole nitrate) 258
VAGISTAT-1 (tioconazole) 378

B

BACTERIAL PROTEIN SYNTHESIS INHIBITOR
BACTROBAN (mupirocin) 39

BARBITUATE ANESTHETIC
BREVITAL (methohexital sodium) 51

BARBITURATE
MEBARAL (mephobarbital) 208
NEMBUTAL SODIUM (pentobarbital
  sodium) 235
PHENOBARBITAL 269
SECONAL SODIUM (secobarbital
  sodium) 317

BARBITURATE/ANALGESIC
ESGIC (acetaminophen) 135
ESGIC-PLUS (acetaminophen) 135
FIORICET (acetaminophen) 140
PHRENILIN (acetaminophen) 271

BENZISOXAZOLE DERIVATIVE
RISPERDAL M-TAB (risperidone) 305

BENZODIAZEPINE
ATIVAN (lorazepam) 31
DALMANE (flurazepam HCl) 87
DIASTAT (diazepam) 106
DIAZEPAM INJECTION (diazepam) 106
KLONOPIN WAFERS (clonazepam) 184
LIBRIUM (chlordiazepoxide HCl) 194
TRANXENE-SD HALF STRENGTH
  (clorazepate dipotassium) 362
VALIUM (diazepam) 379
VERSED INJECTION (midazolam HCl) 385
VERSED SYRUP (midazolam HCl) 386

BENZODIAZEPINE ANTAGONIST
ROMAZICON (flumazenil) 311

BENZYLAMINE ANTIFUNGAL
LOTRIMIN ULTRA (butenafine HCl) 202
MENTAX (butenafine HCl) 210

BETA$_2$ AGONIST
ACCUNEB (albuterol sulfate) 2
ALUPENT (metaproterenol sulfate) 214
FORADIL (formoterol fumarate) 149
MAXAIR AUTOHALER (pirbuterol
  acetate) 207
PROAIR HFA (albuterol sulfate) 283
PROVENTIL (albuterol sulfate) 14
PROVENTIL HFA (albuterol sulfate) 292
SEREVENT (salmeterol xinafoate) 321

TERBUTALINE (terbutaline sulfate) 347
VENTOLIN HFA (albuterol sulfate) 384
VOSPIRE ER (albuterol sulfate) 398
XOPENEX (levalbuterol HCl) 403
XOPENEX HFA (levalbuterol tartrate) 403

BETA-BLOCKER (group II/III antiarrhythmic)
BETAPACE (sotalol HCl) 44
BETAPACE AF (sotalol HCl) 45

BETA-GLUCOCEREBROSIDASE
CEREZYME (imiglucerase) 62

BIGUANIDE
GLUCOPHAGE (metformin HCl) 157

BILE ACID SEQUESTRANT
QUESTRAN LIGHT (cholestyramine) 295

BIOLOGICAL RESPONSE MODIFIER
INTRON A (interferon alfa-2b) 177
ROFERON-A (interferon alfa-2a,
  recombinant) 310

BOWEL CLEANSER
TRILYTE (polyethylene glycol 3350) 249

BROAD-SPECTRUM ANTHELMINTIC
ALBENZA (albendazole) 14
MEBENDAZOLE 209

BROAD-SPECTRUM ANTIFUNGAL
LOPROX TS (ciclopirox) 200

BROAD-SPECTRUM PENICILLIN
PIPERACILLIN (piperacillin sodium) 272

**BROAD-SPECTRUM PENICILLIN/
BETA-LACTAMASE INHIBITOR**
TIMENTIN (clavulanate potassium) 354

BUTYROPHENONE
HALDOL DECANOATE (haloperidol) 161

C

**CALCIUM CHANNEL BLOCKER
(dihydropyridine)**
NORVASC (amlodipine besylate) 243

**CALCIUM CHANNEL BLOCKER/HMG-COA
REDUCTASE INHIBITOR**
CADUET (atorvastatin calcium) 53

CARBAMATE DERIVATIVE
MILTOWN (meprobamate) 218

CARBAMATE DERIVATIVE/SALICYLATE
EQUAGESIC (meprobamate) 130

CARBAPENEM
INVANZ (ertapenem sodium) 178
MERREM (meropenem) 212

CARBONIC ANHYDRASE INHIBITOR
TRUSOPT (dorzolamide HCl) 368

**CARBONIC ANHYDRASE INHIBITOR/
NONSELECTIVE BETA-BLOCKER**
COSOPT (timolol maleate) 81

CARBOXAMIDE ANTICONVULSANT
CARBATROL (carbamazepine) 54
TEGRETOL-XR (carbamazepine) 345

CARBOXYLIC ACID DERIVATIVE
DEPACON (valproate sodium) 96
DEPAKENE (valproic acid) 97

CARDIAC GLYCOSIDE
LANOXICAPS (digoxin) 188

I-19

Therapeutic Class Index

CATION-EXCHANGE RESIN
KAYEXALATE (sodium polystyrene sulfonate) 181

CELL METABOLISM INHIBITOR
MYAMBUTOL (ethambutol HCl) 227

CENTRAL ALPHA-ADRENERGIC AGONIST
METHYLDOPA 215
METHYLDOPATE HCL 216

CENTRAL MUSCLE RELAXANT/ANALGESIC
SOMA CMPD/CODEINE (codeine phosphate) 325
SOMA COMPOUND (carisoprodol) 326

CEPHALOSPORIN (1st generation)
ANCEF (cefazolin) 25
DURICEF (cefadroxil monohydrate) 118
KEFLEX (cephalexin) 182
PANIXINE (cephalexin) 260

CEPHALOSPORIN (2nd generation)
CEFACLOR 56
CEFACLOR ER (cefaclor) 56
CEFTIN (cefuroxime axetil) 58
CEFZIL (cefprozil) 58
MEFOXIN (cefoxitin sodium) 57

CEPHALOSPORIN (3rd generation)
CEDAX (ceftibuten) 55
CEFIZOX (ceftizoxime) 57
CEPTAZ (ceftazidime) 61
CLAFORAN (cefotaxime sodium) 69
FORTAZ (ceftazidime) 149
OMNICEF (cefdinir) 252
ROCEPHIN (ceftriaxone sodium) 309
SPECTRACEF (cefditoren pivoxil) 326
SUPRAX (cefixime) 334
TAZICEF (ceftazidime) 343
TAZIDIME (ceftazidime) 344
VANTIN (cefpodoxime proxetil) 381

CEPHALOSPORIN (4th generation)
MAXIPIME (cefepime HCl) 208

CHOLINESTERASE INHIBITOR
PHOSPHOLINE IODIDE (echothiophate iodide) 271

CLASS I ANTIARRHYTHMIC
NORPACE CR (disopyramide phosphate) 242

CLASS IA ANTIARRHYTHMIC/SCHIZONTICIDE ANTIMALARIAL
QUINIDINE GLUCONATE INJECTION (quinidine gluconate) 296

CLASS IC ANTIARRHYTHMIC
TAMBOCOR (flecainide acetate) 341

CNS DEPRESSANT
XYREM (sodium oxybate) 406

COPPER CHELATING AGENT
DEPEN (penicillamine) 82

CORTICOSTEROID
ACLOVATE (alclometasone dipropionate) 3
AEROBID-M (with menthol) (flunisolide) 11
ASMANEX (mometasone furoate) 29
AZMACORT (triamcinolone acetonide) 36
BECONASE (beclomethasone dipropionate) 42
BETAMETHASONE DIPROPIONATE 44
CLOBEVATE (clobetasol propionate) 73
CORDRAN SP (flurandrenolide) 77
CORMAX SCALP (clobetasol propionate) 78
CORTEF (hydrocortisone) 78
CUTIVATE (fluticasone propionate) 83
CYCLOCORT (amcinonide) 84
DERMA-SMOOTHE/FS (fluocinolone acetonide) 101
DESONATE (desonide) 103
DIPROLENE AF (betamethasone (augmented) dipropionate) 111
ELOCON (mometasone furoate) 124
EMBELINE E (clobetasol propionate) 124
EPIFOAM (hydrocortisone acetate) 128
FLONASE (fluticasone propionate) 142
FLOVENT HFA (fluticasone propionate) 142
FLUNISOLIDE NASAL SPRAY (flunisolide) 144
FML FORTE (fluorometholone) 146
HALOG-E (halcinonide) 160
HYDROCORTISONE ACETATE 168
HYTONE (hydrocortisone) 170
HYTONE 1% (hydrocortisone) 170
LIDEX-E (fluocinonide) 194
LOCOID (hydrocortisone butyrate) 198
NASACORT HFA (triamcinolone acetonide) 233
NASAREL (flunisolide) 233
NASONEX (mometasone furoate monohydrate) 234
OLUX (clobetasol propionate) 251
OLUX-E (clobetasol propionate) 251
OMNARIS (ciclesonide) 251
PROCTOCORT CREAM (hydrocortisone) 285
PROCTOCREAM HC (hydrocortisone) 27
PULMICORT FLEXHALER (budesonide) 294
QVAR (beclomethasone dipropionate) 297
RHINOCORT AQUA (budesonide) 303
SOLU-CORTEF (hydrocortisone sodium succinate) 323
SYNALAR (fluocinolone acetonide) 337
TEMOVATE SCALP (clobetasol propionate) 346
TOPICORT LP (desoximetasone) 361
ULTRAVATE (halobetasol propionate) 374
VANOS (fluocinonide) 381
VERAMYST (fluticasone furoate) 385
VERDESO (desonide) 385
WESTCORT (hydrocortisone valerate) 400

CORTICOSTEROID (medium-potency)
DERMATOP (prednicarbate) 101

CORTICOSTEROID/ANESTHETIC
ANALPRAM-HC (hydrocortisone acetate) 25
NOVACORT (hydrocortisone acetate) 244
PRAMOSONE (hydrocortisone acetate) 276
PROCTOFOAM-HC (hydrocortisone acetate) 285

CORTICOSTEROID/ANTI-INFECTIVE
ALCORTIN (hydrocortisone) 15
VYTONE (hydrocortisone) 399

CORTICOSTEROID/BETA$_2$ AGONIST
ADVAIR (fluticasone propionate) 9
ADVAIR HFA (fluticasone propionate) 10
SYMBICORT (budesonide fumarate dihydrate) 335

COUGH SUPPRESSANT
TUSSEND (chlorpheniramine maleate) 369

THERAPEUTIC CLASS INDEX

COUGH SUPPRESSANT/EXPECTORANT
DURATUSS DM (dextromethorphan
  hydrobromide) 118
MUCINEX DM (dextromethorphan
  hydrobromide) 225
MYTUSSIN AC (codeine phosphate) 63
VI-Q-TUSS (hydrocodone bitartrate) 167

**COUGH SUPPRESSANT/EXPECTORANT/
DECONGESTANT**
GUIATUSS DAC (pseudoephedrine
  HCl) 160

**COUGH SUPPRESSANT/EXPECTORANT/
DECONGESTANT**
TUSSEND EXPECTORANT (hydrocodone
  bitartrate) 369

COX-2 INHIBITOR
CELEBREX (celecoxib) 59

CYCLIC POLYPEPTIDE IMMUNOSUPPRESSANT
SANDIMMUNE (cyclosporine) 316

D

DEBRIDING AGENT
GRANULEX (peruvian balsam) 158

DECONGESTANT
SUDAFED (pseudoephedrine HCl) 330
VISINE L.R. (oxymetazoline HCl) 395
VISINE ORIGINAL (tetrahydrozoline
  HCl) 396

DECONGESTANT/ANTIHISTAMINE
VISINE-A (pheniramine maleate) 396

DECONGESTANT/ASTRINGENT
VISINE A.C. (tetrahydrozoline HCl) 394

DECONGESTANT/LUBRICANT
ALL CLEAR (naphazoline HCl) 17
ALL CLEAR AR (naphazoline HCl) 17
VISINE ADVANCED RELIEF
  (tetrahydrozoline HCl) 395

DEOXYGUANOSINE ANALOGUE
ARRANON (nelarabine) 29

DEPIGMENTING AGENT
CLARIPEL (hydroquinone) 70
ELDOQUIN FORTE (hydroquinone) 121
EPIQUIN MICRO (hydroquinone) 128
LUSTRA-AF (hydroquinone) 203
SOLAQUIN FORTE (hydroquinone) 323

DETERGENT CLEANSER
PHISOHEX (hexachlorophene) 271

DIAGNOSTIC DYE
AK-FLUOR (fluorescein sodium) 13
IC-GREEN (indocyanine green) 171

DIBENZAZEPINE
TRILEPTAL (oxcarbazepine) 365

DICARBAMATE ANTICONVULSANT
FELBATOL (felbamate) 138

DICARBOXYLIC ACID ANTIMICROBIAL
AZELEX (azelaic acid) 36
FINEVIN (azelaic acid) 140

**DIHYDROFOLATE REDUCTASE INHIBITOR/
ANTIBIOTIC**
POLYTRIM (trimethoprim sulfate) 275

DIHYDROFOLIC ACID REDUCTASE INHIBITOR
RHEUMATREX (methotrexate sodium) 214

DIHYDROINDOLONE
MOBAN (molindone HCl) 221

DIPHENYLBUTYLPIPERIDINE
ORAP (pimozide) 254

DIRECT ACTING SKELETAL MUSCLE RELAXANT
DANTRIUM (dantrolene sodium) 88
DANTRIUM IV (dantrolene sodium) 88

DNA FRAGMENTATION AGENT
TRISENOX (arsenic trioxide) 367

DOPAMINE AGONIST
SYMMETREL (amantadine HCl) 336

DOPAMINE ANTAGONIST/PROKINETIC
REGLAN INJECTION (metoclopramide
  HCl) 217

DOPAMINE RECEPTOR AGONIST
PARLODEL (bromocriptine mesylate) 260

**DOPAMINE/NOREPINEPHRINE/SEROTONIN
REUPTAKE INHIBITOR**
MERIDIA (sibutramine HCl
  monohydrate) 211

E

ECTOPARASITICIDE/OVICIDE
LINDANE 195

EMOLLIENT
LAC-HYDRIN (ammonium lactate) 186

ENDOGENOUS NUCLEOSIDE
ADENOCARD (adenosine) 7

ENDOTHELIN RECEPTOR ANTAGONIST
TRACLEER (bosentan) 361

ENZYME
MYOZYME (alglucosidase alfa) 230

ERYTHROPOIESIS AGENT
FOLIC ACID 148

ERYTHROPOIESIS STIMULATOR
EPOGEN (epoetin alfa) 130
PROCRIT (epoetin alfa) 284

ESTROGEN/PROGESTOGEN COMBINATION
ESTROSTEP FE (norethindrone
  acetate) 136
TRI-SPRINTEC (ethinyl estradiol) 256
YAZ (ethinyl estradiol) 407

EXPECTORANT
GUAIFENESIN ER (guaifenesin) 118
HUMIBID (guaifenesin) 166
MUCINEX (guaifenesin) 225

EXPECTORANT/DECONGESTANT
DURATUSS (pseudoephedrine HCl) 117
GUAIFENEX PSE 120
  (pseudoephedrine HCl) 127

EXPECTORANT/NASAL DECONGESTANT
MUCINEX D (pseudoephedrine HCl) 225

EXPECTORANT/SYMPATHOMIMETIC
ENTEX LA (phenylephrine HCl) 127

F

**5-AMINOSALICYLIC ACID DERIVATIVE/
SULFAPYRIDINE**
AZULFIDINE (sulfasalazine) 37
AZULFIDINE EN (sulfasalazine) 37

I-21

Therapeutic Class Index

5-HT₃ ANTAGONIST
ANZEMET (dolasetron mesylate) 27
KYTRIL (granisetron HCl) 185
ZOFRAN (ondansetron) 414

FLUORIDE PREPARATION
PREVIDENT 5000 PLUS (sodium
 fluoride) 280

FLUORIDE SUPPLEMENT
LURIDE (sodium fluoride) 203

FLUORINATED PYRIMIDINE NUCLEOSIDE ANTIVIRAL
VIROPTIC (trifluridine) 394

FLUOROQUINOLONE
CILOXAN (ciprofloxacin HCl) 65
CIPRO IV (ciprofloxacin) 67
CIPRO ORAL (ciprofloxacin HCl) 67
FLOXIN OTIC SINGLES (ofloxacin) 143
IQUIX (levofloxacin) 179
NEGGRAM (nalidixic acid) 234
OCUFLOX (ofloxacin) 250
QUIXIN (levofloxacin) 297
VIGAMOX (moxifloxacin HCl) 390
ZYMAR (gatifloxacin) 418

FOLIC ACID ANTAGONIST
DARAPRIM (pyrimethamine) 90

4-HYDROXYPHENYLPYRUVATE DIOXYGENASE INHIBITOR
ORFADIN (nitisinone) 256

FUSION INHIBITOR
FUZEON (enfuvirtide) 151

G

GABA ANALOG
KEMSTRO (baclofen) 38
NEURONTIN (gabapentin) 238

GENERAL ANESTHETIC
AMIDATE (etomidate) 21
DIPRIVAN (propofol) 111

GLUCAGON
GLUCAGON 156

GLUCOCORTICOID
CELESTONE (betamethasone) 60
CELESTONE SOLUSPAN
 (betamethasone sodium phosphate) 60
DECADRON (dexamethasone) 103
DELTASONE (prednisone) 277
DEPO-MEDROL (methylprednisolone
 acetate) 99
MEDROL DOSE PACK
 (methylprednisolone) 209
ORAPRED (prednisolone sodium
 phosphate) 255
PEDIAPRED (prednisolone sodium
 phosphate) 262
PRELONE (prednisolone) 278
SOLU-MEDROL (methylprednisolone
 sodium succinate) 324

GLYCOSAMINOGLYCAN
HEPARIN SODIUM 162

GONADOTROPIN RELEASING HORMONE
SUPPRELIN LA (histrelin acetate) 333

GONADOTROPIN-RELEASING HORMONE ANALOG
SYNAREL (nafarelin acetate) 338

GUANOSINE NUCLEOSIDE ANALOGUE
BARACLUDE (entecavir) 40

H

H₁ ANTAGONIST
ALLEGRA (fexofenadine HCl) 17
CLARINEX REDITABS (desloratadine) 69
CLARITIN REDITAB OTC (loratadine) 70
ELESTAT (epinastine HCl) 122
LIVOSTIN (levocabastine HCl) 198
OPTIVAR (azelastine HCl) 254
PALGIC (carbinoxamine maleate) 258
XYZAL (levocetirizine dihydrochloride) ... 406
ZYRTEC (cetirizine HCl) 418

H₁ ANTAGONIST AND MAST CELL STABILIZER
PATANOL (olopatadine HCl) 261
ZADITOR (ketotifen fumarate) 408

H₁ ANTAGONIST/ALPHA-AGONIST (imidazoline)
NAPHCON-A (pheniramine maleate) 232
OPCON-A (pheniramine maleate) 253

H₁ ANTAGONIST/SYMPATHOMIMETIC AMINE
ALLEGRA-D (pseudoephedrine HCl) 18
CLARINEX-D 24 HOUR
 (pseudoephedrine sulfate) 69
CLARITIN-D OTC (pseudoephedrine
 sulfate) 70

H₁ RECEPTOR ANTAGONIST
EMADINE (emedastine difumarate) 124

H₂ BLOCKER
AXID ORAL SOLUTION (nizatidine) 35
PEPCID AC (famotidine) 266
PEPCID RPD (famotidine) 265
TAGAMET (cimetidine) 66
ZANTAC (ranitidine HCl) 408
ZANTAC 150 (ranitidine HCl) 409

H₂ BLOCKER/ANTACID
PEPCID COMPLETE (magnesium
 hydroxide) 266

HEMATINIC
FERRLECIT (sodium ferric gluconate
 complex) 139

HIPPURIC ACID SALT
HIPREX (methenamine hippurate) 163

HMG-COA REDUCTASE INHIBITOR
LESCOL (fluvastatin sodium) 190
LIPITOR (atorvastatin calcium) 196
MEVACOR (lovastatin) 218
PRAVACHOL (pravastatin sodium) 277
ZOCOR (simvastatin) 413

HOMEOPATHIC COMPLEX
TRAUMEEL (botanical/mineral
 substances) 363
TRAUMEEL TOPICAL (botanical/
 mineral substances) 363

HUMAN CHORIONIC GONADOTROPIN
NOVAREL (chorionic gonadotropin) 244
PREGNYL (chorionic gonadotropin) 278
PROFASI (chorionic gonadotropin) 286

HUMAN GROWTH HORMONE
GENOTROPIN MINIQUICK
 (somatropin) 154
HUMATROPE (somatropin) 165
NORDITROPIN NORDIFLEX
 (somatropin) 241
NUTROPIN AQ (somatropin) 249

THERAPEUTIC CLASS INDEX

OMNITROPE (somatropin) 252
SAIZEN (somatropin) 315
TEV-TROPIN (somatropin) 349

HYDANTOIN
DILANTIN (phenytoin) 109
PHENYTEK (phenytoin sodium) 270

HYDRAZINE DERIVATIVE
MATULANE (procarbazine HCl) 207

HYDROXYBENZOIC ACID DERIVATIVE
PASER (aminosalicylic acid) 261

I

IMIDAZOLIDINEDIONE ANTIBACTERIAL
FURADANTIN (nitrofurantoin) 150
MACROBID (nitrofurantoin
  monohydrate) 204
MACRODANTIN (nitrofurantoin
  macrocrystals) 204

IMMUNE RESPONSE MODIFIER
ALDARA (imiquimod) 15

IMMUNEGLOBULIN
WINRHO SDF (rho (D) immune
  globulin) 400

IMMUNOGLOBULIN
GAMMAR-P (immune globulin) 152
IMOGAM RABIES-HT (rabies immune
  globulin) 172

IMMUNOMODULATORY AGENT
THALOMID (thalidomide) 350

IMMUNOSUPPRESSIVE AGENT
ZENAPAX (daclizumab) 411

INHALATION ANESTHETIC
SUPRANE (desflurane) 333
ULTANE (sevoflurane) 373

INOSINE MONOPHOSPHATE DEHYDROGENASE INHIBITOR
MYFORTIC (mycophenolic acid) 229

INSULIN
HUMALOG (insulin lispro) 165
HUMULIN 50/50 (insulin, human
  (isophane/regular)) 167
HUMULIN R (insulin human, rDNA
  origin) 166
LANTUS (insulin glargine, human) 188
LEVEMIR (insulin detemir, rDNA origin) ... 191
NOVOLIN 70/30 (insulin, human
  (isophane/regular)) 245
NOVOLIN R (insulin human, rDNA
  origin) 245
NOVOLOG (insulin aspart) 246

IRON CHELATING AGENT
EXJADE (deferasirox) 137

IRON SUPPLEMENT
FEOSOL (ferrous sulfate) 139
INFED (iron dextran) 176
NIFEREX (iron) 239

IRON-CHELATING AGENT
DESFERAL (deferoxamine mesylate) 101

IRON/VITAMIN
FERO-GRAD-500 (ferrous sulfate) 139
IROFOL (polysaccharide iron
  complex) 180

ISONICOTINIC ACID HYDRAZIDE
NYDRAZID (isoniazid) 180

ISONICOTINIC ACID HYDRAZIDE/RIFAMYCIN DERIVATIVE/NICOTINAMIDE ANALOGUE
RIFATER (pyrazinamide) 304

L

LAXATIVE
FLEET GLYCERIN LAXATIVES (glycerin) 141

LEPROSTATIC AGENT
DAPSONE 89

LEUKOTRIENE INHIBITOR
ZYFLO (zileuton) 417

LEUKOTRIENE RECEPTOR ANTAGONIST
ACCOLATE (zafirlukast) 1
SINGULAIR (montelukast sodium) 322

LINCOMYCIN DERIVATIVE
CLEOCIN (clindamycin HCl) 71
CLEOCIN T (clindamycin phosphate) 72
CLEOCIN VAGINAL OVULES
  (clindamycin phosphate) 72
CLINDAGEL (clindamycin phosphate) 72
EVOCLIN (clindamycin phosphate) 137

LINCOSAMIDE DERIVATIVE/RETINOID
ZIANA (clindamycin phosphate) 412

LIPASE INHIBITOR
XENICAL (orlistat) 401

LOCAL ANESTHETIC
MARCAINE (bupivacaine HCl) 205
MARCAINE WITH EPINEPHRINE
  (bupivacaine HCl) 206
NESACAINE-MPF (chloroprocaine
  HCl) 237
SENSORCAINE-MPF (bupivacaine
  HCl) 318
SENSORCAINE-MPF W/EPINEPHRINE
  (bupivacaine HCl) 319
XYLOCAINE-MPF (lidocaine HCl) 403
XYLOCAINE-MPF WITH EPINEPHRINE
  (lidocaine HCl) 405

LOOP DIURETIC
LASIX (furosemide) 151

LUBRICANT
VISINE FOR CONTACTS (hydroxypropyl
  methylcellulose) 395
VISINE TEARS (hydroxypropyl
  methylcellulose) 396

LYMPHOCYTE-SELECTIVE IMMUNOSUPPRESSANT
ATGAM (lymphocyte immune globulin,
  anti-thymocyte globulin (equine)) 30

M

MACROCYCLIC LACTONE IMMUNOSUPPRESSANT
RAPAMUNE (sirolimus) 297

MACROLACTAM ASCOMYCIN DERIVATIVE
ELIDEL (pimecrolimus) 122

MACROLIDE
AZASITE (azithromycin) 36
ERYTHROMYCIN OPHTHALMIC
  (erythromycin) 135

MACROLIDE ANTIBIOTIC
BIAXIN (clarithromycin) 46
E.E.S. (erythromycin ethylsuccinate) 119
ERYC (erythromycin) 131

I-23

Therapeutic Class Index

ERYPED (erythromycin
  ethylsuccinate) 132
ERY-TAB (erythromycin) 132
ERYTHROCIN (erythromycin stearate) 133
ERYTHROMYCIN 134
ERYTHROMYCIN BASE (erythromycin) 134
PCE (erythromycin) 262
ZITHROMAX (azithromycin) 412

MACROLIDE ANTIBIOTIC/SULFONAMIDE
PEDIAZOLE (erythromycin
  ethylsuccinate) 264

MACROLIDE IMMUNOSUPPRESSANT
PROGRAF (tacrolimus) 286
PROTOPIC (tacrolimus) 291

MAST CELL STABILIZER
ALAMAST (pemirolast potassium) 14
ALOCRIL (nedocromil sodium) 19
ALOMIDE (lodoxamide tromethamine) 19
INTAL (cromolyn sodium) 177
OPTICROM (cromolyn sodium) 254

METHYLXANTHINE
CAFCIT (caffeine citrate) 54

MONOBACTAM
AZACTAM (aztreonam) 35

MONOCLONAL ANTIBODY/IGE-BLOCKER
XOLAIR (omalizumab) 402

MONOCLONAL ANTIBODY/IL-2R ALPHA (CD25) blocker
SIMULECT (basiliximab) 321

MONOCLONAL ANTIBODY/RSV F-PROTEIN BLOCKER
SYNAGIS (palivizumab) 337

MONOCLONAL ANTIBODY/TNF-ALPHA RECEPTOR BLOCKER
REMICADE (infliximab) 300

MULTIPLE VITAMIN/FLUORIDE SUPPLEMENT
POLY-VI-FLOR (multiple vitamin) 275

MUSCULAR ANALGESIC (central-acting)
ROBAXIN INJECTION
  (methocarbamol) 307
SKELAXIN (metaxalone) 322

N

NAPHTHOIC ACID DERIVATIVE (retinoid-like)
DIFFERIN (adapalene) 108

NAPTHOQUINONE ANTIPROTOZOAL
MEPRON (atovaquone) 211

NARCOTIC AGONIST ANALGESIC
ACTIQ (fentanyl citrate) 4

NASAL DECONGESTANT AND EXPECTORANT
GUAIFED-PD (phenylephrine HCl) 159

NEURAMINIDASE INHIBITOR
RELENZA (zanamivir) 300
TAMIFLU (oseltamivir phosphate) 341

NEUROLEPTIC BUTYROPHENONE
INAPSINE (droperidol) 173

NICOTINAMIDE ANALOGUE
PYRAZINAMIDE 295

NIPECOTIC ACID DERIVATIVE
GABITRIL (tiagabine HCl) 152

NITROGEN MUSTARD ALKYLATING AGENT
CYTOXAN (cyclophosphamide) 86
NEOSAR (cyclophosphamide) 235

NITROIMIDAZOLE
FLAGYL (metronidazole) 140

NITROSOUREA ALKYLATING AGENT
CEENU (lomustine) 56

NONBARBITURATE ANESTHETIC
KETAMINE (ketamine HCl) 183

NON-NARCOTIC ANTITUSSIVE
TESSALON (benzonatate) 348

NON-NUCLEOSIDE REVERSE TRANSCRIPTASE INHIBITOR
RESCRIPTOR (delavirdine mesylate) 301
SUSTIVA (efavirenz) 335
VIRAMUNE (nevirapine) 393

NONSELECTIVE BETA-BLOCKER
INDERAL (propranolol HCl) 174

NSAID
ACULAR (ketorolac tromethamine) 5
ALEVE (naproxen sodium) 16
DOLOBID (diflunisal) 113
EC-NAPROSYN (naproxen) 232
MECLOFENAMATE (meclofenamate
  sodium) 209
MOBIC (meloxicam) 221
MOTRIN (ibuprofen) 223
MOTRIN IB (ibuprofen) 224
MOTRIN, INFANTS (ibuprofen) 224
TOLECTIN (tolmetin sodium) 359

NSAID (fenamate derivative)
PONSTEL (mefenamic acid) 275

NSAID (indole derivative)
INDOCIN (indomethacin) 175
INDOCIN I.V. (indomethacin sodium
  trihydrate) 174

NSAID (propionic acid derivative)
DAYPRO (oxaprozin) 90

NSAID (pyranocarboxylic acid derivative)
LODINE XL (etodolac) 199

NSAID (pyrrolo-pyrrole derivative)
TORADOL (ketorolac tromethamine) 183

NUCLEOSIDE ANALOG COMBINATION
TRIZIVIR (abacavir sulfate) 367

NUCLEOSIDE ANALOGUE
COMBIVIR (zidovudine) 75
EMTRIVA (emtricitabine) 125
EPIVIR (lamivudine) 129
EPIVIR-HBV (lamivudine) 129
REBETOL (ribavirin) 298
RETROVIR (zidovudine) 303
TYZEKA (telbivudine) 372
VALTREX (valacyclovir HCl) 379
VIDEX EC (didanosine) 389
VIRAZOLE (ribavirin) 394
ZOVIRAX (acyclovir) 416

NUCLEOSIDE ANALOGUE ANTIVIRAL
VITRASERT (ganciclovir) 397
ZOVIRAX CREAM (acyclovir) 416

O

OPIOID AGONIST-ANTAGONIST ANALGESIC
TALWIN NX (pentazocine HCl) 340

OPIOID ANALGESIC
BUPRENEX (buprenorphine HCl) 52
DEMEROL INJECTION (meperidine HCl) 94

THERAPEUTIC CLASS INDEX

DEMEROL ORAL (meperidine HCl) 95
DURAGESIC (fentanyl) 117
LORTAB (hydrocodone bitartrate) 201
REPREXAIN (hydrocodone bitartrate) 389
SUBLIMAZE (fentanyl citrate) 329
SUFENTA (sufentanil citrate) 331
SYNALGOS-DC (dihydrocodeine
  bitartrate) 337
TYLENOL WITH CODEINE (codeine
  phosphate) 372
ULTIVA (remifentanil HCl) 373

OPIOID ANTAGONIST
NARCAN (naloxone HCl) 231

OPIOID ANTITUSSIVE
CODICLEAR DH (hydrocodone
  bitartrate) 159
ENTEX HC (hydrocodone bitartrate) 126
HISTUSSIN D (hydrocodone bitartrate) 164

OPIOID ANTITUSSIVE/ANTIHISTAMINE
TUSSIONEX PENNKINETIC
  (chlorpheniramine polistirex) 370

OPIOID/ANTICHOLINERGIC
LONOX (diphenoxylate HCl) 200

ORGANOPHOSPHATE/CHOLINESTERASE INHIBITOR
OVIDE (malathion) 257

ORNITHINE DECARBOXYLASE INHIBITOR
VANIQA (eflornithine HCl) 381

OSMOTIC LAXATIVE
MIRALAX (polyethylene glycol 3350) 221

OXAZOLIDINONE CLASS ANTIBACTERIAL
ZYVOX (linezolid) 419

P

PANCREATIC ENZYME SUPPLEMENT
COTAZYM (protease) 81
PANCREASE MT (protease) 259
VIOKASE (protease) 392
ZYMASE (protease) 418

PARTIAL OPIOID AGONIST/OPIOID ANTAGONIST
SUBUTEX (buprenorphine) 329

PENICILLIN
BICILLIN C-R (penicillin G benzathine) 46
BICILLIN C-R 900/300 (penicillin G
  benzathine) 47
BICILLIN L-A (penicillin G benzathine) 47
PERMAPEN (penicillin G benzathine) 267
PFIZERPEN (penicillin G potassium) 268

PENICILLIN (penicillinase-resistant)
DICLOXACILLIN (dicloxacillin sodium) ... 107

PENICILLIUM-DERIVED ANTIFUNGAL
GRIFULVIN V (griseofulvin) 158
GRIS-PEG (griseofulvin) 158

PEPTIDE SYNTHESIS INHIBITOR
TRECATOR (ethionamide) 364

PERIPHERAL VASODILATOR
MINOXIDIL 220

PHENOTHIAZINE
CHLORPROMAZINE 64
PERPHENAZINE 267

PHENOTHIAZINE DERIVATIVE
COMPRO (prochlorperazine) 76

PHENERGAN INJECTION
  (promethazine HCl) 269
PROMETHEGAN (promethazine HCl) 287

PHENOTHIAZINE DERIVATIVE/ SYMPATHOMIMETIC
PROMETHAZINE VC (phenylephrine
  HCl) 288

PHENOTHIAZINE DERIVATIVE/ANTITUSSIVE
PROMETHAZINE DM
  (dextromethorphan HBr) 288
PROMETHAZINE W/CODEINE (codeine
  phosphate) 289

PHENOTHIAZINE DERIVATIVE/ANTITUSSIVE/ SYMPATHOMIMETIC
PROMETHAZINE VC/CODEINE
  (phenylephrine HCl) 288

PHENYLTRIAZINE
LAMICTAL CD (lamotrigine) 186

PIPERAZINE ANTIHISTAMINE
ATARAX (hydroxyzine HCl) 169
VISTARIL (hydroxyzine pamoate) 170

PIPERAZINE PHENOTHIAZINE
TRIFLUOPERAZINE HCL 364

PIPERIDINE PHENOTHIAZINE
THIORIDAZINE (thioridazine HCl) 352

PLATELET-DERIVED GROWTH FACTOR (recombinant human)
REGRANEX (becaplermin) 299

PLATELET-REDUCING AGENT
AGRYLIN (anagrelide HCl) 12

PLEUROMUTILIN ANTIBACTERIAL
ALTABAX (retapamulin) 20

POLYENE ANTIFUNGAL
ABELCET (amphotericin B (lipid
  complex)) 1
AMBISOME (amphotericin B) 20
AMPHOTEC (amphotericin B cholesteryl
  sulfate) 23
MYCOSTATIN TOPICAL (nystatin) 228
NYSTOP (nystatin) 250

POLYENE ANTIFUNGAL/CORTICOSTEROID
MYCOLOG-II (triamcinolone
  acetonide) 228

POLYPEPTIDE ANTIBIOTIC
COLY-MYCIN M (colistimethate
  sodium) 75

PROSTAGLANDIN E$_1$
PROSTIN VR PEDIATRIC (alprostadil) 291

PROTEASE INHIBITOR
AGENERASE (amprenavir) 11
FORTOVASE (saquinavir) 150
INVIRASE (saquinavir mesylate) 178
KALETRA (ritonavir) 180
NORVIR (ritonavir) 243
VIRACEPT (nelfinavir mesylate) 392

PROTEIN SYNTHESIS INHIBITOR
ONCASPAR (pegaspargase) 253

PROTEIN-TYROSINE KINASE INHIBITOR
GLEEVEC (imatinib mesylate) 156

PROTON PUMP INHIBITOR
NEXIUM (esomeprazole magnesium) 239
PREVACID SOLUTAB (lansoprazole) 279
PRILOSEC (omeprazole) 281

Therapeutic Class Index

PSORALEN
OXSORALEN (methoxsalen) 258

PURIFIED NEUROTOXIN COMPLEX
BOTOX (botulinum toxin type A) 50

PURINE ANALOG
PURINETHOL (mercaptopurine) 294
THIOGUANINE 352

PURINE NUCLEOSIDE ANTIVIRAL
VIRA-A (vidarabine) 392

PYRANOQUINOLINE ANTI-INFLAMMATORY AGENT
TILADE (nedocromil sodium) 353

PYRETHROID PEDICULICIDE
NIX (permethrin) 240

PYRETHROID SCABICIDAL AGENT
ACTICIN (permethrin) 4
ELIMITE (permethrin) 122

PYRIMIDINE SYNTHESIS INHIBITOR
MALARONE PEDIATRIC (proguanil HCl) 205

PYRIMIDINEDIONE DERIVATIVE
MYSOLINE (primidone) 231

PYRROLIDINE DERIVATIVE
KEPPRA (levetiracetam) 182

Q

QUININE DERIVATIVE
PLAQUENIL (hydroxychloroquine sulfate) 273

QUINOLINEMETHANOL DERIVATIVE
LARIAM (mefloquine HCl) 189

R

RECOMBINANT URATE-OXIDASE ENZYME
ELITEK (rasburicase) 123

RETINOIC ACID DERIVATIVE
RETIN-A MICRO (tretinoin) 302
TAZORAC (tazarotene) 345

RETINOID
AMNESTEEM (isotretinoin) 2
VESANOID (tretinoin) 387

REVERSE TRANSCRIPTASE INHIBITOR
HIVID (zalcitabine) 164

RIFAMYCIN DERIVATIVE
PRIFTIN (rifapentine) 280
RIFADIN (rifampin) 304

S

SALICYLATE
BAYER ASPIRIN EXTRA STRENGTH (aspirin) 42
BAYER ASPIRIN REGIMEN WITH CALCIUM (aspirin) 41
ECOTRIN (aspirin) 120

SALICYLATE (non-acetylated)
TRILISATE (choline magnesium trisalicylate) 366

SELECTIVE ALPHA$_2$ AGONIST
ALPHAGAN P (brimonidine tartrate) 20

SELECTIVE NOREPINEPHRINE REUPTAKE INHIBITOR
STRATTERA (atomoxetine HCl) 326

SELECTIVE SEROTONIN REUPTAKE INHIBITOR
FLUVOXAMINE MALEATE (fluvoxamine maleate) 145
PROZAC (fluoxetine HCl) 293
ZOLOFT (sertraline HCl) 415

SEMISYNTHETIC AMPICILLIN DERIVATIVE
AMOXIL (amoxicillin) 22
DISPERMOX (amoxicillin) 112

SEMI-SYNTHETIC PENICILLIN DERIVATIVE
AMPICILLIN 23

SEMISYNTHETIC PENICILLIN/BETA LACTAMASE INHIBITOR
UNASYN (ampicillin Sodium) 374

SEMI-SYNTHETIC RIFAMPIN ANALOG
XIFAXAN (rifaximin) 402

SEROTONIN/HISTAMINE ANTAGONIST
CYPROHEPTADINE (cyproheptadine HCl) 84

SKELETAL MUSCLE RELAXANT (central-acting)
FLEXERIL (cyclobenzaprine HCl) 141
SOMA (carisoprodol) 325

SKELETAL MUSCLE RELAXANT (depolarizing)
ANECTINE (succinylcholine chloride) 26

SKELETAL MUSCLE RELAXANT (nondepolarizing)
NIMBEX (cisatracurium besylate) 239
PANCURONIUM (pancuronium bromide) 259
TRACRIUM (atracurium besylate) 362
VECURONIUM (vecuronium bromide) 383
ZEMURON (rocuronium bromide) 410

SMOOTH MUSCLE ANTISPASMODIC
URISPAS (flavoxate HCl) 378

STIMULANT LAXATIVE
DULCOLAX (bisacodyl) 116
FLEET BISACODYL (bisacodyl) 141
SENOKOT (senna) 318

STOOL SOFTENER
COLACE (docusate sodium) 74

STOOL SOFTENER/LAXATIVE COMBINATION
PERI-COLACE (docusate sodium) 266

STREPTOGRAMIN
SYNERCID (quinupristin) 339

***STREPTOMYCES* DERIVED BACTERIOSTATIC AGENT**
SUMYCIN (tetracycline HCl) 332

***STREPTOMYCES LINCOLNENSIS* DERIVATIVE**
LINCOCIN (lincomycin HCl) 195

SUCCINIMIDE
CELONTIN (methsuximide) 61
ZARONTIN (ethosuximide) 409

SULFAMATE-SUBSTITUTED MONOSACCHARIDE ANTIEPILEPTIC
TOPAMAX (topiramate) 360

SULFONAMIDE
AK-SULF (sulfacetamide sodium) 48
GANTRISIN PEDIATRIC (sulfisoxazole) 153
KLARON (sulfacetamide sodium) 184
ROSULA NS (sulfacetamide sodium) 314
SULFAMYLON (mafenide acetate) 332

THERAPEUTIC CLASS INDEX

SULFONAMIDE ANTICONVULSANT
ZONEGRAN (zonisamide) 416

SULFONAMIDE/CORTICOSTEROID
BLEPHAMIDE S.O.P. (sulfacetamide sodium) 49

SULFONAMIDE/SULFUR COMBINATION
CLENIA (sulfacetamide sodium) 71
PLEXION SCT (sulfacetamide sodium) 274
ROSAC (sulfacetamide sodium) 313
ROSULA (sulfacetamide sodium) 313
SULFACET-R (sulfacetamide sodium) 331
ZETACET (sulfacetamide sodium) 411

SULFONAMIDE/TETRAHYDROFOLIC ACID INHIBITOR
BACTRIM DS (sulfamethoxazole) 39
SULFATRIM PEDIATRIC (sulfamethoxazole) 320

SYMPATHOMIMETIC
NEO-SYNEPHRINE OPHTHALMIC (phenylephrine HCl) 237

SYMPATHOMIMETIC AMINE
ADDERALL (amphetamine salt combo) 6
ADDERALL XR (amphetamine salt combo) 6
CONCERTA (methylphenidate HCl) 76
DAYTRANA (methylphenidate) 91
DESOXYN (methamphetamine HCl) 103
DEXEDRINE SPANSULES (dextroamphetamine sulfate) 104
DEXTROSTAT (dextroamphetamine sulfate) 105
FOCALIN (dexmethylphenidate HCl) 147
FOCALIN XR (dexmethylphenidate HCl) 147
METADATE CD (methylphenidate HCl) 213
METADATE ER (methylphenidate HCl) 213
METHYLIN ER (methylphenidate HCl) 216
RITALIN SR (methylphenidate HCl) 306
TENUATE DOSPAN (diethylpropion HCl) 347

SYMPATHOMIMETIC AMINE
VYVANSE (lisdexamfetamine dimesylate) 399

SYMPATHOMIMETIC CATECHOLAMINE
EPIPEN JR. (epinephrine) 128
TWINJECT (epinephrine) 371

SYNTHETIC ACTH
CORTROSYN (cosyntropin) 80

SYNTHETIC CARBOCYCLIC NUCLEOSIDE ANALOGUE
ZIAGEN (abacavir sulfate) 412

SYNTHETIC GONADOTROPIN RELEASING HORMONE ANALOG
LUPRON DEPOT-PED (leuprolide acetate) 203

SYNTHETIC PENICILLIN
AMPICILLIN INJECTION (ampicillin sodium) 23

SYNTHETIC THYMIDINE NUCLEOSIDE ANALOGUE
ZERIT (stavudine) 411

SYNTHETIC VASOPRESSIN ANALOG
DDAVP RHINAL TUBE (desmopressin acetate) 92
DESMOPRESSIN ACETATE 102

T

TETRACYCLINE DERIVATIVE
DECLOMYCIN (demeclocycline HCl) 92
DORYX (doxycycline hyclate) 115
DYNACIN (minocycline HCl) 119
MINOCIN (minocycline HCl) 219
MONODOX (doxycycline monohydrate) 223
SOLODYN (minocycline HCl) 323
VIBRAMYCIN IV (doxycycline hyclate) 388
VIBRA-TABS (doxycycline hyclate) 387

TETRAHYDROFOLIC ACID INHIBITOR
PRIMSOL (trimethoprim HCl) 283

THIAZIDE DIURETIC
DIURIL (chlorothiazide) 113
HYDROCHLOROTHIAZIDE 168

THIENAMYCIN/DEHYDROPEPTIDASE I INHIBITOR
PRIMAXIN I.M. (cilastatin) 282
PRIMAXIN I.V. (cilastatin) 282

THIOUREA-DERIVATIVE ANTITHYROID AGENT
PROPYLTHIOURACIL 289

THIOXANTHENE
NAVANE (thiothixene) 234

THROMBOLYTIC AGENT
CATHFLO ACTIVASE (alteplase) 55

THYROID HORMONE SYNTHESIS INHIBITOR
TAPAZOLE (methimazole) 342

THYROID REPLACEMENT HORMONE
ARMOUR THYROID (thyroid) 28
CYTOMEL (liothyronine sodium) 85
LEVOTHROID (levothyroxine sodium) 192
LEVOXYL (levothyroxine sodium) 193
SYNTHROID (levothyroxine sodium) 339
THYROLAR (liotrix) 353
TIROSINT (levothyroxine sodium) 355
UNITHROID (levothyroxine sodium) 376

TNF RECEPTOR BLOCKER
ENBREL (etanercept) 126

TOPICAL CORTICOSTEROID
CLODERM (clocortolone pivalate) 73

TOPICAL IMMUNOMODULATOR
RESTASIS (cyclosporine) 302

TOXOID
TETANUS TOXOID ADSORBED (tetanus toxoid) 349

TOXOID COMBINATION
TETANUS & DIPHTHERIA TOXOIDS ADSORBED (diphtheria toxoid) 349

TREMATODICIDE
BILTRICIDE (praziquantel) 48

TRIAZOLE ANTIFUNGAL
DIFLUCAN (fluconazole) 108
MYCELEX TROCHE (clotrimazole) 227
NOXAFIL (posaconazole) 246

TRICHLOROACETALDEHYDE MONOHYDRATE
CHLORAL HYDRATE 64

TRICYCLIC ANTIDEPRESSANT
ANAFRANIL (clomipramine HCl) 24
SURMONTIL (trimipramine maleate) 334
TOFRANIL (imipramine HCl) 358
TOFRANIL-PM (imipramine pamoate) 359
VIVACTIL (protriptyline HCl) 397

I-27

Therapeutic Class Index

TRICYCLIC GLYCOPEPTIDE ANTIBIOTIC
VANCOCIN (vancomycin HCl) 380
VANCOCIN ORAL (vancomycin HCl) 380

TYPE II TOPOISOMERASE INHIBITOR
VUMON (teniposide) 398

TYROSINE HYDROXYLASE INHIBITOR
DEMSER (metyrosine) 95

U

URICOSURIC
PROBENECID 283

URINARY TRACT ANALGESIC
PROSED DS (hyoscyamine sulfate) 290

V

VACCINE
ACTHIB (haemophilus B conjugate) 3
ADACEL (pertussis vaccine acellular, adsorbed) 5
DAPTACEL (pertussis vaccine acellular, adsorbed) 89
DRYVAX (smallpox vaccine, dried) 115
FLUMIST (influenza virus vaccine Live) 144
FLUVIRIN (influenza virus vaccine) 145
FLUZONE (influenza virus vaccine) 146
GARDASIL (human papillomavirus recombinant vaccine, quadrivalent) 153
HAVRIX (hepatitis A vaccine (Inactivated)) 162
IMOVAX RABIES VACCINE (rabies vaccine) 172
MENACTRA (meningococcal polysaccharide diptheria toxoid conjugate vaccine) 210
MERUVAX II (rubella vaccine live) 212
MUMPSVAX (mumps virus vaccine live) 226
PNEUMOVAX 23 (pneumococcal vaccine) 274
PROQUAD (varicella virus vaccine live) 290
RECOMBIVAX HB PEDIATRIC/ADOLESCENT (hepatitis B (recombinant)) 299
ROTATEQ (rotavirus vaccine, live) 314
VAQTA (hepatitis A vaccine (inactivated)) 382
YF-VAX (yellow fever vaccine) 407

VACCINE/TOXOID COMBINATION
BOOSTRIX (pertussis vaccine, acellular) 50
INFANRIX (pertussis vaccine, acellular) 176
PEDIARIX (poliovirus vaccine, inactivated) 263
TRIPEDIA (pertussis vaccine, acellular) 366

VALPROATE COMPOUND
DEPAKOTE (divalproex sodium) 97
DEPAKOTE ER (divalproex sodium) 98

VASODILATOR
HYDRALAZINE (hydralazine HCl) 168

VENOM SPECIFIC IMMUNOGLOBULIN FAB FRAGMENT
CROFAB (crotalidae polyvalent immune fab (ovine)) 82

VERMICIDAL AND/OR VERMIFUGAL AGENT
MINTEZOL (thiabendazole) 220

VINCA ALKALOID
VINBLASTINE (vinblastine sulfate) 390
VINCRISTINE SULFATE 391

VITAMIN B COMPLEX
POTABA (potassium p-aminobenzoate) 276

VITAMIN D ANALOG
ROCALTROL (calcitriol) 308
ZEMPLAR IV (paricalcitol) 410

VITAMIN K DERIVATIVE
PHYTONADIONE 272

W

WAKEFULNESS-PROMOTING AGENT
PROVIGIL (modafinil) 292

X

XANTHINE BRONCHODILATOR
THEO-24 (theophylline) 351
THEOLAIR (theophylline) 351
UNIPHYL (theophylline) 375

XANTHINE OXIDASE INHIBITOR
ALOPRIM (allopurinol sodium) 19
ZYLOPRIM (allopurinol) 417

Visual Identification Guide

VISUAL PRODUCT IDENTIFICATION GUIDE*

ACCUNEB

RX (albuterol sulfate)
DEY

0.63 mg/3 mL

1.25 mg/3 mL

ACCUTANE

RX (isotretinoin)
ROCHE

10 mg

20 mg

40 mg

AEROBID INHALER SYSTEM

RX (flunisolide)
FOREST

250 mcg/inhalation
7g, 100 metered inhalations

AEROBID-M INHALER SYSTEM

RX (flunisolide)
FOREST

250 mcg/inhalation
7g, 100 metered inhalations

ADDERALL

C-II (mixed salts of a single-entity amphetamine product) (dextroamphetamine saccharate/dextroamphetamine sulfate/amphetamine aspartate/amphetamine sulfate)
SHIRE

5 mg

7.5 mg

10 mg

12.5 mg

15 mg

20 mg

30 mg

ADDERALL XR

C-II (mixed salts of a single-entity amphetamine product) (dextroamphetamine saccharate/dextroamphetamine sulfate/amphetamine aspartate/amphetamine sulfate)
SHIRE

5 mg

10 mg

15 mg

20 mg

25 mg

30 mg

Extended-Release Capsules

ADVAIR DISKUS

RX (fluticasone propionate/salmeterol inhalation powder)
GLAXOSMITHKLINE

100 mcg-50 mcg/blister
60 blisters

Also available in a 28-blister institutional pack.

250 mcg-50 mcg/blister
60 blisters)

500 mcg-50 mcg/blister
60 blisters

*Other dosage forms and strengths may be available

VISUAL PRODUCT IDENTIFICATION GUIDE

ALLEGRA
RX (fexofenadine HCl)
SANOFI-AVENTIS

30 mg | 60 mg | 180 mg

ALLEGRA-D 12 HOUR
RX (fexofenadine HCl/pseudoephedrine HCl)
SANOFI-AVENTIS

60 mg/120 mg
Extended-Release Tablets

ALLEGRA-D 24 HOUR
RX (fexofenadine HCl/pseudoephedrine HCl)
SANOFI-AVENTIS

180 mg/240 mg
Extended-Release Tablets

AMOXIL
RX (amoxicillin)
GLAXOSMITHKLINE

500 mg

500 mg

875 mg

AMOXIL CHEWABLE TABLETS
RX (amoxicillin)
GLAXOSMITHKLINE

200 mg | 400 mg

AMOXIL FOR ORAL SUSPENSION
RX (amoxicillin)
GLAXOSMITHKLINE

200 mg/5 mL
100 mL

Refer to product information section for other strengths and bottle sizes.

AMOXIL PEDIATRIC DROPS FOR ORAL SUSPENSION
RX (amoxicillin)
GLAXOSMITHKLINE

50 mg/mL
30 mL

ATROVENT HFA
RX (ipratropium bromide HFA)
BOEHRINGER INGELHEIM

17 mcg/inh | 12.9 g

ATROVENT INHALATION SOLUTION
RX (ipratropium bromide)
BOEHRINGER INGELHEIM

0.02% per 2.5 mL

ATROVENT NASAL SPRAY
RX (ipratropium bromide)
BOEHRINGER INGELHEIM

0.03% 30 mL | 0.06% 15 mL

VISUAL PRODUCT IDENTIFICATION GUIDE

AUGMENTIN

RX (amoxicillin/clavulanate potassium)
GLAXOSMITHKLINE

250 mg/125 mg

500 mg/125 mg

875 mg/125 mg

AUGMENTIN CHEWABLE TABLETS

RX (amoxicillin/clavulanate potassium)
GLAXOSMITHKLINE

125 mg/31.25 mg   200 mg/28.5 mg

250 mg/62.5 mg   400 mg/57 mg

AUGMENTIN ES-600

RX (amoxicillin/clavulanate potassium)
GLAXOSMITHKLINE

600 mg-42.9 mg/5 mL   600 mg-42.9 mg/5 mL   600 mg-42.9 mg/5 mL
75 mL   125 mL   200 mL

AUGMENTIN POWDER FOR ORAL SUSPENSION

RX (amoxicillin/clavulanate potassium)
GLAXOSMITHKLINE

125 mg-31.25 mg/5 mL   200 mg-28.5 mg/5 mL
150 mL   100 mL

250 mg-62.5 mg/5 mL   400 mg-57 mg/5 mL
150 mL   100 mL

Refer to product information section for other bottle sizes.

AUGMENTIN XR

RX (amoxicillin/clavulanate potassium)
GLAXOSMITHKLINE

1000 mg/62.5 mg
Extended-Release Tablets

AXID ORAL SOLUTION

RX (nizatidine)
BRAINTREE

15 mg/mL

AZMACORT INHALATION AEROSOL

RX (triamcinolone acetonide)
KOS

60 mg/20 gram inhaler
100 mcg/inh

V3

VISUAL PRODUCT IDENTIFICATION GUIDE

CONCERTA

C-II (methylphenidate HCl)
MCNEIL

| 18 mg | 27 mg |
| 36 mg | 54 mg |

Extended-Release Tablets

CORTISPORIN-TC

RX (colistin sulfate/neomycin sulfate/
thonzonium bromide/hydrocortisone
acetate otic suspension)
KING

3 mg - 3.3 mg - 0.5 mg - 10 mg/mL

DAYTRANA

C-II (methylphenidate transdermal system)
SHIRE

| 10 mg/9 hr | 15 mg/9 hr |
| 20 mg/9 hr | 30 mg/9 hr |

DEPAKOTE

RX (divalproex sodium)
ABBOTT

| 125 mg | 250 mg | 500 mg |

Delayed-Release Tablets

DEPAKOTE ER

RX (divalproex sodium)
ABBOTT

| 250 mg | 500 mg |

Extended-Release Tablets

DEPAKOTE SPRINKLE CAPSULES

RX (divalproex sodium coated particles)
ABBOTT

125 mg

DEXEDRINE

C-II (dextroamphetamine sulfate)
GLAXOSMITHKLINE

15-mg Spansule®

Also available as 5-mg Spansule®
and 10-mg Spansule® capsules.

5 mg

DEXTROSTAT

C-II (dextroamphetamine sulfate)
SHIRE

5 mg

10 mg

E.E.S. 400 FILMTAB

RX (erythromycin ethylsuccinate)
ABBOTT

400 mg

VISUAL PRODUCT IDENTIFICATION GUIDE

HAVRIX
RX (Hepatitis A Vaccine, Inactivated)
GLAXOSMITHKLINE

720 EL.U./0.5 mL single-dose vial

720 EL.U./0.5 mL prefilled, disposable Tip-Lok® syringe

1440 EL.U./mL single-dose vial

1440 EL.U./mL prefilled, disposable Tip-Lok® syringe

INFANRIX
RX (Diphtheria and Tetanus Toxoids and Acellular Pertussis Vaccine Adsorbed)
GLAXOSMITHKLINE

0.5 mL single-dose vial

Single-dose, prefilled, disposable Tip-Lok® Syringe

IMODIUM A-D
OTC (loperamide HCl)
MCNEIL

1 mg/7.5 mL   1 mg/7.5 mL   2 mg Caplet

IMODIUM ADVANCED
OTC (loperamide HCl/simethicone)
MCNEIL

2 mg/125 mg Caplet   2 mg/125 mg Chewable Tablet

KEPPRA
RX (levetiracetam)
UCB

250 mg   500 mg

750 mg   1000 mg

KEPPRA
RX (levetiracetam)
UCB

100 mg/mL

KEPPRA
RX (levetiracetam)
UCB

500 mg/5 mL vial

KYTRIL
RX (granisetron HCl)
ROCHE

K1
1 mg

V7

VISUAL PRODUCT IDENTIFICATION GUIDE

MALARONE PEDIATRIC TABLETS

RX

(atovaquone/proguanil HCl)
GLAXOSMITHKLINE

62.5 mg/25 mg

METADATE CD

C-II

(methylphenidate HCl, USP)
UCB

10 mg

20 mg

30 mg

40 mg

50 mg

60 mg

Extended-Release Capsules

MOBIC

RX

(meloxicam)
BOEHRINGER INGELHEIM

7.5 mg

15 mg

MOBIC ORAL SUSPENSION

RX

(meloxicam)
BOEHRINGER INGELHEIM

7.5 mg/5 mL

MOTRIN IB

OTC

(ibuprofen)
MCNEIL

200 mg
Caplets and Tablets

CHILDREN'S MOTRIN ORAL SUSPENSION

OTC

(ibuprofen)
MCNEIL

100 mg/5 mL

Berry (also available as dye-free),
Bubble Gum, Grape and Tropical Punch Flavors

CONCENTRATED MOTRIN INFANTS' DROPS

OTC

(ibuprofen)
MCNEIL

50 mg/1.25 mL
Berry Flavor

50 mg/1.25 mL
Dye-Free
Berry Flavor

JUNIOR STRENGTH MOTRIN

OTC

(ibuprofen)
MCNEIL

100 mg Chewable Tablet
Orange and Grape Flavors

100 mg
Caplet

NASONEX

RX

(mometasone furoate monohydrate)
SCHERING

50 mcg/actuation
17 g, 120 sprays

V9

VISUAL PRODUCT IDENTIFICATION GUIDE

NEXIUM
RX (esomeprazole magnesium)
ASTRAZENECA LP

20 mg

40 mg

Delayed-Release Capsules

OMNICEF FOR ORAL SUSPENSION
RX (cefdinir)
ABBOTT

250 mg/5 mL   125 mg/5 mL

OMNICEF
RX (cefdinir)
ABBOTT

300 mg

PCE DISPERTAB TABLETS
RX (erythromycin particles)
ABBOTT

333 mg

500 mg

PEDIARIX
RX [Diphtheria and Tetanus Toxoids and Acelluar Pertussis Adsorbed, Hepatitis B (Recombinant) and Inactivated Poliovirus Vaccine Combined]
GLAXOSMITHKLINE

0.5 mL single-dose vial

0.5 mL single-dose, prefilled, disposable Tip-Lok® syringe

PROAIR HFA
RX (albuterol sulfate)
TEVA SPECIALTY

108 mcg/inh
8.5 g canister
200 actuations

PREVACID
RX (lansoprazole)
TAP

15 mg   30 mg

Delayed-Release Oral Suspension

VISUAL PRODUCT IDENTIFICATION GUIDE

TEGRETOL

RX (carbamazepine USP)
NOVARTIS

200 mg

TEGRETOL-XR

RX (carbamazepine)
NOVARTIS PHARMACEUTICALS

100 mg 200 mg 400 mg

(With the presence of a release portal)
Extended-Release

TOPAMAX

RX (topiramate)
ORTHO-MCNEIL NEUROLOGICS

25 mg

50 mg

100 mg

200 mg

TOPAMAX SPRINKLE

RX (topiramate)
ORTHO-MCNEIL

15 mg 25 mg

CHILDREN'S TYLENOL MELTAWAYS

OTC (acetaminophen)
MCNEIL

80 mg

Grape Punch, Wacky Watermelon and Bubblegum Burst Flavors

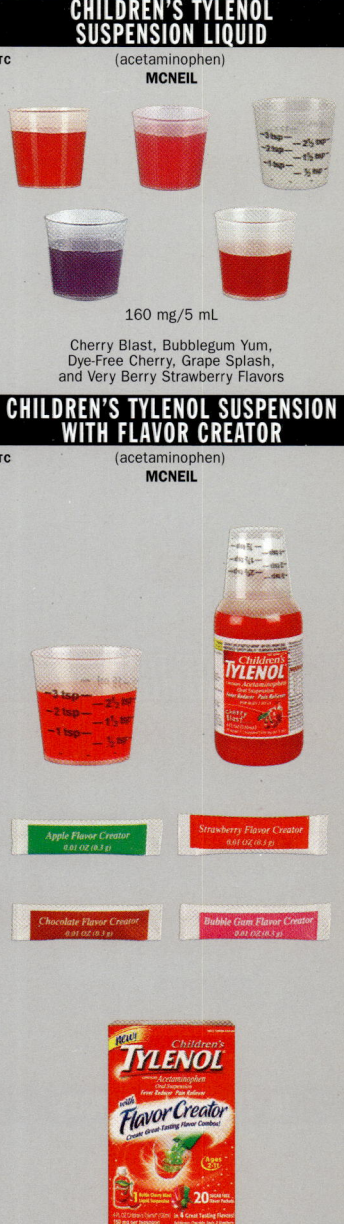

CHILDREN'S TYLENOL SUSPENSION LIQUID

OTC (acetaminophen)
MCNEIL

160 mg/5 mL

Cherry Blast, Bubblegum Yum, Dye-Free Cherry, Grape Splash, and Very Berry Strawberry Flavors

CHILDREN'S TYLENOL SUSPENSION WITH FLAVOR CREATOR

OTC (acetaminophen)
MCNEIL

160 mg/5mL

Contains (1) 4 fl. oz Cherry Blast Liquid plus 20 sugar-free flavor packets in 4 flavors (apple, strawberry, chocolate and bubble gum)

V13

VISUAL PRODUCT IDENTIFICATION GUIDE

XOLAIR
RX (omalizumab)
GENENTECH

150 mg

XOPENEX
RX (levalbuterol HCl)
SEPRACOR

1.25 mg/0.5 mL
Concentrate

XOPENEX
RX (levalbuterol HCl)
SEPRACOR

0.31 mg/3 mL

0.63 mg/3 mL

1.25 mg/3 mL

XOPENEX HFA
RX (levalbuterol tartrate)
SEPRACOR

45 mcg/inh

YAZ
RX (Each light-pink tablet contains 3 mg drospirenone and 0.02 mg ethinyl estradiol. Each white tablet is inert.)
BERLEX, INC.

ZANTAC 25 EFFERDOSE
RX (ranitidine HCl effervescent)
GLAXOSMITHKLINE

25 mg

ZANTAC SYRUP
RX (ranitidine HCl)
GLAXOSMITHKLINE

15 mg/mL
1 pint

ZOFRAN
RX (ondansetron HCl)
GLAXOSMITHKLINE

4 mg

8 mg

VISUAL PRODUCT IDENTIFICATION GUIDE

ZOFRAN INJECTION

RX (ondansetron HCl)
GLAXOSMITHKLINE

2 mg/mL
2-mL single-dose vial

2 mg/mL
20-mL multi-dose vial

ZOFRAN INJECTION PREMIXED

RX (ondansetron HCl)
GLAXOSMITHKLINE

32 mg/50 mL

ZOFRAN ODT

RX (ondansetron)
GLAXOSMITHKLINE

4 mg

8 mg

Orally Disintegrating Tablets

ZOFRAN ORAL SOLUTION

RX (ondansetron HCl)
GLAXOSMITHKLINE

4 mg/5 mL
50 mL

ZYMAR

RX (gatifloxacin ophthalmic)
ALLERGAN

0.3%
5 mL

ZYRTEC

RX (cetirizine HCl)
PFIZER

5 mg

10 mg

ZYRTEC CHEWABLE TABLETS

RX (cetirizine HCl)
PFIZER

5 mg

10 mg

ZYRTEC-D 12 HOUR

RX (cetirizine HCl/pseudoephedrine HCl)
PFIZER

5 mg/120 mg
Extended-Release Tablets